Comprehensive Management of

HEAD AND NECK CANCER

Comprehensive Management of
HEAD AND NECK CANCER

Editors

Narayana Subramaniam
MS MRCSEd MCh FICRS
Consultant and Assistant Fellowship Director
Department of Head and Neck Oncology and Reconstructive Surgery
Mazumdar Shaw Medical Center, Narayana Health City
Bengaluru, Karnataka, India

Sivakumar Vidhyadharan
MS DNB MCh FICRS FEBORL-HNS
Director
The Head And Neck Centre & Hospital
(THANC Hospital), Chennai
Consultant
Department of Head and Neck Surgical Oncology
Apollo Proton Cancer Centre
Chennai, Tamil Nadu, India

Samskruthi P Murthy
MS MCh FHNO
Assistant Professor
Department of Head and Neck Oncology
Kidwai Memorial Institute of Oncology
Director
Can-C Superspecialty Centre
Bengaluru, Karnataka, India

Foreword

Subramania Iyer

Preface

N Gopalakrishna Iyer

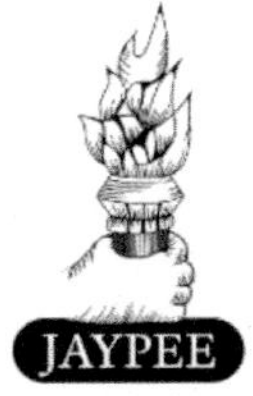

JAYPEE BROTHERS MEDICAL PUBLISHERS
The Health Sciences Publisher
New Delhi | London

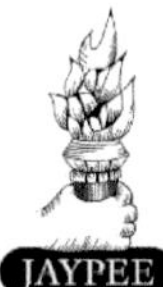

Jaypee Brothers Medical Publishers (P) Ltd.

Headquarters
EMCA House
23/23-B, Ansari Road, Daryaganj
New Delhi 110 002, India
Landline: +91-11-23272143, +91-11-23272703
+91-11-23282021, +91-11-23245672
E-mail: jaypee@jaypeebrothers.com

Corporate Office
Jaypee Brothers Medical Publishers (P) Ltd.
4838/24, Ansari Road, Daryaganj
New Delhi 110 002, India
Phone: +91-11-43574357
Fax: +91-11-43574314
E-mail: jaypee@jaypeebrothers.com

Overseas Office
JP Medical Ltd.
83, Victoria Street, London
SW1H 0HW (UK)
Phone: +44-20 3170 8910
E-mail: info@jpmedpub.com

EU GPSR Authorised Representative
Logos Europe, 9 rue Nicolas Poussin
17000, La Rochelle, France
Phone: +33 (0) 6 67 93 73 78
E-mail: Contact@logoseurope.eu

Website: www.jaypeebrothers.com
Website: www.jaypeedigital.com

Comprehensive Management of Head and Neck Cancer

First Edition: 2021, Reprint: **2026**

ISBN: 978-81-947090-4-6

Printed in India

Dedicated to

All those who have been affected by
head and neck cancer directly or indirectly,
whose struggles inspire us to be better.

Contributors

Adharsh Anand MS MCh
Consultant
Department of Head and Neck Oncology and Reconstructive Surgery
St Gregorios Medical Mission Multi-Specialty Hospital
Parumala, Kerala, India

Akshat Malik MS MCh
Senior Clinical Fellow
Department of Head and Neck Surgery
Imperial College Healthcare NHS Trust
London, UK

Aseem Mishra MS MCh
Assistant Professor
Head and Neck Services
Department of Surgical Oncology
Homi Bhabha Cancer Hospital
Varanasi, Uttar Pradesh, India

Athira Ramakrishnan MS DNB FHNS
Consultant
Department of Otolaryngology and Head and Neck Surgery
Fortis Hospital
Bengaluru, Karnataka, India

Dimpy Sharma MS MCh
Consultant
Department of Plastic Surgery
BPL Nursing Home
Mathura, Uttar Pradesh, India

Dinesh MG MS MCh FMAS FMAO
Senior Consultant
Department of Surgical Oncology
Chief
Department of Minimal Access Surgical Oncology
BGS Gleneagles Global Hospitals
Bengaluru, Karnataka, India

Federico Biglioli MD
Professor and Head
School of Maxillofacial Surgery
University of Milan
Head of Maxillofacial Surgery
San Paolo and San Carlo Hospital
Milan, Italy

Federico Bolognesi MD
Maxillofacial Surgeon
Oral and Maxillofacial Surgery Unit
Department of Head and Neck
S Orsola University Hospital
University of Bologna, Bologna BO, Italy

Gaurav Sundar MD FRCR
Consultant
Department of Radiology
Liverpool University Hospitals NHS Foundation Trust, Merseyside, UK

Hitesh Singhavi MDS
Consultant
Department of Head and Neck Oncology
Fortis Hospital, Mumbai
Former Fellow
Head and Neck Services
Tata Memorial Hospital
Mumbai, Maharashtra, India

Manish Mair MS MCh
Clinical Fellow
Head and Neck Services
University Hospital of Leicester, UK
Ex-Consultant
Head and Neck Services
Tata Memorial Hospital
Mumbai, Maharashtra, India

Narayana Subramaniam
MS MRCSEd MCh FICRS
Consultant and Assistant Fellowship Director
Department of Head and Neck Oncology and Reconstructive Surgery
Mazumdar Shaw Medical Center
Narayana Health City
Bengaluru, Karnataka, India

Naveen BS MDS FHNS
Associate Consultant
Department of Head and Neck Surgical Oncology
VPS Lakeshore Hospital
Kochi, Kerala, India

Nikita Oza MD
Consultant
Department of Histopathology
SRL Diagnostics Centre of Excellence
Mumbai, Maharashtra, India

PC Jacob
MDS Cert Maxillofacial Prosthetics (UCLA)
Consultant
Department of Head and Neck Oncology
Mazumdar Shaw Medical Center
Narayana Health City, Bengaluru
Chief Executive
Ora-Care Dental Clinic
Bengaluru, Karnataka, India

Pranothi Srinivasalu
MSc MRes CDE
Nutrition Counselor and Certified Diabetes Educator
Owner, Eden Nutrizion
Bengaluru, Karnataka, India

Radhika Kapahtia MS MCh
Specialist Senior Resident
Department of Plastic and Reconstructive Surgery
Tata Memorial Centre
Mumbai, Maharashtra, India

Samskruthi P Murthy
MS MCh FHNO
Assistant Professor
Department of Head and Neck Oncology
Kidwai Memorial Institute of Oncology
Director
Can-C Superspecialty Centre
Bengaluru, Karnataka, India

Saurabha Kumar MD
Consultant
Department of Radiation Oncology
Mazumdar Shaw Medical Center
Narayana Health City
Bengaluru, Karnataka, India

Shabala Paul
MD Fellowship in Transplant Anesthesia
Consultant Anesthesiologist
Mazumdar Shaw Medical Center
Narayana Health City
Bengaluru, Karnataka, India

Shashikant Limbachiya MS MCh
Consultant
Department of Head and Neck
Oncology and Reconstructive Surgery
Narayana Multispeciality Hospital
Ahmedabad, Gujarat, India

Sivakumar Vidhyadharan
MS DNB MCh FICRS FEBORL-HNS
Director
The Head And Neck Centre & Hospital
(THANC Hospital), Chennai
Consultant
Department of Head and
Neck Surgical Oncology
Apollo Proton Cancer Centre
Chennai, Tamil Nadu, India

Smita Mathias MSc PhD
Senior Therapist
Department of Speech and
Swallow Therapy
Mazumdar Shaw Medical Center
Narayana Health City
Bengaluru, Karnataka, India

Smitha Chinmay Kulkarni
DNB FEBNM FANMB MNAMS
Assistant Professor
Department of Nuclear Medicine and
Molecular Imaging
Amrita Institute of Medical Science
Kochi, Kerala, India

Soudhamini Shastry
MD MRCPsych
Core Psychiatry Trainee
Health Education England
North West, UK

Suman Bhasker MD
Professor
Department of Radiation Oncology
All India Institute of Medical Sciences
New Delhi, India

Sushma Mehta MDS MFDS FHNS
Honorary Surgeon
Department of Head and Neck Surgery
Rangadore Memorial Hospital and
Fortis Hospital
Bengaluru, Karnataka, India

Trupti Kolur
MDS Fellowship in Oral Oncology
Consultant
Department of Head and Neck Oncology
Mazumdar Shaw Medical Center
Narayana Health City
Bengaluru, Karnataka, India

Vidita Powle MS MRCSEd FHNS
Honorary Consultant
Department of Head and Neck Surgery
Jehangir Hospital and Aditya Birla
Memorial Hospital, Pune
Saifee Hospital and Research Centre
Mumbai, Maharashtra, India

Vidya Bhushan R MS DNB FHNS FUICC
Consultant
Department of Head and Neck
Oncology and Reconstructive Surgery
Mazumdar Shaw Medical Center
Narayana Health City
Bengaluru, Karnataka, India

Vijay Kumar Srinivasalu
MD DM ECMO (PhD)
Consultant
Department of Medical Oncology
Mazumdar Shaw Medical Center
Narayana Health City
Bengaluru, Karnataka, India

Vijay Pillai
MDS MBBS FHNS AO Fellow
Consultant and Head
Fellowship Director
Department of Head and Neck
Oncology and Reconstructive Surgery
Mazumdar Shaw Medical Center
Narayana Health City
Bengaluru, Karnataka, India

Vinay Kumar MD
Assistant Professor
Department of Radiation Oncology
Kidwai Memorial Institute of Oncology
Bengaluru, Karnataka, India

Vineeth Sukrithan MD
Assistant Professor
Department of Medicine
Division of Medical Oncology
Ohio State University and Arthur G
James Comprehensive Cancer Center
Columbus, Ohio, USA

Vivek Shetty MS FHNS
Consultant
Department of Head and Neck
Oncology and Reconstructive Surgery
Mazumdar Shaw Medical Center
Narayana Health City
Bengaluru, Karnataka, India

Foreword

While considering the cancers affecting the body, head and neck cancers are distinct; they are different from others with several subsites having unique features, diverse and varied pathologies and they require a multidisciplinary treatment for their cure. These cancers, though amongst the most common in several parts of the world, often fare the worst due to the lack of an organized treatment delivery system, with ownership being distributed unevenly among various surgical and oncological specialties. The lack of trained and dedicated professionals required to form a multidisciplinary treatment team is often reflected in the poor outcomes associated with head and neck cancer.

The head and neck surgical oncologist fits in well as the leader of this multidisciplinary team, as a majority of the cases need primary surgical treatment or continued involvement of the surgeon either to establish a diagnosis or subsequently in post-treatment surveillance or salvage therapy. Only recently have the avenues of structured training in head and neck surgical oncology opened up, paving the way to create a talent pool to fill this void.

A reference book was essential for these trainees, and this book aptly titled *Comprehensive Management of Head and Neck Cancer* will be a great boon to them. With its well-conceived structure, methodical layout of each chapter and stress on supportive care, rehabilitation and clinical research, I am sure it will soon become a reference book to all those who are interested in head and neck cancer.

Subramania Iyer
MCh FRCS
Chairman
Head and Neck Surgical Oncology and
Reconstructive Surgery
Amrita Institute of Medical Sciences
Amrita Vishwa Vidyapeetham
Kochi, Kerala, India

Preface

Life is short, and art long, opportunity fleeting,
experimentations perilous, and judgment difficult.

– Hippocrates

The last three decades have seen a dramatic shift in paradigms in the management of head and neck malignancies. This shift is reflected in our scientific understanding that encompasses the etiology, pathogenesis, pathologic manifestations and therapeutic strategies that continue to evolve and shape current and future clinical trials. However, the same shift has also forced a change in the art of managing these patients, towards a more holistic approach in dealing with individuals, and their future with the disease or when they are free of disease.

This textbook takes a comprehensive view that attempts to distill the salient issues in each of these topics, and that's what makes it different from many other, more focused, manuscripts currently available to lifelong learners involved in the treatment of these patients.

Each clinical chapter is presented in a systematic manner, to incorporate the most recent evidence-based practice guidelines, while also presenting the controversies in a succinct manner. The addition of chapters that encompass genetics, molecular pathway and translational biology direct the reader to consider current concepts of precision and personalized therapy. Management principles are also presented as a continuum of care, for example in planning surgical resection and reconstruction, or surgical planning in anticipation of radiation or chemotherapy. Furthermore, there is an expanded emphasis on the understanding of anesthesia, nuclear medicine and interventional radiology, and its application to management of various clinical scenarios.

Yet, the art is not lost. Chapters that cover issues surrounding nutrition, speech and swallowing therapy, pain management and psychology support the increasing role the rehabilitation team plays in the holistic management of some of our patients. This emphasis extends beyond treatment and into the realm of quality of life and survivorship, with additional chapters on chronic pain management, long-term psychosocial issues, body self-image (e.g., facial nerve function) and general well-being.

Apart from figures and tables summarizing each relevant section, the book has also included key algorithms and protocols and standardized questionnaires that are useful in planning audits and research protocols, apart from day-to-day management.

The ability to bring all elements of the art and science in managing these patients, who present from all walks of life, is what makes this book stand out from existing textbooks, and also makes it a delight to read and reference.

N Gopalakrishna Iyer
MBBS (Hons) PhD (Cantab) FRCSEd FAMS
Head, Department of Head and Neck Surgery
Singapore General Hospital and National Cancer Centre
Head, Division of Medical Sciences
Humphrey Oei Institute of Cancer Research
Professor, Duke-NUS Medical School, Singapore

Acknowledgments

Writing this book has been a rewarding experience because of the inspiring co-editors and contributors who were instrumental in completing the book.

We are grateful to our teachers who have been a constant source of motivation and have always been supportive throughout our professional journey.

We would like to extend our gratitude to our publishing team for their excellent work editing the text and providing brilliant illustrations. Ms Nikita Chauhan (Senior Development Editor) in particular has added great value to this book. Thank you to our colleagues and our students who propel us to do more. We would also like to thank Dr S Rajasekaran for his guidance and support in bringing this idea to fruition.

We are indebted to our patients who place their faith in us to treat them and embolden us to further our skills, research and care.

We would like to thank our families for their unparalleled support and love and our parents who provided us with an opportunity to follow our dreams. Last but not the least, thank you to our friends for their belief in us.

We also like to thank Shri Jitendar P Vij (Group Chairman), Mr Ankit Vij (Managing Director), Mr MS Mani (Group President), Ms Chetna Malhotra Vohra (Associate Director—Content Strategy), Ms Pooja Bhandari (Production Head), and the staff of M/S Jaypee Brothers Medical Publishers (P) Ltd, New Delhi, India.

Contents

SECTION 5 POST-TREATMENT CARE AND REHABILITATION

CHAPTER 1

Head and Neck Cancer Treatment: Past, Present and Future

Vijay Pillai

HISTORICAL ASPECTS

The evolution of head and neck surgery encapsulates the evolution of a specialty. From the confines of general surgery, otolaryngology, plastic and reconstructive surgery and maxillofacial surgery, the specialty has carved out a niche of its own.

The history of development of head and neck surgery also parallels the developments seen in medicine and surgery such as advances in anesthesia, antisepsis, transfusion and hemostasis; this had led to development of major extirpative procedures.

The brief description that follows is neither exhaustive nor all inclusive, but summarizes various key developments in head and neck cancer therapy.

The earliest mention of cancer dates back to the medical documents of the Edwin Smith Papyrus and the Ebers Papyrus. A description of an "eating ulcer on the gums" treated with a mixture of cinnamon, gum, honey and oil seems to be the first treatment described for oral cancer.[1]

The Greek Physician Hippocrates (460 BC) was the first to use the term carcinoma and describe skin cancers and its treatment with cautery and caustic pastes. Aurelius Cornelius Celsus (30 AD) treated cancer of the face and lip with excision. Galen in 200 AD advocated the humoral theory of disease and neoplasms due to excess black bile that needed to be treated with diet and purging.[2]

The medieval age was characterized by a general lack of progression of any scientific developments and it was with the Renaissance (1500–1760 AD) that knowledge started to develop with Vesalius' anatomical studies. As the use of tobacco reached the European and American continents we find the mention of cancer and also its related treatments.

Table 1 summarizes key milestones and developments in the evolution of head and neck cancer.

EVOLUTION OF HEAD AND NECK SURGERY

Oral Cancer Surgery

As a better understanding of the biology and pathways of spread of oral cancer developed, contributions have been made to access and management of these tumors, which form the principles of current practice. In addition various studies demonstrated the involvement of the mandible in oral cancer and founded the principles of mandible resection in oral malignancies.

It is worthwhile mentioning the early pioneering surgeons and their contributions:

- Lip-split approach with a mandibular division developed by von Langenbeck and Billroth
- Wedge excision for tongue tumors with lingual artery control by von Langenbeck
- Roux described the cervical approach to the oral cavity
- Kocher cervical approach for oral cavity and lateral mandibular osteotomies
- Theodore Billroth described bilateral mandibular osteotomies

Neck Dissection

Management of the neck is an integral part of head and neck surgery of any site. Neck dissection itself is an operation that evolved from a radical surgery (as proposed by Crile and Hayes Martin) to selective neck dissection (preserving function); we are now in the era of superselective neck dissection and sentinel lymph node biopsy.

George Crile was the first person to describe the enbloc resection of the cervical lymphatics in 1906.[3] Hayes Martin reported his experience at the Memorial Sloan Kettering Cancer Center from 1928 to 1950 describing radical neck dissections. This was the procedure of choice for clinically positive necks with the sacrifice of the internal jugular vein, spinal accessory and sternomastoid

Table 1: Key milestones and developments in the evolution of head and neck cancer.

Year	*Contributor and role*
1740	Jean Godinot established the first cancer hospital in Reims, France
1790	Onuigbo described nodal metastases: A sign of incurability
1801–1878	Johannes Müller and Alfred Donne did the pioneering work in histopathology
1805–1906	Manuel Garcia described indirect laryngoscopy
1815–1856	Horace Wells, William Morton and John Warren introduced general anesthesia
1821–1902	Rudolph Virchow developed the concept of cellular pathology putting aside Galen's humoral theory
1851	Gurdon Buck described laryngofissure, later reported by Cohen
1865–1867	Thiersch and Waldeyer proposed the origin of cancer from the epithelial surface and stromal invasion
1873	Billroth performed the first laryngectomy
1885–1893	General Grant's oropharyngeal cancer and President Cleveland's oral cancer gave impetus to the development of histopathologic examination
1895–1900	Description of frozen section by Nezelof and its popularization by Thomas Stephen Cullen
18th century	First reports of neck dissection and its importance in disease control: Butlin demonstrated efficacy of neck dissection for tongue cancer, Jawdynski from Poland performed a block dissection of the neck
1905–1906	George Crile described the block dissection of the neck popularized subsequently by Hayes Martin
1919	Coutard developed external beam irradiation
1922	Gluck and Soerensen standardized the technique of laryngectomy
1924	Giacomo Puccini an Italian opera artist received brachytherapy using the Columbia apparatus at Brussels
1938	Hayes Martin at Memorial Hospital described the commando operation
1939	Justo Alonso (Uruguay) performed horizontal partial laryngectomy
1965	Bakamjian introduced the two-stage pharyngoesophageal reconstruction with the deltopectoral flap
1979–1980	Stephen Ariyan described the pectoralis major myocutaneous flap
1983	Yang and David Soutar described the radial forearm flap
1989	Hidalgo described the free fibula flap first introduced by Taylor in 1977
2000	Anterolateral thigh flap first described by Song popularized by Wei and colleagues

muscle along with the clearance of levels I-V. He was not a proponent of prophylactic dissection of the clinically negative neck. Starting in 1938 at Memorial Sloan Kettering Cancer Center, the group published their results of 665 radical neck dissections performed in 599 patients in 1959.[4] Due to the extensive morbidity of the removal of the nonlymphatic structures Suarez in 1952, described the modified radical neck dissection preserving the nonlymphatic structures.[5] Ballantyne from the MD Anderson Cancer Center demonstrated comparable results of modified radical neck dissection with radical neck dissections with removal of only those lymph nodes having the highest risk of metastases.[6] The concept of functional neck dissection developed with the work of Bocca and Suarez in the 1960s and 1970s.

The pioneering clinical evidence that changed the radicality of neck dissection toward a selective approach was the work of Byers from MD Anderson in 428 patients[7] and the series of 1,081 patients by Shah from the Memorial Sloan Kettering Cancer Center that studied the progression of cervical metastasis from primaries of the oral cavity, oropharynx, larynx and hypopharynx.[8]

Thyroid Surgery

Thyroid surgery advances classically reflect the development of our specialty. Initially in the domain of the general surgeon, advances in understanding the anatomy of the parathyroids, the recurrent and external laryngeal nerve, techniques of intraoperative nerve monitoring, imaging and histology acquisition, with high-quality ultrasound, surgery has moved into the head and neck surgeon's armamentarium. From its earliest descriptions in 200 BC for goiter (gutter), with the first surgery being performed in 1646, significant advances and refinements have been made. Kocher, Billroth and Wells made significant contributions in the early century. Rapid strides have been made in the staging system with dynamic risk stratification and personalized approaches in the management of thyroid malignancies.[9] Similarly, parathyroid surgery made rapid advances with the use of radioimmunometric assays and intraoperative delineation with radionuclide scans.[10]

Laryngeal Surgery

The initial total laryngectomies were considered highly morbid and thus the role of radiotherapy was envisaged as an excellent alternative. However, radiotherapy had its limitations in advanced cancer. Improvements in the understanding of the anatomy and the lymphatic drainage led Pressman to elaborate the importance of subtotal laryngectomies.[11] Open cordectomy, vertical partial laryngectomy, supracricoid laryngectomy and supraglottic laryngectomy were less radical but were able to achieve cure.[12,13] With the introduction of the CO_2 laser in the 1970 it was demonstrated that oncologic cure rates similar to radiotherapy could be achieved in early lesions. Jako and colleagues from the United States,[14] and Kleinsasser and Steiner[15] from Germany developed endoscopic laser excision of laryngeal tumors thus creating a paradigm shift in the management approach. Robot-assisted supraglottic laryngectomy with and without CO_2 laser has expanded the indication for transoral laryngeal cancer resection.[16] Voice restoration after laryngectomy was first described by Singer and Blom in 1980. Tracheoesophageal puncture and valve prosthesis is the standard of care for voice rehabilitation after laryngectomy.[17] The future hold exciting scope with the possibility of laryngeal transplantation.

Salivary Gland Surgery

Salivary gland surgery has developed with a better understanding of the anatomy of the facial nerve, intraoperative nerve monitoring, better rehabilitative measures for the paralyzed face (both dynamic and static), histology driven management of the primary and neck, and adjuvant treatment. The role of molecular profiling in recurrent tumors has enabled use of targeted agents. Surgical extirpation of advanced tumors necessitated the use of various lateral skull-base approaches.

Skull-base Surgery

Alfred Ketchum from the National Institute of Health was the first person to describe a craniofacial approach that permitted an enbloc resection of the cribriform plate with the ethmoid complex.[18] Subsequently this concept was extended by Terz et al.[19] Using the concepts of endoscopic sinus surgery, Kassam, Carrau and Synderman used these to develop transnasal approaches to the management of skull-base tumors.[20] Lewis reported innovative techniques with hypotensive anesthesia, high speed drills and repair of the surgical defect reducing operative mortality to 5%.[21] Lateral skull-base surgery was advanced by the development of the three Fisch approaches that gave access to lesions in the infratemporal space in relation to the petrous carotid, venous sinuses and the facial nerve.[22]

Reconstructive Surgery

In the last 40–50 years major strides have been made in reconstructive surgery as this was able to overcome the morbidity associated with extensive ablations, ensure timely commencement of adjuvant therapy and better quality of life and function. From the use of skin grafts, local flaps, diversion conduits, axial pattern flaps, the advent of pedicled flaps such as the deltopectoral and pectoralis major was a major hallmark in head and neck reconstruction.[23,24] By the 1970s reconstructive microsurgery had developed as a specialty and was evident in the application of various free flaps in head and neck reconstruction.[25-27] Currently, the reconstructive armamentarium is so extensive that one can choose from a reconstructive elevator rather than a reconstructive ladder.

Prosthodontics and Implantology

As the reconstructive armamentarium improved to include free flaps, osseous reconstruction has heralded a new finesse in final outcomes. The use of virtual planning, cutting guides and customized implants has significantly brought in precision, reduced surgical time and enables optimal functional rehabilitation. Primary dental implantation has also been proven to be safe in the settings of adjuvant radiotherapy. Craniofacial implants and obturators are the other aspects of rehabilitation.[28]

EVOLUTION OF RADIOTHERAPY

This brief description will give insights to the development of radiotherapy in head and neck along with different fractionation schedules and delivery modalities, the details of which will be covered in the relevant sections.

The role of radiation therapy in head and neck cancer emerged in the early 1900s with initially single fraction treatments with subsequent multifraction treatment schedules developed in Europe.[29] Advancements were made in the field to incorporate radiation in the postoperative setting in the early 1950s by Fletcher and colleagues at MD Anderson and expanding it to the definitive setting by Million and colleagues (University of Florida) and Wang (Harvard) over the 1960s to 1980s.[30]

Fletcher's work defined the indications for postoperative radiotherapy and its benefits in improving locoregional control. It also showed differences between aryepiglottic fold lesions and false vocal cord lesions and refined the techniques of radiation delivery, precise data recording and reporting, radiobiology and time-dose factors and preservation of larynx function. The development of protocols enabled its use in organ preservation protocols for tumors of the oropharynx, larynx, hypopharynx and nasopharynx.

The use of radiation was evaluated in different settings in well-designed randomized trials and meta-analysis.

- *Definitive setting:* Evidence for use of radiotherapy with chemotherapy in the definitive setting was in organ preservation trials of appropriately selected patients with larynx and hypopharynx cancer. This was evidenced from the results of the RTOG 91-11 and EORTC HPX trials.[31-33]
- *Altered fractionation:* Accelerated repopulation is known to cause locoregional failure in patients experiencing delay in commencement of treatment and in patients with extended overall radiation treatment times. Altered fractionation regimens can be either hyperfractionation or accelerated fractionation. The EORTC trial demonstrated that hyperfractionation in oropharynx improved local control with a strong trend toward improved survival and no difference in late effects.[34] Similarly the Danish group (DAHANCA) also reported improved local control at 5 years by 10% for patients treated with 6 fractions per week, but with no difference in overall survival.[35] The meta-analysis suggested that altered fractionation regimens delivered without chemotherapy improved locoregional control and survival (6.4% and 3.4%) at 5 years.[36]
- *Concomitant chemoradiation:* MACH-NC demonstrated a 5-year 4.5% absolute survival benefit of adding chemotherapy to radiation which was most evident in the concurrent setting, with a 6.5% absolute benefit (HR 0.81, 95% CI 0.78–0.86).[37]
- *Postoperative chemoradiotherapy:* Randomized trials conducted by the EORTC and RTOG demonstrated an improvement in local control, disease free survival and overall survival with the addition of cisplatin to postoperative radiotherapy. The presence of positive margins and extranodal extension of tumor were the common indications.[38-40]

Refinements in Radiation Delivery

From the initial two dimensional clinical and plain radiograph-based findings that would delineate the regions for risk to deliver radiotherapy, progress has been made to three dimensional CT-based conformal approaches. These use parallel opposed fields to deliver radiation.

Era of intensity modulated radiotherapy (IMRT): By modulating the intensity of the beam and allowing it to conform to the shape of the target tissue, it was possible to significantly reduce the dose to critical structures. By using multiple radiation beams from different directions with a steep dose gradient and highly conformal dose distribution it was possible to have better coverage of tumor and high risk target areas.

Inverse planning is used to define the target dose for the tumor. It allows for the delivery of simultaneous integrated boost without treatment field modifications.[41,42] Variations have been developed in the delivery of IMRT such as step and shoot fields: Multileaf collimator (MLC) does not move, sliding window fields (MLC moves), volumetric arc therapy (VMAT: gantry and MLC move), tomotherapy (gantry, couch and MLC move).

Brachytherapy: Radioactive sources were placed within the tumor and combined with an external beam to boost the primary to a higher dose while still minimizing exposure to surrounding tissues. This was commonly employed for tumors of the lip, tongue, floor of mouth, recurrent nasopharyngeal cancers and recurrent tumors of the head and neck.[43,44] This along with intraoperative radiotherapy (IORT) done with electrons or high dose rate low energy photon source allows steep dose fall-off sparing normal tissues.[45]

Stereotactic radiosurgery (SRS): A highly conformal form of radiotherapy allowing delivery of high dose radiation to the tumor in small fractions. First described for the palliation of skull-base recurrences, has been proven to be effective and well tolerated in the palliative setting.[46] The Cyberknife (Accuracy Inc., Sunnyvale CA) is a smaller 6MV X-band accelerator mounted on a robotic arm allowing greater degrees of movement freedom. It can track implanted fiducial markers and has six degrees of freedom. It is mostly used for reradiation.

Proton therapy: Proton therapy aims at reducing the incidental dose to nontarget structures. This has a direct bearing on outcomes as the toxic effects follow a dose-response relationship. A focused beam created by a particle accelerator allows the protons to travel fast through the body with minimal interactions and then increase the interactions as the velocity is reduced with maximal energy deposited resulting in the "Bragg peak" and no exit dose. The dosimetric advantage can translate to clinical benefits. Treatment can be delivered by using passive or active scanning techniques. The active or intensity modulated proton therapy (IMPT) is the most commonly used. Skull-base chordomas, chondrosarcomas, paranasal malignancies are indications for proton therapy post-resection. The use of protons for oropharyngeal and nasopharyngeal cancers can minimize the treatment toxicity. Adenoid cystic carcinoma which are unresectable and periorbital tumors are also indications for proton therapy. Reirradiation is also another avenue for proton treatment. Reported toxicity includes reduced rate of feeding tube dependence, malnutrition, lower mucositis, nausea and dysgeusia though the skin toxicity is higher.[47]

EVOLUTION OF CHEMOTHERAPY

Dating back to the 1940s the first chemotherapeutic agents were developed from nitrogen mustard. Teropterin was the first folic acid antagonist to be used in advanced nasopharyngeal carcinoma. Gradually the role of platinum-based components came in as a radiosensitizer and predictor of radiosensitivity. The development of chemotherapy has been from a point when it was initially used in the palliative setting with intra-arterial methotrexate to neoadjuvant, concomitant with radiation and in the adjuvant settings. A variety of cytotoxic agents has been used, the common ones being cisplatin, carboplatin, paclitaxel, docetaxel, 5-fluorouracil, methotrexate, ifosfamide, hydroxyurea. Targeted agents that are in vogue are cetuximab [(antiepidermal growth factor receptor (EGFR)], imatinib, gefitinib and erlotinib, though the evidence of benefit for the latter two is lacking. The concept of metronomic chemotherapy is gaining significance in the recurrent and metastatic setting.[48]

Refinements in Chemotherapy

Platinum-based chemotherapeutic regimens are the cornerstone in the concomitant and adjuvant settings. Multiple phase 3 trials of induction chemotherapy followed by locoregional treatment compared to locoregional treatment alone have shown variable results with regards to survival and decreasing distant metastasis. A meta-analysis showed that induction chemotherapy conferred a nonsignificant survival improvement of 2% at 5 years (HR, 0.95 95% CI 0.88–1.01, $p = 0.10$).[49] The addition of a taxane to cisplatin plus 5-flurouracil-based induction regimen has been shown to improve survival.[50,51]

Organ Preservation Therapy

The use of organ preservation therapy in head and neck cancer was introduced because of poor functional outcomes with surgery. Surgical organ preservation protocols use transoral robotic surgery (TORS) or transoral laser microsurgery (TLMS) or open partial laryngeal surgeries. However, this discussion would primarily be on nonsurgical options. Curative chemoradiotherapy has been established as the standard of care which showed an absolute decrease in 5-year mortality of 6.5% with decreased locoregional failures.[37,52] RTOG 91-11 established concurrent chemoradiotherapy for locoregional control and organ preservation in patients with resectable Stage III or IV glottic or supraglottic disease.[31,32] This modality is preferred in advanced laryngeal or hypopharyngeal cancers without cartilage involvement. High dose cisplatin (100 mg per square meter of body surface area) given intravenously every 21 days for 3 cycles concurrent with radiotherapy is the standard of care.[37] Patients with poor performance status may have carboplatin substituted for cisplatin though it is less effective as definitive therapy.[53]

Bonner in 2006 showed that cetuximab with radiotherapy provided better locoregional control and overall survival compared to radiotherapy alone, however there was no comparison with cisplatin radiotherapy regimen. This has been borne out by the data from recent randomized trials.[54-56]

Induction Chemotherapy

The role of induction chemotherapy remains controversial and is recommended by the guidelines in a clinical trial setting. Taxane-based chemotherapy in the TAX 324 and EORTC TAX 323 trials showed improved survival but with higher toxic effects and treatment delays.[50,51] However, there is significant heterogeneity in trial design which needs to be cautiously interpreted before it can be used before definitive chemoradiation. Toxic effects from induction chemotherapy can prevent 20–30% patients from completing definitive chemoradiation.[57] Various single institution trials have looked at the role of induction chemotherapy in advanced oral cancer with borderline resectability, as a bioselection tool to guide treatment decision.

FUTURE AVENUES

Personalized Therapy

The treatment modalities of head and neck cancer include surgery, radiation, chemotherapy, and targeted therapy (most recently the checkpoint inhibitors). A common denominator for all these modalities is the toxicity profile. Biomarker driven treatment strategies are an exciting avenue of clinical research. Existing markers are for human papilloma virus (HPV) in oropharyngeal carcinoma, and Epstein-Barr virus (EBV) in nasopharyngeal carcinoma, in addition pathways and markers associated with EGFR downstream signaling abnormalities (PI3K/MTOR pathway and PTEN pathway) and immune checkpoint-related markers. Advances in digital genomic technologies, detection of circulating DNA from clinical specimens offer potential predictive biomarkers in head and neck squamous cell carcinoma (HNSCC) therapy.[58] With both pembrolizumab and nivolumab getting accelerated approval by the FDA the future is likely drugs that are biomarker based, have a high clinical efficacy and durable response rate. With increased access to next-generation sequencing and with the TCGA tumor type agnostic therapy is a reality in clinical development and practice.

Vaccinations

Patient specific vaccinations will soon become a reality. With the availability of next generation sequencing, many neoantigens have been identified. The neoantigen with highest affinity are formulated into a peptide or dendritic cell vaccine and delivered as a patient specific vaccine to promote an antitumor response. The presence of neoantigen specific T cells in the blood are used to monitor response. Currently phase I clinical trials are ongoing for vaccines for glioblastoma, melanoma, colon cancer and breast cancer. Viral protein-based vaccines are used in HPV associated HNSCC namely the bivalent HPV 16/18 and the quadrivalent HPV 6/11/16/18.

Robotic Surgery

Transoral robotic surgery for head and neck cancer needs appropriate patient selection with outcomes similar to organ sparing techniques having been reported. It has widespread applications as in treatment of the unknown primary, oropharyngeal cancer (allowing for possible deintensification of treatment and better functional outcomes), supraglottic laryngectomy (with outcomes similar to patients treated by radiotherapy) and advanced applications in nasopharyngeal and parapharyngeal tumors.

Composite Tissue Allotransplantation and Tissue Engineering

There are various groups involved in research of tissue engineered regenerative medicine (TERM) using stem cells to develop bone regenerates. Similarly work is ongoing in the field of stem cell-based tissue engineered larynx and airway constructs and also complex face transplants have been performed.

CONCLUSION

Head and neck oncology has developed over the century with tremendous strides in surgical and nonsurgical modalities of care. From multiple worldwide associations to international cooperative and collaborative groups, the specialty has fostered dedicated training and also integration of multiple disciplines. The future holds exciting prospects in terms of personalized medicine, endoscopic and robotic surgerics and the expanding scope of regenerative medicine, all carving out a distinct niche for themselves in the specialty.

REFERENCES

1. Butterfield WC. Tumor treatment, 3000 BC. Surgery. 1966;60:476-9.
2. Kardinal CG. An outline of the history of cancer. Part 1. Mo Med. 1977;74:662-6.
3. Crile G. Excision of cancer of the head and neck. With special reference to the plan of dissection based on one hundred and thirty two operations. JAMA. 1906;47:1780-6.
4. Martin H, Del Valle B, Ehrlich H, Cahan WG. Neck dissection. Cancer. 1951;4:441-99.
5. Suarez O. El problema de las metastasis linfaticas y alejadas del cancer de laringe e hipofaringe. Rev Otorrinolaringol. 1963;23:83-99.
6. Jesse RH, Ballantyne AJ, Larson D. Radical or modified neck dissection: a therapeutic dilemma. Am J Surg. 1978;136:516-9.
7. Byers RM, Wolf PF, Ballantyne AJ. Rationale for elective modified neck dissection. Head Neck Surg. 1988;10:160-7.
8. Shah JP. Patterns of cervical lymph node metastasis from squamous carcinomas of the upper aerodigestive tract. Am J Surg. 1990;160:405-9.
9. Haugen BR, Alexander EK, Bible KC, Doherty GM, Mandel SJ, Nikiforov YE, et al. 2015 American Thyroid Association Management Guidelines for Adult Patients with thyroid nodules and differentiated thyroid cancer. Thyroid. 2016;26:1-133.
10. Irvin GL 3rd, Dembrow VD, Prudhomme DL. Operative monitoring of parathyroid gland hyperfunction. Am J Surg. 1991;162:299-302.
11. Pressman JJ, Simon MB, Monell CM. Anatomic studies related to the dissemination of cancer of the larynx. Cancer. 1961;14:1131-8.
12. Alonso J. Conservative surgery of the larynx. Am Acad Ophthalmol Otolaryngol. 1947;51:633-42.
13. Weinstein GS, Laccourreye O, Brasnu D, Laccourreye H. Organ preservation surgery for laryngeal cancer. San Diego, Calif: Singular Publishing Group; 2000.
14. Stron MS, Jako GJ. Laser surgery in the larynx. Early clinical experience with continuous CO_2 laser. Ann Otol. 1972;81:791-8.
15. Steiner W, Ambrosch P. Endoscopic laser surgery of the upper aerodigestive tract. Stuttgart-New York: Thieme; 2000.
16. Weinstein GS, O Malley BW Jr, Snyder W, Hocksterin NG. Transoral robotic surgery: supraglottic partial laryngectomy. Ann Otol Rhinol Laryngol. 2007;117: 817-20.

17. Singer MI, Blom ED. An endoscopic technique for restoration of voice after total laryngectomy. Ann Otol Rhinol Laryngol. 1980;89:529-33.
18. Ketcham AS, Chretian PB, Van Buren JM, Hoye RC, Beazley RM, Herdt JR. The ethmoid sinuses: a reevaluation of surgical resection. Am J Surg. 1973;126:469-76.
19. Terz JJ, Young HF, Lawrence W Jr. Combined craniofacial resection for locally advanced carcinoma of the head and neck. Am J Surg. 1980;140:613-24.
20. Snyderman CH, Carrau RL, Kassam AB, Zanation A, Prevedello D, Gardner P, et al. Endoscopic skull base surgery: principles of endonasal oncological surgery. J Surg Oncol. 2008;97:658-64.
21. Lewis JS. Temporal bone resection. Review of 100 cases. Arch Otolaryngol. 1975;101:23-5.
22. Fisch U, Fagan P, Valavanis A. The infratemporal fossa approach for the lateral skull base. Otolaryngol Clin North Am. 1984;17:513-52.
23. Bakamjian VY. A two-stage method for pharyngoesophageal reconstruction with a primary pectoral skin flap. Plast Reconstr Surg. 1965;36:173-84.
24. Ariyan S. The pectoralis major myocutaneous flap. A versatile flap for reconstruction in the head and neck. Plast Reconstr Surg. 1979;63:73-81.
25. Soutar DS, Scheker LR, Tanner NS, Mc Gregor IA. The radial forearm flap: a versatile method for intra-oral reconstruction. Br J Plast Surg. 1983;36:1-8.
26. Hidalgo DA, Rekow A. A review of 60 consecutive fibula free flap mandible reconstruction. Plast and Reconstr Surg. 1995;96:585-96.
27. Song YG, Chen GZ, Song YL. The free thigh flap: a new free flap based on the septocutaneous artery. Br J Plast Surg. 1984;37:149-59.
28. Gilbert RW. Reconstruction of the oral cavity; past, present and future. Oral Oncol. 2020;108:104683.
29. Thames HD, Hendry JH. Fractionation in Radiotherapy. London; New York: Taylor and Francis; 1987. pp. 297.
30. Fletcher GH, Jesse RH, Lindberg RD, Koons CR. The place of radiotherapy in the management of the squamous cell carcinoma of the supraglottic larynx. Am J Roentgenol Radium Ther Nucl Med. 1970;108:19-26.
31. Forastiere AA, Goepfert H, Maor M, Pajak TF, Weber R, Morrison W, et al. Concurrent chemotherapy and radiotherapy for organ preservation in advanced laryngeal cancer. N Engl J Med. 2003;349:2091-98.
32. Forastiere AA, Zhang Q, Weber RS, Maor MH, Goepfert H, Pajak TF, et al. Long term results of RTOG 91-11: a comparison of three nonsurgical treatment strategies to preserve the larynx in patients with locally advanced larynx cancer. J Clin Oncol. 2013;31:845-52.
33. Lefebvre JL, Chevalier D, Luboinski B, Kirkpatrick A, Collette L, Sahmoud T. Larynx preservation in pyriform sinus cancer: preliminary results of a European organization for research and treatment of cancer phase III trial. EORTC Head and Neck Cancer Cooperative Group. J Natl Cancer Inst. 1996;88:890-9.
34. Horiot JC, Le Fur R, N'Guyen T, Chenal C, Schraub S, Alfonsi S, et al. Hyperfractionation versus conventional fractionation in oropharyngeal carcinoma: final analysis of a randomized trial of the EORTC cooperative group of radiotherapy. Radiother Oncol. 1992;25:231-41.
35. Overgaard J, Hansen HS, Specht L, Overgaard M, Grau C, Andersen E, et al. Five compared with six fractions per week of conventional radiotherapy of squamous cell carcinoma of head and neck: DAHANCA 6 and 7 randomised controlled trial. Lancet. 2003;362:933-40.
36. Bourhis J, Overgaard J, Audry H, Ang KK, Saunders M, Bernier J, et al. Hyperfractionated or accelerated radiotherapy in head and neck cancer: a meta-analysis. Lancet. 2006;368: 843-54.
37. Pignon JP, le Maître A, Maillard E, Bourhis J; MACH-NC Collaborative Group. Meta-analysis of chemotherapy in head and neck cancer (MACH-NC); an update on 93 randomised trials and 17,346 patients. Radiother Oncol. 2009;92:4-14.
38. Bernier J, Cooper JS, Pajak TF, van Glabbeke M, Bourhis J, Forastiere A, et al. Defining risk levels in locally advanced head and neck cancers : a comparative analysis of concurrent postoperative radiation plus chemotherapy trials of the EORTC(#22931) and RTOG(#9501). Head Neck. 2005;27: 843-50.
39. Bernier J, Domenge C, Ozsahin M, Matuszewska K, Lefèbvre JL, Greiner RH, et al. Postoperative irradiation with or without concomitant chemotherapy for locally advanced head and neck cancer. N Engl J Med. 2004;350:1945-52.
40. Cooper JS, Pajak TF, Forastiere AA, Jacobs J, Campbell BH, Saxman SB, et al. Postoperative concurrent radiotherapy and chemotherapy for high risk squamous cell carcinoma of the head and neck. N Engl J Med. 2004;350:1937-44.
41. Mendenhall WM, Amdur RJ, Palta JR. Intensity-modulated radiotherapy in the standard management of head and neck cancer: promises and pitfalls. J Clin Oncol. 2006;24: 2618-23.
42. Lee N, Puri DR, Blanco AI, Chao KS. Intensity-modulated radiation therapy in head and neck cancers: an update. Head Neck. 2007;29:387-400.
43. Harrison LB. Applications of brachytherapy in head and neck cancer. Semin Surg Oncol. 1997;13:177-84.
44. Kupferman ME, Morrison WH, Santilaan AA, Morrison WH, Santillan AA, Roberts D, et al. The role of interstitial brachytherapy with salvage surgery for the management of recurrent head and neck cancers. Cancer. 2007;109:2052-7.
45. Debenham BJ, Hu KS, Harrison LB. Present status and future directions of intraoperative radiotherapy. Lancet Oncol. 2013; 11:e457-e464.
46. Voynov G, Heron DE, Burton S, Heron DE, Burton S, Grandis J, et al. Frameless stereotactic radiotherapy for recurrent head and neck carcinoma. Technol Cancer Res Treat. 2006;5: 529-35.
47. Ramaekers BLT, Grutters JPC, Pijls-Johannesma M. Protons in head -and -neck cancer: bridging the gap of evidence. Int J Radiat Oncol. 2013;85:1282-8.
48. Patil VM, Noronha V, Joshi A, Pinninti R, Dhumal S, Bhattacharjee A, et al. Metronomic chemotherapy in platinum-insensitive failures and/or early failures post multimodality management in oral cancers. Indian J Med Paediatr Oncol. 2015;36:161-5.
49. Pignon JP, Bourhis J, Domenge C, Designé L. Chemotherapy added to locoregional treatment for head and neck squamous-cell carcinoma: 3 meta-analyses of updated individual data. MACH-NC Collaborative Group. Met-Analysis of Chemotherapy on Head and Neck Cancer. Lancet. 2000;355:949-55.
50. Posner MR, Hershock DM, Blajman CR, Hershock DM, Blajman CR, Mickiewicz E, et al. Cisplatin and fluorouracil alone or with docetaxel in head and neck cancer. N Engl J Med. 2007;357:1705-15.

51. Vermoken JB, Remenar E, van Herpen C, Gorlia T, Mesia R, Degardin M, et al. Cisplatin, fluorouracil, and docetaxel in unresectable head and neck cancer. N Engl J Med. 2007;357:1695-704.
52. Bourhis J, Blanchard P, Landais C, Petit C, Zhang Q, Grégoire V, et al. Meta-analysis of chemotherapy in head and neck cancer (MACH-NC): An update on 100 randomized trials and 19,248 patients, on behalf of MACH-NC group. Ann Oncol. 2016;(Suppl 6):vi328-vi350.
53. Guan J, Li Q, Zhang Y. A meta-analysis comparing cisplatin-based to carboplatin-based chemotherapy in moderate to advanced squamous cell carcinoma of head and neck (SCCHN). Onco Target. 2016;7:7110-9.
54. Bonner JA, Harari PM, Giralt J, Harari PM, Giralt J, Azarnia N, Shin DM, Cohen RB, et al. Radiotherapy plus cetuximab for squamous-cell carcinoma of the head and neck. N Engl J Med. 2006;354:567-78.
55. Mehanna H, Robinson M, Hartley A, Kong A, Foran B, Fulton-Lieuw T, et al. Radiotherapy plus cisplatin or cetuximab in low-risk human papilloma virus-positive oropharyngeal cancer (De-ESCALate HPV): an open-label randomized controlled phase 3 trial. Lancet. 2019;393:51-60.
56. Gillison ML, Trotti AM, Harris J, Eisbruch A, Harari PM, Adelstein DJ, et al. Radiotherapy plus cetuximab or cisplatin in human papillomavirus-positive oropharyngeal cancer: a randomised, multicenter, non-inferiority trial. Lancet. 2019; 393:40-50.
57. Hadad RJ, Posner M, Hitt R, Cohen EE, Schulten J, Lefebvre JL, et al. Induction chemotherapy in locally advanced squamous cell carcinoma of the head and neck: role, controversy and future directions. Ann Oncol. 2018;29:1130-40.
58. Eze N, Lo YC, Burtness B. Biomarker driven treatment of head and neck squamous cell cancer. Can Head Neck. 2017; 26:1-12.

SECTION 1 Pretreatment Assessment and Evaluation

Radiological Evaluation of Head and Neck Cancer

Gaurav Sundar

INTRODUCTION

The imaging evaluation of head and neck cancers has evolved over the years with advances in imaging technology and changes in cancer management, allowing more cancers to be diagnosed early and improving overall survival.[1]

The radiological evaluation in head and neck cancers serves four primary purposes:

1. A tool to diagnose cancers in potentially "blind" areas to endoscopic and clinical evaluation such as the tongue base and vallecula
2. Staging of malignant cancer and assessment of operability
3. Follow-up or surveillance after completion of cancer treatment
4. Assessment of pertinent comorbidities

Common to all subsites of head and neck cancer, the radiological evaluation must include the:

- Local extent and size of the tumor
- Perineural spread and bone involvement
- Involvement of regional lymph nodes including extracapsular spread
- Presence of distant metastases
- Synchronous primary malignancies[2]

A variety of imaging modalities can be used in the evaluation of head and neck cancer. More than one modality is often needed for the complete evaluation of the cancer as information provided by the different modalities often complements each other. The merits and limitations of the various modalities will be discussed below.

IMAGING MODALITIES

Magnetic Resonance Imaging

In patients with no contraindications to magnetic resonance (MR), it is the primary modality used in the diagnosis and local staging of head and neck cancers. The excellent soft tissue contrast resolution and multi-planar capabilities allow MR to accurately differentiate normal from abnormal tissue for local staging. A standard MR protocol including imaging sequences, plane, and their application is summarized in **Table 1**.

Additional sequences and planes can be added in selected circumstances. For example, sagittal imaging is useful in evaluation of tumors involving the hard palate, nasopharynx, the tongue base, and epiglottis. Diffusion-weighted imaging (DWI) and dynamic contrast enhanced (DCE) MR have application in evaluating lymph nodes

Table 1: Standard magnetic resonance protocols.

Sequence	*Plane*	*Application*
T1 FSE	Axial	• Study the anatomy • Baseline to assess for enhancement
T1 FSE + gadolinium	Axial	Assess for tumor enhancement
T2 SE	Axial and coronal	• Evaluate pathology and extent • High resolution images to evaluate bone
STIR	Axial	• Screen for pathology which will appear bright • Evaluate marrow edema in the mandible (tumor involvement or osteoradionecrosis)

(FSE: fast spin echo; SE: spin echo; STIR: short tau inversion recovery)

and differentiating recurrence within postradiation changes.[3] MR angiography can be useful to delineate arterial involvement **(Figs. 1A to C)**.

Limitations to the use of MR include the relatively longer time of imaging (approximately 30 minutes), artefacts produced by dental amalgams, and patients with contraindication to MR (pacemaker, claustrophobia, and metallic implants).

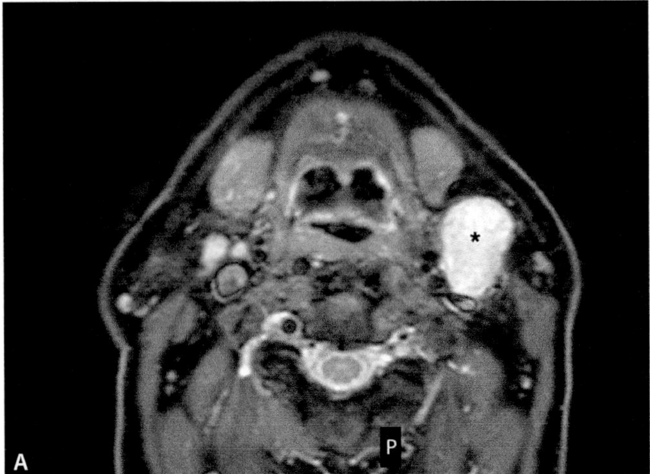

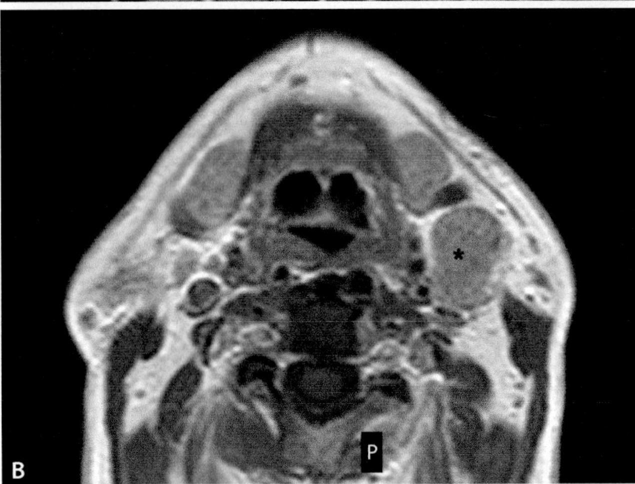

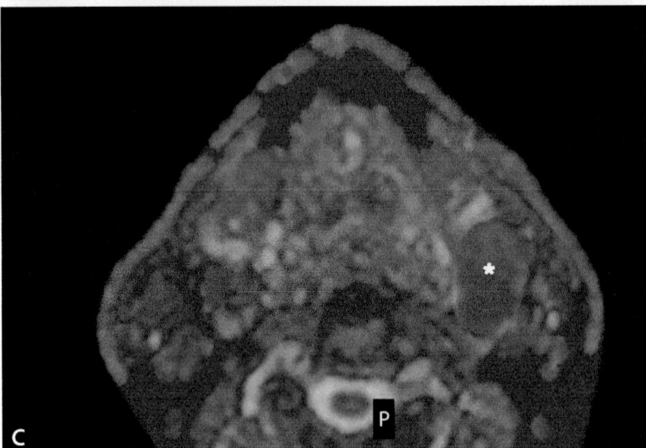

Figs. 1A to C: (A) Gadolinium enhanced T1-weighted sequence; (B) Axial short tau inversion recovery (STIR) sequence showing a necrotic left-sided level II lymph node; (C) Apparent diffusion coefficient (ADC) map from a diffusion-weighted imaging (DWI) MR showing low signal in the corresponding lymph node indicating restricted diffusion from a pathological lymph node. [(*) showing left-sided level II lymph node].

Computed Tomography

Computed tomography (CT) is an alternative and/or synergistic to MR in the local staging of head and neck cancers when there are contraindications to the use of MR. It is relatively inexpensive, quick, and widely available when compared to MR. Both CT and MR are excellent at detecting lymph nodal disease and their extent. CT is particularly useful in the evaluation of bone involvement in the mandible and skull base and screening of the lungs for metastasis. A standard protocol when using CT as a primary diagnostic tool would be to image the entire neck and chest from skull base to the diaphragm after administering intravenous iodinated contrast. The limitations of CT include relatively poor soft tissue contrast resolution, radiation exposure, artefacts from dental amalgams, and need for the use of iodinated contrast.

Ultrasonography

Ultrasound (US) provides an excellent adjunct tool in the evaluation of the superficial structures of the neck. It is the primary modality of choice for the evaluation of the thyroid and salivary glands. It is excellent in the morphological characterization of lymph nodes, detection of microcalcification, necrosis, and extracapsular spread. It is used to improve the accuracy of fine-needle aspiration (FNA) or biopsy. Doppler US is useful in the evaluation of the vessels of the head and neck to detect vascular encasement or thrombosis. Limitations of US include inability to evaluate retropharyngeal and mediastinal lymph nodes. US and FNA are both heavily dependent on operator's skill.

Plain X-ray and Fluoroscopy

Orthopantomograms are routinely used to detect dental disease and treat them prior to radiation treatment for oral cancers to avoid the risk of osteoradionecrosis.

Molecular Imaging and Positron Emission Tomography/Computed Tomography

Fluorodeoxyglucose (FDG) positron emission tomography (PET)/CT has an established role in evaluation and staging of head and neck squamous cell carcinomas.[4] Current indications include:

- Detection of primary lesions with malignant neck lymphadenopathy which is not evidence on clinical examination, panendoscopy and MR.

- Evaluation of distant metastasis in primary malignancy with high risk of dissemination—high grade, locally advanced disease, or high-risk anatomical site like the nasopharynx.
- Assessment of treatment response and in differentiating post-treatment changes from tumor recurrence.
- Differentiating reactive versus metastatic lymphadenopathy.

Some of the limitations that must be remembered are that FDG PET/CT offers no advantage over MR in the local T-staging and that small lesions may be below the threshold for detection in areas with physiological uptake like the tonsils or the vocal cords and larynx if the patient coughs or talks during the uptake phase of imaging. Moreover, diagnostic CT scans are more sensitive in the detection of small lung metastases compared to the low-dose CT used in FDG PET/CT.

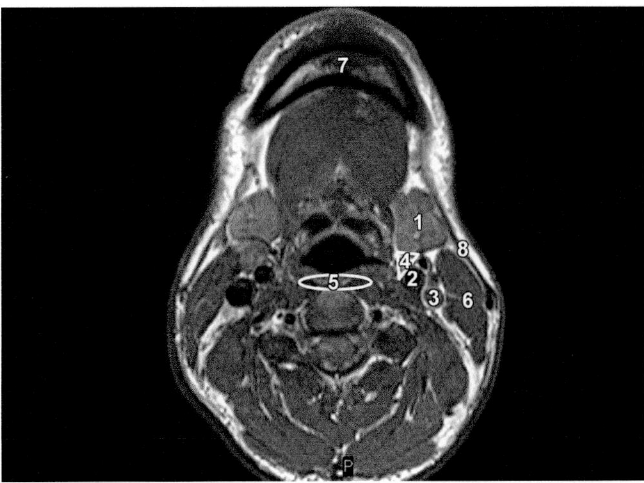

Fig. 2: Axial T1-weighted MR of the suprahyoid neck. 1: Submandibular salivary gland; 2: Carotid artery; 3: Internal jugular vein; 4: Parapharyngeal space; 5: Retropharyngeal space; 6: Sternocleidomastoid; 7: Mandible.

ANATOMY

Knowledge of cross-sectional anatomy of the head and neck is imperative for the head and neck radiologist and surgeon for the accurate staging and assessment of cancer. Although a detailed description of surgical and radiological anatomy is beyond the scope of this chapter, a basic review of clinically relevant anatomy will be discussed here.

Anatomically, the head and neck is divided into multiple spaces by various fascial planes having its own contents and possible pathologies. The hyoid bone bifurcates the neck into the suprahyoid and infrahyoid region on cross-sectional imaging.

The suprahyoid neck comprises the pharyngeal mucosa space, the masticator space, the parapharyngeal space, the parotid space, the carotid space, the retropharyngeal space, and the perivertebral space including the vertebrae **(Fig. 2)**.

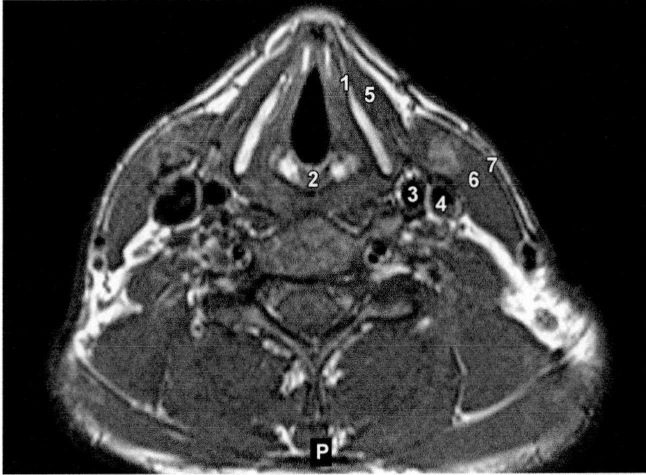

Fig. 3: Axial T1-weighted MR of the infrahyoid neck. 1: Thyroid cartilage; 2: Cricoid cartilage; 3: Carotid artery; 4: Internal jugular vein; 5: Strap muscles; 6: Sternocleidomastoid; 7: Platysma.

The infrahyoid neck spaces consist of the visceral space including the trachea, esophagus, thyroid, and parathyroid glands, the carotid space, the retropharyngeal space, and the perivertebral space which extend downwards from the suprahyoid neck **(Fig. 3)**.

The retropharyngeal space is a potential space which exists between the visceral fascia anteriorly and prevertebral fascia posteriorly. It extends superiorly from the skull base to the level of the carina in the posterior mediastinum inferiorly making it a potential route of spread of infection and tumor from the neck to the mediastinum **(Fig. 4)**.

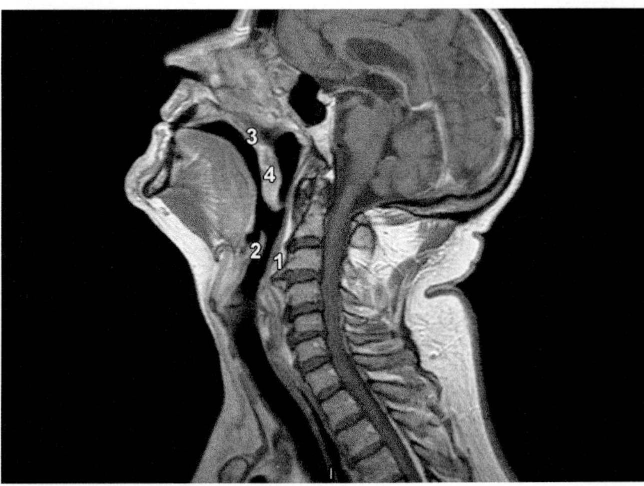

Fig. 4: Sagittal T1-weighted MR of the midline neck. 1: Retropharyngeal space; 2: Epiglottis; 3: Hard palate; 4: Soft palate.

Apart from this anatomical classification that is useful in recognizing the location of the pathology and a possible etiology, the mucosal-lined structures of the

Table 2: Sites and subsites of the head and neck with their lymphatic drainage patterns.

Sites	*Subsites*	*Spread to*
Oral cavity	Lip, anterior tongue, floor of mouth, buccal mucosa, upper and lower alveolar ridge, hard palate, and retromolar trigone	• Level I, II, and III • Bone
Oropharynx	Tonsil, base of tongue, soft palate, and lateral and posterior pharyngeal wall above the hyoid	Level II, III, and retropharyngeal
Hypopharynx	Pyriform sinus, postcricoid area, and posterior pharyngeal wall below the hyoid	• Level II, III, IV, and retropharyngeal • Submucosal spread
Larynx: Supraglottis	Epiglottis, false vocal cords, arytenoid cartilage, and aryepiglottic folds	• Level II, III, and IV • Pre-epiglottic space • Transglottic spread to glottis and subglottis
Larynx: Glottis	True vocal cords and anterior commissure posterior commissure	• Lymph node (LN) spread is rare • Paraglottic space • Transglottic spread to supraglottis or glottis
Larynx: Subglottis	N/A	• Level III, IV, and VI (upper paratracheal) • Transglottic spread to glottis and supraglottis
Nasopharynx	N/A	Level II, III, IV, V, retropharyngeal, and parapharyngeal
Nasal cavity and paranasal sinuses	Maxillary, sphenoid, ethmoidal, frontal, medial maxillary wall, and nasal septum	Orbit, infratemporal fossa, pterygoid plates, and intracranial
Major and minor salivary glands	N/A	Level IA, IB, II, III and V

upper aerodigestive tract have been divided into different sites and subsites **(Table 2)**. This is because the most common pathology affecting this area is cancer and this subdivision is useful to assess for regional lymph nodal spread and for staging and prognostication purposes.

LOCAL T STAGING

In this section, general imaging evaluation that have implications for local T-staging of all head and neck cancers will be considered. Specific features of various subsites will be discussed in a later section.

Tumor Size

The initial T-staging of most head and neck cancers is primarily based on the size of the tumor. Direct and endoscopic evaluation can only visualize the mucosal extent of the tumor and grossly underestimate the submucosal spread. The excellent soft tissue contrast resolution and multiplanar capabilities of MR make it best suited to differentiate abnormal tissue from normal anatomical structure and accurately measure the tumor. The best sequences to use are short tau inversion recovery (STIR) and fat-suppressed contrast-enhanced T1-weighted sequences in both of which tumor stands out as high signal intensity on a background of low signal normal tissue. Measurements must be made in orthogonal transverse and craniocaudal dimensions and the largest measurement used to determine stage.

Anatomical Subsite and Adjacent Site Involvement

Head and neck cancer can involve adjacent structures through contiguous spread. Involvement of more than one anatomical subsite or adjacent anatomical sites upstages cancers. Depending on the site of the primary malignancy, important anatomical sites which are better evaluated with imaging include the retromolar trigones, pterygoid plates, medial and lateral pterygoid muscles, extrinsic tongue muscles, cortical bone of the maxilla and mandible, laryngeal cartilages, carotid vessels, prevertebral space, skull base, and intracranial extension. Mucosal disease extent and identification of vocal cord fixation are better evaluated clinically.

Cortical Bone Involvement

Many oral and pharyngeal tumors have the potential of invading the mandible or hard palate. CT is very sensitive in detecting early cortical erosion and must be evaluated in the appropriate bone window setting. Dedicated dental CT scan equipment (DentaScan) use a cone-beam CT technique to produce higher resolution images which are more sensitive to detect subtle cortical erosions.[5] More advanced tumors involving the marrow or inferior alveolar canal are better evaluated with MR. The normal fat-containing bone marrow has a high signal on T1-weighted imaging and low signal on STIR sequences which contrasts the tumor infiltrating the

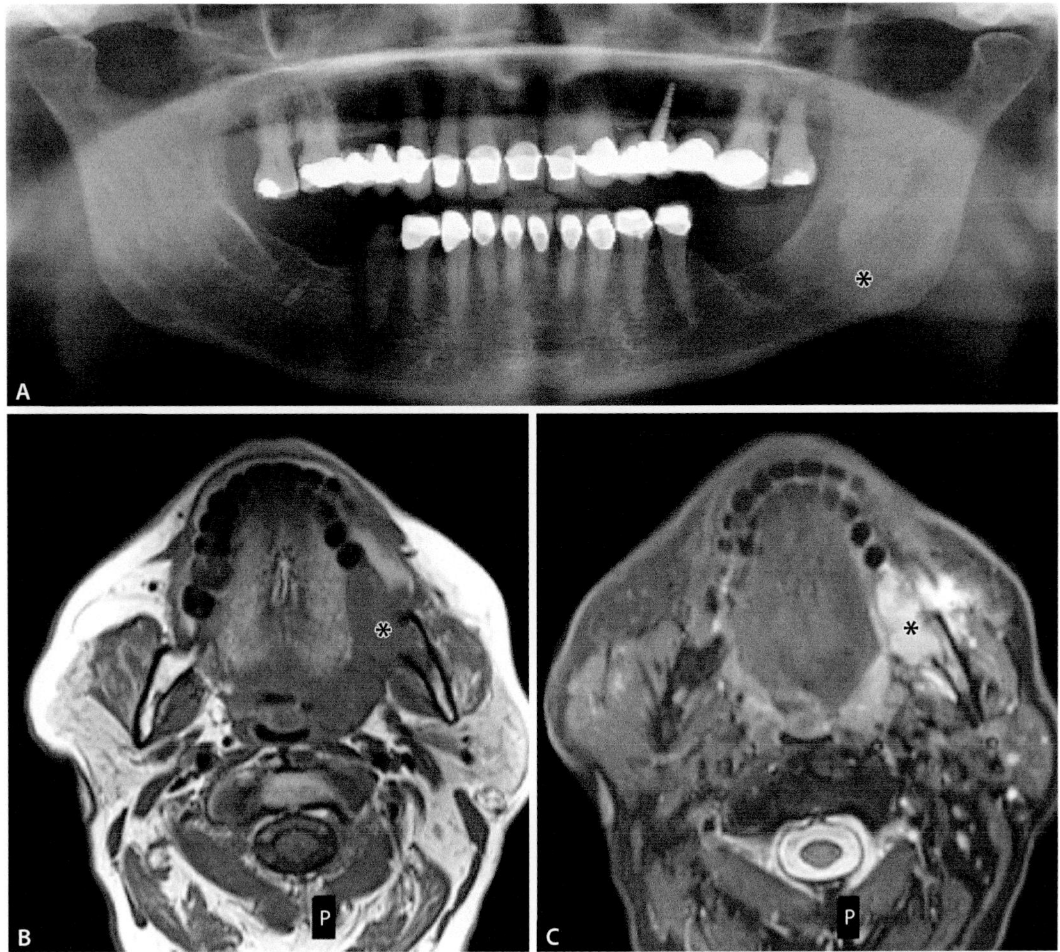

Figs. 5A to C: (A) Orthopantomogram demonstrating bone destruction in left hemimandible; (B and C) Axial STIR and T1-weighted MR confirming a left side tonsil malignancy invading the mandible. Note the replacement of the normal high T1 signal marrow within the mandible with low signal tumor. [(*) showing bone destruction].

marrow which is seen as low signal on T1-weighted images and high signal on STIR sequences. A potential pitfall can arise from recent dental extractions, osteoradionecrosis, and infection that may have similar appearances on MR and careful clinical and historical correlation is needed to avoid this pitfall **(Figs. 5A and B)**.

Carotid Vascular Involvement

Encasement or invasion of the common carotid or internal carotid artery (ICA) by the primary tumor or lymph nodes usually makes them inoperable. CT and MR are accurate in detecting vascular encasement.[6] The only definite imaging feature that indicates vascular involvement is demonstrating direct tumor extension into the vessel. Loss of fat plane between the tumor and the carotid vessels, compression or deformity of the vessel and >180° of vascular encasement by the tumor are other less specific signs of vascular involvement **(Fig. 6)**.

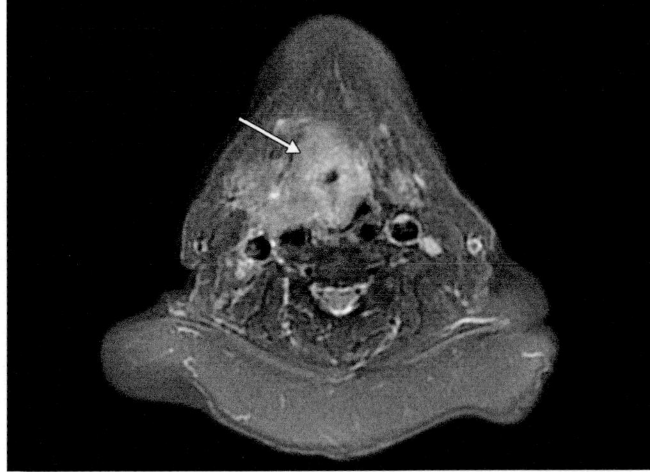

Fig. 6: Axial STIR MR depicting a laryngeal malignancy encasing the right carotid artery over 180°.

Prevertebral Fascia Involvement

This denotes fixation of the tumor to the prevertebral musculature making it inoperable and increases the chance of tumor spread to retropharyngeal lymph nodes that must be carefully sought. Tumors arising from the nasopharynx and posterior pharyngeal wall have a propensity for involving the prevertebral fascia. The normal retropharyngeal space contains fat that is seen as high signal on sagittal T1-weighted images. Because tumors must extend through the retropharyngeal space before invading the prevertebral fascia, preservation of this normal high signal T1 fat stripe is a reassuring indicator of the absence of prevertebral fascia involvement.[7] Signs of prevertebral fascia involvement include abnormal high T2 signal intensity or contrast enhancement within the prevertebral muscles.

Laryngeal Cartilage Involvement

Laryngeal cancers that extend to the paraglottic space can invade the laryngeal cartilages. Early invasion of the cortex of the thyroid cartilage (T3 disease) must be differentiated from through-and-through extension (T4a disease), as this can have major treatment implications in larynx-sparing therapies. Early invasion of the cartilage can be seen as sclerosis on CT.[8] While this is rather reliable in detecting invasion of the cricoid and arytenoid cartilage, diagnosing thyroid cartilage invasion on CT can be notoriously difficult. This is because of variably age-related ossification of the thyroid cartilage. Ossification does not occur uniformly through the entire cartilage making it challenging to differentiate normal ossification from cancer-related sclerosis. As a caveat, areas of erosion adjacent to tumor in an otherwise completely ossified cartilage can be a marker for cartilage invasion. MR is more specific in identifying cartilage invasion and can be seen as a change in the signal intensity within the cartilage matrix (high T2 signal or enhancement on gadolinium). The demonstration of tumor tissue on both sides of the cartilage is a reliable indicator of through-and-through cartilage invasion on both CT and MR.

Pre-epiglottic Fat Invasion

Invasion of the pre-epiglottic fat from supraglottic malignancies is a surrogate marker for the risk of hyoid bone invasion which is crucial in laryngeal-conservation surgery. This is best evaluated on sagittal and axial T1-weighted MR and is marked by invasion of the normally high signal intensity pre-epiglottic fat by low signal intensity tumor.[9]

Dural and Skull-base Invasion

Sinonasal tumors and nasopharyngeal tumors have the potential to extend intracranially through the skull base; either directly through the bone or via one of the numerous skull-base foramina. Early involvement may be in the form of dural thickening and enhancement. It can be difficult to differentiate reactive dural thickening from tumor infiltrating the dura although thickening >5 mm and nodular thickening make malignancy more likely.[10] Extension through the skull-base foramina may be seen as enlargement of the foramen on CT or demonstration of enhancing tumor within the foramen on fat suppressed T1-weighted MR **(Figs. 7A and B)**.

Orbital Invasion

Sinonasal tumors can invade the orbit directly through the orbital floor or the lamina papyracea. Orbital invasion can also occur through the skull-base foramen—the inferior orbital fissure which communicates with the pterygopalatine fossa. Imaging features of early orbital

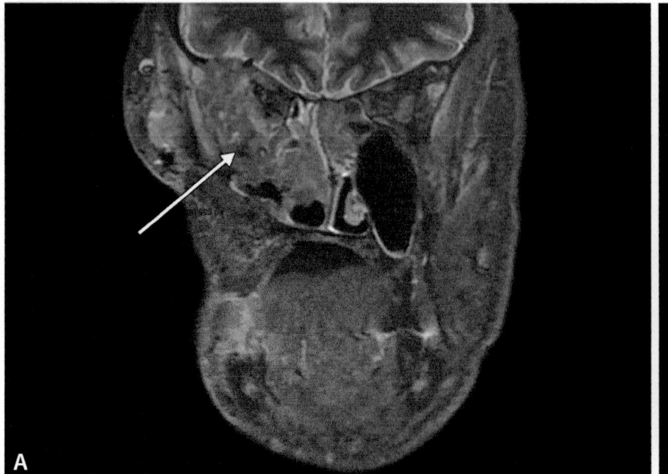

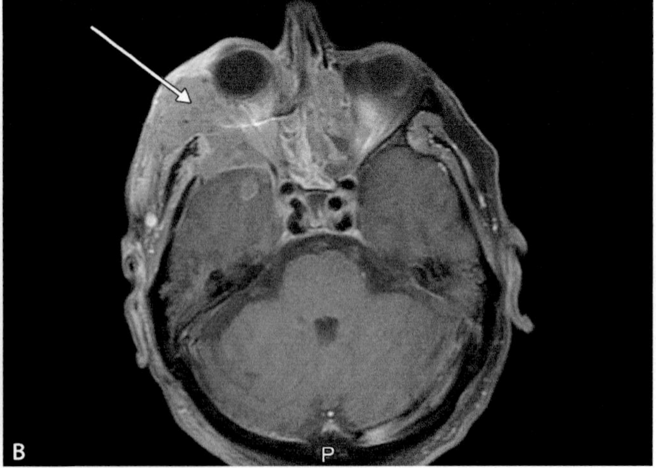

Figs. 7A and B: Coronal T2-weighted (A) and axial postgadolinium fat suppressed T1-weighted MR (B) demonstrating a right-sided maxillary sinus tumor invading the orbit and dural of the middle cranial fossa.

involvement is seen as orbital bone erosion on high-resolution CT images **(Figs. 7A and B)**. More advanced tumors may infiltrate the intraorbital fat, and this is best seen on T1-weighted images as low signal tumor infiltrating the high signal fat or on STIR sequences as high signal tumor infiltrating the low signal fat. Invasion of the extraocular muscles can also be demonstrated on MR.

Perineural Spread of Tumor

Spread of tumor through the perineural lymphatics, perineurium or endoneurium is collectively referred to as perineural spread (PNS). PNS is not infrequently seen in head and neck tumors, can often be clinically silent in the early stages, and diagnosed earlier on imaging. The detection of PNS can have profound therapeutic implications and the failure to diagnose PNS can result in delayed tumor recurrence.

Although all tumors have the potential for PNS, certain tumor subtypes have a greater propensity for this route of spread—adenoid cystic carcinoma, cutaneous melanoma, and mucoepidermoid carcinoma are especially neurotropic.

The most common sites of tumor and the route and nerve through which they spread are listed in **Table 3**.

Imaging features of PNS depends on the location of the primary and the nerve along which the tumor spreads. The pterygopalatine fossa is a common site of PNS and normally contains fat seen as high signal on T1-weighted MR and low density on CT. Replacement of this fat by tumor is seen as enhancing soft tissue on CT and low signal on T1-weighted MR.[11] The pterygopalatine ganglia located within the pterygopalatine fossa provides potential routes of tumor spread as it communicates with the greater and lesser palatine nerves, the V2 division of the trigeminal nerve and the vidian nerve; the latter arising from the greater superficial petrosal nerve, a branch of the facial nerve and thus providing a channel of tumor spread from the VII cranial nerve and V cranial nerve. In general, spread through skull-base foramen and nerve canals can be seen as enlargement of the foramina or canal on CT (when comparing to the contralateral side) or demonstrating enhancing soft tissue within the foramina or canal on CT or MR **(Figs. 8A and B)**.

Table 3: Routes and perineural spread in common head and neck tumors.

Sites	*Route*	*Nerve*
Adenoid cystic tumor of minor salivary glands	Hard palate	Greater and lesser palatine nerve → pterygopalatine fossa → V2
Nasopharyngeal carcinoma	Nasopharynx	• Pterygopalatine fossa → V2 • Masticator space → V3
Primary or metastatic major salivary gland tumor	Parotid gland	• Facial nerve • Auriculotemporal branch → V3
Squamous cell carcinoma (SCC) of oral cavity, lip, or skin	Mandibular invasion	Inferior alveolar nerve → V3

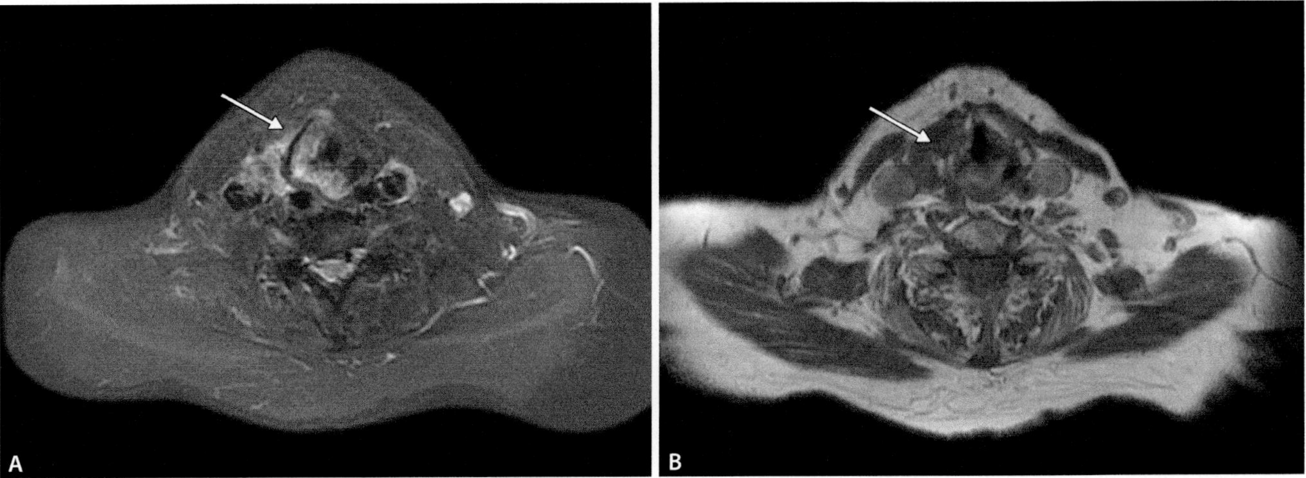

Figs. 8A and B: Axial STIR (A) and axial T1-weighted (B) MR demonstrating a laryngeal malignancy extending through the right thyroid cartilage lamina. On the T1-weighted MR, note the normal high signal in the cartilage on the left side which has been replaced by low signal tumor on the right side.

NODAL STAGING

Anatomy

The lymph nodes in the neck are divided anatomically into seven levels.

Level I

- Below mylohyoid muscle and above the lower margin of the hyoid bone (or at the carotid bifurcation)
- Anterior to the posterior border of the submandibular glands:
  - *Level IA:* Submental nodes, i.e., between the anterior bellies of the digastric muscles
  - *Level IB:* Submandibular nodes, i.e., posterolateral to the anterior belly of the digastric muscles and anterior to the posterior border of the submandibular glands

Level II

- Internal jugular (deep cervical) chain
- Base of the skull to the inferior border of hyoid bone (or the carotid bifurcation)
- Anterior to the posterior border of sternocleidomastoid (SCM) muscle
- Posterior to the posterior border of the submandibular glands:
  - *Level IIA:* Anterior, lateral, medial, or posterior to the internal jugular vein. If the node is posterior to the internal jugular vein, it must be inseparable from it
    - The superior most is the jugulodigastric node
  - *Level IIB:* Posterior to the internal jugular vein but have a fat plane separating the nodes and the vein

Level III

- Internal jugular (deep cervical) chain
- Lower margin of hyoid to lower margin of cricoid cartilage (or the intermediate tendon of omohyoid)
- Anterior to the posterior border of SCM
- Lateral to the medial margin of the common carotid artery (CCA)/ICA

Level IV

- Internal jugular (deep cervical) chain
- Lower margin of cricoid cartilage to level of the clavicle
- Anterior and medial to an oblique line drawn through the posterior edge of SCM and the posterolateral edge of the anterior scalene muscle
- Lateral to the medial margin of the CCA

Level V

- Posterior triangle (spinal accessory) nodes
- Posterior to the back of the SCM muscle and anterior to the trapezius muscle
  - *Level VA:* Superior half, posterior to levels II and III (between base of the skull and inferior border of cricoid cartilage)
  - *Level VB:* Inferior half, posterior to level IV (between the inferior border of cricoid cartilage and the level of clavicles)

Level VI

- Prelaryngeal (Delphian node)/pretracheal
- Anterior to visceral space
- From the inferior margin of hyoid bone to the manubrium
- Anterior to levels III and IV

Level VII

- Superior mediastinal nodes
- Between CCAs, below superior aspect of manubrium to level of the brachiocephalic vein

Other Groups

- *Supraclavicular nodes:* These nodes are identified as those nodes lying medial to the clavicles and lateral to the carotid artery on the axial images where a part of the clavicle can be seen. They include some level IV and level V nodes.
- *Retropharyngeal nodes:* The importance of identifying this nodal group is that their involvement makes most head and neck cancers inoperable.
- *Parotid nodes:* Nodes within the parotid can be involved in malignancies of the scalp, orbit, and nasopharynx.

Criteria for Abnormal Lymph Nodes

- *Size:* This is the simplest but least reliable method to decide if a lymph nodes harbors tumor or not. Large lymph nodes can be benign and small lymph nodes may be malignant. There is also a great variation in criteria used to classify a lymph node as pathological depending on the nodal group involved and whether the measurement was made in the axial or craniocaudal plane and if the measurement is along the short axis or long axis of the lymph node. In routine clinical practice, a cutoff of 10 mm in the short axis is used for most lymph node groups. Nodes in the level II and Ib are more frequently enlarged from reactive benign causes such as infections and inflammatory conditions in the oral cavity or oropharynx and a higher cutoff of 15 mm is used in these two groups to improve the specificity.[12]

- *Morphology:* There are various morphological features which help differentiate benign lymph node enlargement from malignant enlargement. Most morphological characteristics are best visualized on US which can also help guide FNA in equivocal cases **(Figs. 9A and B)**.
  - *Shape:* Benign lymph node enlargement often retains the normal reniform shape of the lymph node while malignant nodes are often round.
  - *Margins:* The evaluation of the lymph node capsule is best done with US although MR can better diagnose invasion of adjacent structures like the muscles and vasculature. Capsular irregularity or frank invasion of adjacent structures is classified as extracapsular spread and upstages nodal disease to N3b in the latest tumor, node, and metastasis (TNM) classification.

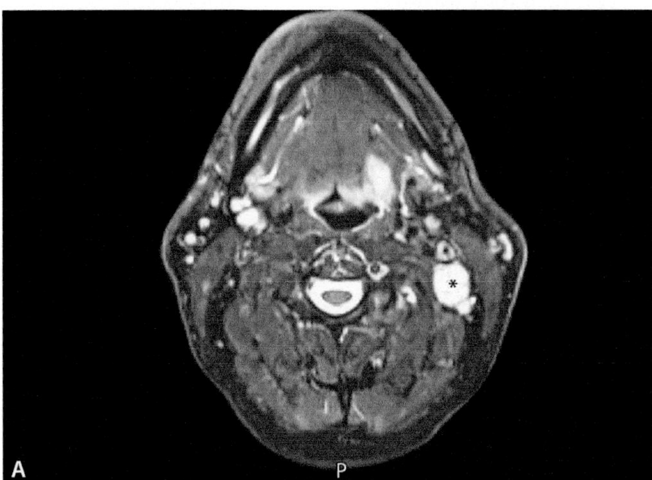

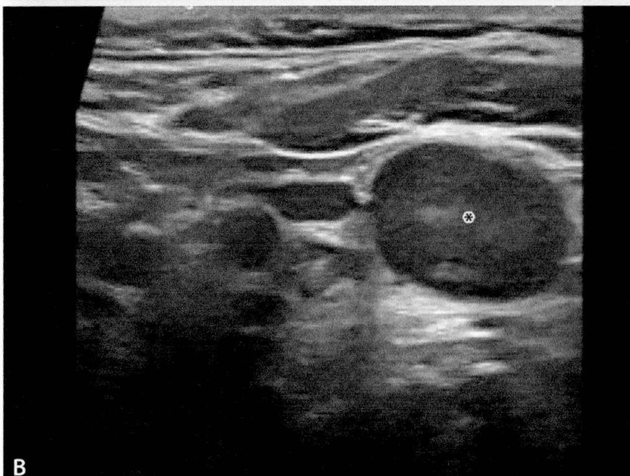

Figs. 9A and B: (A) Axial STIR MRI of the neck showing an enlarged level II lymph node; (B) US of the lymph node showing pathological morphology—round shape, hypoechoic with loss of central fatty hilum. [(*) showing level II lymph node].

  - *Evaluation of the lymph node hilum:* Metastatic disease often first spreads to the hilum which contains the vascular pedicle of the lymph node. This results in replacement of the normal fat-filled hilum with tumor tissue which can easily be identified on US and sometimes even MR.
  - *Central necrosis:* The presence of central necrosis is characteristically associated with malignancy (and some infections like tuberculosis). Necrosis is seen on CT and MR as a nonenhancing central area and is hypoechoic on US. A potential pitfall is that necrotic lymph nodes are often not FDG-avid and can be missed on PET/CT.
  - *Calcification:* Although mediastinal lymph node calcification is often a marker of benign disease, cervical lymph node calcification can be seen in papillary thyroid cancer and treated head and neck cancers. In countries where tuberculosis is endemic, tubercular lymphadenopathy continues to be the most common cause for calcified cervical lymph nodes.
- *Distribution:* While it is common to have scattered subcentimeter lymph nodes in the level II and Ib, the clustering of three or more lymph nodes in the drainage area of a known malignancy must be viewed with suspicion. It is important to evaluate the contralateral side as asymmetrical lymph node enlargement can also be a marker for malignancy.

Role of Imaging in Evaluating Lymph Nodes

For the purpose of staging, the imaging evaluation of nodal disease in head and neck cancers must include the following:

- *Size:* For the purpose of staging, nodal size is measured in the longest dimension (transverse or craniocaudal).
- *Number:* Single or multiple.
- *Laterality:* Ipsilateral or contralateral to the primary tumor. Midline lymph nodes are classified as ipsilateral for the purpose of staging. For midline tumors (like epiglottis), a unilateral lymph node is considered ipsilateral while bilateral lymph nodes are considered contralateral.
- *Extracapsular spread:* Imaging features of extracapsular spread include capsular irregularity, fat stranding, loss of fat-plane with adjacent structures or frank invasion of adjacent structures such as the strap muscles, neck viscera or vasculature.

SPECIFIC TUMOR SITES

In the following subsections, specific clinical questions that can be answered using imaging for the staging of individual cancer subsites in the upper aerodigestive tract, major salivary glands, and paranasal sinuses will be discussed.

Oral Cavity and Oropharynx

Imaging is performed in nearly all cancers except those with obviously clinically superficial tumors and leukoplakia.

Staging objectives include:

- Determine size and volume of tumor that determines T staging.
- Extension to involve the extrinsic or deep tongue muscles, retromolar trigone, submandibular space (oral tumors), and prevertebral space (oropharyngeal tumors) **(Figs. 10A and B)**.
- Cortical and deep bone marrow invasion including invasion of the inferior dental nerve canal which are indicated by replacement of the normal high T1 signal of bone marrow with low T1 signal of tumor, high signal on STIR, and contrast enhancement within the marrow.
- Perineural spread through the inferior alveolar nerve (mandible) or greater palatine nerve (hard palate) which is seen as high STIR signal and enhancement within the expected region of the nerve.
- *T4b disease:* Tumor invades masticator space, pterygoid plates, or skull base, and/or encases ICA
- Lymph nodal disease and evaluation of extracapsular spread.

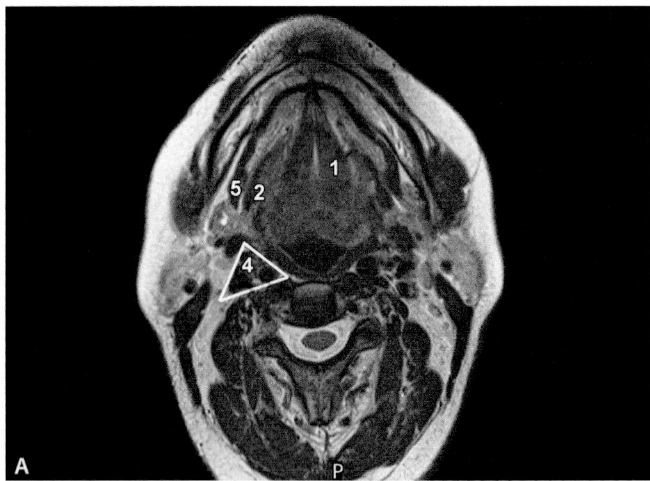

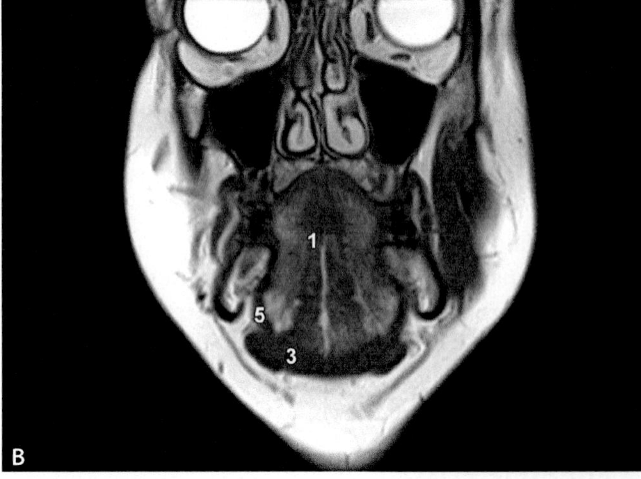

Figs. 10A and B: Axial (A) and coronal (B) T2-weighted MR demonstrating structures related to the oral cavity and oropharynx. 1: Genioglossus; 2: Hyoglossus; 3: Anterior belly of digastric; 4: Carotid triangle; 5: Mylohyoid.

Tips and Tricks

- Always perform any imaging prior to biopsy as postbiopsy changes can upstage tumors on imaging.
- Asking the patient to puff the cheeks or perform Valsalva maneuver is useful in evaluation buccal mucosa tumors.
- Dental amalgam can create substantial artefacts both on CT and MR. Using nonfat suppressed sequences tend to reduce MR artefacts and are hence preferred in oral cavity tumors.
- In evaluation bone invasion, CT is superior to MR in detecting early cortical bone invasion while MR is superior to CT in detecting deeper marrow invasion and PNS.
- The tongue base and tonsils are common sites of occult primary disease in patients presenting with cervical lymph nodal disease. In such cases, FDG PET/CT is very useful in identifying the primary disease but it must be remembered that normal FDG uptake is seen in the palatine and lingual tonsils (base of tongue) and subtle asymmetrical uptake may be the only clue to guide biopsy from these regions.
- Dental disease can mimic bone involvement both on FDG PET/CT and CT and MR, and clinical history is important to differentiate tumor involvement from inflammation and dental infection.

Nasopharynx

Imaging is performed in all patients with known cancer. Because nasopharyngeal cancers often cause eustachian tube obstruction, a unilateral middle ear effusion is sometimes the presenting feature of these tumors. Consequently, many tumors are initially diagnosed on CT evaluation of the temporal bone. Tumors found to be in an advanced stage do not require any further imaging. Most other tumors are best evaluated with MR and FDG PET/CT.

Staging objectives include:

- Evaluation of local extent including skull-base invasion.

- *Lymph nodal involvement*: Retropharyngeal and posterior triangle (level V) lymph nodes are commonly involved.
- Distant metastasis in the lungs, liver, and bone are more common in nasopharyngeal tumors than other head and neck cancers making FDG PET/CT vital in staging.

Tips and Tricks

- Perineural spread through the maxillary division of the trigeminal nerve is common at the skull base and coronal postcontrast MR is the most useful sequence in evaluating for this.
- Supraclavicular lymph nodal involvement confers a poor prognosis and any imaging should cover this region.
- The fossa of Rosenmüller must carefully be evaluated for tumor in all patients with unilateral middle ear effusion.
- The nasopharyngeal "soft tissue" may never completely revert back to normal after radiotherapy and PET/CT is useful to evaluate for residual disease.
- US and FNA is useful in the evaluation of nonenlarged but morphologically suspicious lymph nodes in patients who are to receive focused radiation therapy which will spare these regions.

Hypopharynx

These tumors commonly have bulky submucosal spread resulting in clinical understaging at endoscopy. Imaging is, therefore, indicated in all patients with diagnosed cancer.

Staging objectives include:
- Determine the local size and extent of the tumor including parapharyngeal spread and involvement of the prevertebral fascia.
- Identify midline and contralateral extension, as this will affect surgical resection.
- Identify laryngeal cartilage involvement, extension into the prelaryngeal strap muscles and subcutaneous tissue which upstage disease to T4b and are usually not resectable.
- Postcricoid malignancies can spread to the cervical esophagus, which needs to be evaluated.
- Evaluate lymph nodal disease including superior mediastinal lymph nodes in patients with postcricoid tumors.

Tips and Tricks

- Breathing and swallowing can produce motion artefact and imaging is best done in quite respiration without any swallowing during data acquisition.
- The appearance of the laryngeal cartilages is very variable on CT as ossification is often nonuniform and varies with age. The only definite evidence of cartilage involvement is identifying tumor on either side of the laryngeal cartilage or invasion of the prelaryngeal strap muscles and is best evaluated on MR.
- Remember to evaluate retropharyngeal lymph nodes in patients with posterior pharyngeal wall invasion.

Larynx

Laryngeal cancers often present early and the diagnosis is often made on laryngoscopy. The contribution of imaging is to complement endoscopy and indicated in T2 and higher lesions. Vocal cord fixation upstages all cancers to T3 and this can only be evaluated clinically.

Staging objectives include:
- Assess submucosal and paraglottic spread.
- Evaluate invasion of the pre-epiglottic space and tongue base—best identified on MR.
- Evaluate for laryngeal cartilage invasion.
- Evaluate extent of nodal disease—midline nodal disease is considered to be ipsilateral to the tumor.

Tips and Tricks

- Imaging should be performed in quite respiration and the patient must be instructed not to swallow during image acquisition.
- Patients should be instructed not to talk during the uptake phase of FDG to reduce uptake in the intrinsic muscles of the larynx.
- Radiation therapy can cause significant edema of the laryngeal mucosa and can mimic tumor on all imaging modalities. Imaging should ideally be deferred for 12 weeks after radiotherapy.

Salivary Glands

The majority of salivary gland tumors are benign pleomorphic adenomas. Malignant tumors more commonly arise from the sublingual and submandibular salivary glands and the deep lobe of the parotid gland. They include adenoid cystic tumor and mucoepidermoid carcinoma both of which have a predilection for PNS. The presence of lymph nodes in the parotid gland (but not the submandibular or sublingual gland) makes them a possible site for metastatic disease (from the scalp) and lymphoma.

Staging objectives include:
- Determine local extent of the tumor.
- Identify lymph node disease.
- Identify PNS.

Tips and Tricks

- Intraparotid lymph nodes can mimic tumors on US.
- Normal salivary glands demonstrate moderate FDG uptake and this must not be mistaken for pathology.
- Perineural spread is best identified on MR.

TREATMENT FOLLOW-UP AND IMAGING OF TUMOR RECURRENCE

Almost all patients treated for head and neck cancers have imaging follow-up after treatment:

- To evaluate treatment response
- To detect treatment-related complications
- For early identification of tumor recurrence
- To detect second primaries

The following are the recommendations of the United Kingdom National Multidisciplinary Guidelines:[13]

- Patients should be followed up to a minimum of 5 years.
- Initial follow-up frequency should be 2–3 monthly for the first 2 years and then 3–6 monthly subsequently. Some patients are imaged more frequently depending on the clinical findings, tumor subsite and biology, smoking and human papillomavirus (HPV) status.
- MR with or without PET/CT should be used when recurrence is suspected clinically.

Ideally, MR sequences on follow-up should be identical to that employed at the baseline staging scans to allow for direct comparison. Imaging appearances after treatment depend on the type of treatment received and this must be clearly mentioned in the radiological request. In the initial weeks or months after completion of radiotherapy, there can be edema and inflammation in the radiation field seen on MR. These appearances can mask any residual tumor lying within the radiation field and follow-up imaging will help exclude malignancy as radiation-induced changes often reduce with time. In selected patients, PET/CT can be helpful as it has a high negative predictive value to exclude tumor recurrence but can also give rise to false-positive results if there is infection or inflammation after surgery or chemoradiotherapy (CRT). Recurrence is usually seen as focal nodular areas of FDG uptake or enhancement on MR near the resection margins while inflammatory changes are usually more diffuse. A detailed description of imaging appearances of tumor recurrence and radiation changes is beyond the scope of this chapter.

Finally, follow-up imaging may be needed to exclude treatment-related complications. Of special note is osteoradionecrosis that occurs as a result of radiation-induced injury to the bone marrow, commonly affecting the mandible. It appears as areas of cortical destruction on CT and orthopantomograph (OPG) with surrounding sclerosis and soft-tissue thickening. While osteoradionecrosis is usually a sterile process, there can be secondary infection and osteomyelitis that can be difficult to identify on imaging and requires a clinical diagnosis. The role of imaging is to assess the extent of bone necrosis, presence of pathological fractures, involvement of the inferior alveolar nerve canal, and identify any fistula formation that will affect the surgical management.

REFERENCES

1. Pulte D, Brenner H. Changes in survival in head and neck cancers in the late 20th and early 21st century: a period analysis. Oncologist. 2010;15(9):994-1001.
2. Lewis-Jones H, Colley S, Gibson D. Imaging in head and neck cancer: United Kingdom national multidisciplinary guidelines. J Laryngol Otol. 2016;130(S2):S28-31.
3. Dai YL, King AD. State of the art MRI in head and neck cancer. Clin Radiol. 2018;73(1):45-59.
4. Olliff J, Richards P, Connor S, Wong WL, Beale T, Madani G, et al. Recommendations for cross-sectional imaging in cancer management. London: The Royal College of Radiologist; 2014.
5. Uribe S, Rojas LA, Rosas CF. Accuracy of imaging methods for detection of bone tissue invasion in patients with oral squamous cell carcinoma. Dentomaxillofac Radiol. 2013; 42(6):20120346.
6. Lodder WL, Lange CA, Teertstra HJ, Pameijer FA, van den Brekel MW, Balm AJ. Value of MR and CT imaging for assessment of internal carotid artery encasement in head and neck squamous cell carcinoma. Int J Surg Oncol. 2013; 2013:968758.
7. Hsu WC, Loevner LA, Karpati R, Ahmed T, Mong A, Battineni ML, et al. Accuracy of magnetic resonance imaging in predicting absence of fixation of head and neck cancer to the prevertebral space. Head Neck. 2005;27(2):95-100.
8. Becker M, Zbären P, Delavelle J, Kurt AM, Egger C, Rüfenacht DA, et al. Neoplastic invasion of the laryngeal cartilage: reassessment of criteria for diagnosis at CT. Radiology. 1997;203(2):521-32.
9. Loevner LA, Yousem DM, Montone KT, Weber R, Chalian AA, Weinstein GS. Can radiologists accurately predict preepiglottic space invasion with MR imaging? Am J Roentgenol. 1997;169(6):1681-7.
10. Eisen MD, Yousem DM, Montone KT, Kotapka MJ, Bigelow DC, Bilker WB, et al. Use of preoperative MR to predict dural, perineural, and venous sinus invasion of skull base tumors. Am J Neuroradiol. 1996;17(10):1937-45.
11. Ginsberg LE. MR imaging of perineural tumor spread. Neuroimaging Clin N Am. 2004;14(4):663-77.
12. Schwartz LH, Bogaerts J, Ford R, Shankar L, Therasse P, Gwyther S, et al. Evaluation of lymph nodes with RECIST 1.1. Eur J Cancer. 2009;45(2):261-7.
13. Simo R, Homer J, Clarke P, Mackenzie K, Paleri V, Pracy P, et al. Follow-up after treatment for head and neck cancer: United Kingdom National Multidisciplinary Guidelines. J Laryngol Otol. 2016;130(S2):S208-11.

CHAPTER 3

Pathology of Head and Neck Tumors

Nikita Oza, Narayana Subramaniam

INTRODUCTION

Accurate pathological examination forms the foundation for diagnosis and management of head and neck tumors. In addition to histological examination, several advanced techniques are used routinely in the management of this complex and diverse spectrum of disorders; a thorough knowledge is of utmost importance for anyone treating these patients. This chapter is a brief overview of processing of specimens for gross and microscopic histology, advanced diagnostic procedures and head and neck squamous cell carcinoma and its histological variants.

HISTOPATHOLOGY OF HEAD AND NECK TUMORS[1,2]

Histology is microscopic study of normal body tissue. The term histology is derived from Greek word "histos" (tissue) and "logos" (study), coined by Mayer in 1819. Histopathology is the science of studying disease-related structural changes in the human body. Several steps are required before the tissue is ready for a diagnosis. An optimum thickness is required for preparation of slides for accurate interpretation. Histotechnology is the branch of pathology that deals with processing and preparation of tissues to ensure a good quality for interpretation. Techniques routinely performed are paraffin embedding technique, exfoliative cytology, fine-needle aspiration cytology (FNAC), fine-needle aspiration biopsy (FNAB), frozen section, immunohistochemistry (IHC), fluorescence technique, tissue microarray and molecular techniques.

Specimen Processing

Tissue specimens received require documentation relating to the patient, tissue of origin and clinical details. Giving them a number that will identify each specimen as belonging to a particular patient accessions the specimens. A pathologist, assistant, or resident then examines specimens. Gross examination involves a description of the specimen and placing all or parts of it into small plastic cassettes while they are being processed to a paraffin block. When the case is suspected to be malignant, all the relevant surfaces are inked (with different colors) in order to be able to determine margins. The colored ink can be seen on microscopy as well.

Fixation

It is a series of chemical changes in order to reduce the risk of further alterations in cellular morphology. Fixation prevents degenerative changes due to autolysis and putrefaction, causing coagulation of proteins to maintain the cellular architecture without a change in relation of groups of cells to one another. It also results in a less friable semisolid state that can easily be manipulated without tissue damage and disruption. Commonly used fixatives are 10% buffered formalin, ethyl alcohol, mercuric chloride, acetone, potassium dichromate, picric acid and osmium tetroxide.

The time necessary for fixation is important routinely 10% buffered formalin at room temperature takes 4–6 hours for small specimens; whereas big specimens are fixed for 8–12 hours. Excessive prolonged fixation can have deleterious effect on immunohistochemistry. An ideal tissue thickness (3–5 mm) is important to allow adequate and even penetration of the fixative.

The purpose of fixation is to preventing autolysis and bacterial infection, to fix tissue to avoid changes in volume or shape during processing, to prepare tissue and leave it in a condition as close to their living state as possible with no small molecule loss.

Decalcification

This is the process in which insoluble calcium salts are removed from the tissue in order to allow sectioning and study. Several agents have been used for this purpose, each with their own advantages and disadvantages. Typically specimens are decalcified with hydrochloric or formic acid in the ratio of 20:1. The entire volume of this solution is replaced on a daily basis until the process is complete. The duration required for decalcification is highly variable, from a day to several weeks, dependent on the size of the specimen and the density of the calcium deposits. Typically, large bony specimens are immersed in 10% buffered formalin (90 mL) and nitric acid (10 mL) for simultaneous fixation and decalcification. The tissue is then decalcified using 10% nitric acid kept at 37°C. For firm tissues such as tracheal cartilage that require mild decalcification, the mixture of 10% buffered formalin (95 mL) and nitric acid (5 mL) for simultaneous fixation and decalcification. The tissue is then decalcified with 5% nitric acid solution for 5–6 hours.

After achieving decalcification, the tissue is rinses in running tap water (30 minutes for smaller tissues and 3–4 hours for bigger tissues). The tissues are then put in 70% alcohol for 30 minutes to completely remove any acid; otherwise the tissue will not acquire the hematoxylin stain.

Machine Processing

Once fixation is complete, the tissue needs further processing in order to take a form in which it can be easily slices into thin sections for staining and interpretation. The most common technique used in embedding within paraffin blocks, which allows for sectioning between 3 and 10 µm. This process during which the tissue is embedded in paraffin is known as processing.

This ensures that the tissue, through this embedding, is pliable enough to cut but formidable enough to prevent a loss of shape and distortion. The stages of tissue processing are:

- *Dehydration:* Wet fixed tissues are water-soluble and cannot be embedded in paraffin. This water must first be removed through dehydration, with alcohol of 70–100% strength. Formalin may also be added to alcohol. The time period required for dehydration is variable. Tissue blocks 1 mm thick require 30 minutes of exposure while those 5 mm thick need 90 minutes of dehydration. Tissues may be held and stored indefinitely in 70% ethanol without harm.
- *Clearing:* This process involves replacing the dehydrating fluid with a fluid that is totally miscible with both the dehydrating fluid and the embedding medium, commonly xylene.
- *Embedding:* When the alcohol in the tissue has been replaced with xylene, it can then be embedded in paraffin. The tissue is placed in a paraffin bath at 60°C. The paraffin is changed twice or thrice to ensure that the tissue is saturated with it.

Staining

The staining process makes use of dyes that have the ability to stain components of the tissue differentially in order to better delineate their anatomy. The most commonly used stain is hematoxylin and eosin (H&E). Other stains are referred to as "special stains" because they are employed in specific situations according to the diagnostic need (Periodic Acid Schiff's stain, Gomori's methenamine silver stain and Ziehl–Neelsen for highlighting microorganisms and Congo red stain for amyloidosis). An automated stainer is commonly used. Frozen sections are stained by hand, because this is faster than undergoing the entire process. The stain is referred to as "progressive" stain when the staining process continues until the desired tint is achieved. Cover slides are used to protect the tissue from being scratched, to provide better optical quality for viewing under the microscope, and for better preservation.

GENERAL CONSIDERATIONS IN GROSSING OF HEAD AND NECK ONCOLOGY SPECIMENS

- Orient the specimen and describe the type of resection (e.g., mandibulectomy, glossectomy, laryngopharyngectomy). Record the number of teeth and their appearances
- Weigh the specimen and measure the dimensions
- Carefully examine the external surface, locate the tumor and mention the anatomic site of origin (examples include buccal mucosa, gingivobuccal sulcus, retromolar trigone, anterior two-thirds tongue)
- Determine the extent of the tumor and its spread to adjacent structures on the mucosal surface
- Describe the color and appearance of the tumor, i.e., whether ulcerative, ulceroinfiltrative/proliferative, polypoidal, verrucous-like
- Measure the tumor in two dimensions in fresh state
- Ink the mucosal and soft tissue cut margins with India ink and/or colored ink. Fix the specimen with glacial acetic acid solution
- Carefully note the distance of the tumor from mucosal cut margins, skin cut margins and bony cut margins

when present. Submit the cut margins radially one by one
- The tumor is sectioned perpendicularly to the mucosa and the thickness is measure accurately. During the same time, note the appearances and consistency of the cut surface of tumor. Note the distance of the tumor from base/deep margin
- Measure the skin flap if resected and described whether it is grossly involved or free. Submit the section from the skin irrespective of gross impression
- Note the invasion of tumor in different tissue planes such as soft tissue and muscles
- Examine the non-neoplastic mucosa and comment on the presence of any other lesion. Record the distance of the second lesion from primary and closest margin
- If the tumor appears to abut or grossly involves the mandible, cut the mandible through and through with electric saw and fix the specimen. Extract teeth if the tumor appears to involve the dentulous area
- On cutting the bone, describe the appearance of bone and measure the distance between tumor in the bone and bony cut margins
- Submit at least one section of the mandible with overlying tumor irrespective of the gross impression
- **Figures 1 and 2** show the gross specimens following a retromolar trigone cancer and multinodular goiter respectively.

Sections to be submitted for reporting

- Minimum of four tumor sections have to be taken. If tumor is small such that four sections cannot be taken, then the tumor is to be completely embedded
- Attempt to take normal mucosa on both sides along with the tumor in the same section. Tumor host interface needs to be sampled extensively to assess perineural invasion, lymphovascular emboli and patterns of invasion. Preferably, entire slice of tumor along with at least 1 cm of the adjoining non-tumorous stroma is to be embedded
- Radial mucosal and skin cut margins
- Underlying and/or overlying bone with bony cut margins
- Overlying skin (when present)
- Adjacent soft tissue
- Lymph nodes
    - Nodes have to be embedded without completely stripping of the fat
    - Nodes ≤5 mm to be embedded completely, nodes ≤1 cm to be bisected while nodes >1 cm to be serially sliced perpendicular to the long axis at an interval of 2–5 mm and completely embedded if no gross tumor focus is identified
    - If gross tumor focus is identified then the focus with the largest tumor nodule to be embedded along with the surrounding fat

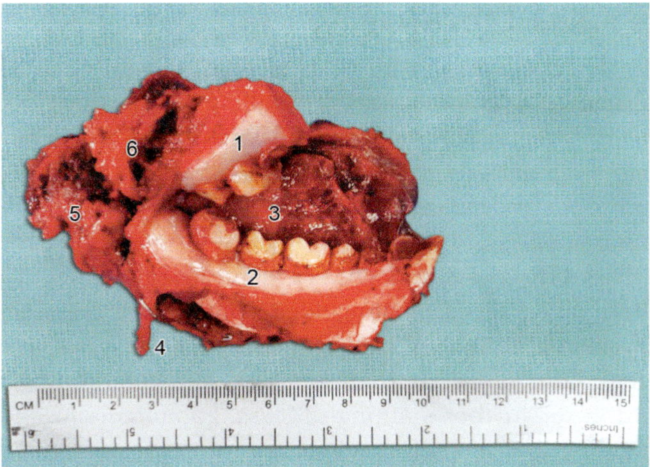

Fig. 1: Fresh surgical excision of a left retromolar trigone tumor en bloc showing maxilla: 1; mandible: 2; tumor: 3; lingual nerve: 4; masseter: 5; medial pterygoid: 6.

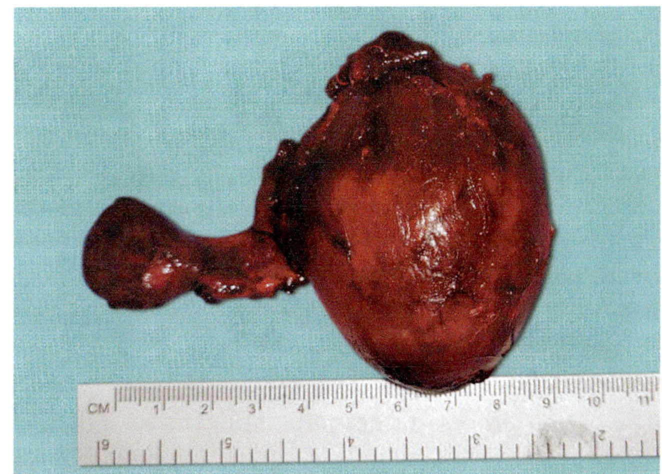

Fig. 2: Total thyroidectomy specimen showing left lobe follicular carcinoma thyroid.

EXFOLIATIVE CYTOLOGY[3]

In this method, cells are collected after they have been either spontaneously shed by the body (spontaneous exfoliation) or manually scraped/brushed off from a surface in the body (mechanical exfoliation). This fluid can be subjected to examination. Examples of mechanical exfoliation include Pap smears, where cervical cells which are scraped off are subjected to microscopy, or oral lesion brushings, where brushing cells from its surface and subjecting them to cytopathologic analysis study a visible lesion in the oral cavity.

FINE-NEEDLE ASPIRATION[4]

In this technique, a thin needle (by convention ≥22 G) is inserted into the mass for sampling of cells that after being stained will be examined microscopically. They are invaluable in head and neck cancer as they are rapid, accurate and relatively noninvasive. They are used in management of neck swellings, lymphadenopathy, thyroid disorders and salivary gland lesions. They can be image-guided or nonguided. The smears are then evaluated for on-site adequacy using 1% toluidine blue stain. The slides are then wet fixed in alcohol and air dried for further staining process. Papanicolaou and May Grunwald Giemsa stains are routinely performed for cytology specimens. When they are nondiagnostic they can be added or core biopsy can be performed. A diagnosis of lymphoma can be very hard to establish on fine-needle aspiration; core-needle biopsy can allow for immunohistochemistry, however fine-needle aspiration with flow cytometry is being more commonly used in this setting. Open biopsy must be performed with caution in suspected malignancy, especially in cases that will not be planned for curative intent surgery; spillage can reduce cure rates. In patients who are planned for curative intent surgery, open biopsy may necessitate excision of the previous surgical tract and scar. Fine-needle aspiration in individual subsites has been covered in detail in respective chapters.

IMMUNOHISTOCHEMISTRY[5]

This is the process of detecting antigens in cells of a tissue section with complementary binding antibodies. As part of this process, paraffin blocks comprising hundreds of separate tissue cores are assembled; hollow needles can remove small cores of tissue which are then reinserted into a recipient paraffin block where they are cut into fine sections with a microtome, stained and studied. Each of these microarray blocks can be further sectioned into hundreds of thin slices. **Table 1** shows commonly performed immunohistochemical markers employed in poorly differentiated carcinoma.

Table 1: Immunohistochemical markers commonly used in poorly differentiated carcinoma.

Histology	*Markers*
Basaloid squamous cell carcinoma	P63, P40, P16, HMWCK
Small cell carcinoma	Chromogranin, CD56, C-Kit, AE1, Mib-1
Neuroendocrine tumors	Chromogranin, Synaptophysin, CD56
Myoepithelial carcinoma	P63, Calponin, CD10, S100
Poorly differentiated adenocarcinoma	CK-7, CEA, P63

FLUORESCENT IN SITU HYBRIDIZATION[6]

In situ hybridization is the method of localizing and detecting specific nucleotide sequences in morphologically preserved tissue sections or cell preparations by hybridizing the complementary strand of a nucleotide probe against the sequence of interest. Fluorescent probes are then used as indicators that this binding has occurred. If nucleic acids are preserved in a histological specimen, they can be detected by using a complementary probe. Unlike classical cytogenetics (karyotyping), fluorescent in situ hybridization (FISH) does not require metaphase preparation of the cells of interest. It also requires less tissue and can be performed more rapidly than southern blot and polymerase chain reaction. It is commonly used for human papillomavirus (HPV) deoxyribonucleic acid (DNA) or messenger ribonucleic acid (mRNA) detection in HPV-associated oropharyngeal carcinoma, HPV DNA for HPV-associated carcinoma with adenoid cystic such as features, EWSR1 detection for break-apart hyalinizing clear cell carcinoma, ETV6 break-apart detection for secretory carcinoma and PLAG1 and HMGA2 break-apart detection for pleomorphic adenoma.

NEXT GENERATION SEQUENCING[7]

It is a high-throughput process that determines the DNA sequence of a given tissue sample. This method is highly scalable—it can be applied to both a small subset of genes or the entire genetic code. In principle, the concept behind next generation sequencing (NGS) technology is similar to Sanger sequencing. The process involved here is DNA polymerase catalyzes nucleotides that are labeled with fluorescence into a template strand for DNA synthesis. The fluorophore labels allow for the nucleotides used to be identified. The process is rapid and can allow for sequencing of the whole genome within a day.

Unlike with earlier techniques where the genome was fragmented into several fragments that were sequenced individually, NGS allows for simultaneous processing of million fragments in parallel, reducing the time taken and cost. Additionally, this process has a high sensitivity, allowing for detection of mutations in even 5% of a tumor DNA sample. This allows for identification of mutations with prognostic and therapeutic implications, and is being used more commonly to identify candidates for clinical trials.

MARGIN ASSESSMENT

Completeness of surgical excision is an important prognostic determinant in patients of head and neck cancer. Although the final surgical margins are confirmed by microscopic examination of the fixed histopathological specimens, there are several tools that aid the surgeon in performing an adequate resection. Ravi et al.[8] described a working classification for oral squamous cell carcinoma that is largely applicable to other sites in the head and neck.

Preoperative Assessment

- *Vital staining:*[9,10] This is an in vivo technique that uses staining using dyes such as toluidine blue, iodine and indigo carmine with Congo red to distinguish between benign and malignant tissue. Used extensively in colposcopy to direct site of biopsies in field change, it is now more commonly being used in oral cancer screening. In curative intent surgery it can be used to map out field change more accurately to ensure good mucosal margins. Indigo carmine and Congo red have also been used for deeper margins, to direct suspicious areas for frozen section.
- *Fluorescent visualization:*[11] Malignant transformation results in loss of normal autofluorescence. Under fluoroscopic visualization, normal oral mucosa emits pale green autofluorescence and areas of malignant transformation lack this; hence it can be used to map out areas of involvement for adequate clearance.

Intraoperative Assessment

- *Examination of resected margins:* Detailed examination of the specimen and its circumferential margins immediately after resection, with the help of the pathologist can aid complete resection. The pathologist can often mark the margins and section the specimen to measure radial margins; close margins can be revised immediately. Chaturvedi et al.[12] showed that if a margin was 7 mm on gross examination, the likelihood of a final positive margin was low, potentially obviating the routine need for frozen section.
- *Frozen section analysis:* This is an important technique that can aid adequacy of tumor excision. The main instrument required is the cryostat, which is a fine microtome. Although the preparation is much more rapid than conventional formalin fixed tissue, the technical quality of the sections is lower. In head and neck, frozen section can be used to identify margin adequacy, evaluate benign versus malignant tissue, evaluate lymph node spread, identification of the parathyroid glands and to determine if further testing is required (such as in lymphoma).[13] In the context of head and neck pathology, it has been shown to have a diagnostic accuracy of 95–98%, and a 2–4% error rate.[14,15] Although very popular in the United States, its use varies widely with the availability of resources and expertise. When compared to margins taken from the tissue bed after resection, it is reasonable to expect that margins derived from the specimen itself are more reliable. This is because of the reduced chance of a nonrepresentative margin, the ability to measure the distance of the margin from the tumor as opposed to labeling it as "free" when no tumor is identified, and because pathologists are more likely to identify nests of tumor closer to the core of the tumor.[16]
- *Ultrasonography:*[17] This has been shown to be a reliable method to map out tongue tumors in cross section, allowing identification of the deep margin and confirming adequacy of excision. Although it is an additional tool at the disposal of the surgeon and has potential, it is user dependent and is helpful only for identification of gross tumor spread and not microscopic disease.
- *Touch imprint cytology:*[18,19] This involves touching tissue to a glass slide to allow transfer of cells that can be examined under the microscope after fixation. The diagnostic categories are negative for malignancy, atypical cells present but nondiagnostic for malignancy, atypical cells present, atypical cells present suspicious for malignancy and positive for malignancy. Although attractive, this technique lacks widespread validation in oral cavity.
- *Microendoscopy:*[20,21] Initially popularized to visualize the uterine walls, it allows for rapid and detailed examination of a mucosal surface, with detection of patterns specific for malignancy. It allows magnification of up to 150X. This technique can also been adapted to flexible fiberoptic probes and can be used in conjunction with fluorescence. Like other techniques it can map out mucosal margins with reasonable accuracy. Although it has been used in oral cancer, validation on a large scale is lacking.
- *Optical coherence tomography:*[22] This is a form of imaging that uses light to allow cross-sectional imaging of living tissues. As light passes through tissue, the natural turbidity provided split the light, which is passed through a polarized controller, an interferometer, dispersed by diffraction grating and finally focused on to an indium gallium arsenide line

camera to form a 2D image. The patterns in these images determine the likelihood of malignancy. Full-field optical coherence tomography allows for clearer images up to a few hundred micrometers depth. It is hoped that this technology will be mature enough to replace frozen section.

Postoperative Assessment

Moh's micrographic surgery:[23,24] This is considered the gold-standard technique for locally invasive cutaneous malignancies, especially over cosmetically important areas, like the face. It enables extensive horizontal sectioning of margins using a Moh's map, with a low recurrence rate in experienced hands. Margins can either be assessed using frozen section or formalin fixed for definitive interpretation.

Molecular Assessment and Gene Signature[25,26]

These are advanced tests that can be performed on margins that look for altered gene signatures or molecular markers that indicate premalignant or malignant transformation of the surrounding tissue even earlier than invasive neoplastic cells appear. These markers include p53, EGFR and K-RAS mutations and p16 promoter hypermethylation. These are still being validated and have not become widespread practice.

PATHOLOGY OF HEAD AND NECK SQUAMOUS CELL CARCINOMA[27]

Conventional head and neck squamous cell carcinoma (HNSCC) comprises variable degrees of squamous differentiation. Well-differentiated tumors resemble normal squamous epithelium except for keratin pearls and invasion of basement membrane with well-differentiated tumor cells, while poorly differentiated tumors have no resemblance to the normal squamous epithelium. As with other tumors, SCC shows several hallmarks of cancer such as disorganized growth, a loss of polarity, dyskeratosis, intercellular bridges, an increased nuclear to cytoplasmic ratio, nuclear chromatin irregularities, prominent eosinophilic nucleoli and increased mitotic figures (including atypical forms). As differentiation reduces, there is an increase in mitotic figures and necrosis. Broder's grading system is used to classify differentiation, where well, moderately, poorly and undifferentiated tumors have ≥75%, 50–74%, 25–49% and <25% differentiated tumor cells respectively. **Table 2** shows the histological variants of HNSCC.

Table 2: Histological variants of head and neck squamous cell carcinoma (HNSCC).[28-30]

Feature	*Verrucous*	*Spindle cell (sarcomatoid)*	*Basaloid*	*Adenosquamous*	*Papillary/exophytic*
Macroscopic	Broad-based warty and fungating mass	Polypoid mass	Firm to hard with central necrosis	Indurated submucosal nodule	Polypoid, exophytic, bulky, papillary, fungiform
Microscopic	Well differentiated neoplastic cells with bland cytology and minimal cellular atypia. Principally exophytic, and endophytic growth pattern. Vertical church-spire like keratinization and parakeratin plugging are the hallmark of the tumor	Biphasic; SCC present, but ulcerated; blended/ transition with atypical spindle cell population, hypercellular, variable patterns of spindle-cell growth, pleomorphism, opacified cytoplasm, increased mitotic figures	Biphasic; invasive, lobular, basaloid component most prominent, palisaded, high N/C ratio, abrupt squamous differentiation (metaplasia, dysplasia, carcinoma in situ or invasive), mitotic figures, comedo necrosis, hyaline material	Biphasic; SCC and adenocarcinoma, undifferentiated component, separate or intermixed with areas of transition, infiltrative, mitotic figures, sparse inflammatory infiltrate	More than 70% exophytic or papillary architecture; "cauliflower-like" vs. "celery like", unequivocal cytomorphologic malignancy, surface keratinization, invasive, but difficulty to demonstrate, koilocytic atypia
Ancillary studies	HPV identified. Strong expression of p53, Ki67 and p63. Negative for E cadherin, Integrin α6 and less expression of Laminin 5γ2	70% positive with epithelial markers	Keratin, EMA, CK7 and *34βE12*	Mucin positive adenocarcinoma cells	None
Differential diagnosis	Verrucous hyperplasia, SCC	Benign and malignant mesenchymal processes, melanoma, synovial sarcoma	Adenoid cystic carcinoma, neuroendocrine carcinoma (small-cell carcinoma)	Basaloid SCC, mucoepidermoid carcinoma, adenocarcinoma with squamous metaplasia	In situ SCC, squamous papilloma, reactive hyperplasia

REFERENCES

1. Layton C, Bancroft JD, Suvarna SK. Fixation of tissues. Bancroft's Theory and Practice of Histological Techniques E-Book. Amsterdam: Elsevier; 2018. pp. 40.
2. Rosai J. Rosai and Ackerman's Surgical Pathology e-book. Amsterdam: Elsevier Health Sciences; 2011.
3. Ogden GR, Cowpe JG, Wight AJ. Oral exfoliative cytology: review of methods of assessment. J Oral Pathol Med. 1997; 26(5):201-5.
4. Orell SR, Sterrett GF, Whitaker D, Vielh P. Techniques of FNA cytology. In: Orell SR, Sterrett GF, Whitaker D (Eds). Fine Needle Aspiration Cytology, 5th edition. New Delhi: Elsevier India Pvt. Ltd.; 2011. pp. 8-27.
5. Wenig BM. Atlas of Head and Neck Pathology. Amsterdam: Elsevier Health Sciences; 2015.
6. Wang MB, Alavi S, Engstrom M, Lee J, Namazie A, Moatamed F, et al. Detection of chromosome 11q13 amplification in head and neck cancer using fluorescence in situ hybridization. Anticancer Res. 1999;19(2A):925-31.
7. Loyo M, Li RJ, Bettegowda C, Pickering CR, Frederick MJ, Myers JN, et al. Lessons learned from next-generation sequencing in head and neck cancer. Head Neck. 2013; 35(3):454-63.
8. Ravi SB, Annavajjula S. Surgical margins and its evaluation in oral cancer: a review. J Clin Diagn Res. 2014;8(9): ZE01.
9. Kerawala CJ, Beale V, Reed M, Martin IC. The role of vital tissue staining in the marginal control of oral squamous cell carcinoma. Int J Oral Maxillofac Surg. 2000;29(1):32-5.
10. Missmann M, Jank S, Laimer K, Gassner R. A reason for the use of toluidine blue staining in the presurgical management of patients with oral squamous cell carcinomas. Oral Surg Oral Med Oral Pathol Oral Radiol Endod. 2006;102(6): 741-3.
11. Poh CF, Zhang L, Anderson DW, Durham JS, Williams PM, Priddy RW, et al. Fluorescence visualization detection of field alterations in tumor margins of oral cancer patients. Clinl Can Res. 2006;12(22):6716-22.
12. Chaturvedi P, Datta S, Nair S, Nair D, Pawar P, Vaishampayan S, et al. Gross examination by the surgeon as an alternative to frozen section for assessment of adequacy of surgical margin in head and neck squamous cell carcinoma. Head Neck. 2014;36(4):557-63.
13. Harrison LB, Sessions RB, Hong WK. Head and neck cancer: a multidisciplinary approach. Philadelphia: Lippincott Williams & Wilkins; 2009.
14. Ikemua K, Ohya R. The accuracy and usefulness of frozen-section diagnosis. Head Neck. 1990;12:298.
15. Gandour-Edwards R, Donald PJ, Wiese D. The accuracy and clinical utility of frozen section in head and neck surgery. Evidence at a university medical center. Head Neck. 1993; 15:33.
16. Robbins KT, Triantafyllou A, Suárez C, López F, Hunt JL, Strojan P, et al. Surgical margins in head and neck cancer: intra- and postoperative considerations. Auris Nasus Larynx. 2019;46(1):10-7.
17. Tarabichi O, Bulbul MG, Kanumuri VV, Faquin WC, Juliano AF, Cunnane ME, et al. Utility of intraoral ultrasound in managing oral tongue squamous cell carcinoma: systematic review. Laryngoscope. 2019;129(3):662-70.
18. Klimberg VS, Westbrook KC, Korourian S. Use of touch preps for diagnosis and evaluation of surgical margins in breast cancer. Ann Surg Oncol. 1998;5(3):220-6.
19. Creager AJ, Shaw JA, Young PR, Geisinger KR. Intraoperative evaluation of lumpectomy margins by imprint cytology with histologic correlation: a community hospital experience. Arch Pathol Lab Med. 2002;126(7):846-8.
20. Upile T, Fisher C, Jerjes W, El Maaytah M, Singh S, Sudhoff H, et al. Recent technological developments: in situ histopathological interrogation of surgical tissues and resection margins. Head Face Med. 2007;3(1):13.
21. Hamdoon Z, Jerjes W, McKenzie G, Jay A, Hopper C. Assessment of tumour resection margins using optical coherence tomography. Head Neck Oncol. 2010;2(S1):O7.
22. Nguyen FT, Zysk AM, Chaney EJ, Kotynek JG, Oliphant UJ, Bellafiore FJ, et al. Intraoperative evaluation of breast tumor margins with optical coherence tomography. Can Res. 2009;69(22):8790-6.
23. Bernstein JA, Hodgin EC, Holloway HW, Hedlund CS, Storey ES, Hubert JD. Mohs micrographic surgery: a technique for total margin assessment in veterinary cutaneous oncologic surgery. Vet Comp Oncol. 2006;4(3):151-60.
24. Kalavrezos N, Bhandari R. Current trends and future perspectives in the surgical management of oral cancer. Oral Oncol. 2010;46(6):429-32.
25. Braakhuis BJ, Bloemena E, Leemans CR, Brakenhoff RH. Molecular analysis of surgical margins in head and neck cancer: more than a marginal issue. Oral Oncol. 2010;46(7): 485-91.
26. De Carvalho AC, Kowalski LP, Campos AH, Soares FA, Carvalho AL, Vettore AL. Clinical significance of molecular alterations in histologically negative surgical margins of head and neck cancer patients. Oral Oncol. 2012;48(3):240-8.
27. Thompson LD. Squamous cell carcinoma variants of the head and neck. Curr Diagn Pathol. 2003;9(6):384-96.
28. Koch BB, Trask DK, Hoffman HT, Karnell LH, Robinson RA, Zhen W, et al. Commission on Cancer at the American College of Surgeons, Chicago, IL, the American Cancer Society, Atlanta, GA. National survey of head and neck verrucous carcinoma: patterns of presentation, care, and outcome. Cancer. 2001;92(1):110-20.
29. Viswanathan S, Rahman K, Pallavi S, Sachin J, Patil A, Chaturvedi P, et al. Sarcomatoid (spindle cell) carcinoma of the head and neck mucosal region: a clinicopathologic review of 103 cases from a tertiary referral cancer centre. Head Neck Pathol. 2010;4(4):265-75.
30. Pathak J, Swain N, Patel S, Poonja LS. Histopathological variants of oral squamous cell carcinoma-institutional case reports. J Oral Maxillofac Pathol. 2014;18(1):143.

Psycho-oncology and Pretreatment Counseling in Head and Neck Cancer

Soudhamini Shastry

INTRODUCTION

Dealing with mental health is a sensitive, integral aspect of care of patients with head and neck cancer. If mental health problems go untreated, patients' adherence to treatment, rehabilitation times, and risk of suicide may all be affected.

Assessment of psychological problems, differentiating "normal" from "abnormal" reactions, deciding when to refer to psychiatric services—while these tasks seem challenging at first, it helps to remember that being an attentive, empathic listener is a good place to start.

Additionally, positive treatment experience built on a good rapport with the treating team contributes to building resilience among patients—both survivors who experience remission, as well as the less fortunate patients facing prospects of palliation.

PRETREATMENT PSYCHOLOGICAL ASSESSMENT

Receiving the diagnosis of cancer or the news of its relapse can be a considerable source of stress;[1] patients understandably go through a difficult time, experiencing a mixture of emotions and thoughts. Specifically, the management of head and neck cancer may involve procedures that result in noticeable scars/disfigurement and difficulties with essential bodily functions such as swallowing and speech.[2]

An Austrian study found that oncologists were not very good at identifying their patients' emotional distress and need for counseling; unfortunately, this was worse among doctors treating patients with head and neck cancer.[3]

The Edmonton Symptom Assessment System[4] (ESAS; **Fig. 1**) is a scale that screens for symptoms routinely seen in patients with cancer, particularly those receiving palliative care. The Hospital Anxiety and Depression Scale[5] (HADS; **Fig. 2**) is a psychometric scale that was designed to measure the severity of psychiatric symptoms, for use specifically in nonpsychiatric hospital settings. Such tools possess the advantage of objectivity to an extent, but often, they require clinical expertise to interpret results meaningfully.[6]

A past history or family history of psychiatric illness and suicidal attempts can provide clues to the patient's coping reserve and current psychological state. Understandably, patients with the personality trait of health anxiety (existent prior to receiving cancer diagnosis) may face considerable anxiety/fear of cancer recurrence after treatment.

Even if mental health issues are not severe enough to warrant a formal psychiatric referral, it is prudent to record baseline and periodic assessments of mental state.

Depression, Anxiety and Adjustment Disorders

Depression, anxiety and adjustment disorders are commonly encountered psychiatric disorders in patients with cancer, with a prevalence of about 30–40% in hospital settings.[7] Remarkably, depression has been reported to be more prevalent in patients with head and neck cancers than in other types of cancer, perhaps partly due to reasons discussed in the previous section.[8]

Depression independently worsens morbidity and elevates mortality in patients with cancer,[9] an effect observed in other physical illnesses such as heart disease[10] and stroke[11] as well.

The International Statistical Classification of Diseases and Related Health Problems 10th Revision (ICD-10) diagnostic criteria used to diagnose depression are fairly straightforward **(Box 1)**.

The ICD-10 subdivides *anxiety disorders* into generalized anxiety disorder, panic disorder, phobic disorders, etc. (please refer the ICD-10 DCR for the diagnostic criteria of the individual conditions.)

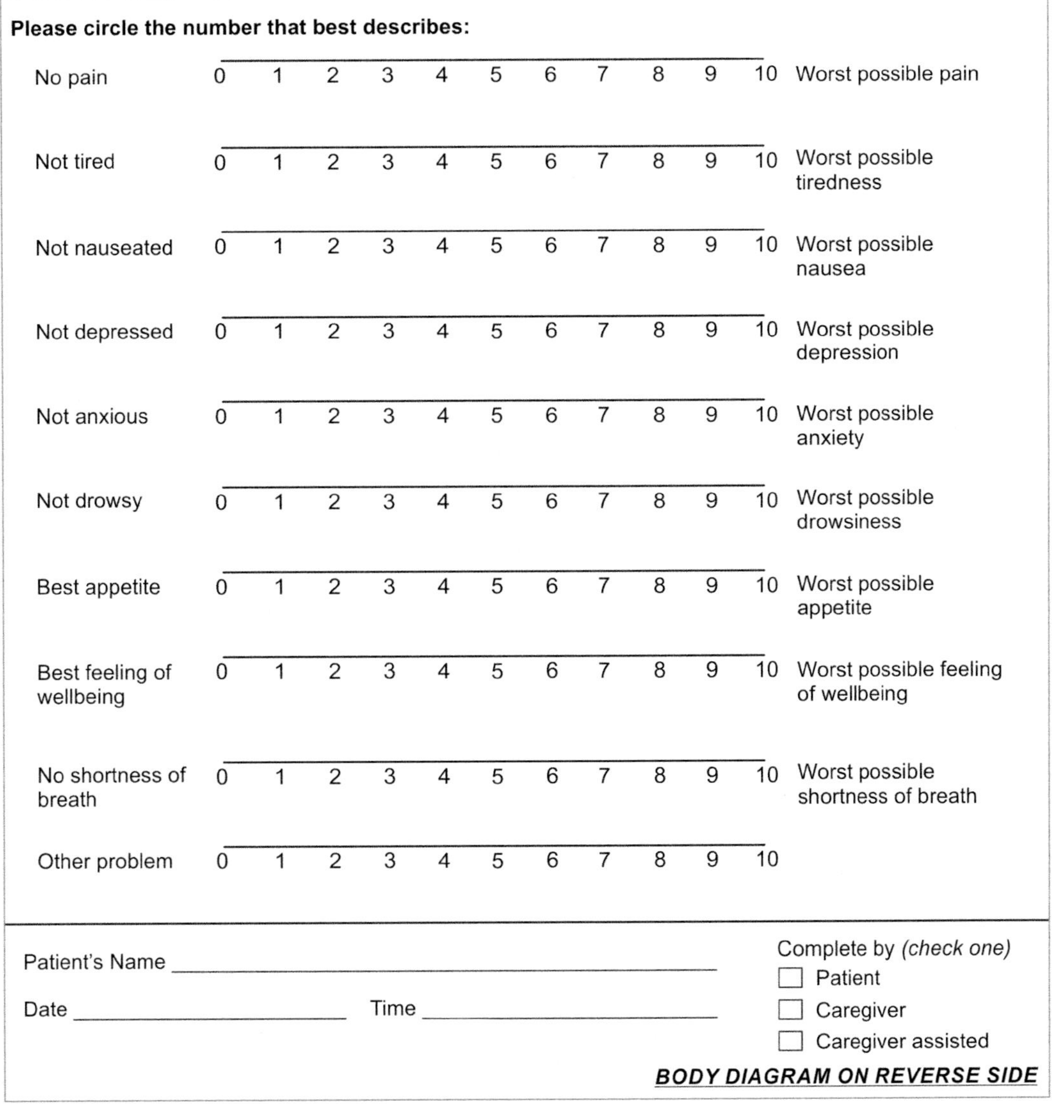

Please circle the number that best describes:

No pain	0	1	2	3	4	5	6	7	8	9	10	Worst possible pain
Not tired	0	1	2	3	4	5	6	7	8	9	10	Worst possible tiredness
Not nauseated	0	1	2	3	4	5	6	7	8	9	10	Worst possible nausea
Not depressed	0	1	2	3	4	5	6	7	8	9	10	Worst possible depression
Not anxious	0	1	2	3	4	5	6	7	8	9	10	Worst possible anxiety
Not drowsy	0	1	2	3	4	5	6	7	8	9	10	Worst possible drowsiness
Best appetite	0	1	2	3	4	5	6	7	8	9	10	Worst possible appetite
Best feeling of wellbeing	0	1	2	3	4	5	6	7	8	9	10	Worst possible feeling of wellbeing
No shortness of breath	0	1	2	3	4	5	6	7	8	9	10	Worst possible shortness of breath
Other problem	0	1	2	3	4	5	6	7	8	9	10	

Patient's Name ______________________

Date ______________ Time ______________

Complete by *(check one)*
- ☐ Patient
- ☐ Caregiver
- ☐ Caregiver assisted

BODY DIAGRAM ON REVERSE SIDE

Fig. 1: The Edmonton Symptom Assessment System (ESAS): Numerical Scale.

Adjustment disorder is a term used to denote a psychiatric condition arising as a result of a stressor, characterized by a clinically significant impairment, deemed to be in excess of a normal reaction to the stressor in question. However, the symptom profile is not sufficient to meet the criteria for the diagnosis of major syndromes such as depression or anxiety.

Irrespective of the diagnosis—a simple, comprehensive and holistic approach to mental health assessment is exploring the biological, psychological and social dimensions, also known as "biopsychosocial model".[12]

- *Biological,* e.g., disruptions in sleep, appetite, energy levels, attention and concentration; physical symptoms of anxiety (sympathetic overactivity), etc.
- *Psychological,* e.g., disturbance of mood, apprehensions and anxious thoughts, diminished motivation to carry out activities of daily living, drop in the level of confidence, thoughts of helplessness, hopelessness, etc.
- *Social,* e.g., seeming quiet, withdrawn, impaired social functioning.

Irrespective of the diagnosis, red flags requiring further assessment and referral to psychiatric department include:

- Very severe biological symptoms
- Excessive guilt, feelings of worthlessness, suicidal ideation/plans
  - Asking about suicidal ideation does not induce/increase suicidality, so it is very important to ask patients about this
- *Psychotic symptoms:* These patients have a disturbed sense of reality and impaired insight, i.e., hearing voices, harboring delusions, or suffering from incongruent elated mood.

Tick the box beside the reply that is closest to how you have been feeling in the past week.
Do not take too long over you replies; your immediate is best

D	A		D	A	
		I feel tense or 'wound up':			**I feel as if I am slowed down:**
	3	Most of the time	3		Nearly all the time
	2	A lot of the time	2		Very often
	1	From time to time, occasionally	1		Sometimes
	0	Not at all	0		Not at all
		I still enjoy the things I used to enjoy:			**I get a sort of frightened feeling like 'butterflies' in the stomach:**
0		Definitely as much		0	Not at all
1		Not quite so much		1	Occasionally
2		Only a little		2	Quite often
3		Hardly at all		3	Very often
		I get a sort frightened feeling as if something awful is about to happen:			**I have lost interest in my appearance:**
	3	Very definitely and quite badly	3		Definitely
	2	Yes, but not too badly	2		I do not take as much care as I should
	1	A little, but it does not worry me	1		I may not take quite as much care
	0	Not at all	0		I take just as much care as ever
		I can laugh and see the funny side of things:			**I feel restless as I have to be on the move:**
0		As much as I always could		3	Very much indeed
1		Not quite so much now		2	Quite a lot
2		Definitely not so much now		1	Not very much
3		Not at all		0	Not at all
		Worrying thoughts go through my mind:			**I look forward with enjoyment to things:**
	3	A great deal of the time	0		As much as I ever did
	2	A lot of the time	1		Rather less than I used to
	1	From time to time, but not too often	2		Definitely less than I used to
	0	Only occasionally	3		Hardly at all
		I feel cheerful:			**I get sudden feelings of panic:**
3		Not at all		3	Very often indeed
2		Not often		2	Quite often
1		Sometimes		1	Not very often
0		Most of the time		0	Not at all
		I can sit at ease and feel relaxed:			**I can enjoy a good book or radio or TV program:**
	0	Definitely	0		Often
	1	Usually	1		Sometimes
	2	Not often	2		Not often
	3	Not at all	3		Very seldom

Please check you have answered all the questions

Scoring:

Total score: Depresion (D) ________________ Anxiety (A) ____________________

0–7 = Normal

8–10 = Borderline abnormal (borderline case)

11–21 = Abnormal (case)

Fig. 2: Hospital Anxiety and Depression Scale (HADS).

A psychiatrist plans the treatment of anxiety, depression and adjustment disorders along the biopsychosocial dimensions.

- *Biological:* Treatment of cancer; treatment of contributory physical causes of depression such as underactive thyroid, B_{12}/folate deficiencies; treatment with antidepressants, benzodiazepines (short-term), hypnotics (short-term); ECT, and so on.
- *Psychological:* Counseling, cognitive behavioral therapy (CBT), mindfulness, etc., preferred in mild

Box 1: The ICD-10 diagnostic criteria of depression.

Major symptoms: At least one of these has to have been present for a diagnosis of depression
- Pervasive low mood
- Loss of interests and enjoyment
- Increased fatigability and diminished activity

Minor symptoms:
- Reduced concentration and attention
- Reduced self-esteem and self-confidence
- Ideas of guilt and unworthiness
- Bleak and pessimistic views of the future
- Ideas or acts of self-harm or suicide
- Disturbed sleep
- Diminished appetite

A combination of major and minor symptoms has to have been present on most days, most of the time for at least *2 weeks*

Mild depression: Four symptoms

Moderate depression: Five to six symptoms

Severe depression: Seven or more symptoms, further qualified as with or without psychotic symptoms

and moderate cases, depending on the availability of trained therapist.
- *Social:* Improving support by involving family and friends, referral to support groups such as Cancer Sahyog, which also offers financial support to patients in need.

Caregivers are also significantly affected by head and neck cancer—they may experience high levels of anxiety, worries of recurrence and may be affected by the patient's sense of well-being (and their own sense of well-being may reciprocally affect the patient too).[13] Hence, it is vital that caregivers are supported throughout the process of treatment too.

TOBACCO AND ALCOHOL CESSATION

Over three-quarters of head and neck cancers can be attributable to the combination of tobacco and alcohol use.[14] This staggering contribution signifies that cessation efforts among patients with head and neck cancer have numerous paybacks:
- The broad range of general improvements in physical health seen in all other individuals giving up tobacco and alcohol use
- The specific benefits in patients with cancer include:
  - A potential reduction in disease recurrence and incidence of new primaries
  - Improved response to cancer treatments
  - Improved quality of life[15]

Tobacco Cessation

When overall mortality among newly diagnosed head and neck cancer patients is compared: continuing smokers > quitters and former smokers > never smokers. India has a higher burden of oral cancers associated with the use of smokeless tobacco, which is available in myriad forms.[16] Hence, tobacco cessation interventions should be integrated into standard cancer treatment plans.[17]

The Cochrane Tobacco Addiction Group publishes evidence and guidelines on managing smoking cessation. Brief advice against smoking is defined as "verbal instructions to stop smoking with or without added information about the harmful effects of smoking." It is one of the most economical interventions in medicine and it can be carried out as a part of routine care by any health professional in 1–2 minutes.

Suggested phrasing for giving brief advice to smokers from "ABC of smoking cessation" by Tim Coleman:[18]
- The best thing you can do for your health is to stop smoking and I would advise you to stop as soon as possible.
- Tobacco is very addictive, so it can be very difficult to give up, and many people have to try several times before they succeed. Your chances of succeeding are much greater if you make use of counseling support, which I can arrange for you, and either nicotine replacement therapy or the antismoking drug bupropion, which I can prescribe for you.
- How do you feel about your smoking?
- How do you feel about tackling your smoking now?

Smokers who are highly motivated to quit may be supported by trained counselors who deliver intensive behavioral support to individuals or to groups. These counselors may focus on past smoking history, identify triggers for smoking behavior, set target quit dates, review progress periodically, etc.

The most effective methods to help smokers quit often combine drug treatment and specialist support. The combined treatment effects multiply rather than add up! Medications such as varenicline, bupropion, nortriptyline and clonidine have all been found to have varying levels of effectiveness in the treatment of tobacco dependence, but their use may be limited by side effects.

Nicotine replacement therapy, as the name suggests, attempts to eliminate withdrawal symptoms **(Fig. 3)**. It is available in many forms and all forms are effective. Prescribing practices depend on the availability of these forms as well as the individual patient characteristics/preferences.
- The use of inhalers very closely resembles the use of cigarettes, with respect to the act of smoking
- The use of oral chewing gums, again, resembles the use of smokeless forms of tobacco
- Patches ensure a constant level of nicotine in the bloodstream
- Nasal sprays can satisfy cravings/urges as they supply higher doses of nicotine rapidly[19]

Alcohol Cessation

Individuals may consume alcohol socially without developing dependence (a less common occurrence with tobacco use), hence it is important to avoid assumptions and inappropriate stereotypes. The issue of safe drinking limits is a contentious one, with different organizations issuing different standards. Tools such as CAGE and AUDIT may be used to screen all patients for harmful use of alcohol and dependence is defined by the ICD-10 diagnostic criteria. Useful markers that indicate heavy drinking include altered liver function tests, and more severe physical complications such as delirium tremens, alcohol withdrawal seizures, and alcoholic liver cirrhosis.

Prochaska and DiClemente proposed a model of stages of change[20] **(Fig. 4)** to understand the process of change for problematic behaviors. Motivational interviewing is an evidence-based intervention with the aim of enhancing motivation, guiding the patient through the stages of change.[21] Most clinicians can

Fig. 3: Fagerström test for nicotine dependence.

1. How soon after you wake up do you smoke your first cigarette?

Within 5 minutes	(3 points)
5 to 30 minutes	(2 points)
31 to 60 minutes	(1 point)
After 60 minutes	(0 point)

2. Do you find it difficult not to smoke in places where you should not, such as in church or school, in a movie, at the library, on a bus, in court or in a hospital?

Yes	(1 point)
No	(0 point)

3. Which cigarette would you most hate to give up; which cigarette do you treasure the most?

The first one in the morning	(1 point)
Any other one	(0 point)

4. How many cigarettes do you smoke each day?

10 or fewer	(0 point)
11 to 20	(1 point)
21 to 30	(2 points)
31 or more	(3 points)

5. Do you smoke more during the first few hours after waking up than during the rest of the day?

Yes	(1 point)
No	(0 point)

6. Do you still smoke if you are so sick that you are in bed most of the day, or if you have a cold or the flu and have trouble breathing?

Yes	(1 point)
No	(0 point)

Scoring: 7 to 10 points = highly dependent; 4 to 6 points = moderately dependent; less than 4 points = minimally dependent.

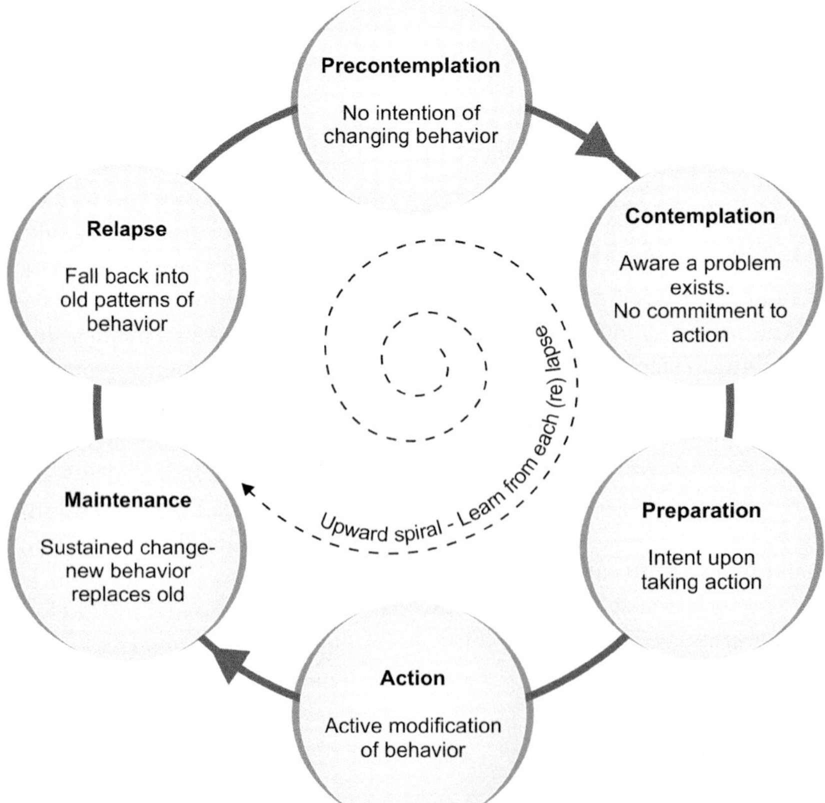

Fig. 4: The stages of change model.

Box 2: FRAMES model.

- *Feedback:* Regarding personal impairment following assessment of substance use problems. The diagnosis of cancer may offer the opportunity of a "teachable moment" to encourage behavior change
- *Responsibility:* For the patient and for change is placed on the patient, respecting their autonomy
- *Advice:* About the importance of changing patterns of substance use is presented in a nonjudgmental manner, specifically the adverse consequences of continued substance use
- *Menu:* Menu of self-directed change options is offered to the patient, allowing them to choose the approach that suits them best
- *Empathy:* Showing warmth, respect and understanding is more effective than a confrontational or coercive style
- *Self-efficacy:* Instilling a sense of optimism in the patient, that the goals are achievable

deliver this effective brief intervention, comprising the following elements popularly known by the acronym *FRAMES* **(Box 2)**.

Patients may be referred to mental health professionals to receive more specialized treatments that fall under the umbrella of cognitive-behavioral interventions (such as assertiveness skills training, drink refusal skills training, problem-solving skills training, relaxation training).

The organization of Alcoholics Anonymous (AA) deserves a special mention. AA meetings are led by nonprofessionals and free of charge. AA works by strengthening the social support systems and it can very effective in a subset of patients.

The pharmacological treatment of alcohol dependence includes treatments for alcohol withdrawal as well as relapse prevention. Alcohol withdrawal is treated with thiamine and benzodiazepines. Medications used in relapse prevention are acamprosate, naltrexone, disulfiram, topiramate and baclofen among others.

IMPROVING COMMUNICATION

Try to think of the last time you witnessed excellent, satisfying communication between a doctor and a patient with cancer. Now try to remember the doctor and patient characteristics that determined the nature of that interaction.

Good communication with patients requires doctors to possess/demonstrate

- The right knowledge
- Anticipation of the information needs of patients
- A confident, open, respectful attitude
- An ease with which they switch between different types of communication such as providing verbal explanations, drawing diagrams, handing out leaflets, providing internet links.

Patient factors influencing communication include:

- Age
- Gender
- Level of education
- Socioeconomic level
- Ethnicity[22]

If a doctor could anticipate the information needs of the patient they were about to review, this could make their interaction more productive. A study conducted in the USA aimed at patients just diagnosed with head and neck cancer revealed:

- Most patients wanted further information on treatment options, advice on how to stay healthy after treatment, and how to manage sequelae. Understandably, most of them experienced this need for information at the time of diagnosis, or during early stages of treatment.
- Women sought more information about coping with stress and anxiety than male patients.
- Younger patients were more interested in aspects of functioning like sexuality after treatment than older patients[23]

Breaking Bad News

Many doctors feel uncomfortable when they have to discuss unfavorable prognostic information with their patients, and it does not help that this is a commonly encountered scenario in the field of cancer.

Try to think of the behavior you would expect from your doctor if you were in such this unfortunate situation, and it does not take long to realize the bottom-line: you would appreciate the truth delivered from a doctor who appears to genuinely care about you.

While it is challenging to plan these discussions beforehand, it is useful to have a framework in mind. The SPIKES protocol is an elegant, practical strategy to handle these situations:[24]

- *S: Setting up* the interview, ice-breaking comments, introductions
- *P:* Assessing the patient's *Perception*: how much do they know already?
- *I:* Obtaining the patient's *Invitation*
  - "I am afraid it looks more serious than we had hoped. If it is alright with you, I would like to talk you through it."
  - Some patients may not express a desire for full information about their diagnosis, prognosis and this is a valid psychological coping mechanism. Information must not be "dumped" onto a patient if they do not feel ready to receive it.
- *K:* Giving *Knowledge* and information to the patient
  - Try to use simple, jargon-free language

- *E:* Addressing the patient's *Emotions* with *Empathic* responses
    - This comprises verbal and nonverbal responses
    - Some patients may need time for the news to sink in, long pauses may be necessary
- *S: Strategy* and *Summary*
    - Encourage questions from patients and try to answer them honestly
    - Clarify understanding
    - Work on a collaborative plan

IMPROVING COMPLIANCE TO TREATMENT

Treatment compliance can be an issue among patients with head and neck cancer. Sharma et al. evaluated this among 47 elderly head and neck cancer patients and found that over one-third were noncompliant.[25] Obviously, treatment outcomes and survival are influenced by compliance so making efforts to improve the same are important.

Treatment noncompliance may be a result of the following:
- *Pragmatic reasons:* Expensive treatment regimens, intolerable side effects, etc.
- *Lack of awareness:* Regarding the purpose of treatment, the impact of treatment, etc.
- *Social reasons:* Poor literacy, religious beliefs, lack of social support, stigma
- *Psychological reasons:*
    - Presence of psychological problems, particularly depression may render the patient "hopeless" about the treatment outcome, they may miss appointments
    - Psychological disturbances can be associated with cognitive impairment (problems with attention, concentration) that can affect the patient's understanding of cancer and its treatment.

Strategies to improve patient compliance include:
- Ensure the patient is well informed about the benefits of treatment, address all their concerns and expectations.
- Regularly review compliance, anticipate poor compliance in patients with the indicators listed earlier, and watch out for clues such as lack of response to treatment, missed appointments, etc.
- Simplify treatment regimens and schedule regular follow-ups to review their progress.
- Adopt a multidisciplinary approach—the involvement of nurses, pharmacists, etc., in addition to physicians have been found to improve compliance.

Obtain help from family members and friends where appropriate.[26]

COUNSELING IN END-OF-LIFE CARE/PALLIATION

Dealing with patients with cancer is already a sensitive affair, and for some of them, unfortunate bleak prognoses are inevitable. As doctors, we must approach these situations delicately and sensibly.

It is good practice to assess the level of suffering of patients with cancer whenever there is a change in prognosis. While suffering is often considered in terms of physical symptoms (such as pain—which may warrant palliation treatment), it may also have emotional, social and spiritual significance, particularly at the end of life. Acknowledging these problems and providing adequate support can improve the quality of life of these patients.

While some patients may accept/resign to the prospects of facing death; others may experience denial, worry about pain and other physical symptoms, struggle with the thought of losing control, develop clinical depression, and so on. Hence, end-of-life conversations are difficult to prepare for. A rigid formulaic approach to these conversations may be unsuitable and may make the doctor come across as insensitive. Once again, being an attentive, empathic listener is a good place to start. Remember the features of good communication and try to use them—try to be patient and let the genuine concern you have for your patient show.

A patient-led approach may be practical. Start with—what is worrying this patient the most? What meaning does this prognosis have for them? Discussions on spiritual meaning, existence and purpose may dominate the conversation—the clinician may have to acknowledge their own inexperience in these areas.

There may be dedicated specialists providing emotional support in palliative care in your hospital. It may be necessary to, or sometimes patients may themselves request a referral to psychology department. Therapists may try a variety of interventions based on the recognized needs, e.g., CBT approaches, therapist-guided life review, meaning-centered group psychotherapy, etc.[27]

Supporting ones close to the patient with cancer is equally important, as is addressing their concerns and fears, which may be linked with the patient's own concerns and fears. These individuals are likely to require further support when they attain bereaved status, when they could be referred to cancer bereavement groups in the community.

REFERENCES

1. Holmes TH, Rahe RH. The Social Readjustment Rating Scale. J Psychosom Res. 1967;11(2):213-8.

2. Howren MB, Christensen AJ, Karnell LH, Funk GF. Psychological factors associated with head and neck cancer treatment and survivorship: evidence and opportunities for behavioral medicine. J Consult Clin Psychol. 2013;81(2): 299-317.
3. Sollner W, DeVries A, Steixner E, Lukas P, Sprinzl G, Rumpold G, et al. How successful are oncologists in identifying patient distress, perceived social support, and need for psychosocial counselling? Br J Cancer. 2001;84(2):179-85.
4. Bruera E, Kuehn N, Miller MJ, Selmser P, Macmillan K. The Edmonton Symptom Assessment System (ESAS): a simple method for the assessment of palliative care patients. J Palliat Care. 1991;7(2):6-9.
5. Zigmond AS, Snaith RP. The hospital anxiety and depression scale. Acta Psychiatr Scand. 1983;67(6):361-70.
6. Watanabe S, Nekolaichuk C, Beaumont C, Mawani A. The Edmonton Symptom Assessment System—what do patients think? Support Care Cancer. 2009;17(6):675-83.
7. Mitchell AJ, Chan M, Bhatti H, Halton M, Grassi L, Johansen C, et al. Prevalence of depression, anxiety, and adjustment disorder in oncological, haematological, and palliative-care settings: a meta-analysis of 94 interview-based studies. Lancet Oncol. 2011;12(2):160-74.
8. Massie MJ. Prevalence of depression in patients with cancer. J Natl Cancer Inst Monogr. 2004;32:57-71.
9. Pinquart M, Duberstein PR. Depression and cancer mortality: a meta-analysis. Psychol Med. 2010;40(11):1797-810.
10. Rutledge T, Reis VA, Linke SE, Greenberg BH, Mills PJ. Depression in heart failure a meta-analytic review of prevalence, intervention effects, and associations with clinical outcomes. J Am Coll Cardiol. 2006;48:1527-37.
11. Robinson RG, Jorge RE. Post-Stroke depression: a review. Am J Psychiatry. 2016;173(3):221-31.
12. Engel GL. The need for a new medical model: a challenge for biomedicine. Science. 1977;196:129-36.
13. Longacre ML, Ridge JA, Burtness BA, Galloway TJ, Fang CY. Psychological functioning of caregivers for head and neck cancer patients. Oral Oncol. 2012;48(1):18-25.
14. Curado MP, Boyle P. Epidemiology of head and neck squamous cell carcinoma not related to tobacco or alcohol. Curr Opin Oncol. 2013;25(3):229-34.
15. McCarter K, Martinez U, Britton B, Baker A, Bonevski B, Carter G, et al. Smoking cessation care among patients with head and neck cancer: a systematic review. BMJ Open. 2016; 6(9):e012296.
16. McKay AJ, Patel RK, Majeed A. Strategies for tobacco control in India: a systematic review. PLoS One. 2015;10(4):e0122610.
17. Choi SH, Terrell JE, Bradford CR, Ghanem T, Spector ME, Wolf GT, et al. Does quitting smoking make a difference among newly diagnosed head and neck cancer patients? Nicotine Tob Res. 2016;18(12):2216-24.
18. Coleman T. ABC of smoking cessation. Use of simple advice and behavioural support. BMJ. 2004;328(7436):397-9.
19. Lancaster T, Stead L, Silagy C, Sowden A (for the Cochrane Tobacco Review Group). Effectiveness of interventions to help people stop smoking: findings from the Cochrane Library. BMJ. 2000;321(7257):355-8.
20. Alidosti M, Tavassoli E, Baneshi M, Gharlipour Z. The determination of physical activity among girl adolescents based on Trans-Theoretical Model (TTM). Int J Pediatr. 2017;5(7):5315-26.
21. Miller WR, Rose GS. Toward a theory of motivational interviewing. Am Psychol. 2009;64(6):527-37.
22. Chaturvedi SK, Strohschein FJ, Saraf G, Loiselle CG. Communication in cancer care: psycho-social, interactional, and cultural issues. A general overview and the example of India. Front Psychol. 2014;5:1332.
23. Fang CY, Longacre ML, Manne SL, Ridge JA, Lango MN, Burtness BA. Informational needs of head and neck cancer patients. Health Technol (Berl). 2012;2(1):57-62.
24. Baile WF, Buckman R, Lenzi R, Glober G, Beale EA, Kudelka AP. SPIKES—a six-step protocol for delivering bad news: application to the patient with cancer. The oncologist. 2000;5(4): 302-11.
25. Sharma A, Madan R, Kumar R, Sagar P, Kamal VK, Thakar A, et al. Compliance to therapy—elderly head and neck carcinoma patients. Can Geriatr J. 2014;17(3):83-7.
26. Boyle D, Bubalo J. Enhancing patient adherence to improve outcomes with oral chemotherapy. US Pharm. 2007;32(10) (Oncology Suppl):1-8.
27. Vachon MLS. Counselling and psychotherapy in palliative/hospice care: a review. Palliat Med. 1988;2:36-50.

Preoperative Assessment and Anesthetic Considerations in Head and Neck Cancer Surgery

Shabala Paul, Narayana Subramaniam

INTRODUCTION

Anesthesia for head and neck cancer surgery is posed with unique challenges. Management of the difficult airway, prolonged duration of surgery, potentially life-threatening hemorrhage, nerve monitoring and the risks associated with energy source use in close proximity to the airway are just some of these challenges that anesthetists need to face in these patients. This chapter provides a brief overview of these considerations that all those involved in their surgery need to be aware of.

PREOPERATIVE ASSESSMENT

The preoperative assessment of patients from an anesthetic point of view is essential as this group of patients prove to be different from other subsets of patients presenting to the preanesthesia clinic for evaluation. The major aims of preoperative assessment are to determine if there will be airway difficulties, identifying risks and optimizing physiology and control of comorbid illnesses.[1]

History and Comorbidities

- *Age:* The majorities of these patients are elderly and carry the risks associated with anesthetized geriatric patients.
- *Comorbidities:*
  - Smoking and alcohol—significant cardiorespiratory disease, chronic obstructive pulmonary disease (COPD)
  - *COPD:* Common in head and neck cancer patients and any reversible element should be optimized
- *Preoperative malnutrition:* Discussed in Chapter 6 on Nutrition
- *Sequelae of treatment are described in* ***Box 1****.*

Box 1: Sequelae of treatment.

Radiotherapy:
- Limited neck extension
- Temporomandibular joint (TMJ) ankylosis
- Osteoradionecrosis of mandible
- Hypothyroidism
- Baroreceptor damage
- Carotid artery stenosis
- Delayed wound healing

Maxillectomy and craniofacial resection:
- Difficult mask ventilation
- Difficult nasal access
- Temporalis contracture
- TMJ pseudoankylosis

Tongue, floor of mouth surgery:
- Trismus
- Fixed immobile tongue
- Limited mandibular space
- *Increased tongue:* Oral cavity ratio with flap reconstruction

Laryngeal surgery:
- Laryngeal stenosis
- Impaired swallowing
- Aspiration risk

Neck dissection:
- Damage to IX, X and XII nerves
- Impaired swallowing
- Aspiration risk
- Vocal cord palsy

Airway Evaluation

This requires the assessment of difficulty in mask ventilation, intubation and the feasibility of rescue plans in achieving oxygenation. For example, prior radiotherapy can result in a fibrotic airway due to woody, noncompliant tissue that makes mask ventilation and laryngoscopy difficult.

Before anesthesia, the following issues should be addressed:[2]

- Difficult mask ventilation?

- Direct or indirect laryngoscopy?
- Difficult intubation?
- Aspiration risk?
- Awake or anesthetized control of airway?
- Possibility of cricothyrotomy?
- Difficult extubation and recovery?

Anticipation of Difficult Airway

A number of simple clinical tests have been devised for the identification of a difficult airway prior to anesthesia. Although the statistical value of a single test may not be adequate, they help in achieving vigilance for a potential airway hazard. Prior documentation of a difficult airway also contributes to ensuring a safe control of the patient's airway. A few of these tests have been described here:

- *Mouth opening:* <3 cm opening is a nonreassuring sign. But there are videolaryngoscopes requiring only 1.8–2 cm mouth opening for insertion
- *Modified Mallampati Score:*[3] This is one of the most popular assessment tools **(Fig. 1)**. Among these, Class III and IV are associated with a difficult intubation
- *Thyromental distance (TMD):*[4] A TMD of less than 6.5 cm is nonreassuring
- *Sternomental distance (SMD):* An SMD of less than 12.5 cm is significant for difficulty in laryngoscopy

Preprocedure Imaging

- *Chest X-ray:* It may demonstrate distal obstruction, airway collapse, or gas trapping
- *X-ray neck:* It can help detecting anteroposterior and lateral narrowing
- *CT:* Information from a neck CT may be useful in identifying any narrowing or deviation of the trachea and the diameter to ensure that an appropriate sized endotracheal tube is used, feasibility of a fiberoptic bronchoscopy-aided intubation, early tracheostomy, etc.

Combined airway management planning with surgeons: An early joint discussion with surgeons regarding the plan for airway management helps save valuable time in the operating theaters. Management protocols need to be based on the availability of equipment, technical expertise and skill, and patient presentation. Instituting protocols help save time and prevent unfamiliar techniques. Clear communication and team-oriented approach is important to deal with potentially disastrous situations.

Management of the Airway[5,6]

The preferred techniques are as follows:

A. *Awake fiberoptic intubation:* It requires planning and thorough preparation for ideal conditions:
   - Resuscitation equipment including AMBU bag
   - Monitoring including capnography
   - Intravenous (IV) access and a running IV fluid
   - IV glycopyrrolate 3–4 µg/kg as an antisialagogue to facilitate vision
   - Nasal vasoconstrictors—oxymetazoline, xylometazoline
   - Sedation—with fentanyl, dexmedetomidine infusion, propofol
   - Calculation of maximum local anesthetic dose beforehand
   - Constant communication with the patient at all times

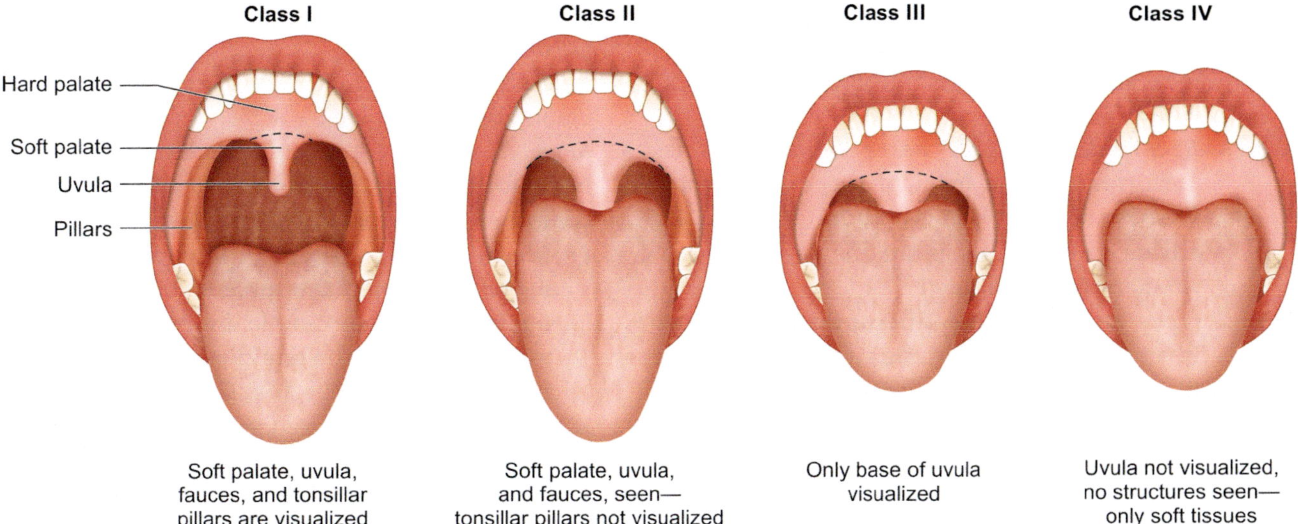

Fig. 1: Modified Mallampati Score for airway assessment.

Anesthetizing the airway:

1. Positioning
2. Identify the patent nasal passage
3. Spray nasal mucosa with vasoconstrictor
4. Nebulize 2 mL of 4% lignocaine (25% absorption)
5. *Nasal packing:* With 2% lignocaine + adrenaline 1:200,000 soaked cotton pledgets/ribbon gauze left in situ for 3 minutes. This anesthetizes the nose and nasopharynx
6. *Four puffs of 10% lignocaine to throat:* Two on either side. This anesthetizes the tongue and oropharynx
7. *Glossopharyngeal nerve block:* It can be blocked using topical spray, lignocaine-soaked pledgets or by nerve block. Intraorally, 5 mL of local anesthetic is injected submucosally (with a 22-gauge needle) at the caudal aspect of the posterior tonsillar pillar.

   The steps described above anesthetize the airway up to the level of the vocal cords. Below the vocal cords, the following steps are performed:

   1. *SAYGO technique: Spray As You Go* during endoscopy. 2% lignocaine can be sprayed along the airway as the endoscope is advanced through the distal airways by attaching a syringe containing it to the working channel of the endoscope.
   2. *Superior laryngeal nerve block:* The superior laryngeal nerve can be blocked in the pyriform fossa where it runs just deep to the mucosa by using Kraus or Jackson forceps to hold a cotton pledget soaked in lignocaine 2% against the mucosa for about 60 seconds. Alternatively, the nerve can be blocked externally where the nerve pierces the thyrohyoid membrane near the greater cornua of the hyoid bone. 2 mL of local anesthesia (LA) is injected into this area with a 25 G needle.
   3. *Recurrent laryngeal nerve block:* This is performed at the level of the cricothyroid membrane. A 20–22 G 10 mL needle is advanced till air is aspirated and 4 mL of LA (4% lidocaine) is injected
   4. Once prepared, the fiberoptic endoscope is advanced gently through the nostril with identification of structures, taking care not to cause any mucosal injury and adequate visualization.
   5. Once the vocal cords and subsequently the carina is seen, the lubricated, preloaded endotracheal tube (ETT) is railroaded over the endoscope and after confirmation of capnography and breath sounds, the patient is induced and muscle relaxant can be given.

B. *Routine GA induction and intubation:* With or without muscle relaxant. Nasal or oral endotracheal depending on the site of surgery

C. *Elective tracheostomy:* Based on level of airway difficulty. It can be done under LA or monitored anesthetic care with mild sedation

D. *Transnasal high-flow rapid insufflation ventilatory exchange (THRIVE):* It is valuable to allow adequate oxygenation during an apneic window, especially when the airway is yet to be secured. THRIVE involves oxygenation during apnea, continuous positive airway pressure, reducing the dead space and ensuring that oxygen saturation is adequate

E. *Inhalational induction:* It may not be a viable alternative in these cases and a backup plan is mandatory before induction. In theory, induction with inhalational agents allows for a slow induction with spontaneous inhalation; if obstruction of the airway occurs, it can be reversed through interruption of supply of the inhaled agents. However, it has been seen that airway obstruction is often sudden and exhalation of gases do not occur, resulting in sudden and often dramatic hypoxia.

GENERAL ANESTHETIC MANAGEMENT[7]

- Supine position with 15–20° head up tilt to improve venous drainage
- *Limited airway access:* Requires long ventilator tubing, vascular lines
- *Protection of eyes:* Use tapes, eye shields
- Pressure points require padding, compression stockings with intermittent pneumatic calf compression are desirable
- *Major resection:* Large bore IV access when significant blood loss is anticipated
- *Monitoring:* Apart from the standard monitors, the need for invasive monitoring is dictated by age, comorbid conditions, and nature of surgery.
  - *Invasive BP monitoring:* Site of arterial line depends on where the surgeon decides to harvest the free flap. For example, in the case of a radial forearm free flap, the side chosen by the surgeon is the nondominant one. In this situation, the arterial line should be inserted on the other hand after ensuring a negative Allen's test.
  - *Central venous catheter:* Useful for longer postoperative access, management of central venous pressure. Femoral or peripherally placed central

catheters can also be used if there is interference with the surgical field.
- *Temperature monitoring:* Patients are prone to development of hypothermia if there is extensive exposure of tissues. Bladder temperature or rectal temperature probes can be used if oral or nasal probes cannot be placed.
- *Cardiac monitoring:* Useful in guiding intraoperative fluid therapy, can prevent fluid overload in free flap transfer. LiDCO or FloTrac are pulse contour-based cardiac output monitors.
- *End tidal CO_2:* The importance of this monitor lies in detecting air embolisms, which are estimated to occur at an incidence of 1–2% in radical neck dissections and thyroidectomies.

▪ *Maintenance of anesthesia:* Total IV anesthesia or inhalational anesthesia with fentanyl, morphine or remifentanil.
- Opioids are added to blunt hemodynamic responses during intense surgical stimulation
- It should be governed by the expected degree of intraoperative stimulation, postoperative pain, duration of surgery, whether the patient is opioid naïve and the individual surgical technique
- Suppresses airway reflexes, reduces requirement of other anesthetic agents and helps in controlled hypotension
- Assists in EEG monitoring, neuromonitoring and helps decrease patient movement
- It allows smooth emergence from anesthesia and helps in postoperative pain control

▪ *Moderate controlled hypotension:* To reduce bleeding and improve visibility
- It involves maintaining the blood pressure at a systolic pressure of 100 mm Hg and a mean arterial pressure (MAP) between 60 and 70 mm Hg
- The need for controlled hypotension and the target BP should be discussed with the surgeon beforehand with due consideration given to the patients comorbidities
- It should be avoided in patients with uncontrolled hypertension, coronary artery disease, chronic renal failure, cerebrovascular disease and advanced liver disease
- Generally, opioids with propofol and inhalational agents are sufficient to induce the intended level of hypotension. Other drugs commonly used for this purpose are sodium nitroprusside, beta-blockers (metoprolol, esmolol, labetalol), calcium channel blockers (nicardipine) and α_2 agonists (clonidine, dexmedetomidine).

▪ *Blood transfusion:*
- Hemoglobin target is a sliding value in head and neck and plastic microvascular surgery
- Use of an osseous free flap for reconstruction versus a nonosseous flap resulted in a higher risk of blood transfusion
- Blood transfusion has been found to correlate with poorer overall survival and recurrence free survival, and with higher postoperative wound infection rates in patients with head and neck cancers who undergo free tissue transfer
- Studies have found no difference in outcome of free flaps with a lower hemoglobin threshold for transfusion. Thus, in patients undergoing free tissue transfer, there is no strict cutoff for transfusion and it remains an arbitrary value
- Increased volume of transfusion was also associated with higher wound infection rates

▪ *Perioperative fluid management, use of vasoactive agents and antithrombotic agents:*
- The anesthetic objective is achieving adequate tissue oxygenation by maintaining adequate cardiac output to optimize flap flow. Although hypotension, often induced by general anesthesia, may endanger flap survival, excessive intraoperative fluid administration has been shown to increase flap failure rates by various mechanisms. Besides hypotension, vasoconstriction caused by hypothermia or pain also has to be taken into account
- The general advice points toward *avoiding high volumes* of fluid replacement. The explanation being that it leads to mechanical stress on the pedicle impairing microcirculation and also damages the endothelial glycocalyx layer causing extravasation. This proceeds to cause counter-pressure on tissues, venous stasis and ultimately thrombosis
- Fluid volume higher than 5,500 mL was associated with an increase in medical and surgical complications
- To achieve optimal blood flow for free tissue transfer a hyperdynamic circulation is essential. This can be achieved by either hypervolemic hemodilution, normovolemic hemodilution, or by decreasing systemic vascular resistance. Besides vessel radius and perfusion pressure, *viscosity* plays a relatively large role in determining blood flow in flap microcirculation. Blood with a reduced hematocrit has a better flow profile than blood with a normal hematocrit

- A hematocrit of 30–40% in normovolemic hemodilution has been recommended. Correction of mild to moderate anemia with blood transfusions potentially may have an adverse effect due to increased blood viscosity and immunosuppression
- Generally, intraoperative fluid administration for maintenance should not exceed 6 mL/kg/h. The ideal type of fluid without serious side effects is still unknown
- Despite some concerns expressed in the literature due to the theoretical risk of peripheral vasoconstriction, there is no clinical evidence against the selective use of vasoactive agents during free flap surgery
- Antithrombotic agents are no substitute for meticulous surgical technique or early detection of flap compromise but are used additionally to prevent anastomotic occlusion. Due to the risk of serious side effects, routine use of dextrans is not warranted. The benefits of additional intraoperative use of systemic or topical heparin remain controversial

- *Glycemic control:* Stress hyperglycemia is common during surgery. There are no clear targets with relationships to outcome at present. General anesthetic protocols for blood sugar control are used
- *Postoperative nausea and vomiting (PONV):* Meticulous care has to be taken to help mitigate the effects of anesthetics causing PONV. A combination of an antiemetic such as ondansetron along with a corticosteroid must be used
- *Antibiotic prophylaxis:* From a number of sources, ampicillin-sulbactam or cefuroxime are the preferred prophylactic antibiotic for major clean-contaminated head and neck procedures. The duration of administration depends on the type of surgery, subsite and other factors
- *Nasogastric tube (NGT) insertion:* Patients with head and neck cancer can have intrinsic issues precluding easy and safe passage of NGTs, including mechanical obstruction due to tumor, reconstruction or edema, previous radiotherapy-induced fibrosis, and distorted anatomy. The effect of general anesthesia on relaxation of smooth muscle in the oropharynx can also contribute to this. There are various techniques that can be used to facilitate NGT insertion including forward displacement of larynx, use of a Magill's forceps, use of videolaryngoscopes and so on. No method is foolproof and it has to be modified for use in individual patients
- *Extubation plan:* The airway after a difficult intubation is at risk of being a difficult extubation. In addition, other surgical factors may contribute to postoperative airway obstruction.

  The causes for postoperative airway obstruction commonly are:
  - Laryngospasm
  - Laryngeal edema (e.g., prolonged Trendelenburg position)
  - Vocal cord paralysis
  - Reduced venous drainage
  - Bleeding into the airway (including clots blocking the inlet)
  - Local infection
  - Neck hematoma
  - Foreign body (e.g., retained throat pack)
  - Obesity/obstructive sleep apnea
  - Inadequate reversal of neuromuscular blocking drug

  The surgeries, which predispose to these complications, are:
  - Neck pathology (bleeding after neck dissection/thyroidectomy; postoperative carotid blow out)
  - Tongue biopsy
  - Tonsillectomy
  - Pan-endoscopy (reactive cord edema)
  - Radical neck dissection [tied internal jugular vein (IJV), likelihood of vocal cord edema attributable to venous congestion]
  - Abnormal airway morphology—tumor still present (biopsy/examination under anesthesia only for diagnosis)
  - Debulking tumor issues—continued oozing/redundant tissue obstructing narrow glottis
  - Edema following surgery—bimaxillary osteotomy, any major airway surgery

  The decision to perform a tracheostomy depends on the need for longer-term airway protection, but may also have been performed if tracheal intubation has failed or has been deemed too hazardous. *There should be a clear bed-head sign to identify whether the airway is a temporary tracheostomy or laryngectomy.* There are clear guidelines for emergency tracheostomy management in both cases. The type of tracheostomy should also be identified (Slit, Bjork flap or percutaneous). **Flowchart 1** shows an algorithm from the Difficult Airway Society for extubation.
- *Use of corticosteroids:*[8] The use of prophylactic corticosteroids before elective extubation is associated with significant reductions in postextubation

Flowchart 1: Difficult Airway Society (DAS) extubation guidelines.

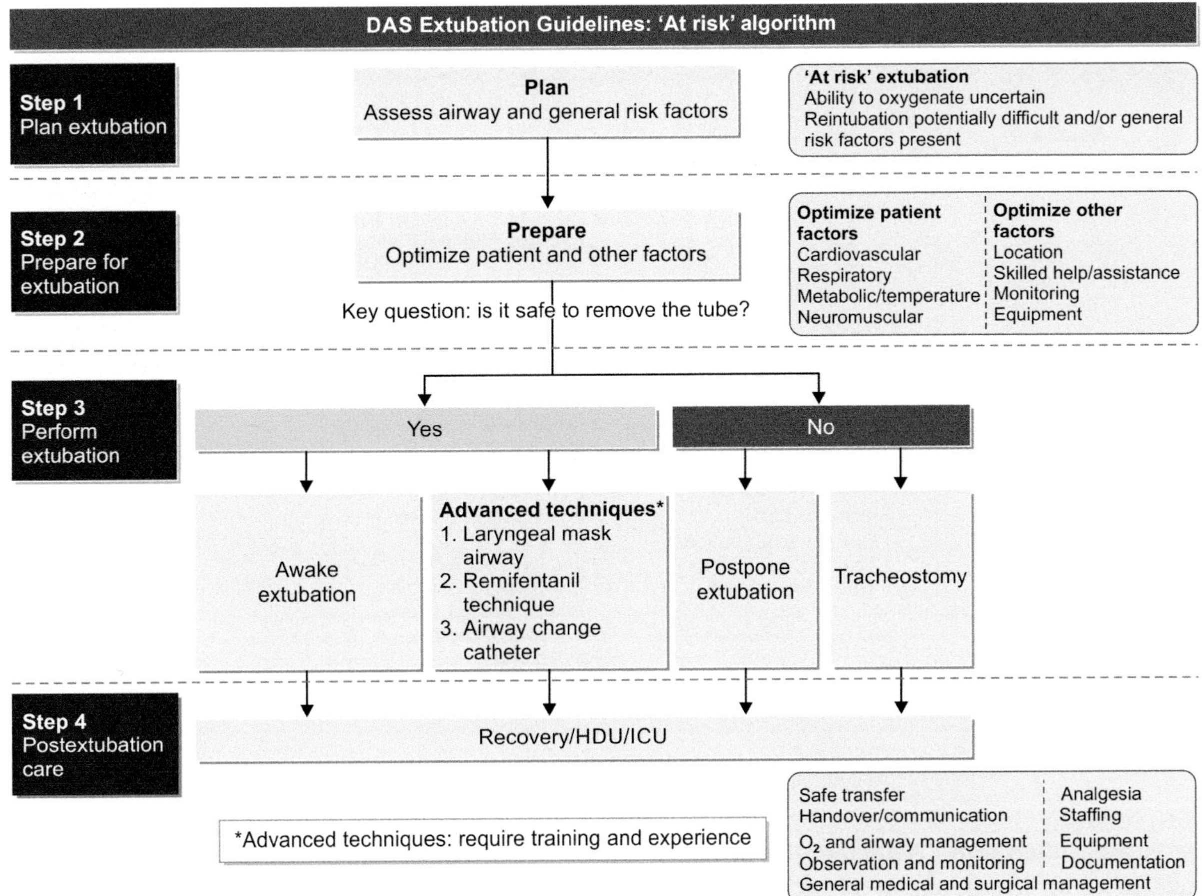

(HDU: high-dependency unit; ICU: intensive care unit)

airway events and reintubation. Various studies have used different glucocorticoids in their regimen, viz., dexamethasone 4–8 mg, methylprednisolone 20–40 mg and hydrocortisone 50–100 mg and different timings sometimes extending postoperatively. Adverse effects found were gastrointestinal (GI) bleeding, hyperglycemia and infections albeit rare.

Management of Complications

- *Bleeding:* Intraoperatively, bleeding can arise from the major vessels in the neck. Valsalva maneuver (VM) is widely used to test cardiac and baroreflex functions in addition to adrenergic system responses. Besides being used for these purposes, the application of VM can help to identify potential bleeding sites after head and neck surgeries. VM helps in hemostasis by increasing internal jugular venous pressure and by causing reflux of venous blood. The limiting factor using this technique is that sustained increased positive expiratory end pressure can cause complications, such as barotrauma. Therefore, the pressure cannot be held for more than a minute limiting the chances of identifying any potential bleeding vessels. A passive VM can be performed under anesthesia by squeezing the reservoir bag of the Bain's breathing circuit to maintain a sustained airway pressure of ≥40 mm Hg for at least 10 seconds.[9,10] Postoperatively, major bleeding or a rapidly expanding hematoma can compromise the airway causing life-threatening hypoxia. In such a situation, removal of surgical clips can relieve the obstruction immediately following which the patient needs to be shifted to the theater and intubated with a smaller sized tracheal tube, anticipating airway edema.
- *Venous air embolism (VAE):* There is a 1–2% risk of venous air embolism in head and neck surgeries namely radical neck dissection and thyroidectomy **(Flowchart 2)**. When VAE is suspected the surgeon should be informed so that the open vessel can be identified and further embolism prevented through packing with saline-soaked gauze. The operating

Flowchart 2: Manifestations of venous air embolism.

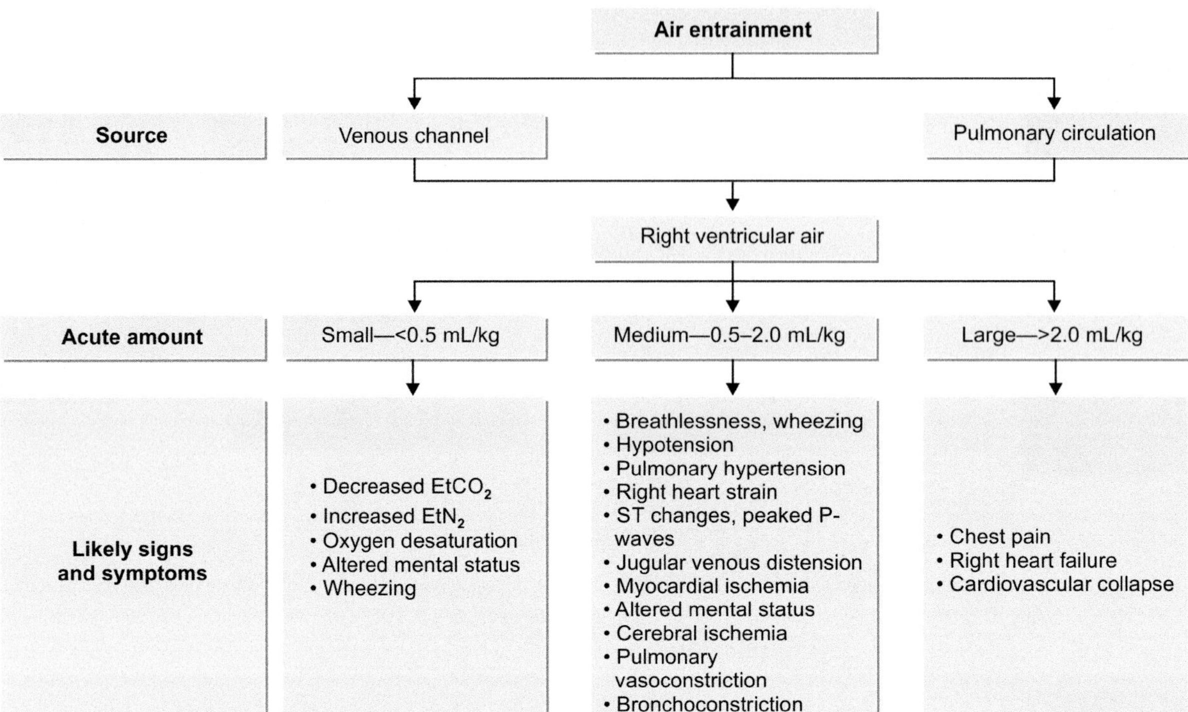

($EtCO_2$: endtidal carbon dioxide analysis; EtN_2: endtidal nitrogen analysis)

table is then tilted into Trendelenburg position to reduce the air pressure gradient **(Flowchart 3)**.

- *Respiratory distress:* Respiratory embarrassment can arise due to a variety of reasons following head and neck surgery. Swelling due to airway edema, blood in the airway, presence of an intraoral flap, tracheostomy tube block are a few causes and each factor requires individualized treatment. General measures that can improve these conditions temporarily are head elevation, nebulized epinephrine, and high-flow nasal oxygen. In these situations, the availability of a surgical airway kit in the vicinity is essential. Constant humidification, regular cleansing and suctioning of the tracheostomy tube is required to prevent blockage of the tube by mucus.
- *Carotid sinus reflex:* Hypotension and bradycardia caused by carotid sinus reflux may occur upon dissection around the carotid bifurcation, pressure on the carotid sinus and even hyperextension of the neck. Occasionally, it has been known to even induce a cardiac arrest. It can be potentiated by the presence of drugs that influence a central vagotonic action and adrenergic blockade. This may be avoided by careful dissection at the carotid bifurcation without manipulation, avoiding direct pressure over the carotid arteries, injection of 2 mL of local anesthetic into the adventitia at the carotid bifurcation between the internal and external carotid arteries, or both.
- *Airway fires:*[11-13] The presence of airway fires is associated with the use of LASERs in surgery as they are highly effective and rapid sources of ignition. The ignition and propagation of fire requires a triad of components: ignition source, fuel, and oxidizer. Anesthesiologists and laser operators must work together to ensure the lowest possible fraction of inspired oxygen (FiO_2) concentration at critical points in all laser procedures. Common sources of fuel in the operating room include the ETT and other plastic items, drapes and towels, and alcohol-based preparation solutions. Less common fuels include hair and skin ointments, which highlight the need for reminding patients to be ready for surgery with the face free of makeup and no products in the hair.
If laser use near the airway is planned, then implementing cuff-protective strategies such as the following is essential:
    - Use saline to fill the cuff. A cuff puncture may extinguish a small fire
    - Tint the saline in the cuff with methylene blue to act as an early marker of cuff puncture
    - Place the cuff as far away as possible (distal in the trachea) from the site of laser use

Flowchart 3: Algorithm for management of venous air embolism.

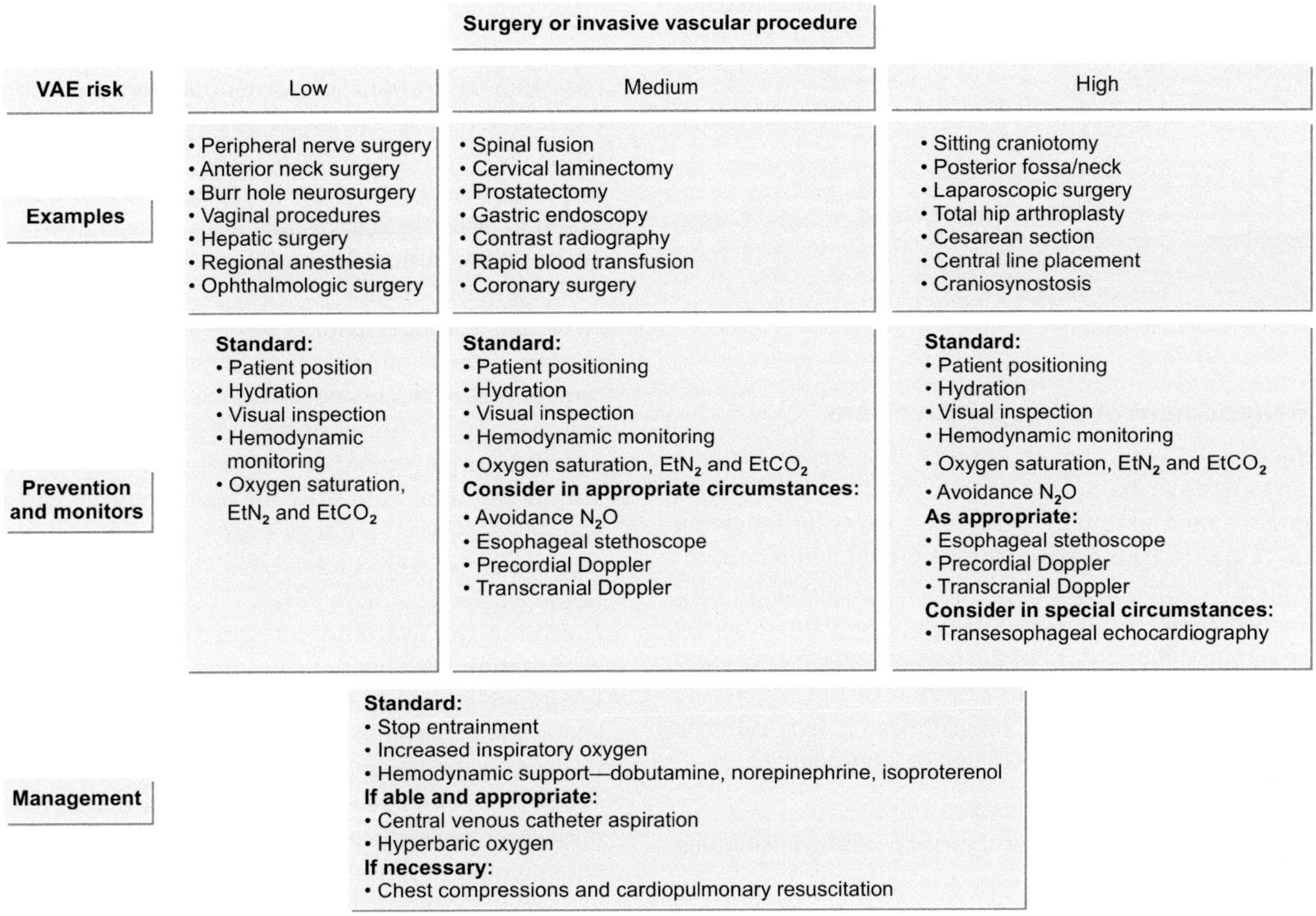

Surgery or invasive vascular procedure

VAE risk	Low	Medium	High
Examples	• Peripheral nerve surgery • Anterior neck surgery • Burr hole neurosurgery • Vaginal procedures • Hepatic surgery • Regional anesthesia • Ophthalmologic surgery	• Spinal fusion • Cervical laminectomy • Prostatectomy • Gastric endoscopy • Contrast radiography • Rapid blood transfusion • Coronary surgery	• Sitting craniotomy • Posterior fossa/neck • Laparoscopic surgery • Total hip arthroplasty • Cesarean section • Central line placement • Craniosynostosis
Prevention and monitors	**Standard:** • Patient position • Hydration • Visual inspection • Hemodynamic monitoring • Oxygen saturation, EtN_2 and $EtCO_2$	**Standard:** • Patient positioning • Hydration • Visual inspection • Hemodynamic monitoring • Oxygen saturation, EtN_2 and $EtCO_2$ **Consider in appropriate circumstances:** • Avoidance N_2O • Esophageal stethoscope • Precordial Doppler • Transcranial Doppler	**Standard:** • Patient positioning • Hydration • Visual inspection • Hemodynamic monitoring • Oxygen saturation, EtN_2 and $EtCO_2$ • Avoidance N_2O **As appropriate:** • Esophageal stethoscope • Precordial Doppler • Transcranial Doppler **Consider in special circumstances:** • Transesophageal echocardiography

Management

Standard:
- Stop entrainment
- Increased inspiratory oxygen
- Hemodynamic support—dobutamine, norepinephrine, isoproterenol

If able and appropriate:
- Central venous catheter aspiration
- Hyperbaric oxygen

If necessary:
- Chest compressions and cardiopulmonary resuscitation

(VAE: venous air embolism; $EtCO_2$: endtidal carbon dioxide; EtN_2: endtidal nitrogen)

- Use moistened cotton pledgets or sponges to cover any exposed cuff. These sponges may seal leaks of oxygen around an ill-fitting ETT cuff, segregating the higher FiO_2 being delivered to the patient from the ambient air above the glottis and may protect the tube from laser strikes by adding a layer of water-saturated protection
- Use of N_2O should be avoided when there is potential risk of fire

Blowtorch scenario: If ignited and combustion breaches the ETT with its centrally flowing reservoir of oxidizer, a *blowtorch* scenario in the airway can occur. The potential for far reaching thermal injury to the pulmonary tract exists. In addition, products of complete and partial combustion including smoldering debris, particulate matter, toxic gases and other compounds may cause further insult.

Endotracheal tube considerations: Among the ETTs available for laser surgeries, the polyvinyl chloride (PVC) type is not only the type that most readily ignited, but it also deposits carbonaceous debris and causes the most severe burns and cellular damage. The PVC ETT also produces more toxic byproducts of combustion, such as hydrochloric acid. The red rubber ETT was more ignition-resistant and produced less debris and tissue inflammation. Silicone ETTs took the longest exposure to ignite, but the finding of silica ash raised concern for possible remote development of silicosis.

The laser resistant ETT available now are given in **Table 1**.

Management of airway fire:

- Remove the tracheal tube or breathing circuit. Hand it off to be extinguished and inspected
- Stop airway gas flow (consider disconnecting the circuit)
- Flammable and burning materials are removed from the patient
- Pour saline or water into the patient's airway (to extinguish the fire and cool the tissues)

Table 1: Available laser resistant endotracheal tubes (ETTs).

Laser-Shield II	Silicone rubber tube wrapped with aluminum and wrapped over with Teflon	CO_2 or KTP lasers
Lasertubus	Soft white rubber reinforced with corrugated copper foil and an absorbent sponge; double cuffed	CO_2 or KTP lasers
Sheridan Laser-Trach	Red rubber design with embossed copper foil and outer covering designed to reduce damage to mucosal surfaces and vocal cords	CO_2 or KTP lasers

Management of Postoperative Pain[14,15]

Head and neck cancer surgery can cause intense postoperative pain, peaking in the first hours after surgery then gradually decreasing over the following 48–72 hours. Pain assessment should take into account difficulty or impossibility of speaking (especially with tracheostomy). Immediate postoperative pain following surgery to the mid-third of the face or oral cavity is often due to deafferentation of a branch of the trigeminal nerve (V2 or V3), in which case there is hypoesthesia leading to discomfort exacerbated by large edema.

Some specific considerations are:

- Due to the long duration of surgery, careful positioning can help prevent pain
- In the immediate postoperative period following head and neck cancer surgery, multimodal analgesia should be prescribed, associated to patient-controlled analgesia with IV morphine (PCA) after titration. In case of re-emergence of pain and intensification persisting beyond 72 hours, a locoregional complication (pharyngostoma, abscess) should be suspected
- Care-related pain should be prevented by prior administration of an analgesic adapted in terms of dosage, action time and route, ensuring optimal administration conditions (professional agreement). This pertains to tracheostomy and Ryles tube care. Changing a tracheotomy cannula is invasive and potentially painful, and must be performed under good conditions: patient in dorsal decubitus, strictly flat, with frontal lighting, a Laborde tracheal dilator, aspiration and the replacement cannula to hand. The irritative cough that accompanies cannulation can be limited by preventive lidocaine pulverization. Tracheal aspiration must not be traumatic
- In chronic pain secondary to facial surgery with or without a cutaneous approach, attention should be paid to facial skin care, preventing edema. Non-aggressive intraoral treatments should be applied several times daily, with mastication and facial motion exercises
- Myofascial pain secondary to surgery-induced muscular and aponeurotic remodeling is notably encountered when a pediculated muscular-cutaneous flap is used for defect reconstruction; it can be limited by sectioning the motor nerve branch of the transposed muscle. Once such pain is established, certain authors recommend botulinum toxin injection, others physical therapy
- Neck and shoulder pain is frequent after neck dissection, directly impairing quality of life. The causes remain poorly elucidated, but partly implicate neural lesions (spinal nerve and cervical plexus roots) inducing involvement of the trapezius and other scapulohumeral belt muscles, which tend to cause shoulder stiffness that may evolve toward retractile capsulitis. Several studies have shown that spinal nerve sparing is a necessary but not sufficient condition for avoiding cervicoscapular pain and dysfunction. When, however, the spinal nerve is sectioned, symptom severity and duration increase; when this is required for oncologic reasons, sparing the cervical plexus roots limits pain. When the spinal nerve is spared, limiting the extension of neck dissection can reduce postoperative pain, especially when lymph nodes in contact with the spinal nerve are spared. Spinal nerve monitoring during neck surgery has failed to show benefit in terms of postoperative pain. Physical therapy, botulinum toxin injection can also help in reduction of pain
- Following flap surgery, immediate postoperative pain should be addressed by the use of a patient controlled analgesia with morphine
- Postoperative pain following sectioning of pectoralis major muscle plane is usually moderate without movement but aggravated by abduction and external rotation of the ipsilateral upper limb, especially when ipsilateral neck dissection was associated
- In latissimus dorsi muscle flap harvesting, postoperative pain is at the muscle-sectioning site and may be aggravated by dynamic lateral dorsal movement or dynamic movement of the ipsilateral shoulder
- In an antebrachial flap, neuropathic pain in the wrist and first three digits may be due to damage to the sensory branch of the radial nerve; the latter should be respected during dissection and dermoepidermal grafting
- In a fibular flap, postoperative pain is due to muscle dissection and distension and to destabilization of the ankle. Active intraoperative drainage reduces

tension in the muscle compartment and prevents hematoma. A local anesthetic such as ropivacaine can be infiltrated into the muscle compartment for up to 48 hours. Edema can be limited by raising the limb. Massage can be used for lymphatic drainage of the limb and to release adherent scar tissue over the longer term. Lower limb rehabilitation is based on passive and active mobilization of the foot and ankle. Walking under weight bearing should be adapted and progressive

- Postoperative pain in anterolateral thigh flap harvesting is due to extensive dissection of the muscle compartment or excessive tension in skin closure. Rotation-plasty or secondary closure may be required to reduce tension. Postoperative rehabilitation by physical therapy and walking aids are recommended
- In digestive flaps, pain is due to penetration of the abdominal cavity. Intraoperatively, curare anesthesia, minimal intestinal loop mobilization, conserving the peritoneal fluid and great care in closing the abdominal wall limit postoperative pain. An abdominal support belt associated to antispasmodics facilitates effort and reduces pain.

ENHANCED RECOVERY AFTER SURGERY

Enhanced recovery after surgery (ERAS) is a multimodal perioperative care pathway designed to reduce perioperative morbidity and reduce morbidity associated with surgery. The specific protocol for patients undergoing head and neck cancer surgery with free flap reconstruction is as follows:[16]

- *Preadmission education:* The psychosocial aspects of undergoing head and neck surgery are believed to have an impact on clinical outcomes. A qualified health practitioner could help provide structured teaching to the patient
- *Perioperative nutritional care:* All patients undergoing major surgery require a formal nutritional assessment. Those identified as being malnourished require intensive rehabilitation prior to surgery. Fasting should be limited as far as possible. Carbohydrate loading prior to surgery may be considered. Tube feeding should be initiated within 24 hours in patients in whom oral feeding is not feasible
- *Thromboembolism prophylaxis:* These patients are at increased risk of venous thromboembolism and should undergo pharmacologic prophylaxis; however, the risk of bleeding must be weighed against the benefits on an individualized basis, especially for those on therapeutic anticoagulation
- *Antibiotic prophylaxis:* As per category (clean/clean-contaminated/contaminated/dirty). The use of topical decontamination of the upper aerodigestive tract with mupirocin and 0.2% chlorhexidine has been shown to reduce pneumonia rates and nosocomial infections in patients in the intensive care unit (ICU)
- *Postoperative nausea and vomiting prophylaxis:* Patients undergoing head and neck cancer surgery are at moderate to high risk of developing PONV; hence they should receive preoperative and intra-operative medications to mitigate it. A combination of corticosteroid and antiemetic such as a 5-HT3-receptor agonist should be considered
- *Preanesthetic medication:* Patients should receive short acting anxiolytics
- *Standard anesthetic protocol:* Avoidance of too deep anesthesia, especially in elderly patients, is recommended
- *Preventing hypothermia:* Normothermia should be maintained intraoperatively. Monitoring of temperature during these long procedures is imperative. A core temperature of less than 36°C can be associated with cardiac morbidity, bleeding and wound infections
- *Perioperative fluid management:* Fluids should be managed in a goal-directed manner, avoiding over and under hydration
- *Routine postoperative intensive care admission:* Routine ICU admission may not be indicated. Low-risk uncomplicated patients may be managed in a high dependency unit or specialist ward with adequate equipment and expertise. Risk factors for complications include bilateral neck dissection, an APACHE II score >10, massive blood transfusion, early postoperative complications requiring further operation under general anesthesia, smoking history, and perioperative antibiotic choice
- *Pain management:* As described earlier
- *Postoperative flap monitoring:* At least hourly for the first 24 hours postoperatively. Monitoring should be continued for the duration of the patient's stay with tapering of intensity after the first 24 hours. Method of monitoring should include, at a minimum, clinical examination by experienced staff with adjunct monitoring techniques where available
- *Postoperative mobilization:* Early mobilization on day 1
- *Postoperative wound care:* There is strong evidence to support polyurethane film for use at skin graft donor sites with reductions in patient pain and discomfort

relative to other dressing types. Vacuum-assisted closure may be used for complex wounds in the neck or flap donor sites. Polyurethane film or hydrocolloid dressings should be used on the skin graft donor sites
- *Urinary catheterization:* To be removed as soon as feasible, ideally within a day of surgery
- *Tracheostomy care:* Decannulation after tracheostomy and stoma closure is recommended so as to help in the respiratory and swallowing rehabilitation. Surgical closure of the tracheostomy site should be performed. The decision to perform a tracheotomy is dependent on the presence of severe comorbidities, tumor stage and location, alcohol consumption, extent of resection, and whether or not a bilateral neck dissection was performed.
- *Postoperative pulmonary physical therapy:* Chest physiotherapy should be initiated as early as possible after head and neck reconstructions to avoid atelectasis and pneumonia. The type of physical therapy consists usually of incentive spirometry, intermittent positive pressure breathing, and deep breathing exercises

NEUROMONITORING IN ANESTHESIA[17,18]

Intraoperative neuromonitoring (IONM) is a relatively recent advance in electromyography (EMG) applied to head and neck surgery. Its purpose is to allow real-time identification and functional assessment of vulnerable nerves during surgery. The nerves most often monitored in head and neck surgery are the motor branch of the facial nerve (VII), the recurrent or inferior laryngeal nerves (X), the vagus nerve (X), and the spinal accessory nerve (XI), with other cranial lower nerves monitored less frequently.

The goal in providing anesthesia during these procedures is to allow adequate depth of anesthesia while accomplishing neuromonitoring. The specific modality of IONM is EMG, both spontaneous and evoked. Spontaneous and evoked EMGs are "cousins" to a modality anesthesiologists commonly use while administering routine anesthetics: neuromuscular junction (NMJ) monitoring. In an evoked EMG, the nerve innervating a muscle is stimulated with a supraphysiologic voltage and current (of the order of 0.5 mA). This helps in spatial identification of nerves to preserve them from injury, usually during operations. Nerves commonly monitored during head and neck surgery are:

- The superior laryngeal, recurrent laryngeal, and vagus nerves during thyroidectomy, parathyroidectomy, neck dissection, carotid endarterectomy, and other surgeries in the anterior cervical region
- The motor branch of the facial nerve during tympanic, mastoid, parotid, and other otologic surgeries
- Other cranial or cervical spinal nerves and branches during neck dissection
- The lower cranial or cervical spinal nerve during lateral skull-base surgery.

Peripherals, or data inputting devices, used in IONM are stimulating electrodes shaped such as probes, needles, or surgical instruments. They may even be especially designed and insulated surgical instruments such as drills that are used to stimulate nerves and muscles during dissection. Needle electrodes placed in target muscles are the most commonly used recording devices used. Their wires or leads connect to the recording hardware.

The general anesthetic technique followed is a total intravenous technique, with a short-acting narcotic through infusion combined with propofol, is generally considered. Nitrous oxide and volatile agents may also be used. The main drug categories to be avoided are the neuromuscular blocking agents and local anesthetics. The neuromuscular blocking drugs are used at induction and intubation as long as their effects have cleared by the time IONM begins.

Nerve integrity monitor (NIM) tube monitoring during thyroid surgery:
The overall goals are to:

- Provide for a quick induction, intubation, and positioning, including neck extension. Intubation should be with a dry styletted NIM tube of the largest practical size possible to allow for good contact between the electrodes and the tracheal mucosa. After induction, lightening or partial emergence from the induction dose, and optimal placement of the NIM tube, the patient must be maintained at a certain depth of anesthesia. It must be deep enough to assure that no spontaneous EMG activity occurs in the vocalis muscles, but not too deep to prevent hypotension or delayed emergence.
- Allow partial emergence or lightening immediately after intubation so that respiratory variation in the vocalis muscle is seen (i.e., accurate tube placement with good electrical contact).
- Quickly deepen the patient with intravenous anesthetic such as propofol to prevent any movement of the tube from coughing. This can be done with a 0.25–1 mg/kg bolus of propofol and increasing the inspired concentration of volatile agent. An alternative approach to the use of the specialized NIM tube or applied electrodes involves continuous intraoperative observation of vocal cord movement

using laryngeal mask airway (LMA) and fiberoptic bronchoscope. To facilitate accurate placement, the NIM tube has an embedded blue dye stripe (or lettering stripe) oriented anteriorly (12 o'clock) along the shaft of the tube. Located at 9 o'clock (left) and 3 o'clock (right) are the embedded wire electrodes contacting the vocal cords and underlying vocalis muscles. The tube placement itself is critical because small displacements (rotation or insertion/removal) can cause large changes in impedance and evoked responses. The tube depth of insertion is very important, because the embedded electrodes are of finite length and must be apposed to the vocal cords for optimal readings. After induction and intubation, and before incision, or intraoperatively, these position adjustments may be made to optimize otherwise unsatisfactory baseline readings. These adjustments may be performed with plain visualization of the face and tracheal tube using conventional laryngoscopy, fiberoptic laryngoscopy, or GlideScope laryngoscopy. The GlideScope is becoming widely used for precise insertion and manipulation of the embedded electrode or tubes with adhesive electrodes. The advantage of the GlideScope is that the surgeon may use the device to assist and confirm placement of the tube, which expedites the procedure because correct initial placement usually avoids the need for further manipulation.

The tube may move during surgery due to:

- Blunt and sharp dissection and retraction involves manipulating the larynx and, indirectly, the tube stimulating the recurrent laryngeal nerve causes adduction of the cords and small displacements result
- Some surgeons, as a means of showing nerve integrity, stimulate the recurrent laryngeal nerve and simultaneously palpate for vocal cord adduction, and
- Patient movement may occur because muscle relaxation is contraindicated and anesthetic depth may not be excessive.

It has been observed that a very high standard of expertise is required for placing the tubes. Respiratory variation in the EMG indicates a lighter than desirable intraoperative plane of anesthesia. Deepening of anesthesia is usually necessary. The goal is timely deepening to avoid coughing on and displacement of the tube.

Another patient safety issue in head and neck surgery is extension of the head and neck. Severe neck extension during anterior neck surgery has been reported to cause trauma to the brainstem or spinal cord, or hypoperfusion of the posterior circulation. Fortunately, it can be detected earlier with movement of the embedded electrode tube.

Facial Nerve Monitoring

The facial nerve is vulnerable to injury during parotidectomies, tympanomastoidectomies and other head and neck procedures during dissection. The recording electrodes (surface gel or needle) are placed either awake or after induction and intubation in or overlying the orbicularis oculi and orbicularis oris muscles. These are the two positive channels. A scalp electrode may be used for grounding the patient, or the ground may be placed elsewhere. The frontalis muscle may be monitored in addition to the standard two channels. The stimulating electrode may be a monopolar or bipolar fine-tipped probe, or incorporated into surgical instruments like the rotary burr. Stimulating near the facial nerve will result in a characteristic waveform or audio signal. Based on the latency and amplitude of the waveform, the facial nerve is identified and avoided during surgery. Nerve function is tested, first as a means of localizing it, then during the procedure when the operative site is in proximity to the nerve, and at the end of the procedure to prove retained function.

CONCLUSION

Improvements in perioperative monitoring and management have largely been responsible for significant advancements in patient outcomes with surgical techniques remaining relatively unchanged. Understanding the principles behind safe and effective perioperative care will contribute to enhanced recovery and reduced patient morbidity.

REFERENCES

1. Charters P, Ahmad I, Patel A, Russell S. Anaesthesia for head and neck surgery: United Kingdom National Multidisciplinary guidelines. J Laryngol Otol. 2016;130(S2):S23-7.
2. Crawley SM, Dalton AJ. Predicting the difficult airway. BJA Educ. 2015;15(5):253-7.
3. Mallampati SR, Gatt SP, Gugino LD, Desai SP, Waraksa B, Freiberger D, et al. A clinical sign to predict difficult tracheal intubation; a prospective study. Can Anaesth Soc J. 1985;32(4):429-34.
4. Khan ZH, Mohammadi M, Rasouli MR, Farrokhnia F, Khan RH. The diagnostic value of the upper lip bite test combined with sternomental distance, thyromental distance, and interincisor distance for prediction of easy laryngoscopy and intubation: a prospective study. Anesth Analg. 2009;109(3):822-4.
5. Gupta S, Sharma R, Jain D. Airway assessment: predictors of difficult airway. Indian J Anaesth. 2005;49(4):257-62.

6. Bellhouse CP, Dore C. Criteria for estimating likelihood of difficulty of endotracheal intubation with the Macintosh laryngoscope. Anaesth Intens Care. 1988;16(3):329-37.
7. Mishra S, Bhatnagar S, Jha RR, Singhal AK. Airway management of patients undergoing oral cancer surgery: a retrospective study. Eur J Anaesthesiol. 2005;22(7):510-4.
8. Kuriyama A, Umakoshi N, Sun R. Prophylactic corticosteroids for prevention of postextubation stridor and reintubation in adults: a systematic review and meta-analysis. Chest. 2017;151(5):1002-10.
9. Rawlinson WA, Edmonds-Seal J, Adams AP. Anaesthesia and the Valsalva manoeuvre. A test of circulatory responses in neurosurgical patients including those in the sitting position. Anaesthesia. 1979;34(6):534-42.
10. Tokaç M, Dumlu EG, Bozkurt B, Öcal H, Aydın C, Yalçın A, et al. Effect of intraoperative Valsalva maneuver application on bleeding point detection and postoperative drainage after thyroidectomy surgeries. Int Surg. 2015;100(6):994-8.
11. Rogers ML, Nickalls RW, Brackenbury ET, Salama FD, Beattie MG, Perks AG. Airway fire during tracheostomy: prevention strategies for surgeons and anaesthetists. Ann Royal Coll Surg Engl. 2001;83(6):376.
12. Akhtar N, Ansar F, Baig MS, Abbas A. Airway fires during surgery: management and prevention. J Anaesthesiol Clin Pharmacol. 2016;32(1):109.
13. Yao D. Laser Surgery of the Airway. In: Anesthesiology. Cham: Springer; 2017. pp. 305-11.
14. Bianchini C, Malago M, Crema L, Aimoni C, Matarazzo T, Bortolazzi S, et al. Post-operative pain management in head and neck cancer patients: predictive factors and efficacy of therapy. Acta Otorhinolaryngol Ital. 2016;36(2):91.
15. Espitalier F, Testelin S, Blanchard D, Binczak M, Bollet M, Calmels P, et al. Management of somatic pain induced by treatment of head and neck cancer: postoperative pain. Guidelines of the French Oto-rhino-laryngology-head and neck surgery society (SFORL). Eur Ann Otorhinolaryngol Head Neck Dis. 2014;131(4):249-52.
16. Dort JC, Farwell DG, Findlay M, Huber GF, Kerr P, Shea-Budgell MA, et al. Optimal perioperative care in major head and neck cancer surgery with free flap reconstruction: a consensus review and recommendations from the enhanced recovery after surgery society. JAMA Otolaryngol Head Neck Surg. 2017;143(3):292-303.
17. Dillon FX. Electromyographic (EMG) neuromonitoring in otolaryngology-head and neck surgery. Anesthesiol Clin. 2010;28(3):423-42.
18. Sarnthein J, Hejrati N, Neidert MC, Huber AM, Krayenbühl N. Facial nerve motor evoked potentials during skull base surgery to monitor facial nerve function using the threshold-level method. Neurosurg Focus. 2013;34(3):E7.

Nutritional Assessment and Considerations in Head and Neck Cancer Therapy

Pranothi Srinivasalu, Narayana Subramaniam

INTRODUCTION

Cachexia and anorexia, the two most commonly seen complications during the final stage in malignancy and could be used to identify early signs of cancer. Cancer patients with malnutrition are on the rise, and most studies have placed it at an estimate of 40–80%.[1] Malnutrition is of utmost importance since it aggravates infection and lowers the treatment outcome, thereby affecting life expectancy. Nutritional issues can cause increased mortality and treatment-related morbidity in this population. The primary result of malnutrition is weight loss, which is a significant problem causing mortality and morbidity in patients diagnosed with cancer. The purpose of this chapter is to summarize the literature on nutritional assessment and considerations in patients with head and neck cancer to optimize their treatment and limit morbidity in this vulnerable population.

PRETREATMENT NUTRITIONAL ASSESSMENT AND SCREENING

The two common tools used for pretreatment nutritional assessment and screening are the Subjective Global Appraisal (SGA) **(Fig. 1)** and Malnutrition Universal Screening Tool (MUST) **(Flowchart 1)**. As the SGA is more rigorous and extensive, the MUST is preferred in most outpatient settings.[2] The SGA focuses on several domains, weight change, dietary intake, gastrointestinal symptoms, functional capacity, comorbidities related to nutritional needs and a physical examination. Patients are classified as very mild risk to well-nourished, mild-moderate risk of malnourishment or severely malnourished. MUST focuses on body mass index (BMI), weight loss score (over the preceding 3–6 months) and short-term poor nutritional intake (>5 days). Based on this assessment, they are classified as low, medium or high-risk categories with corresponding recommendations.

CANCER CACHEXIA

Cachexia, also known as wasting syndrome, is a disorder associated with exhaustion, loss of weight, loss of appetite, and muscle atrophy. This is metabolically mediated and may be independent of caloric intake and nutritional adequacy. These patients classically present as thin and wasted, however in the context of a high general incidence of obesity, making a diagnosis may not be very straightforward. The major mediators of cachexia are believed to TNF-α and IL-6. Tumor-related factors also include other proinflammatory cytokines such as lipid mobilizing factor, myostatin and stress hormones like glucocorticoids. Host factors include decreased food intake, hypermetabolism and hypoalbuminemia. Additionally, there may be additional metabolic disruptions such as an exaggerated insulin response to a carbohydrate load resulting in hyperglycemia and hypertriglyceridemia. The principal diagnosis of the disease includes weight loss to more than 5% within 13 months or less.[3] The pathophysiology and clinical course are shown in **Figure 2.**[4] Treatment of cancer cachexia is through aggressive nutritional supplementation wherever possible. This may be insufficient in isolation, however; appetite stimulants such as megestrol acetate (400 mg/day increased to 600–800 mg/day) are of benefit. Other appetite stimulants such as corticosteroids have also shown some benefit. Omega-3 fatty acids such as eicosapentaenoic acid (EPA) can prevent lipolysis. Thalidomide (100 mg/day) has also been used to increase caloric intake, improve appetite and decrease nausea. It may also lead to attenuation of weight loss and lean body mass, however literature on its use is still limited.[5]

ESTIMATING NUTRITIONAL REQUIREMENTS

Patients with cancer often lose significant weight and suffer a nutritional deficit. This complicates the

<table>
<tr><th colspan="2">SUBJECTIVE GLOBAL ASSESSMENT RATING FORM</th></tr>
<tr><td colspan="2">Patient Name: ID #: Date:</td></tr>
<tr><th colspan="2">HISTORY</th></tr>
<tr><td>WEIGHT/WEIGHT CHANGE:
1. Baseline wt: ________(Dry weight from 6 months ago)
Current wt: ________(Dry weight today)
Actual wt loss/past 6 months: ________%loss: _______(actual loss from baseline or last SGA)
2. Weight change over 2 weeks: ______No change _______Increase ______Decrease</td><td>Rate 1–7</td></tr>
<tr><td>DIETARY INTAKE No Change________(Adequate) No Change________(Inadequate)
1. Change: Suboptimal intake: ______ Protein _______ Keal ______ Duration ________
Full liquid: ___________ Hypocaloric liquid __________ Starvation __________</td><td></td></tr>
<tr><td>GASTROINTESTINAL SYMPTOMS
Symptom: Frequency: Duration:
__________None __________ __________
__________Anorexia __________ __________
__________Nausea __________ __________
__________Vomiting __________ __________
__________Diarrhea __________ __________
Never, daily, 2–3 times/week, 1–2 times/week >2 weeks, <2 weeks</td><td></td></tr>
<tr><td>FUNCTIONAL CAPACITY
Description Duration:
___________ No dysfunction ___________
___________ Change in function ___________
___________ Difficulty with ambulation ___________
___________ Difficulty with activity (Patient specific “normal”) ___________
___________ Light activity ___________
___________ Bed/chair ridden with little or no activity ___________
___________ Improvement in function ___________</td><td>b</td></tr>
<tr><td>DISEASE STATE/COMORBIDITIES AS RELATED TO NUTRITIONAL NEEDS
Primary diagnosis ______________________Comorbidities ________________________
Normal requirements ______ Increased requirements _______ Decreased requirements _____
Acute metabolic stress: ______ None ______Low _______Moderate _______ High</td><td></td></tr>
<tr><th colspan="2">PHYSICAL EXAMINATION</th></tr>
<tr><td>________ Loss of subcutaneous fat (Below eye, triceps, biceps, chest) ______ Some areas _____All areas
________ Muscle wasting (Temple, clavicle, scapula, ribs, quadriceps, calf, knee, interosseous ______ Some areas _____All areas
________ Edema (Related to undernutrition/use to evaluate weight change)</td><td></td></tr>
<tr><th colspan="2">OVERALL SGA RATING</th></tr>
<tr><td>Very mild risk to well-nourished = 6 or 7 most categories or significant, continued improvement.
Mild-moderate = 3, 4, or 5 ratings. No clear sign of normal status or severe malnutrition.
Severely malnourished = 1 or 2 rating in most categories/significant physical signs of malnutrition.</td><td></td></tr>
</table>

Fig. 1: Subjective Global Appraisal (SGA) for Nutritional Assessment.

estimation of nutritional requirements are presentation. It has been shown that patients with cancer have an excess energy expenditure of 138–289 kcal/day, which may increase substantially when the patient is on treatment.[6]

- For the nonobese patient, total energy expenditure and protein requirement based on body weight is calculated as 30-35 kcal/kg/day and 1.2 g/kg/day, respectively
- However, a more accurate estimation comes from estimated energy requirement (EER).[7] This is the more accurate individualized estimate based on weight, sex, energy expenditure, physical activity and height. The units are height in meter, age in years, and weight in kilograms
  - For men, EER = [662 – (9.53 × age)] + PA × [(15.91 × weight) + (539.6 × height)]
  - For women, EER = [354 – (6.91 × age)] + PA × [(9.36 × weight) + (726 × height)]

Here, PA is physical activity constant, as shown in **Table 1**.

Flowchart 1: Malnutrition Universal Screening Tool for Nutritional Assessment.

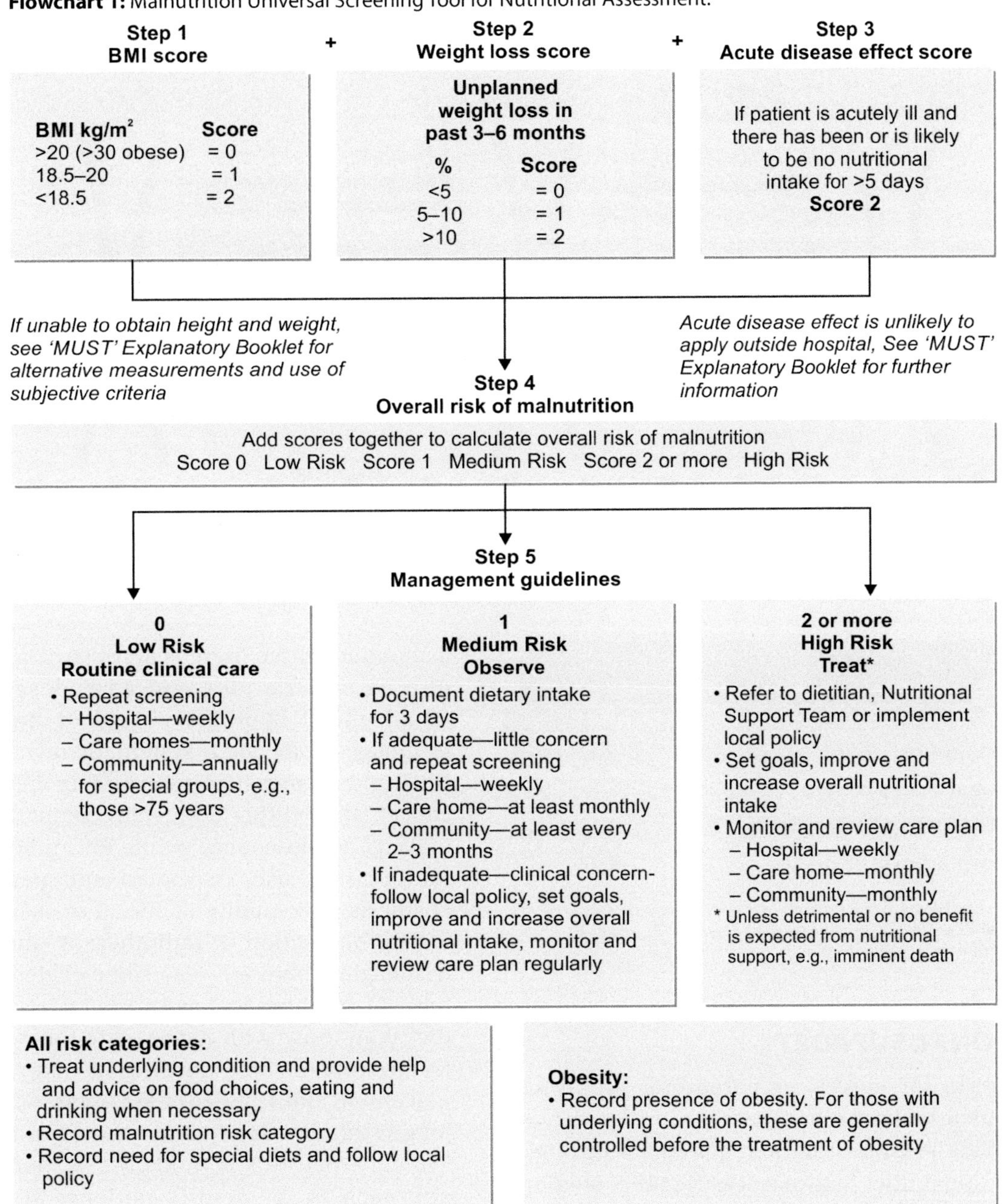

REFEEDING SYNDROME[8,9]

This refers to the metabolic disruption that occurs on re-establishing nutrition in patients with long-standing malnourishment or starvation. Typically within the first 4–7 days after initiating feeding support, the patient develops fluid and electrolyte imbalances (typically hypomagnesemia and hypophosphatemia) with complications that can involve the neurological, pulmonary, cardiac and neuromuscular systems. During prolonged fasting, the body switches its major fuel source to fatty acids and amino acids. During refeeding, insulin is released as a result of spike in blood sugar levels that results in synthesis of glycogen, protein and fat. This process results in depletion of phosphates, potassium and magnesium that are utilized during this synthetic phase. There is also an intracellular fluid shift that results in further electrolyte imbalance. If untreated this can result in arrhythmias, seizures, multiorgan dysfunction and even death. Although most cases are mild, severe cases (where phosphate levels are <2 mg/dL) require ICU admission for monitoring and correction. Daily doses of vitamins (especially thiamine) and minerals are required. Caloric intake should be reduced to 480 kcal/day for at least 2 days while electrolytes are replenished.

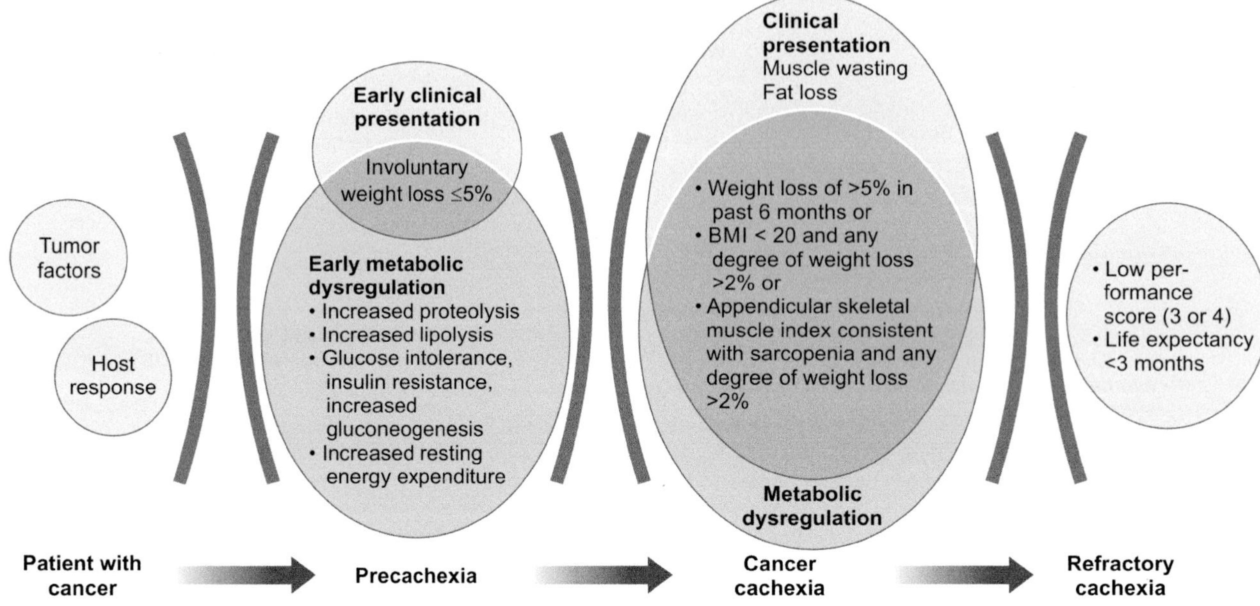

Fig. 2: Pathophysiology of cancer cachexia.

Table 1: Physical activity (PA) constant used in the prediction of estimated energy requirement (EER).

Daily physical activity levels	*PA factor in men*	*PA factor in women*
Sedentary: Activities of daily living	1	1
Low active: 30–60 minutes of daily activities	1.12	1.12
Active: ≤60 minutes or less of moderate daily activities	1.25	1.27
Very active: ≥60 minutes of vigorous activity or 120 minutes of moderate activities	1.48	1.45

NUTRITIONAL SUPPORT

This is the term for enteral or parenteral supply of nutrients to treat malnutrition. Enteral nutrition refers to delivery of the person's caloric requirement through the gastrointestinal tract (e.g., nasogastric tube, feeding jejunostomy, percutaneous endoscopic gastrostomy tubes), while parenteral nutrition refers to delivery of nutrients intravenously. The three types of nutritional support that are provided to patients are:

1. *Enteral nutritional support:* This refers to the insertion of feeding tubes into patients who have a functional gut but are incapable of eating adequate amounts to meet their requirements. This is preferred over parenteral feeding as it conserves the integrity of the gut, is more affordable and easier to administer feeds. For short term (<30 days) a nasogastric or nasojejunal tube is used, whereas for longer periods, a percutaneous endoscopic gastrostomy (PEG) is used. A feeding jejunostomy performed through laparoscopic or open surgery is usually reserved for a situation where there is an obstruction to passage of a nasogastric tube and an endoscope, such as in advanced hypopharyngeal or upper cervical esophageal cancers. A systematic review comparing PEG and nasogastric tube use in head and neck cancer showed that both were comparable in terms of weight maintenance; while PEG tubes were better for long-term use, associated with greater mobility, cosmesis and quality of life, they were associated with prolongation of radiotherapy, more pain and dysphagia. There was also some evidence that those on PEG may have less motivation to return to an oral diet than those with nasogastric tubes.[10] This belief has prompted some oncologists delay feeding tube placement until patients are symptomatic, fearing long-term tube dependency, however there is some evidence that this is unlikely.[11] A more reasonable approach is to identify patients at high-risk of requiring support and proceed with feeding tube placement, however motivate patients to continue swallowing as long as feasible. In the absence of aspiration, allowing patients to continue swallowing with the tube in place can be helpful.
2. *Parenteral nutritional support:* This is where nutrients in the form of a fluid are administered intravenously through either a peripheral or central line. The formulations available differ based on the caloric requirement. These are not usually used except when there is concomitant gut surgery or the patient is unable to tolerate enteral feeding. However, it is not without the risk of complications, including phlebitis, electrolyte imbalance, transaminitis, coagulation disturbances and renal dysfunction.

3. *Immune-enhancing nutrition*[12]: This refers to the use of specialized formulations that include nutrients such as glutamine, omega-3 fatty acids and alanine, which help to regulate the response of the body in illness or injury. They are recommended in high-risk patients and may not have a routine role in head and neck cancer management.

Nutritional Considerations in Specific Situations

- *Perioperative:* A preoperative nutritional assessment is critical to prevent issues with recovery, refeeding syndrome, wound healing-related issues and significant postoperative morbidity. If patients are high-risk, surgery should be deferred where possible to allow nutritional support. If a patient is unable to eat, enteral feeding support with a nasogastric or nasojejunal tube can be used for 1–2 weeks prior to surgery. Postoperatively, feeding should be initiated as soon as possible. If the patient has a feeding tube placed, premature removal with inadequate oral intake can be problematic and should be avoided. Chyle leak should be managed with a fat-free diet with medium chain triglyceride supplementation. Consultation with a swallowing therapist and nutritionist can ensure that the patient receives adequate nutrition in spite of limitations in quantity and consistency of food that the patient tolerates.
- *Radiotherapy ± chemotherapy:* This results in weight loss even when the patient has adequate oral intake and nutritional counseling. Weekly assessment is important to identify issues such as severe mucositis and dysphagia that can hamper swallowing and cause breaks in treatment, compromising cure. Regular weight measurement is crucial to identify early nutritional issues. Tube feeding should be initiated early in patients who are unlikely to be able to maintain adequate oral intake during their treatment. To deal with disruptions in salivation, patients are advised to increase drinking fluids and food moisture. Patients are also advised to consume calorie-dense foods (oils, groundnuts, ghee) to compensate for reduction in the quantity they eat.
- *End-of-life care:* In terminal patients, quality of life is of utmost importance. Feeding tube placement should be performed if oral feeding is not feasible or successful. It may also be helpful in administration of medication, which will otherwise not be feasible. Caloric requirement is the primary consideration in nutritional planning. If patients wish to continue to eat orally, this should be encouraged except in cases of aspiration risk.

CONCLUSION

Nutritional management in head and neck cancer is an important yet often overlooked consideration. Malnutrition can interrupt therapy, worsen treatment-related morbidity and hasten clinical deterioration and even death. Nutritionists remain an invaluable part of the multidisciplinary team, however a basic knowledge of these concepts and principles is important for any one treating cancer.

REFERENCES

1. Palliative Care Australia. Standards for providing quality palliative care for all Australians. Deakin West, ACT: Palliative Care Australia; 2005.
2. Wiseman M. The second world cancer research fund/ American Institute for Cancer Research expert report. Food, nutrition, physical activity, and the prevention of cancer: A global perspective: Nutrition society and BAPEN medical symposium on 'nutrition support in cancer therapy'. Proc Nutr Soc. 2008;67(3):253-6.
3. Saunders J, Smith T. Malnutrition: causes and consequences. Clin Med. 2010;10(6):624.
4. Gorenc M, Kozjek NR, Strojan P. Malnutrition and cachexia in patients with head and neck cancer treated with (chemo) radiotherapy. Rep Pract Oncol Radiother. 2015;20(4): 249-58.
5. Dodson S, Baracos VE, Jatoi A, Evans WJ, Cella D, Dalton JT, et al. Muscle wasting in cancer cachexia: clinical implications, diagnosis, and emerging treatment strategies. Ann Rev Med. 2011;62:265-79.
6. Talwar B, Donnelly R, Skelly R, Donaldson M. Nutritional management in head and neck cancer: United Kingdom National Multidisciplinary Guidelines. J Laryngol Otol. 2016;130(S2):S32-40.
7. Poslusna K, Ruprich J, de Vries JH, Jakubikova M, van't Veer P. Misreporting of energy and micronutrient intake estimated by food records and 24 hour recalls, control and adjustment methods in practice. Br J Nutr. 2009;101(S2): S73-85.
8. Mehanna HM, Moledina J, Travis J. Refeeding syndrome: what it is, and how to prevent and treat it. Br Med J. 2008; 336(7659):1495-8.
9. Doig GS, Simpson F, Heighes PT, Bellomo R, Chesher D, Caterson ID, et al. Restricted versus continued standard caloric intake during the management of refeeding syndrome in critically ill adults: a randomised, parallel-group, multicentre, single-blind controlled trial. Lancet Respir Med. 2015;3(12):943-52.
10. Wang J, Liu M, Liu C, Ye Y, Huang G. Percutaneous endoscopic gastrostomy versus nasogastric tube feeding for patients with head and neck cancer: a systematic review. J Radiat Res. 2014;55(3):559-67.
11. Brown T, Banks M, Hughes BG, Lin C, Kenny LM, Bauer JD. Impact of early prophylactic feeding on long term tube dependency outcomes in patients with head and neck cancer. Oral Oncol. 2017;72:17-25.
12. Pollock GR, Van Way CW III. Immune-Enhancing Nutrition in Surgical and Critical Care. Mo Med. 2012;109(5): 388-92.

Management of Head and Neck Cancer

CHAPTER 7

Strategies in Oral Cancer Prevention

Shashikant Limbachiya, Samskruthi P Murthy, Narayana Subramaniam, Sivakumar Vidhyadharan

INTRODUCTION

Oral cancer is one of the most common cancers in Indian men. Most oral cancers are preventable as they are associated with proven risk habits such as tobacco and alcohol consumption. Although there have been declines in oral cancer incidence, survival has remained relatively unchanged over three decades. The most attractive strategy to improve outcome in oral cancer is prevention; the oral cavity is easily accessible for visualization, making it an ideal site for various prevention strategies. Best outcomes can be achieved through chemoprevention (agents that can halt malignant transformation or reverse the process), lifestyle modifications (cessation of high-risk habits such as smoking, alcohol consumption, tobacco/betel nut chewing) and regular screening of patients at high-risk of developing invasive cancers.

LEVELS OF PREVENTION

Oral cancer is highly prevalent in India. Even though there has been a small decline in the incidence of 6.4% when compared to 1996–2006,[1] 90% of the patients present in advanced stages with modest survival.[2] With South East Asia contributing to 90% of the global oral cancer load,[3] the only reasonable approach is risk mitigation and prevention. Oral cancer is caused by a series of mutagenic insults by known high-risk habits such as tobacco and alcohol consumption. The prevention strategies can be classified as primordial, primary, secondary and tertiary based on the timing of intervention **(Fig. 1)**.

- *Primordial prevention:* Aimed to prevent social and cultural patterns in society that increase the possibility of disease occurrence. One such example is the National Tobacco Control Program (NTCP) of India. More than 275 million adults consume tobacco in India and 85% of them start this habit before they reach 18 years of age.[4] The Cigarettes and Other Tobacco Products Act (COTPA) was passed by the Indian Parliament in May 2003, following which Government of India launched the National Tobacco Control Program in 2007. The objectives of the program are to increase awareness regarding harmful effects of tobacco, to effectively implement the COTPA, control tobacco consumption and minimize deaths caused by it. The NTCP is implemented by the three-tier system at a central, state and district level. The program is aimed at children and young adults to prevent habituation of smoking.

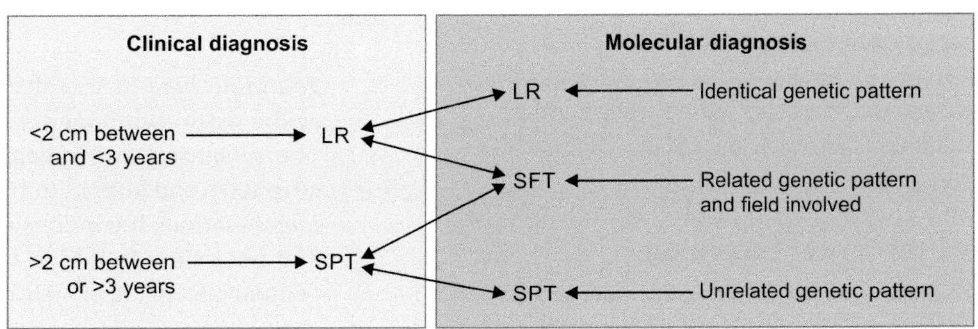

Fig. 1: Second primary and second field tumors. (LR: local recurrence, SPT: seond primary tumor, SFT: second field tumor)

The program is currently implemented in 36 states and 612 districts.

- *Primary prevention:* Aimed at cessation/control of high-risk factors that play a vital role in disease causation. The risk of cancer is high even after cessation of habits. Stopping the habit may not be enough, but sustained abstinence is paramount to reduce the risk compared to the normal population. It takes 20 years to reduce the risk of cancer to normal population after cessation of smoking and alcohol consumption.[5,6] Studies have shown that NTCP has resulted in the reduction of incidence of tobacco consumption with sustained cessation seen in patients who are counseled.[7]
- *Secondary prevention:* Aimed at identifying patients at risk of developing cancer by screening or detection; this can be achieved by screening programs to identify and manage premalignant lesions and chemoprevention. These strategies are detailed subsequently.
- *Tertiary prevention:* Aimed at prevention of occurrence of second primary tumors in a patient after the management of primary cancer. This can be achieved by regular follow-up and chemoprevention. There is a 20–30% risk of developing a second primary tumor in 20 years after management of primary head and neck cancer.[2] Tertiary prevention plays a vital role in improving the long-term outcome of patients.

PART A: ORAL CANCER SCREENING

Screening programs for a disease are aimed at those with high incidence and significantly impact the population with regard to mortality and morbidity and pose financial burden. Most oral cancer patients present at an advanced stage, where survival is as low as 3% at 5 years, while survival in early stages is as high as 54%.[8] When the cost of lost productivity due to premature cancer mortality was calculated in Brazil, China, South Africa and India, India spent $46.3 billion in 2012 alone; India spent the highest cost per case of oral cancers.[9] The impact of oral cancer on mortality, morbidity and resultant lost cost of productivity and quality of life is significant. Oral cancer serves as an ideal subsite for screening due to accessibility, its known risk factors, identifiable premalignant lesions and evidence that early detection improves survival.[10]

Tests Used for Oral Cancer Screening

Various tests are available for oral cancer screening. Sensitivity is defined as efficacy of the test to detect those with disease and specificity is defined as the ability of the test to report negative when the disease is absent. More than statistical parameters, the acceptability of the test among the test population is paramount. The tests can be broadly classified as mucosal, salivary and combined tests based on the sample used for testing.

1. Mucosal tests
   a. *Nontargeted:* These include methods that visualize whole of oral cavity without any specific aids to identify at-risk lesions
      i. *Conventional oral examination (COE):* It is the gold standard test currently available for oral cancer screening. The test utilizes white light to examine the oral cavity to identify suspected lesions, which are biopsied for histological evaluation. The sensitivity and specificity of COE are 88.7% and 60.9%, respectively.[11] COE is advantageous as it is associated with high validity and can be applied in a primary setting. It requires minimum examination time per patient once personnel are efficiently trained. It can be repeated with no morbidity and no special instruments are needed. Even a primary health worker can be trained to perform COE; it does not require a doctor to conduct. The test is subject to variability with its validity wholly based on the examiner skill and ability to identify suspected lesions. Due to the invasiveness of the procedure, the test acceptability may be low.[12]
      ii. *Mouth self-examination:* Breast self-examination is a well-known strategy for early detection of breast cancer. Likewise, mouth self-examination presents an attractive strategy. The test has a low sensitivity of 18%, while the specificity is 99.9%.[12] Subjects can easily identify red patches but find it difficult to identify white patches. Compliance is a major drawback.
   b. *Targeted:* Lesion targeted tests are those that are used to either supplement COE or enhance identification and evaluate high-risk suspicious lesions
      i. *Dyes:*[13-15]
         - *Toluidine blue:* It is a dye with affinity to acidic tissue component like nucleic acids. The sensitivity and specificity range from 40 to 100% and from 31 to 100%, respectively.
         - *Lugol's iodine:* It contains elemental iodine and potassium iodide. It reacts with intracellular glycogen, which results in brown color change. The diagnostic value is low, as Lugol's iodine results in nonspecific staining.

ii. *Light-based approaches:*
   - *Chemoluminescence:* Commercially available as ViziLite system by Zila Pharmaceuticals, Phoenix, Arizona, this technique aids in better visualization of suspected lesions. The ViziLite system utilizes chemoluminescent light (wavelengths of 490–510 nm) after oral gargle with 1% acetic acid. The acetic acid wash dehydrates tissue and enhances their reflectance with chemiluminescent light. Suspicious lesions appear acetowhite, while normal mucosa appears blue.[16] The test sensitivity and specificity are similar to COE.[17]
   - *Wide field autofluorescence imaging:* Commercially available as VELscope by LED Dental, Inc., White Rock, British Columbia, Canada. Cellular structures (such as collagen and keratin), metabolites [such as nicotinamide adenine dinucleotide hydride (NADH)], and flavin adenine dinucleotide (FAD) impart tissue autofluorescence.[18] Due to cellular changes in premalignant and malignant lesions, lose autofluorescence that can be visualized under light. The test sensitivity and specificity for the VELscope range from 30 to 98% and 15 to 100%, respectively.
   - *Reflectance confocal microscopy:* Commercially available as Vivascope microscopes, they provide optical visualization noninvasively at the cellular level by utilizing focused laser illumination. A depth of 200–300 mm can be evaluated with 0.5–1 mm resolution. The cellular changes such as increased nuclear density, disorganized cellular morphology are picked up by reflectance confocal microscopy.[19-22] This technology, named as the Dermascope, is used in triaging skin lesion for biopsy in high-risk patients for skin cancer.

iii. *Molecular targeted approaches:*
   - *Lectins targeting sialic acid:* Glycosylation is significantly altered in tumor cells. Lectins bind to glycolipids and glycoproteins that are overly expressed in cancer cells. Lectins are inexpensive and have low toxicity profile. It has a sensitivity of 100 and 81% to detect malignant and dysplastic lesions, respectively. The lower sensitivity for dysplastic lesions is due to a slightly higher rate of false positivity for chronic inflammatory lesions.[23,24]
   - *Glucose metabolism:* The Warburg effect is a process where cancer cells show an increase in glucose metabolism, which is exploited in fluorodeoxyglucose positron emission tomography computed tomography (FDG PET CT) imaging systems. FDG PET has low space configuration of 0.3 cm^2, hence may miss out small suspicious lesions. Hence 2-NBDG (2-[N-(7-nitrobenz-2-oxa-1,3-diazol-4-yl) amino]-2-deoxy-D-glucose), an FDG analog, is used to detect areas of malignancy. Further studies are required to explore its validity and safety.[25]
   - *Porphyrins:* 5-aminolevulinic acid is a precursor of protoporphyrin IX, which is photosensitive. Hence administration of 5-aminolevulinic acid increases production of protoporphyrin IX, which is photosensitive and can be utilized for fluorescence imaging. The same property is exploited for photodynamic therapy. The sensitivity and specificity are 99% and 60%, respectively.
   - *Poly (ADP-ribose) Polymerase:* Poly (ADP-ribose) polymerase 1 (PARP1) is a DNA repair enzyme that is highly expressed by cancer cells. Feasibility studies have shown promising results, but further studies are required to assess their validity.[26-29]

2. *Salivary tests:* Salivary biomarkers arose as a noninvasive alternative with a high theoretical acceptability among a test population. Various biomarkers consisting of salivary constituents, proteomic, transcriptomic, genomic, and metabolomic analyses have been explored as a potential biomarker for cancerous and precancerous lesion. Description and validity of each biomarker is exhaustive, as more than 150 biomarkers are described and studied. The salivary biomarker approach is limited due to lack of standardized method for saliva collection and processing, and absence of cut off value for levels of biomarkers in normal, inflammatory, precancerous and cancerous environments.[30]
3. *Combined tests:*
   a. *Brush cytology:* Commercially available as OralCDx, this is a noninvasive technique in which oral rinse, saliva or scraping from the lesion can be used to attain a sample for testing. As the test is noninvasive, it can be performed repeatedly. As only cytological evaluation is done, if atypia is present in the sample, it will need to be confirmed with a histopathological examination of the lesion.[31]

b. *Spectroscopy:* This technique is based on the principle that when light interacts with matter, a spectroscopic signature is captured based on absorption, emission and reflectance by the substance that is tested. The signature attained can be analyzed, and even a nonexpert can achieve an objective diagnosis. The signature is dependent on the microscopic changes and changes in tissue morphology. Fluorescence, infrared and Raman spectroscopy are various spectroscopic methods. Raman spectroscopy is one of the most common methods used. Raman spectroscopy does not need any reagents and only based on the biochemical composition of the tissue examined. It can be used for cells, biofluid and tissues. It also has high spatial resolution with increased depth of penetration than other methods of spectroscopy.[31]

Screening Programs

Screening programs are population-based, where all the subjects in a geographical area are screened, or opportunistic, when aimed at those with a high risk of developing malignancy. The effectiveness of a screening program was assessed by a randomized trial conducted in Thiruvananthapuram,[32] conducted in 13 clusters (intervention group had 7 clusters and 96,517 subjects while the control group had 6 clusters and 95,536 individuals). The trial consisted of 3 yearly visual inspections and guided biopsies by trained workers between 1996 and 2004. The referral compliance was 63%. 96% of oral cancer deaths occurred in tobacco/alcohol users. There was a 34% reduction in cancer-related mortality among high-risk group (tobacco/alcohol users), while there was no survival benefit in low risk group or subjects with no habits. The reduction in mortality was consistent even in the follow-up study at 15 years follow-up.[33] The cost of visual inspection in the trial was $6 (USD) and cost per life saved was $835 (USD).[34] The findings from the trial established the efficacy of visual inspection and the effectiveness of the screening program.

In another study, the efficacy of mouth self-examination among 34,766 high-risk subjects was studied. The study reported an increased awareness of 80% among participants however the compliance was poor (32%). However, mouth self-examination showed a very low sensitivity of 18% and a high specificity of 99.9%.[12] Population-based screening in Taiwan evaluated visual inspection and directed biopsies in 2,334,299 subjects who were smokers/betel nut chewer or both between 2004 and 2009.[35] 55.1% were effectively screened. The study showed an increased rate of early-stage cancers in the screened group than the nonscreened group (46.5% vs. 39.6%, $p < 0.01$). The incidence of oral cancer was also significantly higher in nonscreened group than the screened group. The screening program showed a stage shift of 45% and the efficacy of visual inspection strategy in high-risk group.

The national screening program conducted since 1984 in Cuba and follow-up evaluation at 15 years showed no significant improvement in oral cancer mortality.[36] The findings of this screening program emphasizes on the importance of organized workflow with appropriate coverage to include high-risk group subjects and referral systems for an effective screening program aimed to reduce cancer-related mortality.

Visual/clinical oral examination with directed biopsies is the current gold standard of oral cancer screening. The available evidence has proven the efficacy of COE in the screening program to reduce oral cancer morbidity in high-risk group subjects. Various noninvasive techniques have shown promising results but need further standardization and validation to be implemented in a screening program.

PART B: PREMALIGNANT LESIONS OF THE ORAL CAVITY

Introduction

Carcinogenesis of oral cancer is a multistep process that occurs over time by accumulation of various genetic and epigenetic changes. The concept of "field cancerization" proposed by Slaughter highlights the fact that a person with an existing premalignant lesion or oral cancer in a subsite has a tendency to recur and is at an increased risk of second malignancy due to the exposure of the entire upper aerodigestive tract to carcinogens.[37]

Definition

The World Health Organization (WHO) classifies oral precancerous/potentially malignant disorders into two general groups, as follows:

1. *Premalignant lesion or precancerous lesion* is defined as morphologically altered tissue in which cancer is more likely to occur than in its apparently normal counterpart. These precancerous lesions include leukoplakia, erythroplakia, and the palatal lesions of reverse smokers.
2. *A precancerous condition* is a generalized state associated with significantly increased risk of cancer.

The precancerous conditions include submucosal fibrosis, lichen planus, epidermolysis bullosa, and discoid lupus erythematous.

The potentially premalignant lesion is an alternative term that is keeping with the concept that not all lesions will have any potential to progress to malignancy and that the clinician is faced with a mucosal change that is only potentially premalignant lesion.[37]

At a WHO workshop in 2007, it was recommended that the distinction between potentially malignant lesions and conditions be abandoned in favor of a common term oral potentially malignant disorders (OPMDs), which is now accepted in the new classification.[38]

Oral Potentially Malignant Disorders

Oral Leukoplakia

Leukoplakia is defined as a white plaque of questionable risk having excluded (other) known diseases or disorders that carry no increased risk for cancer **(Fig. 2)**.[39,40]

Diagnosis of oral leukoplakia (OL) is by exclusion; it is a clinical diagnosis and needs histological confirmation. The prevalence of OL ranges from 1 to 5% and malignant transformation rate of 3–17%.[41-43]

The conditions that need to be excluded are oral candidiasis, lichen planus, leukoedema, healing aphthous ulcers, white sponge nevus and frictional keratosis. The rate of malignant transformation is dependent on the characteristics of the OL lesion. A homogeneous OL has very low risk of malignant transformation, while nonhomogeneous lesions have a higher risk of malignant transformation; in proliferative verrucous leukoplakia (PVL) this is 40–75% and erythroleukoplakia it is 21%.[41,42] Nonhomogeneous lesions have a 7-fold higher risk than homogeneous lesions when large sized.[42,43] The risk of transformation is also dependent on the degree of dysplasia with increased risk for severe dysplasia. Active intervention with surgical excision is dependent on characteristics such as nonhomogeneity and grade of dysplasia.

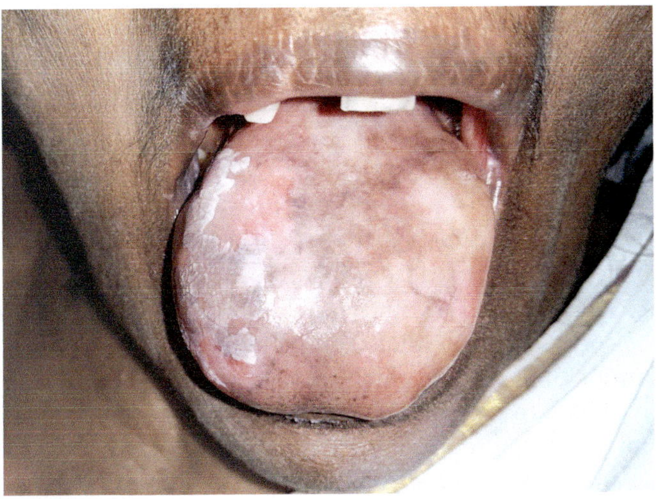

Fig. 2: Leukoplakia.

Oral Erythroplakia

Oral erythroplakia (OE) is defined as the red velvety plaque that cannot be attributed to any other disease. The rate of malignant transformation is as high as 50%. They are associated with invasive carcinoma in 51% and carcinoma in situ at presentation in 40% of cases.[44] Hence, surgical excision must be offered with a depth of excision up to superficial muscle layer in tongue and the submucosal layer in other oral subsites.

Oral Submucosal Fibrosis

Oral submucosal fibrosis (OSMF) is a condition characterized by progressive fibrotic disease of the oral cavity **(Table 1)**. This condition is highly prevalent in Asian countries that have higher rate of areca nut chewing such as India, Pakistan, Taiwan, Sri Lanka and Nepal. Various etiologic factors have been described earlier such as micronutrient deficiency, autoantibodies, capsaicin in chilli, but the International Agency for Research on Cancer (IARC) by way of epidemiological and in vitro studies has shown that areca nut is the sole etiological factor.[45-47] The association of areca nut consumption is dose-dependent with increased risk directly associated with increased longer duration of use and higher daily consumption.

The primary pathophysiology of OSMF is through increased collagen deposition and reduced collagen breakdown. The pathognomonic change in OSMF is subepithelial deposition of type 1 collagen fibers due to fibroblast activation and proliferation. Polyphenols in the areca nut also cause cross-linking between collagen fibers, which makes them resistant to degradation by collagenases. Arecoline also induces various growth factors such as TGF beta, fibroblast growth factor and insulin-like growth factor. Matrix metalloproteinases (MMP) are responsible for the degradation of fibrillar collagen. The MMPs are underexpressed in OSMF. The copper in areca nut increases salivary copper levels and serum copper levels that could upregulate copper-dependent enzyme—lysyl oxidase, which results in collagen cross-linking. In advanced stages, progressive trismus is mainly due to changes in the extracellular matrix,

Table 1: Classification of oral submucous fibrosis.

Grading/staging	*Clinical*	*Functional*	*Histopathological*	*Treatment*	*Prognosis*
Grade 1	• Involvement of less than one-third of the oral cavity • Mild blanching, burning sensation, recurrent ulceration, and stomatitis • Dryness of mouth	Mouth opening up to 35 mm	*Stage of inflammation:* Fine edematous collagen, congested blood vessels, abundant neutrophils along with lymphocytes with myxomatous changes in subepithelial, connective tissue layer of epithelium	Cessation of habit, nutritional supplement, antioxidants, topical steroid ointment	Excellent
Grade 2	• Involvement of one-third to two-thirds of the oral cavity • Blanching of oral mucosa with mottled and marble like appearance, fibrotic bands palpable and involvement of soft palate and premolar area	• Mouth opening 25–35 mm • Cheek flexibility reduced by 33%	*Stage of hyalinization:* • Juxta-epithelial collagen hyalinization with lymphocytes, eosinophils • Dilated and congested blood vessels • Less fibroblastic activity • Granulation changes in muscle layer with reduced inflammatory cells in subepithelial layer	• Habit cessation, nutritional supplement, intralesional injection of placental extracts, hyaluronidase, steroid therapy • Physiotherapy	• Good • Recurrence rate is low
Grade 3	• Involvement of greater than two-thirds of the oral cavity • Severe blanching. Broad thick fibrous palpable bands at cheeks and lips and rigid mucosa, depapillated tongue and restricted tongue movement and shrunken bud lite uvula • Floor of the mouth involvement and lymphadenopathy	• Mouth opening 15–25 mm • Cheek flexibility reduced by 66%	*Stage of fibrosis:* • Complete collagen hyalinization without fibroblast and edema • Obliterated blood vessels • Plasma cells and lymphocytes are present • Extensive fibrosis with hyalinization from subepithelial to superficial muscle layers with atrophic, degenerative changes	Surgical treatment including band excision and reconstruction with BFP or split thickness graft bilateral temporalis myotomy and coronoidectomy	• Fair • Recurrence rate is high
Grade 4	• Leukoplakia changes, erythroplakia • Ulcerating and suspicious malignant lesion	Mouth opening <15 mm or nil	*Stages of malignant transformation:* Erythroplakia changes into squamous cell carcinoma	Surgical treatment and biopsy of suspicious lesion	Poor, malignant transformation

where elastin is replaced by type 1 collagen resulting in reduced elasticity. Even though there is evidence to support a dose-dependent association between OSMF and areca nut consumption, younger patients with lesser exposure to areca nut chewing are diagnosed with OSMF. Polymorphism of *Cytochrome P450 3A* gene causes increased susceptibility to OSMF.[48] The disease in early stages is characterized by the formation of vesicles and ulcers. Intolerance to spicy food is one of the earliest and most specific symptoms of OMSF. The rate of malignant transformation ranges from 7 to 30%.[41] A grading system of OSMF was proposed by Warnakulasuriya[49] where the five grades are:

- *Grade 1:* Burning, depapillation, blanching or leathery mucosa (disease triad for OSMF) with mouth opening, >35 mm
- *Grade 2:* Burning, depapillation, blanching or leathery mucosa with fibrous bands and moderate limitation of mouth opening 20–35 mm
- *Grade 3:* Severe OSMF and limitation of opening <20 mm
- *Grade 4A:* OSMF with other potentially malignant disorder
- *Grade 4B:* OSMF with oral epithelial dysplasia
- *Grade 5:* OSMF with invasive squamous cell carcinoma (SCC)

The treatment strategy of OSMF is multifold. In early stages, the primary aim must be to halt disease progression which is achieved by cessation of betel nut chewing, enzymatic degradation with hyaluronidase, collagenase, and chymotrypsin, immune modulators such as corticosteroids, interferon-gamma, placental extracts, antioxidant therapy such as beta carotene, vitamin E, lycopene to eliminate oxygen radicals and correction of micronutrient deficiency. In advanced stage, treatment is aimed at management of trismus by surgical excision of fibrotic bands with appropriate reconstruction to prevent further postsurgical fibrosis.

Oral Lichen Planus

Oral lichen planus (OLP) is a systemic autoimmune disorder that affects mucosal and cutaneous surfaces. The disorder has a strong female predilection. Various forms of lichen planus are present, but the reticular form is the most common intraoral presentation, which appears as an interconnecting lace-like pattern with raised thin white lines called Wickham striae. The rate of transformation is 0–5%.[41] The management is most often conservative with immune modulators.

Clinical Prognostic Determinants of Progression to Cancer

- *Site:* Location of lesions within the oral cavity is related to the etiological factors and therefore may vary with geographical location as well as local habits, however it may influence risk of malignancy. For example, betel quid chewers have lesion involving buccal mucosa, whereas reverse smokers will have lesions involving palate. The lateral border of tongue and floor of the mouth is the most common site for oral potentially malignant disorders and oral cancer due to pooling of saliva and prolonged exposure to dissolved carcinogens.[50]
- *Clinical appearance:* The clinical appearance of OL is characterized as homogeneous and nonhomogeneous. There is consensus in the literature that nonhomogeneous lesions have a greater risk of malignant transformation compared with homogeneous lesions.[51] The highest rates of malignant change were noted in lesions that were described as speckled, erosive or as erythroleukoplakia, emphasizing that these lesions are not, in fact, true leukoplakias (white plaques) but have a red component.
- *Size:* Lesions greater than 200 mm^2 were more likely to progress to malignancy compared with smaller lesions.[52] It is found that the risk of transformation was six times greater in patients with large confluent lesions that extended over more than one anatomic site compared with those with smaller localized lesions.
- *Patient age and duration of lesion:* The risk of malignant change is higher within the first 5 years after diagnosis of OPMD, although the condition is chronic and persistent. The transformation rates are higher in older individuals.[53] Studies from India show that premalignant lesions are likely to develop and progress to cancer in older individuals due to high incidence of leukoplakia in young age groups.[54]
- *Sex:* Females have a higher risk of malignant transformation of lesions as compared to men, despite the fact that OPMD are less common in female.[54] It is still unclear why women are more predisposed to malignant transformation compared with men. In large Indian studies, females were found to be much less likely to have lesions, but this was related to the fact that they were less likely to use tobacco.[55]
- *Habits:* Tobacco use and consumption of alcohol are well-established etiologic factors for the development of OPMDs with malignant transformation seen with continuous and persistent use of these habits. Lesions in nonsmokers (sometimes referred to as "idiopathic leukoplakia") seem to be at a higher risk of progression to cancer. This suggests that although tobacco is the major etiological cause, there is a genetic predisposition in cases of nonsmokers.[56] The use of betel quid and areca nut are also risk factors.

Histologic Determinants of Progression to Cancer

Epithelial Dysplasia

The gold standard diagnostic procedure for diagnosing epithelial dysplasia is biopsy and histologic examination, which enables to rule out other specific diagnosis and evaluate any tissue change, most significant of which are features of cytologic atypia and distorted epithelial architecture, which together are referred to as oral epithelial dysplasia (OED).[57]

Oral epithelial dysplasia is a histologically diagnosis and can clinically manifest as or in OLP, OL and OSMF. The rate of malignant transformation ranges 6–36% depending on the grade of dysplasia.[41] The average time to malignant transformation is 7.5 years, and hence long-term following even after surgical excision is mandated. The latest 2017 WHO classification system uses a combination of architectural and cytologic features in an attempt to provide a more objective approach to the diagnosis and grading of OED **(Table 2)**.[58]

Many pathologists grade lesions into mild, moderate, and severe dysplasia on the basis of the extent and degree of the changes. Mild dysplasia defines a lesion in which the architectural and cytologic changes are minimal and limited to the lower third of the epithelium. Moderate dysplasia demonstrates changes involving up to two-thirds of the full thickness of the epithelium. Severe dysplasia displays more marked changes, which may extend beyond the lower two-thirds of the epithelium. Carcinoma in situ (CIS) is regarded as the most severe form of severe dysplasia and involves changes

Table 2: Cytological and architectural diagnostic criteria for oral epithelial dysplasia.[58]

Architectural changes	*Cytological changes*
Irregular epithelial stratification	Abnormal variation in nuclear size (anisonucleosis)
Loss of polarity of basal cells	Abnormal variation in nuclear shape (nuclear pleomorphism)
Drop-shaped rete ridges	Abnormal variation in cell shape (cellular pleomorphism)
Increased number of mitotic figures	Increased nuclear/cytoplasmic ratio
Abnormally superficial mitotic figures	Atypical mitotic figures
Premature keratinization in single cells (dyskeratosis)	Increased number and size of nucleoli
Keratin pearls within rete ridges	
Loss of epithelial cell cohesion	
Hyperchromasia	

through the entire epithelial thickness, but in the oral cavity, even these lesions may show a degree of surface keratinization.

In an attempt to improve the reliability of grading, a number of authors have developed a binary grading scheme, which is supported by the WHO, although it is recognized that further validation and evidence from clinical studies are needed.[58] The binary system divides lesions into "high risk" and "low risk" on the basis of the number of features identified on histologic examination. High-risk lesions show at least four architectural features and five cytologic features, while low-risk lesions show fewer changes.

The main goal of OED diagnosis and binary grading is to provide better management of the patients; patients with moderate to severe OED require clinical intervention whereas regular follow-up is adopted in patients with mild dysplasia. As it stands, the grade of OED is still the most important prognostic factor for malignant transformation. The rate of malignant transformation varies considerably, even in cases of severe dysplasia, which depends on the population in the study. The binary system may have better prognostic value and superior reproducibility compared with the current more widely used 3-scale grading system. With further evaluation, it is believed that the binary system will become the standard grading scheme.

Biomarkers as Predictors of Progression

The most common biomarkers to be analyzed were p53, followed by proliferation markers (Ki67 and PCNA). Other markers include cell cycle proteins, loss of heterozygosity (LOH), and a range of cell surface and stromal proteins. Analysis of DNA content (ploidy) provides a simple measure of gross genetic aberrations and is known to be highly associated with malignancy.

Analysis of DNA aneuploidy may be one potentially useful biomarker that has yet to be fully exploited. Aneuploid dysplastic lesions have a higher risk of malignant progression. Aneuploidy can now be measured by using image cytometry, and its application to cytology samples may soon result in rapid and reliable noninvasive tests for risk assessment of oral lesions.[59,60]

Human Papillomavirus-associated Epithelial Dysplasia

In a meta-analysis of studies up to 1997, Miller and Johnstone found that human papillomavirus (HPV) was more likely to be detected in precancerous lesions than in normal oral mucosa. HPV was detected in 10% of normal tissues compared with 22.2% of nondysplastic leukoplakias and 26.2% of dysplastic lesions. Subsequently, the relationship between high-risk HPV and oropharyngeal SCC has become well established, but the role of HPV in OPMDs remains uncertain.[61] Proliferative verrucous leukoplakia is the most common presentation with high transformation rates to malignancy. They are commonly associated with women, >60 years of age and nonsmokers.

Human papillomavirus-associated epithelial dysplasia consistently shows an association with infection by high-risk HPV (HPV-16). The gold standard for diagnosis is to demonstrate HPV infection by in situ hybridization (ISH), but p16 expression may be a good surrogate marker for high-risk HPV types. However, although p16 expression is sensitive, it is not specific because HPV-negative epithelial dysplasia may be p16 positive. Although p16 is now accepted as a surrogate for HPV expression in oropharyngeal carcinoma, further work is needed to determine its value in the diagnosis of HPV-associated epithelial dysplasia. As these lesions have high propensity of malignant transformation, they have to be excised.

Approach to Clinical Risk Assessment and Management

Assessing the risk of malignant change in OPMDs can be difficult because any decision at each stage of the management pathway is not binary, and the clinician may be faced with a number of options. The process of undertaking a clinical assessment can be considered in three stages: (1) clinical history, (2) clinical examination, and (3) surgical biopsy with histopathologic evaluation.

Flowchart 1 graphically presents the features encountered at each stage that may be associated with risk. The starting point is the identification of a suspicious lesion, which, for this purpose, is defined as a lesion that cannot be diagnosed as a specific disorder on clinical examination. Specific lesions, such as lichen planus or OSMF, have defined risks and are not illustrated. In **Flowchart 1**, the features encountered at each stage are given a risk profile: white, gray, or black, indicating low, medium, or high risk, respectively.

History taking is the first stage of clinical assessment, and here, female nonsmokers would be regarded as being at higher risk compared with males. At clinical examination, erythroplakia has a higher risk compared with leukoplakia, but nonhomogeneous lesions have a higher risk compared with homogeneous lesions, and speckled lesions are at a higher risk compared with verrucous lesions.

Histopathological evaluation is paramount and is considered critical for making the final informed decision about management. Combined the three stages of evaluation is essential to achieve optimal outcomes in the risk assessment of OPMDs. The risk factors based on demographic and clinical data are helpful when a clinically patient presents with high-risk features while histology reports low risk, then such patients may benefit from aggressive management. With biopsy-proven grade of dysplasia, further management decision with respect to observation or surgical excision can be planned. The management recommendation for low-grade dysplasia is controversial where observation and excision can both be recommended. Moderate grade dysplasia can be managed with excision while all severe dysplasia/carcinoma in situ must be surgically excised with adequate margins.

Flowchart 1: Management of a suspicious oral lesion.

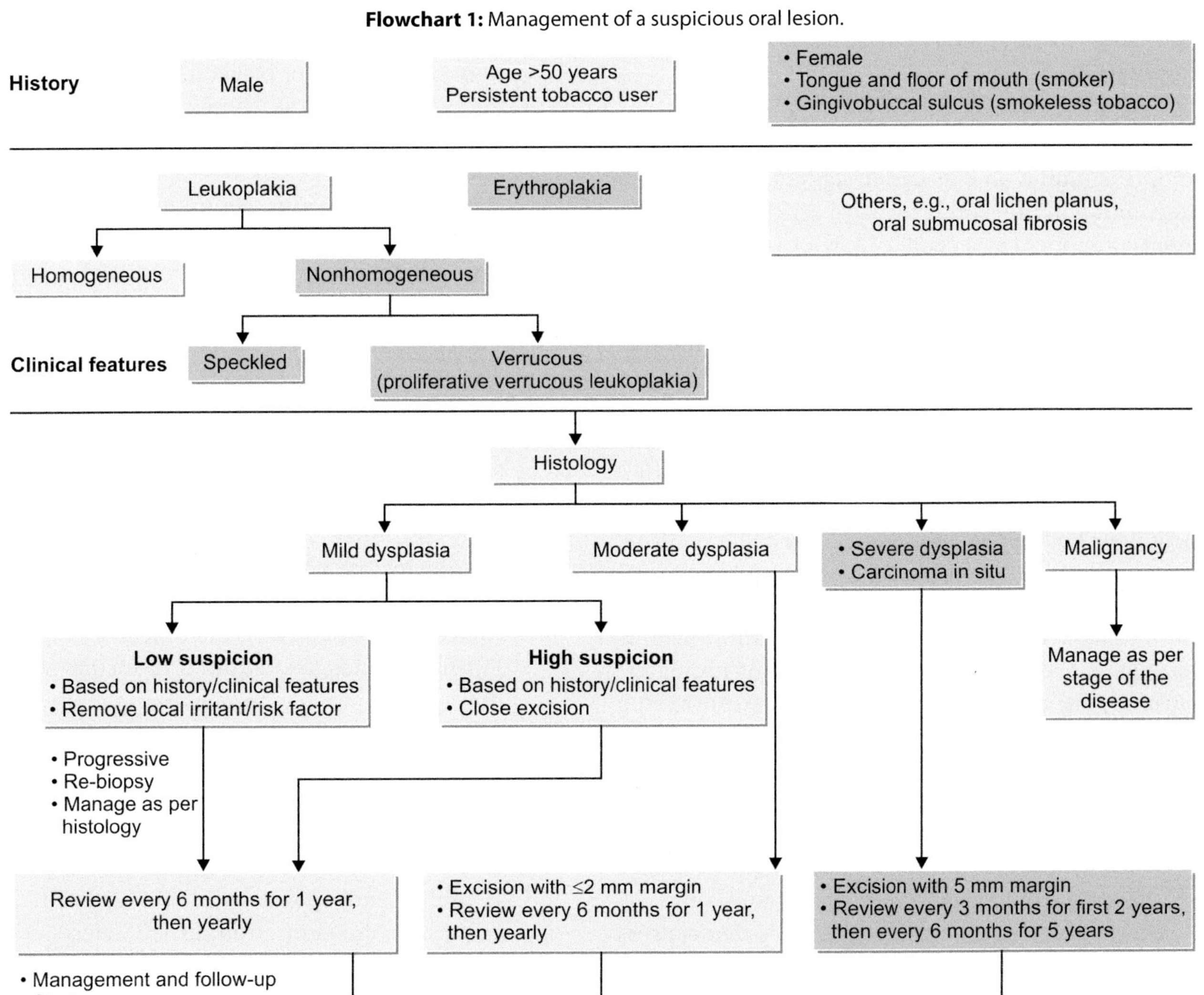

Flowchart 2: Oral chemoprevention strategies.

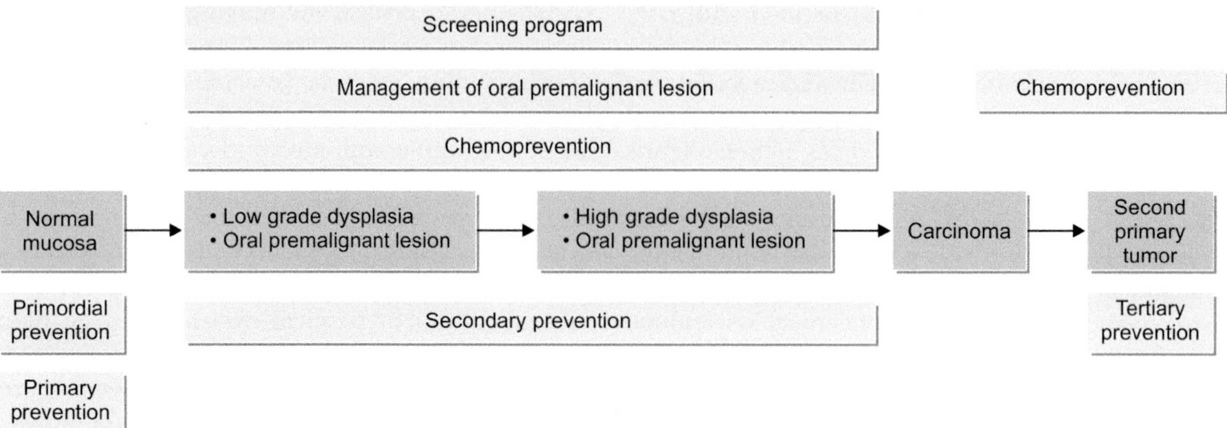

Follow-up strategy: Average time to malignant transformation is 7.5 years, and hence long-term follow-up even after surgical excision is mandated. Cases with severe dysplasia/CIS changes must be followed up as stage I oral carcinoma. The rest of the follow-up strategy is depicted in **Flowchart 2**.

PART C: CHEMOPREVENTION

Chemoprevention is an effective strategy at various levels of intervention in preventing invasive cancer. It forms an essential component of secondary and tertiary prevention strategies. Chemoprevention is employed to halt or reverse the carcinogenic process by using synthetic or natural products.[62] The multiple risk factors and multiple processes that play a part in the causation of oral cancer, make it difficult to identify a single agent that can halt carcinogenic transformation.[63] Even though various trials and agents have been evaluated, their routine use in clinical practice is not recommended. Based on the action of chemoprevention agent, they can broadly be classified as antimutagenic, antiproliferative agents and others.

1. *Antimutagens:* The mechanisms of action of antimutagens are directed at prevention of mutagen/carcinogen effect on DNA or by suppressing mutations that are generated by the mutagen/carcinogen effect.[63]
   i. *N-acetyl-cysteine:* N-acetyl-l-cysteine (NAC) prevents epidermal growth factor receptor (EGFR)-induced phosphorylation. In vitro studies have shown that NAC promotes apoptosis and cell cycle arrest in oral cancer cell lines that express EGFR.[64,65] About 80% of oral cancers express EGFR, making it a potential chemoprevention strategy. The EUROSCAN multicentric trial studied the effect of chemoprevention in preventing second primary tumor in treated cases of head and neck cancer and lung cancer **(Fig. 1)**. The study included four arms to receive vitamin A (300,000 IU/day followed by 150,000 IU/day in the 2nd year), NAC (600 mg/day for 2 years), both compounds, or placebo. Following a median period of 49 months, there was no difference in event-free survival among intervention arms and placebo.[66]
   ii. *Topical bleomycin:* Bleomycin is a known chemotherapeutic agent, commonly used in the management of lymphoma. Using topical application can increase local concentrations and effect of bleomycin with reduced systemic effects. Chau et al. studied the effects of topical bleomycin in management of oral premalignant lesions. The study used topical bleomycin in serial concentrations of 1%, 0.5% and 0% (placebo) for a mean duration of 2 weeks. Complete response with respect to no clinical or histological response was seen 40.2%, 25% and 8% in serial concentrations of 1%, 0.5% and 0% (placebo) respectively of topical bleomycin.[67] Further studies are required to further validate the use of topical bleomycin.
   iii. *Polyphenols:* Polyphenols primarily consists of plant extracts that are protective against reactive oxygen species. Commonly studied polyphenols are green tea extracts and curcumin.
      a. *Green tea extracts:* Green tea consists of polyphenol epigallocatechin 3-gallate (EGCG) in high concentration. EGCG arrests cells in G1/G0 phase and inhibits angiogenesis by preventing VEGF secretion by tumor cells.[68,69] A phase II trial by Tsao et al. who studied the efficacy of green tea extract in high-risk oral

premalignant lesion showed a dose-dependent response rate in complete/partial response of oral premalignant lesion, but the response rate did not reach statistical significance.[70] Further evidence for routine use is awaited.

b. *Curcumin:* Curcumin is a polyphenol found in curcumin longa. Curcumin is a potent inhibitor of NF-κB/COX-2.[71,72] The potential of chemopreventive abilities of curcumin has been explored in various cancers of oral cavity, colon, breast and prostate. Phase I trial by Cheng et al. proved the biological safety of high dose (8 g/day) of curcumin as a chemopreventive agent. The study consisted of precancerous lesions from various systems and included only 13 patients of oral premalignant lesion.[73] Promising results were showed by phase IIB trial in 2016. The study randomized 223 patients into curcumin 3.6 g/day and a placebo arm. A significant response was seen in the curcumin arm (HR: 0.50, 95% CI: 0.27–0.92, p = 0.02). However, continuation of curcumin in partial responders beyond 6 months did not show any benefit, with the trial showing a good safety profile of curcumin with 3.6 g/day.[74] Further studies with long-term follow-up are required to translate the benefit of curcumin to clinical practice.

2. *Antiproliferatives:* Antiproliferatives are chemopreventive agents that prevent the proliferation of cells.

i. *Vitamins and their analogues:* The chemopreventive role of naturally occurring vitamin A, vitamin E, beta-carotene and synthetic retinoids has been studied extensively. Various trials as chemopreventives before the occurrence of invasive tumor from premalignant lesions (primary chemoprevention) and in the prevention of second primary after management of primary invasive cancer (secondary chemoprevention) have been conducted since 1957.

a. *Primary chemoprevention:* The first report of efficacy of vitamin A as a chemopreventive agent was established in 1957.[75] High response rates with vitamin A precursor—beta-carotene were seen in further studies. A double-blinded placebo-controlled trial was conducted in 160 fisherwomen in India who were administered with vitamin A (300,000 IU per week) + beta-carotene (360 mg per week) or placebo for a year showed a response rate of 52% in vitamin A-arm, 33% in beta-carotene arm but most of the responders relapsed after discontinuation of the agent.[76] Two placebo-controlled studies evaluated the efficacy of alpha-tocopherol, beta-carotene, both or placebo did not show any response in subjects with risk of head and neck cancer.[77,78] Based on findings from these studies, a randomized placebo-controlled study was designed to determine the efficacy of isotretinoin (1 or 2 mg per day) versus placebo in 44 patients with leukoplakia.[79] The advantage of the trial was that histological response was also studied and showed an overall response rate with isotretinoin to be 67% versus 10% with placebo. However, the toxicity associated with a high dose of 2 mg/day resulted in dose reduction in as many as 46% of the patients. About 50% of responders relapsed within 3 months of discontinuation of the treatment. A subsequent trial also used induction high dose isotretinoin (1.5 mg/kg per day) for 3 months followed by continuation phase for 9 months with low dose isotretinoin (0.5 mg/kg per day) or beta-carotene (30 mg/day). The trial showed a 95% response rate with isotretinoin, but with significant side effects with isotretinoin.[80]

b. *Secondary chemoprevention:* Evidence in secondary chemoprevention has been disappointing. The largest study included 1,190 patients with stage I/II head and neck cancer patients were assigned to isotretinoin 30 mg/day versus placebo showed no benefit.[81] Relatively higher doses of isotretinoin have shown a reduction in secondary cancers but included a small number of patients in the trial, while the role of beta-carotene and alpha-tocopherol studied has shown a detrimental effect with increased rate of second primary tumors (HR 1.86, 95% CI) in one of the trials.[82]

ii. *Nonsteroidal anti-inflammatory drugs (NSAIDs):* The rationale of using NSAIDs as chemopreventive drugs in head and cancer is due to increased prostaglandin secretion and overexpression of COX-2 receptors in these cancers.[83] COX-2 aids in carcinogenesis by immunosuppression and angiogenesis. Increased expression of COX-2 is seen even in leukoplakia patches. The meta-analysis by Shi et al., who reviewed studies evaluating the association of NSAIDs with the risk of developing head and neck cancers,

Table 3: Randomized trials of significance in chemoprevention of head and neck cancer.[88]

Study	*Number of patients*	*Intervention*	*Summary*	*Intent of chemoprevention*
Hong et al.	44	13-cis-retinoic acid (13-cRA) placebo	54% response rate	Primary
Hong et al.[94]	103	13-cRA placebo	24% risk reduction in second primary tumor	Secondary
Sankaranarayanan et al.[15]	160	Vitamin A, beta-carotene placebo	Vitamin A 52% and beta-carotene 33% response rate	Primary
van Zandwijk et al.[15]	2592	Retinyl palmitate, N-acetyl cysteine, both or placebo	No risk reduction	Secondary
Mayne et al.[95]	264	Beta-carotene, placebo	No effect	Primary
Bairati et al.[21]	540	Alpha-tocopherol, beta-carotene	Detrimental effect	Secondary
Khuri et al.[20]	1190	Isotretinoin placebo	No effect	Secondary
Papadimitrakopoulou et al.[26]	50	Celecoxib, placebo	No effect	Primary
Kuriakose et al.[13]	223	Curcumin, placebo	Better response with curcumin (HR: 0.50, 95% CI: 0.27–0.92, $p = 0.02$)	Primary

revealed a statistically significant risk reduction in those taking NSAIDs.[84] The association was dose-dependent and seen most with aspirin and COX-2 inhibitors. Aspirin is a nonselective COX inhibitor resulting in inhibition of prostaglandin synthesis. Aspirin has shown to reduce the risk of death by head and neck cancer by 25%.[85] However, randomized trials studying the effect of topical/systemic COX-2 inhibitors such as celecoxib have not demonstrated any significant benefit. A high dose of COX inhibitor administration is associated with increased cardiovascular risk.[86,87]

iii. *Ligands of peroxisome proliferator-activated receptor gamma (PPAR-γ):* Activation of PPAR-γ results in antiproliferative and proapoptotic action.[88] A retrospective study analysis has shown a significant reduction in the incidence of head and neck cancer in those who took thiazolidinediones (TZDs) than those who did not.[89] TZDs are a commonly prescribed drug to treat diabetes mellitus. A phase III trial evaluating the effects of TZDs in leukoplakia in nondiabetic patients is underway.

3. *Others:*
   i. *Molecular targets:* EGFR is expressed in most of the head and neck cancers, making it a potential target for chemoprevention. The phase III trial—erlotinib prevention of oral cancer trial, compared between erlotinib and placebo in patients with leukoplakia.[90] This is one of the first trials to have cancer-free survival as their endpoint. Even though there was no difference in cancer-free survival, they validated the loss of heterozygosity as a potential marker for tumor progression. A combination of erlotinib and celecoxib has been evaluated in a small number of patients, has shown a response rate of 63% and also down-regulation of EGFR and p-ERK suggesting these markers as surrogate markers for response evaluation in further studies.[91,92]
   ii. *Immune modulation:* The role of HPV and vaccination in the oropharynx is well documented. But the role of HPV vaccine in reducing the risk of HPV-related oral cancer is not established. There is rising evidence of the role of immunotherapy in various cancers. Anti-PD1 treatment is associated with a rise in CD B and FOXP3 cells which are known to secrete antitumoral factors such as IFNg and granzyme.[93] Use of immunotherapy in preventing invasive cancer transformation from OPL seems theoretically valid but further in vitro and in vivo studies are required **(Table 3)**

Conclusion

Chemoprevention is an attractive strategy for reducing the risk of oral cancer. The available literature has shown variable response rates, which are not sustained after cessation of the chemopreventive agent. The lag period for OPL to turn malignant takes several years, while most studies have limited follow-up period ranging from 12 days to 14 months, making interpretation of the data difficult. The response rates are mostly with high doses of the chemopreventive agent, which is associated with high toxicity profile limiting their prolonged use. Hence, use of natural agents such as green tea extract and curcumin in which high doses are well tolerated and hold future promise, but need further validation.

PART D: TOBACCO CESSATION

The effects of tobacco consumption on overall health, cancer-related outcomes are well documented. Tobacco consumption during and after treatment of cancer leads to lower response rate to treatment, higher risk of recurrence and increased risk of second primary. Tobacco cessation plays a vital role in preventing risk of malignancy, at every level from primary to tertiary intervention. A meta-analysis has shown that even after excising a high-grade oral premalignant lesion, the risk of malignancy is reduced but not completely eliminated,[96] with continuation of tobacco consumption in these patients further worsening outcomes **(Flowchart 3)**. A phase II trial showed a reduction in risk of malignant transformation of oral premalignant lesion in both curcumin and placebo arm as, the trial included tobacco cessation strategies in both arms.[74] Tobacco cessation forms the core in management of patients with either premalignant lesion or invasive cancer.

Burden of Tobacco Use

Tobacco is consumed in various forms from cigars, cigarettes, and *beedis* to smokeless forms such as *khaini, gutkha, paan masala, mawa, gul, bajjar, gudakhu,* and snuff. Over 1,100 million smokers exist in the world and carry a tobacco-related mortality rate of 5 million deaths each year that is approximately 1 out 10 deaths among adults globally.[97] India is the third-largest country growing tobacco and second-largest consumer of tobacco, with 700,000 tobacco-related death every year.[98] The oral cancer (related to tobacco) incidence is 10 per 100,000 adult men.[99]

Nicotine Dependence

Addiction to tobacco is exerted by the effect of nicotine, which is a major component of tobacco. Nicotine is absorbed by mucosal surfaces of the oral cavity and respiratory tract. Nicotine binds to prototypic nicotinic acetylcholine receptor (nAChR) agonist that enhances cognition and also releases neurotransmitters such as acetylcholine, glutamate, dopamine, norepinephrine, serotonin and GABA. Acute nicotine consumption leads to enhanced cognition and also mild euphoria, but with chronic use, the neuroadaptations lead to tolerance to these effects. As a result, within hours of nicotine cessation, withdrawal symptoms emerge.[100]

Nicotine withdrawal is characterized by irritability, anger, impatience, difficulty in concentrating and craving. Nicotine/tobacco dependence is defined as a cluster of behavioral, cognitive and physiological phenomena that develop after repeated tobacco use and that typically include a strong desire to use tobacco, difficulties in controlling its use, persistence in tobacco use despite harmful consequences, a higher priority given to tobacco use than other activities and obligations, increased tolerance and sometimes a physical withdrawal state.[101]

Various questionnaires are used to quantify nicotine dependence, but one of the commonly used is the Fagerström Test for Nicotine Dependence (Refer Section 1 Chapter 4).[102] It is important to assess the level of nicotine dependency as among smokers, 70% want to quit, while only 4–7% quit successfully.[103]

Flowchart 3: Tobacco-induced carcinogenesis.

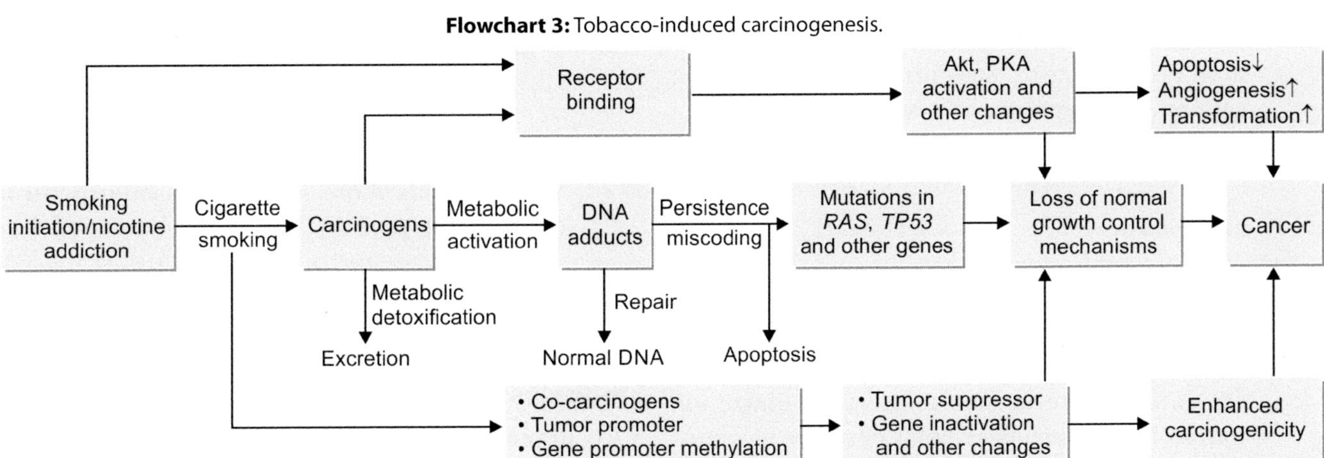

Management Strategy

1. *Psychosocial intervention*: Counseling and motivating the patient to continue cessation of smoking is essential in maintaining long-term success. The counseling intervention may be different for every person with time per session, number of sessions, and mode of counseling being different for every case.
   a. *Brief interventions in primary clinical setting:* The patient comes in contact with primary health physician at first, who plays an important role in identifying the patient, in counseling and triaging the patient who needs further psychosocial support and/or pharmaceutical support to maintain nicotine abstinence. The strategy for tobacco cessation counseling consists of 5A's: ask, advise, assess, assist and arrange,[104] which must be included in every session with a primary care health provider or counseling sessions at specialty tobacco clinics. This approach is restricted by the time that can be given by the primary physician to each patient but has shown success as identification, and further referral is based on the first physician-patient consults. The primary physician refers to the point of first contact, and may be the dentist who first encounters any oral pathology. If required the patient can be then referred to a specialty clinic.
   b. *Specialty tobacco clinic intervention:* Counseling by a psychiatrist/psychologist who is trained specifically in tobacco cessation counseling techniques must be involved in patients likely to relapse. The intensity and frequency of counseling is more in these patients and is most often combined with pharmacotherapy to sustain tobacco abstinence.
   c. *Quit lines:* Telephone-based helplines for a patient willing to quit are helpful as the potential outreach is immense. Due to anonymity of the subject maintained, more patients may utilize this service. But telephonic counseling is challenging, pharmacotherapy cannot be administered and counselor–patient bond is weaker in this service.

2. *Pharmacotherapy:*
   a. *Nicotine replacement therapy (NRT):* NRT is aimed at reducing the withdrawal symptoms and eliminating the craving for tobacco during the abstinent period. Various forms of nicotine replacement are available. On an average, all forms of NRT reach peak levels of serum nicotine, 20 minutes after consumption.[105]
      A. *Nicotine oral absorption*
      Gum: available in 2 or 4 mg, in ion resin base buffered in alkaline pH to increase absorption via buccal mucosa.[106] Instructions during their usage are to "chew and park"' and to not consume foods that alter oral pH. 25% of released nicotine gets ingested. Cessation maintenance rate with oral gum is 50–70%.[107]
      Lozenges: Deliver 25% more dose than gum and lesser frequency of usage (7–8 per day) is enough to gain benefit.[108]
      Sublingual tablets: They release less nicotine than gum and needs to be taken more frequently.
      B. *Nicotine patch:* Nicotine transdermal patches maintain a steady and constant blood nicotine level. Increases chance of abstinence by 1.5–2 fold than placebo.[108]
      C. *Nasal sprays:* These have the fastest and highest level of serum nicotine attained. These help in better titration of dosing for effective control. Each spray consists of 0.5 mg. A single dose of nicotine spray is one spray in each nostril, so that a total of 1 mg is delivered. Spray is given every hour. A maximum of 40 mg/day can be administered.[108]
   b. *Bupropion:* Craving associated with nicotine is primarily attributed to dopamine release by the nicotine. Bupropion is an antidepressant with dopaminergic and noradrenergic properties. Due to dopaminergic action, craving for nicotine is lost.[102] Bupropion is started as a 150 mg daily dose for first 3–7 days then gradually increased to 300 mg per day (as tolerated). The treatment is continued for 12 weeks and started 1–2 weeks before decision to quit tobacco is made. A side effect is the risk of having a seizure (0.1%).
   c. *Varenicline:* Administration of varenicline is also to eliminate craving. They act by strongly binding to $\alpha4\beta2$ and $\alpha7$ nicotinic cholinergic receptors and release dopamine mimicking the action of nicotine. The dose ranges from 0.5 to 2 mg per day and continued use up to 3–6 months is recommended. Varenicline is more potent than bupropion in controlling nicotine craving.[102] Second-line drugs such as nortriptyline (0.15–0.75 mg/day for 3–10 weeks) or clonidine (75–100 mg per day for 12 weeks) can be prescribed.

Smokeless Tobacco

A Cochrane systematic review includes 34 randomized trials that have studied the efficacy of tobacco cessation strategies in a total of 16,000 smokeless tobacco users.[109] The review concluded that varenicline is a more potent drug to maintain smokeless tobacco abstinence (risk reduction 2.31) and abstinence rate sustained at 6 months was higher with smokeless tobacco than smokers. Among nicotine replacement therapy, oral lozenges were more effective than other preparation among smokeless tobacco users. Behavioral changes by counseling can increase tobacco cessation rates in smokeless tobacco, which was not evident in the review due to the heterogeneity of the trials.

Precision Medicine

Patients with high nicotine metabolism rate have a higher rate of success with tobacco cessation. *CYP2A6* gene encodes for cytochrome P450 that converts nicotine to cotinine in liver and is further metabolized to 3-hydroxycotinine also mediated by *CYP2A6*. The hydroxycotinine/cotinine ratio, is known as the nicotine metabolite ratio (NMR), is a validated marker for nicotine metabolism.[110] Patients with high NMR benefit with varenicline than nicotine replacement therapy and patients with low NMR show equal efficacy with varenicline and nicotine replacement therapy.[102] Routine genetic testing is not recommended in the management of nicotine dependence. The nicotinic receptor subunit *CHRNA5/A3/B4* gene (variant rs1051730) has been associated with increased risk of nicotine dependence, but their implication in management strategy for nicotine dependence is unknown.

Conclusion

Tobacco is one of the leading causes of preventable death. Tobacco cessation plays an important role in the management strategy of oral premalignant lesions and also in head and neck cancer. Triaging patients based on the extent of nicotine dependence and form of tobacco consumption helps in planning a successful tobacco cessation program. Sustained abstinence rates are very low if not accompanied by counseling and pharmacotherapy.

REFERENCES

1. Pulte D, Brenner H. Changes in survival in head and neck cancers in the late 20th and early 21st century: a period analysis. Oncologist. 2010;15:994-1001.
2. Ernest and Young Report. Call for Action: Expanding Cancer Care in India. Ernest and Young Report; 2015. [online] Available from: https://www.ey.com/call-for-action-expanding-cancer-care-in-india-earnest-and-young-report. [Last accessed July, 2020].
3. Warnakulasuriya S. Global epidemiology of oral and oropharyngeal cancer. Oral Oncol. 2009;45:309-16.
4. Pandey AK, Singh RJ, Lal P, Gopalan B, Tripathi GK, Sharma R. Ten years of India's National Tobacco Control Programme: achievements, challenges and the way forward. Tobacco Ind Dis. 2018;16(1):439.
5. Foy JP, Bertolus C, William Jr WN, Saintigny P. Oral premalignancy: the roles of early detection and chemo-prevention. Otolaryngol Clin N Am. 2013;46:579-97.
6. Warnakulasuriya S. Living with oral cancer: epidemiology with particular reference to prevalence and life-style changes that influence survival. Oral Oncol. 2010;46:407-10.
7. Mangalath U, Aslam SA, Khadar AH, Francis PG, Mikacha MSK, Kalathingal JH. Recent trends in prevention of oral cancer. J Int Soc Prev Community Dent. 2014;4(3):131-8.
8. Sankaranarayanan R, Swaminathan R, Brenner H, et al. Cancer survival in Africa, Asia, and Central America: a population-based study. Lancet Oncol. 2010;11:165-73.
9. Pearce A, Sharp L, Hanly P, Barchuk A, Bray F, de Camargo Cancela M, et al. Productivity losses due to premature mortality from cancer in Brazil, Russia, India, China, and South Africa (BRICS): A population-based comparison. Cancer Epidemiol. 2018;53:27-34.
10. Speight PM, Epstein J, Kujan O, Lingen MW, Nagao T, Ranganathan K, et al. Screening for oral cancer-a perspective from the Global Oral Cancer Forum. Oral Surg Oral Med Oral Pathol Oral Radiol. 2017;123(6):680-7.
11. Fuller C, Camilon R, Nguyen S, Jennings J, Day T, Gillespie MB. Adjunctive diagnostic techniques for oral lesions of unknown malignant potential: systematic review with meta-analysis. Head Neck. 2015;37(5):755-62.
12. Elango KJ, Anandkrishnan N, Suresh A, Iyer SK, Ramaiyer SK, Kuriakose MA. Mouth self-examination to improve oral cancer awareness and early detection in a high-risk population. Oral Oncol. 2011;47(7):620-4.
13. Allegra E, Lombardo N, Puzzo L, Garozzo A. The usefulness of toluidine staining as a diagnostic tool for precancerous and cancerous oropharyngeal and oral cavity lesions. Acta Otorhinolaryngo. 2009;29(4):187-90.
14. Fedele S. Diagnostic aids in the screening of oral cancer. Head Neck Oncol. 2009;1:5.
15. Epstein JB, Silverman S Jr, Epstein JD, Lonky SA, Bride MA. Analysis of oral lesion biopsies identified and evaluated by visual examination, chemiluminescence and toluidine blue. Oral Oncol. 2008;44(6):538-44.
16. De Veld DC, Witjes MJ, Sterenborg HJ, Roodenburg JL. The status of in vivo autofluorescence spectroscopy and imaging for oral oncology. Oral Oncol. 2005;41(2):117-31.
17. Lane PM, Gilhuly T, Whitehead P, Zeng H, Poh CF, Ng S, et al. Simple device for the direct visualisation of oral-cavity tissue fluorescence. J Biomed Opt. 2006;11(2):024006.
18. Awan KH, Morgan PR, Warnakulasuriya S. Evaluation of an autofluorescence based imaging system (VELscope) in the detection of oral potentially malignant disorders and benign keratoses. Oral Oncol. 2011;47(4):274-7.
19. Farah CS, McIntosh L, Georgiou A, McCullough MJ. Efficacy of tissue autofluorescence imaging (VELScope) in the visualisation of oral mucosal lesions. Head Neck. 2012;34(6):856-62.
20. Amirchaghmaghi M, Mohtasham N, Delavarian Z, Shakeri MT, Hatami M, Mozafari PM. The diagnostic value of the native fluorescence visualisation device for early detection of premalignant/malignant lesions of the oral cavity. Photodiagnosis Photodyn Ther. 2017;21:19-27.

21. Rajadhyaksha M, Anderson RR, Webb RH. Video-rate confocal scanning laser microscope for imaging human tissues in vivo. Appl Opt. 1999;38(10):2105-15.
22. Maitland KC, Gillenwater AM, Williams MD, El-Naggar AK, Descour MR, Richards-Kortume RR. In vivo imaging of oral neoplasia using a miniaturised fiber optic confocal reflectance microscope. Oral Oncol. 2008;44(11):1059-66.
23. Mody R, Antaram Joshi SH, Chaney W. Use of lectins as diagnostic and therapeutic tools for cancer. Journal of pharmacological and toxicological methods. 1995;33(1):1-10.
24. Baeten J, Johnson A, Sunny S, Suresh A, Birur P, Uma K, et al. Chairside molecular imaging of aberrant glycosylation in subjects with suspicious oral lesions using fluorescently labeled wheat germ agglutinin. Head Neck. 2018;40(2): 292-301.
25. Nitin N, Carlson AL, Muldoon T, El-Naggar AK, Gillenwater A, Richards-Kortum R. Molecular imaging of glucose uptake in oral neoplasia following topical application of fluorescently labeled deoxyglucose. Int J Cancer. 2009;124(11):2634-42.
26. Yang X, Palasuberniam P, Kraus D, Chen B. Aminolevulinic acid based tumor detection and therapy: molecular mechanisms and strategies for enhancement. Int J Mol Sci. 2015;16(10):25865-80.
27. Leunig A, Betz CS, Mehlmann M, et al. Detection of squamous cell carcinoma of the oral cavity by imaging 5-aminolevulinic acid-induced protoporphyrin IX fluorescence. Laryngoscope. 2000;110(1):78-83.
28. Staibano S, Pepe S, Lo Muzio L, Somma P, Mascolo M, Argenziano G, et al. Poly(adenosine diphosphate-ribose) polymerase 1 expression in malignant melanomas from photo exposed areas of the head and neck region. Human Pathol. 2005;36(7):724-31.
29. Mascolo M, Ilardi G, Romano MF, Celetti A, Siano M, Romano S, et al. Overexpression of chromatin assembly factor-1 p60, poly(ADP-ribose) polymerase 1 and nestin predicts metastasising behaviour of oral cancer. Histopathology. 2012;61(6):1089-105.
30. Kaur J, Jacobs R, Huang Y, Salvo N, Politis C. Salivary biomarkers for oral cancer and pre-cancer screening: a review. Clin Oral Investig. 2018;22(2):633-40.
31. Singh SP, Ibrahim O, Byrne HJ, Mikkonen JW, Koistinen AP, Kullaa AM, et al. Recent advances in optical diagnosis of oral cancers: Review and future perspectives. Head Neck. 2016;38(S1):E2403-11.
32. Sankaranarayanan R, Ramadas K, Thomas G, Muwonge R, Thara S, Mathew B, et al. Effect of screening on oral cancer mortality in Kerala, India: a cluster-randomised controlled trial. Lancet. 2005;365:1927-33.
33. Sankaranarayanan R, Ramadas K, Thara S, Muwonge R, Thomas G, Anju G, t al. Long term effect of visual screening on oral cancer incidence and mortality in a randomised trial in Kerala, India. Oral Oncol. 2013;49(4):314-21.
34. Subramanian S, Sankaranarayanan R, Bapat B, Somanathan T, Thomas G, Mathew B, et al. Cost-effectiveness of oral cancer screening: results from a cluster randomised controlled trial in India. Bull World Health Organ. 2009;87:200-6
35. Chuang SL, Su WW, Chen SL, Yen AM, Wang CP, Fann JC, et al. Population-based screening program for reducing oral cancer mortality in 2,334,299 Taiwanese cigarette smokers and/or betel quid chewers. Cancer. 2017;123(9):1597-609.
36. World Health Organization. (2011). Mortality database. [online] Available from: http://www-dep.iarc.fr/WHOdb/WHOdb.htm. [Last accessed July, 2020].
37. Jaiswal G, Jaiswal S, Kumar R, Sharma A. Field cancerization: concept and clinical implications in head and neck squamous cell carcinoma. J Exp Ther Oncol. 2013;10:209-14.
38. Sarode SC, Sarode GS, Karmarkar S, Tupkari JV. Oral (mucosal) potentially malignant disorders. Oral Oncol. 2012;48:e35-6.
39. Warnakulasuriya S, Johnson NW, van der Waal I. Nomenclature and classification of potentially malignant disorders of the oral mucosa. J Oral Pathol Med. 2007;36:575-80.
40. Brouns ER, Baart JA, Bloemena E, Karagozoglu H, van der Waal I. The relevance of uniform reporting in oral leukoplakia: definition, certainty factor and staging based on experience with 275 patients. Med Oral Patol Oral Cir Bucal. 2013;18(1):e19-26.
41. Panwar A, Lindau R, Wieland A. Management for premalignant lesions of the oral cavity. Expert Rev Antican Ther. 2014;14(3):349-57.
42. Amagasa T, Yamashiro M, Uzawa N. Oral premalignant lesions: from a clinical perspective. Int J Clin Oncol. 2011;16(1):5-14.
43. Watabe Y, Nomura T, Onda T, Yakushiji T, Yamamoto N, Ohata H, et al. Malignant transformation of oral leukoplakia with a focus on low-grade dysplasia. J Oral Maxillofac Surg Med Pathol. 2016;28(1):26-9.
44. Reddi SP, Shafer AT. Oral premalignant lesions: management considerations. Oral Maxillofac Surg Clin North Am. 2006;18:425-33.
45. International Agency on Research for Cancer. IARC monographs on the evaluation of the carcinogenic risk of chemicals to humans (Vol. 37). Tobacco habits other than smoking: betel quid and areca nut chewing; and some related nitrosamines. Lyon: IARC; 1985.
46. International Agency on Research for Cancer. IARC monographs on the evaluation of carcinogenic risks to humans, (Vol. 85). Tobacco habits other than smoking: betel quid and areca-nut chewing. Lyon: IARC; 2004.
47. International Agency on Research for Cancer. IARC monographs on the evaluation of carcinogenic risks to humans (Vol. 100E), personal habits and indoor combustion. Lyon: IARC; 2012.
48. Tilakaratne WM, Klinikowski MF, Saku T, Peters TJ, Warnakulasuriya S. Oral submucous fibrosis: review on aetiology and pathogenesis. Oral Oncol. 2006;42(6):561-8.
49. Warnakulasuriya S. Semiquantitative clinical description of oral submucous fibrosis. Ann Dent. 1987;46:18-21.
50. Jaber MA, Porter SR, Speight PM, Eveson JW, Scully C. Oral epithelial dysplasia: clinical characteristics of western European residents. Oral Oncol. 2003;39:589-96.
51. World Health Organization Collaborating Centre for Oral Precancerous lesions. Definition of leukoplakia and related lesions: an aid to studies on oral precancer. Oral Surg Oral Med Oral Pathol. 1978;46:518-39.
52. Holmstrup PP, Vedtofte PP, Reibel J, Stoltze K. Long-term treatment outcome of oral premalignant lesions. Oral Oncol. 2006;42:461-74.
53. Napier SS, Cowan CG, Gregg TA, Stevenson M, Lamey PP, Toner PG. Potentially malignant lesions in Northern Ireland: size (extent) matters. Oral Dis. 2003;9:129-37.
54. Schepman KP, van der Meij EH, Smeele LE, van der Waal I. Malignant transformation of oral leukoplakia: a follow-up study of a hospital-based population of 166 patients with oral leukoplakia in The Netherlands. Oral Oncol. 1998;34: 270-5.
55. Mehta FS, Shroff BC, Gupta PC, Daftary DK. Oral leukoplakia in relation to tobacco habits: a ten-year follow-up study of

Bombay policemen. Oral Surg Oral Med Oral Pathol. 1972; 34(3):426-33.
56. Reibel J. Prognosis of oral pre-malignant lesions: significance of clinical, histopathological, and molecular biological characteristics. Crit Rev Oral Biol Med. 2003;14:47-62.
57. Warnakulasuriya S, Reibel J, Bouquot J, Dabelsteen E. Oral epithelial dysplasia classification systems: predictive value, utility, weaknesses and scope for improvement. J Oral Pathol Med. 2008;3:127-33.
58. Reibel J, Gale N, Hille J. Oral potentially malignant disorders and oral epithelial dysplasia. In: El-Naggar AK, Chan JKC, Grandis JR, Takata T, Slootweg PPJ (Eds). WHO Classification of Head and Neck Tumours, 4th edition. Lyon, France: IARC; 2017. pp. 112-5.
59. Warnakulasuriya S. Lack of molecular markers to predict malignant potential of oral precancer. J Pathol. 2000;190(4):407-9.
60. Alaizari NA, Sperandio M, Odell EW, Peruzzo D, Al-Maweri SA. Meta-analysis of the predictive value of DNA aneuploidy in malignant transformation of oral potentially malignant disorders. J Oral Pathol Med. 2018;47(2):97-103.
61. Miller CS, Johnstone BM. Human papillomavirus as a risk factor for oral squamous cell carcinoma: a meta-analysis, 1982-1997. Oral Surg Oral Med Oral Pathol Oral Radiol Endodontol. 2001;91(6):622-35.
62. Fotedar V, Fotedar S, Seam RK, Gupta MK. Oral cancer and chemoprevention. Int J Pharm Sci Invent. 2013;2(2):16-20.
63. Bauman JE, Grandis J. Oral cancer chemoprevention—the end of EPOC, the beginning of an epoch of molecular selection. JAMA Oncol. 2016;2(2):178-9.
64. Bhattacharya S. Natural antimutagens: a review. Res J Med Plant. 2011;5(2):116-26.
65. Tsai JY, Dillon JK. Chemoprevention in Oral Cancer. In: Improving Outcomes in Oral Cance. Cham: Springer; 2020. pp. 13-22.
66. van Zandwijk N, Dalesio O, Pastorino U, de Vries N, van Tinteren H. EUROSCAN, a randomized trial of vitamin A and N-acetylcysteine in patients with head and neck cancer or lung cancer. J Natl Cancer Inst. 2000;92(12):977-86.
67. Chau L, Jabra JT, Lai W, Svider PF, Warner BM, Lin HS, et al. Topical agents for oral cancer chemoprevention: a systematic review of the literature. Oral Oncol. 2017;67:153-9.
68. Ding Y, Yao H, Yao Y, Fai LY, Zhang Z. Protection of dietary polyphenols against oral cancer. Nutrients. 2013;5:2173-91.
69. Gomes de Moura CF, Noguti J, Pacheco de Jesus GP, Ribeiro FA, Garcia FA, Gollucke AP, et al. Polyphenols as chemopreventive agent in oral carcinogenesis: putative mechanisms of action using in-vitro and in-vivo test systems. Eur J Cancer Prev. 2013;22:467-72.
70. Tsao AS, Liu D, Martin J, Tang XM, Lee JJ, El-Naggar AK, et al. Phase II randomized, placebo-controlled trial of green tea extract in patients with high-risk oral premalignant lesions. Cancer Prev Res. 2009;2(11):931-41.
71. Rai B, Kaur J, Jacobs R, Singh J. Possible action mechanism for curcumin in pre-cancerous lesions based on serum and salivary markers of oxidative stress. J Oral Sci. 2010;52(2): 251-6.
72. Patel JB, Shah FD, Joshi GM, Patel PS. Clinical significance of inflammatory mediators in the pathogenesis of oral cancer. J Can Res Ther. 2016;12:447-57.
73. Cheng AL, Hsu CH, Lin JK, Hsu MM, Ho YF, Shen TS, et al. Phase I clinical trial of curcumin, a chemopreventive agent, in patients with high-risk or pre-malignant lesions. Anticancer Res. 2001;21:2895-900.
74. Kuriakose MA, Ramdas K, Dey B, Iyer S, Rajan G, Elango KK, et al. A Randomized Double-Blind Placebo-Controlled Phase IIB Trial of Curcumin in Oral Leukoplakia. Cancer Prev Res. 2016;9(8):683-91.
75. Wulf K. Zur Vitamin A-Behandlung der Leukoplakien. Archiv für klinische und experimentelle Dermatologie. 1957;206(1):495-8.
76. Sankaranarayanan R, Mathew B, Varghese C, Sudhakaran PR, Menon V, Jayadeep A, et al. Chemoprevention of oral leukoplakia with vitamin A and beta carotene: an assessment. Oral Oncol. 1997;33:231-6.
77. Liede K, Hietanen J, Saxen L, Haukka J, Timonen T, Hayrinen-Immonen R, et al. Long-term supplementation with alpha-tocopherol and beta-carotene and prevalence of oral mucosal lesions in smokers. Oral Diseases. 1998;4(2):78-83.
78. Wright ME, Virtamo J, Hartman AM, Pietinen P, Edwards BK, Taylor PR, et al. Effects of α-tocopherol and β-carotene supplementation on upper aerodigestive tract cancers in a large, randomized controlled trial. Cancer. 2007;109(5): 891-8.
79. Hong WK, Endicott J, Itri LM, Doos W, Batsakis JG, Bell R, et al. 13-cis-retinoic acid in the treatment of oral leukoplakia. New Engl J Med. 1986;315(24):1501-5.
80. Lippman SM, Batsakis JG, Toth BB, Weber RS, Lee JJ, Martin JW, et al. Comparison of low-dose isotretinoin with beta carotene to prevent oral carcinogenesis. N Engl J Med. 1993;328(1):15-20.
81. Khuri FR, Lee JJ, Lippman SM, Kim ES, Cooper JS, Benner SE, et al. Randomized phase III trial of low-dose isotretinoin for prevention of second primary tumors in stage I and II head and neck cancer patients. J Natl Cancer Inst. 2006;98(7): 441-50.
82. Bairati I, Meyer F, Gélinas M, Fortin A, Nabid A, Brochet F, et al. A randomized trial of antioxidant vitamins to prevent second primary cancers in head and neck cancer patients. J Natl Cancer Inst. 2005;97(7):481-8.
83. Lin DT, Subbaramaiah K, Shah JP, Dannenberg AJ, Boyle JO. Cyclooxygenase-2: a novel molecular target for the prevention and treatment of head and neck cancer. Head Neck. 2002;24:792-9.
84. Shi J, Leng W, Zhao L, Xu C, Wang J, Chen X, et al. Nonsteroidal anti-inflammatory drugs using and risk of head and neck cancer: a dose-response meta-analysis of prospective cohort studies. Oncotarget. 2017;8(58):99066-74.
85. Jayaprakash V, Rigual NR, Moysich KB, Loree TR, Nasca MA, Menezes RJ, et al. Chemoprevention of head and neck cancer with aspirin: a case-control study. Arch Otolaryngol Head Neck Surg. 2006;132(11):1231-6.
86. Mushine JL, Atkinson JC, Greer RO, Papadimitrakopoulou VA, Van Waes C, Rudy S, et al. Randomized, double-blind, placebo-controlled phase IIB trial of the cyclooxygenase inhibitor ketorolac as an oral rinse in oropharyngeal leukoplakia. Clin Cancer Res. 2004;10:1565-73.
87. Papadimitrakopoulou VA, William W, Dannenberg AJ, Lippman SM, Lee JJ, Ondrey FG, et al. Pilot randomized phase II study of celecoxib n oral premalignant lesions. Clin Cancer Res. 2008;14(7):2095-101.
88. Burotto M, Szabo E. PPARγ in head and neck cancer prevention. Oral Oncol. 2014;50(10):924-9.
89. Govindarajan R, Siegel ER. The effect of exposure to thiazolidinediones on the development of head-and-neck cancer in patients with diabetes mellitus. Transl Res Oral Oncol. 2017;2:1-5.

90. William WN, Papadimitrakopoulou V, Lee JJ, Mao L, Lin H, Martin AM, et al. Randomized placebo-controlled trial (RCT) of erlotinib for prevention of oral cancer (EPOC) (abstract 6007) [2014 American Society of Clinical Oncology (ASCO) meeting]. J Clin Oncol. 2014;32(15 Suppl):1-9.
91. Kreimer AR, Chaturvedi AK. HPV-associated oropharyngeal cancers—are they preventable? Cancer Prev Res. 2011; 4(9):1346-9.
92. Saba NF, Hurwitz SJ, Kono SA, Yang CS, Zhao Y, Chen Z, et al. Chemoprevention of head and neck cancer with celecoxib and erlotinib: results of a phase Ib and pharmacokinetic study. Cancer Prev Res. 2014;7(3):283-91.
93. Gutkind JS, Bui JD. The Next Frontier: Head and Neck Cancer Immunoprevention. Cancer Prev Res. 2017;10: 681-3.
94. Hong WK, Lippman SM, Itri LM, Karp DD, Lee JS, Byers RM, et al. Prevention of second primary tumors with isotretinoin in squamous-cell carcinoma of the head and neck. N Engl J Med. 1990;323:795-801.
95. Mayne ST, Walter M, Cartmel B, Goodwin WJ Jr, Blumberg J. Supplemental betacarotene, smoking, and urinary F2-isoprostane excretion in patients with prior early stage head and neck cancer. Nutr Cancer. 2004;49:1-6.
96. Mehanna HM, Rattay T, Smith J, McConkey CC. Treatment and follow-up of oral dysplasia—a systematic review and meta-analysis. Head Neck. 2009;31(12):1600-9.
97. Rao V, Chaturvedi P. Tobacco and health in India. Ind J Cancer. 2010;47(5):3.
98. Chaly PE. Tobacco control in India. Ind J Dent Res. 2007; 18(1):2.
99. Gajalakshmi V, Peto R, Kanaka TS, Jha P. Smoking and mortality from tuberculosis and other diseases in India: retrospective study of 43,000 adult male deaths and 35,000 controls. Lancet. 2003;362(9383):507-15.
100. Shiffman S, West RJ, Gilbert DG. Recommendation for the assessment of tobacco craving and withdrawal in smoking cessation trials. Nicotine Tob Res. 2004;6(4):599-614.
101. Bhatnagar D, Jain DC. Tobacco dependence treatment Guidelines. National Tobacco Control Programme, India; 2011.
102. Heatherton TF, Kozlowski LT, Frecker RC, Fagerstrom KO. The Fagerstrom test for nicotine dependence: a revision of the Fagerstrom Tolerance Questionnaire. Br J Addict. 1991;86:1119-27.
103. Li MD. Management, Pharmacotherapies, and Precision Medicine for Smoking Cessation. In: Tobacco Smoking Addiction: Epidemiology, Genetics, Mechanisms, and Treatment. Singapore: Springer; 2018. pp. 339-49.
104. Use T. Dependence Clinical Practice Guideline Panel, Staff and Consortium Representatives. A clinical practice guideline for treating tobacco use and dependence: a US Public Health Service report. JAMA. 2000;283(24):3244-54.
105. Silagy C. Nicotine replacement therapy for smoking cessation (Cochrane Review). The Cochrane Library. 2003;3.
106. Fernö O, Lichtneckert SJ, Lundgren CE. A substitute for tobacco smoking. Psychopharmacologia. 1973;31(3):201-4.
107. Benowitz NL, Jacob III P, Savanapridi C. Determinants of nicotine intake while chewing nicotine polacrilex gum. Clin Pharmacol Therap. 1987;41(4):467-73.
108. Shaik SS, Doshi D, Bandari SR, Madupu PR, Kulkarni S. Tobacco use cessation and prevention-a review. J Clin Diagn Res. 2016;10(5):ZE13.
109. Ebbert JO, Elrashidi MY, Stead LF. Interventions for smokeless tobacco use cessation. Cochrane Database Syst Rev. 2015(10):CD004306.
110. Allenby CE, Boylan KA, Lerman C, Falcone M. Precision medicine for tobacco dependence: development and validation of the nicotine metabolite ratio. J Neuroimm Pharmacol. 2016;11(3):471-83.

CHAPTER 8

Premalignant Lesions of the Larynx

Shashikant Limbachiya, Samskruthi P Murthy, Narayana Subramaniam, Sivakumar Vidhyadharan

INTRODUCTION

Laryngeal cancer comprises of 2.4% of all cancers worldwide, with glottis being the most common site involved.[1] Premalignant lesions of the larynx also more commonly affect the glottis than other subsites. The mucosal changes resulting from the change causes early voice change, and hence most patients present early. The lag period between occurrence of premalignant disease and invasive cancer is several years, which affords enough time to diagnose and treat premalignant disease, and to prevent recurrence.[2,3] Alteration of the mucosal surface is variable, and a histological diagnosis is almost always required to assess the malignant potential of the laryngeal lesions.[4] The contemporary management of early laryngeal premalignant and malignant lesions must establish equipoise between oncologic success and minimal treatment morbidity. Changes in voice or other symptoms such as dysphagia or referred otalgia often direct the initial evaluation of the larynx.

CLASSIFICATION

The terminologies to describe premalignant lesions of the larynx have been varied. Various terms and classifications are proposed which are subject to interobserver variability and make comparison between studies difficult. The terms squamous metaplasia, parakeratosis, and keratosis do not imply premalignant potential, while terms such as dysplasia, atypia, and carcinoma in situ demonstrate premalignant potential.[5]

Leukoplakia is described as a white patch or plaque that cannot be characterized clinically or pathologically as any other disease.[6] The term leukoplakia, like in the oral cavity, is a clinical term. The histology of the leukoplakia patch may be variable and hence the potential to turn malignant varies. The diagnosis of leukoplakia is always by exclusion.[7] Dysplasia is defined as altered epithelium with increased likelihood for progression to squamous cell carcinoma (SCC).[6] They are most prevalent epithelial precursor lesions.[8,9]

The various classification systems lack consensus, while most studies follow one of the following classification systems **(Table 1)**.

Table 1: Classification systems for premalignant lesions of the larynx.

World Health Organization (WHO) classification[10]	*Squamous intra-epithelial neoplasm (SIN)*[9]	*Ljubljana classification squamous intra-epithelial lesions (SIL)*[8]
Mild dysplasia	SIN-1	Basal/parabolas cell hyperplasia
Moderate dysplasia	SIN-2	Atypical hyperplasia
Severe dysplasia	SIN-3	Atypical hyperplasia
Carcinoma in situ	SIN-3*	Carcinoma in situ

*Combined severe dysplasia and carcinoma in situ.

NATURAL HISTORY

The rate of malignant transformation for mild dysplasia and moderate dysplasia were 0–11.5% and 0–45%, respectively. This risk is significantly higher for severe dysplasia, with values ranging from 46.5 to 63%.[11]

DIAGNOSIS

Premalignant lesions of larynx hinge on a high degree of suspicion in at-risk patient. This includes patients with a known history of exposure to carcinogens and change in voice for >3 weeks. Visualization of mucosal abnormalities and visually directed biopsies and histological correlation is necessary before confirming the diagnosis. These modalities may prove to be useful in diagnosis and surveillance of patients with premalignant lesions:

- *Autofluorescence endoscopy (AFE):* AFE has a specificity, sensitivity, and accuracy of 84%, 91%, and 88%, respectively.[12] It is based on the variability of emission of white light by biological structures such as mitochondria and lysosomes following absorption of light. Systemic or local fluorescent marker called fluorophore is used. Induced fluorescence endoscopy (IFE) has a sensitivity, specificity, and accuracy of 95%, 62%, and 76%, respectively. White light endoscopy (WLE) has sensitivity, specificity, and accuracy of 72%, 79%, and 77%, respectively.

- *Narrow band imaging (NBI):* NBI has promising application in investigations aimed at the identification of suspicious mucosal lesions. The technique relies on the use of blue and green light with wavelengths corresponding to 415 and 540 nanometer, respectively, which are preferentially absorbed by hemoglobin. The light penetrates through the thin mucosal lining and highlights the submucosal microvascular pattern. Alterations in these patterns due to neoangiogenesis may help identify premalignant and malignant lesions.[13] Ni et al.[14] proposed classification system based on microvascular characteristics and intraepithelial papillary capillary loops (IPCLs), which is represented in the **Table 2**. They described that type I–III was associated with benign, type IV–V with premalignant lesion, and malignant lesion always expressed pattern type combining NBI with WLE increased the diagnostic sensitivity to 100% for identification of malignant lesions. The calculated sensitivity, specificity, and positive predictive value and negative predictive values were 100%, 71.43%, 92%, and 100%, respectively with NBI. The technique is easy, fast, and obviates the need for additional staining. It provides a two-dimensional (2D) assessment of lesions with abnormal submucosal vascular patterns, but cannot provide an assessment of depth of abnormal tissue. The overall diagnostic gain attained concerning margins and suspicious of malignancy with NBI ranges between 18 and 27%.[15,16] Overall, current recommendations for diagnosis and routine surveillance should include the use of direct laryngoscopy with mapping biopsies as standard practice.

Table 2: Ni's classification of premalignant lesions of the larynx based on narrow band imaging.

Type of lesion	*Submucosal vascular patterns [intraepithelial papillary capillary loop (IPCL)]*
Type I lesions	To thin, oblique, and arborescent vessels without any IPCL
Type II lesions	Enlarged, oblique, and arborescent vessels without any IPCL
Type III lesions	Vessels are obscured or seen indistinctly by white mucosa
Type IV lesions	IPCL can be recognized as regular, small, and dark brown spots
Type V lesions	
Type Va lesions	IPCL appears solid or hollow, with a brownish, speckled pattern, and of various shapes
Type Vb lesions	Irregular, tortuous, and line-like shapes
Type Vc lesions	Brownish speckles or tortuous, line-like shapes with irregular distribution, and scattered on tumor surface

TREATMENT

The principles of management of premalignant epithelial lesions of the larynx are based on maintaining a high index of suspicion in the predisposed patient population. The overall appearance of the lesion is considered to be the most essential factor in determining further management. The management decision must be based on various factors:[17]

- *Patient factors:* The lifestyle of the patient concerning smoking and alcohol consumption must be taken into consideration. Treating a patient who refuses to quit smoking is challenging, as they are more prone to recurrence and progression to invasive carcinoma. The patient's general condition, fitness for surgery, physiological age, and comorbidity must also be considered before managing a treatment decision.
- *Tumor factors:* The extent and focality of the lesion is important. Extensive lesion may be difficult to excise with negative margins. Histopathological mapping of the lesion with multiple biopsies should be performed, followed by staged resection, if feasible.

Surgical excision of the lesion by microlaryngeal surgery with carbon dioxide (CO_2) laser or cold steel instruments is the current standard of treatment in premalignant lesions of the larynx. It may be challenging to assess which lesions need active intervention and which are those for active surveillance. The various factors mentioned above must be factored in before decision making.[17]

Using frozen section to differentiate between benign and malignant lesions is not recommended as the correlation between frozen section and histopathology was only 63%.[18] Hence a preoperative biopsy is mandatory in cases with multiple lesions, extensive superficial lesions, and when extensive surgical excision is planned.

The extent of surgery is vital in achieving good control rates. The cordectomy classification of European Laryngological Society is used to describe the extent

Table 3: Outcomes after excision of premalignant lesions of the larynx.

Study	*Outcome*	*Type of surgery*	*Remarks*
Mild to moderate dysplasia			
Dispenza et al.[20]	Recurrence rate of 13% low-grade dysplasia 29% for moderate dysplasia	Type I cordectomy for low-grade dysplasia type II for moderate dysplasia	
Minni et al.[21]	Recurrence rate of 12% low-grade dysplasia 8% for moderate dysplasia	Type I cordectomy for low-grade dysplasia type II for moderate dysplasia	
Severe dysplasia			
Damm et al.[23]	83% local control rate	Superficial and subligamental cordectomy	
Le et al.[24]	80% local control rate at 10 years follow-up	Vocal cord stripping and extensive excision (not defined)	This study includes hemilaryngectomy and radiotherapy as salvage in recurrent cases; hence the control rate does not present only microlaryngeal surgery outcomes
Gallo et al.[25]	Recurrence rate of 18.7% in LIN-3 Progression to malignancy 9.7% in LIN-3	Vocal cord stripping	One of the studies largest numbers, but the rate of recurrence is higher probably because only vocal cord stripping was the treatment modality

of resection.[19] Type I (subepithelial cordectomy) is performed for mild dysplasia, type II (subligamental cordectomy) or type I for moderate dysplasia,[20,21] while severe dysplasia may need extensive resection of up to type III (transmuscular cordectomy) for good local control.[22] The efficacy of CO_2 laser excision is validated by many studies, which are summarized in **Table 3**.

Photodynamic therapy (PDT) is a nonsurgical modality that utilizes light of specific wavelength, which activates the absorbed sensitizing agent, which is concentrated by tumor. The advantage of PDT is that the continuity of vocal cord mucosa is well preserved, which leads to better voice outcome.[26] Studies assessing safety of PDT in the management of prelaryngeal lesions of the larynx are limited. Their advantage lies with the management of large extensive superficial lesions, which might be subject to significant voice change if surgically excised. The main disadvantage lies with the fact that there is no tissue diagnosis available with this procedure.

Radiation therapy may offer some benefit when resection of the broad area would be necessary and would result in considerable morbidity or when recurrence has occurred despite multiple resections and there is concern for organ preservation. While most of the studies have included carcinoma in situ cases, the control rate cannot be directly compared with surgical excision.[27,28] The role of radiotherapy as upfront treatment modality even for severe dysplasia is not recommended.

Voice Outcomes

Postsurgical excision and change in voice often persists for 3–6 months.[29,30]

Postoperative Instructions and Follow-up

All patients should be counseled regarding measures to reduce risk factors, especially to stop smoking or alcohol intake. Symptomatic patients with laryngopharyngeal reflux should also be counseled about the potential risks, and they should be offered antireflux treatment. Low-risk patients with low-moderate dysplasia need follow-up of 6 months to 2 years and after that if symptoms persist. Patients with severe dysplasia must be followed up as in early laryngeal carcinoma with follow-up to 4–6 years.[31]

CHEMOPREVENTION

Chemoprevention presents as a valuable strategy in controlling carcinogenesis in head and neck region. Unlike oral cavity, studies pertaining to chemoprevention strategies for larynx are limited. A prospective non-randomized study by Papadimitrakopoulou et al. reported a histological response of 48% and clinical response of 57% at 12 months in patients with premalignant lesion in upper aero digestive tract.[32] Chemoprevention regime in the study consisted of administration of oral isotretinoin, oral alpha tocopherol, and subcutaneous interferon alpha for 12 months. Hong et al. demonstrated a reduction in the incidence of second malignancy in SCC of larynx/pharynx/oral cavity with 13-cis-retinoic acid.[33] The current literature is limited to recommend routine use of chemoprevention strategy in larynx; further studies are required to test the efficacy profile of chemoprevention in premalignant lesions of the larynx. The role of human papillomavirus (HPV) in the causation of premalignant lesions of the larynx is not substantiated. Molecular markers such as amplification of cyclin D1, PTEN inactivation, and loss of heterogeneity[34-36] have been associated with the progression of premalignant lesions to invasive carcinoma in the larynx, but their routine use is not recommended. Further studies may guide individualized management of lesions in the future.

CONCLUSION

Management strategy of premalignant lesions of the larynx is based on various factors and all factors (patient and tumor factors) must be taken into account during the decision-making process. The available studies on management of premalignant lesions of larynx are difficult to interpret, as they are not uniformly represented. Directed biopsies, surgical excision, and control of high-risk habits form the primary treatment strategy. The evidence for utility of chemoprevention agents in larynx is limited, and future studies are required to recommend their routine use.

REFERENCES

1. Waghmare CM, Agarwal J, Bachher GK. Quality of voice after radiotherapy in early vocal cord cancer. Expert Rev Anticancer Ther. 2010;10(9):1381-8.
2. Miller AH, Fisher HR. Clues to the life history of carcinoma in situ of the larynx. Laryngoscope. 1971;81(9):1475-80.
3. Weller MD, Nankivell PC, McConkey C, Paleri V, Mehanna HM. The risk and interval to malignancy of patients with laryngeal dysplasia; a systematic review of case series and meta-analysis. Clin Otolaryngol. 2010;35(5):364-72.
4. Isenberg JS, Crozier DL, Dailey SH. Institutional and comprehensive review of laryngeal leukoplakia. Ann Otol Rhinol Laryngol. 2008;117(1):74-9.
5. Ferlito A, Devaney KO, Woolgar JA, Slootweg PJ, Paleri V, Takes RP, et al. Squamous epithelial changes of the larynx: diagnosis and therapy. Head Neck. 2012;34(12):1810-6.
6. Gale N, Westra WH, Pilch BZ. Epithelial precursor lesions. In: Barnes L, Eveson JW, Reichart, P Sindransky D (Eds). World Health Organization Classification of Tumors: Pathology and Genetics of Head and Neck Tumors. Lyon: IARC; 2005. pp. 177-9.
7. Warnakulasuriya S, Johnson NW, Van der Waal I. Nomenclature and classification of potentially malignant disorders of the oral mucosa. J Oral Pathol Med. 2007;36(10): 575-80.
8. Kambič V, Gale N, Ferluga D. Laryngeal hyperplastic lesions, follow-up study and application of lectins and anticytokeratins for their evaluation. Pathol Res Pract. 1992; 188(8):1067-77.
9. Crissman JD. Laryngeal keratosis and subsequent carcinoma. Head Neck Surg. 1979;1(5):386-91.
10. Eveson JW. Pleomorphic adenoma. Pathology and Genetics of Head and Neck Tumors. Geneva: WHO; 2005.
11. Sadri M, McMahon J, Parker A. Management of laryngeal dysplasia: a review. Eur Arch Otorhinolaryngol. 2006;263(9): 843-52.
12. Arens C, Dreyer T, Glanz H, Malzahn K. Indirect autofluorescence laryngoscopy in the diagnosis of laryngeal cancer and its precursor lesions. Eur Arch Otorhinolaryngol. 2004;261(2):71-6.
13. Piazza C, Del Bon F, Peretti G, Nicolai P. Narrow band imaging in endoscopic evaluation of the larynx. Curr Opin Otolaryngol Head Neck Surg. 2012;20(6):472-6.
14. Ni XG, He S, Xu ZG, Gao L, Lu N, Yuan Z, et al. Endoscopic diagnosis of laryngeal cancer and precancerous lesions by narrow band imaging. J Laryngol Otol. 2011;125(3):288-96.
15. Piazza C, Cocco D, Del Bon F, Mangili S, Nicolai P, Majorana A, et al. Narrow band imaging and high definition television in evaluation of oral and oropharyngeal squamous cell cancer: a prospective study. Oral Oncol. 2010;46(4):307-10.
16. Piazza C, Cocco D, De Benedetto L, Del Bon F, Nicolai P, Peretti G. Narrow band imaging and high definition television in the assessment of laryngeal cancer: a prospective study on 279 patients. Eur Arch Otorhinolaryngol. 2010;267(3):409-14.
17. Hakeem AH, Hakeem IH, Pradhan SA. Premalignant lesions of the larynx and their management. Otorhinolaryngol Clin. 2010;2(3):161-5.
18. Jin YJ, Jeong WJ, Paik JH, Ahn SH. Role of Frozen Biopsy in Glottic Premalignant Lesions. Pathol Oncol Res. 2017;23(3): 519-23.
19. Remacle M, Eckel HE, Antonelli A, Brasnu D, Chevalier D, Friedrich G, et al. Endoscopic cordectomy. A proposal for a classification by the Working Committee, European Laryngological Society. Eur Arch Otorhinolaryngol. 2000; 257(4):227-31.
20. Dispenza F, De Stefano A, Marchese D, Martines F, Dispenza C. Management of laryngeal precancerous lesions. Auris Nasus Larynx. 2012;39(3):280-3.
21. Minni A, Barbaro M, Rispoli G, Diaferia F, Bernardeschi D, Filipo R. Treatment with laser CO_2 cordectomy and clinical implications in management of mild and moderate laryngeal precancerosis. Eur Arch Otorhinolaryngol. 2008;265(2):189-93.
22. Johnson FL. Management of advanced premalignant laryngeal lesions. Curr Opin Otolaryngol Head Neck Surg. 2003; 11(6):462-6.
23. Damm M, Sittel C, Streppel M, Eckel HE. Transoral CO_2 laser for surgical management of glottic carcinoma in situ. Laryngoscope. 2000;110(7):1215-21.
24. Le QT, Takamiya R, Shu HK, Smitt M, Singer M, Terris DJ, et al. Treatment results of carcinoma in situ of the glottis: an analysis of 82 cases. Arch Otolaryngol Head Neck Surg. 2000;126(11):1305-12.
25. Gallo A, de Vincentiis M, Della Rocca C, Moi R, Simonelli M, Minni A, et al. Evolution of precancerous laryngeal lesions: A clinicopathologic study with long-term follow-up on 259 patients. Head Neck. 2001;23(1):42-7.
26. Rigual NR, Thankappan K, Cooper M, Sullivan MA, Dougherty T, Popat SR, et al. Photodynamic therapy for head and neck dysplasia and cancer. Arch Otolaryngol Head Neck Surg. 2009;135(8):784-8.
27. Spayne JA, Warde P, O'Sullivan B, Payne D, Liu FF, Waldron J, et al. Carcinoma-in-situ of the glottic larynx: results

of treatment with radiation therapy. Int J Radiat Oncol Biol Phys. 2001;49(5):1235-8.

28. Garcia-Serra A, Hinerman RW, Amdur RJ, Morris CG, Mendenhall WM. Radiotherapy for carcinoma in situ of the true vocal cords. Head Neck. 2002;24(4):390-4.
29. Xu W, Han D, Hou L, Zhang L, Yu Z, Huang Z. Voice function following CO_2 laser microsurgery for precancerous and early-stage glottic carcinoma. Acta Otolaryngol. 2007;127(6):637-41.
30. Chu PY, Hsu YB, Lee TL, Fu S, Wang LM, Kao YC. Longitudinal analysis of voice quality in patients with early glottic cancer after transoral laser microsurgery. Head Neck. 2012;34(9): 1294-8.
31. Mehanna H, Paleri V, Robson A, Wight R, Helliwell T. Consensus statement by otorhinolaryngologists and pathologists on the diagnosis and management of laryngeal dysplasia. Clin Otolaryngol. 2010;35(3):170-6.
32. Papadimitrakopoulou VA, Clayman GL, Shin DM, Myers JN, Gillenwater AM, Goepfert H, et al. Biochemoprevention for dysplastic lesions of the upper aerodigestive tract. Arch Otolaryngol Head Neck Surg. 1999;125(10):1083-9.
33. Hong WK, Lippman SM, Itri LM, Karp DD, Lee JS, Byers RM, et al. Prevention of second primary tumors with isotretinoin in squamous-cell carcinoma of the head and neck. N Engl J Med. 1990;323(12):795-801.
34. Panwar A, Lindau R, Wieland A. Management of premalignant lesions of the larynx. Expert Rev Anticancer Ther. 2013;13(9): 1045-51.
35. Califano J, Van Der Riet P, Westra W, Nawroz H, Clayman G, Piantadosi S, et al. Genetic progression model for head and neck cancer: implications for field cancerization. Cancer Res. 1996;56(11):2488-92.
36. Freier K, Joos S, Flechtenmacher C, Devens F, Benner A, Bosch FX, et al. Tissue microarray analysis reveals site-specific prevalence of oncogene amplifications in head and neck squamous cell carcinoma. Cancer Res. 2003;63(6): 1179-82.

CHAPTER 9

Management of the Neck

Akshat Malik, Aseem Mishra, Samskruthi P Murthy, Narayana Subramaniam, Sivakumar Vidhyadharan

INTRODUCTION

All head and neck malignancies, depending upon the tumor biology, subsite, and the extent of the tumor, are capable of metastasis to cervical lymph nodes. Head and neck squamous cell carcinoma (HNSCC) comprises the majority of malignant tumors in head and neck, and hence the following section focuses on the management strategy in its histology. Management of clinicoradiologically node-negative (N0) and node-positive (N+) varies considerably and has been controversial. In this chapter, we cover an overview of key topics related to the management of the neck and their application in clinical practice.

BIOLOGICAL BASIS OF LYMPH NODE METASTASIS

Lymphangiogenesis is the first step in the initiation of lymph nodal metastasis. Lymphangiogenetic cytokines like vascular endothelial growth factor C/D initiate genesis of lymphatic vessels in peritumoral and intratumoral area.[1] The interaction between lymphatic endothelial cells and tumor cells is paramount for progression of lymphatic spread. Common lymphatic endothelial and vascular endothelial receptor-1 (CLEVER-1), mannose receptor, lymphatic vascular endothelial protein-1 (LYVE-1) expressed by lymphatic endothelial cells act as tumor adhesion receptors. Disconnected tumor cells express metalloprotease-9 that aid in tumor invasion and interact with adhesion receptors on lymphatic endothelium and drain to sentinel lymph node (SLN) via afferent lymphatic vessels.[2]

LEVELS OF LYMPH NODE AND PATTERNS OF SPREAD

The head and neck region has a rich plexus of lymphatics and lymph nodes. Rouviere[3] originally described the levels of lymph nodes; however, this description has undergone several stages of evolution. The current of nodal stations in the neck are represented in **Table 1**. Levels I–VI are commonly encountered during neck dissection of various sites, but additional nodal levels are important especially while planning target volumes during radiotherapy.

The pattern of lymphatic spread is vital to plan the extent of nodal basin treatment either with neck dissection or with inclusion in the radiation field. The pattern of spread was initially described by

Table 1: Nodal levels of head and neck region.[4]

IA	Submental group
IB	Submandibular group
II	Upper jugular group
III	Middle jugular group
IVA	Lower jugular group
IVB	Medial supraclavicular group
V	Posterior triangle group
VA	Upper posterior triangle nodes
VB	Lower posterior triangle nodes
VC	Lateral supraclavicular group
VI	Anterior compartment group
VIA	Anterior jugular nodes
VIA	Prelaryngeal, pretracheal, and paratracheal nodes
VII	Prevertebral compartment group
VIIA	Retropharyngeal nodes
VIIB	Retrostyloid nodes
VIII	Parotid group
IX	Buccofacial group
X	Posterior skull group
XA	Retroauricular and subauricular nodes
XB	Occipital nodes

Table 2: Percentage of metastatic nodes in different head and neck subsites.[5]

		Level I	Level II	Level III	Level IV	Level V
Oral cavity	Elective	58	51	26	9	2
	Therapeutic	61	57	44	20	4
Oropharynx	Elective	7	80	60	27	7
	Therapeutic	17	85	50	33	11
Hypopharynx	Elective	0	75	75	0	0
	Therapeutic	10	78	75	47	11
Larynx	Elective	14	52	55	24	7
	Therapeutic	8	68	70	35	5

Shah et al. based on nodal metastases from radical neck dissection specimen of various subsites of head and neck.[5] The patterns of spread is represented in **Table 2**.

LYMPH NODE STAGING

Staging of the lymph node is crucial as it determines the overall treatment plan. Tumor, node, and metastasis (TNM) staging for the lymph node metastasis is the most accepted staging system. The presence of extranodal extension (ENE) is an essential factor affecting survival, and thus the 8th edition of TNM has included in it the staging. Presence of ENE is included in the nodal staging; the clinical lymph node staging is enlisted in **Table 3**.[6]

Pathological node staging differs from the clinical staging as the presence of ENE in a single node <3 cm will be staged N2a. Presence of multiple nodes with ENE or a single node >3 cm with ENE will be staged as N3b.

Table 3: Lymph node staging in HPV-negative HNSCC.

Nx	Regional lymph nodes cannot be assessed
N0	No regional lymph node metastasis
N1	Metastasis in a single ipsilateral lymph node, 3 cm or smaller in greatest dimension and ENE-negative
N2	Metastasis in a single ipsilateral lymph node larger than 3 cm but not larger than 6 cm in greatest dimension and ENE-negative; or metastases in multiple ipsilateral lymph nodes, none larger than 6 cm in greatest dimension and ENE-negative; or metastasis in bilateral or contralateral lymph nodes, none larger than 6 cm in greatest dimension and ENE-negative
N2a	Metastasis in a single ipsilateral lymph node larger than 3 cm but not larger than 6 cm in greatest dimension and ENE-negative
N2b	Metastasis in multiple ipsilateral lymph nodes, none larger than 6 cm in greatest dimension and ENE-negative
N2c	Metastasis in bilateral or contralateral lymph nodes, none larger than 6 cm in greatest dimension and ENE-negative
N3	Metastasis in a lymph node larger than 6 cm in greatest dimension and ENE-negative; or metastasis in any lymph node(s) and clinically overt ENE-positive
N3a	Metastasis in a lymph node larger than 6 cm in greatest dimension and ENE-negative
N3b	Metastasis in any node(s) and clinically overt ENE-positive

(ENE: extranodal extension; HNSCC: head and neck squamous cell carcinoma; HPV: human papillomavirus)

Various alternate staging systems have been proposed. They are:

- *Lymph node density:* Ratio of excised positive nodes to the total number of excised nodes[7]
- Number of positive nodes[8,9]
- *Log odds of positive lymph nodes (LODD):* Log ratio of positive nodes to negative nodes.[10]

A recent comparative analysis has evaluated the efficacy of various nodal staging system against American Joint Committee on Cancer (AJCC) "N-staging" (8th edition) in oral cancer patients and concluded that positive nodes and lymph node density predicted overall survival and disease-free survival more accurately than AJCC "N-staging" (8th edition).[11] However, AJCC "N-staging" (8th edition) is the most widely accepted and widely used staging system.

PROGNOSTIC VALUE OF EXTRANODAL EXTENSION

Extranodal extension is defined as an extension of tumor beyond the capsule of the lymph node. The prognostic implication of ENE is immense; it is associated with significantly lower 5-year disease-specific survival and overall survival, as well as higher locoregional recurrence.[12,13] Patients with ENE have a 10-fold increase in the risk of distant metastasis.[14] When analyzed retrospectively, implementation of ENE into TNM staging has shown a 30% upstaging in N category. The stage discrimination with respect to 5-year disease-specific survival and overall survival was also significant.[15] However, ENE is not associated with negative impact in human papillomavirus (HPV)-associated oropharyngeal carcinoma. Hence, the N categorization for HPV associated oropharyngeal carcinoma is based on the number of nodes involved.[16]

CLINICAL EXAMINATION

Clinical examination of the neck should be done systematically with the patient in the sitting position and relaxed. Palpation should be done using the flat of the fingers, starting from the level IA proceeding posteriorly to the submandibular area. Palpation of the jugular chain of lymph nodes should be done with the neck turned to the ipsilateral side. Completing the neck examination with the posterior triangle palpation, contralateral neck must also be palpated carefully. The size and number of the lymph nodes should be recorded. Involvement of the surrounding structure and fixity to the carotid artery should be assessed for the presence of clinical ENE. Carotid artery involvement is suspected with restricted vertical movement of the node and correlates well with pathological involvement of carotid artery.[17] Studies evaluating the accuracy of clinical examination for neck node metastasis have shown a sensitivity of clinical examination for assessment of cervical lymph node metastasis of around 60–70%.[18,19]

IMAGING EVALUATION FOR NODAL DISEASE IN THE NECK

Accuracy of Image Modalities

Several imaging modalities have been described for staging the neck in HNSCC. However, till date, there has been no single imaging modality which can secure a 100% diagnosis. A meta-analysis by Liao et al. had analyzed the accuracy of various imaging modalities in N0 head and neck tumors. It showed a sensitivity of 50–66% and specificity of 78–83% among various modalities, with no significant benefit of one over the other.[20,21] Another meta-analysis by Kyzas et al. evaluated the role of positron emission tomography (PET) fused with contrast-enhanced computerized tomography (CT) (CE CT) in the clinically N0 neck. It showed a sensitivity of 50%.[21] In recently concluded Sentinel European Node Trial (SENT) evaluating the sentinel node biopsy,[22] patients accrued in the study were extensively worked up in the preoperative period, despite which 23% were node positive after examination of the sentinel node.

The sensitivity of contrast-enhanced CT in the N0 neck is 60–75%. For ultrasonography (USG), the reported sensitivity is as high as 88% and as low as 14%, since reporting is intrinsically user-dependent. PET-CT has a sensitivity of around 60–70%. CT is more specific compared to USG for evaluating an N0 patient.[23,24]

As several imaging modalities (CT, MRI, PET-CT, and USG) have a similar sensitivity and specificity, the site of the primary tumor would also direct the choice of imaging. For a carcinoma of the tongue or oropharynx, an MRI would be the investigating modality of choice, as it would accurately predict the soft tissue extension and the depth of the tumor. For carcinoma of the gingivobuccal sulcus complex, larynx or hypopharynx, a CT would be the investigation of the choice, as it would appropriately stage the primary and would also provide relevant information regarding the neck nodes.

Imaging Characteristics of Metastatic Node

- *Size:* Size criteria are among the first to be considered during image reporting. Various size cutoff values with variable sensitivity and specificity are reported in the literature. Nodes measuring 1.5 cm in greatest diameter in level I/II and greater than 1 cm in other nodal stations are considered to harbor metastasis, with 80% accuracy.[25] However, the cutoff 11 mm has also been suggested for level II, with a metastasis detection rate of 75%.[26] A retropharyngeal node measuring over 6–8 mm is considered abnormal.[27] Nodal grouping defined as three or more nodes in continuity with each other are considered to be metastatic even if the size or shape criteria is achieved, especially if they are in the known lymphatic drainage path.[28]
- *Shape:* Rounded nodes are considered metastatic. The shape definition is subjective hence the Solbiati index has been proposed as an objective method of nodal shape assessment; it is the ratio of maximal diameter/minimal diameter, which when <2 is considered a metastatic rounded node.[29]
- *Density:* Nodal necrosis characterized by focal central hypodensity with nodal rim enhancement on CT scan is considered almost pathognomonic of metastatic node. Gadolinium-enhanced T1-weighted image on MRI will show central focal defect, and hyperintense on fat-suppressed T2 image is considered on MRI image reporting. Detection of central necrotic area with sensitivity and specificity of 91%/93% and 93%/89% on CT scan and MRI, respectively.[30] Central necrosis in smaller nodes is difficult to identify.
- *Extranodal extension*: Identification and reporting of ENE is paramount for adequate staging of the patient. Imaging criteria that define ENE are indistinct nodal margin, infiltration to adjacent structures, and irregular nodal enhancement, in combination, is known to improve specificity and positive predictive value.[31] Irregular nodal border is the most characteristic

with a CT sensitivity and specificity of 61% and 95%, respectively and MRI sensitivity and specificity of 40% and 97%, respectively.[32]

- *Carotid involvement:* CT scan will show contiguous or encasing of the carotid artery when involved. MRI features are loss of fascial plane between mass and carotid artery on T2-weighted images.[33] The tumor seldom involves the lumen of the carotid artery; most postsurgical specimens show involvement of adventitia to have an incidence of 37.5–43%.[34,35] Degree of circumferential carotid artery encasement must be assessed. 270° encasement of carotid artery predicts artery involvement with sensitivity and specificity of 92–100% and 88–93%, respectively.[36,37] Various degrees of encasement (>90° and >180°) have been described, but have a very low false-negative rate.[38,39]

PATHOLOGY

Thorough pathological evaluation is vital, as further treatment and prognostication is dependent on the pathological reporting. The guidelines for handling and reporting a neck dissection specimen as per the Royal College of Pathologists are discussed here.[40]

Specimen Handling and Block Selection

Nodal yield in neck dissection specimen is an important parameter that is dependent on surgeon factors and pathologist factors. Handling and sectioning of the specimen is important to count and assess the number of nodes involved. The specimen can be sent as a whole with specimen corked on board with level identification or sectioned into respective nodal stations. The specimen must be stored for 24–48 hours in 10% formalin with formalin 10 times the volume of the specimen in an adequately sized container.

Lymph node identification is usually made by inspection and palpation around vein, submandibular gland then into fatty tissue. All nodes >3 mm must be examined. Each node with pericapsular adipose tissue can be dissected and subjected for examination. Large palpable nodes are dissected into half, and the section with the largest dimension of the tumor is selected for examination. When nodes appear negative, then all slices must be processed. An alternative method is serially sectioning the whole specimen and embedding all tissue. This method is ideal for selective neck dissection specimen. Care must be taken not to count a large node twice. Reporting of core and noncore data is essential, and **Table 4** lists the features to be included in the reporting.

Table 4: Summary of the Royal College of Pathologists reporting of nodal specimens.[40,41]

The Royal College of Pathologists summary of nodal specimen reporting	
Core elements	*Noncore elements*
• Specimen submitted • Histologic tumor type • Number of nodes examined (per level) • Number of nodes positive (per level) • Maximum dimension of the largest involved lymph node • Maximum dimension of the largest metastatic deposit (for each side of neck, if applicable) • ENE (present/not identified; major or minor) • Soft tissue metastasis (present/not identified) • Regional lymph node • Categorization	• Operative procedure • Primary tumor site • Margin status • Ancillary studies • Nonlymphatic structures involved by ENE • Greatest extent of ENE, mm • Number of nodes with ENE

(ENE: extranodal extension)

Extranodal Extension

Pathologically, ENE >2 mm is considered significant.[42] Lewis et al. proposed an ENE grading system which includes five grades:[43]

- *Grade 0:* Tumor is confined within nodal tissue with adjoining lymphoid tissue between tumor and capsule
- *Grade 1:* Tumor reaches the capsule of a node with no adjacent tissue between tumor and capsule
- *Grade 2:* Tumor extends to perinodal tissue, limited to ≤1 mm beyond capsule
- *Grade 3:* Tumor extends >1 mm beyond the capsule of node
- *Grade 4:* It is soft tissue metastasis with no identifiable nodal tissue or architecture.

Number of Nodes

With the inclusion number of metastatic nodes in oropharyngeal carcinoma, the accuracy of nodal counting is vital. Nodal count is subject to interpathologist variability and is dependent on various factors such as use of fat clearing solutions, block selection method used, and processing fresh versus formalin-fixed nodal tissue.[44]

TREATMENT

Surgical Treatment of Nodal Disease

Evolution of Neck Dissection

Surgeons knew the fact that head and neck cancers can metastasize to cervical nodes in the mid-19th century.

It was understood that such lesions were advanced and required removal of primary as well as the neck nodes.[45] Jawdynski gave the first description of neck dissection in Polish in 1888. In 1906, George Washington Crile described a systematic approach to addressing neck nodes in an en-bloc manner. He described the removal of all lymphatic structures between the superficial and deep cervical fascia along with sternocleidomastoid muscle, internal jugular vein, the tail of parotid, submandibular gland, and spinal accessory nerve. It became known as radical neck dissection.[46] In 1951, Hayes Martin published details of radical neck dissection with a step-by-step approach.[47] Suarez published on functional neck dissection in 1963. Here he preserved the nonlymphatic structures (sternocleidomastoid, internal jugular vein, and spinal accessory nerve) while performing proper nodal clearance. Bocca[48] further popularized it. With further knowledge about the pattern of lymph node metastasis given by Lindberg in 1972 and Shah in 1990, selective neck dissections were carried out more commonly.[5,49] Here the low-risk nodal levels were not addressed.[50] As there were several overlapping terminologies prevalent world over, American Academy of Otolaryngology-Head and Neck Surgery (AAO-HNS) standardized the neck dissection terminologies. These were given in 1991 and further revised in 2002 and updated in 2008.[51] Present classification identified four categories of neck dissections—(1) radical neck dissection (level I–V and the three nonlymphatic structures are removed), (2) modified radical neck dissection (level I–V are addressed with preservation of at least one of the three nonlymphatic structures), (3) selective neck dissection (one or more lymph node levels may be preserved along with nonlymphatic structures), and (4) extended radical neck dissection (involves removal of additional lymphatic or nonlymphatic structures such as level VII nodes, retropharyngeal lymph nodes, skin, etc.). Another term, which has been used, is super selective neck dissection where only one or two contiguous lymph node levels are addressed.

Lateral Neck Dissection: Subtypes

Lateral neck dissection refers to removal of level II–IV nodes, generally recommended for hypopharyngeal or laryngeal primaries with clinically node-negative (cN0) neck. Anterolateral neck dissection refers to removal of level I–IV nodes, also called extended supraomohyoid neck dissection and most often used for oral cavity cancers. Supraomohyoid neck dissection addresses level I–III nodes for oral cavity cancers. Posterolateral neck dissection addresses level II–V and may be used for parotid and cutaneous malignancies.

Central Compartment Neck Dissection: Limited and Extended

Central compartment dissection refers to the dissection of the level VI lymph nodes. The compartment extends between both common carotid arteries laterally, and from the hyoid bone superiorly to the innominate artery inferiorly. The central compartment nodes are the first echelon nodes in thyroid carcinoma. Metastasis to the central compartment is also of considerable significance in laryngeal and hypopharyngeal cancers. Meticulous dissection of the level VI should be performed in these cancers as residual disease in this area leads to recurrence after thyroidectomy in differentiated thyroid cancer and stomal recurrence in squamous carcinoma of larynx and hypopharynx. A study by Weber et al. has shown that the presence of positive lymph node in the level VI is associated with significantly reduced survival in laryngeal cancer.[52] Metastasis to the central compartment nodes can also be associated with metastasis to the upper mediastinal nodes. An extensive dissection of the level VI and VII is to be done in differentiated thyroid cancers with clinicoradiological nodes in the upper mediastinum.[53]

Surgical Description of Neck Dissection

Comprehensive neck dissection refers to excision of all the fibrofatty, lymph nodes, and lymph bearing tissue from levels I–V. The subplatysmal flaps are raised after appropriate incision planning. All the fibrofatty tissue in the submental triangle is removed (level IA). The submandibular triangle is dissected after identifying and preserving the marginal mandibular nerve. Facial artery and vein are clipped at the lower border of the mandible. Dissection is continued over the hyoglossus muscle. The hypoglossal nerve is identified and preserved, and the level IB is dissected out along with submandibular gland. The anterior border of the sternocleidomastoid is delineated, and all the tissue is dissected along the carotid sheath from the posterior belly of digastric to the transverse cervical artery inferiorly. Posterior triangle dissection is performed after identifying and preserving the spinal accessory nerve. It exits 1 cm above the Erb's point and enters into the anterior border of trapezius inferiorly. Meticulous dissection of the posterior triangle should be performed, and the cervical nerve roots should be preserved where possible; this is achieved by dissecting parallel to them. Meticulous clearance of the level VA should be performed above the point of exit of the spinal accessory nerve, as this is one of the common routes of spread into the posterior triangle from the level II in the N+ neck.

For a selective neck dissection, a limited dissection is performed from levels I–III in a supraomohyoid neck dissection and levels I–IV in an extended supraomohyoid dissection. The surgical steps are similar, as described above. However, a selective dissection does not require a vertical limb incision and would avoid dissection of the posterior triangle.

Complications:

- *Neural complications:* One of the most critical complications of neck dissection is the shoulder morbidity. This is associated with injury to the spinal accessory nerve. The shoulder dysfunction significantly affects quality of life as various activities of daily life are affected.[54,55] Spinal accessory nerve-sparing neck dissection is associated with better shoulder function.[56,57] However, some amount of shoulder dysfunction occurs even when the nerve is preserved.[58] Employing early shoulder exercise and physiotherapy at the earliest is necessary to improve shoulder mobility. The exercises are aimed at promoting function, improve scapular stability, reduce pain by maintaining the length of muscles, range of movements, and prevent frozen shoulder.[59] Damage to the marginal mandibular nerve is one of the most neglected complication of neck dissection, which is associated with reduced functional and cosmetic outcome. The cervical portion of marginal mandibular nerve as most vulnerable to injury.[60] Various retrospective studies have shown that classical Hayes Martin maneuver may not be oncologically safe as prefacial nodal clearance is compromised.[61,62] After 6 months, static procedures can be used to correct the lip deformity.[60]
- *Chyle leak:* There is a risk of chyle leak secondary to injury to the thoracic duct and or lymphatic channels at the root of the neck. The incidence of chyle leak in neck dissection is 2–8%.[63-66] Early diagnosis and treatment is essential as chylous extravasation causes dehydration, malnutrition electrolyte imbalances, and immune suppression. Low output leaks (<500 mL/day) can be conservatively managed while high output leaks (>500 mL/day) most often needs surgical intervention.[67]
- *Bilateral internal jugular vein ligation:* Bilateral internal jugular vein ligation may need to be performed in rare cases. Sacrificing both bilateral internal and external jugular vein can lead to intracranial hypertension, blindness, and neurological sequelae. Staged contralateral ligation of internal jugular may be well tolerated as the venous collaterals from brain are diverted to vertebral venous plexus.[68]
- *Other complications:* Other complications such as hematoma formation, delayed wound healing, and injury to the tail parotid, which poses a significant risk of development of parotid fistula, can occur. All complications are avoidable with meticulous dissection and intraoperative vigilance.

Sentinel Lymph Node Biopsy

Technique: Preoperative lymphoscintigraphy allows assessment of the individual lymphatic drainage pattern of each patient. About 1–2 mL of patent blue V and ^{99m}Tc sulfur colloid dye is injected around the tumor, and an incision is made in line with neck dissection incision (in case it is required subsequently). A handheld gamma probe is used to identify radioactive sentinel nodes. Suspected nodes are excised and gamma probe radioactive count is confirmed ex vivo. Sentinel nodes are fixed and sectioned with step-serial sections at intervals of approximately 150 µm. If the nodes still appear negative after histologic examination, an adjacent section from each level is examined by immuno-cytochemistry [immunohistochemistry (IHC)] using the multicytokeratin antibody AE1/AE3. Detection of micrometastasis (0.2–2 mm) is associated with poor survival.[69]

Sentinel lymph node biopsy (SLNB) is useful in early oral/pharyngeal cancers. The SENT conducted in multiple centers in Europe found that in cT1-T2N0 oral cancers, SLNB had a sensitivity of 86% and negative predictive value (NPV) of 95%.[22] Their preoperative evaluation utilized CT/MRI with or without USG. SLNB detected occult metastasis in 23% of patients. 53.3% of false negatives could be salvaged with neck dissection subsequently. In another study by Chung et al. on cN0 oral tongue cancers, occult false negatives were seen in 11.7% patients in the application phase.[70] In a meta-analysis of 66 studies in 2016, Liu et al. found that sensitivity was 87% and NPV was 94%. SLNB with IHC was shown to have a significantly higher sensitivity.[71] SLNB is more cost-effective than elective neck dissection (END) when adjusted per quality-adjusted life years (QALYs), as reported by Hernando and Govers.[72] Van der Linden also found it to be more cost-effective when compared with USG-guided fine-needle aspiration cytology (FNAC). Hernando found that SLNB group had significantly better shoulder function, less scar length, lesser chances of developing orocervical communication and neck hematoma as compared to the END group.[73] Fen et al. in a long-term study have shown that overall survival and cervical recurrence-free survival were similar at 10 years for SLNB and the END group.[74]

Current recommendations for sentinel node biopsy in oral cancer: The current standard of care is END; there are no prospective trials that have compared SLNB with END. Hence, SLNB can be performed under strict guidelines and in an experienced set up. The 8th International Symposium on Sentinel Node Biopsy has recommended the following additional guidelines.[75]

- *Patient selection criteria:*
  - The primary tumor must be resected with adequate margins without need for entry into the neck for reconstruction purposes.
  - Depth of invasion alone must not be taken as an indicator to choose SLNB over END.
- *Technique criteria:*
  - Optical tracers such as indocyanine green, patent blue V sodium, isosulfan, or methylene blue must be used adjunct to radionuclide. Optical tracers alone must not be used, especially patent blue V sodium, isosulfan, or methylene blue as they have a high washout rate.
  - Unexpected nodal areas located on imaging must also be explored during SLN retrieval. Knowledge of the common drainage pathway helps in easier retrieval of nodes.
  - Tumors of floor of mouth commonly result in shine-through effect, making SLN identification difficult. The shine-through effect can be avoided by identification of SLN by gamma probe after dissecting surrounding fat from level IB or SLNB identified after tumor excision.
  - SLNB must not be performed as a staged procedure, after excision of tumor. Significant scarring in the excised area and tissue rearrangements will interfere with SLNB as a staged procure.
  - SLN must be considered significant when the gamma count is 10 times the background or 10% of the hottest node.
  - Pathologically, isolated tumor cells must be considered as positive.
- *Outcomes and management:*
  - The role adjuvant therapy after neck dissection is based on the pathology report. The consensus regarding adjuvant therapy in an SLNB negative patient with tumor adverse features warranting adjuvant therapy is not defined.
  - SLNB negative patients must be followed up with ultrasound every 3 months for the first 12–18 months after which regular protocol as per the primary tumor is followed.
  - False omission rate of SLNB must not exceed the neck recurrence rate after END (pN0). False omission rate is used to test the accuracy of the test from that particular center as a quality check.

Management of the cN0 Neck

The management of the cN0 neck in head neck cancer patients has been controversial. According to a study by Weiss et al. using a complex mathematical analysis, it was concluded that END should be considered for patients in whom chances of occult metastasis was more than 20%.[76] The principle of treating N0 neck is based on known pathways of lymphatic spread that is unique to each subsite.

- *Oral cavity:* In oral cancers, tumor thickness has often been associated with the risk of nodal metastasis. In a meta-analysis by Huang et al., it was seen that the risk of nodal metastasis increased significantly between 4 (4.5%) and 5 mm (16.6%).[77] The treatment modality of choice for advanced (T3–T4) tumors is surgery of the primary and END. The dilemma of performing a neck dissection arises in early oral cavity cancers. However, the debate has been answered to a significant extent by the trial by D'Cruz et al., which showed the advantage of END over therapeutic neck dissection. About 500 patients were included in the analysis. The END arm showed improved overall survival (80% vs. 67.5%) and disease free survival (69.5% vs. 45.9%) when compared to the therapeutic neck dissection arm.[78] A meta-analysis by Ren et al. has evaluated five studies and shown that END has better overall and disease free survival as compared to observation and therapeutic neck dissection in cN0 oral cancers.[79] Supraomohyoid neck dissection is generally advised for N0 oral cancer patients. Byers el at. reported 15.8% skip metastasis to level IV in tongue cancers[80] and suggested doing an extended supraomohyoid neck (levels I–IV) dissection for these patients. However, the results of this study were controversial. A trial by Brazilian Head and Neck Group has showed that level I–III neck dissection was adequate for cN0 patients.[81] Whether level IIB is to be addressed in the elective setting is also controversial. Lea et al. in their meta-analysis of nine studies have found that a 6.04% occult metastasis to this level in oral cancer patients.[82] Another meta-analysis by Kou et al. has shown 6% metastasis to this level for cN0 and cN+ oral cancer patients. In a prospective study on 583 patients by Pantvaidya et al., multivariate analysis identified presence of level IIA metastasis as the single most important factor to predict metastasis at level IIB. Level IIB and III positivity were also statistically significant factors predicting level V metastasis. Skip metastasis to levels IV and V were never observed in the absence of metastasis to levels I–III.[83]

- *Oropharyngeal cancer:* Level II–IV neck dissection is recommended for oropharyngeal cancers. These cancers have rich lymphatic supply and have high chances of nodal metastasis. According to Moore et al., contralateral neck nodes may be seen if multiple ipsilateral neck nodes are present or in midline tumors or those involving the posterior tonsillar pillar.[84] Almeida et al. in a meta-analysis of 12 studies on transoral robotic surgery (TORS) noted that neck dissections were concurrent in 61% and staged in 39% times.[85] They also noted an incidence of pharyngocervical fistula in 2.5% of the cases. Mockelman in a study on assessing the best time for neck dissection for patients undergoing TORS found that no difference in complications or oncologic results between the concurrent and the sequential neck dissection group. Staged neck dissection patients had a longer hospital stay.[86]
- *Laryngeal and hypopharyngeal cancer:* END in hypopharyngeal and laryngeal cancers will also encompass levels II–IV. Contralateral neck nodes will need to be addressed if ipsilateral neck nodes are positive or if the disease is not lateralized. A recent systematic review by Sanabria et al. has assessed the rate of occult metastasis in laryngeal cancer.[87] The overall rate of occult metastasis is 19.9% and 8% in supraglottic and glottis cancer, respectively. The rate of occult metastasis to level I, V, and IIB in laryngeal cancer were 2.4%, 2%, and 0.4%, respectively. The incidence of occult metastasis is higher in T3/T4 tumors of the larynx.

Management of the N+ Neck

- *Oral cavity:* Various studies have shown that the risk of lymph node metastasis in carcinoma of the oral cavity is highest in levels I–III. In a clinically positive neck, a selective neck dissection is advisable from levels I–V. However, the study by Pantvaidya, which prospectively evaluated 583 neck dissection specimens,[83] concluded that 91% of metastasis was concentrated in levels I–III and 96% in levels I–IV. There was no skip metastasis to the level IV or V, with the incidence of metastasis to level V in the N+ neck around 3.6%. They also evaluated the factors predicting level V metastasis and showed that metastasis to level IIB and III are the most significant factors affecting level V metastasis. Therefore, in N+ oral cavity cancer, selective neck dissection (I–IV) can be safely undertaken if level II is negative for metastasis. The incidence of metastasis to levels IIB and V is low. Shah et al. have shown that the incidence of level V metastasis is around 2–5%.[5] Hence in an oral cavity cancer with no significant level II lymph node metastasis, a comprehensive neck dissection may be avoided.
- *Oropharynx/larynx/hypopharynx carcinoma:* In oropharyngeal cancer, a comprehensive neck dissection of level I–V is recommended. In carcinoma of the hypopharynx and the bilateral larynx, dissection of level II–V is recommended in N+ neck. Ipsilateral dissection of central compartment nodes should be undertaken in all patients of laryngeal and hypopharyngeal cancers.

Nonsurgical Treatment of Nodal Disease

The management of neck is based on treatment modality chosen for primary tumor. With the advent of organ preservation protocols, recent decades have shown an increase in radiation and chemoradiation therapy to treat laryngeal and pharyngeal diseases. When radiotherapy alone is used to treat for early-stage tumors, then elective neck irradiation is planned, which has shown excellent control rates of 90–97%. With larger primary tumors and bulkier nodal disease, multimodality treatment with concurrent chemoradiotherapy (CCRT) is indicated.

Primary CCRT is increasingly used in the treatment of the neck in patients with oropharyngeal, laryngeal, and hypopharyngeal cancer. These tumors show good response at the primary site in comparison to the neck nodes. Wee et al. have shown that after a complete response at the neck nodes after primary CCRT, there is a less than 5% risk of recurrence.[88] Complete response rates range from 80% in N1 disease to 40% in N3 nodes.[89] Therefore, in patients with N2–N3 nodes, surveillance with PET-CT is indicated; if PET-CT shows residual disease, then a salvage neck dissection should be performed. Mehanna et al. have shown in the PET-NECK trial, that PET-CT has a high NPV; a follow-up PET-CT showing no uptake in the neck can be observed in a clinically evident node. However, a careful follow-up and presence of viable tumor cells should be ruled out in these patients.[90]

Postoperative Radiotherapy for Nodal Disease

The advantage of postoperative radiotherapy (PORT) has been shown in multiple retrospective studies where good control rates were observed after neck dissection and adjuvant radiotherapy for N1/N2 patients, but not for N3.

The Radiation Therapy Oncology Group (RTOG) 73-03 trial has shown that PORT had better survival and locoregional control when compared to preoperative radiotherapy for patients undergoing definitive surgery for the primary site.[91] Peters et al., in a randomized trial, showed that at a dose of at least 63 Gy was required as PORT for good locoregional control; any further increase in dose was not found to be beneficial.[92] Ang et al. showed that overall treatment time less than 11 weeks led to better disease control and survival.[93] The intergroup 0034 study found that addition of sequential chemotherapy between surgery and radiotherapy improved locoregional control and survival in high-risk patients only (close/positive margins and ENE) though the association was not found to be significant. Role of adjuvant chemoradiotherapy has been proven by individual studies from Bernier and Cooper and further confirmed by their combined analysis.[94] Bernier's study showed improved locoregional control, disease-free survival, and overall survival, whereas Cooper's study showed significant improvement only in locoregional control. In their combined analysis, adjuvant chemoradiotherapy was shown to improve survival in patients with positive margins and those having nodes with extracapsular spread.[95]

Management of Carotid Artery Involvement

Nodal disease involving carotid artery portends poor prognosis with a 24% rate of distant metastasis.[33] Sacrifice and reconstruction of the carotid artery is challenging. Patients who undergo carotid ligation have a high rate of neurological complications. Preoperative assessment with balloon occlusion test, normal single-photon emission computed tomography (SPECT) or satisfactory backpressure >70 mm Hg during balloon occlusion is associated with significantly less thromboembolic complications. Peeling off tumor from the carotid artery does not obey oncologic principles and should not be performed.[96]

Carotid artery sacrifice and appropriate reconstruction is beneficial in select group of patients after adequate preoperative evaluation. The recent meta-analysis, which included 24 studies with a total of 357 patients who underwent sacrifice of extracranial carotid artery in head and neck cancer, has shown a 1-year survival of 65.4%.[97] The rate of complications such as permanent cerebrovascular complications and carotid blowout was 3.6% and 1.4%, respectively.

Management of Recurrent Neck Disease

Recurrent neck disease is associated with a higher rate of distant metastasis. Hence, all cases with recurrent neck disease must be evaluated for distant metastasis. If the recurrent can be resected then nodal clearance is the most appropriate option. Reirradiation is associated with various complications, can be considered when an interval between previous treatment is >2 years.[98] Unresectable nodal disease is difficult to manage. Palliative chemotherapy can be administered based on the general condition of the patient. A fungating neck mass must be palliated with hemostatic strategy and control of infection.

CONCLUSION

Lymph nodal metastasis in head and neck cancer is the most significant prognosticator of survival. Management of nodal disease was surrounded by controversy, but with recent prospective trials, there are clear guidelines in the management of nodal disease. END is the current standard of treatment for N0 disease of the oral cavity. Treatment of N+ disease is dictated by treatment of choice for primary tumor.

REFERENCES

1. Shintani S, Li C, Ishikawa T, Mihara M, Nakashiro KI, Hamakawa H. Expression of vascular endothelial growth factor A, B, C, and D in oral squamous cell carcinoma. Oral Oncol. 2004;40(1):13-20.
2. Teymoortash A, Werner JA. Current advances in diagnosis and surgical treatment of lymph node metastasis in head and neck cancer. GMS Curr Top Otorhinolaryngol Head Neck Surg. 2012;11:Doc04.
3. Rouviere H. Anatomie des lymphatiques de l'homme. Paris: Masson et Cie; 1932.
4. Thomas Robbins K. Standardizing neck dissection terminology. Arch Otolaryngol Head Neck Surg. 1991;117:601-5.
5. Shah JP. Patterns of cervical lymph node metastasis from squamous carcinomas of the upper aerodigestive tract. Am J Surg. 1990;160(4):405-9.
6. Amin MB, Greene FL, Edge SB, Compton CC, Gershenwald JE, Brookland RK, et al. The eighth edition AJCC cancer staging manual: continuing to build a bridge from a population-based to a more "personalized" approach to cancer staging. CA Cancer J Clin. 2017;67(2):93-9.
7. Gil Z, Carlson DL, Boyle JO, Kraus DH, Shah JP, Shaha AR, et al. Lymph node density is a significant predictor of outcome in patients with oral cancer. Cancer. 2009;115(24):5700-10.
8. Roberts TJ, Colevas AD, Hara W, Holsinger FC, Oakley-Girvan I, Divi V. Number of positive nodes is superior to the lymph node ratio and American Joint Committee on Cancer N staging for the prognosis of surgically treated head and neck squamous cell carcinomas. Cancer. 2016;122(9):1388-97.
9. Lydiatt WM, Patel SG, O'Sullivan B, Brandwein MS, Ridge JA, Migliacci JC, et al. Head and neck cancers—major changes in the American Joint Committee on cancer eighth edition cancer staging manual. CA Cancer J Clin. 2017;67(2):122-37.
10. Lee CC, Ho HC, Su YC, Lee MS, Hung SK, Chen YL. The prognostic ability of log odds of positive lymph nodes in oral cavity squamous cell carcinoma. Medicine (Baltimore). 2015;94(27):e1069.

11. Subramaniam N, Balasubramanian D, Kumar N, Murthy S, Vijayan SN, Nambiar A, et al. Lymph node staging systems in oral squamous cell carcinoma: a comparative analysis. Oral Oncol. 2019;97:92-8.
12. Suton P, Salaric I, Granic M, Mueller D, Luksic I. Prognostic significance of extracapsular spread of lymph node metastasis from oral squamous cell carcinoma in the clinically negative neck. Int J Oral Maxillofac Surg. 2017;46(6):669-75.
13. Jose J, Coatesworth AP, Johnston C, MacLennan K. Cervical node metastases in squamous cell carcinoma of the upper aerodigestive tract: the significance of extracapsular spread and soft tissue deposits. Head Neck. 2003;25(6):451-6.
14. Ho AS, Kim S, Tighiouart M, Gudino C, Mita A, Scher KS, et al. Metastatic lymph node burden and survival in oral cavity cancer. J Clin Oncol. 2017;35(31):3601.
15. Matos LL, Dedivitis RA, Kulcsar MA, de Mello ES, Alves VA, Cernea CR. External validation of the AJCC Cancer Staging Manual, in an independent cohort of oral cancer patients. Oral Oncol. 2017;71:47-53.
16. Mermod M, Tolstonog G, Simon C, Monnier Y. Extracapsular spread in head and neck squamous cell carcinoma: a systematic review and meta-analysis. Oral Oncol. 2016; 62:60-71.
17. Yoo GH, Hocwald E, Korkmaz H, Du W, Logani S, Kelly JK, et al. Assessment of carotid artery invasion in patients with head and neck cancer. Laryngoscope. 2000;110(3): 386-90.
18. Anand N, Chaudhary N, Mittal MK, Prasad R. Comparison of the efficacy of clinical examination, ultrasound neck and computed tomography in detection and staging of cervical lymph node metastasis in head and neck cancers. Indian J Otolaryngol Head Neck Surg. 2007;59(1):19-23.
19. Kallalli BN, Rawson K, Kumari V, Patil S, Singh A, Sulaga S. Comparison between clinical examination, ultrasonography, and computed tomography in assessment of cervical lymph node metastasis in oral squamous cell carcinoma. J Indian Acad Oral Med Radiol. 2016;28(4):364-9.
20. Liao LJ, Lo WC, Hsu WL, Wang CT, Lai MS. Detection of cervical lymph node metastasis in head and neck cancer patients with clinically N0 neck—a meta-analysis comparing different imaging modalities. BMC Cancer. 2012;12(1):236.
21. Kyzas PA, Evangelou E, Denaxa-Kyza D, Ioannidis JP. 18F-fluorodeoxyglucose positron emission tomography to evaluate cervical node metastases in patients with head and neck squamous cell carcinoma: a meta-analysis. J Natl Cancer Inst. 2008;100(10):712-20.
22. Schilling C, Stoeckli SJ, Haerle SK, Broglie MA, Huber GF, Sorensen JA, et al. Sentinel European Node Trial (SENT): 3-year results of sentinel node biopsy in oral cancer. Eur J Cancer. 2015;51(18):2777-84.
23. Chaturvedi P, Datta S, Arya S, Rangarajan V, Kane SV, Nair D, et al. Prospective study of ultrasound-guided fine-needle aspiration cytology and sentinel node biopsy in the staging of clinically negative T1 and T2 oral cancer. Head Neck. 2015;37(10):1504-8.
24. Chaukar D, Dandekar M, Kane S, Arya S, Purandare N, Rangarajan V, et al. Relative value of ultrasound, computed tomography and positron emission tomography imaging in the clinically node-negative neck in oral cancer. Asia Pac J Clin Oncol. 2016;12(2):e332-8.
25. Som PM. Detection of metastasis in cervical lymph nodes: CT and MR criteria and differential diagnosis. AJR Am J Roentgenol. 1992;158(5):961-9.
26. Sumi M, Ohki M, Nakamura T. Comparison of sonography and CT for differentiating benign from malignant cervical lymph nodes in patients with squamous cell carcinoma of the head and neck. Am J Roentgenol. 2001;176(4):1019-24.
27. Mancuso AA, Harnsberger HR, Muraki AS, Stevens MH. Computed tomography of cervical and retropharyngeal lymph nodes: normal anatomy, variants of normal, and applications in staging head and neck cancer. Part II: pathology. Radiology. 1983;148(3):715-23.
28. Van den Brekel MW, Stel HV, Castelijns JA, Nauta JJ, Van der Waal I, Valk J, et al. Cervical lymph node metastasis: assessment of radiologic criteria. Radiology. 1990;177(2):379-84.
29. Solbiati L, Rizzatto G, Bellotti E, Montali G, Cioffi V, Croce F. High-resolution sonography of cervical lymph nodes in head and neck cancer: criteria for differentiation of reactive versus malignant nodes. Radiology. 1998;169:113.
30. King AD, Tse GM, Ahuja AT, Yuen EH, Vlantis AC, To EW, et al. Necrosis in metastatic neck nodes: diagnostic accuracy of CT, MR imaging, and US. Radiology. 2004;230(3):720-6.
31. Carlton JA, Maxwell AW, Bauer LB, McElroy SM, Layfield LJ, Ahsan H, et al. Computed tomography detection of extracapsular spread of squamous cell carcinoma of the head and neck in metastatic cervical lymph nodes. Neuroradiol J. 2017;30(3):222-9.
32. Almulla A, Noel CW, Lu L, Xu W, O'Sullivan B, Goldstein DP, et al. Radiologic-pathologic correlation of extranodal extension in patients with squamous cell carcinoma of the oral cavity: implications for future editions of the TNM classification. Int J Radiat Oncol Biol Phys. 2018;102(4): 698-708.
33. Freeman SB, Hamaker RC, Borrowdale RB, Huntley TC. Management of neck metastasis with carotid artery involvement. Laryngoscope. 2004;114(1):20-4.
34. Huvos AG, Leaming RH, Moore OS. Clinicopathologic study of the resected carotid artery: analysis of sixty-four cases. Am J Surg. 1973;126(4):570-4.
35. McCready RA, Miller SK, Hamaker RC, Singer MI, Herod GT. What is the role of carotid arterial resection in the management of advanced cervical cancer? J Vasc Surg. 1989;10(3): 274-80.
36. Yousem DM, Hatabu H, Hurst RW, Seigerman HM, Montone KT, Weinstein GS, et al. Carotid artery invasion by head and neck masses: prediction with MR imaging. Radiology. 1995;195(3):715-20.
37. Gritzmann N, Grasl MC, Helmer M, Steiner E. Invasion of the carotid artery and jugular vein by lymph node metastases: detection with sonography. AJR Am J Roentgenol. 1990;154(2):411-4.
38. Langman AW, Kaplan MJ, Dillon WP, Gooding GA. Radiologic assessment of tumor and the carotid artery: correlation of magnetic resonance imaging, ultrasound, and computed tomography with surgical findings. Head Neck. 1989;11(5):443-9.
39. Rothstein SG, Persky MS, Horii S. Evaluation of malignant invasion of the carotid artery by CT scan and ultrasound. Laryngoscope. 1988;98(3):321-4.
40. Lee JA. Datasets for histopathology reports on head and neck carcinomas and salivary neoplasms. London: Royal College of Pathologists; 2005.
41. Bullock MJ, Beitler JJ, Carlson DL, Fonseca I, Hunt JL, Katabi N, et al. Data Set for the Reporting of Nodal Excisions and Neck Dissection Specimens for Head and Neck Tumors: Explanations and Recommendations of the Guidelines

From the International Collaboration on Cancer Reporting. Arch Pathol Lab Med. 2019;143(4):452-62.
42. Covello P, Kim DD. Current Updates in Staging and Prognosis in Oral Cancer. Improving Outcomes in Oral Cancer. Switzerland: Springer; 2020. pp. 33-43.
43. Lewis JS, Carpenter DH, Thorstad WL, Zhang Q, Haughey BH. Extracapsular extension is a poor predictor of disease recurrence in surgically treated oropharyngeal squamous cell carcinoma. Mod Pathol. 2011;24(11):1413-20.
44. Sherbeck JP, Zhao L, Lieberman RW. High variability in lymph node counts among an international cohort of pathologists: questioning the scientific validity of node counts. J Natl Compr Canc Netw. 2018;16(4):395-401.
45. Gross SD. System of Surgery: Pathological, Diagnostic, Therapeutic, and Operative, 5th edition. Philadelphia: Henry C Lea's Son; 1872.
46. Crile G. Excision of cancer of the head and neck: with special reference to the plan of dissection based on one hundred and thirty-two operations. JAMA. 1987;258(22):3286-93.
47. Martin H, Del Valle B, Ehrlich H, Cahan WG. Neck dissection. Cancer. 1951;4(3):441-99.
48. Bocca E, Pignataro O. A conservation technique in radical neck dissection. Ann Otol Rhinol Laryngol. 1967;76(5): 975-87.
49. Lindberg R. Distribution of cervical lymph node metastases from squamous cell carcinoma of the upper respiratory and digestive tracts. Cancer. 1972;29(6):1446-9.
50. Shah JP, Andersen PE. The impact of patterns of nodal metastasis on modifications of neck dissection. Ann Surg Oncol. 1994;1(6):521-32.
51. Robbins KT, Shaha AR, Medina JE, Califano JA, Wolf GT, Ferlito A, et al. Consensus statement on the classification and terminology of neck dissection. Arch Otolaryngol Head Neck Surg. 2008;134(5):536-8.
52. Weber RS, Marvel J, Smith P, Hankins P, Wolf P, Goepfert H. Paratracheal lymph node dissection for carcinoma of the larynx, hypopharynx, and cervical esophagus. Otolaryngol Head Neck Surg. 1993;108(1):11-7.
53. Woo JH, Park KN, Lee JY, Lee SW. Predictive factors of superior mediastinal nodal metastasis from papillary thyroid carcinoma—a prospective observational study. PloS One. 2016;11(2): e0148420.
54. Van Wilgen CP, Dijkstra PU, Van der Laan BF, Plukker JT, Roodenburg JL. Shoulder and neck morbidity in quality of life after surgery for head and neck cancer. Head Neck. 2004;26(10):839-44.
55. Rogers SN, Ferlito A, Pellitteri PK, Shaha AR, Rinaldo A. Quality of life following neck dissections. Acta Otolaryngol. 2004;124(3):231-6.
56. Remmler D, Byers R, Scheetz J, Shell B, White G, Zimmerman S, et al. A prospective study of shoulder disability resulting from radical and modified neck dissections. Head Neck Surg. 1986;8(4):280-6.
57. El Ghani F, Van Den Brekel MW, De Goede CJ, Kuik J, Leemans CR, Smeele LE. Shoulder function and patient well-being after various types of neck dissections. Clin Otolaryngol Allied Sci. 2002;27(5):403-8.
58. Erisen L, Basel B, Irdesel J, Zarifoglu M, Coskun H, Basut O, et al. Shoulder function after accessory nerve-sparing neck dissections. Head Neck. 2004;26(11):967-71.
59. Van Wilgen CP, Dijkstra PU, van der Laan BF, Plukker JT, Roodenburg JL. Morbidity of the neck after head and neck cancer therapy. Head Neck. 2004;26(9):785-91.
60. Murthy SP, Paderno A, Balasubramanian D. Management of the marginal mandibular nerve during and after neck dissection. Curr Opin Otolaryngol Head Neck Surg. 2019; 27(2):104-9.
61. Riffat F, Buchanan MA, Mahrous AK, Fish BM, Jani P. Oncological safety of the Hayes-Martin manoeuvre in neck dissections for node-positive oropharyngeal squamous cell carcinoma. J Laryngol Otol. 2012;126(10):1045-8.
62. Tirelli G, Marcuzzo AV. Lymph nodes of the perimandibular area and the hazard of the Hayes Martin maneuver in neck dissection. Otolaryngol Head Neck Surg. 2018;159(4):692-7.
63. Dhiwakar M, Nambi GI, Ramanikanth TV. Drain removal and aspiration to treat low output chylous fistula. Eur Arch Otorhinolaryngol. 2014;271(3):561-5.
64. Nussenbaum B, Liu JH, Sinard RJ. Systematic management of chyle fistula: the southwestern experience and review of the literature. Otolaryngol Head Neck Surg. 2000;122(1):31-8.
65. Langford RJ, Daudia AT, Malins TJ. A morphological study of the thoracic duct at the jugulo-subclavian junction. J Craniomaxillofac Surg. 1999;27(2):100-4.
66. Crumley RL, Smith JD. Postoperative chylous fistula prevention and management. Laryngoscope. 1976;86(6):805-13.
67. Delaney SW, Shi H, Shokrani A, Sinha UK. Management of chyle leak after head and neck surgery: review of current treatment strategies. Int J Otolaryngol. 2017;2017:8362874.
68. Ven BK. Venous outflow of the brain after bilateral complete jugular ligation. Turk Neurosurg. 2008;18(1):56-60.
69. Cho JH, Lee YS, Sun DI, Kim MS, Cho KJ, Nam IC, et al. Prognostic impact of lymph node micrometastasis in oral and oropharyngeal squamous cell carcinomas. Head Neck. 2016;38(S1):E1777-82.
70. Chung MK, Lee GJ, Choi N, Cho JK, Jeong HS, Baek CH. Comparative study of sentinel lymph node biopsy in clinically N0 oral tongue squamous cell carcinoma: long-term oncologic outcomes between validation and application phases. Oral Oncol. 2015;51(10):914-20.
71. Liu M, Wang SJ, Yang X, Peng H. Diagnostic efficacy of sentinel lymph node biopsy in early oral squamous cell carcinoma: a meta-analysis of 66 studies. PLoS One. 2017;12(1):e0170322.
72. Hernando J, Villarreal P, Álvarez-Marcos F, García-Consuegra L, Gallego L, et al. Sentinel node biopsy versus elective neck dissection. Which is more cost-effective? A prospective observational study. J Craniomaxillofac Surg. 2016;44(5):550-6.
73. van der Linden N, Flach GB, de Bree R, Uyl-de Groot CA. Cost-utility of sentinel lymph node biopsy in cT1-T2N0 oral cancer. Oral Oncol. 2016;53:20-6.
74. Fan SF, Zeng ZY, Peng HW, Guo ZM, Wang SL, Zhang Q. Sentinel lymph node biopsy versus elective neck dissection in patients with cT1-2N0 oral tongue squamous cell carcinoma. Oral Surg Oral Med Oral Pathol Oral Radiol. 2014;117(2):186-90.
75. Schilling C, Stoeckli SJ, Vigili MG, de Bree R, Lai SY, Alvarez J, et al. Surgical consensus guidelines on sentinel node biopsy (SNB) in patients with oral cancer. Head Neck. 2019;41(8): 2655-64.
76. Weiss MH, Harrison LB, Isaacs RS. Use of decision analysis in planning a management strategy for the stage N0 neck. Arch Otolaryngol Head Neck Surg. 1994;120(7):699-702.
77. Huang SH, Hwang D, Lockwood G, Goldstein DP, O'Sullivan B. Predictive value of tumor thickness for cervical lymph-node involvement in squamous cell carcinoma of the oral cavity: a meta-analysis of reported studies. Cancer. 2009;115(7):1489-97.

78. D'Cruz AK, Vaish R, Kapre N, Dandekar M, Gupta S, Hawaldar R, et al. Elective versus therapeutic neck dissection in node-negative oral cancer. N Engl J Med. 2015;373(6): 521-9.
79. Ren ZH, Xu JL, Li B, Fan TF, Ji T, Zhang CP. Elective versus therapeutic neck dissection in node-negative oral cancer: evidence from five randomized controlled trials. Oral Oncol. 2015;51(11):976-81.
80. Byers RM, Weber RS, Andrews T, McGill D, Kare R, Wolf P. Frequency and therapeutic implications of "skip metastases" in the neck from squamous carcinoma of the oral tongue. Head Neck. 1997;19(1):14-9.
81. Pereira RN, Ikeda MK, Andrade RP, Magrin J, Miguel RE, Santos CR, et al. Results of a prospective trial on elective modified radical classical versus supraomohyoid neck dissection in the management of oral squamous carcinoma. Am J Surg. 1998;176(5):422-7.
82. Lea J, Bachar G, Sawka AM, Lakra DC, Gilbert RW, Irish JC, et al. Metastases to level IIb in squamous cell carcinoma of the oral cavity: a systematic review and meta-analysis. Head Neck. 2010;32(2):184-90.
83. Pantvaidya GH, Pal P, Vaidya AD, Pai PS, D'Cruz AK. Prospective study of 583 neck dissections in oral cancers: implications for clinical practice. Head Neck. 2014;36(10): 1503-7.
84. Moore EJ, Olsen KD, Martin EJ. Concurrent neck dissection and transoral robotic surgery. Laryngoscope. 2011;121(3): 541-4.
85. De Almeida JR, Byrd JK, Wu R, Stucken CL, Duvvuri U, Goldstein DP, et al. A systematic review of transoral robotic surgery and radiotherapy for early oropharynx cancer: a systematic review. Laryngoscope. 2014;124(9):2096-102.
86. Möckelmann N, Busch CJ, Münscher A, Knecht R, Lörincz BB. Timing of neck dissection in patients undergoing transoral robotic surgery for head and neck cancer. Eur J Surg Oncol. 2015;41(6):773-8.
87. Sanabria A, Shah JP, Medina JE, Olsen KD, Robbins KT, Silver CE, et al. Incidence of occult lymph node metastasis in primary larynx squamous cell carcinoma, by subsite, T classification and neck level: a systematic review. Cancers (Basel). 2020;12(4):1059.
88. Wee JT, Anderson BO, Corry J, D'Cruz A, Soo KC, Qian CN, et al. Management of the neck after chemoradiotherapy for head and neck cancers in Asia: consensus statement from the Asian Oncology Summit 2009. Lancet Oncol. 2009; 10(11):1086-92.
89. Karakaya E, Yetmen O, Oksuz DC, Dyker KE, Coyle C, Sen M, et al. Outcomes following chemoradiotherapy for N3 head and neck squamous cell carcinoma without a planned neck dissection. Oral Oncol. 2013;49(1):55-9.
90. Mehanna H, Wong WL, McConkey CC, Rahman JK, Robinson M, Hartley AG, et al. PET-CT surveillance versus neck dissection in advanced head and neck cancer. New Engl J Med. 2016;374(15):1444-54.
91. Tupchong L, Phil D, Scott CB, Blitzer PH, Marcial VA, Lowry LD, et al. Randomized study of preoperative versus postoperative radiation therapy in advanced head and neck carcinoma: long-term follow-up of RTOG study 73-03. Int J Radiat Oncol Biol Phys. 1991;20(1):21-8.
92. Peters LJ, Goepfert H, Ang KK, Byers RM, Maor MH, Guillamondegui O, et al. Evaluation of the dose for post-operative radiation therapy of head and neck cancer: first report of a prospective randomized trial. Int J Radiat Oncol Biol Phys. 1993;26(1):3-11.
93. Ang KK, Trotti A, Brown BW, Garden AS, Foote RL, Morrison WH, et al. Randomized trial addressing risk features and time factors of surgery plus radiotherapy in advanced head-and-neck cancer. Int J Radiat Oncol Biol Phys. 2001;51(3):571-8.
94. Laramore GE, Scott CB, Al-Sarraf M, Haselow RE, Ervin TJ, Wheeler R, et al. Adjuvant chemotherapy for resectable squamous cell carcinomas of the head and neck: report on Intergroup Study 0034. Int J Radiat Oncol Biol Phys. 1992;23:705-13.
95. Bernier J, Cooper JS. Chemoradiation after surgery for high-risk head and neck cancer patients: how strong is the evidence? Oncologist. 2005;10(3):215-24.
96. Loré Jr JM, Boulos EJ. Resection and reconstruction of the carotid artery in metastatic squamous cell carcinoma. Am J Surg. 1981;142(4):437-42.
97. Bäck LJ, Aro K, Tapiovaara L, Vikatmaa P, de Bree R, Fernández-Álvarez V, et al. Sacrifice and extracranial reconstruction of the common or internal carotid artery in advanced head and neck carcinoma: Review and meta-analysis. Head Neck. 2018;40(6):1305-20.
98. Paleri V, Urbano TG, Mehanna H, Repanos C, Lancaster J, Roques T, et al. Management of neck metastases in head and neck cancer: United Kingdom National Multidisciplinary Guidelines. J Laryngol Otol. 2016;130(S2):S161-9.

CHAPTER 10

Carcinoma of Unknown Primary

Naveen BS, Sivakumar Vidhyadharan, Samskruthi P Murthy, Narayana Subramaniam

INTRODUCTION

Cancer of unknown primary (CUP), metastatic cervical cancer of unknown primary (MCCUP) or metastasis of unknown origin (MUO) or is an uncommon clinical situation accounting for up to 3–5% of all head neck cancers.[1] It is defined as histological diagnosis of metastasis within the lymph node without detection of a primary tumor. Comes et al. further suggested that for the diagnosis to be established there should be no previous history of any malignancy, no definite symptoms related to specific organ, no clinical, no radiological evidence of primary tumor or cytological proven carcinoma.[2]

Squamous cell carcinoma accounts for about 53–77% of cervical node metastasis, particularly when nodes are present in upper and mid neck.[3-5] Other uncommon histological subtypes include adeno-carcinoma, undifferentiated carcinoma, lymphoma, melanoma and differentiated thyroid malignancies. Anatomically, upper and mid neck nodes have primary in head neck region while lower neck nodes (often the supraclavicular region) have infraclavicular primary and are mainly adenocarcinomas.[6] Most commonly affected nodes are level II, followed by level III and bilateral nodal involvement accounting for less than 10%.[3,5-9] Clinically, majority of the cases are staged N2, with mean node size of 3.5-5 cm.[3,7-11] The average time interval between node appearance and establishing a diagnosis ranges between 2 and 5 months.[3,5,12]

ETIOLOGY

Some of the theories behind development of CUP are as follows:

- Proliferation of squamous elements of branchial remnants within cervical lymph nodes
- Small indolent primary tumors in the tonsil or tongue base not clinically demonstrable may be associated with nodal metastasis
- The primary tumor may have regressed by the time the nodal disease presents due to a good immune response
- Small primary tumors may have a slower growth rate when compared to nodal deposits, or a necrotic primary tumor may have sloughed off

CLINICAL HISTORY

Cancer of unknown primary is mostly commonly seen in men aged 55–65 years old. In the present era, there is an increasing trend of CUP in younger, nonsmoking patients, which is one of the manners in which human papilloma virus (HPV) associated oropharyngeal cancers present.[13] History of hoarse voice, dysphagia, hemoptysis, earache, nasal block, nasal bleeding should be elicited. A history of skin lesions in the head and neck or their removal is important. Current or past usage of tobacco or related products and alcohol consumption should be elicited to determine carcinogen exposure.[3,5,8,9] Exposure to radiation, drug history or previous disease should be also recorded.

CLINICAL EXAMINATION

The location of cervical lymphadenopathy may suggest the possible location of the primary tumor.[6,14] Oral cavity or lip primaries are likely to involve levels I-III, while oropharynx, larynx, hypopharynx and thyroid primaries are likely to involve levels II-IV. Nasopharyngeal primary tumors and cutaneous malignancies need to be ruled out if level V nodes are involved. Bilateral node metastases are common in primaries of the nasopharynx, base tongue and hypopharyngeal primaries.[14] Examination of axilla and inguinal nodes also required examination where generalized lymphadenopathy may occur, such as lymphoma. Examination of the nodal disease comprises size, extent, consistency and potential involvement of adjacent structures, which may help establish a diagnosis or prognosticate the patient.

After detailed examination of the neck, a meticulous evaluation of the head and neck and upper aerodigestive tract is performed. Examination of the scalp is crucial to detect hidden skin cancers. Meticulous examination of the oral cavity and pharynx are performed, which may present with subtle abnormalities such as mucosal thickening, irregularity or leukoplakia. In squamous CUP, the nasopharynx, hypopharynx and oropharynx are often the location of the primary tumor. Flexible endoscopic examination is crucial to thoroughly visualize the fossae within the nasopharynx, the base of tongue and the valleculla, along with the larynx and hypopharynx. The hidden areas that require special attention are the laryngeal surface of the epiglottis, ventricle, subglottis, apex of the pyriform sinus and base of tongue. Specialized maneuvers such as modified Valsalva may enable this. Detailed examination of the oropharynx, with palpation of the tonsils and the base of the tongue are also important, as these primary tumors may be submucosal. Evaluation of the nasal cavity is also a routine part of this examination. A brief but systematic general examination may reveal clinical evidence of metastatic disease, which has a major impact on management.

ESTABLISHING A PATHOLOGICAL DIAGNOSIS

If the initial clinical examination fails to lead to a probable primary site, fine needle aspiration cytology (FNAC) of the nodal mass is the next step in establishing a diagnosis. It is efficient, not very painful, noninvasive and carries negligible risk of tumor seeding.[15] Core biopsy as compared to FNAC requires local anesthesia and has higher risk for bleeding and fistula formation, and is hence reserved for cases where repeated FNACs are nondiagnostic or when a core of tissue is required for immunohistochemical evaluation, such as lymphomas or undifferentiated tumors.[15,16] Ultrasound guidance may not be indicated in a clinically palpable node unless it is cystic or suspicious for necrosis, necessitating representative sampling. Excision biopsy should be attempted only after FNAC, core biopsy and ultrasound-guided biopsies are inconclusive or in patients suspicious for lymphoma,[17] with the incision planned so that the scar can be excised during neck dissection if required subsequently. Immunohistochemistry is often used to differentiate tumor origin, especially when undifferentiated.

In head and neck squamous cell carcinoma (HNSCC), earlier reports suggested local recurrence and poor survival with excision biopsy of nodal metastases,[18,19] however newer reports suggest if biopsy was followed by either radiation or comprehensive neck node dissection with excision of involved scars there was no difference in disease outcomes when compared with those who underwent appropriate primary treatment.[20,21]

RADIOLOGICAL EVALUATION

Contrast-enhanced computed tomography (CECT) scan covering from the base of skull to the thoracic inlet is routinely advised in evaluation of CUP. It has the advantages of being quick and noninvasive with good spatial resolution. It provides information on extent of nodes, extranodal extension and relation of nodes to vital anatomic structures. CECT can be complemented or supplanted by a gadolinium contrast enhanced magnetic resonance imaging (MRI), as it has better soft tissue resolution. The possibility of identifying a primary cancer ranges between 9.3 and 23%[4,22-24] and rises to 60% when radiology directed endoscopic biopsy is taken from suspicious sites.[17] However with increased availability of PET scan, isolated use of CT/MRI scan is diminishing in this context.

Misdiagnosis of malignant cysts in the neck may cause delay in diagnosis, a violated neck, tumor spillage, and spread. Differences in radiographic criteria can guide clinical decision-making in the patient with a neck mass. A study by Goyal et al. indicated that the CT characteristics of branchial cleft cysts varied considerably from those of cystic lymph node metastases. Branchial cleft cysts have a tendency to be more homogeneous and larger and unlikely are to exhibit septations or extranodal extension, in contrast with metastatic lymph nodes.[25] However, an FNA is necessary to confirm the diagnosis. Som et al. explained imaging features that are frequently observed with metastatic nodes, namely central necrosis, nodal grouping, and size of the nodules.[26]

Curtin et al. performed a multi-institutional study to ascertain the sensitivity and specificity of several size and radiographic criteria that regulate nodal metastasis and showed that CT functioned better than MRI, and there was 84% negative predictive value and 50% positive predictive value using a size criterion of 1 cm or the presence of an internal abnormality. They also reported that exploiting internal abnormality with size did not significantly improve sensitivity or specificity.[27] It is also to be noted that branchial cleft cysts are likely to be larger, and this correlates with the low positive predictive value linked with size criteria. There was a significant divergence in the age distribution of the two populations, with those having branchial cleft cysts being much younger than those having malignancy. In evaluating cystic masses, it is crucial not only to have a high suspicion for malignancy but also to be able to exclude masses that are congenital or secondary to inflammation or infection. It is especially important among the non-smoking population of under 40 years old, because the incidence of a malignant lymph node imitating a benign neck mass is higher.[25,27]

Positron Emission Tomography

Positron emission tomography (PET) has a routine role in staging, assessing treatment response and in disease surveillance. In case of failure to identify origin based clinical and cytological examination, PET in combination with CECT (PET-CT) is an apt investigation to identification the primary tumor, extent of disease, and distant metastasis, often altering the course and intent of treatment.[28] The advantage of PET-CT scan over other imaging modalities is that it is a single stage procedure that covers the full body. Apart from detecting disease, it yields functional and prognostic information. Rushthoven et al. in their meta-analysis reported a primary tumor detection rate with PET-CT of 25%.[29] A more recent study by Kwee et al. reported a primary tumor detection rate of 37%,[26,30] with both studies suggesting high false positive rate for oropharyngeal primaries. Al-Ibraheem et al. suggested primary detection rate of 28.3% with false positive rates of about 37%.[31] Potential drawbacks of PET scan include higher false positive rates, exposure to radiation and poor identification of small primaries (<5 mm). The likelihood of a primary to appear subsequently after a negative PET-CT and pan endoscopy is around 6%,[32] reiterating the high negative predictive value of PET-CT of about 86%, with an overall accuracy of 69% and positive predictive value of 56%.[32]

Narrow Band Imaging

Narrow band imaging (NBI) endoscopy is useful for detecting primary tumors in patients of CUP, particularly for superficial and small carcinomas of the upper aerodigestive tract. Hayashi T et al. reported that an identification rate of 35% with a true positive rate of 64% when NBI was used in the context of CUP.[33] Ryu et al. showed that NBI endoscopy detected occult primary tumors in 13.3% of patients with squamous CUP, with the identified primary tumor and nodal disease appearing histologically similar.[34]

A distinct brown region and an irregular microvascular pattern on NBI are characteristic features of superficial HNSCC. Ryu et al. also established that use of NBI imaging criteria ruled out malignancy in 80% of ambivalent lesions, and could have a role in reducing unnecessary biopsies and wastage of time. It is also shown to be cost-effective relatively to other diagnostic imaging techniques such as CT, MRI, and PET-CT.[33,34]

Panendoscopy and Biopsy

Thorough evaluation of nasopharynx, oral cavity, oropharynx, larynx, hypopharynx and esophagus is performed under general anesthesia when office examination yields no information. Cianchetti reported successful identification of primary in about 29% after other initial modalities failed to identify primary tumors.[17] Mendenhall reported a positive yield of 17% when there was no clinical or radiological evidence of malignancy, with figures increasing to 56% and 58% when either radiological or clinically suspected sites were biopsied.[35]

Another directed procedure, ipsilateral tonsillectomy, yielded tumor detection rates of 18–44.6%.[10,36] Waltonen et al. showed tonsillectomy resulted in a higher rate of detecting occult tumors when compared to deep tonsil biopsies in the absence of visible or palpable lesions (29.5% and 3.2% respectively).[37] Evidence supporting bilateral tonsillectomy is less convincing, with tumor detection rates varying from 10 to 23%.[38,39] Although most series discussing this subject do not include ipsilateral tonsillectomy in their diagnostic protocol, many authors recommend removal of the entire tonsil as part of the diagnostic workup. This allows focused therapy, reduced morbidity, and improved follow-up. In the case of previous tonsillectomy, any residual tonsil tissue should be removed (if present), or the tonsil fossa should be biopsied. Lapeyre et al. found carcinoma in 26% of tonsil specimen after tonsillectomies.[40] Identifying a tonsillar primary has major advantage over treating the patient for CUP, which is the reduction in the field of radiotherapy and resultant treatment-related morbidity.[41] This is because radiation fields in a tonsil cancer regimen do not regularly include the nasopharynx and most of the parotid gland can be shielded. The contralateral tonsil will also be spared since the treatment volume is adjusted just to treat the ipsilateral tonsil. In the case of true CUP, treatment encompasses coverage of the at-risk mucosa (nasopharynx, oropharynx, hypopharynx) to 60 Gy using opposed lateral ports, creating substantial xerostomia.[41]

Dziegielewski et al. in their retrospective review of patients who underwent transoral robotic surgery (TORS) for known tonsillar cancer found that 10% of the patients had synchronous bilateral HPV+ SCC of the tonsil on final histopathology, which were not detected on clinical examination or PET-CT. They opined that this may be becuase contralateral tonsillar tumors may be more indolent or missed on imaging, and recommended that all patients undergoing primary TORS for tonsillar squamous cell carcinoma require a contralateral tonsillectomy to obtain a definitive tissue diagnosis.[42]

It has been argued that routine contralateral tonsillectomy does not appear to increase rates of morbidity or complications, and the subsequent symmetric palatal arch could supposedly enhance cancer surveillance and identification of recurrence.[43] Rokkjaer et al. performed a retrospective review concluding that bilateral tonsillectomy must be recommended in all patients with suspected or biopsy-proven unilateral or bilateral tonsillar SCC and in patients with CUP,[44] however this view is still controversial. It is also imperative to note that these findings reflect a population where HPV-related cancers predominant and cannot be extrapolated to a population where tobacco related cancers predominate. **Flowchart 1** shows approach to CUP using TORS.

In the situations where either the results of multiple FNACs followed by a core-needle biopsy are inconclusive, or when a neck lump is clinically and histologically doubtful for lymphoma, an open cervical lymph node biopsy must be performed to obtain adequate tissue for a conclusive result. Also, among 92% of patients with malignant lymphoma, an ultrasound-guided core needle biopsy is a substitute to an open biopsy, wherein complete subclassification of the lymphoma is achievable.[45,46] Martin et al. and other researchers stated that open biopsy was a needless procedure because

Flowchart 1: Intraoperative decision-making algorithm for cancer of unknown primary (CUP) treated with transoral robotic surgery (TORS).

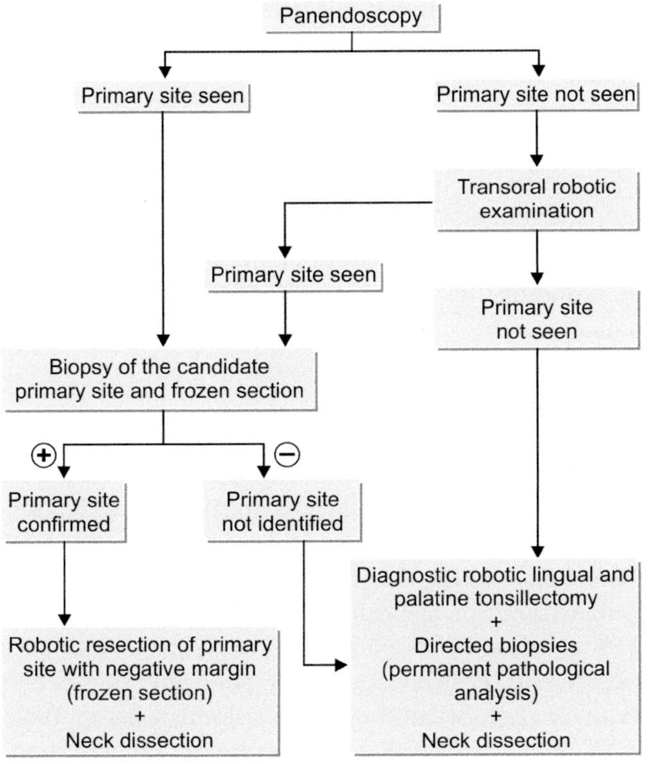

of its probability of recurrence, high rates of local complications and systemic spread.[18,19,47] However, later studies reported no worsening of regional neck control or survival following open neck node biopsy.[20,21,48] It is imperative, however, that an open neck node biopsy must not be implemented prior to an undertaking of a comprehensive clinical, radiological, and endoscopic examination for the primary tumor.[45]

Along with panendoscopy, directed biopsies, and PET-CT, the feasibility and efficiency of using either TORS or transoral laser microsurgery (TLM) in the diagnosis and management of CUP in the head and neck have been established. In a select group of patients, application of either TORS or TLM during an examination under anesthesia, both detects and treats the primary and may also reduce the number of patients requiring wide-field irradiation.[49-51] Despite thorough evaluation, 2–8% of patients with cervical metastases ultimately have no primary tumor site identified.

Molecular Studies

Human papilloma virus and Epstein-Barr virus (EBV) has been studied and found to be associated with oropharyngeal and nasopharyngeal cancers, respectively. Begum et al. have demonstrated HPV 16 virus in metastatic nodes and from primary oropharynx malignancy using in situ hybridization (ISH).[52] Desai et al. similarly reported presence of HPV virus using polymerase chain reaction with high positivity of about 44.4% with oropharyngeal primaries.[53] EBV has been proven to cause undifferentiated nasopharyngeal cancers. Sensitivity and specificity of about 90% have been reported for EBV detection in FNAC samples.[54,55] ISH is more sensitive and specific than PCR in detecting EBV;[56] sensitivity and specificity of using circulating EBV DNA for detecting nasopharyngeal cancer with PCR are about 96% and 93%, respectively.[57] Micro-RNA (miRNA) is involved in regulating pathways associated with development, differentiation and tumorigenesis.[58] Barker et al. also hypothesized that their expression determined by PCR could predict site of metastatic disease.[59] Other molecular methods still under development are image cytometry and fluorescence-guided screening and evaluation in detection of primary tumors.[60,61]

Zhang et al. investigated the prospect of defining the site of the primary tumors by identifying HPV-related carcinomas, by using ISH and morphology in metastatic cervical lymph nodes. They were able to identify high-risk HPV by ISH, using ethanol-fixed and Papanicolaou-stained smears from FNA biopsies. They reported that nonkeratinizing SCC in metastatic cervical lymph nodes predicted positive HPV-ISH and was strongly suggestive of an oropharyngeal primary tumor. The presence of nonkeratinizing SCC correlated well with HPV positivity; 70% of them were HPV positive while only 15% of keratinizing SCC were HPV positive.[62]

Begum et al. showed HPV16-ISH outcomes from 77 FNA biopsies paraffin-embedded, formalin-fixed cell block sections. Although tumors of nonoropharyngeal origin were negative, they detected HPV16 DNA integration in 10 of 19 oropharyngeal carcinomas and in 3 of 10 squamous cancers with unknown primary.[52-63] The role of HPV in nonoropharyngeal cancers is less clear; Umudum et al. reported HPV DNA integration in one patient with a nasopharyngeal primary and in 1 patient with an oral cavity primary, after performing HPV-ISH with ethanol-fixed smears on 11 cervical lymph nodes with metastatic HNSCC.[64]

Assessing Distant Metastasis

To establish the intent of treatment it is necessary to rule out distant metastasis. Reports suggest distant metastasis in about 14% of patients with MCCUP.[4] The most routinely used modality is CT thorax. A low sensitivity and specificity in detecting systemic metastases (73% and 80%) paved the way for routine use of PET-CT. Xu et al. compared PET and PET-CT for initial systemic assessment of patients with head neck cancer and concluded that PET-CT tends to have higher diagnostic accuracy.[65]

Prognostically CUP can be classified into two groups **(Table 1)**, with a majority falling within the poor-risk CUP group, representing adenocarcinoma metastasizing to bone, brain, and/or viscera.[45,66] Absolute responses are rarely observed with median survival ranges between 7 and 11 months with platinum-based combination chemotherapy regimens, with or without new generation cytotoxic drugs.[6,67] Of the 15–20% of patients with CUPs within the favorable prognostic subgroup, the biological behavior of the metastatic disease is akin to other major known tumor types (for example, germ cell tumors, adenocarcinoma of the breast or ovary, or squamous cell carcinoma of head and neck). Histologically, SCC accounts for three-fourths of patients, but other tissue types such as adenocarcinoma, undifferentiated carcinoma, lymphoma, melanoma, papillary thyroid carcinoma, and central nervous system tumors should be considered.[7,45]

Table 1: Cancer of unknown primary prognostic grouping.[45]

Group/tumor type	*Frequency*	*Survival*
Favorable prognosis • Extragonadal germ cell syndrome • Metastatic adenocarcinoma • Head and neck squamous cell carcinoma	15–20%	Variable, potentially curable in the absence of distant metastases
Unfavorable prognosis • Adenocarcinoma metastatic to bone, brain or viscera	80–90%	Poor median survival of 7–11 months

MANAGEMENT

Treatment should be based on the outcomes of diagnostic evaluation. If a primary tumor is found, then management is as per guidelines related to the specific subsite. The guidelines below refer to treatment for carcinoma of an unknown primary (histologically SCC).

Surgery, radiotherapy or chemoradiotherapy remain the main stay of treatment. For early stage disease single modality either surgery or radiation is adequate with adjuvant chemoradiotherapy reserved for extranodal extension.[52] Treatment-related morbidity is an important determinant of treatment, especially in the context of wide field mucosal irradiation. 5-year disease free survival is about 85% and 58% in disease single node involvement and multiple node involvement respectively, emphasizing the role of multimodality treatment in advanced disease. Response assessment should be performed and surgery (planned/salvage neck dissection) should be reserved for patients showing partial response or residual disease after chemoradiotherapy for advanced disease.[52] Treatment recommendations for squamous cell carcinoma of an unknown primary are summarized here.[68]

T0N1

Irrespective of the type of primary treatment these patients usually fare well. A majority of the patients will either undergo either a neck dissection alone or radiation therapy alone, both of which give good outcomes.

T0N2a

This is the most common stage in which patients with CUP usually present. Those with a favorable risk factor profile (p16+, smoking history <10 pack-years, with absent clinical and/or radiographic evidence of extranodal extension) could undergo single modality treatment with surgery or radiotherapy alone. Patient who are p16- or p16+with associated smoking history >10 pack-years could receive surgery with adjuvant radiotherapy. Primary chemoradiotherapy is administered to T0N2a patients with clinical and/or radiographic extranodal extension. Neck dissection as a primary treatment modality in the presence of extranodal extension is not warranted, as adjuvant chemoradiotherapy would likely be required, resulting in treatment with three modalities instead of two, with the concomitant additional treatment-related morbidity. Hence primary chemoradiotherapy without prior surgery is adequate. Among patients in whom a complete metabolic response is not achieved as determined by PET-CT after 10–12 weeks of completing treatment, a salvage neck dissection is indicated.

T0N3

This stage is another common presentation of squamous cell carcinoma of an unknown primary that should be managed with primary chemoradiotherapy because N3 nodes are likely to have extranodal extension. Alternatively, patients can be treated with a neck dissection followed by adjuvant radiation, provided there is no suspicion of extranodal extension on imaging or physical examination. However this is an unlikely scenario as histopathology is likely to reveal extranodal extension, necessitating adjuvant chemoradiotherapy. Patients must be treated with primary chemoradiotherapy if clinical or radiographic examinations are strongly suggestive of extranodal extension. Data is absent with regards to different treatment regimens for microscopic extranodal extension on a p16+ pathology report. In most centers, the standard of care is to also radiate the contralateral neck and probable mucosal subsite.[68]

Additional Considerations

Surgery

After thorough workup, a patient with a single, mobile node <3 cm in diameter may undergo surgery as the only modality. The type of neck dissection depends based on the location of node, however selective neck node dissection should suffice. Jesse et al. in their largest series of 104 patients reported 13% recurrence with N1 disease in ipsilateral side and 32% for patients with N2-3 disease.[69] Data shows that mucosal progression and contralateral neck failure are uncommon in low-risk patients even without adjuvant radiotherapy.[7,70-73]

Irradiation Fields

The potential benefit versus morbidity should be weighed when opting for bilateral neck radiation. Suspected tumor in nasopharynx, base of tongue, multiple neck nodes, N3 nodes having risk of higher chances of contralateral nodes metastasis should be considered for bilateral radiation. Nieder et al. reported better regional control after nodal resection followed by adjuvant bilateral neck radiation.[74] On the contrary, other studies have reported no benefit from more extensive radiation.[7,9,75,76] Neider reported mucosal primary appearance rates of 8% for unilateral radiotherapy and 9.5% after bilateral radiotherapy.[49] Sinnathamby concluded that after thorough workup, the chance of missing a primary is small and most emerging primary lesions are unrelated to the index tumor, debating the role of elective mucosal radiation.[77] Intensity modulated radiotherapy is preferred if total mucosal irradiation is contemplated as it has good control rates and less toxicity than with conventional techniques.[78] Preliminary data has shown that pharyngeal sparing radiotherapy when diagnostic TORS has helped rule out an oropharyngeal primary may reduce morbidity without compromising local control, but any deviations from standard recommendations require multidisciplinary consensus and careful consideration.[79]

CONCLUSION

Cancer of unknown primary is an uncommon occurrence but is a challenging scenario that requires high-quality multidisciplinary care to balance disease control with morbidity. Recent advances have allowed more focused and accurate detection of the primary tumor. It is important to refine treatment protocols in CUP through more robust prognostication and understanding individual patient perspectives and expectations from treatment.

REFERENCES

1. Talmi YP, Wolf GT, Hazuka M, Krause CJ. Unknown primary of the head and neck. J Laryngol Otol. 1996;110:353-6.
2. Comes MS, Beahrs OH, Dockerty MB. Cervical metastasis from occult carcinoma. Surg Gynecol Obstet. 1957;104:607-13.
3. Strojan P, Anicin A. Combined surgery and postoperative radiotherapy for cervical node metastasis from unknown primary tumour. Radiother Oncol. 1998;49:33-40.
4. Regelink G, Brouwer J, de Bree R, Pruim J, van der Laan BF, Vaalburg W, et al. Detection of unknown primary tumours and distant metastases in patients with cervical metastases: value of FDG-PET versus conventional modalities. Eur J Nucl Med Mol Imaging. 2002;29:1024-30.
5. Issing WJ, Taleban B, Tauber S. Diagnosis and management of carcinoma of unknown primary in the head and neck. Eur Arch Otorhinolaryngol. 2003;260:436-43.
6. Saha AR, Rinaldo A, Ferlito A. Metastatic squamous carcinoma in the neck from an occult primary. In: Ferlito A, Robbins KT, Silver CE (Eds). Neck dissection management of regional disease in head and neck cancer. San Diego: Plural Publishing; 2010. pp. 307-17.
7. Grau C, Johansen LV, Jakobsen J, Geertsen P, Andersen E, Jensen BB. Cervical lymph node metastases from unknown primary tumours: results from a national survey by the Danish Society for Head and Neck Oncology. Radiother Oncol. 2000;55:121-9.
8. Aslani M, Sultanem K, Young T, Hier M, Niazi T, Shenouda G. Metastatic carcinoma to the cervical nodes from an unknown

head and neck primary site: is there a need for neck dissection? Head Neck. 2007;29:585-90.
9. Ligey A, Gentil J, Crehange G, Montbarbon X, Pommier P, Peignaux K, et al. Impact of target volumes and radiation technique on loco-regional control and survival for patients with unilateral cervical node metastasis from an unknown primary. Radiother Oncol. 2009;93:483-7.
10. Boscolo-Rizzo P, Da mosto MC, Gava A, Marchiori C. Cervical lymph node metastasis from occult squamous cell carcinoma: analysis of 82 cases. ORL J Otorhinolaryngol Relat Spec. 2006;68:189-94.
11. Chen AM, Farwell DG, Lau DH, Li BQ, Luu Q, Donald PJ. Radiation therapy in the management of head neck cancer of unknown primary origin: how does the addition of concurrent chemotherapy affect the therapeutic ratio? Int J Radiat Oncol Bio Phys. 2011;81(2):346-52.
12. Nguyen C, Shenuda G, Black MJ, Voung T, Donath D, Yassa M. Metastatic squamous cell carcinoma to the cervical lymph nodes from unknown primary mucosal sites. Head Neck. 1994;16:58-63.
13. D'souza G, Zhang HH, D'souza WD, Meyer RR, Gillison ML. Moderate predictive value of demographic and behavioural characteristics for a diagnosis of HPV16 positive and HPV 16 negative head and neck cancer. Oral Oncol. 2010;46:100-4.
14. Werner JA, Dunne AA, Myeers JN. Functional anatomy of the lymphatic drainage system of the upper aerodigestive tract and its role in metastasis of squamous cell carcinoma. Head Neck. 2003;25:322-32.
15. Layfield LJ. Fine needle aspiration in the diagnosis of head and neck lesions: a review and discussion of problems in differential diagnosis. Diag Cytopatol. 2007;35:798-805.
16. Pfeiffer J, Kayser L, Ridder GJ. Minimal-invasive core, needle biopsy of head and neck malignancies: clinical evaluation for radiation oncology. Radiother Oncol. 2009;90:202-7.
17. Cianchetti M, Mancuso AA, Amdur RJ, Werning JW, Kirwan J, Morris CG, et al. Diagnostic evaluation of squamous cell carcinoma metastatic to cervical lymph nodes from an unknown primary site. Laryngoscope. 2009;119:2348-54.
18. Mcguirt WF, Mccabe BF. Significance of node biopsy before definitive treatment of cervical metastatic carcinoma. Laryngoscope. 1978;88:594-7.
19. Ikeda Y, Kubota A, Furukawa M, Tsukuda M. Cervical lymph node metastasis from an unknown primary tumour. Nippon Jibiinkoka Gakkai Kaiho. 2000;103:524-8.
20. Robbins KT, Cole R, Marvel J, Fields R, Wolf P, Goepfert H. The violated neck: cervical node biopsy prior to definitive treatment. Otolaryngol Head Neck Surg. 1986;94:605-10.
21. Ellis ER, Mendenhall WM, Rao PV, McCarty PJ, Parsons JT, Stringer SP, et al. Incisional or excisional neck node biopsy before definitive radiotherapy alone or followed by neck dissection. Head Neck. 1991;13:177-83.
22. Waltonen JD, Ozer E, Hall NC, Schuller DE, Agrawal A. Metastatic carcinoma of the neck of unknown primary origin: evaluation and efficacy of the modern workup. Arch Otolaryngol Head Neck Surg. 2009;135:1024-9.
23. Muraki AS, Mancuso AA, Harnsberger HR. Metastatic cervical adenopathy from tumours of unknown origin: the role of CT. Radiology. 1984;152:749-53.
24. Freudenberg LS, Fischer M, Antoch G, Jentzen W, Gutzeit A, Rosenbaum SJ, et al. Dual modality of 18 F-fluorodeoxyglucose-positron emission tomography/computed tomography in patients with cervical carcinoma of unknown primary. Med Princ Pract. 2005;14:155-60.
25. Goyal N, Zacharia TT, Goldenberg D. Differentiation of branchial cleft cysts and malignant cystic adenopathy of pharyngeal origin. Am J Roentgenol. 2012;199(2):W216-21.
26. Som PM. Detection of metastasis in cervical lymph nodes: CT and MRI criteria and differential diagnosis. Am J Roentgenol. 1992;158:961-9
27. Curtin HD, Ishwaran H, Mancuso AA, Dalley RW, Caudry DJ, McNeil BJ. Comparison of CT and MR imaging in staging of neck metastases. Radiology. 1998;207:123-30.
28. Wong WL, Saunders M. The impact of FDG PET on the management of occult primary head neck tumours. Clin Oncol. 2003;15:461-6.
29. Rusthoven KE, Koshy M, Paulino AC. The role of fluorodeoxyglucose positron emission tomography in cervical lymph node metastases from an unknown primary tumour. Cancer. 2004;101:2641-9.
30. Kwee TC, Kwee RM. Combined FDG-PET/CT for the detection of unknown primary tumours: systematic review and meta-analysis. Eur Radiol. 2009;19:731-44.
31. Al-Ibraheem A, Buck A, Krause BJ, Scheidhauer N. Clinical applications of FDG PET and PET/CT in head and neck cancer. J Oncol. 2009;2009:208725.
32. Miller FR, Karnad AB, Eng T, Hussey DH, Mc Guff HS, Otto RA. Management of the unknown primary carcinoma: long term follow-up on a negative PET scan and negative panendoscopy. Head Neck. 2008;30:28-34.
33. Hayashi T, Muto M, Hayashi R, Minashi K, Yano T, Kishimoto S, et al. Usefulness of narrow-band imaging for detecting the primary tumor site in patients with primary unknown cervical lymph node metastasis. Jpn J Clin Oncol. 2010;40(6):537-41.
34. Ryu IS, Choi SH, Kim DH, Han MW, Roh JL, Kim SY, et al. Detection of the primary lesion in patients with cervical metastases from unknown primary tumors with narrow band imaging endoscopy: preliminary report. Head Neck. 2013;35(1):10-4.
35. Mendenhall WM, Mancuso AA, Amdur RJ, Stringer SP, Villaret DB, Cassisi NJ. Squamous cell carcinoma metastatic to the neck from an unknown head and neck primary site. Am J Otolaryngol. 2001;22:261-7.
36. Haas I, Hoffmann TK, Engers R, Ganzer U. Diagnostic strategies in cervical carcinoma of unknown primary (CUP). Eur Arch Otorhinolaryngol. 2002;259:325-33.
37. Waltonen JD, Ozer E, Schuller DE, Agarwal A. Tonsillectomy vs deep tonsil biopsies in detecting occult tonsil tumours. Laryngoscope. 2009;119:102-6.
38. Koch WM, Bhatti N, Williams MF, Eisele DW. Oncologic rationale for bilateral tonsillectomy in head and neck squamous cell carcinoma of unknown primary source. Otolryngol Head Neck Surg. 2001;124:331-3.
39. Kothari P, Randhawa PS, Farrell R. Role of tonsillectomy in the search for a squamous cell carcinoma from an unknown primary in the head and neck. Br J Oral Maxillofac Surg. 2008;46:283-7.
40. Lapeyre M, Malissard L, Peiffert D, Hoffstetter S, Toussaint B, Renier S, et al. Cervical lymph node metastasis from an unknown primary: is a tonsillectomy necessary? Int J Radiation Oncology Biol Phys. 1997;39:291-6.
41. Randall DA, Johnstone PA, Foss RD, Martin PJ. Tonsillectomy in diagnosis of the unknown primary tumor of the head and neck. Otolaryngol Head Neck Surg. 2000;122(1):52-5.
42. Dziegielewski PT, Boyce BJ, Old M, Teknos TN, Agrawal A, Patwa H, et al. Transoral robotic surgery for tonsillar cancer: addressing the contralateral tonsil. Head Neck. 2017;39:2224-31.
43. Kim CM, St John MA. Should the contralateral tonsil be removed in cases of HPV-positive squamous cell carcinoma of the tonsil? Laryngoscope. 2019;129(6):1257-8.

44. Rokkjaer MS, Klug TE. Prevalence of synchronous bilateral tonsil squamous cell carcinoma: a retrospective study. Clin Otolaryngol. 2018;43:1-6.
45. Strojan P, Ferlito A, Medina JE, Woolgar JA, Rinaldo A, Robbins KT, et al. Contemporary management of lymph node metastases from an unknown primary to the neck: I. A review of diagnostic approaches. Head Neck. 2013;35(1):123-32.
46. Pfeiffer J, Kayser G, Ridder GJ. Sonography-assisted cutting needle biopsy in the head and neck for the diagnosis of lymphoma: can it replace lymph node extirpation? Laryngoscope. 2009;119:689-95.
47. Martin H, Morfit HM. Cervical lymph node metastasis as the first symptom of cancer. Surg Gynecol Obstet. 1944;78:133-59.
48. Colletier PJ, Garden AS, Morrison WH, Goepfert H, Geara F, Ang KK. Postoperative radiation for squamous cell carcinoma metastatic to cervical lymph nodes from an unknown primary site: outcomes and patterns of failure. Head Neck. 1998;20:674-81.
49. Durmus K, Rangarajan SV, Old MO, Agrawal A, Teknos TN, Ozer E. Transoral robotic approach to carcinoma of unknown primary. Head Neck. 2014;36(6):848-52.
50. Nagel TH, Hinni ML, Hayden RE, Lott DG. Transoral laser microsurgery for the unknown primary: role for lingual tonsillectomy. Head Neck. 2014;36(7):942-6.
51. Karni RJ, Rich JT, Sinha P, Haughey BH. Transoral laser microsurgery: a new approach for unknown primaries of the head and neck. Laryngoscope. 2011;121(6):1194-201.
52. Begum S, Gillison ML, Ansari-Lari MA, Shah K, Westra WH. Detection of human papillomavirus in cervical lymph nodes: a highly effective strategy for localizing site of tumor origin. Clin Cancer Res. 2003;9(17):6469-75.
53. Desai PC, Jaglal MV, Gopal P, Ghim SJ, Miller DM, Farghaly H, et al. Human papilloma virus in metastatic squamous carcinoma from unknown primaries in the head and neck: Retrospective 7 year study. Exp Mol Pathol. 2009;87:94-8.
54. Macdonald MR, Freeman JL, Hui MF, Cheung RK, Warde P, McIvor NP, et al. Role of Epstein-Barr virus in fine needle aspirates of metastatic neck nodes in the diagnosis of nasopharyngeal carcinoma. Head Neck. 1995;17:487-93.
55. Lei ZX, Liu QR, Yuan P. Detection of Epstein-Barr virus DNA in fine needle aspiration specimen from cervical lymph nodes with polymerase chain reaction. Lin Chuang Er Bi Yan Hou Ke Za Zhi. 2000;14:454-5.
56. Lee WY, Hsiao JR, Jin YT, Tsai ST. Epstein-Barr virus detection in neck metastases by in-situ hybridization in fine-needle aspiration cytologic studies: an aid for differentiating the primary site. Head Neck. 2000;22:336-40.
57. Chan KC, Lo YM. Circulating EBV DNA as a tumour marker for nasopharyngeal carcinoma. Semin Cancer Biol. 2002;12:489-96.
58. Lin JC, Wang WY, Chen KY, Wei YH, Liang WM, Jan JS, et al. Quantification of plasma Epstein-Barr virus DNA in patients with advanced nasopharyngeal carcinoma. N Engl J Med. 2004;350:2461-70.
59. Barker EV, Cervigne NK, Reis PP, Goswami RS, Xu W, Weinreb I, et al. Micro RNA evaluation of unknown primary lesions in the head and neck. Mol Cancer. 2009;8:127.
60. Palcic B. Nuclear texture: can it be used as a surrogate endpoint marker? J Cell Biochem Suppl. 1994;19:40-6.
61. Kulapaditharom B, Boonkitticharoen V, Kunachak S. Fluorescence-guided biopsy in the diagnosis of an unknown primary cancer in patients with metastatic cervical lymph nodes. Ann Otol Rhinol Laryngol. 1999;108:700-4.
62. Zhang MQ, El-Mofty SK, Dávila RM. Detection of human papillomavirus-related squamous cell carcinoma cytologically and by in situ hybridization in fine-needle aspiration biopsies of cervical metastasis. A tool for identifying the site of an occult head and neck primary. Cancer (Cancer Cytopathol). 2008;114:118-23.
63. Begum S, Gillison M, Nicol TL, Westra WH. Detection of human papillomavirus-16 in fine-needle aspirates to determine tumor origin in patients with metastatic squamous cell carcinoma of the head and neck. Clin Cancer Res. 2007;13:1186-91.
64. Umudum H, Rezanko T, Dag F, Dogruluk T. Human papillomavirus genome detection by in situ hybridization in fine-needle aspirates of metastatic lesions from head and neck squamous cell carcinomas. Cancer. 2005;105:171-7.
65. Xu GZ, Zhu XD, Li MY. Accuracy of whole body PET and PET CT in initial M staging of head neck cancer: a meta-analysis. Head Neck. 2011;33:87-94.
66. Pentheroudakis G, Briasoulis E, Pavlidis N. Cancer of unknown primary site: missing primary or missing biology? Oncologist. 2007;12:418-25.
67. Golfinopoulos V, Pentheroudakis G, Salanti G, Nearchou AD, Ioannidis JP, Pavlidis N. Comparative survival with diverse chemotherapy regimens for cancer of unknown primary site: multiple-treatments meta-analysis. Cancer Treat Rev. 2009;35:570-3.
68. Galloway TJ, Ridge JA. Management of squamous cancer metastatic to cervical nodes with an unknown primary site. J Clin Oncol. 2015;33(29):3328-37.
69. Jesse RH, Perez CA, Fletcher GH. Cervical lymph node metastasis: unknown primary cancer. Cancer. 1973;31:854-9.
70. Wang RC, Goepfert H, Barber AE, Wolf P. Unknown primary squamous cell carcinoma metastatic to the neck. Arch Otolaryngol Head Neck Surg. 1990;116:1388-93.
71. Iganej S, Kagan R, Anderson P, Rao A, Tome M, Wang R, et al. Metastatic squamous cell carcinoma of the neck from an unknown primary: management options and patterns of relapse. Head Neck. 2002;24:236-46.
72. Coker DD, Casterline PF, Chambers RG, Jaques DA. Metastasis to lymph nodes of the head and neck from an unknown primary site. Am J Surg. 1977;134:517-22.
73. Coster JR, Foote RL, Olsen KD, Jack SM, Schaid DJ, DeSanto LW. Cervical nodal metastasis of squamous cell carcinoma of unknown origin: indications for withholding radiation therapy. Int J Radiat Biol Phys. 1992;23:743-9.
74. Nieder C, Gregoire V, Ang KK. Cervical lymph node metastases from occult squamous cell carcinoma: cut down a tree to get an apple? Int J Radiat Oncol Biol Phys. 2001;50:727-33.
75. Lu X, Hu C, Ji Q, Shen C, Feng Y. Squamous cell carcinoma metastatic to cervical lymph nodes from an unknown primary site: the impact of radiotherapy. Tumori. 2009;95: 15-190.
76. Weir L, Keane T, Cummings B, Goodman P, O'Sullivan B, Payne D, et al. Radiation treatment of cervical node metastases from an unknown primary: an analysis of outcome by treatment volume and other prognostic factors. Radiother Oncol. 1995;35:206-11.
77. Sinnathamby K, Peters LJ, Laidlaw C, Hughes PG. The occult head and neck primary: to treat or not to treat? Clin Oncol (R Coll Radiol). 1997;9:322-9.
78. Richards TM, Bhide SA, Miah AB, Del Rosario L, Bodla S, Thway K, et al. Total mucosal irradiation with intensity-modulated radiotherapy in patients with head and neck carcinoma of unknown primary: a pooled analysis of two prospective studies. Clin Oncol. 2016;28(9):e77-84.
79. Grewal AS, Rajasekaran K, Cannady SB, Chalian AA, Ghiam AF, Lin A, et al. Pharyngeal-sparing radiation for head and neck carcinoma of unknown primary following TORS assisted work-up. Laryngoscope. 2020;130(3):691-7.

CHAPTER

11 Cancers of the Oral Cavity

Narayana Subramaniam, Samskruthi P Murthy, Sivakumar Vidhyadharan

INTRODUCTION

Surgically, the boundaries of the oral cavity are the lips anteriorly, the faucial pillars of the oropharynx posteriorly, the buccal mucosa laterally, the palate superiorly, and the floor of the mouth inferiorly. It has been further subdivided into oral cavity proper and vestibule by the dentoalveolar arch.[1] The oral cavity has been divided into distinct subsites based on anatomical location—oral tongue, buccal mucosa, floor of mouth, gingiva, hard palate, and retromolar trigone.[2]

The term "gingivobuccal complex cancers" is an important descriptive term from an Asian perspective; it refers to cancers of the buccal mucosa, lower gingiva, gingivobuccal sulcus, and retromolar trigone, which account for around 40% of the oral cancer burden in Southeast Asia and only 10% of those in the western countries,[3] due to the prolonged exposure of the lower gingivobuccal sulcus to chewing tobacco and betel quid.[4] It is important to note that although none of these water-tight compartments, especially in advanced oral cancer where there can be involvement of multiple contiguous subsites and there are significant biological differences between them that are likely to be prognostically relevant.[5-7]

Functionally, the oral cavity is the entrance of the digestive tract, responsible for the commencement of digestion through salivation, mastication, and propulsion of the bolus into the oropharynx. It also functions as secondary conduit for respiration, articulation for speech, and chemosensory for taste.[8] Lip function is intrinsically linked to a number of other functions, such as production of speech, singing, whistling, playing of musical instruments, and nonverbal communication (kissing and smiling), impairment of which can significantly impact a patient's quality of life.[9]

Cancers of the oral cavity are a heterogeneous group of disorders, with variable etiology, pathogenesis, tumor biology, clinical behavior, and treatment. It is estimated that approximately 90% of all malignancies affecting the oral cavity are squamous cell carcinoma;[10] the only subsite with a higher preponderance for nonsquamous histology is hard palate, where only around 50% of tumors are squamous in origin.[11] The remainder can arise from other epithelial, salivary, hematopoietic, or mesenchymal cells.

Oral cancer is a significant global health problem; oral cancer is associated with around 145,000 deaths annually, with the International Agency for Research on Cancer (IARC), estimating that the cancer burden in developing countries such as India is set to increase by around 70% in the next 20 years.[12] Oral cancer is a significant source of morbidity to survivors, with significant disturbances to speech, swallowing, and cosmesis, either as a result of the disease itself or its treatment. Recent trends have shown improved outcomes in the treatment of oral cancer, likely to be due to better standards of care, earlier detection of disease, and global tobacco cessations efforts.[13] Additional directed efforts are required to optimize treatment; a better comprehension of disease biology and personalization of treatment would afford a better balance of cancer therapy with quality of life concerns.

EPIDEMIOLOGY

Oral squamous cell carcinoma (OSCC) has typically been described as a disease that affects males in the age group of 60–80 years with a history of heavy tobacco and alcohol abuse.[14] However, more recent literature would indicate that it also affects younger patients, with an incidence of up to 27% in patients aged 45 years or younger,[15,16] with tongue being the most common subsite involved in these patients. Epidemiological trends have shown an increasing number of women being affected by oral cancer as well.[12] It is imperative not to dismiss the possibility of oral cancer in younger patients even with no history of tobacco exposure; OSCC has been described in patients as young as 15. The developing world accounts for around 75% of the deaths associated with oral cancer, likely due to advanced stage of presentation and poor access to appropriate care.

RISK FACTORS

Tobacco and alcohol are associated with oral cancer in up to 75% of cases.[17] Studies by the IARC have shown as many as 72 carcinogenic substances in cigarettes.[18] Data exists primarily for smoking, as it can be quantified in terms such as pack years. Other forms of tobacco, common in Asia, include betel quid (a combination of tobacco, betel leaf, areca nut, and catechu powder), gutkha (powdered tobacco, areca nut, slaked lime, catechu, and other condiments), khaini (tobacco with slaked lime), zarda (tobacco boiled in water and slaked lime and spices), kiwam (a thick paste of tobacco with spices), and snuff (fine tobacco powder for inhalation). These are likely to be associated with a higher carcinogenic potential as the components added to tobacco in these preparations (such as areca nut and slaked lime) are also independent carcinogens.[18,19]

Studies have shown that the risk of developing head and neck cancer was 50% higher than healthy individuals for those with <10 pack years exposure, and 300% higher in those with >30 pack year exposure. Tobacco and alcohol are multiplicative risk factors; those with significant exposure to both are expected to have a risk of developing cancer 10–20 times than those with no exposure to either. Alcohol is an independent risk factor for head and neck cancer in the absence of tobacco exposure when consumption exceeds 15 units per week.[4] For those who quit smoking, the risk reduction at 1–4 years is estimated to be 30%, taking over 20 years to have a likelihood of developing cancer equivalent to those who never smoked. For alcohol use, a significant risk reduction was only noted after over 20 years of cessation.[20]

Potentially malignant and premalignant diseases are an important set of conditions linked to oral cancer, and have been described as a separate chapter. Poor oral hygiene and nutrition have been linked to a higher risk of oral cancer but have been poorly quantified, as they often co-exist with tobacco, alcohol, and other carcinogen exposure.[21] The role of infections with human papillomavirus, herpes virus, and candida has also been postulated to be causative factor; however, the quality of evidence is insufficient.[22] Chronic mucosal trauma due to ill-fitting dentures or sharp teeth has also been described as a risk factor for oral cancer.[23] Other associated risk factors include prolonged UV exposure in carcinomas of the lip,[24] previous radiotherapy for diseases such as Hodgkin's lymphoma,[25] and immunosuppressant therapy for conditions such as renal transplantation.[26]

FIELD CANCERIZATION

First described by Slaughter in 1953 in his study of over 700 cases of oral and oropharyngeal squamous cell carcinoma, this refers to the generalized and progressive onset of molecular alterations in the epithelium of the upper aerodigestive tract (UADT) occurring due to chronic exposure to carcinogens.[27] As a result of the exposure of the entire mucosa of the UADT to carcinogens from inhaled smoke, promoted by the action of saliva and alcohol as solvents, there is similar carcinogen-induced damage to the epithelium, resulting in the presence of multiple dysplastic tumors, some of which may undergo malignant transformation to form second primary tumors (SPTs), either synchronously or metachronously. This has been demonstrated by the presence of similar genetic alterations in multiple dysplastic lesions in the same patient.

Based on Vogelstein's model of a multistep pathogenesis for colorectal cancer that showed at least four mutations in oncogenes and tumor suppressor genes being required for malignant transformation,[28] Califano described a "Vogelogram" for head and neck squamous cell carcinoma (HNSCC) that linked molecular alterations to specific histological changes in oral mucosa.[29] He described the phenomenon of "clonal cancerization", where multiple lesions arise from a constant clonal origin with the number of variations in the mutations and tumor suppressor genes determine the extent of progression from premalignant disease to invasive malignancy **(Fig. 1)**. This reiterated the belief that since oral epithelium is constantly being renewed and replaced, the insult to the cell occurs at a basal level to the epithelial stem cells, with transformed stem cells forming a parent clonal unit to form a patch (like leukoplakia), which finally acquires further genetic alternations and mutations either through carcinogen exposure or trauma to form invasive malignancy. There is then spread through lateral migration of the cells, or inoculation via saliva to a distant site within the UADT.

The risk of SPT in HNSCC is estimated to be 9–16%, with the risks being higher for male patients under 60 years, oral cavity and laryngeal tumors, those with smaller index tumors at diagnosis, and those with no lymph nodal spread at presentation. The outcomes associated with SPT were reasonable; the 5-year survival for those who developed SPT was 26%.[30] Lung was also a common site of SPT for those with head and neck cancers,

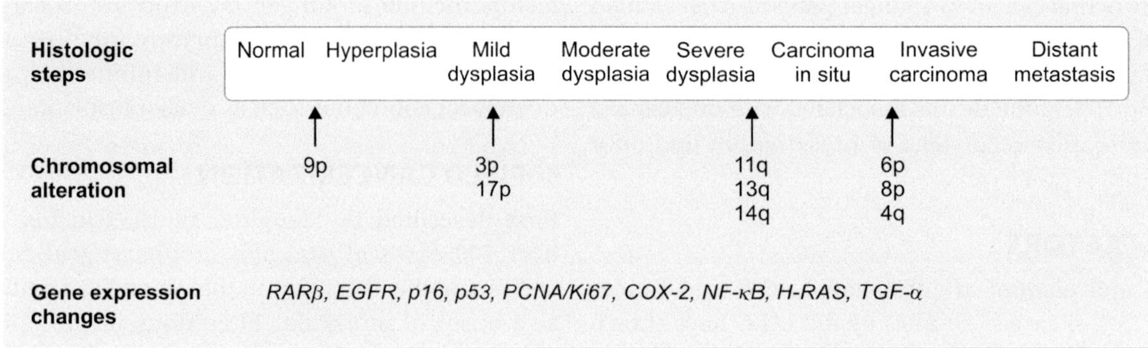

Fig. 1: Progression of premalignant disease to invasive disease and distant metastasis.

followed by esophagus.[31] Interestingly, up to 20% of SPT may occur outside the UADT. The cumulative incidence is estimated to be around 4% per year.[32]

CLINICAL EVALUATION AND EXAMINATION

Although the oral cavity is one of the most accessible sites for examination, oral cancers can present in a number of ways, leading to diagnostic confusion. The most common presentations are a lesion in the oral cavity that may or may not be associated with pain. Patients may have a history of blood-tinged saliva, dysphagia or odynophagia, restriction of tongue movement, trismus due to inflammatory spasm or malignant infiltration of the muscles of mastication, loosening of teeth, or cervical lymphadenopathy. The degree and severity of pain may vary significantly. Pain may range from mild pain due to superficial ulceration of the tumor to severe intractable pain due to trigeminal nerve involvement. Referred otalgia is common; for pain referred to the helix, tragus, skin of the external auditory canal and temporal region, pain transmission is through the auriculotemporal nerve, which is referred through the lingual nerve. For deep ear pain, the pathway involved is the tympanic nerve of Jacobson, which is referred through the glossopharyngeal nerve as they run through the jugular foramen. In posterior otalgia, pain is experienced behind the pinna and the posterior wall of the external auditory canal, with pain referred through Arnold's nerve (auricular branch of the vagus), referred through the superior laryngeal branch of the vagus nerve, which also traverses the jugular foramen.

Lesions are typically visible, with the morphology ranging from proliferative growths seen in well-differentiated or verrucous tumors to ulceroindurative growth seen in poorly differentiated or aggressive tumors. They may be associated with leukoplakia or erythroplakia of the overlying mucosa or the surrounding mucosa in a case of field cancerization. Features of oral submucous fibrosis, such as fibrotic bands, may necessitate simultaneous management during surgery. A thorough evaluation of the UADT, including a laryngoscopy or nasopharyngoscopy, may be advisable at diagnosis to avoid missing a synchronous SPT (estimated incidence of 3–15%).[33] A clinical assessment of tumor extent is crucial for further management. Palpation of extent of induration helps to identify submucosal spread beyond the visible edges of the tumor **(Figs. 2A to F)**.

In tongue tumors, extension to the base tongue, tonsillar pillars, floor of mouth extrinsic muscles, and lingual cortex of the mandible may be appreciated clinically. Lip tumors may involve partial or full thickness of the lip, and may involve the underlying alveolus or the external skin. Floor of the mouth tumors may also involve the mandible to a variable extent, necessitating a marginal or segmental mandibulectomy. Evaluation of mandible involvement can be performed by checking for movement of the tumor in relation to the mandible, or through bidigital palpation for cortical expansion or erosion. Gingivobuccal complex cancers can involve the upper or lower alveolus and the need for a marginal or segmental mandibulectomy for complete surgical clearance needs to be planned. Skin involvement can also be determined preoperatively by assessment for fixity, edema, nodules, or ulceration. Retromolar trigone tumors are difficult to assess clinically and can often erode the mandibular ramus early and disseminate through the infratemporal fossa. Hard palate lesions are palpated for mucosal extent, underlying bony erosion and extension into the soft palate.

Detailed examination of the cranial nerves may give additional information on the tumor extent. Topical xylocaine may aid detailed examination in cases with significant pain or tenderness. Patients with severe trismus may require endoscopic evaluation. For patients likely to require postoperative radiotherapy, a detailed dental examination, including planning of extractions,

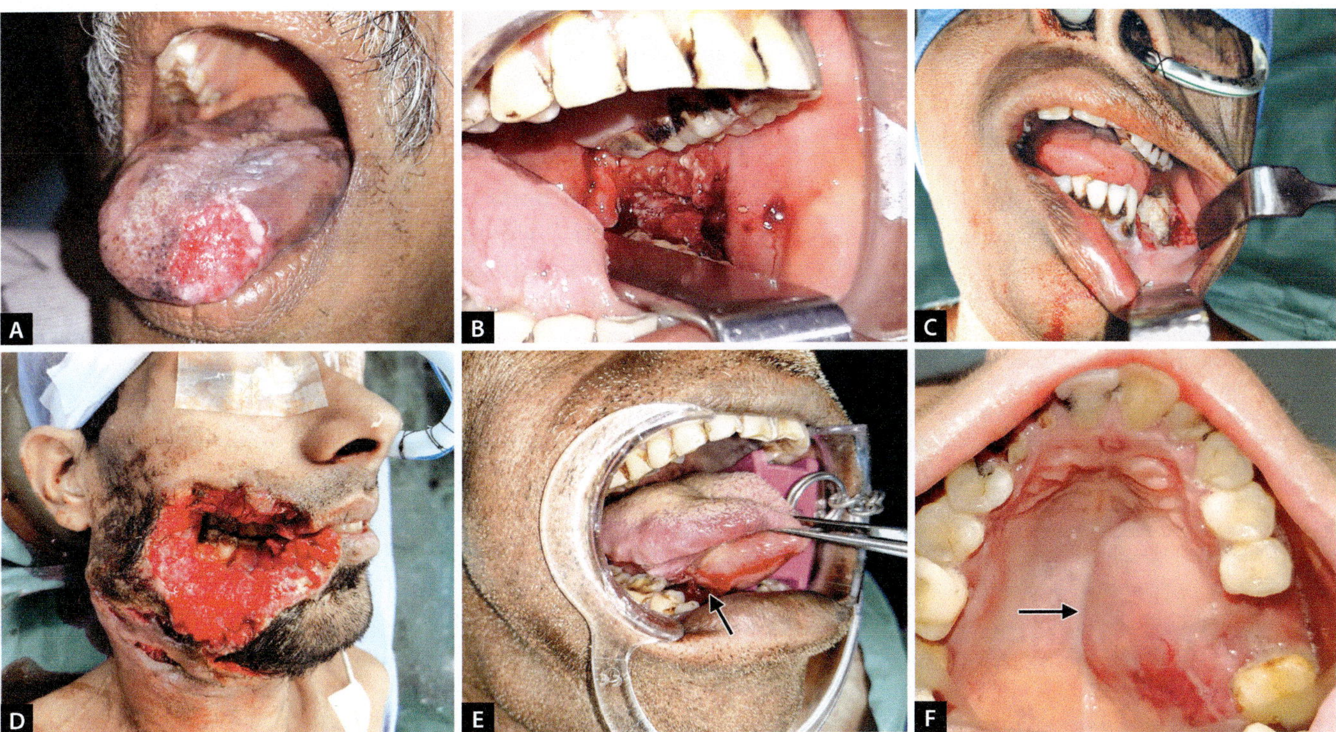

Figs. 2A to F: Varied clinical picture of oral cancer. (A) Left lateral tongue ulcerative tongue lesion on a background of dorsal tongue lichen planus; (B) Left retromolar trigone ulcerative lesion; (C) Left lower alveolar ulceroproliferative lesion; (D) Very advanced right buccal carcinoma with an orocutaneous fistula; (E) Right ventral tongue ulceroindurated lesion; (F) Nonsquamous oral cancer left hard palate.

needs to be performed to avoid delays in starting adjuvant radiotherapy. Preoperative improvement of oral hygiene may reduce postoperative surgical infection rates by reducing the salivary bacterial load.[34]

Careful examination of the bilateral cervical lymph node stations (levels I–V) is critical to identify ipsilateral or contralateral spread. Fixity to adjacent structures, such as sternocleidomastoid, prevertebral fascia, skin and mandible, and assessment of carotid pulse may help to identify signs of inoperability or the need for a radical neck dissection for adequate disease clearance. In cases of radical neck dissection, the interposition of well-vascularized soft tissue between the surgical bed and skin, such as a pectoralis major myocutaneous flap, is advisable to protect the common carotid artery from exposure and catastrophic bleeding in the event of a wound dehiscence or breakdown, and this needs planning.[35] Systemic examination is usually unremarkable; however, frank pulmonary or bony metastases or aspiration pneumonia may be identified.

Staging

The American Joint Committee on Cancer (AJCC), 8th edition/Union for International Cancer Control staging[36] represents a paradigm shift by incorporating depth of invasion (DOI) into the staging of oral cancer **(Table 1)**. This was an acknowledgement that DOI was a better predictor of disease-specific survival than tumor diameter alone,[37] and that a deeply invasive tumor with a small proliferative component has a worse prognosis than a superficial tumor with a significant proliferative component. Additionally, it is the first system to incorporate extranodal extension (ENE), for better prognostication.

Criticisms of the previous AJCC staging, however, persist. Invasion of the masticator space **(Fig. 3)** is considered a vague terminology, and early involvement of the medial pterygoid by gingivobuccal cancers for example, cannot be grouped in pT4b with pterygoid plate involvement or internal carotid artery encasement. Compartmental resection of the infratemporal fossa for en bloc resection of oral cancer via transmandibular approach has been demonstrated in several series,[38-40] enabling good clearance and outcomes. Liao et al. demonstrated that involvement above mandibular notch was a better predictor of poor outcomes for those with infratemporal fossa involvement;[41] patients with infranotch involvement had clinical outcomes similar to other pT4a tumors.

Another area of contention is bone involvement. Although very early cortical erosion of bone is not

Table 1: American Joint Committee on Cancer (AJCC), 8th edition/Union for International Cancer Control (UICC) staging for oral cancer.

Tx	Primary tumor cannot be assessed
Tis	Carcinoma in situ
T1	Tumor ≤2 cm, ≤5-mm depth of invasion (DOI)
T2	Tumor ≤2 cm, DOI > 5 mm and ≤10 mm or tumor >2 cm but ≤4 cm, and DOI ≤ 10 mm
T3	Tumor >4 cm or any tumor with DOI > 10 mm but ≤20 mm
T4a	*Moderately advanced local disease*: (Lip) Tumor invades through cortical bone or involves inferior alveolar nerve, floor of mouth or skin of face; (oral cavity) tumor involves adjacent structures such as cortical bone of maxilla or mandible, maxillary sinus, or skin of face or depth of invasion >20 mm
T4b	Very advanced local disease; tumor invades masticator space, pterygoid plates, skull base, and/or encases the internal carotid artery
Nx	Regional lymph nodes cannot be assessed
N0	No nodal metastasis
N1	Metastases to single lymph node, 3 cm or less in greatest diameter
N2a	Metastases to single ipsilateral node 3–6 cm in size or metastases to a single lymph node <3 cm in size with ENE
N2b	Metastases to multiple ipsilateral nodes 3–6 cm in size
N2c	Metastases to bilateral nodes 3–6 cm in size
N3a	Metastases to nodes >6 cm in size without ENE
N3b	Metastases to any node >3 cm in size with ENE
M0	No metastases
M1	Metastatic disease

(ENE: extranodal extension)

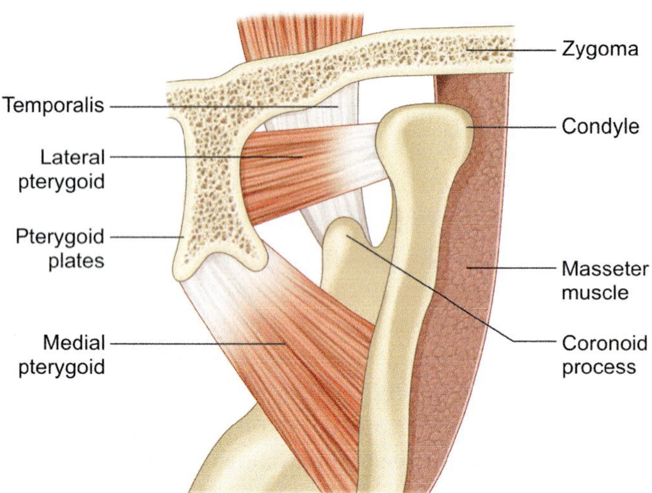

Fig. 3: Anatomy of the masticator space.

classified as pT4a disease, there has been evidence that even gross cortical bone involvement is not prognostically relevant and only medullary involvement is associated with reduced overall and disease-specific survival.[42] Interestingly, the pattern of failure in patients with medullary involvement was distant. Furthermore, the outcome of oral cavity tumors involving the bone is intrinsically linked to tumor diameter; it has also been shown that smaller pT4a tumors (diameter <4 cm) with cortical bone erosion have outcomes similar to pT2 tumors,[43] which bolsters this argument. Bone involvement is intrinsically linked to the proximity of the tumor to the maxilla or mandible, and hence generalizations regarding bone involvement are difficult.

Imaging

The ideal imaging modality should give an accurate assessment of the tumor and the neck nodes. A thorough evaluation for oral cancer would include tumor diameter and depth, bones invasion, lymphadenopathy, extranodal extension of lymph nodes, perineural spread, an SPT, and distant metastases. The most popular cross-sectional imaging modalities are CT or MRI with intravenous (IV) contrast, with both being complementary.[44] PET-CT is also a popular modality used in the preoperative workup; however, its limitations are cost, availability, and poor anatomic resolution.[45] With technological advancements and fusion of PET with MRI, it is expected to become more popular.

CT Imaging of Oral Cancer

This is typically the first imaging modality used for evaluation of oral cancer. The use of IV contrast is recommended unless the patient has a contraindication to iodinated contrast. OSCC typically appears as a lesion with either homogeneous or heterogeneous enhancement on contrast, often with peripheral enhancement of the lesion because of improved vascularity. However, lesions with necrosis will not enhance uniformly on contrast administration and appear hypodense with enhancement only of the periphery. When compared to benign lesions, malignant lesions are more likely to be irregular, nodular, and lacking clear delineation from the surrounding tissue. CT is the ideal imaging modality to determine early and subtle cortical bone erosion or periosteal reaction. A "puffed-cheek" maneuver can be used to better delineate gingivobuccal complex cancers, as this interposes air as a contrast medium between the mucosal surfaces of the gingiva and the buccal mucosa; this cannot be performed in MRI due to inability of patients to hold their breath during the longer image acquisition time. The soft-tissue delineation and determination of extent, however, is inferior to MRI, due to similar attenuation of the tumor and the surrounding tissues. Also, CT is associated with streak artifacts from dental amalgam, which can obscure visualization; this can be partially corrected through image acquisition in a plane at a different angle. The principles of PET–CT interpretation are identical; the additional information conveyed is avidity for 18-fluorodeoxyglucose.

MRI of Oral Cancer

Magnetic resonance imaging has the distinct advantage of improved soft-tissue delineation and characterization when compared to CT. It can also better identify marrow invasion by tumor without gross cortical disruption; hence, it is often advised that CT and MRI are used together to accurate assessment of bony involvement. MRI is also better for identifying perineural spread, which is a common route of spread for gingivobuccal complex and alveolar cancers. On conventional T1-weighted (T1W) images without fat-saturation, OSCC is generally hypointense or isointense when compared to muscles of the tongue and floor of mouth.[46] In spite of this, the enhancement and disruption of normal tissue architecture can help accurately identify tumor extent **(Fig. 4)**. On T2-weighted (T2W) images, OSCC is heterogeneous and hyperintense to muscle; however, there is poor discrimination of inflammation and edema, making overestimation of tumor extent common.[47] Perineural spread can have a varied presentation depending on the stage of spread. Early spread with infiltration of the nerve sheath by tumor is identified with T1W fat-suppressed images. With deposition of tumor within the nerve sheath and widening of the diameter, there is obliteration of the perineural fat at the foramina that can be seen on T1W non-fat-suppressed images or CT. Finally, when there is bony erosion or destruction at the foramina, it is best identified by the bone algorithm of CT.[48]

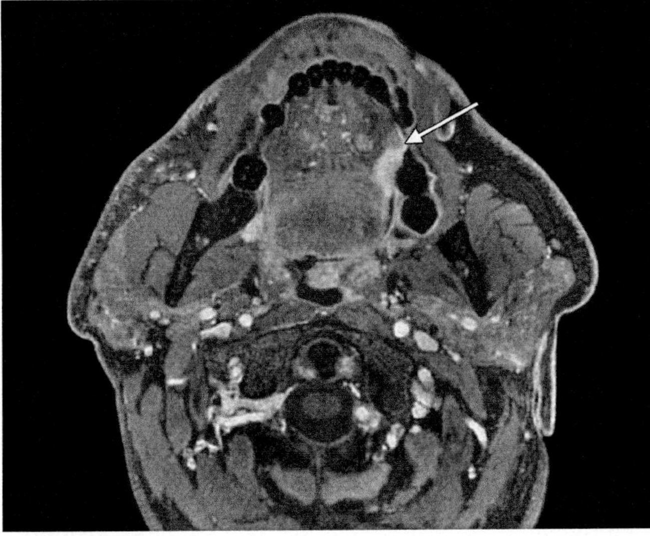

Fig. 4: T1+C MR showing left lateral tongue malignancy (arrow).

Additional Modalities

Ultrasound imaging of the tongue has been shown to give an accurate assessment of tumor thickness, especially in tumors under 5 mm.[49] It has also been shown to help to guide adequacy of surgical resection intraoperatively.[50] Other imaging modalities include orthopantomogram, bone scintigraphy, and DentaScan (reformation of maxillary and mandibular CT in axial, panoramic, and oblique sagittal planes); however, they have all been superseded by CT and MRI and are not used routinely.

Imaging of Individual Subsites (Table 2)

- *Oral tongue:* The routes of spread are dependent on tumor location. Lateral lesions can spread medially to invade tongue musculature, spreading along neurovascular bundles, intrinsic or extrinsic muscles, sometimes all the way up to the point of their attachment. Dorsal lesions may involve

Table 2: Imaging considerations in oral cancer.

Oral tongue	Location and extent, depth of invasion, proximity to midline, submucosal spread, extent of extrinsic muscle involvement, involvement of neurovascular bundles, floor of mouth involvement, mandible involvement, involvement of vallecula and pre-epiglottic space, tonsil/oropharyngeal involvement, and nodal status
Floor of mouth	Location and extent, depth of invasion, proximity to midline, submucosal spread, mandible involvement, neurovascular bundle involvement, sublingual space involvement, involvement of intrinsic and extrinsic muscles of tongue, breach of the mylohyoid, base tongue involvement, and submental skin involvement
Retromolar trigone	Location and extent, depth of invasion, submucosal spread, involvement of buccal mucosa, involvement of upper or lower alveolus, involvement of base of tongue or oropharynx, infratemporal fossa extension, perineural spread, extension into pterygopalatine fossa and orbit
Buccal mucosa	Location and extent, depth of invasion, submucosal spread, buccinator and skin involvement, gingivobuccal sulcus and alveolar involvement, parotid duct and gland involvement, infratemporal fossa involvement and perineural spread
Alveolar ridge	Location and extent, depth of invasion, early cortical bone erosion or periosteal reaction, soft tissue extension to buccal mucosa, lip, floor of mouth or retromolar trigone, extent of cortical destruction and medullary involvement, maxillary sinus involvement, and perineural spread
Hard palate	Location and extent, depth of invasion, submucosal extension, extension to soft palate, bony erosion, maxillary sinus involvement, and perineural spread
Lip	Location and extent, depth of invasion, submucosal spread, upper and lower alveolus involvement, and perineural spread

floor of mouth or mandible. Posterior lesions can spread submucosally and invade base tongue and oropharynx. The fat content of the tongue musculature affects the appearance of tumor on MRI; when the tongue has a significant fat component, the tumor is less intense and identification on T1W images is more difficult, T2W imaging is preferred.

- *Floor of mouth:* These tumors may initially spread horizontally or superiorly as the musculature of the floor of mouth acts as a relative barrier to tumor spread. The mandible may be involved anteriorly, most commonly where the tumor abuts the bone. Tumor may be associated with significant submucosal spread, involvement of the neurovascular bundle, and the sublingual spaces, which communicate below the frenulum and may allow spread contralaterally. There may be obstruction of the submandibular duct ostia leading to duct dilatation and sialadenitis. Larger tumors may involve the intrinsic and extrinsic muscles of the tongue or breach the mylohyoid.
- *Retromolar trigone:* This area is at the junction of oral cavity and oropharynx, with complex patterns of spread. Tumors can involve the ascending ramus of the mandible, lower and upper alveolus, buccal mucosa, base of tongue, floor of mouth, infratemporal fossa, tonsillar pillar, and soft palate through direct extension. Tumors can also spread to the pterygopalatine fossa via the pterygomandibular raphe, which communicates with the middle cranial fossa, orbit, and nasopharynx **(Fig. 5)**. Perineural invasion along the lingual nerve is also common. Oblique reformation with CT is advantageous for imaging as the entire retromolar trigone can be seen in entirety.[51]

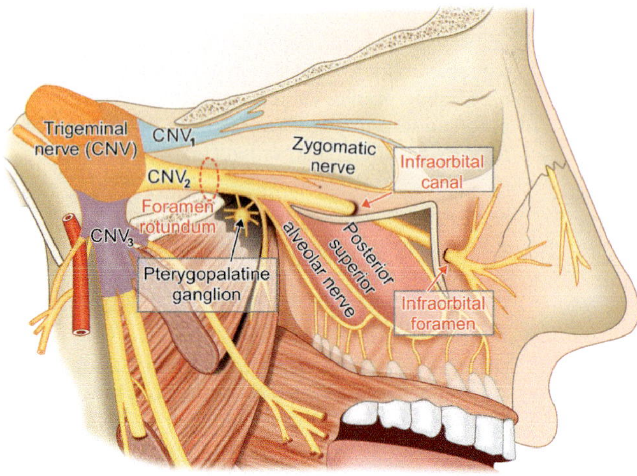

Fig. 5: Pterygopalatine fossa.

- *Buccal mucosa:* A lack of anatomical barriers to spread allows several distinct patterns of spread in these tumors. Through deep invasion, there can be involvement of the buccal fat pad, buccinator muscle, parotid gland, or cheek skin. Involvement of the retromolar trigone and infratemporal fossa can occur early depending on the anatomical location of the tumor. Extension in the superior or inferior directions can result in involvement of the gingivobuccal sulcus and the alveoli, which is well-demonstrated with a puffed-cheek technique on CT. Perineural spread can occur as in retromolar trigone tumors.
- *Gingiva or alveolar ridge:* These are tumors arising from the mucoperiosteum of the upper and lower alveoli. For early lesion, bone erosion is important to determine the extent of surgery. In advanced lesion, the soft tissue extent and bony extent are equally important. Soft tissue extension may occur to the buccal mucosa and lip, floor of mouth, palatal mucosa, or retromolar trigone. Determination of bony extent includes the length of cortical erosion or destruction and medullary canal involvement, which may not always correspond. Upper gingival tumors may involve have extensive maxillary sinus involvement. Perineural spread through the lingual or inferior alveolar nerve is crucial to identify to ensure complete resection.
- *Hard palate:* These tumors can spread to involve significant areas of hard palate mucosa, soft palate, and underlying bone. Significant destruction of maxillary sinus may occur. Perineural spread via the greater and lesser palatine nerves to the pterygopalatine fossa is known.
- *Lip:* Imaging has limited role in early lesions. It is valuable in advanced lesions, especially when significant soft tissue spread precludes an accurate clinical assessment. Perineural spread may involve the mental nerve and via this the marrow of the mandible. MRI and CT have a complementary role here; MRI better delineates soft tissue extent and perineural spread while CT better delineates early cortical erosion and periosteal reaction.

OUTCOMES

The 5-year disease-specific survival estimate for OSCC is shown in **Table 3**. These figures are aggregate values of 5-year disease-specific survival (DSS) quoted in large series in literature;[52-98] however, it is to be noted that an accurate estimation is difficult due to the significant heterogeneity in terminology (certain studies considering

Table 3: 5-year disease-specific survival estimate for oral squamous cell carcinoma (OSCC).

	5-year disease-specific survival estimate							
	Stage I		*Stage II*		*Stage III*		*Stage IV*	
Subsites of the oral cavity	*S*	*RT*	*S*	*RT*	*S*	*RT*	*S*	*RT*
Oral tongue[52-57]	89%	82%	75%	65%	65%	54%	38%	22%
Floor of mouth[58-61]	88%	85%	80%	83%	66%	42%	52%	21%
Retromolar trigone[62-66]	88%	84%	75%	68%	74%	52%	58%	43%
Buccal mucosa[67-72]	85%	79%	70%	63%	62%	41%	38%	15%
Alveolar ridge[73-80]	86%	76%	74%	62%	65%	44%	50%	29%
Hard palate[81-85]	87%	84%	78%	72%	55%	24%	35%	12%
Lip[86-98]	92%	89%	86%	77%	74%	43%	52%	35%

curative radiotherapy include surgical salvage in the survival estimates while others do not), the fact that studies often span over several decades with heterogeneity in treatment policy and quality and marked changes in the staging system with time. It is also relevant to note that some of these studies have treated stage III/IV disease with chemoradiotherapy, while others have used only radical radiotherapy, and fractionation is far from standardized. The most accurate assessment of survival for individual patients is through nomograms; however, their results are not standardized for OSCC.[99] What is clear, however, is the difference in outcomes between subsites, which likely stems from a basic difference in tumor biology, propensity for lymph nodal metastases, and other features. According to the Surveillance Epidemiology and End Results (SEER) Program data from the United States, lip carcinomas have the best 5-year cancer-specific survival (88%) and floor of mouth the worst (54%).[100] "S" refers to patient treated with surgery as the primary modality, and postoperative radiotherapy in stage III/IV, while "RT" refers to treatment with curative intent radiotherapy, with or without surgical salvage.

NONSQUAMOUS CANCERS OF THE ORAL CAVITY

Nonsquamous cancers of the oral cavity are relatively rare, with OSCC accounting for over 90% of oral cancer.[101] They are most commonly minor salivary gland tumors, mucosal melanomas, and sarcomas arising from the bone or soft tissue. Among minor salivary gland tumors, the most common are mucoepidermoid carcinoma, followed by low-grade adenocarcinoma and adenoid cystic carcinoma.[102] Sarcomas involving the oral cavity are rare but can be varied in clinical presentation depending on cell of origin.[103] Diagnosis needs to be established with biopsy and often immunohistochemistry. Nonsquamous cancers, cell or origin, and prognosis are shown in **Table 4**.

Table 4: Nonsquamous cancers, cell or origin, and prognosis.

Tumor type	*Age group*	*Prognosis*
Salivary gland tumors:		
Mucoepidermoid carcinoma	Young adults or adults	Good
Polymorphous low-grade adenocarcinoma	Young adults or adults	Good
Adenoid cystic carcinoma	Adults	Intermediate to poor
Acinic cell carcinoma	Adults	Good to intermediate
Carcinoma ex pleomorphic adenoma	Adults	Poor
Adenocarcinoma	Adults	Poor
Epithelial myoepithelial carcinoma	Adults	Intermediate
Clear cell carcinoma	Adults	Intermediate
Salivary duct carcinoma	Adults	Poor
Sarcomas:		
Fibrosarcoma or malignant fibrous histiocytoma	Young adults or adults	Intermediate
Malignant peripheral nerve sheath tumor	Adults	Poor
Liposarcoma	Adults	Intermediate
Synovial sarcoma	Young adults	Poor
Angiosarcoma	Elderly	Poor
Osteosarcoma	Children and young adults	Intermediate
Chondrosarcoma	Adults	Intermediate

Although the oncological principle of three-dimensional en bloc resection and appropriate reconstruction are similar to OSCC, there are significant differences in the management of these tumors. Margin adequacy and the indications for adjuvant therapy are discussed in the respective chapters on salivary gland

Table 5: Evidence for elective management of the neck in non-squamous tumors of the oral cavity.

Tumor	*Indications for neck dissection in the node-negative neck*
Salivary gland tumors:	
Mucoepidermoid carcinoma	High grade, by Armed Forces Institute of Pathology or WHO grading[104,105]
Adenoid cystic carcinoma	Elective neck treatment is required as occult metastasis in adenoid cystic carcinoma of oral cavity occurred in 22%; unclear whether neck dissection or neck irradiation is superior[106]
General guidelines for salivary gland tumors[107]	• High-grade histology • High-risk (angioinvasive) subtype • Advanced T stage (T3/4)
Sarcomas	• Routinely addressing the node-negative neck not indicated; Incidence of nodal metastases reported as 4%[108] • Lymph node spread occurs in rhabdomyosarcoma, angiosarcoma, epithelioid sarcoma, malignant fibrous histiocytoma, and leiomyosarcoma[109] • Elective neck dissection *may* have a role in synovial sarcoma due to the high risk of nodal metastases[110,111]
Mucosal melanoma	Elective neck dissection indicated in oral cavity mucosal melanoma[112,113]

tumors, tumors of the skin, and soft tissue sarcomas. Neck metastases require therapeutic neck dissection in all nonsquamous cancers; however, elective neck management is unclear in view of the low incidence and paucity of literature available. It is to be remembered that elective irradiation to the node-negative neck, if the primary site requires radiotherapy, is a rational approach that may be associated with less morbidity than elective neck dissection. **Table 5** shows the evidence for elective management of the neck in these tumors. However, in patients undergoing free flap reconstruction (which requires cervicotomy), patients unlikely to be compliant for follow-up and tumors with which nodal recurrences are likely to portend a poor prognosis, elective neck dissection is still a reasonable approach, even if the incidence of occult nodal metastases is low.

TREATMENT PRINCIPLES

As per the National Comprehensive Cancer Network guidelines, early stage disease (I/II) is usually sufficiently treated with single modality treatment while advanced stage disease (III/IV) requires multimodality treatment.[114]

- For T1-2N0 disease, surgery is the first choice of treatment, and radiotherapy is an alternative.
- For T3/T4 disease or any node-positive disease, surgery is the choice of treatment, followed by adjuvant therapy as guided by the adverse features on histopathological examination.
- Unresectable disease is treated as per the patient's performance status.

Early Stage Disease (T1-2N0-1)

Surgery

Surgery is the treatment of choice for early stage OSCC. Surgical treatment comprises wide local excision of the primary and elective neck dissection, with reconstruction as required. Wide excision of the primary tumor has traditionally entailed a 1-cm circumferential gross margin, aiming for a microscopic margin of at least 5 mm;[115-117] however, these teachings have been challenged by recent studies, which have shown that smaller margins are adequate for local control. Recent retrospective studies have suggested that margins as little as 2.2 mm may be sufficient in oral tongue carcinoma,[118] while another has suggested that margins of 1 mm, essentially negative margins, were sufficient for local control.[119] The complex interplay of margins with other adverse pathological features[120] makes a definitive consensus in the absence of prospective data improbable.

Elective neck dissection has been shown to improve overall survival and disease-specific survival in early stage node-negative OSCC, and is to be taken as the standard of care.[121] Supraomohyoid neck dissection (levels I-III) is adequate in node-negative disease; however, tongue has been shown to be associated with skip metastases to level IV,[122] necessitating dissection of level IV in oral tongue carcinoma. Prospective randomized data has shown that supraomohyoid neck dissection (levels I-III) had comparable locoregional control and survival when compared to modified radical neck dissection (levels I-V) in node-negative OSCC, even when the stage of the primary was advanced (T3/4).[123] Sentinel lymph node biopsy is also considered an alternate approach to staging of the neck, and is attractive in view of the significantly lower morbidity;[124] however, it is mandatory to note that head-to-head comparisons with elective neck dissection do not exist.

Radical Brachytherapy

Brachytherapy uses shielded radioisotopes to provide localized radiation around the tumor with minimal doses to the surrounding normal tissues, usually with cesium or iridium, in the form of loops or seeds. It is divided into low-dose rate (LDR), with delivery of <2 gray per hour,

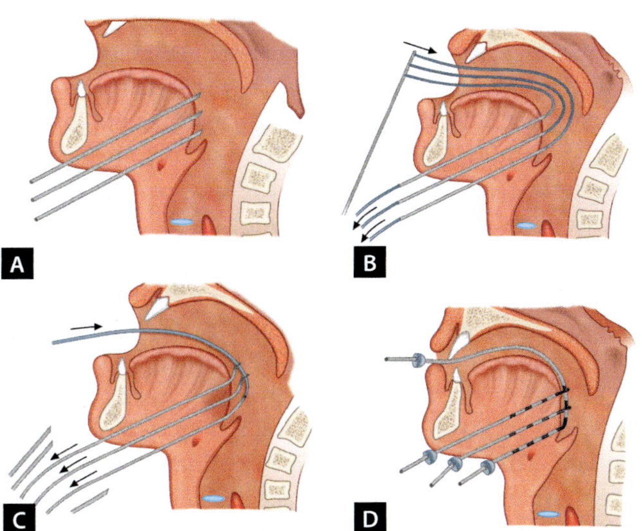

Figs. 6A to D: Brachytherapy catheter placement for oral cancer treatment.

and high-dose rate (HDR) that delivers >12 gray per hour.[125] Insertion of these isotope-loaded catheters or seeds usually requires general anesthesia, with a feeding tube and often a tracheostomy during the treatment period. The technique of insertion is shown in **Figures 6A to D**.

The GEC-ESTRO (Groupe Européen de Curiethérapie–European Society for Therapeutic Radiology and Oncology) recommendations for the use of brachytherapy in OSCC are:[126]

- T1-2N0 oral mucosa <15 mm in thickness
- Oral tongue or floor of mouth lesions must be at least 5 mm away from mandible (to prevent osteoradionecrosis)
- Not suitable for advanced lesions, especially T4 tumors and those abutting mandible

The choice of brachytherapy has been controversial in the past; HDR was preferred in view of the shorter duration of therapy and better safety for the medical professionals handling the isotopes but previous studies showed that LDR brachytherapy was associated with better control and survival.[127] However, a recent meta-analysis of clinical trials showed that both had a comparable cure rate.[128] It is important to note that brachytherapy has been shown to be inferior to surgery in literature.[129]

The neck needs to be addressed in these patients in view of the risk of occult metastasis, usually with an elective neck dissection; prospective data has shown that elective neck irradiation is clearly inferior to elective neck dissection in node-negative early stage OSCC.[130]

Radical External Beam Radiotherapy

This is also a popular option for treatment of OSCC. Although brachytherapy is preferred, the facilities, infrastructure, and technical expertise required may not be available in all centers. Similar to brachytherapy, it is used for radical treatment of the primary site and neck. However, multiple studies have shown that radiotherapy is associated with inferior locoregional control when compared to surgery as the primary modality for treatment of early oral cancer.[131-133]

Adjuvant Radiotherapy after Surgery

Although early stage disease is typically treated with a single therapeutic modality, there are indications for adjuvant radiotherapy after wide excision and elective neck dissection.

- *High-risk features:* Positive/close margins and extranodal extension are associated with a poor overall survival and are typically treated with adjuvant concurrent chemoradiotherapy based on the combined analysis of two randomized control trials.[134] It is to be noted that "positive" margins (<1 mm) and "close" margins (1–4 mm) are not synonymous; several studies show that close margins may not have the same prognostic implications as positive margins, and may not warrant adjuvant therapy.[135,136] More contemporary literature based on observational data from a large population has suggested that in HPV-negative HNSCC, concurrent chemoradiotherapy was beneficial over radiotherapy in extranodal extension but not positive margins, while in HPV-positive HNSCC, concurrent chemoradiotherapy was beneficial over radiotherapy in positive margins but not in extranodal extension.[137] A relatively recent concept introduced in the AJCC, 8th edition is the degree of extranodal extension; it has now been divided into microscopic (≤2 mm) and macroscopic (>2 mm) depending on the amount of extension into the surrounding soft tissue.[138] This is based on literature that showed ENE ≤1.7 mm was not prognostically relevant;[139] however, the degree of microscopic and macroscopic has been introduced only for descriptive purposes and data collection; there is no recommendation on de-escalation of treatment for those with microscopic ENE.
- *Intermediate-risk features:* Perineural invasion has been shown to significantly impact locoregional control and survival.[140-144] Literature has shown that perineural invasion is further impacted by the size of nerve involved[135] and whether adjuvant radiotherapy improves control or survival in early

oral cancer continues to be a debate likely to be answered only by prospective study. Differentiation is another feature shown to impact survival,[145] and whether poorly-differentiated early stage tumors require adjuvant therapy. Lymphovascular invasion, worst pattern of invasion, cohesiveness of tumor front and budding at the tumor front are also adverse pathological features;[135,146,147] however, whether they mandate adjuvant radiotherapy is unclear. An individualized decision needs to be made for each patient; the morbidity of radiotherapy needs to be carefully balanced against the risk of recurrence. Data suggests that those patients with more than one adverse pathological feature are likely to have aggressive disease[147-149] and should receive adjuvant therapy. Scoring systems that determine the likely risk of recurrence[135,147-150] can also aid in decision-making.

- *Nodal status:* Although early nodal disease (N1) in the presence of early tumor stage (T1-2) is still stage-III disease and by definition mandates multi-modality treatment, involvement of a single node without extranodal extension may still be observed according to the NCCN guidelines,[114] based on the findings of Ang's prospective trial,[151] that showed involvement of two or more nodes was an intermediate-risk feature that required adjuvant radiotherapy for improved locoregional control. However, large population-based observational studies have shown that adjuvant therapy is associated with a survival benefit in N1 disease,[152,153] which reflects the practice in many institutions.

Locally Advanced Disease (T3-4aN0/T1-4N2-3)

Surgery

Surgery is the primary treatment modality in advanced OSCC. The principle of en bloc resection of the tumor with adequate margins and appropriate reconstruction remains the same; however, in view of the confines of the oral cavity, resections required are far more extensive, often with partial or complete resection of the maxilla or mandible and extensive soft-tissue loss. Ipsilateral elective neck dissection is indicated even in node-negative disease. The features associated with a high incidence of occult contralateral neck metastases (>20%) are clinical stage (T3/4), tumor crossing the midline and floor of the mouth involvement.[154] Neck dissection is not without significant morbidity; however, the decision to address the contralateral node-negative neck needs to be made based on the likelihood of occult metastases, which is impacted by subsite, size, and location of tumor. Addressing the truly node-negative neck with elective irradiation is sufficient; however, occult nodal metastases is best treated with neck dissection. Clinical or radiologically positive nodal disease requires therapeutic neck dissection. Although classical teaching recommended modified radical neck dissection (levels I-V) for the node positive neck, the incidence of level V metastases in literature has been consistently low and the shoulder dysfunction associated with level V dissection has led to the recommendation that addressing levels I-IV was sufficient even in the node positive neck,[155,156] with dissection of level V only if clinically or radiologically involved. This approach has been validated in a recent systematic review of all mucosal SCC, which showed that incidence of level V involvement was <3%, and that elective dissection of level V was unlikely to confer any oncological benefit.[157]

Adjuvant Therapy

Advanced stage OSCC by definition requires adjuvant therapy to improve locoregional control. The adverse pathological features requiring adjuvant therapy according to the NCCN guidelines are advanced tumor stage T3/4 or nodal stage N2/3, positive margins, perineural invasion, lymphovascular invasion, or nodal disease in levels IV or V. It is important to note that positive margins is best treated with re-resection to achieve negative margins, however, it is not always feasible; identifying the exact area of margin positivity is difficult and tumors margins may be discohesive, depending on the patterns of invasion, making even serial re-excision preclude complete clearance.

Radical External Beam Radiotherapy or Chemoradiotherapy

Although not the standard of care, literature has shown the increasing use of radiotherapy for treatment of advanced OSCC. However, large population-based studies have shown that radiotherapy is associated with inferior survival outcomes.[158] Chemoradiotherapy has also been used as the primary modality in OSCC; however, large population-based studies have shown that chemoradiotherapy is inferior to surgery with adjuvant therapy in operable OSCC.[159] This has also been shown in a prospective trial comparing surgery with adjuvant radiotherapy and chemoradiotherapy for advanced HNSCC, where OSCC and maxillary SCC treated with surgery and adjuvant therapy had a clear survival benefit over those treated with curative intent chemoradiotherapy.[160]

Radiotherapy still does have a role as the primary modality in oral cancer. The indications for radiotherapy over surgery in OSCC are as follows:[161]

- In early stage to avoid functional and cosmetic defects (especially for subsites like lip)
- Unresectable disease
- High-operative risk
- Recurrent disease after multiple resection where further surgery improbable
- Patient preference

Very Advanced Locoregional Disease (T4b/Unresectable Nodal Disease)

For patients with very advanced locoregional (nonmetastatic disease), the treatment is dependent on the individual patient's performance status. The same applies to those unfit for surgery.

- *European Cooperative Oncology Group (ECOG) status of 0-1:* Patients are treated with concurrent systemic therapy with radiotherapy or induction chemotherapy followed by radiotherapy or concurrent chemoradiotherapy.
- *ECOG status of 2:* Treated with definitive radiotherapy with or without concurrent systemic therapy.
- *ECOG status of 3:* Treated with palliative radiotherapy, single agent chemotherapy or best supportive care.

This is a reflection of the ability of the patient's ability to tolerate therapy; the addition of chemotherapy to radiotherapy, either as induction or concurrently, is associated with a significantly higher toxicity profile. Patients with a poor physiological reserve or co-morbid illnesses such as chronic liver disease or kidney disease should not be advised ambitious courses of treatments their health is unlikely to permit them to complete. For patients with poor performance status, palliation is the aim as patients are unlikely to tolerate any curative intent therapeutic modality.

Surgery for Oral Cancer

There are several approaches to the resection of oral cancer. The preferred approach is determined by two major considerations—the location and extent of the tumor, and the proximity to maxilla or mandible. These can be further complicated by patient-related factors, such as trismus, the need for neck dissection, dentition, and previous incisions. The objectives of surgery for oral cancer are excision of the tumor with adequate margins, to provide adequate reconstruction to minimize aspiration, to avoid pooling of food and saliva, and to allow adequate speech and articulation.

The standard surgical approaches to the oral cavity are:[162]

- *Transoral:* This approach is characteristically for anteriorly placed T1/2 tumors of oral tongue, floor of mouth, alveolus, buccal mucosa, and hard palate. It is usually sufficient for tumors up to 5 cm in the maximum dimension.[163-165]
- *Lower cheek flap:* This is a midline incision that splits the lip and continues laterally into the neck for a neck dissection. It is used for posterolateral tumor of the oral cavity or for mandibulectomies (marginal or segmental). It is performed by a midline full-thickness lip split (variations in incision shown in **Figures 7A to E**) with the vertical limb extended till the hyoid, which is continued along the ipsilateral upper neck crease. The symphysis menti is exposed and the mucosal incision is placed along the gingivobuccal or gingivolabial sulci, lateral to the sulci, or interdental. The lower cheek flap is then raised over the body of the mandible and the masseter muscle attachment is taken down to include it in along with the flap. It can be raised up to the mandibular notch to improve access.
- *Upper cheek flap:* This is an adaptation of the Weber–Ferguson incision; the full-thickness upper lip is split and combined with a lateral rhinotomy incision. It is used for posterolateral lesions of the upper alveolus and for extensive lesions of the hard palate. The mucosal incisions possible are similar to the lower cheek flap.
- *Visor flap:* This avoids mandibulotomy and instead involves release of the paramandibular soft tissue and a gingivolabial incision to deliver the mandible in to the neck. It provides good exposure to the anterior mandible, floor of mouth, and entire tongue; however, both mental nerves need to be sacrificed and there is anesthesia over the chin. Although not strictly a visor flap, another approach is the mandibular lingual release described by Stanley.[166] Here, the skin and soft tissue over the mandible are left intact but the entire oral cavity contents and delivered into the neck through an incision in the gingivolabial sulcus, which is continued subperiosteally.
- *Mandibulotomy:* This involves a planned osteotomy in the mandible to improve access to the oral cavity. It provides excellent exposure to posterolateral tumors without the need for mandibular sacrifice. It can also be used for tumors that extend to the base of tongue. The types of mandibulotomy are lateral, median, or paramedian **(Fig. 8)**. The differences between them are shown in **Table 6** as described by Evans et al.[167] The skin incision varies; it may be used

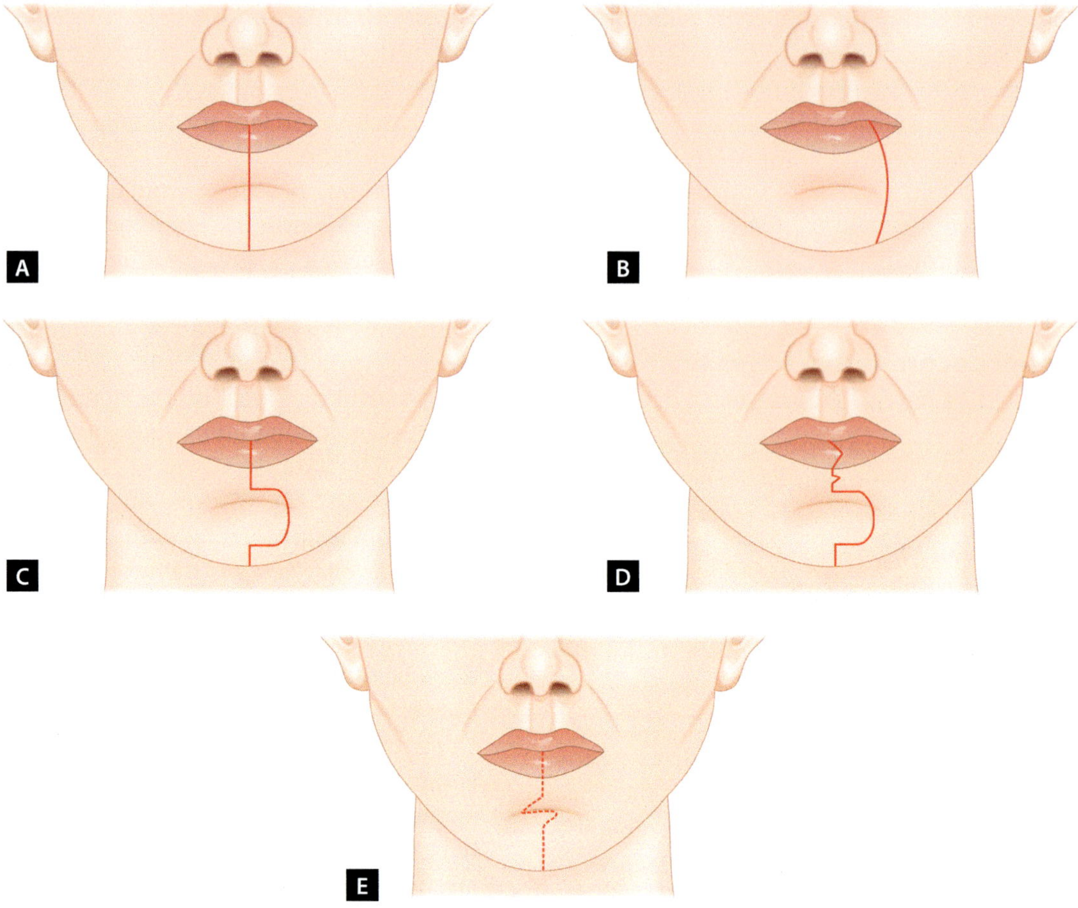

Figs. 7A to E: Lip split incisions. (A) Roux-Trotter incision; (B) Robson incision; (C) McGregor incision; (D) Hayter modification of McGregor incision; (E) Modified 'Z' incision.

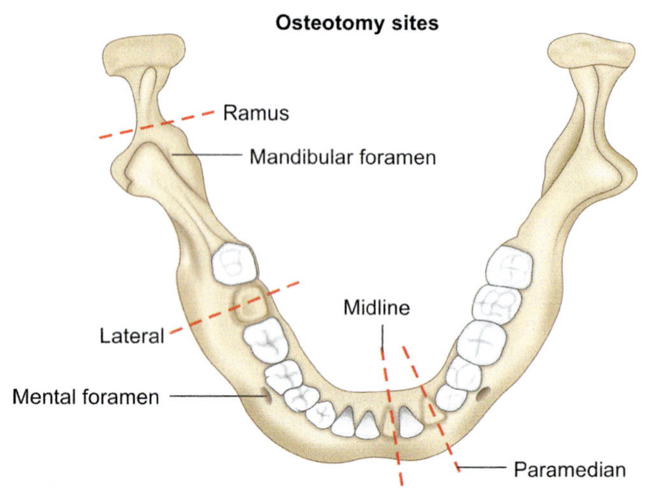

Fig. 8: Mandibulotomy sites.

with a standard cheek flap approach; however, it has been described without the need for a lip-split.[168] The classical technique is a straight-line osteotomy; however, a stair-step modification **(Fig. 9)** has been described as being superior, with less interfragmentary movement with greater resistance to vertical loads.[169] Preplating the mandibulotomy is a must to ensure fixation. To counteract torsion forces at the symphysis, two parallel plates are used, with a minimum of 4–10 mm between them, with at least two screws on either side of the bone segments. The lower plate needs to be fixed first. It has been shown that two 2-mm locking plates provide the greatest resistance to vertical loading.[170] Whether the patient is likely to receive adjuvant radiotherapy is an important consideration; although radiotherapy does not impact postoperative healing, however, rigid fixation is important in reducing the incidence of complications.[171] For patients receiving concurrent chemoradiotherapy, the incidence of plate and osteosynthesis-related complications was significantly higher than with radiotherapy alone,[172] likely to be because of the combined physical, geometric, and radiobiological factors that combine to produce exceptionally high doses of radiotherapy around the metal implant.

Table 6: Types of mandibulotomy.

	Lateral	*Median*	*Paramedian*
Location	Body or angle of mandible	Midline	Between lateral incisor and canine
Exposure	+	++	++
Dental extraction	May be required	Single central incisor	Not required
Inferior alveolar nerve and vessels	Require transection	Spared	Spared
Division of genial muscles	Not required	Required	Not required, only mylohyoid needs division
Mechanical stability	Poor as there is asymmetric muscle pull on two segments	Good	Good
Fixation	May require intermaxillary fixation	Compression mini-plates or steel wire	Compression mini-plates or steel wire
Adjuvant radiotherapy	Osteotomy lies within lateral portal with increased risk of complications	Lies outside lateral portal	Lies outside lateral portal

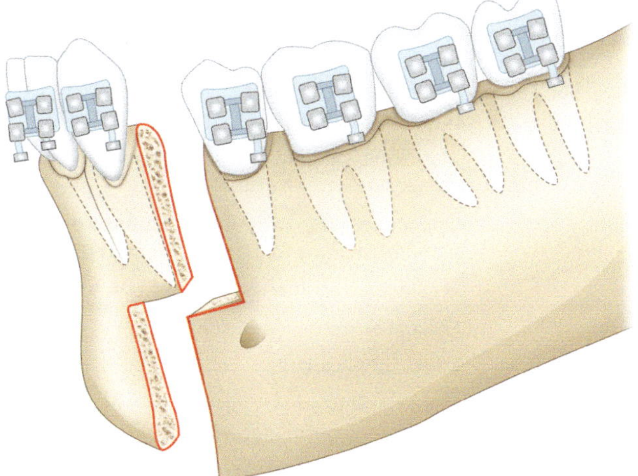

Fig. 9: Stair-step modification.

A comparison of mandible-preserving approaches and mandibulotomy approaches has been shown in **Table 7**. A meta-analysis has shown that there was no difference in recurrence, surgical margins, tongue movement, or speech between the two groups; however, the rate of oral fistula is lower in mandible preservation.[173] A general approach to oral cancer resections is shown in **Table 8**.

MANAGEMENT OF THE MANDIBLE IN ORAL CANCER

Management of the mandible in oral cancer is critical; the requirement and extent of mandible resection need to be determined to ensure adequate three-dimensional margin clearance, but it must be kept in mind that mandible resection has significant impact on the patient's mastication, swallowing, occlusion, and speech.

Historically, it was considered that lymphatic channels from the oral cavity pass through the mandible periosteum to drain into the neck.[175] As a result, the minimal resection of the mandible considered in oral cancer was a segmental mandibulectomy, until Greer first described a marginal mandibulectomy for a floor of mouth cancer.[176] Subsequently, there were studies that demonstrated the safety of this approach by demonstrating that there was no association between mandible periosteum involvement and nodal metastasis.[177] Cortical invasion was also shown to not increase recurrence or survival, and marginal resection was shown to be feasible for lesions abutting the lingual cortex but not extending to the occlusal surface or rim.[178]

More literature began to appear on the mechanism of invasion. McGregor et al. showed that in non-irradiated mandibles, the occlusal route was the nearly 90% of patients, while in irradiated mandibles, the route of entry was much more variable, indicating that conservative surgeries in the irradiated mandible may not be oncologically safe.[179] Cawood and Howell described the relation of the floor of mouth to the crest of the ridge as the mandible resorbs, demonstrating the route of spread in the edentulous or resorbed mandible.[180] Brown in his landmark paper described two discrete patterns of bone invasion: the erosive pattern (where the tumor advances in a broad front with intervening connective tissue layer and an active osteoclastic reaction) and an infiltrative pattern (where there are islands or finger-like projections of tumor into the cancellous spaces of bone with little to no intervening connective tissue or osteoclastic reaction), with the latter being associated with significantly worse disease free survival.[181] He also described seven potential routes of tumor into the mandible:

- Through the occlusal route
- Through the periodontal membrane
- Through the attached gingiva
- Via the mental foramen
- Via the mandibular foramen
- Through abutment of the lower mandible in the neck
- Through cortical bone defects in the edentulous ridge

The evaluation of mandible involvement by oral cancer requires a combination of clinical and radiological assessment for the highest diagnostic reliability.[182]

Table 7: Mandibulotomy versus mandible-sparing approaches.

Characteristic	*Mandibulotomy*	*Mandible-preserving approaches*
Access	++	+
Ease for reconstruction	++	+
Plate-related complication	+	N/A
Mental nerve denervation	N/A	+
Facial scar	+	N/A
Sensory and motor nerve dysfunction	+	++
Ideal subsite	Tongue	Floor of mouth

Table 8: Approaches to oral cancer.

Subsite	*Tumor extent*	*Approach*
Tongue	Resection margin anterior to circumvallate papilla	Per oral
	Resection margin posterior to circumvallate papilla but floor of mouth free	Lip split with mandibulotomy
	Resection margin posterior to circumvallate papilla but floor of mouth involved	Pull-through
Floor of mouth	Anterior or midline lesions not requiring segmental mandibulectomy	Per oral
	Anterior or midline lesions requiring segmental mandibulectomy	Visor
	Posterior lesions or marginal/segmental mandibulectomy	Lower cheek flap
Upper alveolus	Requiring infrastructural maxillectomy	Per oral
	Requiring total maxillectomy	Weber–Ferguson incision
	Requiring total maxillectomy with infratemporal fossa clearance	Weber–Ferguson incision with lower lip slit and mandibulotomy for compartmental resection
Buccal mucosa	Resection margin anterior to tonsillar pillar and up to buccinators	Per oral
	Resection margin posterior to anterior tonsillar pillar	Lower lip split and mandibulotomy or mandibulectomy[174]
	Lower infratemporal fossa involvement	Mandibulotomy or mandibulectomy for compartmental resection[40]
	Pterygoid plate or masticator space involvement	Upper cheek flap with mandibulotomy or mandibulectomy for compartmental resection
	Buccal space involvement	Skin incision as shown in **Figures 10A to E**
Hard palate	Unilateral infrastructural maxillectomy	Per oral or Weber–Ferguson incision
	Bilateral infrastructural maxillectomy	Midfacial degloving
	Total maxillectomy	Weber–Ferguson incision
Lower alveolus	Unilateral marginal or segmental mandibulectomy	Lower cheek flap after making mucosal and lateral soft tissue cuts for adequate margins
	Bilateral marginal or segmental mandibulectomy	Bilateral lower cheek flap after making mucosal and lateral soft tissue cuts for adequate margins

No one radiological investigation can predict mandibular invasion; cross-sectional imaging should be combined with intraoperative periosteal stripping.[183] CT is valuable for cortical erosion, and the reformatted DentaScan can provide accurate evaluation of the buccal and lingual cortical bone with clear visualization of the incisive and inferior alveolar canal;[184] however, patients with fillings or caps may have dental artifacts. MRI has a high negative

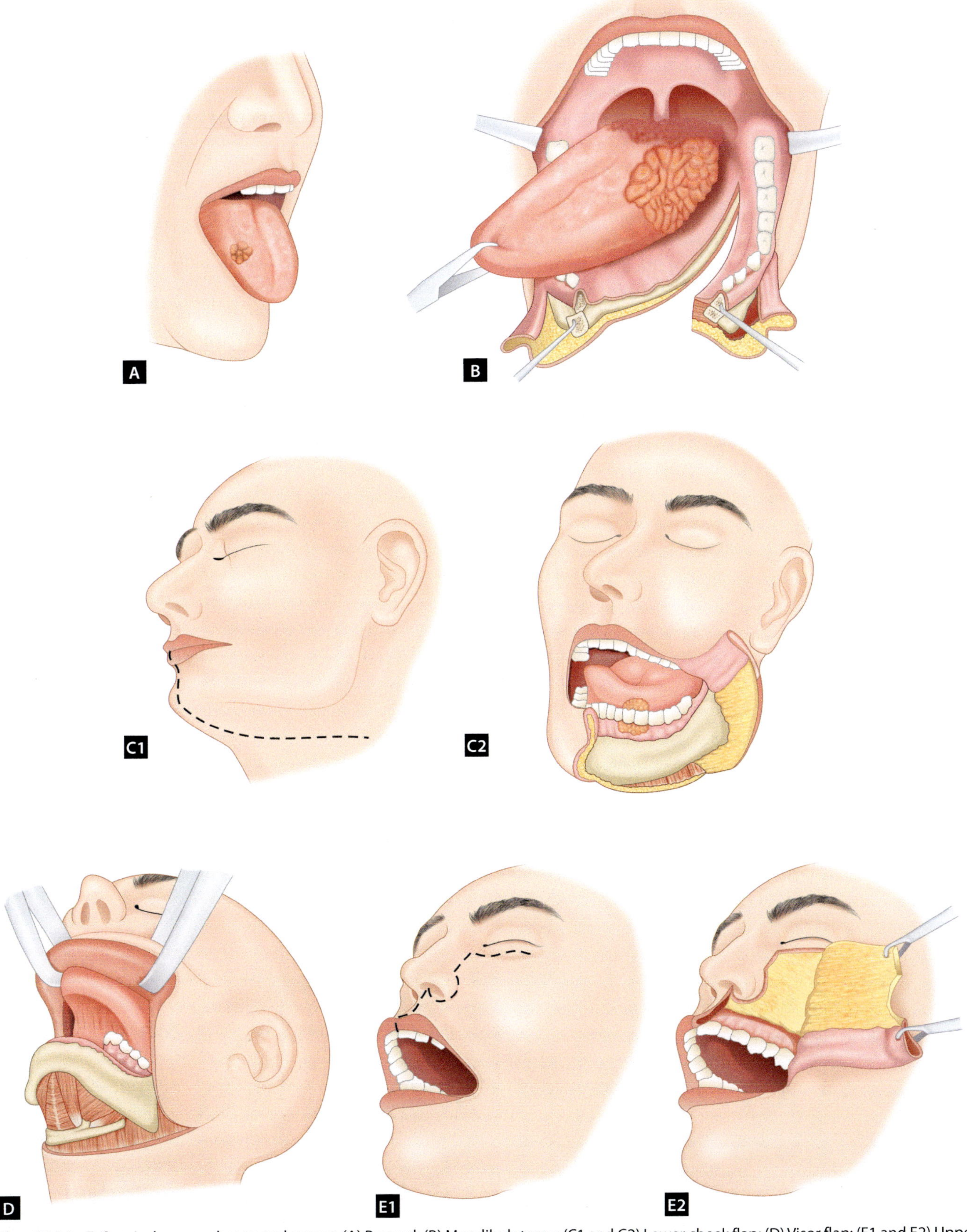

Figs. 10A to E: Surgical approaches to oral cancer. (A) Per oral; (B) Mandibulotomy; (C1 and C2) Lower cheek flap; (D) Visor flap; (E1 and E2) Upper cheek flap.

predictive value; however, specificity is inferior to CT, with a high false-positive rate in dental infection, previous irradiation, or osteoradionecrosis. It is best for assessment of soft tissue involvement adjacent to mandible, perineural spread along the inferior alveolar nerve, and marrow involvement.[185] Nuclear scans, such as technetium, SPECT, and PET, are sensitive for early invasion; however, they are nonspecific with high false-positive rates.[186]

Marginal mandibulectomy is suitable for primary tumor abutting the mandible, those with minimal cortical erosion and minimal involvement of the alveolar process **(Figs. 11A to C)**. This procedure is unsafe, however, in the edentulous mandible (due to high risk of iatrogenic or spontaneous fracture) and in the previously irradiated mandible (due to varied routes of tumor invasion and a higher risk of osteoradionecrosis). Segmental mandibulectomy is suitable for gross invasion, involvement of the medulla, primary mandibular osseous tumors, metastatic tumors to the mandible, paramandibular soft-tissue invasion, and where a marginal resection would leave <1 cm of vertical bone height **(Figs. 12A and B)**.[187]

RECURRENCE AND FOLLOW-UP

Recurrence is defined as the re-emergence of disease after completion of treatment with 6 months having elapsed after complete regression.[188] A majority of recurrences occur within 18 months; hence, the follow-up schedule needs to be more intensive initially. Surveillance protocols vary; the common ones are shown in **Table 9**.

Differentiating between recurrence and SPT is crucial; recurrences are prognostically worse and require aggressive therapy while SPTs are to be treated on their own merit depending on location and stage. Warren and Gates[191] put the first criteria for diagnosis

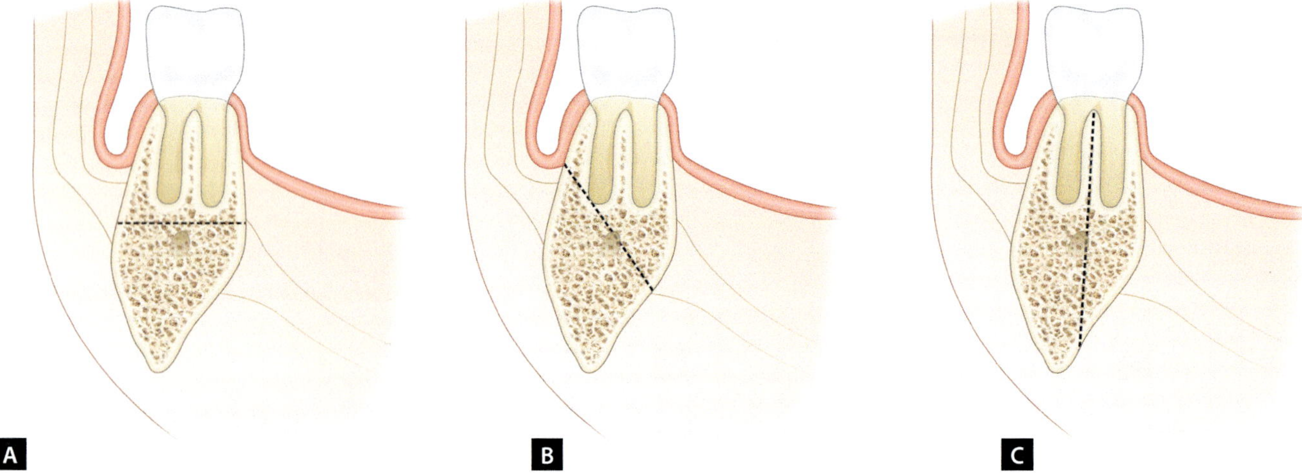

Figs. 11A to C: Marginal mandibulectomy. (A) Horizontal; (B) Oblique; (C) Vertical.

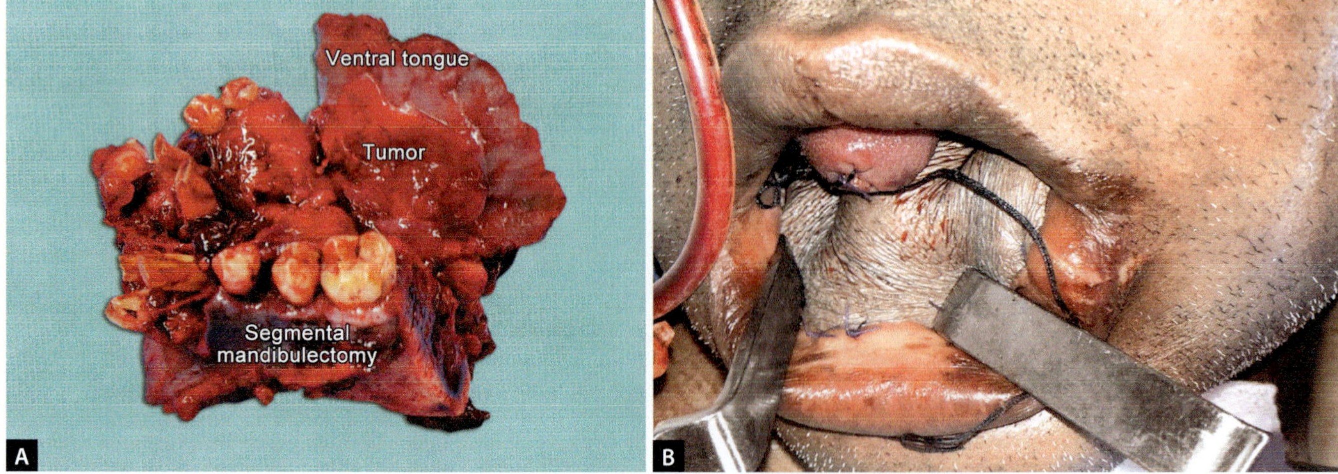

Figs. 12A and B: Floor of mouth malignancy. (A) Excision specimen; (B) Defect reconstructed with fibula free flap.

Table 9: Common surveillance protocols.

National Comprehensive Cancer Network[114]	• Complete clinical examination including fiber-optic examination every 1–3 months for 1st year, 2–6 months for 2nd year, 4–8 months for 3rd–5th year and annually after • Patients with smoking history should be monitored with chest imaging
European Society of Medical Oncology[189]	• Timing of follow-up not specified • Post-treatment baseline imaging of primary and neck recommended
British Association of Head and Neck Oncologists[190]	• Follow-up visits every 4–6 weeks during 1st–2nd year, every 3 months for 3rd year, every 6 months for 4th–5th year • Imaging baseline recommended 3 months after treatment recommended

of SPT forward: (1) both tumors are malignant, (2) two cancers are anatomically separated by normal mucosa, and (3) possibility of one being metastasis from the other is ruled out. Other more sophisticated molecular techniques exist now, such as allelic imbalances in both tumors.[192] SPTs appearing within a 6-month period are synchronous while those appearing later are metachronous; interestingly, one study found that those with synchronous SPTs had significantly worse survival.[193]

CONCLUSION

Although the figures may still seem unimpressive for advanced disease, there has been a considerable improvement in survival for patients with oral cancer over the past two decades, in spite of older age, more advanced disease and a higher rate of distant metastases.[194] This is a reflection of improved standards of surgical and nonsurgical care. Screening and tobacco cessation efforts need to be intensified, especially in the developing world, where these are likely to impact major change. A better understanding of tumor biology is required, to better personalize treatment decisions for optimal outcomes and minimal morbidity. With patients living longer, an emphasis on quality rehabilitative care is paramount for patients to live a fulfilling and productive life.

REFERENCES

1. Snow JB, Wackym PA, Ballenger JJ. Ballenger's Otorhinolaryngology: Head and Neck Surgery, 17th edition. Shelton, Conn; Hamilton, Ont.; London: People's Medical Pub. House/B C Decker; 2009.
2. Sobin LH, Wittekind CH. UICC TNM Classification of Malignant Tumors, 6th edition. New York: Wiley-Liss; 2002.
3. Watkinsom JC, Gaze MN, Wilson JA. Tumors of the lip and oral cavity, Vol 275. London/Oxford: Arnold/Butterworth-Heinemann; 2000. p. 319.
4. Ko YC, Huang YL, Lee CH, Chen MJ, Lin LM, Tsai CC. Betel quid chewing, cigarette smoking and alcohol consumption related to oral cancer in Taiwan. J Oral Pathol Med. 1995;24(10):450-3.
5. Nair S, Singh B, Pawar PV, Datta S, Nair D, Kane S, et al. Squamous cell carcinoma of tongue and buccal mucosa: clinico-pathologically different entities. Eur Arch Otorhinolaryngol. 2016;273(11):3921-8.
6. India Project Team of the International IP, Cancer Genome Consortium. Mutational landscape of gingivo-buccal oral squamous cell carcinoma reveals new recurrently-mutated genes and molecular subgroups. Nat Commun. 2013;4:2873.
7. Vettore AL, Ramnarayanan K, Poore G, Lim K, Ong CK, Huang KK, et al. Mutational landscapes of tongue carcinoma reveal recurrent mutations in genes of therapeutic and prognostic relevance. Genome Med. 2015;7(1):98.
8. Matsuo K, Palmer JB. Anatomy and physiology of feeding and swallowing: normal and abnormal. Phys Med Rehabil Clin N Am. 2008;19(4):691-707.
9. Van De Water T, Staecker H. Basic Science Review for Otolaryngology. New York: Thieme; 2006.
10. Myers JN. Molecular pathogenesis of squamous cell carcinoma of head and neck. In: Myers EN, Syuen JY (Eds). Cancer of Head and Neck. Philadelphia, PA: WB Saunders; 1996. pp. 5-6.
11. Piccirillo JF, Costas I, Reichman ME. Cancers of the head and neck. In: Ries LAG, Young JL, Keel GE, Eisner MP, et al. (Eds). SEER Survival Monograph: Cancer Survival Among Adults: US SEER Program, 1988-2001, Patient and Tumor Characteristics. Bethesda, MD: National Cancer Institute, SEER Program, NIH; 2007.
12. Ferlay J, Soerjomataram I, Ervik M, et al. GLOBOCAN 2012 v1.0, Cancer Incidence and Mortality Worldwide: IARC Cancer Base No. 11. Lyon, France: International Agency for Research on Cancer; 2013. [online] Available from http://globocan.iarc.fr. [Last accessed July, 2020].
13. Simard EP, Torre LA, Jemal A. International trends in head and neck cancer incidence rates: differences by country, sex and anatomic site. Oral Oncol. 2014;50:387-403.
14. Friedlander PL, Schantz SP, Shaha AR, Yu G, Shah JP. Squamous cell carcinoma of the tongue in young patients: a matched-pair analysis. Head Neck. 1998;20(5):363-8
15. Schantz SP, Yu GP. Head and neck cancer incidence trends in young Americans, 1973-1997, with a special analysis for tongue cancer. Arch Otolaryngol Head Neck Surg. 2002; 128(3):268-74.
16. Park JO, Sun DI, Cho KJ, Joo YH, Yoo HJ, Kim MS. Clinical outcome of squamous cell carcinoma of the tongue in young patients: a stage-matched comparative analysis. Clin Exp Otorhinolaryngol. 2010;3:161-5.
17. Petersen PE. Oral cancer prevention and control-the approach of the World Health Organization. Oml Oncol. 2009;45(4-5):454-60.
18. International Agency for Research on Cancer. Tobacco smoke and involuntary smoking. IARC monographs on the evaluation of carcinogenic risks to humans, Vol. 83. Lyon: IARC; 2004. p. 53.
19. Warnakulasuriya S, Trivedy C, Peters TJ. Areca nut use: an independent risk factor for oral cancer: the health problem is under-recognised. Brit Med J. 2002;324(7341):799.
20. Fioretti F, Bosetti C, Thvani A, Franceschi S, La Vecchia C. Risk factors for oral and pharyngeal cancer in never smokers. Oral Oncol. 1999;35(4):375-8.

21. Marron M, Boffetta P, Zhang ZF, Zaridze D, Wünsch-Filho V, Winn DM, et al. Cessation of alcohol drinking, tobacco smoking and the reversal of head and neck cancer risk. Int J Epidemiol. 2009;39(1):182-96.
22. Meurman JH. Infectious and dietary risk factors of oral cancer. Oral Oncol. 2010;46(6):411-3.
23. Singhvi HR, Malik A, Chaturvedi P. The role of chronic mucosal trauma in oral cancer: a review of literature. Indian J Med Paediatr Oncol. 2017;38(1):44.
24. Kademani D. Oral cancer. Mayo Clin Proc. 2007;82:878-87.
25. Toda K, Shibuya H, Hayashi K, Ayukawa F. Radiation-induced cancer after radiotherapy for non-Hodgkin's lymphoma of the head and neck: a retrospective study. Radiat Oncol. 2009;4:21.
26. van Leeuwen MT, Grulich AE, McDonald SP, McCredie MRE, Amin J, Stewart JH, et al. Immunosuppression and other risk factors for lip cancer after kidney transplantation. Cancer Epidemiol Biomarkers Prev. 2009;18:561-9.
27. Slaughter DP, Southwick HW, Smejkal W. "Field cancerization" in oral stratified squamous epithelium; clinical implications of multicentric origin. Cancer. 1953;6(5):963-8.
28. Park BJ, Chiosea SL, Grandis JR. Molecular changes in the multi-stage pathogenesis of head and neck cancer. Cancer Biomark. 2010;9:325-39.
29. Califano J, van der Riet P, Westra W, Nawroz H, Clayman G, Piantadosi S, et al. Genetic progression model for head and neck cancer: implications for field cancerization. Cancer Res. 1996;56(11):2488-92.
30. Jones AS, Morar P, Phillips DE, Field JK, Husband D, Helliwell TR. Second primary tumors in patients with head and neck squamous cell carcinoma. Cancer. 1995;75(6):1343-53.
31. Chuang SC, Scelo G, Tonita JM, Tamaro S, Jonasson JG, Kliewer EV, et al. Risk of second primary cancer among patients with head and neck cancers: a pooled analysis of 13 cancer registries. Int J Cancer. 2008;123(10):2390-6.
32. León X, Quer M, Diez S, Orús C, López-Pousa A, Burgués J. Second neoplasm in patients with head and neck cancer. Head Neck. 1999;21(3):204-10.
33. Davidson J, Gilbert R, Irish J, Witterick I, Brown D, Birt D, et al. The role of panendoscopy in the management of mucosal head and neck malignancy—a prospective evaluation. Head Neck. 2000;22(5):449-54.
34. Meurman JH, Grönroos L. Oral and dental health care of oral cancer patients: hyposalivation, caries and infections. Oral Oncol. 2010;46(6):464-7.
35. Maran AG, Amin M, Wilson JA. Radical neck dissection: a 19-year experience. J Laryngol Otol. 1989;103(8):760-4.
36. Amin MB, Stephen BE, Frederick LG, Byrd DR, Brookland RK, Washington MK, et al. AJCC Cancer Staging Manual, 8th edition. New York: Springer; 2017.
37. Ebrahimi A, Gil Z, Amit M, Yen TC, Liao CT, Chaturvedi P, et al. Primary tumor staging for oral cancer and a proposed modification incorporating depth of invasion: an international multicenter retrospective study. JAMA Otolaryngol Head Neck Surg. 2014;140(12):1138-48.
38. Trivedi NP, Kekatpure V, Kuriakose MA. Radical (compartment) resection for advanced buccal cancer involving masticator space (T4b): Our experience in thirty patients. Clin Otolaryngol. 2012;37(6):477-83.
39. Trivedi NP, Kekatpure VD, Shetkar G, Gangoli A, Kuriakose MA. Pathology of advanced buccal mucosa cancer involving masticator space (T4b). Indian J Cancer. 2015;52(4):611.
40. Chatni SS, Sharan R, Patel D, Iyer S, Tiwari RM, Kuriakose MA. Transmandibular approach for excision of maxillary sinus tumors extending to pterygopalatine and infratemporal fossae. Oral Oncol. 2009;45(8):720-6.
41. Liao CT, Ng SH, Chang JT, Wang HM, Hsueh C, Lee LY, et al. T4b oral cavity cancer below the mandibular notch is resectable with a favorable outcome. Oral Oncol. 2007;43(6):570-9.
42. Ebrahimi A, Murali R, Gao K, Elliott MS, Clark JR. The prognostic and staging implications of bone invasion in oral squamous cell carcinoma. Cancer. 2011;117(19):4460-7.
43. Fried D, Mullins B, Weissler M, Shores C, Zanation A, Hackman T, et al. Prognostic significance of bone invasion for oral cavity squamous cell carcinoma considered T1/T2 by American joint committee on cancer size criteria. Head Neck. 2014;36(6):776-81.
44. Stambuk HE, Karimi S, Lee N, Patel SG. Oral cavity and oropharynx tumours. Radiol Clin N Am. 2007;45:1-20.
45. Kitagawa Y, Nishizawa S, Sano K, Ogasawara T, Nakamura M, Sadato N, et al. Prospective comparison of 18F-FDG PET with conventional imaging modalities (MRI, CT, and 67Ga scintigraphy) in assessment of combined intraarterial chemotherapy and radiotherapy for head and neck carcinoma. J Nucl Med. 2003;44:198-206.
46. Yasumoto M, Shibuya H, Takeda M, Korenaga T. Squamous cell carcinoma of the oral cavity: MR findings and value of T1- versus T2-weighted fast spin-echo images. Am J Roentgenol. 1995;164:981-7.
47. Weber AL, Romo L, Hashmi S. Malignant tumors of the oral cavity and oropharynx: clinical, pathologic, and radiologic evaluation. Neuroimaging Clin N Am. 2003;13:443-64.
48. Ong CK, Chong VH. Imaging of perineural spread in head and neck tumours. Cancer Imaging. 2010;10(1A):S92-8.
49. Shintani S, Yoshihama Y, Ueyama Y, Terakado N, Kamei S, Fijimoto Y, et al. The usefulness of intraoral ultrasonography in the evaluation of oral cancer. Int J Oral Maxillofacial Surg. 2001;30(2):139-43.
50. Songra AK, Ng SY, Farthing P, Hutchison IL, Bradley PF. Observation of tumour thickness and resection margin at surgical excision of primary oral squamous cell carcinoma—assessment by ultrasound. Int J Oral Maxillofacial Surg. 2006;35(4):324-31.
51. Arya S, Chaukar D, Pai P. Imaging in oral cancers. Indian J Radiol Imaging. 2012;22(3):195-208.
52. Quinn MJ. Cancer trends in England and Wales 1950-1999. Studies on medical and population subjects No. 66. London: The Stationery Office; 2001.
53. Conway DI, Stockton DL, Warnakulasuriya KA, Ogdend G, Macphersona LMD. Incidence of oral and oropharyngeal cancer in United Kingdom (1990-1999)—recent trends and regional variation. Oral Oncol. 2006;42(6):586-92.
54. Shiboski CH, Shiboski SC, Silverman S Jr. Trends in oral cancer rates in the United States, 1973-1996. Community Dent Oral Epidemiol. 2000;28(4):249-56.
55. Mroueh R, Haapaniemi A, Grénman R, Laranne J, Pukkila M, Almangush A, et al. Improved outcomes with oral tongue squamous cell carcinoma in Finland. Head Neck. 2017;39(7):1306-12.
56. Ganly I, Patel S, Shah J. Early stage squamous cell cancer of the oral tongue—clinicopathologic features affecting outcome. Cancer. 2012;118(1):101-11.
57. Rusthoven K, Ballonoff A, Raben D, Chen C. Poor prognosis in patients with stage I and II oral tongue squamous cell carcinoma. Cancer. 2008;112(2):345-51.
58. Hicks WL Jr, Loree TR, Garcia RI, Maamoun S, Marshall D, Orner JB, et al. Squamous cell carcinoma of the floor of mouth: a 20-year review. Head Neck. 1997;19(5):400-5.
59. Shaha AR, Spiro RH, Shah JP, Strong EW. Squamous carcinoma of the floor of the mouth. Am J Surg. 1984;148:455-9.

60. Aygun C, Salazar OM, Sewchand W, et al. Carcinoma of the floor of the mouth: a 20-year experience. Int J Radiat Oncol Biol Phys. 1984;10:619-26.
61. Sessions DG, Spector GJ, Lenox J, Parriott S, Haughey B, Chao C, et al. Analysis of Treatment Results for Floor-of-Mouth Cancer. The Laryngoscope. 2000;110(10):1764-72.
62. Kowalski LP, Hashimoto I, Magrin J. End results of 114 extended "commando" operations for retromolar trigone carcinoma. Am J Surg. 1993;166(4):374-9.
63. Huang CJ, Chao KS, Tsai J, Simpson JR, Haughey B, Spector GJ, et al. Cancer of retromolar trigone: long-term radiation therapy outcome. Head Neck. 2001;23(9):758-63.
64. Ayad T, Gélinas M, Guertin L, Larochelle D, Del Vecchio P, Tabet JC, et al. Retromolar trigone carcinoma treated by primary radiation therapy: an alternative to the primary surgical approach. Arch Otolaryngol Head Neck Surg. 2005; 131(7):576-82.
65. Hao SP, Tsang NM, Chang KP, Chen CK, Huang SS. Treatment of squamous cell carcinoma of the retromolar trigone. Laryngoscope. 2006;116(6):916-20.
66. Mendenhall WM, Morris CG, Amdur RJ, Werning JW, Villaret DB. Retromolar trigone squamous cell carcinoma treated with radiotherapy alone or combined with surgery. Cancer. 2005;103(11):2320-5.
67. Diaz EM Jr, Holsinger FC, Zuniga ER, Roberts DB, Sorensen DM. Squamous cell carcinoma of the buccal mucosa: one institution's experience with 119 previously untreated patients. Head Neck. 2003;25(4):267-73.
68. Chhetri DK, Rawnsley JD, Calcaterra TC. Carcinoma of the buccal mucosa. Otolaryngol Head Neck Surg. 2000;123:566-71.
69. Lin CS, Jen YM, Cheng MF, Lin YS, Su WF, Hwang JM, et al. Squamous cell carcinoma of the buccal mucosa: an aggressive cancer requiring multimodality treatment. Head Neck. 2006;28:150-7.
70. Krishnan Nair M, Sankaranarayanan R, Padmanabhan TK. Evaluation of the role of radiotherapy in the management of carcinoma of the buccal mucosa. Cancer. 1988;61(7):1326-31.
71. Fang FM, Wan Leung S, Huang CC, Liu YT, Wang CJ, Chen HC, et al. Combined-modality therapy for squamous carcinoma of the buccal mucosa: treatment results and prognostic factors. Head Neck. 1997;19(6):506-12.
72. Liao CT, Wang HM, Ng SH, Yen TC, Lee LY, Hsueh C, et al. Good tumor control and survivals of squamous cell carcinoma of buccal mucosa treated with radical surgery with or without neck dissection in Taiwan. Oral Oncol. 2006;42(8):800-9.
73. Overholt SM, Eicher SA, Wolf P, Weber RS. Prognostic factors affecting outcome in lower gingival carcinoma. Laryngoscope. 1996;106(11):1335-9.
74. Gomez D, Faucher A, Picot V, Siberchicot F, Renaud-Salis JL, Bussières E, et al. Outcome of squamous cell carcinoma of the gingiva: a follow-up study of 83 cases. J Craniomaxillofac Surg. 2000;28(6):331-5.
75. Hong SX, Cha IH, Lee EW, Kim J. Mandibular invasion of lower gingival carcinoma in the molar region: its clinical implications on the surgical management. Int J Oral Maxillofac Surg. 2001;30(2):130-8.
76. Arduino PG, Carrozzo M, Chiecchio A, Broccoletti R, Tirone F, Borra E, et al. Clinical and histopathologic independent prognostic factors in oral squamous cell carcinoma: a retrospective study of 334 cases. J Oral Maxillofac Surg. 2008;66(8):1570-9.
77. Shingaki S, Nomura T, Takada M, Kobayashi T, Suzuki I, Nakajima T. Squamous cell carcinomas of the mandibular alveolus: analysis of prognostic factors. Oncology. 2002; 62(1):17-24.
78. Beltramini GA, Massarelli O, Demarchi M, Copelli C, Cassoni A, Valentini V, et al. Is neck dissection needed in squamous-cell carcinoma of the maxillary gingiva, alveolus, and hard palate? A multicentre Italian study of 65 cases and literature review. Oral Oncol. 2012;48(2):97-101.
79. Yao M, Chang K, Funk GF, Lu H, Tan H, Wacha J, et al. The failure patterns of oral cavity squamous cell carcinoma after intensity-modulated radiotherapy—the University of Iowa experience. Int J Radiat Oncol Biol Phys. 2007;67(5): 1332-41.
80. De Vicente JC, Recio OR, Pendás SL, López-Arranz JS. Oral squamous cell carcinoma of the mandibular region: a survival study. Head Neck. 2001;23(7):536-43.
81. Yorozu A, Sykes AJ, Slevin NJ. Carcinoma of the hard palate treated with radiotherapy: a retrospective review of 31 cases. Oral Oncol. 2001;37(6):493-7.
82. Ildstad ST, Bigelow ME, Remensnyder JP. Squamous cell carcinoma of the alveolar ridge and palate. A 15-year survey. Ann Surg. 1984;199(4):445-53.
83. Binahmed A, Nason RW, Hussain A, Abdoh AA, Sándor GK. Treatment outcomes in squamous cell carcinoma of the maxillary alveolus and palate: a population-based study. Oral Surg Oral Med Oral Pathol Oral Radiol Endod. 2008;105(6):750-4.
84. Meng FY, Ko JY, Lou PJ, Wang CP, Yang TL, Chang CH, et al. The determining risk factors for treatment outcomes in patients with squamous cell carcinoma of the hard palate. Ann Surg Oncol. 2012;19(6):2003-10.
85. Eskander A, Givi B, Gullane PJ, Irish J, Brown D, Gilbert RW, et al. Outcome predictors in squamous cell carcinoma of the maxillary alveolus and hard palate. Laryngoscope. 2013;123(10):2453-8.
86. de Visscher JG, van den Elsaker K, Grond AJ, van der Wal JE, van der Waal I. Surgical treatment of squamous cell carcinoma of the lower lip: evaluation of long-term results and prognostic factors—a retrospective analysis of 184 patients. J Oral Maxillofac Surg. 1998;56(7):814-20.
87. Antoniades DZ, Styanidis K, Papanayotou P, Trigonidis G. Squamous cell carcinoma of the lips in a northern Greek population. Evaluation of prognostic factors on 5-year survival rate—I. Eur J Cancer Part B: Oral Oncol. 1995;31(5):333-9.
88. Cruse CW, Radocha RF. Squamous cell carcinoma of the lip. Plast Reconstr Surg. 1987;80(6):787-91.
89. Holmkvist KA, Roenigk RK. Squamous cell carcinoma of the lip treated with Mohs micrographic surgery: outcome at 5 years. J Am Acad Dermatol. 1998;38(6):960-6.
90. Vukadinovic M, Jezdic Z, Petrovic M, Medenica LM, Lens M. Surgical management of squamous cell carcinoma of the lip: analysis of a 10-year experience in 223 patients. J Oral Maxillofac Surg. 2007;65(4):675-9.
91. Jovanovic A, Schulten EA, Kostense PJ, Snow GB, van der Waal I. Squamous cell carcinoma of the lip and oral cavity in The Netherlands; an epidemiological study of 740 patients. J Craniomaxillofac Surg. 1993;21(4):149-52.
92. Hasson O. Squamous cell carcinoma of the lower lip. J Oral Maxillofac Surg. 2008;66(6):1259-62.
93. de Visscher JG, Botke G, Schakenraad JA, van der Waal I. A comparison of results after radiotherapy and surgery for stage I squamous cell carcinoma of the lower lip. Head Neck. 1999;21(6):526-30.
94. de Visscher JG, Grond AJ, Botke G, van der Waal I. Results of radiotherapy for squamous cell carcinoma of the vermilion border of the lower lip. A retrospective analysis of 108 patients. Radiother Oncol. 1996;39(1):9-14.

95. Cerezo L, Liu FF, Tsang R, Payne D. Squamous cell carcinoma of the lip: analysis of the Princess Margaret Hospital experience. Radiother Oncol. 1993;28(2):142-7.
96. McCombe D, MacGill K, Ainslie J, Beresford J, Matthews J. Squamous cell carcinoma of the lip: a retrospective review of the Peter Maccallum cancer institute experience 1979–88. ANZ J Surg. 2000;70(5):358-61.
97. Veness MJ, Ong C, Cakir B, Morgan G. Squamous cell carcinoma of the lip. Patterns of relapse and outcome: reporting the Westmead Hospital experience, 1980–1997. J Med Imaging Radiat Oncol. 2001;45(2):195-9.
98. Baker SR, Krause CJ. Carcinoma of the lip. Laryngoscope. 1980;90(1):19-27.
99. Montero PH, Yu C, Palmer FL, Patel PD, Ganly I, Shah JP, et al. Nomograms for preoperative prediction of prognosis in patients with oral cavity squamous cell carcinoma. Cancer. 2014;120(2):214-21.
100. National Cancer Institute (2017). Cancer Stat Facts: Oral Cavity and Pharynx Cancer. National Cancer Institute, Surveillance, Epidemiology and End Result Program. [online] Available from https://seer.cancer.gov/statfacts/html/oralcav.html [Last accessed July, 2020].
101. Montero PH, Patel SG. Cancer of the oral cavity. Surg Oncol Clin. 2015;24(3):491-508.
102. Shoaib T, Soutar DS, MacDonald DG, Camilleri IG, Dunaway DJ, Gray HW, et al. The accuracy of head and neck carcinoma sentinel lymph node biopsy in the clinically N0 neck. Cancer. 2001;91(11):2077-83.
103. Daley T, Darling M. Nonsquamous cell malignant tumours of the oral cavity: an overview. J Can Dent Assoc. 2003;69(9): 577-82.
104. Moss WJ, Coffey CS, Brumund KT, Weisman RA. What is the role of elective neck dissection in low-, intermediate-, and high-grade mucoepidermoid carcinoma? Laryngoscope. 2016;126(1):11-3.
105. Lau VH, Aouad R, Farwell DG, Donald PJ, Chen AM. Patterns of nodal involvement for clinically N0 salivary gland carcinoma: refining the role of elective neck irradiation. Head Neck. 2014;36(10):1435-9.
106. Amit M, Binenbaum Y, Sharma K, Ramer N, Ramer I, Agbetoba A, et al. Incidence of cervical lymph node metastasis and its association with outcomes in patients with adenoid cystic carcinoma. An international collaborative study. Head Neck. 2015;37(7):1032-7.
107. Seethala RR. An update on grading of salivary gland carcinomas. Head Neck Pathol. 2009;3(1):69-77.
108. Weber RS, Benjamin RS, Peters LJ, Ro JY, Achon O, Goepfert H. Soft tissue sarcomas of the head and neck in adolescents and adults. Am J Surg. 1986;152:386-92.
109. Fong Y, Coit DG, Woodruff JM, Brennan MF. Lymph node metastasis from soft tissue sarcoma in adults. Analysis of data from a prospective database of 1,772 sarcoma patients. Ann Surg. 1993;217(1):72.
110. Greager JA, Patel MK, Briele HA, Walker MJ, Das Gupta TK. Soft tissue sarcomas of the adult head and neck. Cancer. 1985;56:820-4.
111. Tran LM, Mark R, Meier R, Calcaterra TC, Parker RG. Sarcomas of the head and neck: prognostic factors and treatment strategies. Cancer. 1992;70:169-77.
112. Umeda M, Shimada K. Primary malignant melanoma of the oral cavity—its histological classification and treatment. Brit J Oral Maxillofac Surg. 1994;32(1):39-47.
113. Mendenhall WM, Amdur RJ, Hinerman RW, Werning JW, Villaret DB, Mendenhall NP. Head and neck mucosal melanoma. Am J Clin Oncol. 2005;28(6):626-30.
114. Pfister DG, Ang KK, Brizel DM, Burtness BA, Busse PM, Caudell JJ, et al. Head and neck cancers, version 2.2013. Featured updates to the NCCN guidelines. J Nat Comprehens Cancer Net: JNCCN. 2013;11(8):917-23.
115. Woolgar JA. Histopathological prognosticators in oral and oropharyngeal squamous cell carcinoma. Oral Oncol. 2006; 42(3):229-39.
116. Yuen PW, Lam KY, Chan AC, Wei WI, Lam LK. Clinicopathological analysis of local spread of carcinoma of the tongue. Am J Surg. 1998;175:242-4.
117. Calabrese L, Giugliano G, Bruschini R, Ansarin M, Navach V, Grosso E, et al. Compartmental surgery in tongue tumours: description of a new surgical technique. Acta Otorhinolaryngol Ital. 2009;29:259-64.
118. Zanoni DK, Migliacci JC, Xu B, Katabi N, Montero PH, Ganly I, et al. A proposal to redefine close surgical margins in squamous cell carcinoma of the oral tongue. JAMA Otolaryngol Head Neck Surg. 2017;143(6):555-60.
119. Tasche KK, Buchakjian MR, Pagedar NA, Sperry SM. Definition of "close margin" in oral cancer surgery and association of margin distance with local recurrence rate. JAMA Otolaryngol Head Neck Surg. 2017;143(12):1166-72.
120. Subramaniam N, Balasubramanian D, Murthy S, Limbachiya S, Thankappan K, Iyer S. Adverse pathological features in early oral squamous cell carcinoma and the role of post-operative radiotherapy—a review. Oral Surg Oral Med Oral Pathol Oral Radiol. 2017;124(1):24-31.
121. D'Cruz AK, Vaish R, Kapre N, Dandekar M, Gupta S, Hawaldar R, et al. Elective versus therapeutic neck dissection in node-negative oral cancer. N Eng J Med. 2015;373(6):521-9.
122. Byers RM, Weber RS, Andrews T, McGill D, Kare R, Wolf P. Frequency and therapeutic implications of "skip metastases" in the neck from squamous carcinoma of the oral tongue. Head Neck. 1997;19(1):14-9.
123. Results of a prospective trial on elective modified radical classical versus supraomohyoid neck dissection in the management of oral squamous carcinoma. Brazilian Head and Neck Cancer Study Group. Am J Surg. 1998;176:422-7.
124. Schilling C, Stoeckli SJ, Haerle SK, Broglie MA, Huber GF, Sorensen JA, et al. Sentinel European Node Trial (SENT): 3-year results of sentinel node biopsy in oral cancer. Eur J Cancer. 2015;51(18):2777-84.
125. Thomadsen BR, Miller R (2005). Brachytherapy Physics. Medical Physical Publishing. [online] Available from https://www.aapm.org/meetings/amos2/pdf/42-11873-3201-79.pdf [Last accessed July, 2020].
126. Mazeron JJ, Ardiet JM, Haie-Méder C, Kovács G, Levendag P, Peiffert D, et al. GEC-ESTRO recommendations for brachytherapy for head and neck squamous cell carcinomas. Radiother Oncol. 2009;91(2):150-6.
127. Umeda M, Komatsubara H, Nishimatsu N, Yokoo S, Shibuya Y, Komori T. High-dose rate interstitial brachytherapy for stage I-II tongue cancer. Oral Surg Oral Med Oral Pathol Oral Radiol Endod. 2000;90(5):667-70.
128. Liu Z, Huang S, Zhang D. High dose rate versus low dose rate brachytherapy for oral cancer–a meta-analysis of clinical trials. PloS One. 2013;8(6):e65423.
129. Umeda M, Komatsubara H, Ojima Y, Minamikawa T, Shibuya Y, Yokoo S, et al. A comparison of brachytherapy and surgery for the treatment of stage I–II squamous cell carcinoma of the tongue. Int J Oral Maxillofac Surg. 2005; 34(7):739-44.
130. Brennan S, Corry J, Kleid S, Porceddu S, Yuen K, Rischin D, et al. Prospective trial to evaluate staged neck dissection or

elective neck radiotherapy in patients with CT-staged T1-2 N0 squamous cell carcinoma of the oral tongue. Head Neck. 2010;32(2):191-8.

131. Murthy V, Agarwal JP, Laskar SG, Gupta T, Budrukkar A, Pai P. Analysis of prognostic factors in 1180 patients with oral cavity primary cancer treated with definitive or adjuvant radiotherapy. J Cancer Res Ther. 2010;6:282-9.
132. Studer G, Zwahlen RA, Graetz KW, Davis BJ, Glanzmann C. IMRT in oral cavity cancer. Radiat Oncol. 2007;2:16.
133. Sowder JC, Cannon RB, Buchmann LO, Hunt JP, Hitchcock Y, Lloyd S, et al. Treatment-related determinants of survival in early-stage (T1-2N0M0) oral cavity cancer: a population-based study. Head Neck. 2017;39(5):876-80.
134. Bernier J, Cooper J, Pajak T, van Glabbeke M, Bourhis J, Forastiere A, et al. Defining risk levels in locally advanced head and neck cancers: a comparative analysis of concurrent post-operative radiation plus chemotherapy trials of the EORTC (22931) and RTOG (9501). Head Neck. 2005;27(10):843-50.
135. Brandwein-Gensler M, Teixeira MS, Lewis CM, Lee B, Rolnitzky L, Hille JJ, et al. Oral squamous cell carcinoma: histologic risk assessment, but not margin status, is strongly predictive of local disease-free and overall survival. Am J Surg Pathol. 2005;29(2):167-78.
136. Ch'ng S, Corbett-Burns S, Stanton N, Gao K, Shannon K, Clifford A, et al. Close margin alone does not warrant post-operative adjuvant radiotherapy in oral squamous cell carcinoma. Cancer. 2013;119(13):2427-37.
137. Ajmani GS, Nocon CC, Wang CH, Bhayani MK. Assessment of adjuvant therapy in resected head and neck cancer with high-risk features. Oral Oncol. 2017;74:15-20.
138. Lydiatt WM, Patel SG, O'Sullivan B, Brandwein MS, Ridge JA, Migliacci JC, et al. Head and neck cancers—major changes in the American Joint Committee on cancer eighth edition cancer staging manual. CA Cancer J Clin. 2017;67(2):122-37.
139. Wreesmann VB, Katabi N, Palmer FL, Montero PH, Migliacci JC, Gönen M, et al. Influence of extracapsular nodal spread extent on prognosis of oral squamous cell carcinoma. Head Neck. 2016;38(S1):E1192-9.
140. O'Brien CJ, Lahr CJ, Soong SJ, Gandour MJ, Jones JM, Urist MM, et al. Surgical treatment of early-stage carcinoma of the oral tongue—would adjuvant treatment be beneficial? Head Neck Surg. 1986;8(6):401-8.
141. Lydiatt DD, Robbins KT, Byers RM, Wolf PF. Treatment of stage I and II oral tongue cancer. Head Neck. 1993;15(4): 308-12.
142. Rahima B, Shingaki S, Nagata M, Saito C. Prognostic significance of perineural invasion in oral and oropharyngeal carcinoma. Oral Surg Oral Med Oral Pathol Oral Radiol Endod. 2004;97(4):423-31.
143. Tai SK, Li WY, Chu PY, Chang SY, Tsai TL, Wang YF, et al. Risks and clinical implications of perineural invasion in T1-2 oral tongue squamous cell carcinoma. Head Neck. 2012; 34(7):994-1001.
144. Tai SK, Li WY, Yang MH, Chu PY, Wang YF, Chang PM. Perineural invasion as a major determinant for the aggressiveness associated with increased tumor thickness in t1-2 oral tongue and buccal squamous cell carcinoma. Ann Surg Oncol. 2013;20(11):3568-74.
145. Sparano A, Weinstein G, Chalian A, Yodul M, Weber R. Multivariate predictors of occult neck metastasis in early oral tongue cancer. Otolaryngol Head Neck Surg. 2004;131(4): 472-6.
146. Close LG, Brown PM, Voitch MF, Reisch J, Schaefer SD. Microvascular invasion and survival in cancer of the oral cavity and oropharynx. Arch Otolaryngol Head Neck Surg. 1989;115(11):1304-9.
147. Almangush A, Bello IO, Keski-Säntti H, Mäkinen LK, Kauppila JH, et al. "Depth of invasion, tumor budding, and worst pattern of invasion: prognostic indicators in early-stage oral tongue cancer." Head Neck. 2014;36(6):811-8.
148. Huang TY, Hsu LP, Wen YH, Huang TT, Chou YF, Lee CF, et al. Predictors of locoregional recurrence in early stage oral cavity cancer with free surgical margins. Oral Oncol. 2010;46(1): 49-55.
149. Al-Rajhi N, Khafaga Y, El-Husseiny J, Saleem M, Mourad W, Al-Otieschan A, et al. Early stage carcinoma of oral tongue: prognostic factors for local control and survival. Oral Oncol. 2000;36:508-14.
150. Low TH, Gao K, Gupta R, Clifford A, Elliott M, Ch'ng S, et al. Factors predicting poor outcomes in T1N0 oral squamous cell carcinoma: indicators for treatment intensification. ANZ J Surg. 2016;86:366-71.
151. Ang KK, Trotti A, Brown BW, Garden AS, Foote RL, Morrison WH, et al. Randomized trial addressing risk features and time factors of surgery plus radiotherapy in advanced head-and-neck cancer. Int J Radiat Oncol Biol Phys. 2001; 51(3):571-8.
152. Shrime MG, Gullane PJ, Dawson L, Kim J, Gilbert RW, Irish JC, et al. The impact of adjuvant radiotherapy on survival in T1-2N1 squamous cell carcinoma of the oral cavity. Arch Otolaryngol Head Neck Surg. 2010;136(3):225-8.
153. Chen MM, Harris JP, Hara W, Sirjani D, Divi V. Association of postoperative radiotherapy with survival in patients with N1 oral cavity and oropharyngeal squamous cell carcinoma. JAMA Otolaryngol Head Neck Surg. 2016;142(12):1224-30.
154. Kowalski LP, Bagietto R, Lara JR, Santos RL, Tagawa EK, Santos IR. Factors influencing contralateral lymph node metastasis from oral carcinoma. Head Neck. 1999;21(2): 104-10.
155. Ambrosch P, Kron M, Pradier O, Steiner W. Efficacy of selective neck dissection: a review of 503 cases of elective and therapeutic treatment of the neck in squamous cell carcinoma of the upper aerodigestive tract. Otolaryngol Head Neck Surg. 2001;124(2):180-7.
156. Pellitteri PK, Robbins KT, Neuman T. Expanded application of selective neck dissection with regard to nodal status. Head Neck. 1997;19(4):260-5.
157. McLean T, Kerr SJ, Giddings CE. Prophylactic dissection of level V in primary mucosal SCC in the clinically N positive neck: A systematic review. Laryngoscope. 2017;127(9):2074-80.
158. Cannon RB, Sowder JC, Buchmann LO, Hunt JP, Hitchcock YJ, Lloyd S, et al. Increasing use of nonsurgical therapy in advanced-stage oral cavity cancer: a population-based study. Head Neck. 2017;39(1):82-91.
159. Spiotto MT, Jefferson G, Wenig B, Markiewicz M, Weichselbaum RR, Koshy M. Differences in survival with surgery and postoperative radiotherapy compared with definitive chemoradiotherapy for oral cavity cancer: A National Cancer Database Analysis. JAMA Otolaryngol Head Neck Surg. 2017;143(7):691-9.
160. Iyer NG, Tan DS, Tan VK, Wang W, Hwang J, Tan NC, et al. Randomized trial comparing surgery and adjuvant radiotherapy versus concurrent chemoradiotherapy in patients with advanced, nonmetastatic squamous cell carcinoma of the head and neck: 10-year update and subset analysis. Cancer. 2015;121(10):1599-607.
161. Hui HS, O'Sullivan B. "Oral cancer: current role of radiotherapy and chemotherapy." Med Oral Patol Oral Cir Bucal. 2013;18(2):e233-40.

162. Shah JP. Surgical approaches to the oral cavity primary and neck. Int J Radiat Oncol Biol Phys. 2007;69(2):S15-8.
163. Battoo AJ, Thankappan K, Ahmad SZ, Hedne N, Balasubramanian D, Trivedi N, et al. Efficacy of per oral access in the surgical management of T2/T3 oral cavity squamous cell carcinoma. Otolaryngol Head Neck Surg. 2012;147(6):1069-75.
164. Sutton DN, Brown JS, Rogers SN, Vaughan ED, Woolgar JA. The prognostic implications of the surgical margin in oral squamous cell carcinoma. Int J Oral Maxillofac Surg. 2003;32(1):30-4.
165. Woolgar JA, Triantafyllou A. A histopathological appraisal of surgical margins in oral and oropharyngeal cancer resection specimens. Oral Oncol. 2005;41(10):1034-43.
166. Stanley RB. Mandibular lingual releasing approach to oral and oropharyngeal carcinomas. Laryngoscope. 1984;94(5): 596-600.
167. Evans PH, Montgomery PQ, Gullane PJ. Principles and practice of head and neck surgery and oncology. CRC Press; 2009.
168. Baek CH, Lee SW, Jeong HS. New modification of the mandibulotomy approach without lip splitting. Head Neck. 2006;28(7):580-6.
169. Steiner T, Raith S, Scherer E, Mücke T, Torsiglieri T, Rohleder NH, et al. Which kind of frontal mandibulotomy is the smartest? A biomechanical study. J Craniomaxillofac Surg. 2015;43(2):199-203.
170. Engroff SL, Blanchaert RH, von Fraunhofer JA. Mandibulotomy fixation: a laboratory analysis. J Oral Maxillofac Surg. 2003;61(11):1297-301.
171. Smeele LE, Slotman BJ, Mens JW, Tiwari R. Local radiation dose, fixation, and non-union of mandibulotomies. Head Neck. 1999;21(4):315-8.
172. Sharan R, Iyer S, Chatni SS, Samuel J, Sundaram KR, Cohen RF, et al. Increased plate and osteosynthesis related complications associated with postoperative concurrent chemoradiotherapy in oral cancer. Head Neck. 2008;30(11):1422-30.
173. Pang P, Li RW, Shi JP, Xu ZF, Duan WY, Liu FY, et al. a comparison of mandible preservation method and mandibulotomy approach in oral and oropharyngeal cancer: A meta-analysis. Oral Oncol. 2016;63:52-60.
174. Tiwari RM, Kodaganur GS, Rao GS. The value of transmandibular approach to total maxillectomy in the management of T3-T4 carcinoma of the maxillary sinus. Eur Arch Otorhinolaryngol. 2010;267(6):951-4.
175. Ward GE, Robben JO. A composite operation for radical neck dissection and removal of cancer of the mouth. Cancer. 1951;4:98-109.
176. Greer DB, Smith RR, Klopp CT. A surgical method of treatment of carcinoma of the floor of the mouth. Surgery. 1953;34(2):279-87.
177. Slootweg PJ, Müller H. Mandibular invasion by oral squamous cell carcinoma. J Craniomaxillofac Surg. 1989;17(2):69-74.
178. Dubner S, Heller KS. Local control of squamous cell carcinoma following marginal and segmental mandibulectomy. Head Neck. 1993;15(1):29-32.
179. McGregor AD, MacDonald DG. Routes of entry of squamous cell carcinoma to the mandible. Head Neck. 1988;10(5): 294-301.
180. Cawood JI, Howell RA. A classification of the edentulous jaws. Int J Oral Maxillofac Surg. 1988;17(4):232-6.
181. Brown JS, Lowe D, Kalavrezos N, D'Souza J, Magennis P, Woolgar J. Patterns of invasion and routes of tumor entry into the mandible by oral squamous cell carcinoma. Head Neck. 2002;24(4):370-83.
182. Brown JS, Griffith JF, Phelps PD, Browne RM. A comparison of different imaging modalities and direct inspection after periosteal stripping in predicting the invasion of the mandible by oral squamous cell carcinoma. Brit J Oral Maxillofac Surg. 1994;32(6):347-59.
183. Brown JS, Lewis-Jones H. Evidence for imaging the mandible in the management of oral squamouscell carcinoma: a review. Brit J Oral Maxillofac Surg. 2001;39(6):411-8.
184. King JM, Caldarelli DD, Petasnick JP. Dentascan—a new diagnostic method for evaluating mandibular and maxillary pathology. Laryngoscope. 1992;102:379-87.
185. Vidiri A, Guerrisi A, Pellini R, Manciocco V, Covello R, Mattioni O, et al. Multi-detector row computed tomography (MDCT) and magnetic resonance imaging (MRI) in the evaluation of the mandibular invasion by squamous cell carcinomas (SCC) of the oral cavity. Correlation with pathological data. J Experiment Clin Cancer Res. 2010;29(1):73.
186. Shaw RJ, Brown JS, Woolgar JA, Lowe D, Rogers SN, Vaughan ED. The influence of the pattern of mandibular invasion on recurrence and survival in oral squamous cell carcinoma. Head Neck. 2004;26(10):861-9.
187. Barttelbort SW, Ariyan S. Mandible preservation with oral cavity carcinoma: rim mandibulectomy versus sagittal mandibulectomy. Am J Surg. 1993;166(4):411-5.
188. Lok BH, Setton J, Ho F, Riaz N, Rao SS, Lee NY. Chapter 41: "Nasopharynx". In: Halperin EC, Brady LW, Perez CA, Wazer DE (Eds). Perez & Brady's Principles and Practice of Radiation Oncology, 6th edition. Philadelphia: Lippincott Williams & Wilkins; 2013. pp. 730-59.
189. Grégoire JL, Licitra LL, Felip E, "Squamous cell carcinoma of the head and neck: EHNS-ESMO-ESTRO clinical practice guidelines for diagnosis, treatment and follow-up." Ann Oncol. 2010;21(Suppl 5):v184-6.
190. British Association of Head and Neck Oncologists. "Practice care guidance for clinicians participating in the management of head and neck cancer patients in the UK. Drawn up by a Consensus Group of Practising Clinicians." Eur J Surg Oncol. 2001;27(Suppl A):S1-17.
191. Warren S, Gates O. Multiple malignant tumors: a survey of literature and statistical study. Am J Cancer. 1932;16: 1358-414.
192. Braakhuis BJM, Tabor MP, Leemans CR, van der Waal I, Snow GB, Brakenhoff RH. Second primary tumors and field cancerization in oral and oropharyngeal cancer: molecular techniques provide new insights and definitions. Head Neck. 2002;24(2):198-206.
193. Panosetti A, Luboinski B, Mamelle G, Richard JM. Multiple synchronous and metachronous cancers of the upper aerodigestive tract: a nine-year study. Laryngoscope. 1989; 99:1267-73.
194. Amit M, Yen TC, Liao CT, Chaturvedi P, Agarwal JP, Kowalski LP, et al. Improvement in survival of patients with oral cavity squamous cell carcinoma: an international collaborative study. Cancer. 2013;119(24):4242-8.

CHAPTER 12

Cancers of the Oropharynx

Samskruthi P Murthy, Sivakumar Vidhyadharan, Narayana Subramaniam

INTRODUCTION

Oropharyngeal cancer forms a significant portion of head and neck cancer and has perhaps undergone the most radical change in etiology, outcome, and treatment over time. Even though there has been an increasing incidence of oropharyngeal cancer over the last three decades, the mortality and the outcomes in oropharyngeal cancer has significantly improved, which is likely to be a reflection of the increasing proportion of human papillomavirus (HPV) in this subsite.[1] The treatment of oropharyngeal cancer has evolved from open resection to organ preservation and now treatment de-escalation strategies. Advances in surgery, radiation, and chemotherapy have significantly improved outcomes in these patients.

ANATOMY

The oropharynx forms a conduit between the respiratory and alimentary tract, as it communicates superiorly with the nasopharyngeal cavity, inferiorly with larynx and hypopharynx and anteriorly with the oral cavity. The boundaries of the oropharynx are the circumvallate papillae of the tongue anteriorly, the junction of hard and soft palate superiorly, the hyoid inferiorly and the pharyngeal wall forming the lateral and posterior perimeter of the oropharynx.[2] The subsites of the oropharynx are base of tongue (BOT), tonsillar complex, soft palate, and posterior pharyngeal wall.

Base of Tongue

Base of tongue is bounded by the circumvallate papillae, base of epiglottis (including the vallecula), and glossopharyngeal sulcus. The substance of BOT consists of musculature, contributed to by the genioglossus, styloglossus, palatoglossus, and hyoglossus muscles. The surface mucosa is lined by squamous epithelium and contains numerous submucosal lymphoid deposits (lingual tonsil) that form a component of Waldeyer's ring. Motor innervation is supplied by the hypoglossal and sensory by the glossopharyngeal nerves. It is important to be familiar with the course of the lingual artery and hypoglossal nerve within the BOT during resection of tumors. The lingual artery branches off from the external carotid at the level of the greater horn of hyoid then passes lateral to middle constrictor muscle, coursing anterolateral to hyoid, and pass deep to hyoglossus muscle. The hypoglossal nerve runs between hyoglossus and stylohyoid and then runs deep to tongue musculature along the superior border of the hyoid. Nodal metastases are primarily to levels II–IV and the retropharyngeal nodes.[2]

Tonsil

The palatine tonsils are lymphoid aggregates lined by a fibrous capsule that rests between palatoglossus and palatopharyngeus muscles. The surface of the tonsil is covered by squamous epithelium and consists of various crypts that are not available for inspection. Sensory innervation is by the maxillary division of the trigeminal nerve (V2). The lateral relations of tonsil are extremely important, especially if tonsillar tumors are planned for surgical resection. The lateral wall of the tonsil is formed by superior and middle constrictor muscle and stylopharyngeus muscle that is traversed by stylopharyngeus, styloglossus, and stylohyoid ligament. The buccopharyngeal fascia forms the division between constrictor and parapharyngeal space. The tonsillar area drains primarily to levels II–II and the retropharyngeal nodes.[2]

Soft Palate

The soft palate is a muscular organ formed by levator veli palatini, tensor veli palatini, palatoglossus, and palatopharyngeus. It is lined by stratified squamous epithelium with motor innervation by the mandibular branch of the trigeminal nerve (V3) and the vagus. The function of the soft palate is crucial for both speech and swallowing as it separates nasopharynx from the oral cavity and oropharynx.[2]

Oropharyngeal Wall

The oropharyngeal wall forms the posterolateral boundary of oropharynx and extends from inferior aspect of the nasopharynx to the level of epiglottis inferiorly. It is lined by squamous epithelium that overlies pharyngeal constrictor muscle, retropharyngeal space, longus capitis and coli muscles, prevertebral fascia and vertebral body posteriorly. It typically is located at the level of C2-C3 vertebra.[2]

EPIDEMIOLOGY

Understanding the epidemiology of oropharynx is vital as the etiological factor affects the final outcome of the disease. The incidence and etiology of oropharyngeal tumors has been subject to demographic changes. The incidence rate has risen from 2.8 to 3.6 per 100,000 population over the last two decades, however the death rate has reduced by 1.77 per 100,000 population.[3] The major increase in incidence is restricted to HPV-related tumors, while the incidence of smoking and alcohol-related oropharyngeal tumors are decreasing. Previously, smoking-related oropharyngeal tumors predominated, with most patients being men in the age group 50–70 years. With a rise in HPV-related tumors, there has been a shift resulting in many younger patients presenting with these tumors. Various lifestyle-related risk factors have been described in oropharyngeal tumors such as sexual habits, oral hygiene, dietary intake of fruits and vegetables, and body mass index.[4] The lifetime risk of oropharyngeal cancer with smoking is 5–12% and 35% for tobacco and alcohol combined.[5] The geographical distribution of HPV-related oropharyngeal cancers is variable with the highest incidence in North America (56%), followed by Australia (45%), Northern, Eastern, and Western Europe (38–39%), Southern Europe (17%), and the rest of the world (13%).[6] High-risk sexual behavior is defined as an increased number of oral sex partners, number of lifetime sexual partners, young age at first coitus, and a history of genital warts. The International Head and Neck Cancer Epidemiology Consortium (INHANCE) reported that with more lifetime and oral sex partners there was an increased risk of oropharyngeal cancer.[7]

Human Papillomavirus in India

The prevalence of HPV in India is difficult to comprehend, as available data with respect to Indian studies is highly variable. The prevalence of HPV-positive head and neck cancer ranges from 7 to 78.7% in Indian studies.[8,9] The variability can be attributed to publication bias, different techniques of HPV detection, and variable sample sizes. HPV-positive oropharyngeal cancer was reported to be 15–22.5%.[8,10] The impact of tobacco usage and alcohol use is important as the prevalence of high-risk behaviors such as tobacco chewing, smoking, chewing and smoking, and alcohol use in HPV-positive head and neck cancer were 53.34%, 47.54%, 47.05%, and 33.48%, respectively.[11] Murthy et al. showed an improved overall survival and cancer specific survival in patients with HPV-positive tumors who were nonsmokers.[12] This survival benefit was lost when the comparison was made between p16-positive and p16-negative head and neck cancer without evaluating the impact of tobacco. Studies have also shown that tobacco use increases the incidence of HPV infection and has an additive effect on carcinogenesis **(Flowchart 1)**.[13]

Carcinogenesis

The main risk factors associated with oropharyngeal carcinoma are tobacco exposure and HPV. The classical progression and initiation of disease has been characterized by chromosomal loss of 9p21, followed by loss of region in chromosome 3p (encodes suppressor gene *FHIT* and *RASSFIA*).[14-17] Later events that drive carcinogenesis are loss of heterozygosity, chromosomal region loss of 17p and p53 mutation.[18] Carcinogen exposure causes genetic events that collectively lead to tumor progression and initiation. Mucosal damage secondary to carcinogen exposure involves an inflammatory cascade that results in a compensatory mechanism, which increases cell proliferation and the risk of mutation.

The association of HPV in oropharyngeal tumors is well recognized. HPV is a circular double-stranded deoxyribonucleic acid (DNA) virus, measuring 55 nm and belongs to the papillomavirus family. Various subtypes (>100) are described, but high-risk subtypes involved in carcinogenesis include 16, 18, 31, and 33.[19] HPV16 is the most common virus identified in oropharynx tumors. HPV commonly affects lingual and palatine tonsils followed by the soft palate and posterior pharyngeal wall.

Flowchart 1: HPV-induced carcinogenesis.

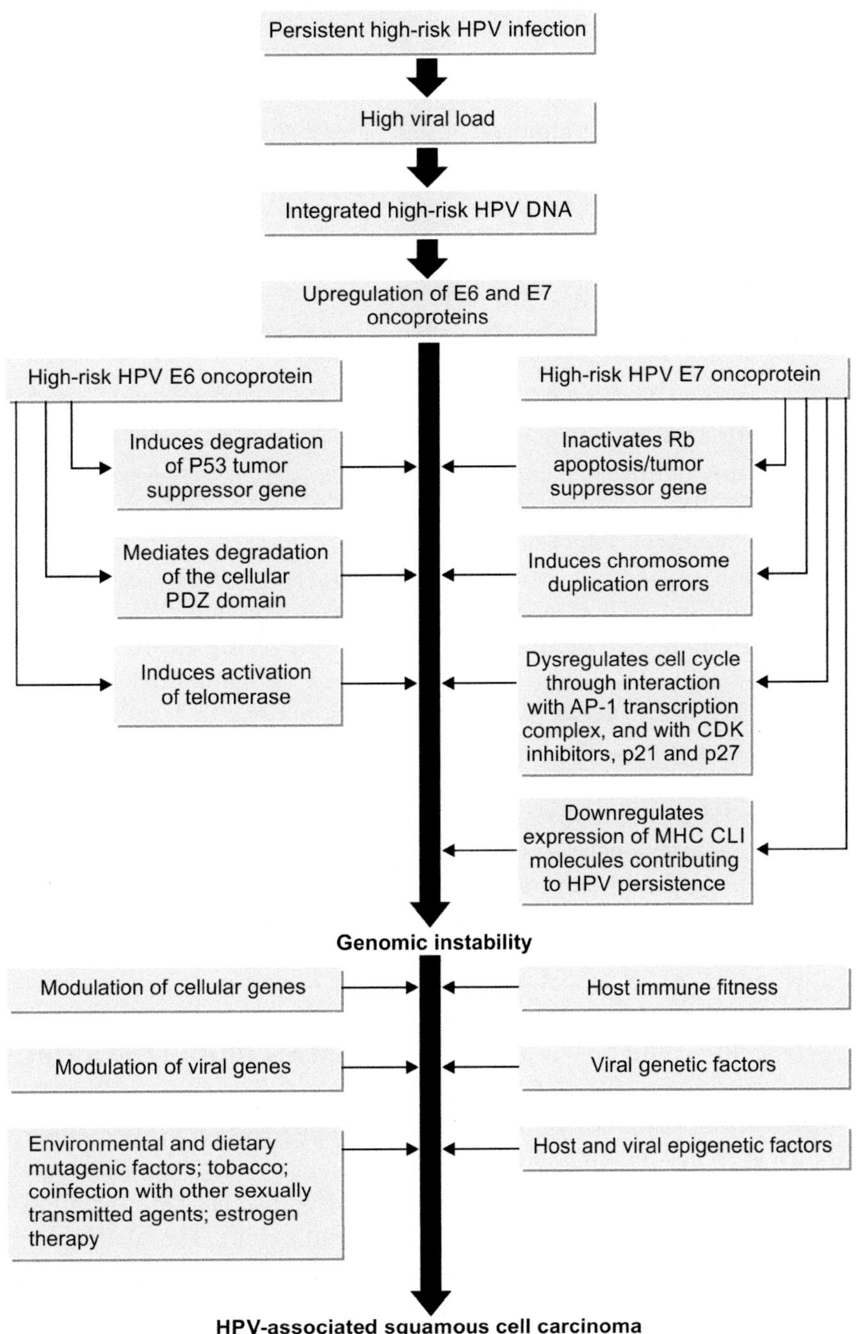

(AP-1: activator protein 1; CDK: cyclin-dependent kinase; DNA: deoxyribonucleic acid; HPV: human papillomavirus)

Tonsillar crypts are analogous to transformation zones of the uterine cervix.[19] Early (E1, E2, E4, E5, E6, and E7) genes and late genes (L1 and L2) are involved in forming structural proteins of the viral capsid.[20]

Heparan sulfate proteoglycans (HSPGs) are located on the cell surface of the keratinocyte that binds to virion via L1 ligand.[21] HPV also binds to cyclophilin B that enables virion uncoating, which is facilitated by L2-N terminal exposure.[22] Cleaved L2 binds annexin A2 heterotetramer that allows internalization of HPV into the keratinocyte.[22] In vitro studies have shown that virion precoated with HSPG growth factor bind to epidermal growth factor receptor (EGFR) of mucosal cell, which in turn activates PIK3CA, AKT, and mTOR pathways.[23] The internalization of HPV occurs by clathrin and caveolin mediated pathways.[20]

After internalization, L2 bound viral DNA escapes from endosomes to reach nucleus along cytoplasmic microtubules.[24] Once inside the nucleus, the viral genome randomly integrates into the host genome.[25] HPV DNA can also be present as an episomal or extrachromosomal particle, as host genome integration occurs in late stages.[26] Transcriptions of viral genomes promote cellular transformation and initiate malignant transformation. E6 and E7 play a crucial role in carcinogenesis. E-associated protein (E6AP) forms complexes with p53 (tumor suppressor gene) that results in p53 degradation via ubiquitin ligase. P53 regulates G1/S and G2/M checkpoints of the cell cycle. E7 protein interferes with the *Rb* gene where degradation of Rb releases E2F, which stimulates S phase of the cell cycle.[20] Each cell consists of 50–100 copies of viral DNA, as the replication process is independent of the cell cycle. When host cell exits cell cycle, the viral gene expression and DNA replication gets further amplified. P16 is a cyclin-dependent kinase inhibitor protein that inhibits pRb phosphorylation by CDK4-cyclin D complex and blocks cell cycle progression. When E7 blocks *Rb* gene, there is overexpression of p16 as a negative feedback mechanism. Thus p16 immunohistochemistry (IHC) is used as a surrogate marker for HPV. Due to the effect of E6/7 on cell cycle regulation, as previously described, there is continued cell cycle progression and inactivation of antiapoptotic pathways that ultimately result in the initiation of invasive tumor.[27]

Human papillomavirus-associated tumors are a distinct entity with respect to molecular signature, pathogenesis, clinical presentation, and final oncologic outcome. HPV-negative tumors show loss of function of TP53, CDKN2A inactivation, and copy number alterations.[28] The difference in molecular characteristics between HPV-positive and HPV-negative tumors is represented in **Table 1**.

Table 1: Genetic alterations in human papillomavirus (HPV)-associated and non-HPV-associated head and neck squamous cell carcinoma (HNSCC).

Genetic alteration	*Non-HPV-associated HNSCC*	*HPV-associated HNSCC*
CDKN2A	Common	Rare
p16^{INK4a} overexpression	Rare	Common
Epidermal growth factor receptor (EGFR)	Common	Rare
p53	Common	Rare (p53 degradation by E6)
pRb	Rare	Rare (pRb degradation by E7)
PIK3CA	Common	Common
TRAF3	Rare	Common

Immune Evasion by Human Papillomavirus

The prevalence of HPV infection is much higher than incidence of HPV-associated oropharyngeal cancer; this stands as evidence that not all who gets infected by HPV develop HPV-associated tumors. Immune evasion is commonly seen in HPV-associated tumors. Patient infected with human immunodeficiency virus (HIV) shows a higher prevalence of HPV-associated tumors and incidence is directly proportional to the levels of CD4 counts.[29] Persistence of HPV in the tissue is essential for malignant transformation. Immune evasion is a property of early proteins (E5, E6, and E7). E7 expression downregulates cell expression of human leukocyte antigen (HLA) class I and transporters associated with antigen processing (TAP).[30] E6 inhibits STAT-1 pathway which plays an essential role in cellular immune response.[31] Programmed death-ligand 1 (PD-L1) and PD1 interaction lead to T cell activation and cytotoxic T cell lysis and hence aids in tumor progression. PD-L1 is expressed by tumor cells and, antigen-presenting cells and PD1 on T cells. 50–60% of head and neck squamous cell carcinoma (HNSCC) express PD-L1.[32] While studies have reported no difference in PD-L1 expression in HPV-positive and HPV-negative tumors, it is evident that HPV evades host immune system to initiate malignant transformation by multiple mechanisms.

HUMAN PAPILLOMAVIRUS TESTING

- *Routine histology:* HPV-positive tumors are characterized by invasion in sheets, lobules or ribbons of cells, absence of strong desmoplastic stromal reaction and with focal keratinization (predominantly non-keratinizing). The histologic picture is 99% specific for HPV infection but lacks sensitivity.[33]
- *Southern blot test:* Southern blot test is a technique that involves enzymatic digestion of viral DNA that is separated by gel electrophoresis and transferred to a membrane. Southern blot test is technically complex and needs fresh frozen sample and hence is impractical to use in a clinical setting.[34]
- *p16 IHC:* p16 is a marker for transcriptional activity for HPV infection. IHC staining of more than 70% is considered positive for p16.[35] Due to its high sensitivity of 94%, low cost, and wide availability has resulted in routine clinical use of p16 IHC.[36] The specificity is low (82%), as up to 20% of p16-positive tumors are HPV-negative on further investigations.[37]

The reliability of interpretation becomes difficult when the IHC staining is weak or equivocal, which happens in less than 5% of cases. When the treatment decision is based on the HPV status of the tumor, then p16 alone is considered inferior and may need an additional test, either polymerase chain reaction (PCR) or DNA/ribonucleic acid (RNA) in situ hybridization (ISH).[37]

- *In situ hybridization:* The principle of ISH is based on the annealing of a labeled probe to target nucleic acids [(DNA/messenger RNA (mRNA)]. The probe consists of complementary sequences to the target nucleic acids. DNA ISH is a clinically available test that can identify integrated HPV. The sensitivity and specificity is around 88%.[36] DNA ISH utilizes formalin-fixed paraffin embedded tissue. The sensitivity of the test may drop when viral load is low and is associated with 11% interobserver discordance.[38] This technique is more widely available in most laboratories. RNA ISH is superior to DNA ISH as it identifies transcriptionally active HPV. RNA ISH is an ideal test as it can amplify low viral signal and has high sensitivity and specificity of 97% and 93%, respectively.[39] However, RNA ISH is a complex procedure, as the procedure is not automated and too laborious.
- *Polymerase chain reaction:* PCR technique can amplify DNA or mRNA target sequences by billions of copies. DNA polymerase is used to synthesize complementary DNA to the offered template with prespecified primer. Reverse transcription PCR (RT-PCR) technique uses reverse transcriptase enzyme to synthesize complementary DNA from target mRNA. Detection of E6/E7 mRNA by RT-PCR is considered the gold standard as it precisely indicates the presence of transcriptionally active HPV **(Table 2)**.[40] PCR to detect HPV DNA is widely available and relatively easier to use. The test is highly sensitive (97%), but the specificity is lower (87%).[41] PCR HPV DNA can be used on formalin-fixed paraffin-embedded tissue. This test can be applied in fine-needle aspiration cytology (FNAC) and saliva samples.

Combination testing is advocated to improve test accuracy. A two-step or three-step testing can be employed. The common two test combinations are p16 IHC with PCR for HPV DNA or p16 IHC with HPV DNA ISH.[35] The transcriptional activity is expressed by p16 positivity that has high sensitivity, and HPV DNA ISH has high specificity and hence complements p16 IHC. This combination of test has been widely used in large epidemiological studies and clinical trials. The combination of p16 IHC with PCR for HPV DNA and p16 IHC with HPV DNA ISH are associated with sensitivities of 97% and 88% and specificities of 94%

Table 2: HPV detection methods.

Method	*Advantages*	*Disadvantages*
HPV DNA		
Consensus and type-specific PCR	High sensitivity	Inability to discern clinically relevant infections from irrelevant infections
Real-time PCR	High sensitivity and specificity, estimation of viral load	Requires complex tissue processing (e.g., microdissection, DNA extraction)
ISH	Optimized for fixed tissues, visualization of viral distribution, highly specific	Reduced specificity at low viral load
Hybrid capture 2	Can be applied to cytologic samples, no need for specimen processing	Further studies are needed to determine overall sensitivity and specificity
HPV RNA		
Reverse transcriptase PCR	Highly sensitive, highly specific	Limited to fresh frozen tissue
HPV proteins		
E6/E7 immunohistochemistry	Visualization of oncoprotein expression	Poor performance
Cellular proteins		
p16 immunohistochemical staining	Optimized for fixed tissues, highly sensitive, strong correlation with HPV interation	Low specificity
Serum antibodies		
Anti-HPV protein antibodies	Minimally invasive, no tissue requirement	Marker of lifetime cumulative exposure to HPV, low sensitivity and specificity as cancer marker

(DNA: deoxyribonucleic acid; HPV: human papillomavirus; ISH: in situ hybridization; PCR: polymerase chain reaction; RNA: ribonucleic acid) and 90%, respectively. The three-test combination is advised for more precision.[38] The algorithm consists of first testing p16 IHC and HPV DNA ISH. PCR is employed only when the sample is p16-positive, but DNA ISH is negative. Using PCR as the third test allowed categorization of HPV into positive/negative in as many as 98% of cases.

Presence of HPV in FNAC aspirate is essential in cases of metastasis of unknown origin. DNA ISH, PCR, and p16 IHC can be used on cell blocks from FNAC aspirate. Due to low sample volume for testing, especially in a cystic node, interpretation of tests is difficult; a lower threshold of p16 IHC staining for FNAC aspirate has been reported to increase the sensitivity and specificity of the test.[35] Liquid-based PCR testing (usually employed for cervical cancer) has been used in FNAC samples of neck nodes with very high sensitivity and specificity of 94.7% and 100%, respectively.[41]

The current recommendation is to use p16 IHC to assess HPV status of the tumor as it is cost-effective and widely available and has high sensitivity. Additional tests such as PCR/DNA ISH can be employed when treatment decision is based solely on HPV status.

HISTORY AND CLINICAL PRESENTATION

Common symptoms are dysphagia or odynophagia, change in voice, hemoptysis or neck lump. Referred otalgia is common in oropharyngeal tumors and is mediated by pharyngeal and tonsillar branches of the glossopharyngeal nerve that traverse petrosal ganglion and synapse with the tympanic nerve of Jacobson which innervate middle ear. The overall rate of lymph node metastases at presentation is 45–78%.[2] Clinical evaluation involves flexible nasopharyngolaryngoscopy and detailed examination of the neck and cranial nerves.

Tumors of the BOT can grow proliferatively into lumen of oropharynx or exhibit submucosal growth. In advanced cases, the tumor can involve deep muscles causing restricted tongue mobility. Most tumors are asymptomatic until advanced stage. Nodal metastases at presentation is 70% ipsilaterally and 10–20% on the contralateral side.[42]

Tumors from tonsil commonly are exophytic or ulcerative **(Fig. 1)**. Submucosal growth is common in advanced tumors. Nodal metastasis occurs at presentation in 69% of patients with tonsillar tumors.[43] Presentation with contralateral nodal metastasis is variable (6–22%).[44]

Tumors that affect the soft palate grow along the mucosal surfaces to adjacent subsites. The lymphatic drainage is to levels II–III and retropharyngeal node with nodal metastasis occurring in 40% of patients.[42]

Tumors of the oropharyngeal wall have a tendency to grow submucosally and hence most often present in advanced stage. About 57% of patients have nodal disease at presentation and bilateral nodal metastasis is common.[42]

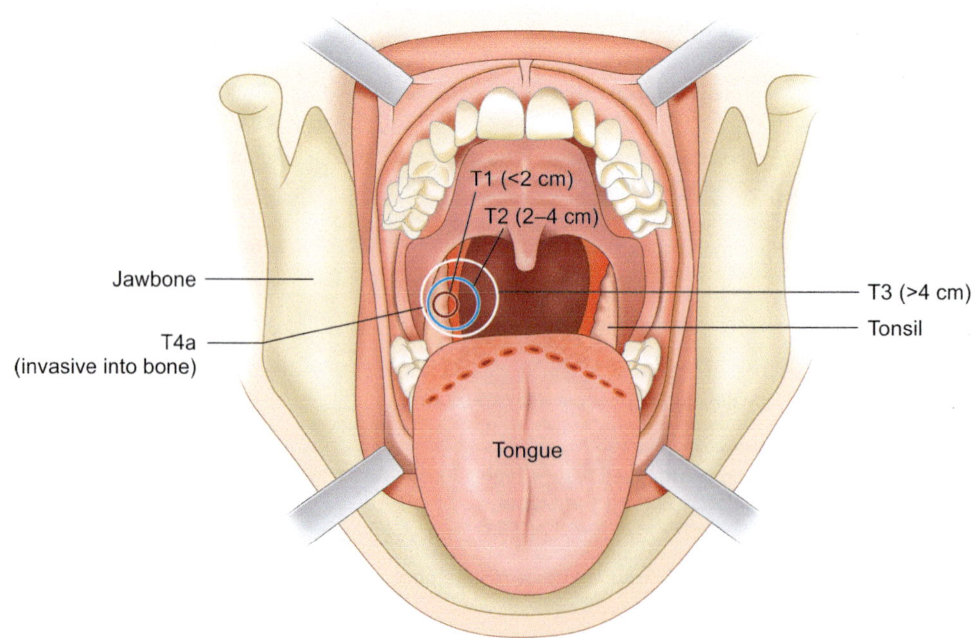

Fig. 1: Clinical staging of tonsil cancer.

EVALUATION

Imaging

The complexity of anatomy in the oropharyngeal region mandates cross-sectional imaging in all cases to assess tumor extent/spread and effectively stage the disease. Various modalities such as contrast-enhanced computed tomography (CT), magnetic resonance imaging (MRI), and positron emission tomography fused with contrast-enhanced computed tomography (PET CT) have been described. Route of spread with respect to adjacent structures; extension to surrounding deep neck spaces, especially parapharyngeal, retropharyngeal, and prevertebral spaces that are in close proximity to oropharyngeal tumors; involvement of lymph nodes; and muscles such as tongue musculature, medial pterygoid muscle, and pharyngeal constrictors must be assessed.

Computed tomography, the most common imaging modality, used due to its wide availability, short acquisition time, fewer motion artefacts, and simultaneous chest screening capability. The tumor extent delineation, bone involvement, and lymph nodal extension can be assessed with accuracy **(Figs. 2A and B)**.

However due to its better soft tissue delineation, MRI is preferred over CT. MRI is superior to CT in the evaluation of early bone involvement, pterygopalatine fossa, prevertebral muscle perineural spread, and extension to the spaces of the neck. The MRI protocols should be high resolution with 3–4 mm slice thickness. The sequences consist of sagittal T1, axial T2 with fat saturation, axial T1, and post-gadolinium with fat saturation.[45] Oropharyngeal carcinomas show intermediate signal on both T1 and T2. Normal lymphoid tissue also shows signal intensity on T1, which tends to be high in T2. Fat planes are crucial in evaluating oropharyngeal tumors. Fat suppression techniques are utilized to neutralize high-intensity fat against tumor margins and are extremely helpful in postcontrast images.[46] CT is inferior in assessing evidence of extra-tonsillar spread to adjacent structures due to poor soft tissue differentiation. The evaluation of soft palate is best described in the coronal and sagittal planes. Perineural spread along lesser palatine nerve can occur. The posterior oropharyngeal wall is in close proximity to the retropharyngeal and prevertebral space. The preserved retropharyngeal fat plane on T1 image has high negative predictive value for tumor involvement.[47,48] BOT is a muscular subsite, and hence tumors of this region is best evaluated with MRI. The inferior extension into preepiglottic fat space can be easily differentiated on MRI. It appears hypointense on sagittal T1 sequence in the background of hyperintense signal from the preepiglottic fat. The extent of fat infiltration plays a major deciding role in cases where surgery is planned. Early mandibular invasion can be assessed by MRI with high accuracy of 93% and a negative predictive value of 96%.[49] The role of PET CT in a primary setting is limited as local tumor extent and identification of lymph nodes

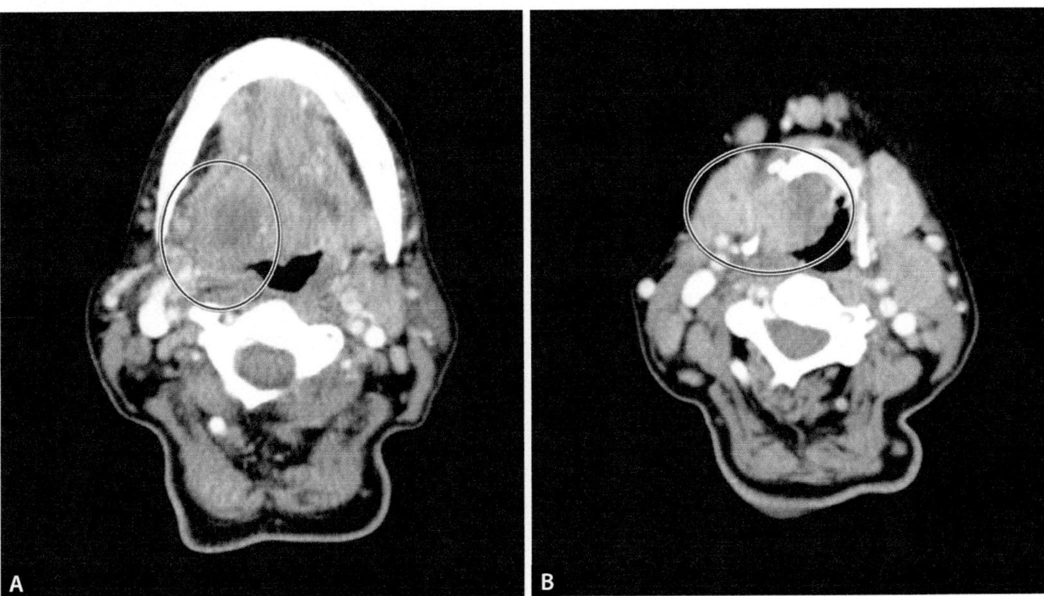

Figs. 2A and B: Axial section of contrast enhanced CT neck in a case of carcinoma base of tongue. (A) Blue circle denotes tumor involving right side of base of tongue, tonsillolingual sulcus, right tonsil up to posterior pharyngeal wall; (B) Blue circle denotes inferior extension of tumor along lateral pharyngeal wall to erode right greater horn of hyoid bone.

can be done accurately with MRI or CT scan. Use of PET CT can be advocated when radiation doses and volume are based on PET detected tumor extension.

Assessment of the nodal size, morphological features, and margination is important to characterize the node as benign or malignant. Lymph nodes measuring over 1 cm which are rounded (Solbiati index <2), central necrosis, peripheral enhancement, loss of fatty hilum, irregular margin, stranding around the node, and irregular rim like enhancement are characteristic of nodal metastasis. Perineural spread can be defined by foraminal thickening, loss of fat around the nerve, increased thickness of the nerve, and appreciating secondary changes in the muscle. A blinded match pair analysis of image characteristic between HPV-positive and HPV-negative tumors of oropharyngeal cancer has shown that HPV-positive tumors are associated with well-defined borders and cystic nodal metastasis while HPV-negative tumors most often demonstrated poorly defined margins and invasion to adjacent muscle.[50]

The indications to evaluate for distant metastasis are patients with lymph node metastasis involving lower regions of the neck and locally advanced cancers (T3/T4 primary and ≥N2 nodal stage).[51] Either PET CT or CT of the chest can be performed to assess mediastinal lymph node involvement and lung metastasis or second primary in the lung. These recommendations are general to all head and neck cancers; there is no separate consensus for recommendation of distant metastasis evaluation with respect to oropharyngeal cancer.

Biopsy

Evaluation under anesthesia is undesirable and not recommended, especially when the treatment plan consists of a nonsurgical modality. The biopsy tissue from the oropharyngeal tumor must be subjected to routine histopathology and p16 IHC. Confirmation of histology can also be performed from the neck nodes. Determination of HPV positivity is important at present because the staging algorithms are different for HPV-positive and HPV-negative oropharyngeal tumors.

Staging

The American Joint Committee on Cancer (AJCC) 8th edition staging systems are shown in **Tables 3 to 5**. The International Collaboration on Oropharyngeal cancer Network for Staging (ICON-S) multicentric data formed the basis that paved the way to changes in tumor, node, and metastasis (TNM) staging in AJCC 8th edition.[52] The cohort included 1,907 patients with HPV-positive oropharyngeal cancer. The overall survival in patients with N1, N2a, and N2b did not significantly defer; hence they were grouped into a single category of ipsilateral node less than or equal to 6 cm.

Table 3: AJCC 8th edition staging for HPV-negative oropharyngeal cancer.

Tx	Primary tumor cannot be assessed
Tis	Carcinoma in situ
T1	Tumor 2 cm or smaller in greatest dimension
T2	Tumor larger than 2 cm but not larger than 4 cm in greatest dimension
T3	Tumor larger than 4 cm in greatest dimension or extension to the lingual surface of epiglottis
T4a	*Moderately advanced local disease:* Tumor invades the larynx, extrinsic muscle of tongue, medial pterygoid, hard palate, or mandible
T4b	*Very advanced local disease:* Tumor invades lateral pterygoid muscle, pterygoid plates, lateral nasopharynx, or skull base or encases carotid artery
Nx	Regional lymph nodes cannot be assessed
N0	No nodal metastasis
N1	Metastasis in a single ipsilateral lymph node, 3 cm or less in greatest dimension and ENE-negative
N2a	Metastasis in a single ipsilateral or contralateral lymph node 3 cm or less in greatest dimension and ENE-positive; or metastasis in a single ipsilateral lymph node more than 3 cm but not more than 6 cm in greatest dimension and ENE-negative
N2b	Metastasis in multiple ipsilateral lymph nodes, none more than 6 cm in greatest dimension and ENE-negative
N2c	Metastasis in bilateral or contralateral lymph nodes, none more than 6 cm in greatest dimension and ENE-negative
N3a	Metastasis in a lymph node more than 6 cm in greatest dimension and ENE-negative
N3b	Metastasis in a single ipsilateral node more than 3 cm in greatest dimension and ENE-positive; or metastasis in multiple ipsilateral, contralateral, or bilateral lymph nodes, with any ENE-positive
M0	No metastases
M1	Metastatic disease

(AJCC: American Joint Committee on Cancer; ENE: extranodal extension; HPV: human papillomavirus)

Another multicentric study that consisted of the p16 positive oropharyngeal cancer who underwent surgical resection showed that patients with four or less metastatic node had a higher 5-year overall survival rates than those with five or more (89% vs. 71%, respectively).[53] The results from this analysis guided the current pathologic staging system for patients with p16 positive oropharyngeal cancer. The modifications to the staging criteria of oropharyngeal p16 positive cancer is based on prognostic models and not on prospective data from clinical trials that will guide in treatment decision-making. The impact of HPV on prognosis and outcome has been

Table 4: AJCC 8th edition staging for HPV-associated oropharyngeal cancer.

Tumor staging	
Tx	Primary tumor cannot be assessed
Tis	Carcinoma in situ
T1	Tumor 2 cm or smaller in greatest dimension
T2	Tumor larger than 2 cm but not larger than 4 cm in greatest dimension
T3	Tumor larger than 4 cm in greatest dimension or extension to the lingual surface of epiglottis
T4	Moderately advanced local disease: Tumor invades the larynx, extrinsic muscle of tongue, medial pterygoid, hard palate, or mandible or beyond
Nodal staging	
Nx	Regional lymph nodes cannot be assessed
N0	No nodal metastasis
A. Clinical	
N1	One or more ipsilateral lymph nodes, none larger than 6 cm
N2	Contralateral or bilateral lymph nodes, none larger than 6 cm
N3	Lymph node(s) larger than 6 cm
B. Pathological	
N1	Metastasis in 4 or fewer lymph nodes
N2	Metastasis in more than 4 lymph nodes
Metastasis staging	
M0	No distant metastases
M1	Metastatic disease

(AJCC: American Joint Committee on Cancer; HPV: human papillomavirus)

Table 5: Combined tumor, node, and metastasis (TNM) staging in oropharyngeal cancer.

p16 positive	*N0*	*N1*	*N2*	*N3*
T0	N/A	I	II	III
T1	I	I	II	III
T2	I	I	II	III
T3	II	II	II	III
T4	III	III	III	III
Any M1 is stage IV				
p16 positive	*N0*	*N1*	*N2a/b/c*	*N3a/b*
T1	I	III	IVA	IVB
T2	II	III	IVA	IVB
T3	III	III	IVA	IVB
T4a	IVA	IVA	IVA	IVB
T4b	IVB	IVB	IVB	IVB
Any M1 is stage IVC				

well-established, and hence various deintensification strategies have been planned.

Ang KK et al. proposed a risk stratification based on p16 positivity and smoking history.[54] The stratification consisted of low-risk group (p16 positive tumors in patients with <10 pack-years of smoking), intermediate-risk group (p16 positive tumors in patients with >10 pack-years of smoking or p16 negative tumors in patients with <10 pack-years of smoking), and high risk group (p16 negative tumors in patients with >10 pack-years of smoking). The overall reduction of death in HPV-positive patients was 58%. The 3-year overall survival in low-, intermediate-, and high-risk group was 93%, 70.8%, and 46.2%, respectively. Most recent trials have utilized these criteria to risk-stratify patients for de-escalation or intensification of treatment.

MANAGEMENT

The current standard of treatment is relatively unchanged as robust data from the de-intensification trials is still awaited. The National Comprehensive Cancer Network (NCCN) recommendations on the management of oropharyngeal cancer are represented in the **Tables 6 and 7.**[51]

ROLE OF RADIOTHERAPY

Radiation therapy (RT) as a single modality or concurrent with chemotherapy [chemoradiotherapy (CRT)] is considered standard of care for curative-intent treatment of oropharyngeal cancer. There is evidence that local control is related to total radiation dose and treatment time. European Organisation for Research and Treatment of Cancer (EORTC) 202791 studied the clinical benefit of altered fractionation which compared hyperfractionation (HR) to conventional radiation[55] and showed that patients with HR had better local control. Based on these findings Radiation Therapy Oncology Group (RTOG) 9003 investigated an altered fractionation

Table 6: NCCN treatment recommendations based on the clinical stage of oropharyngeal tumors (non-HPV associated).[51]

p16 negative	*T1*	*T2*	*T3*	*T4*
N0	RT/resection of primary + ND		CRT/resection of primary + ND with appropriate adjuvant therapy/IC + CCRT or RT	
N1				
N2	CRT/resection of primary + ND with appropriate adjuvant therapy/IC + CCRT or RT			
N3				

(CCRT: concurrent chemoradiotherapy; CRT: chemoradiotherapy; HPV: human papillomavirus; IC: induction chemotherapy; NCCN: National Comprehensive Cancer Network; ND: neck dissection; RT: radiotherapy)

Table 7: NCCN treatment recommendations based on the clinical stage of oropharyngeal tumors (HPV associated).[51]

p16 positive	*T1*	*T2*	*T3*	*T4*
N0	Resection of primary + ND/RT		CCRT/RT/resection of primary + ND with appropriate adjuvant therapy/ IC + CRT or RT	CCRT/RT/resection of primary + ND with appropriate adjuvant therapy/IC + CCRT or RT
N1 (Single node ≤3 cm)	Resection of primary + ND/RT/CCRT			
N1 (Single node >3 cm or 2 or more ipsilateral nodes ≤6 cm)	CRT/resection of primary + ND with appropriate adjuvant therapy/IC + CCRT or RT			
N2				
N3	CCRT/resection of primary + ND with appropriate adjuvant therapy/IC + CCRT or RT			

(CCRT: concurrent chemoradiotherapy; CRT: chemoradiotherapy; HPV: human papillomavirus; IC: induction chemotherapy; NCCN: National Comprehensive Cancer Network; ND: neck dissection; RT: radiotherapy)

scheme that consisted of conventional fractionation of 70 Gy (2 Gy per fractionation delivered once daily) versus split course accelerated fractionation versus concomitant boost fractionation of 72 Gy total dose with a boost of 1.5 Gy hyperfractionated dose during the last 12 days of treatment versus HR.[56] The trial included 1,073 patients, among which oropharyngeal cancer comprised 60%. The study reported that patients with HR and concomitant boost had significantly better locoregional control than other fractionations. The follow-up data showed that HR continued to show improved locoregional control rates than all other altered fractionation. A DAHANCA randomized trial also compared altered fractionation with standard versus altered fractions in treatment of head and neck cancers 28% of patients had pharyngeal tumors, and the study showed benefit with six fractionation per week with improved 5-year local control of 76% and disease-specific survival of 73% versus five fractions per week which showed a lower local control of 54% and disease-specific survival of 66%.[57] These trials support altered fractionation for treating for oropharyngeal cancers.

The current fractionation and target volume dosing recommendations are general and are as represented below:[51]

- *Simultaneous integrated boost technique:* In this technique, 66–72 Gy to gross disease and 44–63 Gy to subclinical disease are delivered either in five fractionations per week or six fractionations per week accelerated schedule.
- *Sequential technique:* It delivers a lower dose during the first 5 weeks, followed by a high boost volume during the sixth and seventh week. This technique uses two to three separate dose plans.
- *Concomitant boost accelerated schedule:* It is a modified sequential technique where dose to the subclinical target is delivered once a day for 6 weeks and a separate boost dose as a second daily fraction is delivered during the last 12 weeks of treatment.

Even though the benefit of HR of 0.83 has been proven, the benefit is not sustained in the context of concurrent chemotherapy. Radiation doses exceeding 72 Gy may lead to unacceptable rates of normal tissue injury, especially in conventional fractionation regime. When elective neck irradiation is planned, then the low-risk site requires 44 Gy and intermediate-risk site requires 63 Gy. During the postoperative period, a dose of 60–66 Gy is rendered with or without systemic therapy with a preferred interval of 6 weeks or less between resection and commencement of RT.

The MARCH meta-analysis, which included 15 randomized trials, showed a survival benefit of 3.4% at 5 years and the updated analysis with 33 trials showed a sustained benefit of HR.[58,59] Most of the trials that have shown the efficacy of concurrent chemoradiotherapy (CCRT) have used conventional fractionation. Based on this, conventional fractionation is considered standard of care, especially in a concurrent setting. RTOG 0129 compared accelerated fractionation with two cycles of cisplatin versus standard fractionation with three cycles of cisplatin showed no significant difference in survival between the two arms, proving that altered fractionation regimen is not beneficial when concurrent with chemotherapy.[60]

Technique of Radiation Therapy

Earlier, conventional radiotherapy with low energy megavoltage or cobalt 60 irradiation was used with a three-field technique where posterior neck electron fields was introduced after 40–42 Gy to protect the spinal cord.[2] Intensity-modulated radiation therapy (IMRT) with three-dimensional (3D) planning and CT/MRI/PET CT based simulations are now considered standard of care for oropharyngeal cancer. IMRT is a 3D conformal radiotherapy which has the capacity to deliver high-dose radiation to the tumor with sparing of nontargeted tissue by steep dose gradient. The advantage of improved target conformity and also ability to produce intentional dose inhomogeneity (dose painting) has made IMRT the standard of care in oropharyngeal tumors.

IMRT is essential due to the presence of various radiosensitive dose-limiting structures in close proximity to the tumor in the oropharyngeal region. IMRT uses multiple fields of up to seven to nine beams of 6 MV photon to target the primary tumor and high-risk regional area. Accurate definition of treatment volume and treatment planning is vital to minimize radiation-related toxicity **(Figs. 3 and 4)**. Radiation planning integrates clinical examination, image findings, known patterns of locoregional spread, and pattern of failure to be incorporated into the treatment planning. Gross tumor volume (GTV) includes tumor and nodal volume of the gross tumor. In the postoperative setting and postinduction chemotherapy setting, the pretreatment imaging and clinical findings are factored into RT planning. The clinical target volume (CTV) is based on the stage of the disease, and the risk of harboring occult disease is integrated into planning. The dose and fractionation of RT is described in **Table 8.**[2]

The RTOG 0022 evaluated the use of IMRT in treating early-stage oropharyngeal cancer to assess feasibility (good target coverage and parotid sparing) and also to assess early and late toxicities.[61] The trial included 69 patients with T1-2N0-1 oropharyngeal cancer patients who were treated with IMRT alone to a dose of 66 Gy in 30 fractions. The authors concluded that IMRT is

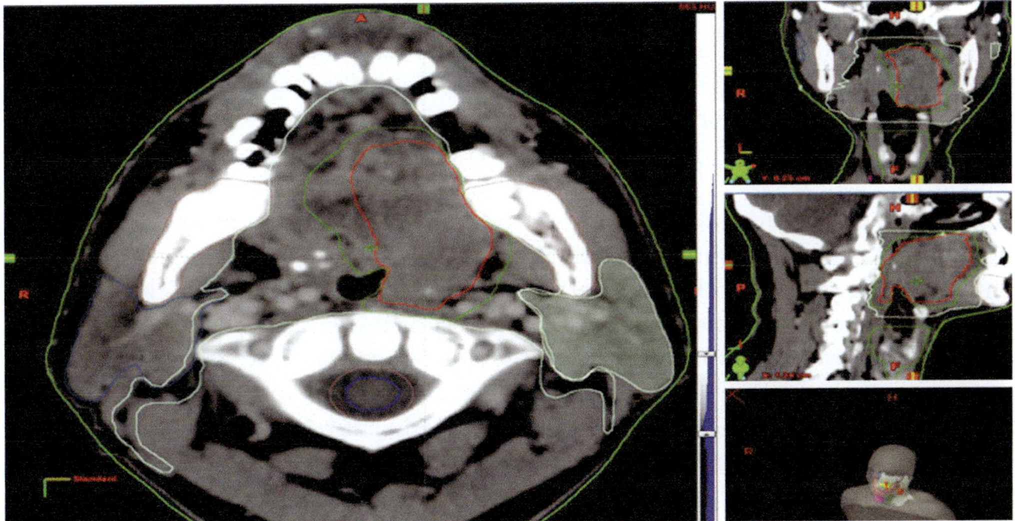

Fig. 3: Intensity-modulated radiation therapy planning for carcinoma base of tongue. Gross tumor volume is marked by red line, high-risk clinical tumor volume by dark green line and intermediate-risk clinical tumor volume by light green line.
Courtesy: Dr Surendra Reddy, Consultant Radiation Oncologist, BGS Gleneagles Global Hospital, Bengaluru.

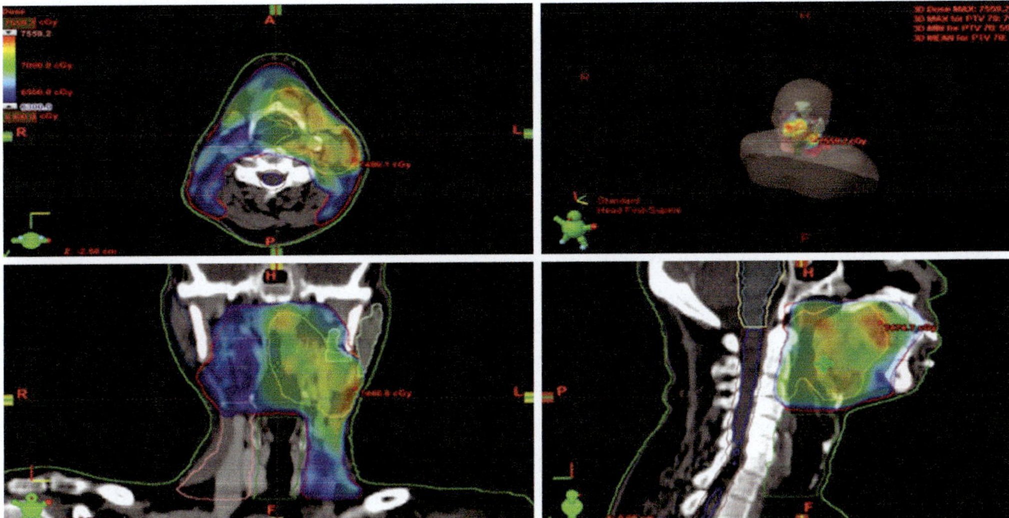

Fig. 4: Dose distribution of intensity-modulated radiation therapy planning for carcinoma base of tongue. High-risk clinical tumor volume receives 70 Gy, intermediate-risk clinical tumor volume 63 Gy and low-risk clinical tumor volume (represented as right lower neck without color wash) receives 56 Gy.
Courtesy: Dr Surendra Reddy, Consultant Radiation Oncologist, BGS Gleneagles Global Hospital, Bengaluru.

Table 8: Radiation dose-volumes in oropharyngeal carcinoma.

Clinical tumor volume (CTV)	*Definition*	*T Stage T1/T2*	*T stage T3/T4*
CTV1	Gross tumor volume with 7–10 mm margin	66 Gy in 30 fractions	69.96 Gy in 33 fractions
CTV2	Adjacent high-risk nodal area including margin around CTV1 and nodal spaces around primary tumor	60 Gy in 30 fractions	63 Gy in 33 fractions
CTV3	Low-risk nodal area	54 Gy in 30 fractions	57 Gy in 33 fractions

feasible with high locoregional control and low radiation toxicity rate. Various single institutional studies have shown high local, regional control with IMRT with rates ranging from 90 to 94%. A randomized phase III trial parotid sparing intensity-modulated versus conventional radiotherapy in head and neck cancer (PARSPORT) was designed to compare conventional radiation and IMRT with a goal of parotid sparing.[62] The trial included 85% of oropharyngeal cancer patients and reported statistically significant improved quality of life (QoL) and reduction in xerostomia with IMRT.

An important aspect of reducing radiation-induced toxicity is accounting for a change in shift of structures and tumor volume during the RT regimen. There is shrinkage of GTV due change in tumor volume and weight loss of the patient which can occur at a rate of 1.8% a day and an approximate of 70% decrease in GTV over the course of RT duration.[63] Due to this shift, there is a possibility of irradiating high doses to organs at risk or inadequate delivery to the tumor volume. To improve locoregional control and reduced toxicity, adaptive image-guided radiotherapy (IGRT) can be utilized. IGRT allows for reassessment and replanning of the RT plan to better accommodate the structural changes during the course of treatment. The role of proton therapy in oropharyngeal cancer is still under evaluation with an ongoing randomized trial comparing IMRT versus intensity-modulated proton therapy (IMPT) is underway (NCT01893307).

ROLE OF CHEMOTHERAPY

The meta-analysis of chemotherapy in head and neck cancer (MACH-NC) includes 87 randomized trials with over 16,000 patients who were treated with chemotherapy either in an induction, concurrent or adjuvant setting. 37% of the patients had oropharyngeal cancer.[64] The maximum benefit of chemotherapy was in a concurrent setting with a hazard ratio for death 0.88, with an absolute benefit of chemotherapy at 5 years of 4.5%. Patients who were administered cisplatin alone or in combination had the most benefit in the concurrent setting. The benefit of concurrent chemotherapy was sustained regardless of fractionation strategy of the RT.

The landmark trial that created paradigms shift from surgery to organ preservation in oropharyngeal cancer was by French head, and neck oncology and radiotherapy group (GORTEC) who investigated 222 patients with stage three or four oropharyngeal cancer were randomized into radiation alone or radiation with three cycles of carboplatin and 5-fluorouracil.[65] They reported a statistically significant locoregional control and overall survival at 5 years of 48% and 22%, respectively. The concurrent arm resulted in an increased rate of grade III/IV complications (56% versus 30%). CCRT is a widely accepted standard of care for locally advanced cases of oropharyngeal cancer.

The role of induction chemotherapy (IC), like in all subsites of head and neck cancers is controversial. EORTC 24971/TAX 323 trial evaluated induction docetaxel, cisplatin, 5-fluorouracil (5-FU) (TPF) and cisplatin and 5-FU (PF) followed by definitive RT.[66] 46% of the patient in each arm of the trial consisted of oropharyngeal cancer. There was a statistically significant increased response to TPF with improved progression-free and overall survival at a median follow-up of 32.5 months. In their follow-up study which consisted of 501 patients (52% were oropharyngeal cancer) compared TPF and PF regimen followed by definitive CCRT which also showed an improved progression-free survival (PFS) and local, regional control at 3 years with TPF regimen. Even though the study has defined the benefit of IC, its benefit has not been compared with standard CTRT. The PARADIGM and DeCIDE trial included 55% of oropharyngeal cancer in each showed no significant difference in overall survival or recurrence-free survival;[67,68] both these trials compared IC to standard CCRT.

ROLE OF SURGERY

Historically, oropharyngeal tumors were managed with surgical resection followed by adjuvant therapy. This fell out of vogue due to the increased functional morbidity that was associated with surgery. Parsons et al. conducted a pooled analysis, including multi-institutional data who underwent surgery with or without adjuvant therapy and radiation.[69] The study included BOT and tonsillar tumors with over 6,000 North American patients and showed that locoregional control, absolute survival, and cause-specific survival were similar in the two treatment modalities. However patients undergoing surgery had four to nine times more frequent rate of severe or fatal complications. For no stage of the disease did the surgical arm perform better than RT in terms of morbidity. Hence the treatment for oropharyngeal cancers shifted over to nonsurgical modalities based on the evidence previously described.

The increasing trend of HPV-associated oropharyngeal cancer has brought in a pool of patients who are much younger in age; various studies have shown long-term complications of radical doses of CRT administered in head and neck cancers. Machtay et al. performed a meta-analysis of RTOG 91-11, RTOG 9703, and RTOG 9914 showed that the toxicity persisting beyond 180 days of treatment was often grade 3 or higher.[70] Inclusion of transoral robotic surgery (TORS) into the treatment strategy allows the clinician to determine adjuvant therapy in patients who would otherwise receive CRT. Studies have shown that upfront TORS deintensified treatment in 76% of stage I/II and 46% of stage III/IV patients, avoiding CCRT. The pathologic staging resulted in 33% of patients who have received CRT received RT alone.[71]

Various prospective studies have shown safety and oncologist efficacy of TORS in HPV-positive and HPV-negative patients. The surgical access to oropharynx is by transoral route or by external cervical route. The transoral route based on instrumentation can be further divided into TORS, transoral laser microsurgery (TLM), and conventional transoral surgery. Open surgeries still have a role in salvage setting and are described later in the chapter.

Transoral Robotic Surgery and Transoral Laser Microsurgery

The advent of advanced retractors and improved magnification with a microscope and an increased precision with the use of laser lead to TLM. The main disadvantage of long rigid equipment used in TLM makes it challenging to reach BOT. Margin assessment, especially at a depth, was difficult due to reduced maneuverability by rigid instruments of TLM.[72] Robotic surgery has various advantages over TLM with 3D panoramic vision, improved range of motion, better optics, and hand tremor filtration, which helps in easier en bloc resection of the tumor **(Fig. 5)**.[72] The advantage of TLM over TORS is with respect to the heat source, where CO_2 laser used in TLM is much more precise in cuts with minimal surrounding tissue thermal damage while TORS results in wider deeper cuts and more thermal damage to surrounding tissues. Oncologic safety of TLM has been proven with 2- and 5-year disease specific survival of 96% and 92%, even in advanced disease.[73]

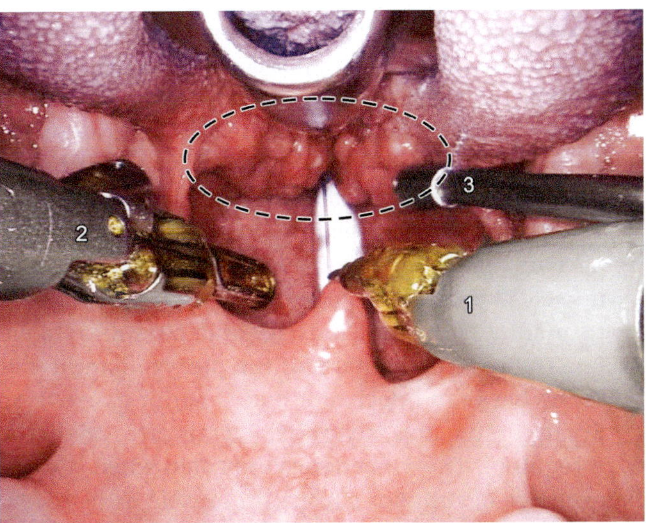

Fig. 5: Central tongue base tumor as seen via robotic console. 1: Cautery spatula; 2: Bipolar Maryland forceps; 3: Suction.

Patient selection is paramount, as complete oncological resection must be achieved with maximum exposure and least surgical morbidity. Patient factors that determine access via TLM can also be utilized for TORS.[72] Various factors such as craniofacial bone abnormalities, mandibular height, hyoid-mental length, and neck circumference can also affect access in TORS. The tumor-related contraindications for TORS as described by Weinstein et al. have roadly classified into vascular functional and oncological factors.[74] They are:

- *Vascular:* Tonsillar involvement with a retropharyngeal carotid artery, tumor located at the midline of the tongue base or vallecula, tumor located adjacent to the carotid bulb or internal carotid artery (ICA), carotid artery enveloped by tumor or metastatic lymph nodes.
- *Functional:* Tumor resection requiring ≥50% of the deep tongue base musculature or posterior pharyngeal wall, resection of the tongue base, and entire epiglottis.
- *Oncological:* Stage T4b, unresectable neck disease, multiple distant metastases, neoplastic-related trismus, prevertebral fascia involvement, mandible or hyoid involvement, tumor extension to lateral neck soft tissues, and involvement of the eustachian tube.

The aim of resection must be to ensure compartmental resection of the tumor. The principles of TORS have been described under the section of robotic surgery. The recent classifications of lateral oropharyngectomy are as follows:[75]

- *Type I* includes resection of palatine tonsils deep to pharyngobasilar fascia with inclusion of palatoglossus arch.

The primary role of type I resection is diagnostic and in patients with severe dysplasia or carcinoma in situ.

- *Type II* includes resection of entire tonsil, palatoglossus, palatopharyngeus and superior constrictor muscle. The deep limit of resection is buccopharyngeal fascia that covers the medial pterygoid muscle.
- *Type III* includes resection of entire tonsil, palatoglossus, palatopharyngeus, superior constrictor muscles, buccopharyngeal fascia with extension to medial pterygoid muscle, and parapharyngeal fat. The dissection starts at the pterygomandibular raphe between buccinator and superior constrictor. Styloglossus and stylopharyngeus are resected, if required. This resection is indicated when there is evidence of superior constrictor muscle involvement on imaging.

Suffixes can be added to notify extensions of resection. Suffix "A" is used when the resection includes soft palate and its muscle up to midline (usually required in tumors involving the superior pole of the tonsil), "B" is used to represent an extension of resection to posterior pharyngeal wall up to the midline, "C" indicates resection of BOT, and "D" is used if the resection margin extends anteriorly towards retromolar trigone area. The resection margin may need to include mandible periosteum and medial pterygoid muscle, if indicated. Validation of this classification is awaited.

Assessment of margin in transoral surgery can be defect driven or specimen driven margins. In TORS due to increased maneuverability, en bloc resection is possible and specimen driven margins are assessed, whereas defect derived margins are employed in TLM. Wide lateral limit of the margin may be difficult to achieve, especially when tumor involves superior constrictor muscle and beyond. Neck dissection must always be performed due to a high rate of occult metastasis in oropharyngeal tumor. Levels II–IV or I–IV are commonly performed, but there is no consensus on the extent of neck dissection. Branches of external carotid artery (ECA), namely lingual, facial, and ascending pharyngeal artery are ligated during neck dissection to reduce the risk of hemorrhage after transoral surgery. Significant controversy revolves around indication for adjuvant therapy after TORS.

Role of Adjuvant Therapy Following TORS/TLM

Role of adjuvant therapy in p16-negative tumors is well defined. Patients with positive margin and extranodal extension (ENE) mandate CCRT based on analysis from RTOG 9501 and EORTC 22931.[76,77] The likely proportion of patients with HPV-positive tumors in these trials was low, in whom ENE is not considered to affect outcomes. The NCCN recommendation for omitting systemic therapy in the adjuvant setting in the presence of ENE is considered as a category B recommendation.[51] The classical margin of 5 mm is difficult to obtain in oropharyngeal subsites, especially during lateral oropharyngectomy. The thickness of constrictor muscle is approximately 2.3 mm. Various studies have shown that a margin of 2 mm is adequate in TORS.[78] Hence patients with positive margin must either be reresected if possible or be considered for adjuvant CCRT until further evidence is available. In HPV-positive tumors with T3/T4 primaries, one positive node more than 3 cm or multiple nodes, perineural invasion, lymphovascular invasion, involvement of level four or five can be considered for adjuvant RT or systemic therapy with RT.[51] A recent retrospective analysis of 4,443 patients based on National Cancer Data Base (NCDB) data has shown that deintensification by using a single primary treatment modality instead of multimodal treatment was associated with worse outcomes, especially in advanced stage tumors that are p16-positive.[79]

Quality of life following TORS was assessed in a review comprising 12 studies showed that patients had chronic gastric tube dependency rate of 0–7%.[80] ADEPT, PATHOS, ECOG 3311, and ORATOR 2 trial are all targeted at defining and determining feasibility of de-escalating adjuvant therapy in HPV-positive tumors. Due to the absence of consensus regarding indication for adjuvant therapy in HPV-positive tumors, the current indications must be derived from RTOG 9501 and EORTC 22931.

Oncologic Outcomes of Transoral Robotic Surgery

Many prospective and retrospective studies have reported excellent oncologic outcomes with TORS for oropharyngeal disease, as shown in **Table 9**.

The randomized phase II trial (ORATOR) was designed to compare RT versus TORS and neck dissection in terms of QoL with respect to swallowing.[89] Participants (oropharyngeal tumors T1-2N0-2 with nodal disease <4 cm) were randomly assigned into two arms. The primary endpoint was to evaluate swallowing-related QoL at one year with the MD Anderson Dysphagia Inventory (MDADI). The study recruited 68 patients and showed that overall survival and PFS in both the groups was excellent without any difference between the groups. p16-positive tumors had markedly improved overall survival and PFS. The QoL assessment for swallowing disability showed that radiotherapy was superior to TORS but did not reach statistical significance. The limitations of the trial must be taken into consideration, such as modest sample size and the fact that the study was not designed to compare survival outcomes. Based on these finding ORATOR 2 trial is being conducted comparing de-escalated radical RT and TORS with de-escalated adjuvant RT.

Table 9: Studies that evaluated safety oncologic outcomes of TORS in oropharyngeal cancer.

Study	*Sample size*	*Median follow-up*	*Survival*
Primary setting			
Weinstein et al.[81]	30	2.7 years	OS 100%
de Almeida et al.[82]	364	20 months	OS 87.1%
Dabas et al.[83]	57	29 months	DFS 89.6% OS 93.8%
Moore et al.[84]	314	3.3 years	OS 86% DFS 94%
Baliga et al.[85]	2,680 (Cancer Registry)	31.4 months	OS 84%
Recurrent setting			
White et al.[86]	64		RFS 74% at 2 years
Dabas et al.[87]	30		RFS 57.5% at 2 years
Paleri et al.[88]	18		RFS 63% at 2 years

(DFS: disease-free survival; OS: overall survival; RFS: recurrence-free survival; TORS: transoral robotic surgery)

Table 10: Reconstruction algorithm following transoral robotic surgery (TORS).[90]

Defect classification	*Subsite*	*Adverse features*	*Reconstruction option*
Class I	1	No	Secondary healing or regional flap
Class II	>1	No	Regional or local flap
Class III	1	Yes	Regional or free flap
Class IV	>1	Yes	Regional or free flap

Adverse features any 1 of exposed internal carotid artery and pharyngocutaneous fistula or >50% of soft palate defect

Reconstruction after Transoral Robotic Surgery

Reconstruction after TORS is dependent on the extent of resection. de Almeida et al. defect classification and reconstruction option algorithm is depicted in **Table 10**.[90]

Class I is defined as involvement of one subsite and class II as involvement of more than one subsite but without adverse features. Class III has at least one of the adverse features with defect restricted to one subsite and class IV as a defect with multiple subsite involvement with one or more adverse feature. The adverse features are ICAs exposure, communication to the neck or >50% soft palate resection. Class I defects can be managed by secondary healing, while class II/III require regional flap and class III/IV can be managed with regional or a free flap. Carotid artery rupture after pharyngeal surgery is seen in 3–14% of cases and pharyngocutaneous fistula in 29%. This classification system and reconstructive algorithm reported good QoL with respect to swallowing using MDADI and velopharyngeal insufficiency assessed by velopharyngeal insufficient QoL.

Management of Recurrent Disease

The proportion of patients receiving CCRT has increased from 15 to 30% between 1985 and 2001.[91] With the advent of newer radiation technology, locoregional recurrence has improved significantly. Given that the vast majority of the patients are treated with definitive CCRT, management of recurrence in these patients is extremely challenging. Open surgical resection is considered a standard of treatment for recurrent or persistent primary disease. Successful salvage is relatively low and recurrence after CCRT, especially with disease free interval of less than 1 year, portends a poor prognosis. Surgical salvage in a previously irradiated field is associated with a high complication rate of 42%.[92] Use of vascularized regional or free flap may improve healing. Patients who present with stage I/II disease at recurrence show a better overall survival of 43.6% as compared to 24.1% in stage III/IV tumors.[92] TORS has also been studied in recurrent oropharyngeal tumors **(Table 9)** and has conclusively proven its role in select group of patients with a significantly lower incidence of tracheostomy and feeding tube dependence.

The role of reirradiation is limited and restricted to cases that cannot be surgically salvaged. RTOG 9610 included 86 patients with recurrent head and neck disease were 34% of them were oropharyngeal tumors.[93] With reirradiation they reported overall survival of 15.2% at 3 years and 3.8% at 5 years. RTOG 9911 enrolled 105 patients (of which 40% had oropharyngeal cancer) who were treated with cisplatin, paclitaxel along with reirradiation, showing a 2-year overall survival of 50.2%.[94] Literature review has shown carotid blow out to be a fatal complication of reirradiation, which is seen in 2.6% of the patients.[95] Patient selection is crucial in reirradiation as outcomes are better when recurrence occurs more than 2 years following definitive treatment.

Role of systemic chemotherapy is confined to patients who are unresectable or not candidates for reirradiation or have distant metastasis. Treatment selection for palliative chemotherapy is similar as other subsites of head and neck cancer. Immunotherapy has proven its efficacy in cisplatin-resistant recurrent tumors of head and neck.[96] Nivolumab has shown a high response rate of 13.3% over standard therapy (single-agent chemotherapy of investigator's choice had a 5.8% response rate). The treatment-related adverse effects were also lower with nivolumab. A third of these patients had pharyngeal tumors. A subset analysis showed a median overall survival of 9.1 months in the nivolumab group with p16-positive tumors while the median overall survival in the same arm for p16-negative tumors was 7.5 months.

Open Approaches to Oropharynx[97]

The role of open surgery is predominantly in the salvage setting. Transoral approach may need to be combined with open approaches for mucosal cuts.

- *Combined transoral transcervical (pull-through) approach:* This approach is best suited for tumors involving BOT without extensive lateral extension to the tonsil. This technique uses a pull-through approach to deliver tongue into the neck for resection under vision. First a neck dissection is performed. Then incisions are made along the ipsilateral tonsillar pillar and continued along the floor of the mouth either leaving a cuff of mucosa laterally on the mandible for closure or by placing a crevicular incision. The entire floor of the mouth incision is continued past the midline. If the patient is edentulous, the incision is placed over the crest of the mandibular arch. When the tumor is not involving the floor of the mouth, the lingual surface of the mandibular periosteum can be preserved, but when the tumor involves floor of the mouth but not the mandible, then the lingual periosteum is included in the specimen. Mucosa with or without periosteum is released anteriorly up to the genial tubercle. The mylohyoid muscle in incised and geniohyoid genioglossus muscle is released from the mandible, and the pterygomasseteric sling is divided. The tongue can then be delivered into the neck. The main limitation of this approach is the involvement of risk to the adjacent neurovascular structures and poor superolateral visualization. During the resection, hypoglossal nerve is most often at risk and may even need to be divided if oncologically indicated. Identification and preservation of superior laryngeal nerve is critical. This approach is contraindicated when there is gross tonsillar involvement where the incision for exposure may encroach on the margin of resection. If required the mandibular lingual release can be extended onto the contralateral side. When bilateral pull-through is performed, preservation of contralateral hypoglossal nerve and the lingual artery is vital to maintain movement and blood supply of the contralateral remnant.
- *Lateral pharyngotomy (LP):* This approach is one of the most frequent approaches used to access the oropharynx. This technique has been well described by Byers. This approach aids in providing access to almost all subsites of the oropharynx. Before commencing, resectability of the tumor must be checked and vascular control has to be attained. LP is performed after the neck dissection. The intermediate tendon of posterior belly of digastric is divided. Stylohyoid and mylohyoid muscles are divided from the hyoid bone. The sternocleidomastoid is retracted laterally to expose the carotid sheath, the common carotid artery, its bifurcation, ICA, and ECA. Ipsilateral facial artery is often tied off during the neck dissection. Ipsilateral hypoglossal nerve and lingual artery are traced from the carotid artery and continued anteriorly. The first branch of the lingual artery is ligated, and descending branch of the hypoglossal nerve is transected so that both these structures can be retracted superiorly. Branching of the ascending pharyngeal artery is identified, and the styloglossus muscle is seen in close relation to it. At this junction, involvement of parapharyngeal space and ICA can be assessed. The involvement of prevertebral fascia can also be assessed by sending frozen sections from here. If the tumor is resectable, then pharyngotomy can be performed. Various route of entry are described based on the location of the tumor. The most frequent entry is through vallecula via suprahyoid access. Entry can be performed at the level of the tonsillar region, which might be challenging to reach, but transection of styloglossus will provide easier access. Ipsilateral floor of the mouth and attachment of medial pterygoid muscle over the mandible may have to be included in the surgical specimen. If the vallecula and tonsillar region are involved by the tumor, then entry can be accessed through the pyriform sinus. Resection of the hyoid bone may be required. Most of the patients will require fasciocutaneous or myocutaneous flap reconstruction. Trotter's modification of LP includes mandibulotomy at the angle of mandible.
- *Transmandibular approaches:*
    - *Mandibular swing:* Mandibular swing is indicated in large tumors of BOT that involve the glossopharyngeal sulcus and tonsil region. A lip-split incision is performed and superiorly-based neck flap is elevated. Lip-split incision over the menti ideally should incorporate a Z-plasty to break the scar. After a lip-split incision, the mucosal incision is continued along gingivolabial sulcus up to the emergence of mental nerve, and the periosteal elevation is restricted to a minimum to prevent devascularization of the mandible. Using a five-hole low profile plate which is bent to the contour of the mandible is plated on the proposed bone cut with bicortical screws.

The plate is removed after appropriate orientation. An oscillating/reciprocating saw is used to cut the bone to prevent bone loss, and the cut is made between the lateral incisor and canine teeth (paramedian mandibulotomy) as the roots diverge with an approximate distance between the two of 2–3 mm. After the bone cut, mucosa along the floor of mouth and mylohyoid muscle is freed from the medial surface of the mandible. The incision along the floor of the mouth is extended up to the proposed anterior margin of the resection. The deep lateral margin may need to include medial pterygoid muscle **(Fig. 6)**. After the resection fasciocutaneous or myocutaneous flap is often required to fill the defect. After the flap inset, the floor of the mouth is closed followed by closure of the mandibulotomy site. The lip and soft tissues are closed in multiple layers without disturbing landmarks of the lip border.

- *Mandibulectomy/composite resection:* The term composite reception was used to describe en bloc removal of oropharyngeal or oral tumor along with mandible and neck dissection. The concept came into vogue based on a belief that tumor cells pass through the periosteum of the mandible on their way to the level I nodal station. This concept was subsequently disproved as there were no malignant cells demonstrable in the periosteum and lymphatics until the tumor involved mandible. Marginal mandibulectomy of the ascending ramus may be required when there is an anterior extension of the tumor to the retromolar area. Composite resection can be performed with the lip-split incision or visor incision. The soft tissue along the lateral aspect of the mandible is freed until the anterior margin of the resection is reached. The bone cuts are made 2 cm away from the tumor or hemimandibulectomy may be required when the marrow is involved. The temporomandibular joint may have to be resected if there is gross infratemporal fossa involvement. Reconstruction with myocutaneous or fasciocutaneous or vascularized bone flap may be required depending on the defect.
- *Medial labiomandibular glossotomy/Trotter's operation:* This approach was originally described as an access to the midline posterior pharyngeal wall. The median mandibulotomy is performed, followed by translingual division along the midline. Identifying the avascular plane of midline lingual septum is essential. The division is continued posteriorly up to vallecula when posterior pharyngeal wall has to be accessed. This approach can be used to resect small tumors of the BOT where the translingual split stops at the anterior margin of resection. In the present day, this approach is rarely done due to increased morbidity and limited access to most of the oropharyngeal subsite.

  To conclude, open oropharyngeal resection is standard only in post-RT salvage setting. Whenever possible, integrity of the mandible must be preserved by utilizing techniques like LP. Composite resection is reserved for patients with cortical or marrow involvement of the mandible. The indications and reconstructive options are represented in **Table 11**.

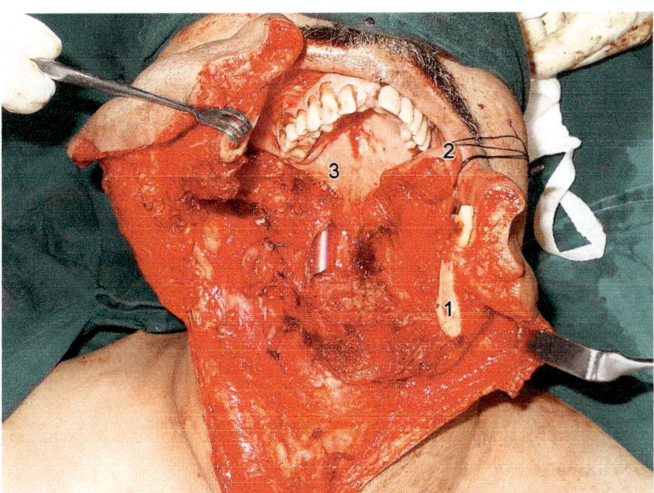

Fig. 6: Mandibulotomy approach to the oropharynx. 1: Paramedian mandibulotomy; 2: Hemiglossectomy defect; 3: Right tonsil and posterior pharyngeal wall defect.

Survival after salvage surgery is modest. Oropharyngeal cancer salvage survival rates range from 13 to 31% at 5 years and a disease-free survival at 5 years of 19–27%.[98] Hence, patient selection is paramount. Contraindications apart from the anatomical extent of the recurrent tumor are a patient with initial stage IV tumor and concomitant local and regional failure. The 2-year overall survival rate in the presence of none, one, and both of these factors is 83%, 49%, and 0% respectively.[99] Outcomes when margins are positive are drastically worse. Postoperative complications, especially pharyngocutaneous fistula, are very common. The outcome of surgical salvage is significantly better when the tumor is HPV-positive, longer time to recurrence, and when completely resected.

Deintensification of Treatment in HPV-associated Oropharyngeal Cancer

With increasing evidence of improved outcomes in HPV-associated oropharyngeal cancer and long-term

Table 11: Open oropharyngeal approaches, indications, and reconstruction options.

Size of the tumor	*Approach*	*Reconstructive option*
Base of the tongue		
Small	Transoral	Secondary healing/regional or local flap
Extensive	Pull-through or lateral pharyngotomy (suprahyoid entry)	Fasciocutaneous flap or myocutaneous flap
Extensive with lateral extension to tonsil	Mandibulotomy	Fasciocutaneous or myocutaneous flap
Mandible involvement	Mandibulectomy	Myocutaneous flap or bony reconstruction or fasciocutaneous
Tonsil and lateral pharyngeal wall		
Small	Transoral	Secondary healing/regional or local flap
Extensive tumor with inferior extension	Lateral pharyngotomy	Fasciocutaneous flap or myocutaneous flap
Extensive tumor with superior extension	Mandibulotomy	Fasciocutaneous or myocutaneous flap
Mandible involvement	Mandibulectomy	Myocutaneous flap or bone reconstruction or fasciocutaneous

toxicity associated with organ preservation protocols has paved the way for treatment regimens that are less intense to achieve similar oncologic outcomes, but with lesser toxicity and improved QoL. This is important in HPV-associated oropharyngeal tumors as these are seen in younger patients who live longer. The main strategies that have been investigated and under investigation for treatment deintensification are described below.

- *Radiation combined with cetuximab:* Cetuximab is a monoclonal antibody against EGFR which is overexpressed in 90% of HNSCC. The rational of replacing cisplatin with cetuximab is based on the study by Bonner et al.[100] They demonstrated improved oncologic outcomes by adding cetuximab to radiation with a survival improvement from 29.3 to 49 months. In the trial, patients with oropharyngeal cancer with small primary, significant nodal involvement, and younger patients benefitted from cetuximab the most. These parameters are characteristic of HPV-driven tumors. Cetuximab is considered less toxic than cisplatin, even though there is no direct comparison. Studies have shown an inverse relation with HPV status and EGFR alteration. Several studies have shown conflicting results on beneficial effects of cetuximab in HPV-positive tumors.[101]

  The RTOG 1016 is a randomized multicentric noninferiority trial designed to assess the effect of RT with cisplatin or cetuximab in HPV-positive oropharyngeal carcinoma.[102] The trial included T1–T2N2a–N3M0 or T3–T4N0–N3M0 tumors which were randomly assigned to cetuximab (loading dose of 400 mg/m^2 5–7 days before RT, followed by cetuximab 250 mg/m^2 weekly for seven doses, total dose 2,150 mg/m^2), or cisplatin (100 mg/m^2 administered on day 1 and 22 of RT, total dose of 200 mg/m^2). Both arms received accelerated RT 70 Gy in 35 IMRT fractions over 6 weeks at six fractions per week. The trial enrolled 849 patients. The median follow-up was 4.5 years. The trial reported 5-year overall survival of 77.9% and 84.6% in the cetuximab and cisplatin arms, respectively. The locoregional rate was significantly lower in the cetuximab arm than cisplatin group (HR 2.05), while the toxicity profile was similar in both arms. This trial showed that cetuximab is inferior to cisplatin and CCRT with cisplatin should be considered the standard of care in HPV-positive tumors.

  The De-ESCALaTE trial is a multicentric phase III trial which included 334 patients with low-risk HPV-positive oropharyngeal cancer were randomized to radiotherapy (70 Gy in 35 fractions) with either intravenous cisplatin (100 mg/m^2 on days 1, 22, and 43 of radiotherapy) or intravenous cetuximab (400 mg/m^2 loading dose followed by 7 weekly infusions of 250 mg/m^2).[103] The trial reported no significant difference in overall toxicity rate. The 2-year overall survival and 2-year recurrence rates for cisplatin and cetuximab were 97.5% versus 89.4%, and 6.0% versus 16.1%, respectively. They concluded that cisplatin is associated with better outcomes than cetuximab in HPV-positive tumors.
- *Less aggressive radiation:* The long-term toxicity secondary to radiotherapy dose received by pharyngeal constrictors, BOT, and supraglottic larynx is well documented. With every 10 Gy raise in RT dose after 55 Gy, rate of dysphagia increases.[104]

Stricture and feeding tube dependency was 50% and 30% respectively when constrictors received 70 Gy. The rate of aspiration was as high as 50% when constrictors receive 65 Gy.[105,106] Hence various strategies are planned to reduce the dose of RT and improve swallowing outcomes.

- *Induction chemotherapy:* IC is used to triage patient who can be administered a reduced dose of RT. The rationale of this approach was drawn by various studies proving IC as a predictor of RT response. As HPV-positive tumors are radio-sensitive, lower radiation doses may be adequate to control disease.

  The ECOG 1308 trial included 80 patients, to receive three chemotherapy cycles (paclitaxel, cisplatin, and cetuximab) as IC, followed by weekly cetuximab and low radiation dose (54 Gy) in complete responders or standard dose (70 Gy) in patients with partial response or stable disease.[107] The trial reported 80% 2-year PFS in complete responders and significantly better swallowing outcome (40% vs. 89%) in complete responders. The trial also showed a significant lower 2-year PFS for patients with T4 and >10 pack-year of smoking and those with <T4N2c) and <10 pack-year of smoking had 2-year PFS of 96%.

  The phase II trial (NCT01716195) was a single-arm trial in which patients received IC with two cycles of paclitaxel and carboplatin followed by RT with paclitaxel.[108] The RT dose was reduced to 54 Gy in complete/partial responders and reduced to 60 Gy in nonresponders. The oncologic outcome with a 15–20% reduction in RT dose was good; 2-year PFS was 92%.

  A phase III trial (Quarterback study-NCT01706939) included 365 patients with p16-positive oropharyngeal tumors, nasopharyngeal tumors, and carcinoma of unknown primary. The induction therapy included docetaxel, cisplatin, and 5-FU followed by RT (56 Gy or 70 Gy) with weekly carboplatin and cetuximab or carboplatin alone. The preliminary results showed 2-year PFS in patients receiving 56 Gy and standard dose to be 87.5% and 83%, respectively. This trial did not include the standard of care treatment arm.

  Villaflor et al. (NCT01133678) designed a trial to evaluate the efficacy of reduced RT volume.[109] The trial was based on the principle that majority of locoregional failures occurred within RT field, particularly in the gross tumor volume; hence elimination of RT volume to an uninvolved area of nodal drainage, especially in lateralized tumors, can further reduce RT volume and translate into improved QoL. The trial investigated IC with cisplatin, paclitaxel, cetuximab ± everolimus. Good responders received 75 Gy (1.5 Gy twice daily every other week) with concurrent RT with a single planning target volume. The trial included locally advanced HNSCC, with 59/94 patients having HPV-positive oropharyngeal carcinoma. HPV-positive oropharyngeal cancers showed a good response to IC and the authors reported that elimination of elective nodal area did not compromise outcome or result in reduced toxicity. Based on these results, a further phase II trial (NCT02258659) is underway.

  The rationale of using IC is relevant in HPV-associated oropharyngeal tumors is that a leading cause of death is distant metastases. Even though these trials did show appreciable oncologic outcomes, most trials have a limited follow-up period ranging from 23 to 30 months.[101] Long-term toxicity profile of these treatment regimens is not defined. Most of these trials lack comparison with standard CCRT with cisplatin.

- *CCRT with reduced RT dose and chemotherapy:* Phase II study (NCT01530997)[110] reported complete pathological response of 86% in low-risk HPV-positive tumors with 60 Gy IMRT (instead of 70 Gy) and concurrent weekly 30 mg/m^2. The trial results were very promising due to good response, which was assessed pathologically. The argument against the trial could be that they included low staged tumors where RT alone would suffice and short follow-up (14.3 months). Based on this preliminary study, a follow-up study is being conducted (NCT02281955) which will utilize the same regimen with use of PET CT to triage patients for surgery, omitting early-stage disease and inclusion of patients with moderate smoking histories.

- *Elimination of chemotherapy:* The phase II trial (HN002) included patients with <10 pack-year of smoking history and T1-T2N1-N2b or T3N0-N2b disease.[111] Patients were randomized to CCRT (60 Gy in 6 weeks with weekly 40 mg/m^2 cisplatin) or moderately accelerated radiotherapy alone (60 Gy in 5 weeks with six fractions per week). The trial accrual is completed, but results are awaited.
- *Less invasive surgery:* The rationale of using TORS in early-stage disease will provide accurate pathological stage that can help in triaging patients to further adjuvant therapy. These strategies are ideal in N0 and N1 disease where risk of neck recurrence is <5%;

Table 12: The role of TORS in de-escalation therapy.

Trial	*Intent*	*Inclusion*	*Therapy*	*Primary endpoint*
"PATHOS" NCT02215265	Reduced-intensity adjuvant treatment in patients undergoing transoral surgery for HPV-positive OPC	HPV-positive cancer (T1-3, N0-2b) treated by transoral surgery and neck dissection Multiple risk stratification based on the pathological report including N status, perineural and/or vascular invasion or close margins, positive margin (<1 mm), extracapsular spread	• Low risk—no adjuvant treatment • Intermediate risk—randomized to: – 50 Gy in 25# – 60 Gy in 30# • High risk—randomized to: – 60 Gy in 30# – 60 Gy in 30# with cisplatin	Patient-reported swallowing outcome
"ADEPT" NCT01687413	Postoperative adjuvant therapy deintensification trial	p16-positive OPSCC with disease resected (with clear margins) by a minimally invasive approach, and ENE +, metastatic lymph nodes +	*Arm 1:* 60 Gy in 30# *Arm 2:* 60 Gy in 30# and cisplatin	• Disease-free survival • Locoregional control
"ECOG 3311" NCT01898494	Transoral surgery followed by low-dose or standard-dose radiation therapy with or without chemotherapy in treating patients	Squamous cell carcinoma or undifferentiated carcinoma of the oropharynx; stage III, IVa, or IVb p16 (HPV)-positive disease	• Low risk—no adjuvant treatment • Intermediate risk—randomized to: – 50 Gy in 25# – 60 Gy in 30# • High risk—chemoradiotherapy	Progression-free survival rate Incidence of grade 3–4 bleeding events during surgery Positive margins after surgery

(ENE: extranodal extension; HPV: human papillomavirus; OPC: oropharyngeal cancer; OPSCC: oropharyngeal squamous cell carcinoma; TORS: transoral robotic surgery)

which raises to 20% in pN2 disease.[101] Hence in patients with adequate margins and N0-1 disease, postoperative adjuvant therapy can be avoided. The studies exploring this rationale are represented in the **Table 12**; however for several trials, results are awaited.

When de-escalation is planned, early-stage disease, HPV-positive, and patients with <10 pack-year of smoking may benefit. Advanced primary (T4), high nodal category (N2c-N3), and a smoking history of 10–20 pack-year are associated with poor outcomes even in HPV-positive oropharyngeal disease; hence patient selection and selection criteria for de-escalation is vital. Tumor control remains the primary aim in oncology practice; de-escalation lies on the narrow edge between tumor control and improved QoL. A recent study has shown that 70% of patients were unwilling to trade off risk of 5% or less drop in survival for CCRT over RT as de-escalation strategy.

The effect of treatment de-escalation in low-risk HPV-positive tumors and intensification in stage III tumors was concluded by a recent analysis of 4,443 patients from NCDB data,[79] which showed worse outcomes in those with single modality treatment over those treated with two or more modalities.

A phase III trial (compARE) is a treatment escalation trial in patients with intermediate and high-risk HPV-positive oropharyngeal cancer. The trial has four arms with arm 1 (receiving CCRT of 70 Gy in 35 fractions with cisplatin ± post-treatment neck dissection), arm 2 (receiving IC with docetaxel, cisplatin, and 5-FU followed by arm 1 treatment), arm 3 (dose-escalated CCRT with 64 Gy in 25 fractions and cisplatin ± post-treatment neck dissection), and arm 4 (resection of primary and selective neck dissection plus postoperative CCRT, where T1-2 receive transoral surgery and T3-4 transoral or open surgery). The primary endpoints of the trial are overall survival and disease-free survival, and its results are awaited.

Oropharyngeal Cancer Prevention Strategies

Primary prevention by HPV immunization that targets L1 capsid protein can be used. The efficacy of prophylactic vaccines to prevent anogenital precancerous lesions is as high as 90–100%. Herrero R et al. conducted a phase III randomized trial included 7,466 subjects, has shown a reduction in oral HPV infection in the vaccine group than placebo group after a follow-up of 4 years.[112] Currently, the bivalent (HPV 16 and 18) Cervarix [GlaxoSmithKline (GSK)], and a quadrivalent vaccine (HPV 16, 18, 6, and 11) Gardasil (Merck) are available.

Screening for HPV positivity for oropharyngeal cancer has been tested with conflicting results.

The screening tests used brush biopsies with PCR testing. Due to the absence of robust data, screening of oropharyngeal cancers is not recommended.

The HPV DNA detection after definitive treatment has been studied as a tertiary prevention strategy. In a preliminary study, persistent HPV DNA after 9, 12, 18, and 24 months after treatment, has shown to be associated with worse survival. However, further validation is required.

FOLLOW-UP STRATEGY

Follow-up schedule is recommended every 1–3 months for the first year, every 2–4 months for the second year, every 4–6 months for 3–5 years, and after 5 years, annual examination must be scheduled. Post-treatment imaging can be recommended as a baseline within 6 months of completion of treatment.[51]

CONCLUSION

Outcomes in oropharyngeal cancer are based on etiologic factors such as HPV and smoking. With the advent of newer technology in surgery and radiation techniques, the oncologic outcomes and QoL in these patients is rapidly improving. Radical changes are being tested in the management of oropharyngeal cancers that in the future may result in a paradigm shift in treatment.

REFERENCES

1. Hay A, Nixon IJ. Recent advances in the understanding and management of oropharyngeal cancer. F1000Res. 2018;7: F1000 Faculty Rev-1362.
2. Beadle BM, Rosenthal DI. Multidisciplinary management of oropharynx carcinomas. Head and Neck Cancer: Multimodality Management, 2nd edition. Germany: Springer International Publishing; 2016. pp. 475-510.
3. Van Dyne EA, Henley SJ, Saraiya M, Thomas CC, Markowitz LE, Benard VB. Trends in human papillomavirus-associated cancers—United States, 1999–2015. Morb Mortal Wkly Rep. 2018;67(33):918-24.
4. Chi AC, Day TA, Neville BW. Oral cavity and oropharyngeal squamous cell carcinoma—an update. CA Cancer J Clin. 2015; 65(5):401-21.
5. Hashibe M, Brennan P, Chuang SC, Boccia S, Castellsaque X, Chen C, et al. Interaction between tobacco and alcohol use and the risk of head and neck cancer: pooled analysis in the International Head and Neck Cancer Epidemiology Consortium. Cancer Epidemiol Biomarkers Prev. 2009;18: 541-50.
6. Forman D, de Martel C, Lacey CJ, Soerjomataram I, Lortet-Tieulent J, Bruni L, et al. Global burden of human papillomavirus and related diseases. Vaccine. 2012;30:F12-23.
7. Heck JE, Berthiller J, Vaccarella S, Winn DM, Smith EM, Shan'gina O, et al. Sexual behaviors and the risk of head and neck cancers: a pooled analysis in the International Head and Neck Cancer Epidemiology (INHANCE) consortium. Int J Epidemiol. 2010;39(1):166-81.
8. Ralli M, Singh S, Yadav SP, Sharma N, Verma R, Sen R. Assessment and clinicopathological correlation of p16 expression in head and neck squamous cell carcinoma. J Cancer Res Ther. 2016;12(1):232-7.
9. Singh AK, Kushwaha JK, Anand A, Sonkar AA, Husain N, Srivastava K, et al. Human Papilloma Virus in Oral Cavity Cancer and Relation to Change in Quality of Life Following Treatment—a Pilot Study from Northern India. Indian J Surg Oncol. 2016;7(4):386-91.
10. Bahl A, Kumar P, Dar L, Mohanti BK, Sharma A, Thakar A, et al. Prevalence and trends of human papillomavirus in oropharyngeal cancer in a predominantly north Indian population. Head Neck. 2014;36(4):505-10.
11. Nair D, Mair M, Singh A, D'Cruz A. Prevalence and impact of human papillomavirus on head and neck cancers: review of Indian studies. Indian J Surg Oncol. 2018;9(4):568-75.
12. Murthy V, Swain M, Teni T, Pawar S, Kalkar P, Patil A, et al. Human papillomavirus/p16 positive head and neck cancer in India: prevalence, clinical impact, and influence of tobacco use. Indian J Cancer. 2016;53(3):387-93.
13. Herrero R, Castellsagué X, Pawlita M, Lissowska J, Kee F, Balaram P, et al. Human papillomavirus and oral cancer: the International Agency for Research on Cancer multicenter study. J Natl Cancer Inst. 2003;95(23):1772-83.
14. Califano J, Van Der Riet P, Westra W, Nawroz H, Clayman G, Piantadosi S, et al. Genetic progression model for head and neck cancer: implications for field cancerization. Cancer Res. 1996;56(11):2488-92.
15. Van Der Riet P, Nawroz H, Hruban RH, Corio R, Tokino K, Koch W, et al. Frequent loss of chromosome 9p21-22 early in head and neck cancer progression. Cancer Res. 1994; 54(5):1156-8.
16. Kisielewski AE, Xiao GH, Liu SC, Klein-Szanto AJ, Novara M, Sina J, et al. Analysis of the FHIT gene and its product in squamous cell carcinomas of the head and neck. Oncogene. 1998;17(1):83-91.
17. Dong SM, Sun DI, Benoit NE, Kuzmin I, Lerman MI, Sidransky D. Epigenetic inactivation of RASSF1A in head and neck cancer. Clin Cancer Res. 2003;9(10):3635-40.
18. Choi S, Myers JN. Molecular pathogenesis of oral squamous cell carcinoma: implications for therapy. J Dent Res. 2008; 87(1):14-32.
19. Gillison ML, Castellsagué X, Chaturvedi A, Goodman MT, Snijders P, Tommasino M, et al. Eurogin Roadmap: comparative epidemiology of HPV infection and associated cancers of the head and neck and cervix. Int J Cancer. 2014;134(3): 497-507.
20. Mallen-St Clair J, Alani M, Wang MB, Srivatsan ES. Human papillomavirus in oropharyngeal cancer: The changing face of a disease. Biochim Biophys Acta. 2016;1866(2):141-50.
21. Sarrazin S, Lamanna WC, Esko JD. Heparan sulfate proteoglycans. Cold Spring Harb Perspect Biol. 2011;3(7):a004952.
22. DiGiuseppe S, Keiffer TR, Bienkowska-Haba M, Luszczek W, Guion LG, Müller M, et al. Topography of the human papillomavirus minor capsid protein L2 during vesicular trafficking of infectious entry. J Virol. 2015;89(20):10442-52.
23. Surviladze Z, Dziduszko A, Ozbun MA. Essential roles for soluble virion-associated heparan sulfonated proteoglycans and growth factors in human papillomavirus infections. PLoS Pathog. 2012;8(2):e1002519.
24. Bergant Marušič M, Ozbun MA, Campos SK, Myers MP, Banks L. Human papillomavirus L2 facilitates viral escape from late endosomes via sorting nexin 17. Traffic. 2012;13(3): 455-67.

25. McKinney CC, Hussmann KL, McBride AA. The role of the DNA damage response throughout the papillomavirus life cycle. Viruses. 2015;7(5):2450-69.
26. Bodelon C, Vinokurova S, Sampson JN, den Boon JA, Walker JL, Horswill MA, et al. Chromosomal copy number alterations and HPV integration in cervical precancer and invasive cancer. Carcinogenesis. 2016;37(2):188-96.
27. Maxwell JH, Khan S, Ferris RL. The molecular biology of HPV-related head and neck cancer. HPV and Head and Neck Cancers. New Delhi: Springer; 2015. pp. 51-63.
28. Cancer Genome Atlas Network. Comprehensive genomic characterization of head and neck squamous cell carcinomas. Nature. 2015;517(7536):576-82.
29. Beachler DC, Weber KM, Margolick JB, Strickler HD, Cranston RD, Burk RD, et al. Risk factors for oral HPV infection among a high prevalence population of HIV-positive and at-risk HIV-negative adults. Cancer Epidemiol Biomarkers Prev. 2012;21(1):122-33.
30. Rautava J, Syrjänen S. Biology of human papillomavirus infections in head and neck carcinogenesis. Head Neck Pathol. 2012;6(1):3-15.
31. Leibowitz MS, Srivastava RM, Andrade Filho PA, Egloff AM, Wang L, Seethala RR, et al. SHP2 is overexpressed and inhibits pSTAT1-mediated APM component expression, T-cell attracting chemokine secretion, and CTL recognition in head and neck cancer cells. Clin Cancer Res. 2013;19(4): 798-808.
32. Gildener-Leapman N, Lee J, Ferris RL. Tailored immunotherapy for HPV positive head and neck squamous cell cancer. Oral Oncol. 2014;50(9):780-4.
33. Lewis Jr JS, Khan RA, Masand RP, Chernock RD, Zhang Q, Al-Naief NS, et al. Recognition of nonkeratinizing morphology in oropharyngeal squamous cell carcinoma—a prospective cohort and interobserver variability study. Histopathology. 2012;60(3):427-36.
34. Venuti A, Paolini F. HPV detection methods in head and neck cancer. Head Neck Pathol. 2012;6(1):63-74.
35. Qureishi A, Mawby T, Fraser L, Shah KA, Møller H, Winter S. Current and future techniques for human papilloma virus (HPV) testing in oropharyngeal squamous cell carcinoma. Eur Arch Otorhinolaryngol. 2017;274(7):2675-83.
36. Schache AG, Liloglou T, Risk JM, Filia A, Jones TM, Sheard J, et al. Evaluation of human papilloma virus diagnostic testing in oropharyngeal squamous cell carcinoma: sensitivity, specificity, and prognostic discrimination. Clin Cancer Res. 2011;17(19):6262-71.
37. Wasylyk B, Abecassis J, Jung AC. Identification of clinically relevant HPV-related HNSCC: in p16 should we trust? Oral Oncol. 2013;49(10):e33-7.
38. Thavaraj S, Stokes A, Guerra E, Bible J, Halligan E, Long A, et al. Evaluation of human papillomavirus testing for squamous cell carcinoma of the tonsil in clinical practice. J Clin Pathol. 2011;64(4):308-12.
39. Bishop JA, Ma XJ, Wang H, Luo Y, Illei PB, Begum S, et al. Detection of transcriptionally active high risk HPV in patients with head and neck squamous cell carcinoma as visualized by a novel E6/E7 mRNA in situ hybridization method. Am J Surg Pathol. 2012;36(12):1874-82.
40. Robinson M, Schache A, Sloan P, Thavaraj S. HPV specific testing: a requirement for oropharyngeal squamous cell carcinoma patients. Head Neck Pathol. 2012;6(1):83-90.
41. Channir HI, Grønhøj Larsen C, Ahlborn LB, van Overeem Hansen T, Gerds TA, Charabi BW, et al. Validation study of HPV DNA detection from stained FNA smears by polymerase chain reaction: improving the diagnostic workup of patients with a tumor on the neck. Cancer Cytopathol. 2016; 124(11):820-7.
42. Lindberg R. Distribution of cervical lymph node metastases from squamous cell carcinoma of the upper respiratory and digestive tracts. Cancer. 1972;29(6):1446-9.
43. Remmler D, Medina JE, Byers RM, Meoz R, Pfalzgraf K. Treatment of choice for squamous carcinoma of the tonsillar fossa. Head Neck Surg. 1985;7(3):206-11.
44. Weber AL, Romo L, Hashmi S. Malignant tumors of the oral cavity and oropharynx: clinical, pathologic, and radiologic evaluation. Neuroimaging Clin N Am. 2003;13(3):443-64.
45. Zima AJ, Wesolowski JR, Ibrahim M, Lassig AA, Lassig J, Mukherji SK. Magnetic resonance imaging of oropharyngeal cancer. Top Magn Reson Imaging. 2007;18(4):237-42.
46. Som PM, Braun IF, Shapiro MD, Reede DL, Curtin HD, Zimmerman RA. Tumors of the parapharyngeal space and upper neck: MR imaging characteristics. Radiology. 1987;164(3):823-9.
47. Hsu WC, Loevner LA, Karpati R, Ahmed T, Mong A, Battineni ML, et al. Accuracy of magnetic resonance imaging in predicting absence of fixation of head and neck cancer to the prevertebral space. Head Neck. 2005;27(2): 95-100.
48. Loevner LA, Ott IL, Yousem DM, Montone KT, Thaler ER, Chalian AA, et al. Neoplastic fixation to the prevertebral compartment by squamous cell carcinoma of the head and neck. AJR Am J Roentgenol. 1998;170(5):1389-94.
49. Bolzoni A, Cappiello J, Piazza C, Peretti G, Maroldi R, Farina D, et al. Diagnostic accuracy of magnetic resonance imaging in the assessment of mandibular involvement in oral-oropharyngeal squamous cell carcinoma: a prospective study. Arch Otolaryngol Head Neck Surg. 2004;130(7): 837-43.
50. Cantrell SC, Peck BW, Li G, Wei Q, Sturgis EM, Ginsberg LE. Differences in imaging characteristics of HPV-positive and HPV-negative oropharyngeal cancers: a blinded matched-pair analysis. Am J Neuroradiol. 2013;34(10):2005-9.
51. National Comprehensive Cancer Network. NCCN Guidelines. [online] Available from http://www.nccn.org/professionals/physician_gls/f_guidelines.asp. [Last accessed July, 2020].
52. O'Sullivan B, Huang SH, Su J, Garden AS, Sturgis EM, Dahlstrom K, et al. Development and validation of a staging system for HPV-related oropharyngeal cancer by the International Collaboration on Oropharyngeal cancer Network for Staging (ICON-S): a multicentre cohort study. Lancet Oncol. 2016;17(4):440-51.
53. Haughey BH, Sinha P, Kallogjeri D, Goldberg RL, Lewis Jr JS, Piccirillo JF, et al. Pathology-based staging for HPV-positive squamous carcinoma of the oropharynx. Oral Oncol. 2016; 62:11-9.
54. Ang KK, Harris J, Wheeler R, Weber R, Rosenthal DI, Nguyen-Tân PF, et al. Human papillomavirus and survival of patients with oropharyngeal cancer. N Engl J Med. 2010; 363(1):24-35.
55. Horiot JC, Le Fur R, N'guyen T, Chenal C, Schraub S, Alfonsi S, et al. Hyperfractionation versus conventional fractionation in oropharyngeal carcinoma: final analysis of a randomized trial of the EORTC cooperative group of radiotherapy. Radiother Oncol. 1992;25(4):231-41.
56. Fu KK, Pajak TF, Trotti A, Jones CU, Spencer SA, Phillips TL, et al. A Radiation Therapy Oncology Group (RTOG) phase III

randomized study to compare hyperfractionation and two variants of accelerated fractionation to standard fractionation radiotherapy for head and neck squamous cell carcinomas: first report of RTOG 9003. Int J Radiat Oncol Biol Phys. 2000; 48(1):7-16.
57. Lyhne NM, Primdahl H, Kristensen CA, Andersen E, Johansen J, Andersen LJ, et al. The DAHANCA 6 randomized trial: effect of 6 vs 5 weekly fractions of radiotherapy in patients with glottic squamous cell carcinoma. Radiother Oncol. 2015;117(1):91-8.
58. Bourhis J, Overgaard J, Audry H, Ang KK, Saunders M, Bernier J, et al. Hyperfractionated or accelerated radiotherapy in head and neck cancer: a meta-analysis. Lancet. 2006;368(9538):843-54.
59. Lacas B, Bourhis J, Overgaard J, Zhang Q, Grégoire V, Nankivell M, et al. Role of radiotherapy fractionation in head and neck cancers (MARCH): an updated meta-analysis. Lancet Oncol. 2017;18(9):1221-37.
60. Nguyen-Tan PF, Zhang Q, Ang KK, Weber RS, Rosenthal DI, Soulieres D, et al. Randomized phase III trial to test accelerated versus standard fractionation in combination with concurrent cisplatin for head and neck carcinomas in the Radiation Therapy Oncology Group 0129 trial: long-term report of efficacy and toxicity. J Clin Oncol. 2014;32(34): 3858-67.
61. Eisbruch A, Harris J, Garden AS, Chao CK, Straube W, Harari PM, et al. Multi-institutional trial of accelerated hypofractionated intensity-modulated radiation therapy for early-stage oropharyngeal cancer (RTOG 00-22). Int J Radiat Oncol Biol Phys. 2010;76(5):1333-8.
62. Nutting CM, Morden JP, Harrington KJ, Urbano TG, Bhide SA, Clark C, et al. Parotid-sparing intensity modulated versus conventional radiotherapy in head and neck cancer (PARSPORT): a phase 3 multicentre randomised controlled trial. Lancet Oncol. 2011;12(2):127-36.
63. Mali SB. Adaptive radiotherapy for head neck cancer. J Maxillofac Oral Surg. 2016;15(4):549-54.
64. Pignon JP, Le Maitre A, Maillard E, Bourhis J, Mach-Nc Collaborative Group. Meta-analysis of chemotherapy in head and neck cancer (MACH-NC): an update on 93 randomised trials and 17,346 patients. Radiother Oncol. 2009;92(1):4-14.
65. Denis F, Garaud P, Bardet E, Alfonsi M, Sire C, Germain T, et al. Final results of the 94-01 French Head and Neck Oncology and Radiotherapy Group randomized trial comparing radiotherapy alone with concomitant radiochemotherapy in advanced-stage oropharynx carcinoma. J Clin Oncol. 2004;22(1):69-76.
66. Vermorken JB, Remenar E, Van Herpen C, Gorlia T, Mesia R, Degardin M, et al. Cisplatin, fluorouracil, and docetaxel in unresectable head and neck cancer. N Engl J Med. 2007;357(17):1695-704.
67. Posner MR, Hershock DM, Blajman CR, Mickiewicz E, Winquist E, Gorbounova V, et al. Cisplatin and fluorouracil alone or with docetaxel in head and neck cancer. N Engl J Med. 2007;357(17):1705-15.
68. Haddad R, O'Neill A, Rabinowits G, Tishler R, Khuri F, Adkins D, et al. Induction chemotherapy followed by concurrent chemoradiotherapy (sequential chemoradiotherapy) versus concurrent chemoradiotherapy alone in locally advanced head and neck cancer (PARADIGM): a randomised phase 3 trial. Lancet Oncol. 2013;14(3):257-64.
69. Parsons JT, Mendenhall WM, Stringer SP, Amdur RJ, Hinerman RW, Villaret DB, et al. Squamous cell carcinoma of the oropharynx: surgery, radiation therapy, or both. Cancer. 2002;94(11):2967-80.
70. Machtay M, Moughan J, Trotti A, Garden AS, Weber RS, Cooper JS, et al. Factors associated with severe late toxicity after concurrent chemoradiation for locally advanced head and neck cancer: an RTOG analysis. J Clin Oncol. 2008;26(21): 3582-9.
71. Gildener-Leapman N, Kim J, Abberbock S, Choby GW, Mandal R, Duvvuri U, et al. Utility of up-front transoral robotic surgery in tailoring adjuvant therapy. Head Neck. 2016;38(8):1201-7.
72. Golusiński W, Golusińska-Kardach E. Current role of surgery in the management of oropharyngeal cancer. Front Oncol. 2019;9:388.
73. Rich JT, Milov S, Lewis Jr JS, Thorstad WL, Adkins DR, Haughey BH. Transoral laser microsurgery (TLM) ± adjuvant therapy for advanced stage oropharyngeal cancer: outcomes and prognostic factors. Laryngoscope. 2009;119(9):1709-19.
74. Weinstein GS, O'Malley BW, Rinaldo A, Silver CE, Werner JA, Ferlito A. Understanding contraindications for transoral robotic surgery (TORS) for oropharyngeal cancer. Eur Arch Otorhinolaryngol. 2015;272(7):1551-2.
75. De Virgilio A, Kim SH, Magnuson JS, Holsinger C, Remacle M, Lawson G, et al. Anatomical-based classification for transoral lateral oropharyngectomy. Oral Oncol. 2019;99:104450.
76. Cooper JS, Pajak TF, Forastiere AA, Jacobs J, Campbell BH, Saxman SB, et al. Postoperative concurrent radiotherapy and chemotherapy for high-risk squamous-cell carcinoma of the head and neck. N Engl J Med. 2004;350(19):1937-44.
77. Bernier J, Domenge C, Ozsahin M, Matuszewska K, Lefèbvre JL, Greiner RH, et al. Postoperative irradiation with or without concomitant chemotherapy for locally advanced head and neck cancer. N Engl J Med. 2004;350(19): 1945-52.
78. Van Loon JW, Smeele LE, Hilgers FJ, van den Brekel MW. Outcome of transoral robotic surgery for stage I–II oropharyngeal cancer. Eur Arch Otorhinolaryngol. 2015;272(1):175-83.
79. Cheraghlou S, Yu PK, Otremba MD, Park HS, Bhatia A, Zogg CK, et al. Treatment deintensification in human papillomavirus-positive oropharynx cancer: outcomes from the National Cancer Data Base. Cancer. 2018;124(4): 717-26.
80. Hutcheson KA, Holsinger FC, Kupferman ME, Lewin JS. Functional outcomes after TORS for oropharyngeal cancer: a systematic review. Eur Arch Otorhinolaryngol. 2015; 272(2):463-71.
81. Weinstein GS, Quon H, Newman HJ, Chalian J, Malloy K. Lin A, et al. Transoral robotic surgery alone for oropharyngeal cancer: an analysis of local control. Arch Otolaryngol Head Neck Surg. 2012;138:628-34.
82. de Almeida JR, Li R, Magnuson JS, Smith RV, Moore E, Lawson G, et al. Oncologic outcomes after transoral robotic surgery: a multi-institutional study. JAMA Otolaryngology Head Neck Surg. 2015;141(12):1043-51.
83. Dabas S, Gupta K, Ranjan R, Sharma AK, Shukla H, Dinesh A. Oncological outcome following de-intensification of treatment for stage I and II HPV negative oropharyngeal cancers with transoral robotic surgery (TORS): a prospective trial. Oral Oncol. 2017;69:80-3.
84. Moore EJ, Van Abel KM, Price DL, Lohse CM, Olsen KD, Jackson RS, et al. Transoral robotic surgery for oropharyngeal carcinoma: surgical margins and oncologic outcomes. Head Neck. 2018;40(4):747-55.

85. Baliga S, Kabarriti R, Jiang J, Mehta V, Guha C, Kalnicki S, et al. Utilization of transoral robotic surgery (TORS) in patients with oropharyngeal squamous cell carcinoma and its impact on survival and use of chemotherapy. Oral Oncol. 2018;86:75-80.
86. White H, Ford S, Bush B, Holsinger FC, Moore E, Ghanem T, et al. Salvage surgery for recurrent cancers of the oropharynx: comparing TORS with standard open surgical approaches. JAMA Otolaryngol Head Neck Surg. 2013;139(8):773-7.
87. Dabas S, Dewan A, Ranjan R, Dewan AK, Shukla H, Sinha R. Salvage transoral robotic surgery for recurrent or residual head and neck squamous cell carcinoma: a single institution experience. Asian Pac J Cancer Prev. 2015;16(17):7-627.
88. Paleri V, Fox H, Coward S, Ragbir M, McQueen A, Ahmed O, et al. Transoral robotic surgery for residual and recurrent oropharyngeal cancers: Exploratory study of surgical innovation using the IDEAL framework for early-phase surgical studies. Head Neck. 2018;40(3):512-25.
89. Nichols AC, Theurer J, Prisman E, Read N, Berthelet E, Tran E, et al. Radiotherapy versus transoral robotic surgery and neck dissection for oropharyngeal squamous cell carcinoma (ORATOR): an open-label, phase 2, randomised trial. Lancet Oncol. 2019;20(10):1349-59.
90. de Almeida JR, Park RC, Genden EM. Reconstruction of transoral robotic surgery defects: principles and techniques. J Reconstr Microsurg. 2012;28(07):465-72.
91. Chen AY, Schrag N, Hao Y, Stewart A, Ward E. Changes in treatment of advanced oropharyngeal cancer, 1985–2001. Laryngoscope. 2007;117(1):16-21.
92. Gonçalves Agra IM, Lopes Carvalho A, Samsonovski Ulbrich F, De Campos OD, Martins EP, Magrin J, et al. Prognostic factors in salvage surgery for recurrent oral and oropharyngeal cancer. Head Neck. 2006;28(2):107-13.
93. Spencer SA, Harris J, Wheeler RH, Machtay M, Schultz C, Spanos W, et al. Final report of RTOG 9610, a multi-institutional trial of reirradiation and chemotherapy for unresectable recurrent squamous cell carcinoma of the head and neck. Head Neck. 2008;30(3):281-8.
94. Langer CJ, Harris J, Horwitz EM, Nicolaou N, Kies M, Curran W, et al. Phase II study of low-dose paclitaxel and cisplatin in combination with split-course concomitant twice-daily reirradiation in recurrent squamous cell carcinoma of the head and neck: results of Radiation Therapy Oncology Group Protocol 9911. J Clin Oncol. 2007;25(30): 4800-5.
95. McDonald MW, Moore MG, Johnstone PA. Risk of carotid blowout after reirradiation of the head and neck: a systematic review. Int J Radiat Oncol Biol Phys. 2012;82(3):1083-9.
96. Ferris RL, Blumenschein Jr G, Fayette J, Guigay J, Colevas AD, Licitra L, et al. Nivolumab for recurrent squamous-cell carcinoma of the head and neck. N Engl J Med. 2016; 375(19):1856-67.
97. Holsinger FC, Laccourreye O, Weber RS. Surgical approaches for cancer of the oropharynx. Oper Tech Otolaryngol. 2005;16(1):40-8.
98. Hamoir M, Schmitz S, Suarez C, Strojan P, Hutcheson KA, Rodrigo JP, et al. The current role of salvage surgery in recurrent head and neck squamous cell carcinoma. Cancers. 2018;10(8):267.
99. Tan HK, Giger R, Auperin A, Bourhis J, Janot F, Temam S. Salvage surgery after concomitant chemoradiation in head and neck squamous cell carcinomas—stratification for postsalvage survival. Head Neck. 2010;32(2):139-47.
100. Bonner JA, Harari PM, Giralt J, Azarnia N, Shin DM, Cohen RB, et al. Radiotherapy plus cetuximab for squamous-cell carcinoma of the head and neck. N Engl J Med. 2006;354(6):567-78.
101. Mirghani H, Blanchard P. Treatment de-escalation for HPV-driven oropharyngeal cancer: where do we stand? Clin Transl Radiat Oncol. 2018;8:4-11.
102. Gillison ML, Trotti AM, Harris J, Eisbruch A, Harari PM, Adelstein DJ, et al. Radiotherapy plus cetuximab or cisplatin in human papillomavirus-positive oropharyngeal cancer (NRG Oncology RTOG 1016): a randomised, multicentre, non-inferiority trial. Lancet. 2019;393(10166):40-50.
103. Mehanna H, Robinson M, Hartley A, Kong A, Foran B, Fulton-Lieuw T, et al. Radiotherapy plus cisplatin or cetuximab in low-risk human papillomavirus-positive oropharyngeal cancer (De-ESCALaTE HPV): an open-label randomised controlled phase 3 trial. Lancet. 2019;393(10166): 51-60.
104. Eisbruch A, Schwartz M, Rasch C, Vineberg K, Damen E, Van As CJ, et al. Dysphagia and aspiration after chemoradiotherapy for head-and-neck cancer: which anatomic structures are affected and can they be spared by IMRT? Int J Radiat Oncol Biol Phys. 2004;60(5):1425-39.
105. Levendag PC, Teguh DN, Voet P, van der Est H, Noever I, de Kruijf WJ, et al. Dysphagia disorders in patients with cancer of the oropharynx are significantly affected by the radiation therapy dose to the superior and middle constrictor muscle: a dose-effect relationship. Radiother Oncol. 2007; 85(1):64-73.
106. Feng FY, Kim HM, Lyden TH, Haxer MJ, Feng M, Worden FP, et al. Intensity-modulated radiotherapy of head and neck cancer aiming to reduce dysphagia: early dose-effect relationships for the swallowing structures. Int J Radiat Oncol Biol Phys. 2007;68(5):1289-98.
107. Marur S, Li S, Cmelak AJ, Gillison ML, Zhao WJ, Ferris RL, et al. E1308: phase II trial of induction chemotherapy followed by reduced-dose radiation and weekly cetuximab in patients with HPV-associated resectable squamous cell carcinoma of the oropharynx—ECOG-ACRIN Cancer Research Group. J Clin Oncol. 2017;35(5):490-7.
108. Chen AM, Felix C, Wang PC, Hsu S, Basehart V, Garst J, et al. Reduced-dose radiotherapy for human papillomavirus-associated squamous-cell carcinoma of the oropharynx: a single-arm, phase 2 study. Lancet Oncol. 2017;18(6): 803-11.
109. Villaflor VM, Melotek JM, Karrison TG, Brisson RJ, Blair EA, Portugal L, et al. Response-adapted volume de-escalation (RAVD) in locally advanced head and neck cancer. Ann Oncol. 2016;27(5):908-13.
110. Chera BS, Amdur RJ, Tepper J, Qaqish B, Green R, Aumer SL, et al. Phase 2 trial of de-intensified chemoradiation therapy for favorable-risk human papillomavirus-associated oropharyngeal squamous cell carcinoma. Int J Radiat Oncol Biol Phys. 2015;93(5):976-85.
111. Yom SS, Torres-Saavedra P, Caudell JJ, Waldron JN, Gillison ML, Truong MT, et al. NRG-HN002: A Randomized Phase II Trial for Patients with p16-positive, Non-Smoking-Associated, Locoregionally Advanced Oropharyngeal Cancer. Int J Radiat Oncol Biol Phys. 2019;105(3):684-5.
112. Herrero R, Quint W, Hildesheim A, Gonzalez P, Struijk L, Katki HA, et al. Reduced prevalence of oral human papillomavirus (HPV) 4 years after bivalent HPV vaccination in a randomized clinical trial in Costa Rica. PloS One. 2013;8(7):e68329.

CHAPTER 13

Cancers of the Larynx

Sivakumar Vidhyadharan, Narayana Subramaniam, Samskruthi P Murthy

INTRODUCTION

Cancer of the larynx is a frequent malignancy of the head and neck region. It has a profound impact on breathing, airway protection, swallowing, and phonation by interfering with the normal structure and functioning of the larynx. Though the larynx may be a potential site for all histological types of neoplasms, laryngeal cancer refers almost exclusively to squamous carcinomas. In this chapter we cover the epidemiology, presentation, and management of laryngeal cancer.

EPIDEMIOLOGY

World over, laryngeal cancer is an important cause of morbidity and mortality. Although its incidence is only about 1.1% of all cancer,[1] it is a potentially devastating disease due to its impact on speech, swallowing, and quality of life (QoL). The commonly described patient of laryngeal cancer is a male in the sixth or seventh decade of life with a history of heavy smoking and alcohol abuse, however this has been changing over time; there is a significant increase in the percentage of women who develop these cancers, especially in the glottis.

RISK FACTORS

Tobacco

Tobacco smoke exposure is the single most important factor in developing laryngeal cancer. There are dozens of carcinogens in tobacco, which have been covered in detail in other sections of this book. These carcinogens in the tobacco smoke are either dissolved in saliva or coat the epithelial cellular surface, are degraded by enzymes into epoxides that bind to deoxyribonucleic acid (DNA) or ribonucleic acid (RNA) and result in their damage, leading to cancer. The odds ratio for tobacco exposure is around 10, with a significant risk reduction after 10 years of abstinence. Additionally, for those who survive 3 or more years after treatment of laryngeal cancer and continue to smoke, the risk of a second primary cancer is seven times higher than those who quit.[2,3]

Alcohol

Alcohol is an independent risk factor for laryngeal cancer, with a dose-dependent risk and a super-multiplicative risk factor when combined with tobacco (viz. the carcinogenic effect of both combined is worse than the sum total of their individual carcinogenic effect). The odds ratio for an intake of 50 g/day and 100 g/day are estimated to be 2 and 4, respectively.[4]

Diet

Case-control studies from multiple centers in Europe revealed that a high and varied intake of fruit, vegetables (particularly rich in carotenes), fish, vegetable oil, and low intake of butter and preserved meats are associated with reduced risk of laryngeal cancers after adjustment for risk factors such as alcohol, tobacco, socioeconomic status, and nutrition. This may be a reflection of the role of micronutrients and antioxidants in carcinogenesis inhibition.[5]

Socioeconomic Status

Due to poor health care, smoking, alcohol consumption, poor dietary habits, and occupational carcinogens, laryngeal cancer has been linked with lower socioeconomic status. There is an increased independent relative risk for people of lower educational standard and unskilled workers as reported by the Heidelberg case-control study, where the incidence of laryngeal carcinoma has shown a gradual increase with increasing deprivation.[3] In developing countries, indoor air pollution by emission products of fossil fuel single stoves is a major risk factor. Burning fossil fuel causes an emission of high concentrations of carcinogenic combustion products such as polycyclic hydrocarbons into the indoor air, the risk increases many fold especially when the emission is in confined spaces.

Viruses

The role of human papillomavirus (HPV) in laryngeal cancers remains contentious. HPV is well established as the cause of recurrent respiratory papillomatosis; types 6 and 11 are most frequently correlated with recurrent respiratory papillomatosis. It is unusual for papillomas of the larynx and lungs to transform into a malignancy even several years after the primary treatment.[6] In resected laryngeal cancer specimens, HPV positivity was found in between 4.4 and 58%, which may represent associated coinfection with the virus and not virus-induced carcinogenesis.

Occupation

Workers exposed to diesel fumes, sulfuric acid fumes, tar products, metal dusts, asbestos, and other inorganic and organic agents may have an increased risk of laryngeal cancer.[7,8] A case-control study from Spain revealed that there was an increased risk of laryngeal cancer among wood-related occupations such as furniture making and woodworking.[9]

Genetic Susceptibility

Egeli et al. reported that among nonsmokers with head and neck cancer (a third had no tobacco exposure) and their first-degree relatives, had high rates of chromosomal aberration and fragile site expression occurred compared with a control group; these aberrations were most often noted in p53.[10] Another report showed that in 74% of the laryngeal cancer patients that they studied, there was loss of heterozygosity in p53.[11] In patients with the Lynch syndrome and Bloom's syndrome, there is an indirect evidence of a genetic predisposition to familial laryngeal cancer.

Ionizing Radiation

It has been associated with the development of carcinomas and sarcomas. Radiation-induced sarcoma may also follow treatment of laryngeal cancer with radiotherapy (RT). The dose at which risk is increased was noted to be over 55 Gy, with doses ranging from 16 to 112 Gy. Low-dose exposure after atomic explosions does not increase this risk.[12-14]

Leukoplakia and Keratosis

These have a relatively low risk of malignant transformation; refer to chapter on premalignant lesions of the larynx for further details.

Chronic Gastroesophageal Reflux

The chronic mucosal irritation resulting from reflux of gastric contents is associated with a risk of malignant transformation. Although not a major risk factor, it is considered to have a significant contribution to the development of laryngeal cancer. A large cohort study comprising nearly 20,000 patients noted that the prevalence of gastroesophageal reflux disease was higher in malignancy (8.9% vs. 4%), and it was an independent risk factor for development of malignancy with an odds ratio of 2.4.[15]

APPLIED ANATOMY[16-18]

The larynx is important for respiration, voice, and deglutition. The larynx is divided anatomically and clinically, into supraglottis, glottis, and subglottis. Embryologically, the supraglottis is derived from the buccopharyngeal anlage of the third and fourth arches, whereas the glottic and subglottic subunit develops from the pulmonary anlages of the fifth and sixth branchial arches.

Supraglottis

The supraglottis, as a laryngeal subunit comprises of the epiglottis, aryepiglottic folds, arytenoids, ventricles, and the false cords. The epiglottis includes the tip, lingual, and laryngeal surfaces. The inferior limit of the supraglottis, as described by the American Joint Committee on Cancer (AJCC), is a horizontal plane traversing across the apex of the ventricle. The anatomic divisional change from the respiratory to squamous epithelium is located at the arcuate line, and is reliably located at the apex. The marginal zone of the supraglottis is recognized for its aggressive clinical biology of carcinomas arising in this region. It is composed of suprahyoid epiglottis and the aryepiglottic fold.

Glottis

The glottic larynx includes true vocal cord, anterior and posterior commissures. According to the AJCC the inferior border of the glottis is a horizontal plane 1 cm inferior to the level of the upper surface of the vocal cord. The strict anatomical definition of the vocal cord is that part of the free edge of the cord covered by squamous epithelium, which has a vertical height of 5 mm, bounded superiorly and inferiorly by the superior and inferior arcuate line. Histologically, the five layers of the vocal fold are: (1) squamous epithelium layer of the mucosa (very thin and helps to hold the shape of the vocal folds however there are no mucous glands located within this epithelium), (2) superficial layer of the lamina propria (consists primarily of loose fibers and matrix and is clinically referred to as Reinke's space; this layer is vital for phonatory function), (3) intermediate layer of the lamina propria (also consists of elastic and collagenous fibers but at a higher concentration than the superficial layer of the lamina propria), (4) deep layer of the lamina propria (consists primarily of a high concentration of collagen bundles, this deep layer is dense and fibrous and together with the intermediate layer forms the vocal ligament) and (5) the vocalis or thyroarytenoid (this muscle provides the main mass of the vocal fold).

Subglottis

This consists of a mobile part from below the true vocal cord to the upper border of the cricoid cartilage (mucosa covering conus elasticus), and a fixed part, which extends up to the inferior border of the cricoid.

CLINICAL EXAMINATION AND PRESENTATION

Clinical examination comprises of a detailed medical history and a physical examination. Physical examination involving close inspection of throat will help find signs of potential malignancy. Direct laryngoscopy is most accurate in evaluating the mucosal surface of the aerodigestive tract. In fact, examination regularly detects superficial carcinomas along the mucosal surface that cannot be detected on MRI. Direct laryngoscopy can be performed either with a flexible or rigid scope. The evaluation of the vocal cord is aided by a flexible laryngoscopy examination in the outpatient clinic. The degree of involvement comprising critical areas, such as the anterior commissure and salivary pooling within the pyriform sinus, which is a subtle sign suggestive of subglottic extension. Videostroboscopy laryngeal examination in the preoperative period, provides an assessment of depth of invasion and thereby potential extent of resection, this would help in the decision-making process.[17-20]

Early glottic cancer is associated with alteration in the tone or quality of voice. Hence, a prompt assessment needs to be performed, if symptoms of hoarseness or a change in voice persist for 3 weeks or longer. Change of voice or hoarseness worsens as the size of tumor increases. Dyspnea and a variable degree of aspiration become evident when one vocal cord fixation occurs. There is a high risk of obstructed airway, presenting with apparent stridor and or possible otalgia as the disease progresses to advanced stages. The primary clinical presentation of neck nodes is unusual in patients with early glottic cancer, unless there is extension or deep invasion of glottic cancer into the supraglottis. In such cases, the patient's presenting complaints may include lymphadenopathy. Patients with early supraglottic cancers may present with globus or foreign body sensation. If the lesion is more exophytic, hemoptysis may become more predominant. A "hot-potato" voice is the frequent voice change in patients with enlarging supraglottic tumors. Hoarseness of voice also occurs as the tumor extends below to involve the vocal cords. Odynophagia, dysphagia, and otalgia are symptoms that commonly arise as the laryngeal tumor spreads laterally.

In contrast to glottic cancers, patients with supraglottic cancers may initially present with neck nodes. All regions above the clavicle are carefully palpated for evidence of metastatic disease or direct extralaryngeal extension. Careful assessment of the midline structures must be documented. Loss of the normal crepitus with side-to-side movement of the laryngeal framework may indicate postcricoid involvement. Complete fixation of the laryngeal complex on clinical examination is also suggestive of prevertebral involvement. Careful palpable assessment of the thyrohyoid membrane, thyroid cartilage, and cricothyroid membrane, as well as the overlying soft tissue of the laryngeal complex may provide a more clinically useful assessment of the tumor than any advanced imaging analysis. Laryngeal carcinoma most frequently metastasizes to nodal levels II, III, and IV in the neck. Supraglottic tumors have the highest rates of occult cervical metastasis (T1, T2, T3, and T4 had 20%, 40%, 60%, and 80% incidence, respectively). Advanced glottic lesions can also present with lymphadenopathy. Subglottic tumors have a significant incidence of extralaryngeal spread because of their proximity to the cricothyroid membrane and the rich postcricoid lymphatics.[21,22]

PATHWAYS OF SPREAD OF LARYNGEAL CANCER[23-26]

The endolaryngeal soft tissues are surrounded within anatomic spaces enclosed typically by fibroelastic membranes. These structures check the spread of early carcinoma to specific compartments, so that small lesions can often be removed with adequate margins by surgery. Once these barriers have been violated, the malignant growth spreads without much resistance into contiguous compartments or into neighboring soft tissue spaces and laryngeal framework. Laryngeal carcinoma may spread from its original site to other portions of the larynx by direct mucosal and submucosal extension, by lymphatic or vascular invasion, by perineural spread or by direct infiltration of the nearby structures. The most important pathways for submucosal tumor dissemination in the larynx occur along the paraglottic space (PGS) and along the pre-epiglottic space (PES). These two spaces also play an important role for the T classification. According to the guidelines of the AJCC, neoplastic invasion of these spaces upstages laryngeal cancer to T3. The PGS is also a potential and symmetrical space filled with fat, present on either side, situated between the laryngeal mucosa and the laryngeal framework. The majority of the PGS within the supraglottic region is filled with fat and there are thin bands of muscle present within fat at the level of false cords. The laryngeal ventricle is encircled by the PGS and merges superiorly with the PES. The anteriorly lying endolarynx is separated from the posteriorly lying piriform sinuses by the aryepiglottic folds. The PGS at the level the glottis is situated between the thyroarytenoid muscle medially and the laryngeal framework which is composed of thyroid and cricoid cartilages laterally. The thyroarytenoid muscle contributes to the volume and provides the outline of the true vocal cord. Another potential space is the PES, a pyramidally shaped space comprising exclusively of fatty tissue. It is bounded anteriorly by the thyrohyoid membrane and thyroid laminae, posteriorly by the infrahyoid epiglottis, cranially by the hyoepiglottic ligament, and caudally by the petiole of the epiglottis. But additional planes may be additionally used to better show the entire craniocaudal extent of a lesion (coronal images for the PGS and sagittal images for the PES). These "pathways of spread" have conventionally been the basis for conservation surgical procedures.

Glottic Tumors

Most glottic cancers arise in the free margin of the anterior two-thirds of the vocal cord. Spread of in situ glottic carcinoma is limited by the basement membrane. Spread of early invasive carcinoma of the mobile cord is limited, by a fibroelastic membrane that comprises of conus elasticus and the vocal ligament with its extension along the floor of the ventricle, the thyroglottic ligament. Glottic cancers that involve the entire length of the true cord, with normal mobility are limited to the mucosa (Reinke's space) without infiltration of the underlying muscle. Vertical spread occurs in the later stages. Anterior spread is limited by the Broyle's ligament, representing the confluence of the vocal ligament, the conus elasticus, and the internal perichondrium of the thyroid ala. The Broyle's ligament is traditionally believed to be resistant to tumor spread. However, once involved, it facilitates subglottic and supraglottic spread along the anterior midline as its fibers extend longitudinally in a superior-inferior direction and so facilitate tumor extension in this axis. Also, the inner perichondrium is dehiscent in the area of the anterior commissure tendon attachment to the thyroid cartilage and so tumors once involving the anterior commissure have a significant propensity for thyroid cartilage invasion. The conus elasticus is believed to be a barrier that limits inferior extension to the subglottis. Deep lateral invasion occurs in the PGS with infiltration of the thyroarytenoid muscle leading to vocal cord fixation. Although the posterior commissure is frequently involved due to advanced tumors from other sites, primary lesions of the posterior glottis are rare.

Supraglottic Tumors

Supraglottic tumors usually spread in an upward direction towards the base of the base of tongue. Proliferative or exophytic tumors commonly arise in the suprahyoid epiglottis. The tumors of the infrahyoid epiglottis tend to grow through the pores in the epiglottic cartilage, into the PES. These tumors spread by encircling the structures of supraglottic larynx and hypopharynx, such as the pharyngoepiglottic fold, aryepiglottic folds, false cords, and the medial wall of the pyriform sinus. PES infiltration occurs early during disease course. The tumors of the false cord spread upwards to involve the epiglottis. Tumors of the arytenoids and the aryepiglottic fold usually spill over into the adjacent pyriform sinus or postcricoid region and are usually referred to as marginal zone carcinomas. They have a propensity for bilateral spread, especially, supraglottic tumors situated at the midline. Structures such as the aryepiglottic fold and arytenoids are areas designated as marginal zone, and tumors in this location have some characteristics of hypopharyngeal tumors, with a higher propensity for lymph node metastasis and poorer prognosis.

Subglottic Tumors

Isolated subglottic tumors are rare and account for less than one percent of all laryngeal tumors. Tumor spread occurs bilaterally and along the entire circumference of the subglottis. The cricoid cartilage is involved early due to the lack of an intervening muscle layer. Early extralaryngeal extension of the carcinoma is through cricothyroid membrane. It is associated with nodal metastasis to level III–IV and to the superior mediastinal nodes.

Transglottic Tumors

Cancer involving both the glottic and supraglottic regions in association with fixation of the true vocal cord is termed transglottic. Kirchner's work suggests that transglottic cancer has a single point of origin, which is most likely deep within the ventricle. Most of the transglottic cancers (65%) invade the laryngeal framework and these tumors are usually not amenable to partial laryngectomy procedures and will necessitate either total or near total laryngectomy (NTL).

IMAGING

Imaging is critical to evaluate the deep extent of laryngeal cancer in order to plan the most conservative radical reliable treatment. Common imaging techniques include computed tomography (CT), magnetic resonance imaging (MRI), and positron emission tomography (PET) scan. The role of imaging in unusual laryngeal and hypopharyngeal tumors is to detect or confirm the presence of a submucosal mass, to determine the deep structures involved and to guide the surgeon to the most appropriate site where to obtain deep aggressive biopsies. Some submucosal masses can be further characterized with regard to their etiology when they display the typical features of chondroid, lipomatous or hypervascularized tissue or those of nontumoral lesions, such as cysts or laryngoceles. The superiority of CT over MRI for laryngeal cancer is debatable, with CT typically demonstrating a higher specificity for identifying thyroid cartilage invasion compared with MRI, but with lower sensitivity. Multidetector computed tomography (MDCT) is the mainstay for local staging but it has its limitations including low sensitivity. On the other hand, MRI is considered for practical and economic reasons (time-consuming and expensive) as a second-level technique and, nevertheless, seems to be affected by a nonsufficient high specificity. T2-weighted MRI allows for excellent visualization of subtle submucosal spread into the PES and PGS.[27]

Computed tomography has a high sensitivity and a high negative predictive value for the detection of cartilage invasion provided that the following criteria are used: sclerosis, erosion, lysis, and extralaryngeal spread. Sclerosis is a sensitive sign for the detection of neoplastic cartilage invasion and enables diagnosis of early or microscopic intracartilaginous tumor spread. It corresponds to bone remodeling and new bone formation induced by the presence of tumor cells in immediate tumor vicinity and sometimes preceding actual invasion. This particular sign is of varying specificity between the laryngeal cartilages with the highest specificity seen in the cricoid (76%) and arytenoid cartilages (79%) and the thyroid cartilage having the lowest specificity (40%). Therefore, if a tumor mass is seen adjacent to a sclerotic cartilage, this does not automatically imply that tumor cells are found within the remodeled marrow cavity. Conversely, failing at surgery to remove a cartilage that exhibits sclerosis on CT carries a 50–60% risk of leaving tumor behind. Minor areas of osteolysis correspond to the CT criteria of erosion, while major areas of osteolysis correspond to the CT criteria of lysis. Histologically, erosion and lysis correspond to destruction of bone due to osteoclastic activity. As a consequence, erosion and lysis can be considered specific criteria for the detection of neoplastic invasion in all cartilages. The overall specificity of erosion and lysis is 93%. However, both of these criteria are not very sensitive as they are bound to the presence of more advanced invasion of laryngeal cartilage.

Extralaryngeal spread upstages a laryngeal tumor as T4 and occurs due to tumor invasion through a cartilage into the extralaryngeal soft tissues. This CT criteria is highly specific (overall specificity, 95%), but because it is only seen very late in the disease process its sensitivity is as low as 44%. By applying the combination of extralaryngeal tumor, sclerosis, and erosion or lysis to all cartilages, one may obtain an overall sensitivity as high as 91%. Because the negative predictive value of this combination is 95%, CT may be considered as an excellent test to exclude cartilage invasion prior to treatment.

The reported sensitivity of MRI for the detection of neoplastic cartilage invasion is 89–94%, the specificity 74–88%, and the negative predictive value 94–96%. Extensive tumor invasion with destruction of cartilage and invasion into extralaryngeal soft tissues can be diagnosed with a high accuracy with MRI. In addition, MRI enables detection of intracartilaginous tumor spread. If tumor is present only adjacent to the inner aspect of a cartilage, the radiologist can differentiate between tumor and nonossified cartilage by comparing the different magnetic resonance (MR) pulse sequences. Cartilage invaded by tumor displays an intermediate to low signal intensity on T1-weighted images, a higher signal intensity on T2-weighted images and areas of enhancement within the cartilage adjacent to the tumor after injection of gadolinium-chelates. If these signs are absent, cartilage infiltration can be ruled out with a high level of confidence, since the negative predictive value of MRI is very high. Unfortunately, the MRI findings suggesting neoplastic cartilage invasion are not as specific as expected initially, but may be false-positive in a considerable number of instances; the positive predictive value (PPV) is only 71%. This is because reactive inflammation, edema, and fibrosis may mimic infiltration of the cartilage by tumor extension. Since inflammatory changes are most common in the thyroid cartilage, the specificity of MRI to detect neoplastic invasion of the thyroid cartilage is only 56%, as opposed to 87% and 95% in the cricoid and arytenoid cartilage, respectively. The positive diagnosis of neoplastic invasion of the thyroid cartilage should, therefore, be made with extreme caution at MRI.

Cartilage invasion is the most investigated topic for both CT and MR. Detection of minor cartilage invasion would be crucial for planning surgical laser resection in T3 tumors. Ryu et al. reported lack of sensitivity for CT in detection of thyroid cartilage penetration and extralaryngeal spread (72% and 73%, respectively) with corresponding PPV of 70% and 80%, respectively. They also reported 50% sensitivity and 63% PPV for arytenoid cartilage destruction and sensitivity of 100% and PPV of 50%, for detection of cricoid invasion.[28] Xia et al. reported sensitivity and PPV of 75% and 80% for cartilage invasion detection, without distinction between minor and major invasion.[29] The inability of MDCT to detect minor cartilage invasion was revealed in the study by Hartl et al., which focused on detection of thyroid cartilage invasion in early laryngeal cancer. Inner cortex invasion was present in 19/236 patients and MDCT was able to demonstrate it just in 13% of them.[30] In addition, Li et al. reported sensitivity of 60% and PPV of 30% in discriminating between major and minor/none cartilage invasion.

Magnetic resonance has the potential to outperform MDCT, at least in demonstrating intracartilaginous spread. This is seen especially well in nonossified cartilage, which displays a homogeneous dark signal on T2-weighted sequences, significantly different from intermediate signal of tumor. Wu et al. reported a series of 26 patients affected by laryngeal cancer involving the anterior commissure, who were studied with MDCT and state-of-the-art MRI before surgery. They reported that MRI staged tumors more accurately than CT with an accuracy of 88.5% and 57.7%, respectively.[31] A precise assessment of PGS and PES invasion is crucial for surgical planning, especially with regard to transoral excision. Ryu et al. utilized MDCT and reported sensitivity, specificity, PPV, and NPV of 87%, 57%, 84%, and 63% for PGS and 83%, 39%, 39%, and 83% for PES in patients affected by locally advanced laryngeal and hypopharyngeal carcinoma. There was no emphasis made on whether there was minor and major invasion of the PES or between the anterior and posterior PGS. This is relevant as in selected cases, minor invasion of the PES or invasion of the anterior PGS without cartilage invasion is amenable to transoral surgery. The potential of MRI [combining T2-weighted and diffusion-weighted imaging (DWI) sequences] can be used, to discriminate tumor invasion of the posterior PGS from peritumoral edema in patients clinically classified as T3 for cord/arytenoid fixation, and also extralaryngeal spread via the inferior PGS route.[28-30]

Tumor volume has been traditionally considered as predictive of local control and survival for head and neck cancer treated with chemoradiotherapy. Rutkowski et al.[32] demonstrated the impact of tumor volume on the outcome of patients with T2 glottic cancer; an analysis of global dose versus initial tumor volume demonstrated that tumors larger than 5 cm^3 needed an extradose of 6.5 Gy to have a local control similar to tumors smaller than 0.5 cm^3. van Bockel et al. found a correlation between tumor volume, local control and survival in a cohort of glottic and supraglottic cancers with different T-categories.[33] Timmermans et al. demonstrated an absence of correlation between tumor volume and outcome in patients with advanced laryngeal cancer treated by RT, chemoradiation, or laryngectomy plus RT.[34] Furthermore, on analyzing the data from the prospective ARCON (accelerated radiotherapy with carbogen and nicotinamide) trial, there was correlation between tumor volume and outcome in both the arms of patients treated by accelerated RT alone and accelerated RT plus carbogen breathing and nicotinamide.[35] In all these studies, tumor volume assessment was performed by contrast-enhanced MDCT, which is still considered the standard for tumor delineation in RT planning. However, it is conceivable that lack in contrast resolution could affect tumor delineation with CT. Caldas-Magalhaes et al. demonstrated that both CT and MR significantly overestimate tumor volume compared to histology (mean volume 7.2 mL at pathology, 14.9 mL for CT, and 18.3 for MR). PET-CT led to lesser overestimation (9.8 mL), but with a worse percentage coverage of tumor (77%) compared to that of CT (85%) and MR (88%).[36]

There is a direct correlation between increasing volume of the primary tumor and increasing rate of local failure. Surgical control rates were found to be associated with tumor volume, where lesions <16 mL in size had 98% control while those larger only had 40% control.[37,38] In comparison, the control rates are better with supraglottic cancers with volume of ≤6 mL based on pretreatment CT and glottic cancers with volumes <3.5 mL (83% and 85%, respectively), than supraglottic cancers >6 mL and glottis cancers >3.5 mL (46% and 22%, respectively).[39,40] Small volume (<5 mL) abnormal signal intensity within the laryngeal cartilage on MRI after RT is considered physiological while larger volumes portend a poor prognosis.[41] DWI sequences could play a role in tumor delineation.

The use of pretreatment PET-CT imaging in known head and neck cancer, changed management in 30.9%, 18%, and 21.6% of the patients reported in the studies by Fleming et al., Schoder et al., and Zanation et al., respectively.[42-44] The information provided by PET-CT led to changes in planned procedures or sparing of previously planned procedure, by detection of synchronous or metastatic disease. It also helped guide biopsy to metabolically active areas within the larynx.[45] Still, there is ambiguity in how PET-CT compares with the fusion of CT, MRI, and/or PET only scan as it is presently used. During treatment, a decreased fluorodeoxyglucose (FDG) activity in the early phase of combined chemoradiotherapy is associated with greater tumor response, survival, and local control.[44]

While PET-CT has found increased use in the pretreatment period, its maximum utility may be in the setting of detecting recurrent cancer after radiation therapy or surgery, where the resultant anatomic changes are difficult to characterize by traditional imaging modalities (CT and MRI) alone.

The best results are obtained when PET-CT is performed 2–3 months after the completion of treatment.[46] Successful RT leads to a substantial reduction of tumor volume within 4 months and treatment failure must be suspected if 50% or more of the tumor mass is still visible after this period.[47-49]

Generally, PET-CT already has a high sensitivity and specificity in detection of recurrences of head and neck cancers. With regards to laryngeal cancer surveillance, a sensitivity of 93.75% and specificity of 91.67% in determining recurrence when the standardized uptake value threshold was set at 3.35 has been demonstrated.[50] On the other hand; PET-CT has low but measurable false-positive rates due to the increased metabolic activity in areas of infection or chronic inflammation. Routine workup for metastatic disease in laryngeal carcinoma involved assessing most frequent sites of distant metastasis which is the lung, followed by liver. Chest radiographs and laboratory investigation of liver function tests (LFTs) with possible liver ultrasonography has been the minimal standard requirement. In patients with high clinical suspicion or an abnormal chest X-ray, a CT of the chest and abdomen may be warranted. At present, a pretreatment PET-CT on patients with advanced stage laryngeal carcinomas has become more frequent practice, but routine use of PET-CT scan for pretreatment work-up of laryngeal malignancies is debatable.

STAGING

The AJCC, 8th edition Cancer Staging Manual bases primary tumor staging for glottic and supraglottic cancers on local extent as well as the presence or absence of vocal cord fixation **(Table 1)**.[25]

DIRECT LARYNGOSCOPY AND PANENDOSCOPY

Preoperative discussion of the airway between the surgeon and the anesthesiologist, and formulation of a primary plan and backup plans to secure the airway is critical in the operative assessment. Depending on the site of lesion, critical assessment of the lesion may only be possible under apneic conditions. As such, communication with competent anesthesiologists is critical. Once the patient is intubated and under anesthesia, a laryngoscope may be used to gain access to the airway. The selection of laryngoscope is largely dependent on surgeon preference and on the patient's anatomy. A variety of scopes exist (Dedo, Hollinger, Lindholm, etc.), each with their own pros and cons and they are often used in combination. It is important to map or photodocument the lesion after completing the endoscopic assessment for synchronous or metachronous lesions. The use of a rigid telescope (0, 30, and 70 degree telescopes) allows for magnification and superior visualization of the subglottis, anterior commissure, and the ventricles and all areas difficult to adequately visualize in the clinic. While vocal fold mobility is best assessed in the office with indirect mirror or fiberoptic examination, palpation of the vocal process in the operating room can help distinguish true vocal fold paralysis from arytenoid fixation. This is critical not only for staging but also to evaluate the cricoarytenoid unit whose function is necessary for many laryngeal conservation procedures. Assessment of the larynx should include both pyriform sinuses and the postcricoid area. Panendoscopy comprising of laryngoscopy, esophagoscopy, and bronchoscopy has been the standard for many years. Nevertheless, with better-quality preoperative imaging some centers do not consider panendoscopy a standard part of the diagnostic workup. Others have encouraged symptom-directed endoscopies based on the fact that most second primaries are discovered by their particular symptoms.

Table 1: AJCC 8th edition staging for laryngeal cancer.

Supraglottis	
T category	*T criteria*
Tx	Primary tumor cannot be assessed
Tis	Carcinoma in situ
T1	Tumor limited to one subsite of supraglottis with normal vocal cord mobility
T2	Tumor invades mucosa of more than one adjacent subsite of supraglottis or glottis or region outside the supraglottis (e.g., mucosa of base of tongue, vallecula, medial wall of pyriform sinus) without fixation of the larynx
T3	Tumor limited to larynx with vocal cord fixation and/or invades any of the following: Postcricoid area, pre-epiglottic space, paraglottic space, and/or inner cortex of thyroid cartilage
T4a	*Moderately advanced local disease:* Tumor invades through the outer cortex of the thyroid cartilage and/or invades tissues beyond the larynx (e.g., trachea, soft tissues of neck including deep extrinsic muscle of the tongue, strap muscles, thyroid, or esophagus)
T4b	*Very advanced local disease:* Tumor invades prevertebral space, encases carotid artery, or invades mediastinal structures.
Glottis	
T category	*T criteria*
Tx	Primary tumor cannot be assessed
Tis	Carcinoma in situ
T1	Tumor limited to the vocal cord(s) (may involve anterior or posterior commissure) with normal mobility
T1a	Tumor limited to one vocal cord
T1b	Tumor involves both vocal cords
T2	Tumor extends to supraglottis and/or subglottis, and/or with impaired vocal cord mobility
T3	Tumor limited to the larynx with vocal cord fixation and/or invasion of paraglottic space and/or inner cortex of the thyroid cartilage
T4a	*Moderately advanced local disease:* Tumor invades through the outer cortex of the thyroid cartilage and/or invades tissues beyond the larynx (e.g., trachea, cricoid cartilage, soft tissues of neck including deep extrinsic muscle of the tongue, strap muscles, thyroid, or esophagus)
T4b	*Very advanced local disease:* Tumor invades prevertebral space, encases carotid artery, or invades mediastinal structures
Subglottis	
T category	*T criteria*
Tx	Primary tumor cannot be assessed
Tis	Carcinoma in situ
T1	Tumor limited to the subglottis
T2	Tumor extends to vocal cord(s) with normal or impaired mobility
T3	Tumor limited to larynx with vocal cord fixation and/or invasion of paraglottic space and/or inner cortex of the thyroid cartilage
T4a	*Moderately advanced local disease:* Tumor invades cricoid or thyroid cartilage and/or invades tissues beyond the larynx (e.g., trachea, soft tissues of neck including deep extrinsic muscles of the tongue, strap muscles, thyroid, or esophagus)
T4b	*Very advanced local disease:* Tumor invades prevertebral space, encases carotid artery, or invades mediastinal structures
Nodal staging	
N category	*N criteria*
NX	Regional lymph nodes cannot be assessed
NO	No regional lymph node metastasis
N1	Metastasis in a single ipsilateral lymph node, 3 cm or smaller in greatest dimension and ENE (–)
N2	Metastasis in a single ipsilateral node, larger than 3 cm but not larger than 6 cm in greatest dimension and ENE (–); or metastases in multiple ipsilateral lymph nodes, none larger than 6 cm in greatest dimension and ENE (–); or metastasis in bilateral or contralateral lymph nodes, none larger than 6 cm in greatest dimension and ENE (–)
N2a	Metastasis in a single ipsilateral node, larger than 3 cm but not larger than 6 cm in greatest dimension and ENE (–)
N2b	Metastases in multiple ipsilateral nodes, none larger than 6 cm in greatest dimension and ENE (–)
N2c	Metastasis in bilateral or contralateral lymph nodes, none larger than 6 cm in greatest dimension and wENE (–)
N3	Metastasis in a lymph node, larger than 6 cm in greatest dimension and ENE (–); or metastasis in any lymph node(s) with clinically overt ENE (+)
N3a	Metastasis in a lymph node, larger than 6 cm in greatest dimension and ENE (–)
N3b	Metastasis in any lymph node(s) with clinically overt ENE (+)
Distant metastases	
M category	*M criteria*
M0	No distant metastasis
M1	Distant metastasis

(AJCC: American Joint Committee on Cancer; ENE: extranodal extension)

DIAGNOSTIC ADJUNCTS

Narrow-band Imaging

Narrow-band imaging (NBI) is a new endoscopic detection technology which utilizes filtered wavelengths (415 nm and 540 nm) to enhance the neoangiogenic microvascular abnormalities related to the preneoplastic and neoplastic transformations of the mucosal epithelium of the upper aerodigestive tract. These neoangiogenic microvascular abnormalities are perpendicular vascular changes (PVCs), which characterize intracapillary papillary capillary loops (IPCLs) and are associated with premalignant and malignant lesions. They grow perpendicularly towards the mucosa due to neoplastic stimuli and are sometimes, also linked to benign lesions such as papillomatosis. The lining epithelium of the larynx and hypopharynx is thin and is composed of nonkeratinized, stratified squamous epithelium that provides easy and reliable inspection by NBI for microvascular abnormalities. In addition to white light endoscopy, NBI allows better and more precise identification of benign vocal cord lesions. Further details are covered in the chapter on premalignant lesions.

Contact Endoscopy

Contact endoscopy (CE) is fundamentally a noninvasive visualization technique which aids in real-time and in situ examination of the vascularization pattern and cellular architecture of the superficial layers of the laryngeal mucosa and various other mucosa.[51] CE without tissue staining can be combined with NBI or Storz Professional Image Enhancement System (SPIES) or i-Scan for the in vivo assessment of superficial vessels with 60X to 150X magnification.[52-55] CE is reported to have an accuracy of 88–94%, a high sensitivity of 90–94.7%, and specificity of 81–100% in diagnosis of lesions of larynx. Assessment of laryngeal mucosa necessitates introduction of contact endoscope via a suspension laryngoscope under general anesthesia. The cellular architecture of the mucosa is reviewed after staining with 1% methylene blue. The methylene blue stain gives the cell's nucleus a dark blue color and light blue color to the cytoplasm. A limitation of CE is that early dysplasia appearing initially within the cells near basement membrane cannot be identified. Because the light and dye are unable to infiltrate deeper than a few superficial layers of the mucosa, there is a delay in identification until the dysplastic cells migrate up to the superficial layers. Another disadvantage due is that since invasive carcinoma is differentiated from carcinoma in situ by angioinvasion or neoangiogenesis at basement membrane level this may not be reliably identified by CE.

TREATMENT APPROACHES

Over the past three decades, there has been considerable technological progress in the rehabilitation of voice, radiation dose delivery, as well as enhancement and acceptance of conservative surgical techniques using different surgical tools. The current philosophy is organ preservation should be the offered wherever oncologically sound and feasible. Patients with early stage tumors have benefited from the success of organ preservation-based surgical approaches. Principles of oncologic surgery in the larynx have evolved significantly as our understanding has grown of the roles played by embryology and anatomy in tumor spread. Regardless of the disease stage and the treatment choice, reducing the incidence of adverse effects with improving QoL are presently thought of important therapeutic objectives.[56,57]

- *Early glottic cancers:* The approach to early glottic cancers is as shown in **Flowchart 1**.[57] Glottic carcinomas represent the majority of laryngeal cancer cases, which is mainly confined to the anterior portion of the vocal cord. Due to lack of lymphatic vessels in the glottic area and the early symptom of hoarseness, glottic tumors can usually be diagnosed at an early stage, and favorable outcomes can be achieved.[58]

Flowchart 1: Approach to early glottic cancers.

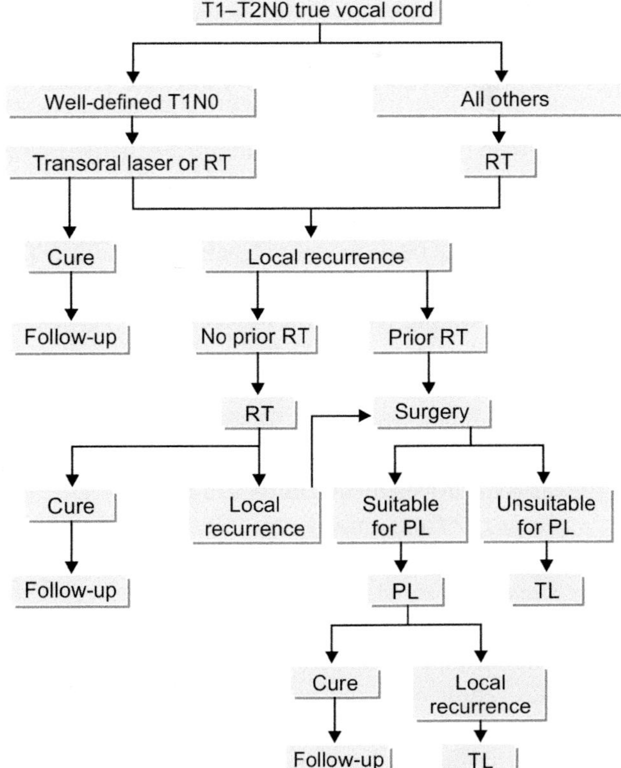

(PL: partial laryngectomy; RT: radiotherapy; TL: total laryngectomy)

Early glottic carcinoma (Tis–T2) are treatable with either transoral CO_2 laser microsurgery (TLM) or RT. There is still much deliberation as to which modality is preferable for both oncological and functional outcomes. Both treatment modalities have advantages and disadvantages. As a general rule, well-defined isolated lesion typically in the mid-cord are ideal for laser excision with adequate margins, while ill-defined diffuse lesions are better treated with RT, especially when the surgeon is not very experienced. One of the most important advantages of TLM as a primary therapeutic modality is the preservation of all treatment options in case of recurrent disease. Generally, patients initially treated with RT cannot be reirradiated and although TLM can be performed after RT, the indication is limited. A Cochrane systematic review update compared RT, open surgery, and endolaryngeal surgery (with or without laser) for early vocal cord carcinoma (glottic T1 and T2a) found no randomized data comparing transoral surgery to RT. They concluded that survival outcomes were comparable and use of any of these modalities was reasonable.[59]

In addition to oncological outcomes, QoL and functional outcomes such as voice and swallowing are also important factors when deciding a primary treatment. A randomized trial comparing TLM with RT focused on assessment of voice quality after treatment of early vocal cord cancer concluded that, overall voice quality between the groups was rated similar, but voice was breathier and the glottal gap was wider in patients treated with laser surgery than in those who received radiation therapy. Patients treated with RT had less voice-related complaints 2 years after completion of treatment.[60] Another consideration is that RT takes weeks of treatment whereas TLM can be limited to one sitting (or more if re-excision is required), and can result in rapid recovery, earlier return to work and less treatment-related costs. O'Hara et al. compared outcomes for T1a and T1b glottic cancers treated with both modalities and concluded that results were comparable with a trend towards improved local control in T1b with RT.

Reports from many studies state that voice outcome in patients treated with TLM are comparable to those treated with RT in Tis-T1a lesions requiring limited subepithelial or subligamental resections. On the other hand, voice outcome for greater sized lesions requiring larger resections is inferior than for smaller lesions.[60-62] There is inadequate comparative data to draw conclusions in T2 glottic carcinoma, however local control rates are comparable; the weighted average laryngeal preservation rate was 88.8%.[58]

A similar classification for glottic carcinomas is shown in **Table 2**:[63] a subepithelial cordectomy (type I), which is resection of the epithelium; a subligamental cordectomy (type II), which is a resection of the epithelium, Reinke's space and vocal ligament; transmuscular cordectomy (type III), which proceeds through the vocalis muscle; total cordectomy (type IV); extended cordectomy, which encompasses the contralateral vocal fold and the anterior commissure (type Va); extended cordectomy, which includes the arytenoid (type Vb); extended cordectomy, which encompasses the subglottis (type Vc); extended cordectomy, which includes the ventricle (type Vd); and for cancers of the anterior commissure, which have extended or not to one or both of the vocal folds, without infiltration of the thyroid cartilage (type VI). Voice outcomes are superior for superficial (ELS type I and II) resections and for extended/deeper resections (ELS type III to VI), RT is associated with better voice outcomes than with TLM.[64]

Anterior commissure involvement in glottic cancer has been an important prognostic determinant of local control, hence whether these patients are better suited for TLM, open partial laryngectomy (OPL) or RT has remained a contentious issue. The potential causes for recurrences in the anterior commissure are the absence of perichondrium at the insertion of vocal ligament to the inner surface thyroid cartilage, the extension of the fibers of

Table 2: European Laryngological Society classification of endoscopic cordectomies for glottic carcinoma.

Definition	*Type*	*Description*
Supepithelial cordectomy	I	Resection of the vocal fold epithelium passing through the superficial layer of the lamina propria
Subligamental cordectomy	II	Resection of the epithelium, Reinke's space and the vocal ligament
Transmuscular cordectomy	III	Resection of the vocal fold down through vocalis muscle
Total cordectomy	IV	Resection of the cord, which extends from the vocal process to the anterior commissure. The depth of the surgical margins reaches or includes the internal perichondrium of the thyroid ala
Extended total cordectomy	Va	Resection includes the contralateral vocal fold and the anterior commissure
	Vb	Resection includes the arytenoids
	Vc	Resection includes the subglottis
	Vd	Resection includes the ventricle and false cords
Anterior commissurotomy	VI	Resection of the anterior commissure with bilateral anterior cordectomy; may include the subglottic mucosa and the cricothyroid membrane

the vocal ligament into the thyroid cartilage, and the network between the intra- and extralaryngeal blood vessels and lymphatics. These have the potential to show occult supraglottic extension to the petiole or subglottic extension, which is actually staged T2. With the delivery of a boost to this area, RT has shown good control rates from T1 lesions extending to the anterior commissure; however, local control rates with surgery have been lower.[65-67] Primary RT has been considered as an effective and voice-preserving treatment modality for glottic carcinoma involving the anterior commissure. Others have advocated OPL due to the achievement of better local control (86–91%) compared to those treated with RT (56–76%).[11,68] TLM has also shown good local control rates in these patients, albeit in experienced hands.[69,70] Endoscopic exposure can be improved at the anterior commissure by transecting the false cords, however this maneuverer would impede the function of the false cords in voice production.

- *Moderately advanced glottic cancers:* This generally refers to lesions associated with vocal cord fixation (T3). Prognostically, these patients can be divided into favorable (≤3.5 mL volume, unilateral with good airway) or unfavorable (diffuse or bilateral disease with airway compromise). Most patients are suitable for radiation-based organ preservation therapy. TLM and open partial laryngectomies are suitable choices in selected patients. Elective treatment of the neck is required, with the same treatment modality as the primary tumor. Further treatment details are described subsequently.
- *Advanced glottic and supraglottic cancers:* For T4 glottic cancers, the crucial determinant of treatment modality of choice is laryngeal cartilage invasion. Patients with invasion of the tumor through the thyroid cartilage (both the inner and outer lamina) are not considered candidates for organ preservation with chemoradiotherapy, and should be considered for total laryngectomy (TL). Patients with significant laryngeal destruction, severe pretreatment laryngeal dysfunction and those with medical comorbidities precluding organ preservation therapy are also considered candidates for surgery. Organ preservation protocols should be avoided in patients with major pre-epiglottic and paraglottic spread, cartilage destruction, massive subglottic disease, and major soft tissue extension. In such situations consideration should be given to TL with postoperative radiation therapy for the best oncologic result. Furthermore organ preservation does not equate with organ function, and patients who have undergone nonsurgical management do have swallowing and vocal quality problems. There are several disadvantages to treating patients with nonsurgical chemotherapy and radiation therapy protocols. These disadvantages include the risk of major mucosal necrosis or chondronecrosis in case endolaryngeal biopsies need to be performed for surveillance. Moreover, surgical salvage after tumor persistence or recurrence requires a TL and can be complex.[71] The complication rate ranges from 33 to 61%, according to some studies.[72,73]
- *Early and moderately advanced supraglottic cancers:* The approach to early supraglottic cancers is as shown in **Flowchart 2.**[57] T1/T2 supraglottic cancers may also be treated with a single modality. Every third patient with supraglottic cancer belongs to an early stage. Early supraglottic carcinomas are described as tumors which do not infiltrate the pre-epiglottic fat, immobilize a vocal cord or metastasize to lymph nodes of the neck. Supraglottic carcinomas with vocal cord fixation with or without invasion of the pre-epiglottic fat, the postcricoid region with or without erosion of the inner cortex of the thyroid cartilage, are classified as T3 tumors. Open supraglottic laryngectomy (SGL), TLM, and

Flowchart 2: Approach to early supraglottic cancers.

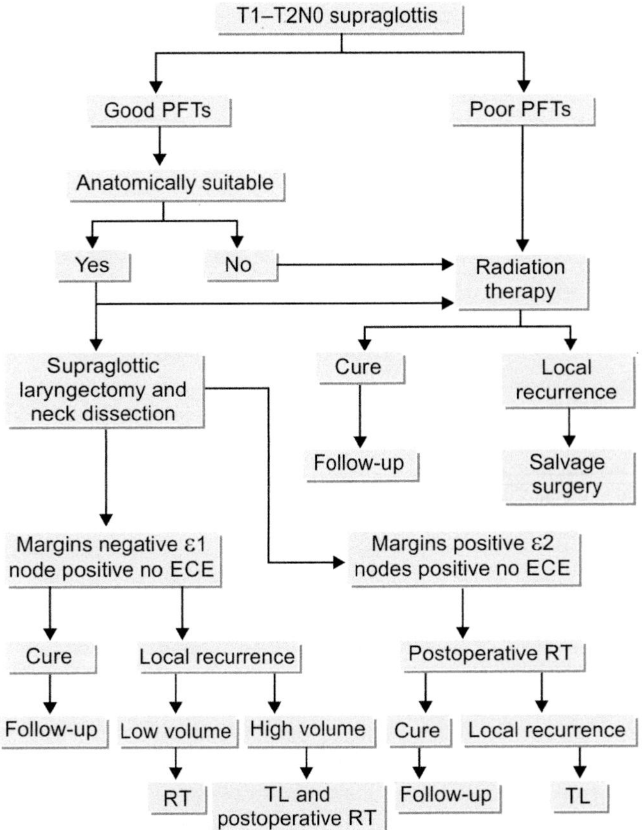

Note: Margins negative <1 node positive, no ENE, margins positive, >2 nodes positive and/or ENE.
(ECE: extracapsular extension; ENE: extranodal extension; PFTs: pulmonary function tests; PL: partial laryngectomy; RT: radiotherapy; TL: total laryngectomy)

supracricoid partial laryngectomy (SCPL) with cricohyoidopexy are some of surgical treatment options for supraglottic carcinomas.[20]

The European Laryngological Society (ELS) proposed classifications of different laryngeal endoscopic cordectomies for supraglottic carcinoma and open partial horizontal laryngectomies for craniocaudal extension of laryngeal carcinoma in order to standardize surgical nomenclature and to better measurement of postoperative outcomes **(Tables 3a and 3b)**.

In their systematic review on transoral surgery versus intensity-modulated RT (IMRT) for early supraglottic cancer, Swanson et al. pointed out the deficiency of high-quality evidence but concluded excellent local control rates of 90% for T1 lesions and 83% for T2 lesions. TLM was associated with better local control than IMRT in T2 lesions (83% vs. 70%).[74]

A Surveillance, Epidemiology, and End Results (SEER) database study of over 2,500 patients with early-stage supraglottic cancer, compared partial laryngeal surgery with neck dissection to definitive RT. In patients with T2N0 cancer, partial laryngeal surgery and neck dissection led to considerably better 5-year disease-specific survival (86% vs. 60%) and overall survival (77% vs. 45%) as compared to RT. The author recognized that occult cervical metastases were probably the reason for the lower survival in the RT group. In spite of the fact that this data predates IMRT, it raises questions as to whether these modalities have comparable survival rates in this setting.[75]

Remacle et al. proposed a classification on behalf of ELS according to which the extents of resections in supraglottic cancers are divided into seven types **(Table 3a)**.[76]

Literature on OPL for early to moderately advanced supraglottic cancer is limited to case series, however in experienced hands, outcomes have been favorable.

Table 3a: European Laryngological Society classification of endoscopic supraglottic laryngectomy.

Definition	*Type*	*Indication and description*
Limited excision	I	Excision of small superficial tumors anywhere on the supraglottis
Medial supraglottic laryngectomy with partial resection of the pre-epiglottic space	IIa	*Tumors of laryngeal surface of epiglottis located above the hyoid bone:* Resection includes the suprahyoid epiglottis
	IIb	*Tumors extending below the hyoid:* Resection includes a total epiglottectomy
Medial supraglottic laryngectomy with resection of the pre-epiglottic space	IIIa	*Tumors extending to petiole of epiglottis:* Resection must include the pre-epiglottic space
	IIIb	*Tumors of the infrahyoid epiglottis extending to the ventricular fold:* Resection includes ventricular folds dissected from the thyroid cartilage
Lateral supraglottic laryngectomy	IVa	*Tumors of the threefold region:* Resection of free edge of the epiglottis, the aryepiglottic fold, pharyngo-aryepiglottic fold, and ventricular fold
	IVb	*Tumor extending to arytenoids:* Resection includes the arytenoids and inner/medial or anterior wall of the piriform fossa

Table 3b: European Laryngological Society classification of supraglottic laryngectomy.

Definition	*Type*	*Description*
Supraglottic laryngectomies	I	Resection of the whole supraglottis, including the pre-epiglottic space and the upper half of the thyroid cartilage *Inferiorly:* Resection encompasses the petiole of the epiglottis, down to the anterior commissure, and the ventricular folds *Posteriorly:* Resection passes in front of the arytenoids, sectioning the ventricular and aryepiglottic folds *Superiorly:* Resection transects the valleculae along the posterior aspect of the hyoid bone Larynx reconstruction is accomplished by a thyrohyoidopexy
Supracricoid laryngectomies	II	Resection of the entire thyroid cartilage, with the inferior limit represented by the upper edge of the cricoid ring
	IIa	Supracricoid laryngectomy with crico-hyoido-epiglottopexy
	IIb	Supracricoid laryngectomy with cricohyoidopexy
Supratracheal laryngectomies	III	Resection of the entire supraglottic, glottic, and part of the subglottic sites, sparing both or at least one functioning cricoarytenoid unit Inferior limit of resection encompasses the cricoid ring and/or part of the cricoid plate and/or the first two tracheal rings
	IIIa	Supratracheal laryngectomy with tracheohyoidoepiglottopexy
	IIIb	Supratracheal laryngectomy with tracheohyoidopexy
Suffix	+ARY	Extension to involve one arytenoid (specify side of resection)
	+BOT	Extension to involve base of tongue
	+PIR	Extension to involve one pyriform sinus (specify side of resection)
	+CAU	Extension to involve one cricoarytenoid unit composed of arytenoid, cricoarytenoid joint, and underlying hemicricoid plate (specify side of resection)

Comparisons between OPL and TLM have shown that TLM has more favorable functional outcomes.[77,78] Based on the current literature it can be concluded that TLM is a suitable alternative to open SGL. Although TLM has lower control rates, survival is comparable. TLM, open SGL, and SCPL show similar results with regard to larynx preservation due to higher secondary laryngectomy rates reported in some series above all after SCPL due to intractable aspiration.[79]

Given the often conflicting literature available it is important to realize that early well-delineated lesions are likely to be successfully resected, while more complex lesions require significant expertise for successful resection. Patients belonging to the latter group are more likely to benefit from standardized RT as incomplete resections are likely to require adjuvant therapy and experience the morbidity associated with two treatment modalities. The patient's priorities, specifically the trade-off between survival and voice quality, if there is one, need to be discussed.

- *Subglottic cancers:* They represent 2% of all laryngeal cancers and hence data is limited. Early subglottic lesions <1 cm under the glottis are candidates for TLM with adequate exposure and expertise. RT offers good local control rates for these lesions in early lesions. External approaches such as hemilaryngectomy and feasible in moderately advanced lesions, while TL is the best treatment option in advanced disease with cartilage invasion. The same principles of organ preservation using chemoradiotherapy apply in this subsite as well.[80]

TRANSORAL LASER MICROSURGERY

Transoral laser microsurgery is a complex adaptive approach to cancer originated by Steiner and built upon the prior work of Jako, Strong, and Vaughan. Steiner's insight was that with a CO_2 laser infiltrative cancer could be resected safely from the larynx in pieces. The limits were the ability to heal by secondary intention, and the resourcefulness of the operator in achieving access and maintaining orientation.[81-83] As an alternative to open partial laryngectomies, the TLM approach, utilizes a phonosurgical narrow cancer-free margin resection for early glottic lesions thereby unimodally removing the tumor or through a more aggressive compartmental resection in case of intermediate to advanced carcinoma of larynx. Piazza et al. emphasized the importance of appropriate preoperative evaluation using the Laryngoscore. It was an objective scoring system centered on several anatomical variables which aimed to predict the event of difficult laryngeal exposure during preoperative counseling and to precisely evaluate the possibility of TLM approach or the need to shift to an alternative treatment approach. The Laryngoscore included 11 parameters to predict difficult laryngeal exposure during operative microlaryngoscopy. When the score was less than 6, favorable laryngeal exposure was observed in 94% of patients. For scores more than 6 and more than 9, difficult or impossible laryngeal exposures were observed in 40 and 67% of patients, respectively.[84]

Technique

Transoral laser microsurgery is performed under microlaryngoscopy using a CO_2 laser coupled with a micromanipulator with superpulse delivery usually in continuous mode (1–2 W). The tumor is resected with a safety margin of 2 mm, using en bloc or piecemeal techniques depending on the site and size of the tumor and the exposure of glottis. Laser vestibulectomy is performed when the lateral or anterior part of the tumor is concealed by the false cord, to obtain sufficient exposure and thereby assess the extent of disease. The tumor extent of the tumor is determined by visual inspection through the operating microscope and by palpation with microforceps. Whenever difficulty is encountered in assessing the lesions through the microscope, intraoperative rigid endoscopy with 0 degree and angled telescopes are used. After completion of the TLM procedure, the anterior, posterior, and deep margins of the surgical specimen are marked with suture knots and ink, and the specimen fixed to a soft board and sent to histopathology. In the situation of piecemeal resections, a diagram of the vocal cord was sent to the pathologist, illustrating how the specimen was removed, and if required a personal review of specimens by the surgeon with the pathologist is usually done. Adequate resection margin in glottic carcinoma has been considered to be unique (limited as 1–2 mm) compared to the general consensus of >5 mm to define an adequate margin in squamous cell carcinoma (SCC) of the head and neck.[85,86]

The extent of laser resection is limited by the patient's ability to regain adequate swallowing function. To avoid postoperative bleeding, which can lead to respiratory compromise, the superior laryngeal artery should be identified and ligated. Tracheostomy is usually not required, due to reduced probability of postoperative edema, even after extensive supraglottic laser resection, unless the patient has pulmonary compromise.[79]

After TLM, the operated endolaryngeal is left to heal by secondary intention, rather than covering the wound with a skin-lined flap. This helps in situations where second-look endoscopies might be required to revisit the primary site. An overhanging anterior glottic scar may hide a salvageable residue and also persistent granulation may signal the need for endoscopic removal to recover voice. Re-epithelialization does not rule out persistent local cancer, nor does a negative finding on a second-look procedure. In situations where no local flaps mobilized or transposed over the defect, even a granuloma could hide a residual tumor. Direct laryngoscopies are helpful in the removal of small, ossified cartilage sequestra that typically occurs, if resection was carried down to the laryngeal framework. Therefore, willingness of a patient to return for a second-look procedure should be discussed before recommending TLM. After many weeks of granulation, healing on the inner aspect of cartilage normally produces thin mucosa on a stiff base. Healing in large endolaryngeal soft tissue wounds produces fibrous scars, often tethered at one or both ends to the rigid framework. Adherence and fibrosis yielded stiffness and rigidity causing hoarseness of voice. Additionally, loss of tissue bulk can potentially create an asymmetric anterior glottic gap, hence occurrence of breathiness. Nevertheless, the persistent anterior glottic gap can be closed with phonosurgery in most cases.

PARTIAL LARYNGECTOMIES

These surgeries are based on a delicate balance between oncological control and functional outcomes. To perform organ preservation surgery, a comprehensive knowledge of the gross and functional anatomy of larynx is required. Surgeons must be able to accurately assess the cancer both clinically and radiologically, know the importance of the cricoarytenoid unit as the basic functional unit, and adhere to standard resection technique to achieve expected functional outcome, even if it involves resection of normal (uninvolved) tissue. A summary of procedures are shown in **Table 4.**

- *Vertical partial laryngectomy (VPL)* ***(Fig. 1)****:* VPL encompasses a range of surgeries, from laryngofissure with cordectomy to extended hemilaryngectomy. The concept of vertical transection of thyroid cartilage and resection extending into the PGS including the glottis is common to all types of VPL. The procedure aims to remove glottic cancers without disrupting the posterior PGS. Therefore, it is most appropriate for early glottic cancer (T1 and some T2 lesions) without fixation of membranous true vocal cords and without anterior commissure involvement. Mooney et al. classified VPL further into subtypes **(Fig. 2)**.[87]
- *Supraglottic laryngectomy* ***(Fig. 3)****:* SGL involves resection of the whole supraglottis such as the epiglottis, the pre-epiglottic fat, and the ventricular folds (false cords) together with the supraglottic part of the thyroid cartilage with or without hyoid bone. The quality of voice is good after SGL, as the vocal cords are preserved.[88,89] Some of the unique issues are the involvement of PESs and PGSs, abundant lymphatic channels, and the need to address the neck due to high risk of occult metastasis in these tumors. Aspiration and failure to develop normal swallow long-term are potential issues **(Tables 3b and 4)**.
- *Supracricoid partial laryngectomy:* SCPL connects the gap between partial open procedures and TL **(Tables 3b and 4)**. SCPL is a viable alternative to TL resulting in excellent and reproducible local control when its indications are adhered to while offering superior QoL for a significant group of patients.[90,91]

Table 4: Summary of partial laryngectomies.

Procedure	*Indications*	*Contraindications*	*Salient steps*
Vertical partial laryngectomy (VPL)	• Large T1 glottic cancer, specifically confined to middle third of vocal cord • Small T2 glottic cancer with a marginal spread into supraglottis or subglottis • Early glottic cancer difficult to attain endoscopic visualize access of entire lesion • Resections requiring extension in both anterior and posterior directions and as well as beyond glottis • Salvage surgical resection for failure of radiation treatment or residual tumor of early and intermediate glottic carcinoma	• Cricoarytenoid joint involvement • Infiltration of the thyroid cartilage • Involvement of more than one-third of the contralateral vocal cord	• Transverse skin incision and subplatysmal flaps are raised • After retraction of the strap muscles, the Delphian nodes and the prelaryngeal soft tissue excised and sent for histology • Midline or paramedian incision for a laryngofissure is created in the thyroid cartilage lamina • Resection in anteroposterior direction includes anterior commissure, membranous cord, and intrinsic muscle • From above below resection is from superior surface of false cord to 5 mm below inferior edge of vocal cord • Petiole of epiglottis sutured anteriorly to prevent prolapse and supraglottic stenosis • Glottic side reconstructed with muscle (sternohyoid), mucosa (false cord), epiglottis or free flap

Contd...

Contd...

Procedure	*Indications*	*Contraindications*	*Salient steps*
Supraglottic laryngectomy	T1, T2, and selected T3 supraglottic carcinomas	• Involvement of cricoid cartilage, with or without thyroid cartilage • Impaired mobility or fixity of vocal cords • Involvement of base of tongue (within 1 cm of circumvallate papilla) • Invasion of cancer to mucosa of both arytenoids • Involvement of the floor of the ventricles or anterior and posterior commissure and extension to glottis	• Transverse skin incision and subplatysmal flaps are raised • Superior half of thyroid cartilage exposed and perichondrium reflected down along with sternothyroid • Inferior constrictor separated from lateral and posterosuperior margins of thyroid cartilage to expose pyriform sinus up to the level of ventricle • Superior laryngeal pedicle preserved • Anterior commissure identified and division is made along oblique line of thyroid cartilage towards superior cornua • Hyoid bone and overlying muscles resected if pre-epiglottic space involved • Entry to the pharynx is made at the vallecula level • Aryepiglottic fold on uninvolved side anterior to arytenoid and dissection is brought anteriorly to plane of thyroid cartilage incision • Tongue base sutured down on to thyroid cartilage like a shelf to prevent aspiration • Sutures placed between perichondrial flap and hyoid bone/infrahyoid muscles
Supracricoid partial laryngectomy	• T1b, T2, T3 glottic. transglottic or supraglottic cancer (when supraglottic laryngectomy is not appropriate) • Supraglottic tumors with limited infiltration of the pre-epiglottic fat • Tumors with fixation of one vocal cord but without fixation of the arytenoid cartilage • Selected T4 carcinoma of larynx with limited invasion of thyroid ala without extension through outer thyroid perichondrium • As salvage after radiotherapy failure	• Involvement of interarytenoid space; posterior commissure; mucosal involvement of bilateral arytenoids • Fixed and immobile arytenoids • Subglottic extension (>10 mm anteriorly or >5 mm posteriorly) • Extralaryngeal spread • Invasion of hyoid bone • Invasion of the pre-epiglottic space [excludes cricohyoidoepiglottopexy (CHEP) but, cricohyoidopexy (CHP) is possible] or tumor originating from the epilarynx	• After elevating the skin flap, tracheostomy, and neck dissection the strap muscles are divided in the midline • Hyoid bone is identified and the thyrohyoid and the sternohyoid muscle are dissected away • Middle and inferior pharyngeal constrictor muscles are released from the cartilage and the thyroid cartilage skeletonized • Cervicomediastinal release of the trachea • Involved arytenoid needs to be excised, preserving its mucosa posteriorly if oncologically feasible, allowing it to assist as a buttress to stabilize the contralateral arytenoid • After making a releasing cut along the lateral edges of thyroid cartilage, disarticulation of the cricothyroid joint is done • Entry is made into the endolarynx via the cricothyroid membrane at the superior border of cricoid to maximize the amount of inferior glottic mucosal margin • For CHEP, the incision on the membrane is transepiglottic • For CHP, the incision on the membrane is just below the hyoid • Superior laryngeal pedicle is preserved • Aryepiglottic folds are divided • Arytenoids are resuspended • Cricopharyngeal myotomy • Pexy is performed with 3–5 impaction sutures 8–10 mm apart inferior to superior • Inferior constrictor reapproximated • Closure with snug dressing to present surgical emphysema

It is based on the principle of preservation of at least one intact cricoarytenoid unit, which allows physiologic speech and sphincteric function during swallow. Aryepiglottic speech is produced by the periodic mucosal wave of the anterior arytenoid cartilage abutting the epiglottis, which is comparable to normal speech in fundamental frequency but less efficient.[92] Swallowing needs intense rehabilitation

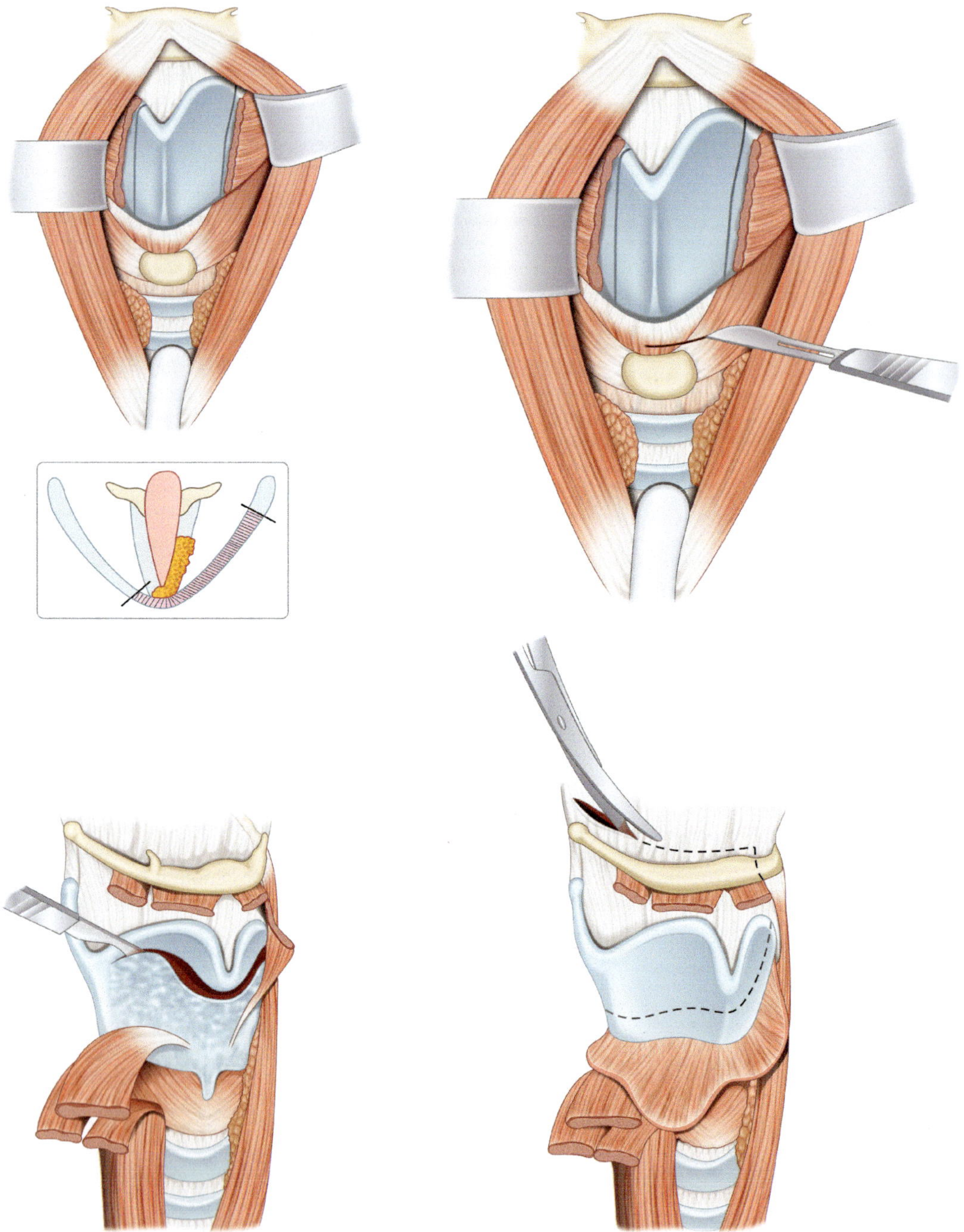

Fig. 1: Vertical partial laryngectomy.

for 2–3 weeks and tube dependence is not uncommon in an irradiated patient. Stenosis, aspiration, and failure to achieve swallowing have been reported. Patients with poor pulmonary function and/or reserve are poor candidates for this procedure. In a large systematic review, open conservative partial laryngectomies showed a 90% control rate in over 5,000 patients and a 91% laryngeal preservation rate in over 3,000 patients.[93]

NEAR TOTAL LARYNGECTOMY (FIGS. 4A TO G)

Near total laryngectomy is a substitute for TL in certain patients with lateralized and locally advanced cancers of the larynx or hypopharynx, who cannot avoid a TL. Although patients end up having a permanent tracheostomy after surgery, NTL is a voice-preserving procedure; speech is powered by

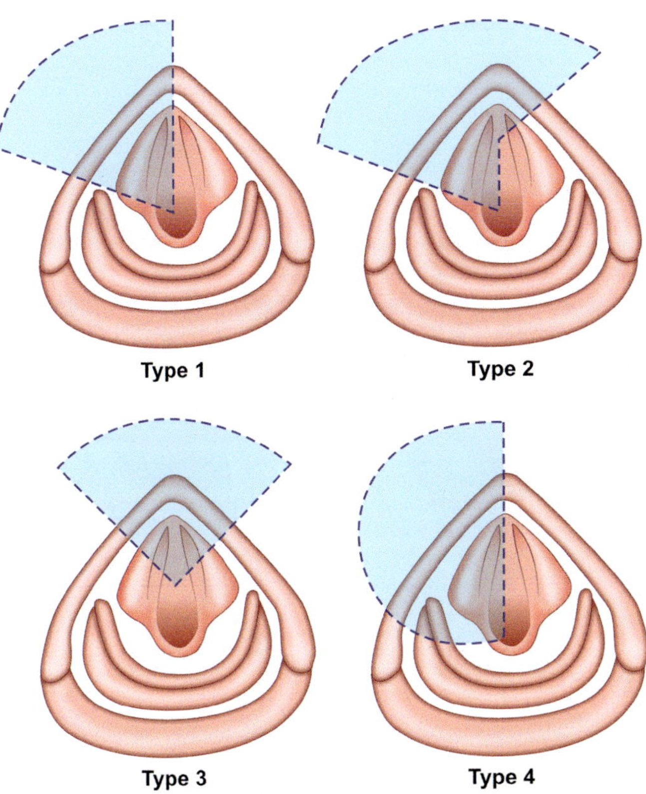

Fig. 2: Classification of vertical partial laryngectomies. Type 1—standard, type 2—frontolateral, type 3—anterofrontal, and type 4—extended partial.

the lungs via a dynamic shunt created from the uninvolved laryngeal tissues. The procedure is reported to have good oncological outcome, with increased success rates. However, due to apparent surgical complexity of the procedure and the required surgical expertise, the technique has not achieved widespread acceptance among surgeons.

The diameter of the constructed shunt must be enough to fit a 14F Foley's catheter. The soft tissue of the uninvolved side, the recurrent laryngeal nerve with the arytenoids, the cricoarytenoid joint along with the segment of the cricoid, and a strip of posterior tracheal wall are preserved to reconstruct a dynamic myomucosal shunt connecting the tracheostome and pharynx. The shunt diverts the air from the lungs and trachea to the pharynx. In addition, it acts like a sphincter and prevents aspiration because it preserves the nerve and mobile cricoarytenoid joint. With good surgical expertise and proper wound healing, the procedure has a high success rate of 90%. The main benefit of the technique is its avoidance of a tracheoesophageal puncture and a prosthesis with its repetitive costs and maintenance. Patient has to occlude the tracheostoma to speak and a successful shunt maybe maintained for life.[94,95]

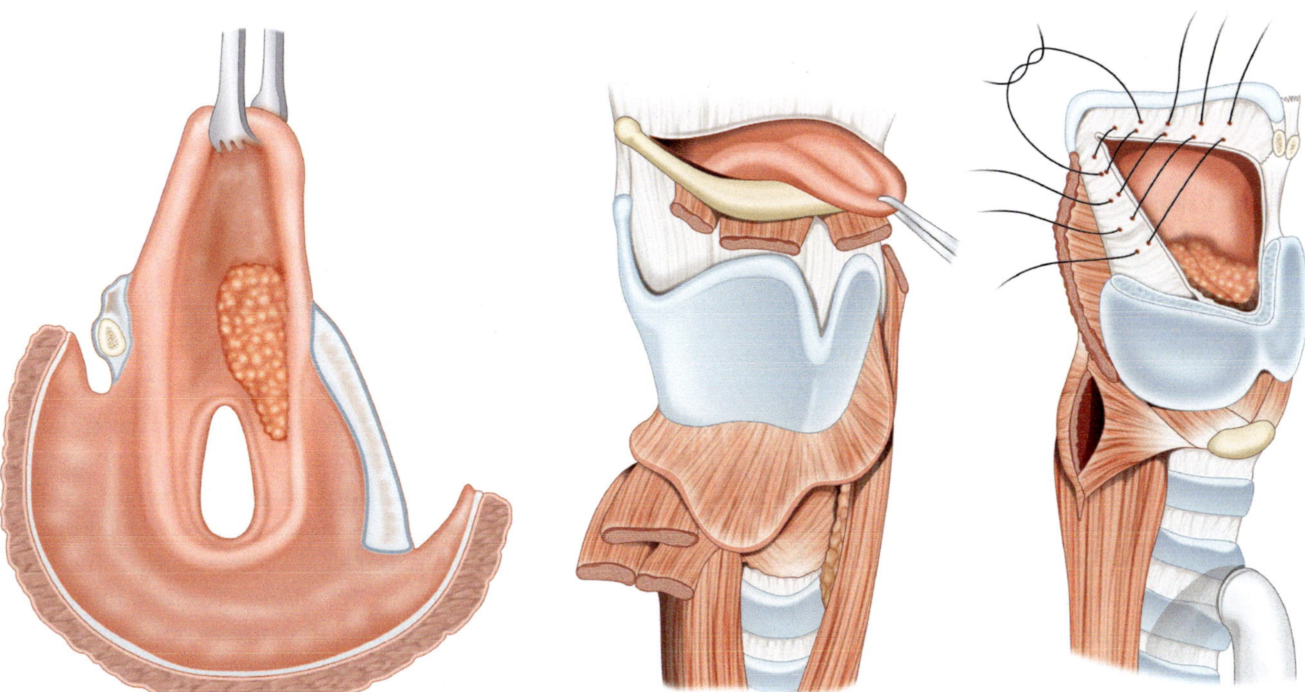

Fig. 3: Supraglottic laryngectomy.

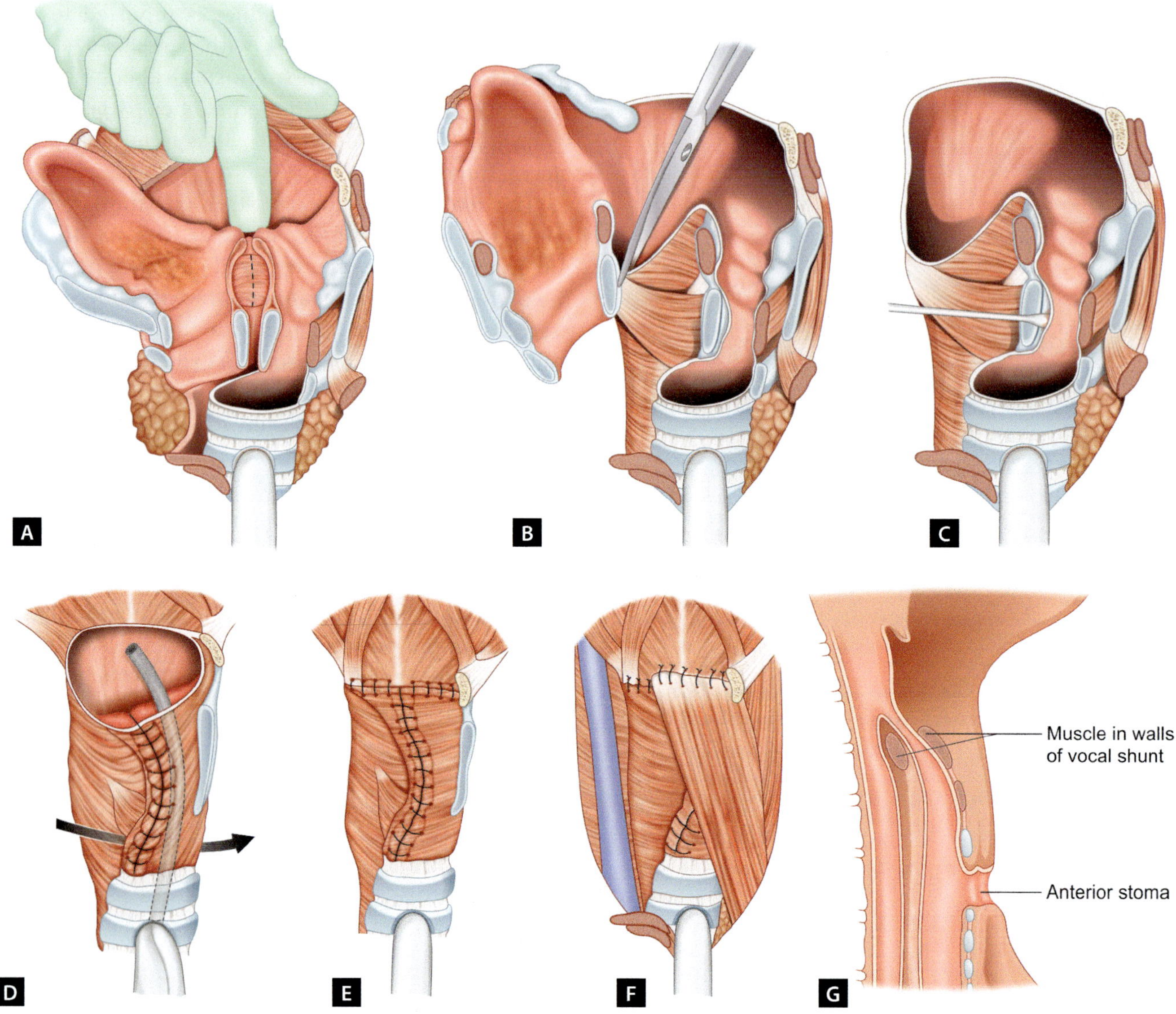

Figs. 4A to G: Near total laryngectomy.

Indications

- T3 and T4 cancers of the larynx and pyriform fossa
- Patients in whom radiotherapy has failed
- Tumors compatible with resection of the pharynx and limited areas of the tongue base, with or without flap reconstruction.

Contraindications

- *Absolute:* Involvement of the interarytenoid and postcricoid areas since, it compromises the oncological safety of the resection.
- *Relative:* Extensive posterior subglottic extension leaves insufficient mucosa to reconstruct the shunt.

TOTAL LARYNGECTOMY

Total laryngectomy with postoperative RT for advanced lesions is the gold standard treatment for advanced carcinoma. It involves the removal of the entire larynx with an end tracheostoma and closure of the pharyngeal mucosa (with or without augmentation) to allow swallowing. Primary TL is indicated in advanced disease that is not amenable to partial laryngectomy, concurrent chemoradiotherapy or RT alone. Tumors infiltrating through cartilage, spread into the extralaryngeal soft tissue of the neck, and extensive involvement of the base of tongue are suitable for TL. Non-neoplastic indications for primary TL include laryngeal dysfunction with life-threatening aspiration or chondroradionecrosis of the larynx. Also, pulmonary status and medical comorbidities and cognitive function may define the treatment options for a given patient. Although TL provides better oncologic outcome and disease-free survival, most patients are averse to undergo surgery with fears of social isolation and depression, due to permanent tracheostoma and loss of speech. Nevertheless, speech rehabilitation with esophageal speech or tracheoesophageal prosthesis (TEP) aids in overcoming the handicap. TL also plays a major role in recurrent or residual cancer after failed organ preservation treatment approaches.

SURGICAL TECHNIQUE[96]

Direct laryngoscopy is performed to confirm the degree of extension of disease and verify the proposed surgical intervention. A Gluck-Sorensen incision or a modified apron or transverse incision is designed incorporating the existing stoma or planning the permanent stoma. This incision may be altered accordingly when performing simultaneous neck dissections. Subplatysmal flaps are raised to the hyoid cartilage superiorly, sternal notch inferiorly, and sternocleidomastoid muscles laterally. The sternocleidomastoid muscles are exposed. The strap muscles are transected 1 cm above the clavicle and elevated from the laryngotracheal complex. The thyroid isthmus is divided; the ipsilateral thyroid gland and paratracheal lymph nodes included with the specimen, especially when there is extralaryngeal disease or subglottic spread. The contralateral thyroid lobe is freed from the trachea and retracted laterally. The superior border of the hyoid cartilage is freed by transecting the suprahyoid musculature. The greater cornu on either side are skeletonized carefully so as not to jeopardize the hypoglossal nerve and lingual artery. The larynx is rotated, and the posterior border of the thyroid cartilage is skeletonized by separating the laryngeal constrictors. The inferior cornu and superior cornu are skeletonized on either side. The superior laryngeal neurovascular structures containing the nerve artery and vein are ligated and cut. The pyriform sinus mucosa is dissected away from the inner thyroid cartilage lamina, if oncologically appropriate. Once the laryngotracheal complex is mobilized, horizontal tracheal cuts are made at a level at least 1 cm below the tumor. The trachea is entered, and an endotracheal tube is placed in the trachea. The anterior tracheal cuts are beveled superiorly, and the posterior wall tracheal cut is placed more cephalad. This provides a larger area for the stoma. The posterior trachea wall then is separated from the cervical esophagus.

A pharyngotomy may be made through the contralateral pyriform sinus or by means of the vallecula. Under direct visualization of the mucosal surfaces, the larynx is resected preserving adequate uninvolved pharyngeal mucosa for closure. Frozen section margins should be assessed. A cricopharyngeal myotomy is performed by sharply dividing the circumferential muscle bands down to the serosal layer. If a TEP is planned, it is performed at this instance. Primary TEP is placed through the common posterior wall, 1 cm below the posterior wall of the free end of the trachea. A temporary catheter or prosthesis is placed to stent the tract. The pharyngeal mucosa is closed using a running inverting suture. This may be done in a T, vertical, or horizontal fashion. The closure should be tension-free. The suture line can be reinforced with a second imbricating suture line if necessary. The use of a linear stapler for pharyngoesophageal closure after TL was depicted by Sofferman and Voronetsky.[97] A bougie may be placed, and a gastrointestinal TA 60 stapler is used to separate the larynx and close the pharynx. Drains are placed in the neopharynx gutter on each side and secured. The tracheal stoma is matured by suturing the end of the trachea to the skin in an interrupted fashion with half vertical mattress sutures. The skin then is closed in layers. Postoperatively, routine care is instituted, including wound care, stoma care, drain care, fluid management, and pain management. Nutritional status and thyroid function should be optimized.

RADIATION-BASED ORGAN PRESERVATION STRATEGIES

Nonsurgical approaches to larynx preservation include either radiation alone, or neoadjuvant chemotherapy with radiation for responders, or concurrent chemotherapy and radiation therapy. There were two pathbreaking trials that paved the way for organ preservation in laryngeal cancer. One study was by the Department of Veterans Affairs (VA) Laryngeal Cancer Study Group and the other was by the Radiation Therapy Oncology Group (RTOG) 91-11.[98,99]

In 1991, VA Laryngeal Cancer Study Group randomly assigned 332 patients with stage III or stage IV laryngeal cancer to receive induction chemotherapy (IC) with two cycles of cisplatin-fluorouracil followed either by a third cycle and then radiation therapy (in responders) or by TL and postoperative radiation (in nonresponders). Patients in the chemoradiotherapy group were treated with salvage laryngectomy when there was either a less than 50% reduction in tumor size or posttreatment persistence of tumor, or tumor recurrence.

In the chemotherapy group, 36% of the patients who did not respond were referred for TL and postoperative radiation therapy. For both the surgery and chemoradiotherapy arms, estimated 2-year survival was 68%. The larynx was preserved in 64% of patients in the chemoradiation group, and 64% of patients in this group were alive and free of disease at 2 years. For this reason, the authors concluded that a positive response to IC may be used as an indication to proceed with radiation therapy instead of surgery. Even though, this study did not prove the survival benefit of chemotherapy because there was no arm for treatment by radiation therapy alone, it was a landmark study for organ preservation treatment.

Follow-up studies to the VA Laryngeal Study Group assessed the functionality of patients treated in the chemoradiation group. This group had better objective speech and only two patients required a tracheostomy.[100,101] After a 10-year follow-up, however, there was no difference in self-reported assessment of speech and swallowing between the two groups.[102]

In 2001 Forastiere et al. published results of the three-arm trial conducted by the RTOG 91-11. In this trial, 547 patients were randomly assigned to one of three arms: IC and RT, concomitant chemoradiotherapy (CCRT), or radiation therapy alone (RT). There was no difference in survival in the three groups at 2 years. Laryngectomy-free survival was longer in CCRT arm (66%) than in IC + RT arm (58%) or RT arm (52%). The laryngeal preservation rates at 2 years mirrored this.

The 10-year update of RTOG 91-11 studied into the long-term effect in these approaches, it was reported that RT alone was significantly inferior to both IC and concurrent chemoradiotherapy arms. Locoregional control and larynx preservation were the best in the CCRT group.[103] An interesting finding was the increase in nononcological deaths were highest in the CCRT group (30.8%), which they believed could be attributed to swallowing dysfunction following silent aspiration. The authors concluded that CCRT is superior to sequential chemoradiotherapy or radiotherapy alone. Also, that simultaneous chemoradiotherapy can be regarded as standard treatment for patients who demand an organ preservation approach. The authors reflect that, primary nonsurgical treatment is feasible for the majority of patients and TL should strictly be reserved for "salvage surgery".

In 2006, Hoffman et al.[104] stated that over the preceding two decades, in contrast to other malignancies, the survival in laryngeal cancer had worsened. They noted that for T3N0 disease, primary surgery with adjuvant RT resulted in the best survival outcomes. In 2007, Chen and Halpern[105] analyzed data comprising 7,019 cases, collected by the national hospital-based cancer registry, found that the risk of death in T3 laryngeal cancer was higher when treated with nonsurgical therapy. Large volumes of population-based data question whether RT should be the standard of care in T3-T4 laryngeal cancer, however this question can only be answered with a randomized trial which is unlikely to happen given the ethical issues with TL in a setting where organ preservation is an acceptable treatment option.

External Beam Radiotherapy Technique

Normally, small glottic cancers are irradiated using two equally weighted parallel-opposed fields, due to their paucity of lymphatic drainage. The dose received by the primary tumor varies between 60 and 70 Gy depending on the clinical stage for a classic fractionation and varies between 70 and 80 Gy in case of multifractioning. A frequently utilized dose-fractionation schedule is 66 Gy for T1 lesions and 70 Gy for T2 cancers given in 2 Gy fractions. Hypofractionated doses are also popular in this setting (60 Gy in 20 fractions). External beam radiation therapy (EBRT) is given over a duration of 6–8 weeks. If supraglottic extension is present, the cervical lymph nodes in levels II–IV of the neck have to be included. Whenever subglottic extension is present, levels II–IV and VI are irradiated together with the larynx. For the neck or locoregional recurrence prevention, it ranges from a prophylactic dose of about 50 Gy when the lymph nodes are clinically negative, to up to 60–70 Gy for the regions with positive lymph nodes. Supraglottic dose is similar to that for glottic carcinoma, however neck treatment of levels II–IV in indicated due to a richer lymphatic drainage as compared to glottic carcinoma. For the clinically N0 neck, selective neck dissection or radiotherapy is recommended. In case of positive cervical nodes a neck dissection with or without adjuvant radiotherapy is advised.

Adjuvant Treatment

After larynx preservation surgery, postoperative or adjuvant radiation therapy is required for patients with locoregionally advanced disease, with or without chemotherapy.[106] Adjuvant chemotherapy comprising of cisplatin 100 mg/m^2 every 21 days concurrent with RT has better local control, progression-free survival, and overall survival than RT alone in patients with high-risk features (positive margins and extranodal extension).[107]

Locally advanced laryngeal cancers (stages III and IV) require radical surgery followed by adjuvant RT. Currently, targeted therapies such as cetuximab can be combined with RT as radical treatment in patients with locally advanced disease. This was investigated in a phase III trial, which compared RT with RT plus cetuximab as a radical treatment in patients with locally advanced disease. The local control was better using the combination treatment (24.4 months vs. 14.9 months), as was overall survival (45.6% vs. 36.4%; hazard ratio, 0.73).[108] It should be noted that the trial was not designed for platinum-ineligible patients; the objective was to evaluate cetuximab in a broad population of patients with locally advanced disease. Trials are ongoing in unresectable disease, but until further data become available, the treatment selection will depend on toxicity and patient fragility.

Induction Chemotherapy

Concurrent chemoradiation is effective for locoregional control, but some trials revealed a poor control in distant disease, especially in patients with an advanced nodal stage. Therefore, IC was developed as an option for functional larynx preservation in locoregionally advanced disease. Usually, the scheme is IC followed by definitive RT; however, this treatment is less effective than CCRT treatment in terms of locoregional control, as demonstrated by RTOG 91-11. The role in unresectable disease is covered in detail in the chapter on multidisciplinary management of unresectable disease.

OUTCOMES

Outcomes in laryngeal cancer are good, irrespective of the primary treatment modality employed. Shown in **Table 5** are the 5-year relative survival rates (likelihood of survival when compared to age-matched controls) for patients of laryngeal cancer treated between 2009 and 2015.[109] Often population-based survival rates are a better reflection of actual patient survival as clinical trial participants are considered "marathon runners"; they are carefully selected patients with good health whose response to treatment and tolerance of side-effects cannot be reliably extrapolated to the general population.

Table 5: Surveillance Epidemiology, and End Results (SEER) 5-year relative survival rates for laryngeal cancer (2009–2015).

Disease status	*Supraglottic*	*Glottic*	*Subglottic*
Localized	61%	83%	60%
Regional	47%	48%	33%
Metastatic	30%	42%	45%
All SEER stages combined	46%	76%	52%

RECURRENT LARYNGEAL CANCER

Recurrent laryngeal cancer occurring after radiation treatment poses numerous challenges as it tends to be more aggressive and associated with poor control rates. Salvage TL is often considered as it a standardized procedure with predictable functional outcomes.[110-112]

Although OPL procedures are less frequently used due to limited expertise and less predictable functional outcomes, they are proven to be oncologically sound procedures in the salvage setting with a high larynx preservation rate. The pooled estimates of 26 studies in a systemic review and meta-analysis assessing the role of open conservation laryngeal surgery in radiorecurrent laryngeal cancers revealed local control rate of 86.9% at 24 months for 560 patients, disease-free survival rate of 91.2% for 352 patients, and overall survival rate was 83.1% for 360 patients.[113]

The role of TLM in the recurrent setting is not well defined. Isolated local recurrences were salvaged with TLM in 86%, regional recurrences in 74% and in multifocal recurrences with infiltration or submucosal extension, salvage was not possible. Margin assessment in a recurrent disease is difficult and recurrence rates can be high as 58% in this setting.[114]

A recent systematic review and meta-analysis have shown that OPL has better salvage rates than TLM. The pooled mean estimate of local control at 24 months after first TLM among 249 patients was 56.9%, which is 30% less than the 24-month local control rates for OPL in recurrent cancers with a relatively lower mean larynx preservation rate of 72.3% for TLM (versus 84% for OPL).[115] Due to the higher locoregional failure following TLM, there is a lower threshold for planning for a TL.[116,117]

STOMAL RECURRENCE[118-120]

This is a specific type of recurrence following TL where local recurrence results in diffuse neoplastic infiltration of the tissue at the junction of the skin and tracheostoma. This occurs more commonly in males and is often presents within 2 years of initial treatment. It is more commonly seen in those with advanced (T4) disease, level VI node involvement, preoperative tracheostomy and subglottic involvement. Stomal recurrence may represent tumor seeding through the tracheostomy, an occult positive margin through subglottic extension or a level VI nodal recurrence. Presentation is with an indurated or ulcerated nodule at the junction of the tracheostoma and skin, which may invade surrounding tissue causing airway obstruction or bleeding. Sisson et al. classified these recurrences in to type I (localized with a discrete nodule in the superior half of the stoma without esophageal involvement), type II (involvement of superior half of stoma with esophageal involvement), type III (involving inferior half of the stoma with direct extension into the mediastinum), and type IV (extension laterally and often under either clavicle). The only potential for cure is extensive surgical resection, which may include removal of skin, mediastinal dissection, removal of manubrium and clavicle heads, pharyngo-esophageal resection and reconstruction and reconstruction. However perioperative mortality is high for type III and IV disease, and careful consideration is required before embarking on such an extensive surgical plan. 2-year survival was 45% in Sisson type I and II and 9% in types III and IV. Avoiding stomal recurrence is the best approach, through adequate clearance of disease (especially in those with subglottic extension) and level VI nodes during TL and including the upper mediastinum in the adjuvant radiotherapy field.

LARYNGEAL CHONDRORADIONECROSIS[121-123]

This is an unusual but potentially devastating complication of radiotherapy to the larynx. Like with osteoradionecrosis, this results due to a disruption of vascularity to the tissue, resulting in arteritis and ischemia, followed by inflammation. It usually presents months to years after completion of treatment and can present with a myriad of symptoms such as pain, voice change, fetor oris, hoarseness, and dyspnea. It can also mimic recurrence with clinical findings such as laryngedema, cartilage exposure, ulceration, new-onset cord fixity, and stridor. Imaging can help in establish a diagnosis; the key findings are cartilage sloughing, erosion, fragmentation, collapse or emphysema. Biopsy may help arrive at a diagnosis; however aggressive biopsy and sampling can worsen clinical symptoms. Mild cases can be treated with symptomatic treatment such as steam inhalation, voice rest, antibiotics, and steroids. Minimal debridement of exposed cartilage may improve symptoms. Severe cases may require laryngectomy.

QUALITY OF LIFE ASSESSMENT

The larynx is functionally and anatomically important in generation of phonation, controlling respiration, protection of the airway protection and contributes to a safe swallow. Either a tumor or its treatment effect may vastly impair the normal functioning of the larynx. Hence focus not only on cure rates but also quality of cure is important when choosing the treatment option for laryngeal cancers. The tumor stage (T), the nodal stage (N), type of treatment approach and duration posttreatment greatly impacts a patient's QoL. For a head and neck site such as the larynx, the influence of a treatment modality on features particular to the larynx such as voice and swallowing have been analyzed by several studies with variable results. A few of the routinely utilized QoL questionnaire tools for head and neck cancers are the University of Washington Quality of Life Questionnaire the European Organization for Research and Treatment of Cancer Quality of Life Questionnaire, these are also used for laryngeal cancers.[124]

Williamson et al. reported that laryngeal cancer patients who underwent definitive RT had the best QoL. The poorest QoL was present among patients with T2 stage and above, those who had undergone CCRT or those who underwent surgery followed by CCRT. Saliva production, taste of food and act of social eating were some of the domains that were impacted.[125]

University of Washington Quality of Life Questionnaire and the Voice Handicap Index (VHI) were used by Azevedo et al. in advanced laryngeal and hypopharyngeal cancer patients to assess and compare health-related QoL voice-specific QoL posttreatment. They concluded that patients with advanced laryngeal or hypopharyngeal cancers show a mild to moderate voice handicap with excellent QoL scores after treatment.[126] Stewart et al. analyzed the emotional and functional subscales following treatment for advanced laryngeal cancer. They noted that the VHI was comparable between those treated with radiotherapy and those who underwent TL with tracheoesophageal puncture, however emotional and functional handicap scores were worse in the radiotherapy group, implying that voice concerns are not the only determinants of QoL in patients of laryngeal cancer.[127] QoL is also affected sociodemographic and socioeconomic factors. Hence, multidisciplinary rehabilitation services can serve to enhance the capacity of laryngeal cancer patients by diminishing acute and chronic treatment-related adverse effects.

REFERENCES

1. Chauhan JPS, Bharti B, Bhadouriya SS, Kumar P, Prem KP, Singh NJ. Laryngeal cancer: a clinicopathological study of 65 cases. Int J Otorhinolaryngol Head Neck Surg. 2018;4(1):163-8.
2. Maier H, Gewelek U, Dietz A, Heller WD. Risk factors of cancer of the larynx: results of the Heidelberg case-control study. Otolaryngol Head Neck Surg. 1992;107(4):577-82.
3. Sokic SI, Adanja BJ, Marinkovic JP. Case controlled study of risk factors in laryngeal cancer. Neoplasma. 1994;41:43-7.

4. Bobdey S, Jain A, Balasubramanium G. Epidemiological review of laryngeal cancer: An Indian perspective. Indian J Med Paediatr Oncol. 2015;36(3):154-60.
5. Dobrossy L. Epidemiology of head and neck cancer: Magnitude of the problem. Cancer Metastasis Rev. 2005;24:9-17.
6. Smith EM, Summersgill KF, Allen J, Hoffman HT, McCulloch T, Turek LP, Haugen TH. Human papillomavirus and risk of laryngeal cancer. Ann Otol Rhinol Laryngol. 2000;109:1069-76.
7. Calvert GM, Ward E, Schnorr TM, Fine LJ. Cancer risks among workers exposed to metalworking fluids: a systematic review. Am J Ind Med. 1998;33:282-92.
8. Tolbert PE. Oils and cancer. Cancer Causes Control. 1997;8: 386-405.
9. Ward EM, Burnett CA, Ruder A, Davis-King K. Industries and cancer. Cancer Causes Control. 1997;8(3):356-70.
10. Egeli U, Ozkan L, Tunca B. The relationship between genetic susceptibility to head and neck cancer with the expression of common fragile sites. Head Neck. 2000;22:591-8.
11. Wight R, Paleri V, Arullendran P. Current theories for the development of nonsmoking and nondrinking laryngeal carcinoma. Curr Opin Otolaryngol Head Neck Surg. 2003; 11:73-7.
12. Narayana A, Vaughan AT, Fisher SG. Second primary tumors in laryngeal cancer: results of long-term follow-up. Int J Rad Oncol Biol Phys. 1998;42:557-62.
13. Brown T, Darnton A, Fortunato L, Rushton L. Occupational Cancer in Britain, Respiratory Cancer sites: larynx, lung and mesothelioma. Br J Cancer. 2012;107:S56-70.
14. Bradley PJ. Radiation-induced tumors of the head and neck. Curr Opin Otolaryngol Head Neck Surg. 2002;10:97-103.
15. El-Serag HB, Hepworth EJ, Lee P. Gastroesophageal reflux disease is a risk factor for laryngeal and pharyngeal cancer. Am J Gastoenterol. 2001;96:2013-8.
16. Sheahan P, Ganly I, Rhys Evans PH, Patel SG. Tumours of the Larynx. In: Montgomery PQ, Rhys Evans PH, Gullane PJ (Eds). Principles and Practice of Head and Neck Surgery and Oncology, 2nd edition. London: Informa Healthcare; 2009. pp. 257-83.
17. Steuer CE, El-Deiry M, Parks JR, Higgins KA, Saba NF. An update on larynx cancer. CA Cancer J Clin. 2017;67(1):31-50.
18. Chu EA, Kim YJ. Laryngeal cancer: diagnosis and preoperative work-up. Otolaryngol Clin North Am. 2008;41(4):673-95.
19. Siddiqui A, Connor SEJ. Imaging of the pharynx and larynx. Imaging. 2013;22:1-27.
20. Siddiq S, Paleri V. Transoral surgery in early-stage laryngeal cancer. J Head Neck Physicians Surg. 2017;5(1):3-12.
21. Breau RL, Suen JY. Management of the N(0) neck. Otolaryngol Clin North Am. 1998;31(4):657-69.
22. Million RR, Cassisi NJ. Radical irradiation for carcinoma of the pyriform sinus. Laryngoscope. 1981;91(3):439-50.
23. Becker M, Burkhardt K, Dulguerov P, Allal A. Imaging of the larynx and hypopharynx. Eur J Radiol. 2008;66(3):460-79.
24. Peretti G, Piazza C, Bolzoni A. Endoscopic Treatment for Early Glottic Cancer: Indications and Oncologic Outcome. Otolaryngol Clin N Am. 2006;39:173-89.
25. Patel SG. Larynx. In: Amin MB (Ed). AJCC Cancer Staging Manual, 8th Edition. Chicago, IL: Springer; 2018. pp. 149-61.
26. Kirchner JA. What have whole organ sections contributed to the treatment of laryngeal cancer? Ann Otol Rhinol Laryngol. 1989;98:661-7.
27. Ravanelli M, Agazzi GM, Farina D, Maroldi R. New Developments in Imaging of Laryngeal Cancer. Curr Otorhinolaryngol Rep. 2017;5:49-55.
28. Ryu IS, Lee JH, Roh JL, Choi SH, Nam SY, Kim SY, et al. Clinical implication of computed tomography findings in patients with locally advanced squamous cell carcinoma of the larynx and hypopharynx. Eur Arch Otorhinolaryngol. 2015;272(10):2939-45.
29. Xia C-X, Zhu Q, Zhao H-X, Yan F, Li S-L, Zhang S-M. Usefulness of ultrasonography in assessment of laryngeal carcinoma. Br J Radiol. 2013;86(1030):20130343.
30. Hartl DM, Landry G, Bidault F. CT-scan prediction of thyroid cartilage invasion for early laryngeal squamous cell carcinoma. Eur Arch Otorhinolaryngol. 2013;270(1):287-91.
31. Wu J-H, Zhao J, Li Z-H, Yang W-Q, Liu Q-H, Yang Z-Y, et al. Comparison of CT and MRI in diagnosis of laryngeal carcinoma with anterior vocal commissure involvement. Sci Rep. 2016;6:30353.
32. Rutkowski T. Impact of initial tumor volume on radiotherapy outcome in patients with T2 glottic cancer. Strahlenther Onkol Organ Dtsch Rontgengesellschaft Al. 2014;190(5): 480-4.
33. van Bockel LW, Monninkhof EM, Pameijer FA, Terhaard CHJ. Importance of tumor volume in supraglottic and glottic laryngeal carcinoma. Strahlenther Onkol Organ Dtsch Rontgengesellschaft Al. 2013;189(12):1009-14.
34. Timmermans AJ, Lange CAH, de Bois JA. Tumor volume as a prognostic factor for local control and overall survival in advanced larynx cancer. Laryngoscope. 2016;126(2):E60-7.
35. Janssens GO, van Bockel LW, Doornaert PA, Bijl HP, van den Ende P, de Jong MA, et al. Computed tomography-based tumor volume as a predictor of outcome in laryngeal cancer: results of the phase 3 ARCON trial. Eur J Cancer. 2014;50(6):1112-9.
36. Caldas-Magalhaes J, Kasperts N, Kooij N. Validation of imaging with pathology in laryngeal cancer: accuracy of the registration methodology. Int J Radiat Oncol Biol Phys. 2012;82(2):e289-98.
37. Mukherji SK, O'Brien SM, Gerstle RJ, Weissler M, Shockley W, Castillo M. Tumor volume: An independent predictor of outcome for laryngeal cancer. J Comput Assist Tomogr. 1999;23:50-4.
38. Mukherji SK, O'Brien SM, Gerstle RJ, Weissler M, Shockley W, Stone JA, et al. The ability of tumor volume to predict local control in surgically treated SCC of the supraglottic larynx. Head Neck. 2000;22:282-7.
39. Freeman DE, Mancuso AA, Parsons JT, Mendenhall WM, Million RR. Irradiation alone for supraglottic larynx carcinoma: Can CT findings predict treatment results? Int J Radiat Oncol Biol Phys. 1990;19:485-90.
40. Lee WR, Mancuso AA, Saleh EM, Mendenhall WM, Parsons JT, Million RR. Can pre-treatment CT findings predict local control in T3 SCC of the glottis treated with radiotherapy alone? Int J Radiat Oncol Biol Phys. 1993;25:683-7.
41. Castelijns JA, van den Brekel MW, Tobi H, Smit EM, Golding RP, van Schaik C, et al. Laryngeal carcinoma after radiation therapy: Correlation of abnormal MR imaging signal patterns in laryngeal cartilage with the risk of recurrence. Radiology. 1996;198:151-5.
42. Fleming AJ Jr, Smith SP Jr, Paul CM. Impact of [18F]-2-fluoro deoxy glucose-positron emission tomography/computed tomography on previously untreated head and neck cancer patients. Laryngoscope. 2007;117(7):1173-9.
43. Schoder H, Yeung HW, Gonen M, Kraus D, Larson SM. Head and neck cancer: clinical usefulness and accuracy of PET/CT image fusion. Radiology. 2004;231(1):65-72.

44. Zanation AM, Sutton DK, Couch ME. Use, accuracy, and implications for patient management of [18F]-2-fluorodeoxyglucose-positron emission/computerized tomography for head and neck tumors. Laryngoscope. 2005;115(7):1186-90.
45. Gordin A, Daitzchman M, Doweck I, Yefremov N, Golz A, Keidar Z, et al. Fluorodeoxyglucose-positron emission tomography/computed tomography imaging in patients with carcinoma of the larynx: diagnostic accuracy and impact on clinical management. Laryngoscope. 2006;116(2):273-8.
46. Andrade RS, Heron DE, Degirmenci B, Filho PA, Branstetter BF, Seethala RR, et al. Post treatment assessment of response using PET-CT for patients treated with definitive radiation therapy for head and neck cancers. Int J Radiat Oncol Biol Phys. 2006;65:1315-22.
47. Mukherji SK, Mancuso AA, Kotzur IM, Mendenhall WM, Kubilis PS, Tart RP, et al. Radiologic appearance of the irradiated larynx. Part 1. Expected changes. Radiology. 1994;193:141-8.
48. Mukherji SK, Mancuso AA, Kotzur IM, Mendenhall WM, Kubilis PS, Tart RP, et al. Radiologic appearance of the irradiated larynx. Part 2. Primary site response. Radiology. 1994;193:149-54.
49. Joshi VM, Wadhwa V, Mukherji SK. Imaging in laryngeal cancers. Indian J Radiol Imaging. 2012;22(3):209-26.
50. Oe A, Kawabe J, Torii K. Detection of local residual tumor after laryngeal cancer treatment using FDG-PET. Ann Nucl Med. 2007;21(1):9-13.
51. Mishra A, Nilakantan A, Datta R, Sahai K, Singh SP, Sethi A. Contact Endoscopy—A promising tool for evaluation of laryngeal mucosal lesions J Laryngol Voice. 2012;2(2):53-9.
52. Davaris N, Lux A, Esmaeili N, Illanes A, Boese A, Friebe M, et al. Evaluation of Vascular Patterns Using Contact Endoscopy and Narrow-Band Imaging (CE-NBI) for the Diagnosis of Vocal Fold Malignancy. Cancers (Basel). 2020;12(1):248.
53. Puxeddu R, Sionis S, Gerosa C, Carta F. Enhanced contact endoscopy for the detection of neoangiogenesis in tumors of the larynx and hypopharynx. Laryngoscope. 2015;125:1600-6.
54. Arens C, Piazza C, Andrea M, Dikker FG, Tjon Pian Gi REA, Voigt-Zimmermann S, et al. Proposal for a descriptive guideline of vascular changes in lesions of the vocal folds by the committee on endoscopic laryngeal imaging of the European Laryngological Society. Eur Arch Otorhinolaryngol. 2016;273:1207-14.
55. Mehlum CS, Rosenberg T, Dyrvig A-K, Groentved AM, Kjaergaard T, Godballe C. Can the Ni classification of vessels predict neoplasia? A systematic review and meta-analysis. Laryngoscope. 2018;128:168-76.
56. Chawla S, Carney AS. Organ preservation surgery for laryngeal cancer. Head Neck Oncol. 2009;1:12.
57. Harrison LB, Sessions RB, Hong WK. Head and neck cancer: a multidisciplinary approach. Philadelphia: Lippincott Williams & Wilkins; 2009. pp. 250-65.
58. Warner L, Lee K, Homer JJ. Transoral laser microsurgery versus radiotherapy for T2 glottic squamous cell carcinoma: a systematic review of local control outcomes. Clin Otolaryngol. 2017;42(3):629-36.
59. Hendriksma M, Heijnen BJ, Sjögren EV. Oncologic and functional outcomes of patients treated with transoral CO_2 laser microsurgery or radiotherapy for T2 glottic carcinoma: a systematic review of the literature. Curr Opin Otolaryngol Head Neck Surg. 2018;26(2):84-93.
60. Aaltonen LM, Rautiainen N, Sellman J, Saarilahti K, Mäkitie A, Rihkanen H, et al. Voice quality after treatment of early vocal cord cancer: A randomized trial comparing laser surgery with radiation therapy. Int J Radiat Oncol Biol Phys. 2014;90:255-60.
61. Sjogren EV, van Rossum MA, Langeveld TP. Voice profile after type I or II laser chordectomies for T1a glottic carcinoma. Head Neck. 2009;31:1502-10.
62. Peretti G, Piazza C, Balzanelli C. Vocal outcome after endoscopic cordectomies for Tis and T1 glottic carcinomas. Ann Otol Rhinol Laryngol. 2003;112:174-9.
63. Remacle M, Eckel HE, Antonelli A, Brasnu D, Chevalier D, Friedrich G, et al. Endoscopic cordectomy. A proposal for a classification by the Working Committee, European Laryngological Society. Eur Arch Otorhinolaryngol. 2000;257(4):227-31.
64. Remacle M, Van Haverbeke C, Eckel H, Bradley P, Chevalier D, Djukic V, et al. Proposal for revision of the European Laryngological Society classification of endoscopic cordectomies. Eur Arch Otorhinolaryngol. 2007;264(6):499-504.
65. Rucci L, Gammarota L, Borghi Cirri MB. Carcinoma of the anterior commissure of the larynx: I. Embryological and anatomic considerations. Ann Otol Rhinol Laryngol. 1996;105:303-8.
66. Rucci L, Gammarota L, Gallo O. Carcinoma of the anterior commissure of the larynx: II. Proposal of a new staging system. Ann Otol Rhinol Laryngol. 1996;105:391-6.
67. Kirchner JA, Carter D. Intralaryngeal barriers to the spread of cancer. Acta Otolaryngol. 1987;103:503-13.
68. Mastronikolis NS, Papadas TA, Goumas PD, Triantaphyllidou IE, Theocharis DA, Papageorgakopoulou N, et al. Head and neck: Laryngeal tumors: an overview. Atlas Genet Cytogenet Oncol Haematol. 2009;13(11):888-93.
69. Chone CT, Yonehara E, Martins JE, Altemani A, Crespo AN. Importance of anterior commisure in recurrence of early glottic cancer after laser endoscopic resection. Arch Otolaryngol Head Neck Surg. 2007;133(9):882-7.
70. Peretti G, Piazza C, Bolzoni A, Mensi MC, Rossini M, Parinello G, et al. Analysis of recurrences in 322 Tis, T1, or T2 glottic carcinoma: a long-term follow-up of 156 cases. Ann Otol Rhinol Laryngol. 2004;113:853-8.
71. Jalisi M, Jalisi S. Advanced laryngeal carcinoma: surgical and non-surgical management options. Otolaryngol Clin North Am. 2005;38(1):47-57.
72. Kraus DH, Pfister DG, Harrison LB, Spiro RH, Strong EW, Zelefsky M, et al. Salvage laryngectomy for unsuccessful larynx preservation therapy. Ann Otol Rhinol Laryngol. 1995;104:936-41.
73. Sassler AM, Esclamado RM, Wolf GT. Surgery after organ preservation therapy: analysis of wound complications. Arch Otolaryngol Head Neck Surg. 1995;121:162-5.
74. Swanson MS, Low G, Sinha UK, Kokot N. Transoral surgery vs. intensity-modulated radiotherapy for early supraglottic cancer: A systematic review. Curr Opin Otolaryngol Head Neck Surg. 2017;25:133-41.
75. Arshad H, Jayaprakash V, Gupta V, Cohan DM, Ambujakshan D, Rigual NR, et al. Survival differences between organ preservation surgery and definitive radiotherapy in early supraglottic squamous cell carcinoma. Otolaryngol Head Neck Surg. 2014;150:237-44.
76. Remacle M, Hantzakos A, Eckel H. Endoscopic supraglottic laryngectomy: a proposal for a classification by the working

committee on nomenclature, European Laryngological Society. Eur Arch Otorhinolaryngol. 2009;266(7):993-8.

77. Bussu F, Almadori G, De Corso E, Rizzo D, Rigante M, Parrilla C, et al. Endoscopic horizontal partial laryngectomy by CO_2 laser in the management of supraglottic squamous cell carcinoma. Head Neck. 2009;31:1196-206.
78. Karatzanis AD, Psychogios G, Zenk J, Waldfahrer F, Hornung J, Velegrakis GA, et al. Evaluation of available surgical management options for early supraglottic cancer. Head Neck. 2010; 32:1048-55.
79. Ambrosch P, Fazel A. Functional organ preservation in laryngeal and hypopharyngeal cancer. GMS Curr Top Otorhinolaryngol Head Neck Surg. 2011;10:1-31.
80. Baron I, Remacle M. Current options in the management of early primary laryngeal cancers. J ENT Mastercl. 2008;1(1): 116-20.
81. Eckel HE. Local recurrences following transoral laser surgery for early glottic carcinoma: frequency, management, and outcome. Ann Otol Rhinol Laryngol. 2001;110:7-15.
82. Steiner W, Ambrosch P, Rödel RM, Kron M. Impact of anterior commisure involvement on local control of early glottic carcinoma treated by laser microresection. Laryngoscope. 2004;114(8):1485-91.
83. Motamed M, Laccourreye O, Bradley PJ. Salvage conservation laryngeal surgery after irradiation failure for early laryngeal cancer. Laryngoscope. 2006;116(3):451-5.
84. Piazza C, Mangili S, Bon FD, Paderno A, Grazioli P, Barbieri D, et al. Preoperative clinical predictors of difficult laryngeal exposure for microlaryngoscopy: the Laryngoscore. Laryngoscope. 2014;124:2561-7.
85. Lee HS, Chun BG, Kim SW. Transoral laser microsurgery for early glottic cancer as one-stage single-modality therapy. Laryngoscope. 2013;123(11):2670-4.
86. Hinni ML, Ferlito A, Brandwein-Gensler MS, Takes RP, Silver CE, Westra WH, et al. Surgical margins in head and neck cancer: a contemporary review. Head Neck. 2013;35(9): 1362-70.
87. Mooney WW, Cole I, Albsoul N, Pearson SA. Salvage vertical partial laryngectomy for radiation failure in early glottic carcinoma. ANZ J Surg. 2002;72:746-49.
88. Myers EN, Alvi A. Management of carcinoma of the supraglottic larynx: evolution, current concepts, and future trends. Laryngoscope. 1996;106(5):559-67.
89. Wein RO, Weber RS. The current role of vertical partial laryngectomy and open supraglottic laryngectomy. Curr Probl Cancer. 2005;29:201-14.
90. Braz DSA, Ribas MM, Dedivitis RA, Nishimoto IN, Barros AP. Quality of life and depression in patients undergoing total and partial laryngectomy. Clinics. 2005;60(2):135-42.
91. Weinstein GS, El-Sawy MM, Ruiz C, Dooley P, Chalian A, El-Sayed MM, et al. Laryngeal preservation with supracricoid partial laryngectomy results in improved quality of life when compared with total laryngectomy. Laryngoscope. 2001;111(1):191-9.
92. Holsinger FC, Weinstein GS, Laccourreye O. Supracricoid partial laryngectomy: An organ preservation surgery for laryngeal malignancy. Curr Probl Cancer. 2005;29:190-200.
93. Thomas L, Drinnan M, Natesh B, Mehanna H, Jones T, Paleri V. Open conservation partial laryngectomy for laryngeal cancer: a systematic review of English language literature. Cancer Treat Rev. 2012;38(3):203-11.
94. Pearson BW. Subtotal laryngectomy. Laryngoscope. 1981;91: 1904-12.
95. D'Cruz AK, Sharma S, Pai PS. Current status of near-total laryngectomy: review. J Laryngol Otol. 2012;126(6):556-62.
96. Agrawal N, Goldenberg D. Primary and salvage total laryngectomy. Otolaryngol Clin North Am. 2008;41(4): 771-80.
97. Sofferman RA, Voronetsky I. Use of the linear stapler for pharyngoesophageal closure after total laryngectomy. Laryngoscope. 2000;110(8):1406-9.
98. Department of Veterans Affairs Laryngeal Cancer Study Group, Wolf GT, Fisher SG, Hong WK, Hillman R, Spaulding M, et al. Induction chemotherapy plus radiation compared with surgery plus radiation in patients with advanced laryngeal cancer. N Engl J Med. 1991;324(24):1685-90.
99. Forastiere AA, Goepfert H, Maor M. Concurrent chemotherapy and radiotherapy for organ preservation in advanced laryngeal cancer. N Engl J Med. 2003;349(22):2091-8.
100. Moyer JS, Wolf GT, Bradford CR. Current thoughts on the role of chemotherapy and radiation in advanced head and neck cancer. Curr Opin Otol Head Neck Surg. 2004;12:82-7.
101. Hillman RE, Walsh M, Wolf GT, Fisher SG, Hong WK. Functional outcomes following treatment for advanced laryngeal cancer: part 1: voice preservation in advanced laryngeal cancer. Ann Otol Rhinol Laryngol. 1998;172:1-27.
102. Terrell JE, Fisher SG, Wolf GT. Long-term quality of life after treatment of laryngeal cancer. The Veterans Affairs Laryngeal Cancer Study Group. Arch Otolaryngol Head Neck Surg. 1998;124(9):964-71.
103. Forastiere AA, Zhang Q, Weber RS, Maor MH, Goepfert H, Pajak TF, et al. Long-term results of RTOG 91-11: a comparison of three nonsurgical treatment strategies to preserve the larynx in patients with locally advanced larynx cancer. J Clin Oncol. 2013;31(7):845-52.
104. Hoffman HT, Porter K, Karnell LH, Cooper JS, Weber RS, Langer CJ, et al. Laryngeal cancer in the United States: changes in demographics, patterns of care, and survival. Laryngoscope. 2006;116(9 Pt 2 Suppl 111):1-13.
105. Chen AY, Fedewa S, Zhu J. Temporal trends in the treatment of early- and advanced-stage laryngeal cancer in the United States, 1985-2007. Arch Otolaryngol Head Neck Surg. 2011;137(10):1017-24.
106. Pignon JP, le Maitre A, Maillard E, Bourhis J, MACH-NC Collaborative Group. Meta-analysis of chemotherapy in head and neck cancer (MACH-NC): An update on 93 randomised trials and 17,346 patients. Radiother Oncol. 2009;92:4-14.
107. Cooper JS, Zhang Q, Pajak TF, Forastiere AA, Jacobs J, Saxman SB, et al. Long-term follow-up of the RTOG 9501/ intergroup phase III trial: Postoperative concurrent radiation therapy and chemotherapy in high-risk squamous cell carcinoma of the head and neck. Int J Radiat Oncol Biol Phys. 2012;84:1198-205.
108. Bonner JA, Harari PM, Giralt J, Cohen RB, Jones CU, Sur RK, et al. Radiotherapy plus cetuximab for locoregionally advanced head and neck cancer: 5-year survival data from a phase 3 randomised trial, and relation between cetuximab-induced rash and survival. Lancet Oncol. 2010;11:21-8.
109. Howlader N, Noone AM, Krapcho M. (2018). SEER Cancer Statistics Review (CSR) 1975-2016. [online] Available from https://seer.cancer.gov/csr/1975_2016/. [Last accessed July, 2020].
110. Rodríguez-Cuevas S, Labastida S, Gonzalez D, Briseño N, Cortes H. Partial laryngectomy as salvage surgery for radiation failures in T1-T2 laryngeal cancer. Head Neck. 1998; 20:630-3.

111. van der Putten L, de Bree R, Kuik DJ, Rietveld DH, Buter J, Eerenstein SE, et al. Salvage laryngectomy: Oncological and functional outcome. Oral Oncol. 2011;47: 296-301.
112. Weber RS, Berkey BA, Forastiere A, Cooper J, Maor M, Goepfert H, et al. Outcome of salvage total laryngectomy following organ preservation therapy: The Radiation Therapy Oncology Group trial 91-11. Arch Otolaryngol Head Neck Surg. 2003;129:44-9.
113. Paleri V, Thomas L, Basavaiah N, Drinnan M, Mehanna H, Jones T. Oncologic outcomes of open conservation laryngectomy for radio recurrent laryngeal carcinoma: A systematic review and meta-analysis of English-language literature. Cancer. 2011;117:2668-76.
114. de Gier HH, Knegt PP, de Boer MF, Meeuwis CA, van der Velden LA, Kerrebijn JD. CO_2-laser treatment of recurrent glottic carcinoma. Head Neck. 2001;23:177-80.
115. Ramakrishnan Y, Drinnan M, Kwong FN, Grant DG, Mehanna H, Jones T, et al. Oncologic outcomes of transoral laser microsurgery for radio recurrent laryngeal carcinoma: A systematic review and meta-analysis of English-language literature. Head Neck. 2014;26:280-5.
116. Johansen LV, Overgaard J, Hjelm-Hansen M, Gadeberg C. Primary radiotherapy of T1 squamous cell carcinoma of the larynx: analysis of 478 patients treated from 1963 to 1985. Int J Radiat Oncol Biol Phys. 1990;18:1307-13.
117. Johansen LV, Grau C, Overgaard J. Supraglottic carcinoma: Patterns of failure and salvage treatment after curatively intended radiotherapy in 410 consecutive patients. Int J Radiat Oncol Biol Phys. 2002;53:948-58.
118. Liang J, Zhu X, Zeng W, Yu T, Fang F, Zhao Y. Which risk factors are associated with stomal recurrence after total laryngectomy for laryngeal cancer? A meta-analysis of the last 30 years. Braz J Otorhinolaryngol. 2020.
119. Mei J, Huang Z, Wu K, Zhao Y, Yang J, Liu Y. Risk Factors of Stomal Recurrence After Laryngectomy: A Systematic Review and Meta-analysis. Ann Otol Rhinol Laryngol. 2017; 126(9):654-68.
120. Wu J, Wu KL, Liu YH, Zhao Y, Wang Y, Wang D. Surgical treatment of stomal recurrence after tracheotomy. Head Neck Surg. 2019;33(8):752-6.
121. Gessert TG, Britt CJ, Maas AM, Wieland AM, Harari PM, Hartig GK. Chondroradionecrosis of the larynx: 24-year University of Wisconsin experience. Head Neck. 2017; 39(6):1189-94.
122. Sebelik ME. Chondroradionecrosis of the larynx in patients treated with organ preservation therapy. Otolaryngol Head Neck Surg. 2004;131(2):P63-4.
123. Farneti D, Fabbri C, Prencipe SR. Chondroradionecrosis of the larynx. Curr Opin Otolaryngol Head Neck Surg. 2019;27(6):463-6.
124. Kolator M, Kolator P, Zatoński T. Assessment of quality of life in patients with laryngeal cancer: A review of articles. Adv Clin Exp Med. 2018;27(5):711-5.
125. Williamson JS, Ingrams D, Jones H. Quality of life after treatment of laryngeal carcinoma: a single centre cross-sectional study. Ann R Coll Surg Engl. 2011;93:591-5.
126. Azevedo EHM, Montoni N, Filho JG, Kowalski LP, de Angelis EC. Vocal Handicap and Quality of Life After Treatment of Advanced Squamous Carcinoma of the Larynx and/or Hypopharynx. J Voice. 2012;26:e63-71.
127. Stewart MG, Chen AY, Stach CB. Outcomes analysis of voice and quality of life in patients with laryngeal cancer. Arch Otolaryngol Head Neck Surg. 1998;124:143-8.

CHAPTER 14

Cancers of the Hypopharynx

Sivakumar Vidhyadharan, Samskruthi P Murthy, Narayana Subramaniam

INTRODUCTION

Cancers of the hypopharynx are relatively infrequent (accounting for 3–5% of all head and neck cancer), but are associated with the worst prognosis among the head and neck squamous cell carcinoma (HNSCC), with a 5-year overall survival in the range of 30–35%. It is believed that this results from the patient's anatomical and disease-related factors rather than poor treatment strategies.[1,2] It also has a recurrence rate as high as 50%, the majority of which occur within the first year after treatment and a high rate of distant metastasis.[3] Often symptoms associated with these tumors are vague and nonspecific, resulting in an advanced stage at diagnosis, compounded by varying degrees of dysphagia and malnutrition believed to be intrinsically linked to this condition.[4] In this chapter, we discuss the clinical features and the evidence on management of these tumors.

EPIDEMIOLOGY

It is a relatively infrequent cancer, with an incidence of <1/100,000 population. They most commonly present in male patients aged 60 years or older, with a history of tobacco and alcohol exposure. Postcricoid carcinoma occurs more commonly in young women, especially in India, Iran, and Japan.[5] These may be associated with sideropenic dysphagia (Paterson–Brown–Kelly syndrome). Most hypopharyngeal cancers are squamous cell carcinoma (SCC). Pyriform sinus tumors are the most common, followed by posterior pharyngeal wall and postcricoid tumors, however the exact percentages vary geographically.[5-7] Since they often present at an advanced stage, 60% of patients present with more than one site involved, making it difficult to identify the site of origin.[8]

RISK FACTORS

The robust data available on etiology of laryngeal cancer is lacking in the hypopharynx; it is often presumed due to similar exposure and anatomical proximity of the subsites that the same general principles apply.

- *Tobacco:* As with development of all other HNSCC, tobacco exposure is a central factor. Cohort and case–control studies have established this risk in hypopharyngeal and cervical esophageal cancers and in India, this exposure can be through smoking, chewing, or snuff.[9-11] It is of interest that in pharyngeal cancer, the risk reduction after cessation of smoking is not as pronounced as with other subsites.[12,13] The risk of developing is twofold even in those with modest tobacco exposure (<10 cigarettes per day).[14]
- *Alcohol:* Alcohol consumption has also been a well-established major risk factor in HNSCC. Interestingly, some studies have shown a higher risk from drinking large quantities over shorter time periods than from sustained exposure to lower quantities.[15] Genetic mutations in the alcohol dehydrogenase enzymes (ADH1B and ALDH2) may also contribute to development of hypopharyngeal cancer. Quitting alcohol was associated with a 40% reduction in the risk of developing head and neck cancer at 20 years when compared to those who continued to drink, however this reduction in pharyngeal cancers is not as pronounced.[13]
- *Occupational factors:* These risks have been historically hard to quantify in isolation from tobacco and alcohol exposure, however there have been studies linking laryngeal and hypopharyngeal cancer to occupational work in the rubber and asbestos industries and other industrial activity like construction, logging, and railway transport.[15,16]
- *Plummer-Vinson syndrome:* Also known as Paterson–Brown–Kelly syndrome or sideropenic dysphagia, this manifests with iron deficiency anemia and dysphagia in women 30–50 years of age without tobacco or alcohol use. Between one- and two-thirds

of postcricoid carcinomas display evidence of Plummer-Vinson syndrome.[17,18]

- *Radiation exposure:* Patients treated with radiotherapy for early laryngeal cancer and non-Hodgkin's lymphoma have been shown to be at an increased risk of developing hypopharyngeal cancer.[15]
- *Miscellaneous factors:* In India, cervical esophageal/hypopharyngeal cancers are reported to occur frequently and this has been attributed to the local practice of drinking boiling hot salt tea with sun-dried vegetables and chilies that shown to result in endogenous nitrosamine production.[12] The role of human papillomavirus (HPV) in nonoropharyngeal cancers is still unclear. HPV deoxyribonucleic acid (DNA) has been seen in esophageal cancer and the belief is that migration of lymphatic tissue from the Waldeyer's ring may play a role.[10] Familial predisposition may play a role in some patients. Morita et al. showed an increase in laryngeal, hypopharyngeal, and esophageal cancer in those with a family history of head and neck cancer independent of other factors. Gastroesophageal reflux may also contribute to cancer risk.[10]

APPLIED ANATOMY[19,20]

The hypopharynx has strict anatomical, functional, and pathologic relationships with the larynx and is a common conduit for both respiration and deglutition, making it an important anatomical site. Since it is a component of the upper aerodigestive tract and tumor in this region presenting at an advanced stage has poor outcomes, the key to improved cure rates is early diagnosis and treatment.

The hypopharynx (or laryngopharynx) is the lowermost segment of the pharynx, extending from the tip of the epiglottis superiorly to the inferior edge of the cricoid cartilage. It is a 5-cm long cone-shaped tube, wider superiorly (almost 4 cm), and narrowing down to about 1.5 cm in the postcricoid and cervical esophagus area. Anteriorly, it communicates with the larynx. The larynx is surrounded by the two funnel-shaped pyriform sinuses and by the postcricoid area, which are the subsites of the hypopharynx. Superiorly, tumors may spread to the lateral pharyngeal wall. Laterally, the hypopharynx is separated from the carotid sheath (the common carotid artery, internal jugular vein, and vagus nerve). Within the lumen of the hypopharynx, the inferior constrictor muscles and the pyriform sinus are bounded medially by the aryepiglottic fold and laterally by the internal surface of the thyroid ala and the thyrohyoid membrane. Posteriorly, the constrictor muscles (superior, middle, and inferior) separate the hypopharynx from the prevertebral fascia and the bodies of the third to the sixth cervical vertebra. Inferiorly, the hypopharynx opens into the esophagus at the level of the upper esophageal sphincter. The inferior constrictor arises anteriorly from the oblique line on the lateral side of the thyroid cartilage and the tendinous arch between the inferior tubercle of the oblique line and the cricoid cartilage. The lower part of the inferior constrictor is known as the cricopharyngeus muscle. The posterior attachment of the inferior constrictor on each side is attached to a thin midline vertical tendon known as the pharyngeal raphe. The cricopharyngeus muscle encircles the hypopharynx in an axial plane, in contrast to the angulated course of the fibers of the other constrictors. It does not have a posterior midline raphe and is continuous from its left to right sides. The cricopharyngeus muscle is the major component of the upper esophageal constrictor and with its tonic contraction, it maintains a constant level of closing pressure. During swallowing, the cricopharyngeus muscle relaxes, permitting passage of the bolus from the hypopharynx into the cervical esophagus.

Three paired muscles (stylopharyngeus, salpingopharyngeus, and palatopharyngeus) contribute to the pharyngeal wall at the level of the oropharynx and help with the craniocaudal movements of the hypopharynx. The stylohyoid and styloglossus muscles are also responsible for pharyngeal elevation during swallowing. The true intrinsic longitudinal muscle in the hypopharynx only begins at the level of the upper esophageal sphincter. Surrounding the hypopharynx are the parapharyngeal and retropharyngeal spaces, which are filled with loose areolar connective tissue, allowing this organ to move freely in relation to the fascia overlying the prevertebral muscles.

The hypopharynx extends from the level of the hyoid bone superiorly to the lower border of the cricoid cartilage inferiorly. The pyriform sinuses on each side, the posterior pharyngeal wall and the postcricoid region, form the three designated anatomical subsites within the hypopharynx. The boundaries of these subsites overlap and their demarcation is fairly arbitrary. The hypopharynx is a mucosal lined tube bounded by constrictor muscles laterally and posteriorly and the laryngeal cartilages anteriorly. The epithelial lining consists of nonkeratinized stratified squamous epithelium. The lamina propria of mucosa contains scattered lymphoid aggregates and mucoserous glands. The hypopharynx gets arterial branches from the ascending pharyngeal (branch of the external carotid) artery and the superior and inferior thyroid arteries. The venous drainage is through a number of small venous channels forming a submucosal plexus that drains into the mid and distal portion of the internal jugular vein. The hypopharynx has a high density of mucosal and submucosal lymphatic channels. This may be the reason for high propensity of tumors of hypopharynx to quickly spread to adjacent lymph nodes, either by a constant retropharyngeal lymph node (Rouvière's node) and then to the deep jugular lymph nodes (levels III-IV) or directly to the latter group. The pyriform sinuses and postcricoid region also drain to the paratracheal lymph nodes (level VI), thus gaining access to the lymphatic system of the thoracic cavity. Branches of the vagus from the superior laryngeal nerve arborize and intercommunicate with branches of the glossopharyngeal nerve to form the pharyngeal plexus. These envelop the constrictor musculature of the pharynx and continue along the esophagus. Disruption of this plexus has deleterious effect on the constrictor activity and sensation of the pharyngeal musculature and mucosa, with subsequent decline of the swallowing function.

CLINICAL EXAMINATION AND PRESENTATION

Dysphagia is a late symptom of postcricoid cancer. Often presentation is delayed until dysphagia has supervened on some other symptom (which may have been present for some time) such as cough, pain, roughness in the throat, halitosis, sore throat, or tightness in the retrosternal region. Productive cough is present even in the absence of signs of bronchitis on auscultation of the chest. Pain may be felt on the side of the neck, often extending upward to the ear due to referred otalgia. Roughness or a sensation of foreign body stuck in the throat seems to be a constant symptom and is often periodic. Halitosis may be present due to food residue in the hypopharynx. Tightness in the retrosternal region is often present and may be first manifestation of dysphagia.[21,22] The appearance of the Plummer-Vinson syndrome may be a precursor of postcricoid cancer. The symptoms of this condition are microcytic anemia, achlorhydria or hyperchlorhydria, a palpable spleen, and dysphagia, which may be periodic. It is uncommon to see all these signs and symptoms in the one patient, with the condition generally manifested by the combination of dysphagia and microcytic anemia. Although the syndrome quickly clears up under iron therapy, the follow-up of these patients is very important as, by frequent examination, cancer in this region may be recognized in its early stage. On examination, it may be associated with postcricoid webs, bands, and strictures that may harbor premalignant lesions. The disorder is a chronic iron-deficiency state and is associated with other deficiencies of vitamins B and C. An impenetrable stricture may form necessitating surgical treatment.

Some of the cardinal symptoms that may be associated with hypopharyngeal tumors are pain (usually lateralized, often radiating to, or most noticeable in the ipsilateral ear), dysphagia (usually constant and progressive; if food "sticks" on swallowing, this must be viewed with extreme suspicion), hemoptysis (this is an unusual, but important symptom which may appear particularly with pyriform fossa tumors), hoarseness (in association with dysphagia and/or referred otalgia, this suggests extension to the larynx), neck mass (should be regarded as a possible nodal metastasis in adults), and weight loss (should be asked about, as it suggests serious disease in the absence of an attempt to lose weight).[23]

Physical examination should include the checking for weight loss, nutrition status, and anemia. The pharynx and larynx may be examined commonly with a flexible fiberoptic nasopharyngoscope that passes through the nose. Obvious swellings or ulceration as well as the presence of Chevalier Jackson's sign (pooling of saliva in the pyriform sinus) and edema of the arytenoids must be identified and photodocumented. In case of tumors situated in the medial wall of pyriform sinus and postcricoid area, evaluation of vocal cord mobility must be performed. Palpation of the neck to determine the presence of enlarged lymph nodes, the mobility of the laryngopharynx in relation to the cervical vertebrae is assessed. The presence of Trotter's sign (tumor extension to the prevertebral muscles causing absent laryngeal crepitus) must be looked for in case of a large tumor. During fiberoptic evaluation, the pyriform sinus may be distended by the patient performing a Valsalva maneuver with the glottis open and pinching the nostrils. Additionally, it is important to examine the posterior pharyngeal wall when the endoscope is being withdrawn.[24,25]

The diagnostic workup and clinical staging of a patient with a suspected hypopharyngeal carcinoma encompasses a history and physical examination followed by imaging and panendoscopy with biopsy. On external examination of the larynx and hypopharynx, a normal crepitus sound is felt or elicited, when the laryngeal cartilage is moved from side to side against the cervical spine. In postcricoid carcinoma, if there is spread within the plane between the laryngeal cartilaginous framework and the cervical spine, there will be an absence of this sensation called Bocca's sign. The hypopharyngeal tumor mass can be visualized by indirect laryngoscopy or video laryngoscopy. If there is pooled saliva within both the pyriform fossa associated with some fullness, then it would indicate the possibility of postcricoid malignancy known as Jackson's sign. Vocal cord palsy should be identified and documented.[25-27]

PATHWAYS OF SPREAD

Hypopharyngeal carcinomas often present with unimpressive mucosal involvement but extensive submucosal extension to involve multiple contiguous subsites, making clinical evaluation difficult. The mucosal component may often show thickening or plaque-like involvement with minimal ulceration, with submucosal involvement on average of 5 mm and 10 mm in the pyriform sinus and postcricoid regions, respectively. The thick laryngeal cartilage provides a robust barrier to resist spread, allowing tumors to preferentially spread along the constrictor muscles. Spread superiorly can result in involvement of the lateral oropharyngeal wall and base tongue in advanced cases. In marginal zone tumors, arising at the junction of the supraglottis and pyriform sinus, tumors can spread through the constrictor muscle of the hypopharyngeal wall in most cases, but the laryngeal cartilages resist invasion and involved in a small number of cases. Involvement of the oropharynx and the base of the tongue through superior spread is not uncommon in advanced cases. Carcinomas of the pyriform sinuses, particularly those involving the medial wall or the marginal zone (between pyriform fossa and supraglottis), have early spread into the supraglottic or glottis larynx. Tumors can also penetrate the cricothyroid membrane with less resistance than the laryngeal cartilages, resulting in extralaryngeal spread. Vocal cord fixation can occur due to invasion of the nerve, disruption of the cricoarytenoid joint or the cricothyroid muscle.[3,5] **Figure 1** shows gross pathology of a typical pyriform fossa sinus cancer.

Around 80% of posterior hypopharyngeal wall tumors are exophytic and are often large (>5 cm) at presentation, involving the posterior oropharyngeal wall. Postcricoid carcinomas tend to grow anteriorly to involve the posterior cricoarytenoid muscle and may extend into the trachea through the cricoid cartilage or inferiorly to involve the esophagus and trachea. The thyroid gland is often involved by hypopharyngeal carcinoma because of the proximity of the superior part of thyroid lobes to the lateral wall of the hypopharynx; this may an alternative route of lymph node spread. The internal jugular vein is frequently invaded and drawn anterior to the common carotid artery and becomes adherent to the pharyngeal wall.

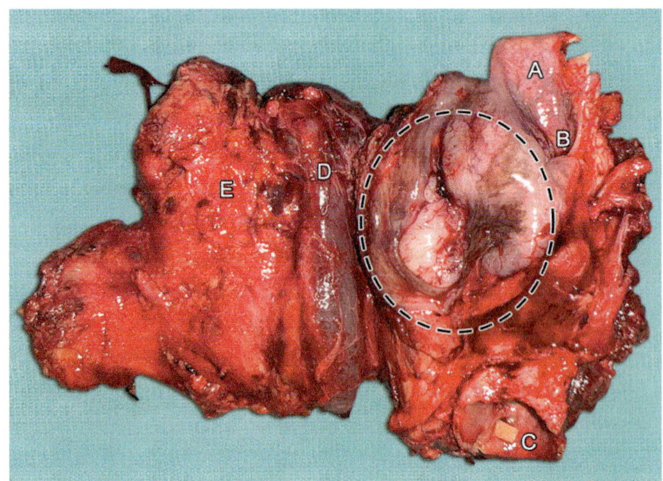

Fig. 1: En bloc resection specimen of left pyriform fossa cancer (circled) and radical neck dissection. A: Epiglottis; B: Laryngeal inlet; C: Trachea; D: Left internal jugular vein; E: Left radical neck dissection specimen.

Regional nodal spread occurs initially in the group of lymph nodes lying in close proximity to the internal jugular vein between the posterior belly of the digastric and the anterior belly of the omohyoid muscles; these nodes receive lymph from the hypopharynx through the supraglottic pedicle. Although the tumor is limited to one-half of the hypopharynx, contralateral nodal spread is known to occur through decussating lymphatic channels. There is a high (>50%) risk of occult nodal metastasis in even small (T1-T2) pyriform sinus carcinomas and may present with enlarged nodes. In patients with a clinically N0 neck, bilateral metastatic neck disease is common with neck dissection specimens containing positive nodes in around 56% of ipsilateral and 47% of contralateral sides of neck. Pyriform sinus carcinomas spread frequently to level II nodes, with level III and IV nodes being involved particularly in clinically node-positive patients and level V involvement occurs in 11%. Retropharyngeal involvement may occur in up to 40% of patients with posterior pharyngeal wall.[26]

Postcricoid carcinomas have a lower incidence (30%) of nodal metastasis than other hypopharyngeal carcinomas and spread to mid and lower cervical nodes and paratracheal nodes and bilateral involvement in 18%. Distant metastases in the lungs, mediastinum, bone, liver, or skin occur in 20–40% of patients within 9 months of diagnosis and survival is usually not >1 year after these are detected. The incidence of distant metastases at presentation is higher in hypopharyngeal carcinomas (17–24%) than for all other head and neck sites (11%).[5]

INVESTIGATIONS

Imaging includes contrast-enhanced computed tomography (CT) or magnetic resonance imaging (MRI) of the neck and superior mediastinum to ascertain local extension and cervical, paratracheal, retropharyngeal, or mediastinal nodal disease. CT is useful in evaluating invasion of the thyroid and cricoid cartilages as well as assessing adenopathy. MRI has better soft tissue definition and the probability to identify occult submucosal disease, invasion of the intrinsic laryngeal musculature or the paraglottic space, and tumor spread along the superior neurovascular pedicle. CT and MRI are complementary imaging modalities in treatment planning; often an inadequacy of one modality can be supplemented with another. Thoracic CT is important for accurate clinical staging and treatment planning in the search for distant metastasis. Functional imaging with positron emission tomography combined with CT (PET-CT) is utilized as an additional staging tool which could assist in assessment of the extent of the primary tumor as well as evaluation of second primaries, distant metastases, and extent of cervical lymphadenopathy. However, it is limited by cost, availability, and the false-positive rates as a consequence of inflammation and other factors.[27]

Under a general anesthetic, panendoscopy is helpful in determining the mucosal extent of the tumor, involvement of adjacent structures, presence of deep fixation, to investigate the possibility of a second primary malignancy, and biopsy of the primary tumor. In patients with postcricoid lesions or cervical esophageal involvement, flexible esophagoscopy is preferred over rigid esophagoscopy technique to reduce the risk of perforation and to assess the distal extent of the tumor. Biopsies of laryngeal and hypopharyngeal tumors are potentially possible under local anesthetic in the outpatient clinic by utilizing a transnasal esophagoscope with a biopsy port. In the manifestation of palpable nodal disease, a fine-needle aspiration may be obtained to confirm suspicion of a metastatic node.[4]

Imaging

Carcinoma of the pyriform sinus is readily detected with endoscopy while very early superficial spreading tumors that are limited to the mucosa may be invisible at cross-sectional imaging. Staging accuracy for tumors of the hypopharynx by clinical examination alone is 55–64%. Adding MRI can improve this substantially from 70 to 87%.[28-30] Knowledge of the site of the primary tumor before imaging is important because it can help the radiologist to obtain a more focused study with both CT and MRI. Unlike the modern, multislice CT machines, MRI acquisition is relatively slow and thus very susceptible to motion artifact. It is very important that the patient does not swallow, cough, or move during MRI acquisition and careful instructions must be given to the patient to remain still. Motion artifacts greatly reduce image quality and they can ruin the ability to accurately assess tumor extent. Nondiagnostic MRI incidence ranges between 10 and 15% and motion artifact is a principle cause of imaging failures.[28,31,32]

In T1-weighted (T1W) MR images, tumor and muscle are low intensity compared with fat, which help in identifying the tumor tissue when it invades fat. In the postcontrast T1W images, the tumor enhances well but has signal intensity similar to fat. Fat suppression, which darkens the fat signal, can make the distinction between fat and tumor more obvious. In precontrast T1W images, fat suppression has a negative effect in detection of head and neck tumors; it is in the postcontrast T1W image that adding fat suppression enhances detection of tumors. Tumors have prolonged T2 relaxation time and can be difficult to distinguish from inflammation, which also show high signal on T2. Fat also shows a high signal in turbo spin-echo (TSE) T2-weighted images, however this can be overcome by using fat saturation.[28,31,32]

Most patients with pyriform sinus tumors present with advanced lesions and diagnosis at CT or MRI is straightforward. Because the pyriform sinus is usually collapsed during quiet respiration, the exact tumor location (medial wall vs. lateral wall) may be difficult to determine radiologically and a very close communication between the radiologist and surgeon is essential.

Postcricoid carcinoma is uncommon but is observed in patients with the Plummer-Vinson syndrome or those at risk. Postcricoid carcinoma often spread submucosally inferiorly toward the cervical esophagus. Because tumor growth is mainly submucosal, the true extent only becomes apparent with axial or sagittal MR images. Carcinoma of the posterior pharyngeal wall commonly involves both the oropharynx and hypopharynx. On axial MR images, these tumors appear as asymmetrical thickening of the posterior pharyngeal wall. At initial presentation, invasion of the prevertebral muscles is unusual. As the tumor advances in stage, these cancers may invade the prevertebral muscles, CT and MRI have a high true-negative but also high false-positive rate in diagnosing such posterior tumor spread. Hsu et al. conducted a study to determine the preoperative accuracy of preservation of the retropharyngeal fat plane on MR images in predicting the absence of fixation or extension of head and neck carcinomas to the prevertebral space. The retropharyngeal fat is clearly visualized as high signal intensity between the pharyngeal mucosa and the prevertebral musculature. They had preservation of the fat plane in 40 patients, of which 39 were found to have resectable tumors, resulting in a negative predictive value of 97.5%.[33] **Figures 2 and 3** show imaging in a typical postcricoid and hypopharyngeal sinus cancer respectively.

In hypopharyngeal and advanced laryngeal cancer patients with equivocal prevertebral space involvement but no other contraindications for surgery, evaluation of fixity of tumor to the prevertebral fascia and muscles is ascertained by side-to-side manipulation of larynx by hand during the examination under anesthesia. Surgical assessment of resectability is through by opening the neck is performed via contralateral side of neck uninvolved by tumor; when tumor involves both sides, access is obtained via the side with less volume of disease. Surgical resection is performed if the tumor is freely mobile in a side-to-side direction and aborted in favor of other modalities of treatment if the tumor is fixed to the prevertebral compartment.

CT thorax seems justified in advanced stages of the primary tumor and/or bulky neck disease. In borderline but resectable disease, PET-CT may be considered to

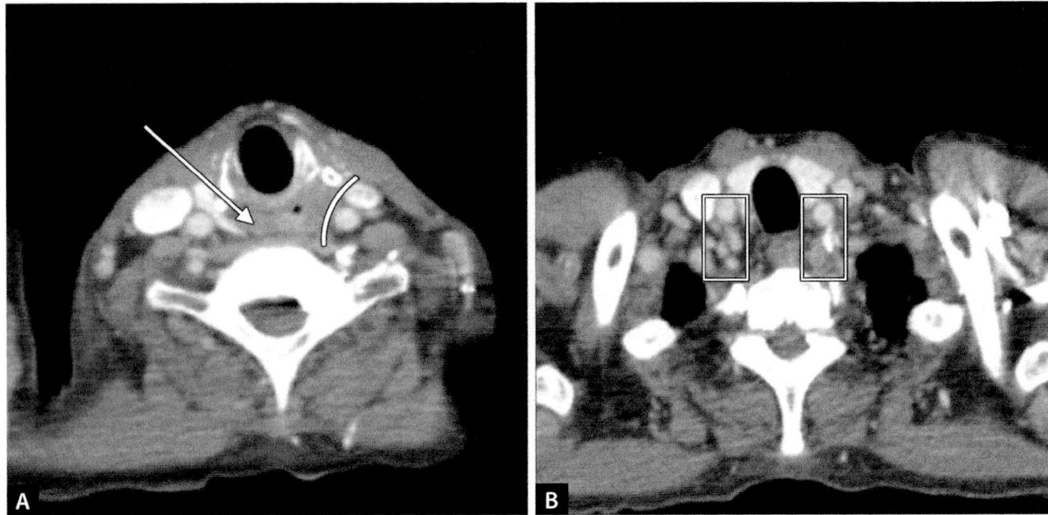

Figs. 2A and B: Axial section of contrast enhanced CT of neck in a case of T4 carcinoma postcricoid region. (A) Arrow denotes tumor involving postcricoid region with extrapharyngeal extension (curved line); (B) Lymph nodal involvement in bilateral level VI (rectangles).

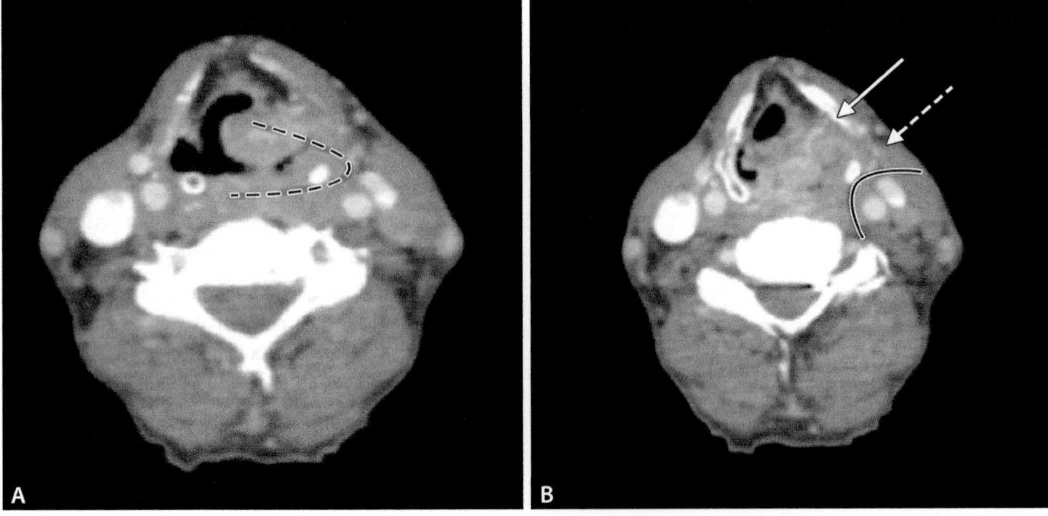

Figs. 3A and B: Axial section of contrast enhanced CT of neck in a case of T4 carcinoma pyriform fossa (left). (A) Curved dotted line depicts tumor involving left pyriform fossa, left aryepiglottic fold and up to posterior pharyngeal wall; (B) Arrow shows left thyroid cartilage widening and dotted arrow denotes invasion of thyroid cartilage. The extrapharyngeal extension of tumor is represented by curved line and note loss of plane between tumor and common carotid artery.

exclude occult distant disease. Distant metastasis is frequently present at presentation, most commonly to the lungs or mediastinum (about 30%) and liver (about 15%).[34]

Endoscopically, the extent of hypopharyngeal and supraglottic carcinomas is often underestimated because of the tendency to spread beneath an intact mucosa. In contrast, submucosal extension can be equally well-evaluated with MR or CT. Although the evaluation of the apex of the pyriform sinus can usually be done by direct laryngoscopy, CT phonation scans or a double contrast pharyngographic barium study may help better define caudal tumor extension in case of bulky endoluminal tumor masses causing a troublesome endoscopic passage. These subregions are better evaluated with CT rather than with MR because it is much easier to perform phonation or Valsalva maneuver during the shorter time of data acquisition. The esophageal inlet is an important landmark to be addressed because an infiltration would need partial esophagectomy in addition to laryngopharyngectomy. A tumor extension below the inferior margin of the cricoid cartilage can be regarded as an esophageal infiltration that can be better assessed with imaging rather than at endoscopy, especially in case of submucosal tumor spread. Anterior extension of tumors of the pyriform sinus into the paraglottic fat can be visualized on axial CT or MR sections.[35]

Tumor volume: Emphasis has been placed on stratifying patients into high- or low-risk groups based on outcome; of these, the most important criteria have been volume of the tumor and cartilage involvement. Pameijer et al. found two important prognostic factors for T1 and T2 pyriform sinus cancers treated with radiation therapy alone, tumor volume, and amount of disease at the pyriform sinus apex. Although this study was conducted based on CT imaging findings, the same or similar results are expected for MR imaging. The authors defined pyriform sinus apex disease as minimal apical disease if the tumor was <10 mm in diameter at the level of the base of the arytenoid cartilage and upper 3 mm of the cricoid cartilage or as bulky apical disease if the diameter was ≥10 mm. Their results characterized three different patient groups with the following criteria and local control rates if treated with radiation therapy alone:

1. *Low-risk group:* Patients with tumor volume <6.5 mL and no or minimal apical disease showed a local control rate of 94%
2. *Moderate-risk group:* Patients with tumor volume of <6.5 mL and bulky apical disease or tumor volume ≥6.5 mL and no or minimal apical disease demonstrated local control rates of 50%
3. *High-risk group:* None of the patients survived with tumor volume of ≥6.5 mL and bulky apical disease.

Hence, reporting of tumor volume and apical disease should be done for all T1 and T2 stage pyriform sinus cancers.[36,37]

STAGING

The American Joint Committee on Cancer (AJCC) 8th edition tumor, node, and metastasis (TNM) staging is given in **Table 1**.

TREATMENT APPROACHES

Patients with hypopharyngeal cancers often present with an advanced stage of disease, comorbid illnesses, and nutritional issues, making decision-making difficult. Although organ preservation approaches are attractive, there are several differences between hypopharyngeal and laryngeal tumors that make extrapolation of these principles complex; submucosal spread of disease and nodal metastases occur more common in hypopharyngeal cancers, necessitating wide margins and concomitant neck dissection, which compound morbidity. The location of these tumors also makes surgery more morbid with respect to swallowing dysfunction and aspiration than most glottic or supraglottic tumors. Additionally, outcomes with any modality are modest to poor, with a clear treatment preference only in certain clinical scenarios. The evidence available on hypopharyngeal cancer is often represented by organ preservation strategies with radiotherapy and/or chemotherapy or surgical case series with head-to-head comparisons except for single randomized trials. Treatment of individual patients requires multidisciplinary input, consideration of the patient's expectations, and expertise available.

- *Early hypopharyngeal cancers:* T1-2N0 disease in this subsite is relatively rare. However, in these patients, radical radiotherapy or surgery [most commonly transoral laser microsurgery (TLM)] is recommended. Often decision-making is based on tumor and patient-related factors. Small well-delineated lesions may be good candidates for surgery while those with suspicion of submucosal spread and adjacent mucosal abnormalities are better candidates for radiotherapy. Inadequate margins require adjuvant radiotherapy, resulting in treatment-related morbidity from both. Resultant swallowing morbidity after surgery needs to be anticipated; patients unlikely to tolerate a period of postoperative aspiration are poor surgical candidates.

Table 1: TNM staging according to the American Joint Committee on Cancer (AJCC) 8th edition.

T category	*T criteria*
Tx	Primary tumor cannot be assessed
Tis	Carcinoma *in situ*
T1	Tumor limited to one subsite of hypopharynx and/or 2 cm or smaller in greatest dimension
T2	Tumor invades more than one subsite of hypopharynx or an adjacent site or measures larger than 2 cm but not larger than 4 cm in greatest dimension without fixation of hemilarynx
T3	Tumor larger than 4 cm in greatest dimension or with fixation of hemilarynx or extension to esophagus
T4a	*Moderately advanced local disease:* Tumor invades thyroid/cricoid cartilage, hyoid bone, thyroid gland, esophageal muscle, or central compartment soft tissue
T4b	*Very advanced local disease:* Tumor invades prevertebral fascia, encases carotid artery, or involves mediastinal structures
N category	*N criteria*
NX	Regional lymph nodes cannot be assessed
N0	No regional lymph node metastasis
N1	Metastasis in a single ipsilateral lymph node, 3 cm or smaller in greatest dimension and ENE (–)
N2	Metastasis in a single ipsilateral node, larger than 3 cm but not larger than 6 cm in greatest dimension and ENE (–) *or* metastases in multiple ipsilateral lymph nodes, none larger than 6 cm in greatest dimension and ENE (–) *or* metastasis in bilateral or contralateral lymph nodes, none larger than 6 cm in greatest dimension and ENE (–)
N2a	Metastasis in a single ipsilateral node, larger than 3 cm but not larger than 6 cm in greatest dimension and ENE (–)
N2b	Metastases in multiple ipsilateral nodes, none larger than 6 cm in greatest dimension and ENE (–)
N2c	Metastasis in bilateral or contralateral lymph nodes, none larger than 6 cm in greatest dimension and ENE (–)
N3	Metastasis in a lymph node, larger than 6 cm in greatest dimension and ENE (–) *or* metastasis in any lymph node(s) with clinically overt ENE (+)
N3a	Metastasis in a lymph node, larger than 6 cm in greatest dimension and ENE (–)
N3b	Metastasis in any lymph node(s) with clinically overt ENE (+)
M category	*M criteria*
M0	No distant metastasis
M1	Distant metastasis

(ENE: extranodal extension; TNM: tumor, node, and metastasis)

- *Advanced hypopharyngeal cancers:* Surgery was long considered the treatment of choice in advanced (stage III/IV) hypopharyngeal cancers, which was traditional total laryngectomy and hypopharyngectomy with neck dissection. However, with the success of organ preservation approaches in the larynx, nonsurgical treatment has become increasingly common. As discussed in the earlier chapter on laryngeal tumors, population-based data has shown poorer survival with nonsurgical therapies in these patients, often due to nononcological causes. However, the central premise of organ preservation is preserving functional speech and swallowing with radiotherapy and reserving surgery as salvage modality, which are functions many patients with advanced hypopharyngeal cancer do not have. It is considered unlikely that patients with a dysfunctional larynx (dysphagia required nonoral feeding, tracheostomy for respiration, and no voice) will regain function after nonsurgical treatment. Additionally, a significant proportion of patients cannot tolerate concurrent chemotherapy, which results in reduced cure rates with nonsurgical treatment. More recent data would suggest that in T3 disease, surgical and nonsurgical treatment results in comparable survival rates while in T4 disease, patients treated with surgery first had better survival.[38,39] There is no one-size-fits-all approach in these patients; hence, multidisciplinary evaluation is crucial to ensure reasonable chance of cure and good functional outcomes following treatment.

Transoral Laser Microsurgery

Adequate visualization is paramount for transoral laser microsurgical partial laryngopharyngectomy. A carbon dioxide (CO_2) laser coupled to the operating microscope is used and the focus diameter of the micromanipulator is about 0.5 mm with the delivered laser energy about 2,080–3,900 W/cm^2. The CO_2 laser coagulates vessels ≤1 mm in diameter. Bleeding from large vessels can be controlled by electrocautery with clipping of exceptionally large vessels. Steiner's adjustable laryngopharyngoscope is used for TLM in the pyriform sinus. This allows resection of the tumor bit-by-bit from cranial to caudal direction. The design of the laryngoscope allows convenient readjustment for ideal exposure at each step. Pyriform sinus cancer can be resected block wise and aided by frozen section to ensure complete resection with preservation of normal tissue for best functional outcomes. These lesions are excised systematically in blocks to ensure adequate margins. Judicious use of frozen section can allow adequate clearance while sacrificing as little healthy tissue as possible.[40]

Pyriform sinus tumors are resected with a margin of at least 5 mm for small superficial tumors and 5–10 mm for larger tumors and those with a deeply infiltrating growth pattern and with submucosal spread. The resected specimens are histopathologically examined by a technique of step serial sections. In cases of exposed or resected thyroid cartilage, a perioperative antibiotic prophylaxis such as penicillin is administered along with an intraoperative dose of corticosteroids.[41]

Results

Steiner et al. treated 129 patients of pyriform sinus SCC with TLM, ranging from pT1 to T4.[42] They also received neck dissection and had nodal metastases in 68%. Advanced patients received adjuvant therapy. Recurrence-free survival rates were 95% for early stage and 69% for advanced stage at 5 years, with all regaining normal swallowing function.[41] They published another series of patients showing a local control rate was 84% for pT1 lesions, 70% for pT2 lesions, 75% for pT3 lesions, and 57% for pT4a lesions at 5 years.[40] Rudert et al. showed a 28% local recurrence rate in their series of 29 T1/T2 hypopharyngeal SCC treated with TLM and showed that nodal metastasis resulted in survival falling from 74 to 34%.[43] Karatzanis et al. studied 119 patients of early hypopharyngeal carcinomas and showed a 5-year disease-specific survival of 78% and 70% for pT1 and pT2 patients, respectively, with 5% needing permanent tracheostomy or percutaneous endoscopic gastrostomy (PEG) feeding.[44] Although outcomes are excellent, it is important to note that these are retrospective series from individual institutions and experienced surgeons, hence these outcomes cannot be extrapolated to the general population operated on by surgeons with limited experience.

Partial Laryngectomies

Laryngeal preservation surgery can be performed with excellent functional results, for a particular group of patients with early-stage hypopharyngeal cancer. Care has to be taken to prevent the risk of chronic or life-threatening aspiration after operation. For small and easily accessible tumors, transoral endoscopic approach is most appropriate. For posterior pharyngeal or small lateral pharyngeal tumors, a lateral or transhyoid pharyngotomy can give good access for a partial pharyngectomy. A partial laryngopharyngectomy can be performed for tumors of the pyriform sinus invading the lateral wall of the hypopharynx.[44]

Conservative surgery is seldom considered to be suitable in pyriform sinus carcinoma because of either oncologic reasons or patient factors such as inadequate pulmonary reserve and postoperative swallowing disorders.[45,46] Only small tumors confined to the lateral wall of the pyriform sinus are amenable to conservative partial pharyngectomy. The technique of partial supraglottic laryngopharyngectomy, described by Ogura et al., is indicated for early tumors preserving vocal cord mobility, limited to the medial wall of the pyriform sinus with possible extension to the aryepiglottic fold.[47,48] Supracricoid hemilaryngopharyngectomy (SCHLP) has been performed for tumors involving the aryepiglottic fold and the medial and anterior wall of the pyriform sinus. The contraindications to laryngeal preservation surgery are invasion of the pyriform sinus apex or postcricoid region, invasion of the posterior hypopharyngeal wall, or fixation of the ipsilateral vocal cord.

Supracricoid Hemilaryngopharyngectomy

The principle of SCHLP is to remove the tumor together with the pyriform sinus and the ipsilateral hemilarynx above the cricoid cartilage. After ipsilateral neck dissection is performed, the ipsilateral thyroid cartilage and half of the hyoid bone are resected. The infrahyoid muscles are dissected and rotated caudally and the larynx is opened by incision in the vallecula and glossoepiglottic folds. The epiglottis and preepiglottic fat are then dissected in the vertical plane. The upper rim of the cricoid cartilage demarcates the caudal resection margin. After removal of the vocal fold and the ventricle, under direct vision, the posterior resection line is demarcated. Following mobilization of the pharynx from the deep cervical fascia, suturing the pharynx to infrahyoid muscles, laryngeal remnant, and vallecula closes the defect. The supraglottic hemilaryngopharyngectomy is a modification of the SCHLP with preservation of both vocal folds.

Results

Ogura achieved a 3-year survival rate of 53% in resection for selected patients with early pyriform sinus carcinoma (mobile vocal cords, no tumor involvement of the apex of the pyriform sinus, postcricoid region, or thyroid cartilage).[48] However, due to local tumor recurrence, 34% of patients required a secondary total laryngectomy.[49] Laccourreye et al. reported on 240 patients who underwent SCHLP for early pyriform sinus carcinomas; local recurrences developed in around 5%, tracheostomy was required in 8% and 15% suffered from dysphagia.[50] Chevalier et al. published results of 31 patients with T1/T2 pyriform sinus carcinomas who underwent SCHLP with radical neck dissection and postoperative radiotherapy followed-up for 15 years. Although local recurrences occurred only in 2%, survival was poor especially in T2 due to neck recurrences and distant metastases.[51] Foucher et al. reported on a small cohort patients with early hypopharynx carcinomas treated with partial pharyngolaryngectomy and elective neck dissection with no adjuvant therapy, showing locoregional control rates over 80%.[52]

Induction chemotherapy followed by SCHLP and adjuvant radiotherapy was another approach. Laccourreye et al. treated 118 patients of T1-T4a hypopharyngeal carcinoma with cisplatin and 5-fluorouracil followed by surgery and adjuvant radiotherapy in almost half of the patients. Laryngeal preservation rate was over 90% and 5-year survival rate was over 50%. Postoperative mortality was 3.7%.[40,52]

Studies on the use of SCHLP had been performed on 147 patients over a 19-year period. The 5-year actuarial local control rate was 90% and the overall laryngeal preservation rate was 91%, showing that the procedure is safe with good functional and oncological outcome for patients with early hypopharyngeal cancer.[44]

Primary partial laryngectomy (PL) with neck dissection is an important treatment option for locally advanced lesions. It is important to note that surgical salvage does not appear to improve survival; it is important to understand the goal of treatment before embarking on them. Improved locoregional control may represent a better quality of life, however consideration of the surgical morbidity and recovery in the context of the recurrent patient's performance status are essential. The patients treated with PL as a primary option revealed a better 5-year disease-free survival than the patients who performed surgery as a salvage procedure (35.8% vs. 11.7%, respectively; $p < 0.05$). Salvage surgery is also associated with higher complication rates and morbidity.[53] Siegel et al. showed that in advanced laryngeal tumors treated with nonsurgical therapies, early survival rates are excellent but these rates decline over time.[54]

Total Laryngectomy with Pharyngectomy

For large tumor involving the posterior wall or the postcricoid region, resection with adequate margins results in a circumferential defect. The continuity of the upper digestive tract between the oropharynx and the esophagus is interrupted and the resultant defect is circumferential. A pharyngolaryngoesophagectomy is required when tumors extend to the cervical esophagus. The defect is usually reconstructed by gastric pull-up where there is only a single anastomosis in the upper neck.[44]

Thomas VT et al. found that laryngectomy improved 5-year overall survival when compared to treatment with chemoradiotherapy (41.5% vs. 18.5%). Although the chemoradiotherapy included unresectable patients, they concluded that surgery resulted in more favorable outcomes.[55] Similar results were seen in another study by Harris et al.[56]

Despite advances in diagnostic methods and treatment, the prognosis of advanced hypopharyngeal cancer remains poor. Though there are various options for treating moderately advanced cancers of the hypopharynx that are candidates for extended total laryngectomy or total laryngopharyngectomy: radical surgery alone, neoadjuvant chemotherapy, and the introduction of molecular therapies, but none have shown better results in terms of survival to surgery plus radiation therapy. A multidisciplinary approach is essential in selecting the best possible treatment specific to each individual patient and to improve the design of future clinical trials. Total laryngectomy is considered the gold standard in advanced hypopharyngeal cancers; the main complication of this procedure is a pharyngocutaneous fistula with an incidence of 37% in this setting.[57] Despite technical advances and the use of prophylactic antibiotics, postoperative fistula is still a major problem for these patients and is the main cause for prolonged hospital stay and postoperative morbidity. Total laryngectomy extended to the pharynx with adjuvant radiation therapy offers good oncological outcomes in terms of locoregional control of disease and survival for locally advanced hypopharyngeal cancer and therefore organ preservation protocols should achieve similar oncological results to those demonstrated for laryngectomy for them to be considered a valid alternative.[58]

Although surgery with postoperative radiotherapy is usually considered to provide higher cure rates for patients with cancer of the hypopharynx than any other treatment modality, in the past, a major cohort of patients were not eligible for surgical treatment.[59-61] However, the ability to reconstruct even extended circular pharyngeal defects by means of innovative and dependable reconstructive surgical techniques significantly expanded the ability to resect even locally advanced primaries. Local control, even at the price of a sacrificed larynx, is probably more important for the patients' well-being than organ preservation. Patients with stage IV disease have a poor prognosis because advanced lymph node metastases which commonly represent systemic spread of the tumor beyond the limits of localized cancer treatment (radiation and surgery) and predictable local or regional control of the disease is the best palliation, if cure cannot be achieved.[62,63]

Surgery as the initial treatment can be an option if the following conditions are present:

- Primary tumor and regional metastases appear to be completely resectable
- Distant metastases not detected during preoperative evaluation
- Coexisting malignancies do not preclude a curative approach
- General health status that is considered sufficient to withstand operative trauma
- Patient is motivated to undergo surgery and capable of dealing with the consequences of such treatment.

Manubrium Resection and Mediastinal Tracheostomy

In the presence of locally advanced tumor with major esophageal or tracheal invasion, or in those patients with level VI nodal metastasis, or when tumors recur in the parastomal region after previous surgery, manubrium resection provides a better exposure to ensure complete tumor clearance with better marginal control. With attention to surgical details, it is a useful adjunct to tumor resection with minimal morbidities. When the remaining stump of the trachea is short, relocation inferior to the innominate artery allows the terminal tracheostome to be fashioned with less tension. Furthermore, the pectoralis major myocutaneous flap can be used to reconstruct the posterior tracheal wall if necessary and the muscle of the flap protects the exposed great vessels from exposure or damage when anastomotic leakage occurs.[44]

RADIATION-BASED ORGAN PRESERVATION STRATEGIES

In early stage (T1/T2) carcinomas of the pyriform sinus, primary radiotherapy (RT) results in excellent locoregional control rates and disease-specific survival rates, however these decline for tumors >6.5 mL in volume.[64] In addition to oncological results, the increase in tumor size results in increasing likelihood of a dysfunctional larynx. Pameijer et al. reported a good control rates in early hypopharynx carcinoma and in addition to a tumor volume of 6.5 mL, involvement of the pyriform sinus apex was also a negative prognostic factor.[38] Wang et al. also showed 5-year local control rates of around 75%.[65]

In patients with locally advanced carcinomas of the hypopharynx (stage III/IVA), primary radiotherapy is normally administered in combination with chemotherapy. Although concurrent chemoradiotherapy (CCRT) has improved locoregional control rates when compared to radiotherapy alone, the toxicity rates are significantly higher.[66,67]

Almost half of those with locally advanced hypopharyngeal carcinomas develop local recurrences after primary CCRT and the 5-year survival rate ranges between 5 and 30%.[66-69] Also, severe functional disabilities result in about 30% of patients. Many studies have observed side effects of CCRT such as swallowing difficulties due to impaired motility, strictures of the hypopharynx or upper esophagus.[70-72]

Induction chemotherapy with cisplatin and 5-fluorouracil combined with radiotherapy is another nonsurgical organ-preservation approach in head and neck cancer. A meta-analysis did not shown any clear benefit of induction chemotherapy in terms of locoregional control, survival, or control of distant metastases.[40]

The European Organization for Research and Treatment of Cancer (EORTC) 24891 studied hypopharynx carcinomas; induction chemotherapy followed by radical RT was compared with primary laryngopharyngectomy followed by postoperative RT in two arms. About half of patients with chemotherapy had complete responses in both the primary and nodal disease. Patients who did not respond to chemotherapy underwent total laryngectomy with partial pharyngectomy and postoperative RT. Those with residual or recurrent cancer underwent salvage surgery. Local and regional control rates were similar in both arms. The 5-year disease-specific survival rate was 36% in the surgery arm and 29% in the chemotherapy arm. Their final analysis revealed the likelihood of living with a functional larynx 5 years after treatment was 22%.[73] They concluded that induction chemotherapy followed by radiotherapy offered good organ preservation without a significant compromise in survival. However, a critical analysis showed that only 52 out of 100 patients completed their chemotherapy cycles according to the study protocol due to several reasons, which resulted in a relatively small number for the final evaluation. There were two treatment-related deaths noted. Although almost all patients had stage III/IV disease, 38 patients had T2 primary tumors with intact vocal cord mobility who may have been candidates for partial laryngectomies.[40]

In the EORTC trial 24954 by Lefebvre et al., 450 patients with untreated, nonmetastatic, and resectable T2-T4N0-N2 laryngeal or hypopharyngeal cancers were randomly assigned to sequential chemotherapy with radiation therapy arm (two cycles of induction chemotherapy with cisplatin/5-fluorouracil, followed in case of response by two additional cycles, followed on day 80 by conventional external beam radiotherapy to a dose of 70 Gy in 35 fractions over 7 weeks) or to alternating chemoradiotherapy arm [cisplatin/5-fluorouracil cycle in weeks 1, 4, 7, and 10, alternated with external beam radiotherapy (20 Gy in 10 fractions) during the three 2-week intervals]. Nonresponders were treated with surgery and postoperative RT. The primary endpoint was survival with a functional larynx. At a median follow-up of 6.5 years, overall survival (median 4.4 and 5.2 years) and progression-free survival (median 3 and 3.1 years) were similar for both arms. At 3 years, the cumulative incidence of larynx events was 46% in control arm and 38% in experimental arm (p = 0.09). They concluded that an 8% difference in larynx function preservation rate at 3 years favoring alternating chemoradiotherapy over sequential chemoradiotherapy did not translate into statistically significant differences.[74]

Alternative approaches have included modifications of chemotherapy regimens and changes in RT fractionation. In a phase II study, induction chemotherapy with paclitaxel or cisplatin followed by concomitant boost RT was achieved in patients with larynx or hypopharynx cancer who had responded to chemotherapy; 3-year survival rate with preserved and functional larynx was 43% with acceptable late toxicity.[75] The reasons very low 5-year survival rates (15–45%) in stage III/IV hypopharyngeal SCC are related to multiple factors other than lymphatic and systemic spread such as a susceptibility to develop secondary malignancies, repeated association with major alcohol abuse, associated comorbidities, and frequent nutritional deficiencies.

In early-staged hypopharyngeal cancer, the overall survival and disease-specific survival rates achieved with radical RT are comparable to that after surgery. However, for advanced staged disease, the results of radical RT followed by salvage surgery for residual or recurrent tumors are inferior to those after primary surgery with adjuvant RT. It must be emphasized that many chemoradiotherapy trials had different mix of patients with laryngeal and hypopharyngeal cancers, making interpretation and meaningful comparisons difficult.

Lefebvre et al. reported a result from phase III study conducted by the EORTC randomly treating 194 patients with stage II-IV hypopharyngeal SCC treated with either surgery and postoperative RT or induction chemotherapy, followed by radical RT for patients with complete response and surgery for nonresponders. The survival at 5 years was about a third of patients, with survival comparable in both arms. This trial was a landmark one that established radiation-based organ preservation strategies in hypopharyngeal cancer.[76] Another randomized control trial by Beauvillain et al. compared the results of surgical and nonsurgical therapy for resectable hypopharyngeal tumors. They established two groups, the first was treated with induction chemotherapy followed by radical surgery with postoperative RT and the second was treated with induction chemotherapy followed by RT. The authors found an overall survival of 37% in the first group compared to 19% in the second group. In terms of response to induction chemotherapy, they observed better statistically significant survival with a complete or partial response to induction chemotherapy in patients in the radical surgery group with a 40% survival compared to 20% survival in the RT group. However, no statistically significant differences were observed in the patients who did not respond to chemotherapy, with 22% survival in the first group and 12.5% in the second group.[77]

A retrospective single-institution review by Harris et al. found greater survival in patients with hypopharyngeal tumors treated with radical surgery followed by adjuvant RT as compared to definitive CCRT, but was not statistically significant (66.3% vs. 41.3%). A large population-based study comparing surgical and nonsurgical therapies showed comparable survival for patients with T3 disease (40% vs. 39%; p = 0.475), but not for patients with T4 disease (29% vs. 24%; p = 0.039).[39] However, the Surveillance, Epidemiology, and End Results (SEER) database analysis did not find a survival difference for T4 patients between surgical and nonsurgical treatments (29.9% vs. 26.1%; p = 0.439).[1]

Although CCRT is the most popular option and acknowledged to be efficient in the larynx (at the expense of more toxic effects), no trial has clearly demonstrated it to be superior to neoadjuvant chemotherapy in hypopharyngeal carcinomas. The preservation of laryngeal form and function is possible in a majority of patients with hypopharyngeal cancers with primary nonsurgical approach is currently an accepted notion. It is still not very clear whether planned early surgical salvage following chemoradiotherapy can be considered comparable to surgery followed by adjuvant therapy in terms of survival.[78]

The presence of a tracheostomy can impact survival in nonsurgical organ preservation-based approaches; it increases the predisposition aspiration, perichondritis and chondroradionecrosis, radiodermatitis, and dysphagia. However, all patients with tracheostomy are not at high risk of these complications; in the absence of demonstrable laryngeal dysfunction and care of the tracheostomy, it can result in favorable outcomes.[79]

OUTCOMES

Outcomes in hypopharyngeal cancer are modest due to the reasons explained earlier. **Table 2** shows the 5-year relative survival rates (likelihood of survival when compared to age-matched controls) for patients of laryngeal cancer treated between 2009 and 2015.[80] Often population-based survival rates are a better reflection of actual patient survival as clinical trial participants have much better survival than those in the general population.

SALVAGE SURGERY

Surgery is reserved as a salvage option in failed organ preservation protocols, except in T4 cancers where it is the primary treatment modality. Pharyngocutaneous fistula (PCF) is the most significant complication after a laryngectomy and it is most often associated with other wound-related complications and previous radiotherapy. PCF rates as high as 65% have been reported and with the advent of free visceral and fasciocutaneous flaps, the rates have considerably decreased.[81-83]

Although in general, it is imperative to obtain a tissue diagnosis before embarking on salvage surgery, in rare exceptions surgical salvage can be performed without repeatedly waiting for a definite histopathology report. Salvage laryngectomy after three consecutive negative biopsies in clinical residual or recurrent carcinoma of larynx/hypopharynx can be indicated when:

- Clinical and radiological residual or recurrent disease with life-threatening symptoms to justify immediate salvage surgery without a positive histopathological report
- Persistent postradiation edema with life-threatening symptoms of other radiation sequelae such as severe aspiration or bronchopneumonia
- Clinically or radiologically evident progressive disease significantly involving the hypopharynx preventing the tumor from progression toward inoperability
- No definite tumor residue or recurrence, clinically and radiologically present, but (a) severely mutilated endolarynx with no useful voice production and chronic aspiration and (b) severe painful perichondritis with chondronecrosis of the entire laryngeal framework not responding to conservative management.

When surgical ablation is possible, treatment approach is usually a total laryngopharyngectomy. When tumor extends circumferentially to the whole hypopharyngeal mucosa or involves the pharyngoesophageal junction, a circular total laryngopharyngectomy (CTLP) with reconstruction is required. Surgical decisions are made based on multidisciplinary planning meetings focusing on tumor resectability, neck fibrosis, presence of massive neck invasion, vascular conditions, and the patient's opinion. Particularly in patients with postradiation fibrosis, with regard to pedicled musculocutaneous flaps such as pectoralis major or latissimus dorsi flaps, the flaps bulkiness often limits tubing of the flap.

The results of salvage treatment after chemoradiotherapy are poor and many of those patients do not qualify for surgery.[84-87] In a report by Taki et al., only 12/41 patients with a recurrence could undergo surgery, of which 7/12 were considered successful.[88]

In advanced hypopharyngeal cancers, including primary and salvage treatment, 5-year overall survival ranges from 17 to around 50%.[89,90] Salvage surgery remains the only curative option for treatment of recurrent hypopharyngeal SCC. Its objective is to obtain tumor control and satisfactory quality of life. However, selection of patients eligible for this type of surgery are important because long-term survival is clearly correlated with the presence of clear margins and the absence of free flap failure. Thus, this treatment should not be

Table 2: Surveillance, Epidemiology, and End Results (SEER) 5-year relative survival rates for laryngeal cancer (2009–2015).

Disease status	*Hypopharyngeal cancer*
Localized	59%
Regional	33%
Metastatic	21%
All SEER stages combined	32%

considered as "palliative" or "debulking" surgery. Fakhry et al. in their study reported that all patients presenting with positive margins died within the year following salvage surgery.[91]

Postcricoid tumors may invade the cricoid, recurrent laryngeal nerves, and upper esophagus. Total esophagectomy and gastric pull-up are preferred for such tumors or those arising in the cervical esophagus. Total esophagectomy may also better treat esophageal skip lesions. Skip lesions are thought to be second primaries and are particularly common (16–18%) in relation with hypopharynx and upper esophageal tumors.[92]

REFERENCES

1. Garneau JC. Hypopharyngeal cancer: a state of the art review. Oral Oncol. 2018;86:244-50.
2. Day D. Hypopharyngeal cancer: looking back, moving forward. Curr Oncol. 2016;23:221-2.
3. Hall SF, Groome PA, Irish J, O'Sullivan B. The natural history of patients with squamous cell carcinoma of the hypopharynx. Laryngoscope. 2008;118:1362-71.
4. Goldstein DP, Kim JJ, Gullane PJ, Montgomery PQ. Tumors of the hypopharynx. In: Montgomery PQ, Evans PH, Gullane PJ (Eds). Principles and Practice of Head and Neck Surgery and Oncology, 2nd edition. London: Informa Healthcare; 2009. pp. 233-41.
5. Helliwell TR. Evidence-based pathology: squamous carcinoma of the hypopharynx. J Clin Pathol. 2003;56:81-5.
6. Mura F, Bertino G, Occhini A, Benazzo M. Surgical treatment of hypopharyngeal cancer: a review of the literature and proposal for a decisional flowchart. Acta Otorhinolaryngol Ital. 2013;33:299-306.
7. Barnes L, Johnson JT. Pathologic and clinical considerations in the evaluation of major head and neck specimens resected for cancer. Part I. Pathol Annu. 1986;21:173-250.
8. Michaels L. Squamous carcinoma of the hypopharynx. In: Michaels L, Hellquist HB (Eds). Ear Nose and Throat Histopathology. London: Springer-Verlag; 1987. pp. 459-63.
9. Kaur T, Sebastian P. Consensus Document for Management of Larynx and Hypopharynx Cancers: Outcome of ICMR Subcommittee on Larynx and Hypopharynx Cancers. New Delhi: Division of Publication and Information; 2017. pp. 1-4.
10. Popescu CR, Bertesteanu SVG, Mirea D, Grigore R, Ionescu D, Popescu B. The epidemiology of hypopharynx and cervical esophagus cancer. J Med Life. 2010;3:396-401.
11. Sapkota A, Gajalakshmi V, Jetly DH, Roychowdhury S, Dikshit RP, Brennan P, et al. Smokeless tobacco and increased risk of hypopharyngeal and laryngeal cancers: a multicentric case-control study from India. Int J Cancer. 2007;121:1793-8.
12. Mishra A, Meherotra R. Head and neck cancer: global burden and regional trends in India. Asian Pacific J Cancer Prev. 2014;15:537-50.
13. Marron M, Boffetta P, Zhang ZF, Zaridze D, Wünsch-Filho V, Winn DM, et al. Cessation of alcohol drinking, tobacco smoking and the reversal of head and neck cancer risk. Int J Epidemiol. 2010;39:182-96.
14. Wyss A, Hashibe M, Chuang SC, Lee YC, Zhang ZF, Yu GP, et al. Cigarette, cigar, and pipe smoking and the risk of head and neck cancers: pooled analysis in the International Head and Neck Cancer Epidemiology Consortium. Am J Epidemiol. 2013;178:679-90.
15. Bradley PJ, Eckel HE. Hypopharyngeal Cancer. Basel: Karger Publishers; 2019. pp. 1-14.
16. Berrino F, Richiardi L, Bofetta P, Estève J, Belletti I, Raymond L, et al. Occupation and larynx and hypopharynx cancer: a job-exposure matrix approach in an international case-control study in France, Italy, Spain and Switzerland. Cancer Causes Control. 2003;14:213-23.
17. Larsson LG, Sandstorm A, Westling P. Relationship of Plummer-Vinson Disease to Cancer of the Upper Alimentary Tract in Sweden. Cancer Res. 1975;33:3308-16.
18. Jacobs A. Anemia and post-cricoid carcinoma. Br J Cancer. 1961;15:736-44.
19. Piazza C, Ribeiro J, Bernal-Sprekelsen M, Paiva A, Peretti G. Anatomy and physiology of the larynx and hypopharynx. In: Anniko M, Bernal-Sprekelsen M, Bonkowsky V, Bradley P, Iurato S (Eds). Otorhinolaryngology, Head and Neck Surgery. Berlin: Springer; 2010. pp. 165-73.
20. Belafsky PC, Lintzenich CR. Development, anatomy, and physiology of the pharynx. In: Shaker R, Belafsky PC, Postma GN, Easterling C (Eds). Principles of Deglutition: A Multidisciplinary Text for Swallowing and its Disorders. New York: Springer; 2013. pp. 165-73.
21. Raven RW. Post-cricoid carcinoma. J Laryngol Otol. 1958; 72:385-96.
22. Byrnes CK. Post-cricoid cancer. Ir J Med Sci. 1950;293:236-43.
23. Islam MN, Siddiqui MM, Ahmed S. Hypopharyngeal carcinoma: a review. J Curr Adv Med Res. 2016;3:26-30.
24. Hillel AD, Schwartz AN. Trumpet maneuver for visual and CT examination of the pyriform sinus and retrocricoid area. Head Neck. 1989;11:231-6.
25. Trotter W. Malignant disease of the hypopharynx and its treatment by excision. Br Med J. 1932;1:510-3.
26. Badwal JS. Pathways of invasion in laryngeal cancer: The concept behind the strategy of surgical management. World J Pharm Med Res. 2017;3:183-7.
27. Wenig BL, Ziffra KL, Mafee MF, Schild JA. MR imaging of squamous cell carcinoma of the larynx and hypopharynx. Otolaryngol Clin North Am. 1995;28:609-19.
28. Jackson CL, Blady JV. Criteria for the selection of treatment of cancer of the larynx. Arch Otolaryngol. 1943;37: 672-9.
29. Lumley JSP, D'Cruz AK, Hoballah JJ. Nose and throat. In: Lumley JSP, D'Cruz AK, Hoballah JJ, Scott-Connor CE (Eds). Hamilton Bailey's Demonstrations of Physical Signs in Clinical Surgery, 19th edition. Boca Raton, Florida: CRC Press, Taylor & Francis Group; 2016. pp. 377-90.
30. Wycliffe ND, Grover RS, Kim PD, Simental A. Hypopharyngeal cancer. Top Magn Reson Imaging. 2007;18:243-58.
31. Zbären P, Becker M, Läng H. Pretherapeutic staging of hypopharyngeal carcinoma. Clinical findings, computed tomography, and magnetic resonance imaging compared with histopathologic evaluation. Arch Otolaryngol Head Neck Surg. 1997;123:908-13.
32. Zbären P, Becker M, Läng H. Staging of laryngeal cancer: endoscopy, computed tomography and magnetic resonance versus histopathology. Eur Arch Otorhinolaryngol. 1997; 254:S117-22.
33. Becker M, Zbären P, Läng H. Neoplastic invasion of the laryngeal cartilage: comparison of MR imaging and CT with histopathologic correlation. Radiology. 1995;194:661-9.

34. Castelijns JA, van den Brekel MW, Hermans R. Imaging of the larynx. Semin Roentgenol. 2000;35:31-41.
35. Hsu WC, Loevner LA, Karpati R, Ahmed T, Mong A, Battineni ML, et al. Accuracy of magnetic resonance imaging in predicting absence of fixation of head and neck cancer to the prevertebral space. Head Neck. 2005;27:95-100.
36. Hermans R. Imaging of hypopharyngeal and cervical oesophageal cancer. Cancer Imaging. 2003;4:7-9.
37. Schmalfuss IM. Imaging of the hypopharynx and cervical esophagus. Magn Reson Imaging Clin North Am. 2002;10: 495-509.
38. Pameijer FA, Mancuso AA, Mendenhall WM, Parsons JT, Mukherji SK, Hermans R, et al. Evaluation of pretreatment computed tomography as a predictor of local control in T1/T2 pyriform sinus carcinoma treated with definitive radiotherapy. Head Neck. 1998;20:159-68.
39. Petersen JF, Timmermans AJ, van Dijk BAC, Overbeek LIH, Smit LA, Hilgers FJM, et al. Trends in treatment, incidence and survival of hypopharynx cancer: a 20-year population-based study in the Netherlands. Eur Arch Otorhinolaryngol. 2018;275:181-9.
40. Cheng CT, Lin CY, Hung-Chun CS, Lin YP, Lim LC, Pennarun N, et al. Survival benefit of surgical approach for advanced oropharyngeal and hypopharyngeal cancer: a retrospective analysis. Head Neck. 2017;39:2104-113.
41. Ambrosch P, Fazel A. Functional organ preservation in laryngeal and hypopharyngeal cancer. GMS Curr Top Otorhinolaryngol Head Neck Surg. 2011;10:1-31.
42. Steiner W, Ambrosch P, Hess CF, Kron M. Organ preservation by transoral laser microsurgery in piriform sinus carcinoma. Otolaryngol Head Neck Surg. 2001;124:58-67.
43. Rudert HH. The CO_2 laser in the management of hypopharyngeal cancer. Curr Opin Otolaryngol Head Neck Surg. 2002;10:118-22.
44. Karatzanis AD, Psychogios G, Waldfahrer F, Zenk J, Hornung J, Velegrakis GA, et al. T1 and T2 hypopharyngeal cancer treatment with laser microsurgery. J Surg Oncol. 2010;102:27-33.
45. Chan JYW, Wei WI. Current management strategy of hypopharyngeal carcinoma. Auris Nasus Larynx. 2013;40:2-6.
46. Mendenhall WM, Parsons JT, Cassisi NJ, Million RR. Squamous cell carcinoma of the pyriform sinus treated with radical radiation therapy. Radiother Oncol. 1987;9:201-8.
47. Ho CM, Ng WF, Lam KH, Wei WJ, Yuen AP. Submucosal tumor extension in hypopharyngeal cancer. Arch Otolaryngol Head Neck Surg. 1997;123:959-65.
48. Ogura J, Jurema A, Watson R. Partial laryngopharyngectomy and neck dissection for pyriform sinus cancer. Conservation surgery with immediate reconstruction. Laryngoscope. 1960;70:1399-417.
49. Ogura JH, Marks JE, Freemann RB. Results of conservation surgery for cancers of the supraglottis and pyriform sinus. Laryngoscope. 1980;90:591-600.
50. Laccourreye H, St Guily JL, Brasnu D, Fabre A, Menard M. Supracricoid hemilaryngopharyngectomy. Analysis of 240 cases. Ann Otol Rhinol Laryngol. 1987;96:217-21.
51. Chevalier RJ, Watelet JB, Darras JA, Piquet JJ. Supraglottic hemilaryngopharyngectomy plus radiation for the treatment of early lateral margin and pyriform sinus carcinoma. Head Neck. 1997;19:1-5.
52. Foucher M, Poissonnet G, Rame JP, Toussaint B, Védrine PO, Dassonville O, et al. T1-T2 N0 hypopharyngeal cancers treated with surgery alone. A GETTEC study (French Neck Study Group). Ann Otolaryngol Chir Cervicofac. 2009;126:203-7.
53. Rodrigues J, Breda E, Monteiro E. Surgically-Treated Locoregionally Advanced Hypopharyngeal Cancer: Outcomes. Int Arch Otorhinolaryngol. 2018;22:443-8.
54. Siegel R, Naishadham D, Jemal A. Cancer statistics, 2013. CA Cancer J Clin. 2013;63:11-30.
55. Thomas VT, Nittala MR, Bhanat E, Albert AA, Vijayakumar S. Management of Advanced-stage Hypopharyngeal Carcinoma: 25-Year Experience from a Tertiary Care Medical Center. Cureus. 2020;12:e6679.
56. Harris BN, Biron VL, Donald P, Farwell DG, Luu QC, Bewley AF, et al. Primary surgery vs. chemoradiation treatment of advanced-stage hypopharyngeal squamous cell carcinoma. JAMA Otolaryngol Head Neck Surg. 2015; 141:636-40.
57. Virtaniemi JA, Kumpulainen EJ, Hirvikoski PP, Johansson RT, Kosma VM. The incidence and etiology of postlaryngectomy pharyngocutaneous fistulas. Head Neck. 2001;23:29-33.
58. García-Cabo HP, Fernández-Vañes L, Álvarez FL, Marcos CA, Llorente JL, Rodrigo JP. Results of total laryngectomy as treatment for locally advanced hypopharyngeal cancer. Acta Otorrinolaringol Esp. 2017;68:328-35.
59. Eckel HE, Staar S, Volling P, Sittel C, Damm M, Jungehuelsing M. Surgical treatment for hypopharynx carcinoma: feasibility, mortality, and results. Otolaryngol Head Neck Surg. 2001; 124:561-9.
60. Kleinsasser O, Glanz H, Kimmich T. Treatment of carcinoma of the piriform sinus. HNO. 1989;37:460-4.
61. Axon PR, Woolford TJ, Hargreaves SP, Yates P, Birzgalis AR, Farrington WT. A comparison of surgery and radiotherapy in the management of post-cricoid carcinoma. Clin Otolaryngol Allied Sci. 1997;22:370-4.
62. de Vries EJ, Stein DW, Johnson JT, Wagner RL, Schusterman MA, Myers EN, et al. Hypopharyngeal reconstruction: a comparison of two alternatives. Laryngoscope. 1989;99:614-7.
63. Julieron M, Germain MA, Schwaab G, Marandas P, Bourgain JL, Wibault P, et al. Reconstruction with free jejunal autograft after circumferential pharyngolaryngectomy: eighty-three cases. Ann Otol Rhinol Laryngol. 1998;107:581-7.
64. Mendenhall WM, Morris CG, Amdur RJ, Hinerman RW, Mancuso AA. Parameters that predict local control after definitive radiotherapy for squamous cell carcinoma of the head and neck. Head Neck. 2003;25:535-42.
65. Wang CC. Carcinoma of the hypopharynx. In: Wang CC (Ed). Radiation Therapy for Head and Neck Neoplasms. New York: John Wiley & Sons, Inc.; 1998. pp. 205-20.
66. Prades JM, Schmitt TM, Timoshenko AP, Simon PG, de Cornulier J, Durand M, et al. Concomitant chemoradiotherapy in pyriform sinus carcinoma. Arch Otolaryngol Head Neck Surg. 2002;128:384-8.
67. Khan A, Spiro JD, Dowsett R, Greenberg BR. Sequential chemotherapy and radiotherapy for organ preservation in advanced resectable nonlaryngeal head and neck cancer. Am J Clin Oncol. 1999;22:403-7.
68. Jones AS. Tumors of the hypopharynx. In: Jones AS, Philipps DE, Hilgers FJ (Eds). Diseases of the Head and Neck, Nose and Throat. New York: Oxford University Press, Inc.; 1998. pp. 230-49.
69. Bahadur S, Thakar A, Mohanti BK, Lal P. Results of radiotherapy with, or without, salvage surgery versus combined surgery and radiotherapy in advanced carcinoma of the hypopharynx. J Laryngol Otol. 2002;116:29-32.
70. Lazarus CL, Logemann JA, Pauloski BR, Colangelo LA, Kahrilas PJ, Mittal BB, et al. Swallowing disorders in head and

neck cancer patients treated with radiotherapy and adjuvant chemotherapy. Laryngoscope. 1996;106:1157-66.
71. Kotz T, Abraham S, Beitler J, Wadler S, Smith RV. Pharyngeal transport dysfunction consequent to an organ-sparing protocol. Arch Otolaryngol Head Neck Surg. 1999;125: 410-3.
72. Lazarus C, Logemann JA, Shi G, Kahrilas P, Pelzer H, Kleinjan K. Does laryngectomy improve swallowing after chemoradiotherapy? A case study. Arch Otolaryngol Head Neck Surg. 2002;128:54-7.
73. Lefebvre JL, Chevalier D, Luboinski B, Traissac L, Andry G, de Raucourt D. Is laryngeal preservation (LP) with induction chemotherapy (ICT) safe in the treatment of hypopharyngeal SCC? Final results of the phase III EORTC 24891 trial. J Clin Oncol. 2004;14:5531.
74. Lefebvre JL, Horiot JC, Rolland F, Tesselaar M, Leemans CR, Geoffrois L, et al. Phase III study on larynx preservation comparing induction chemotherapy and radiotherapy versus alternating chemoradiotherapy in resectable hypopharynx and larynx cancers. EORTC protocol 24954-22950. J Clin Oncol. 2007;18:6016.
75. Dietz A, Rudat V, Dreyhaupt J, Pritsch M, Hoppe F, Hagen R, et al. Induction chemotherapy with paclitaxel and cisplatin followed by radiotherapy for larynx organ preservation in advanced laryngeal and hypopharyngeal cancer offers moderate late toxicity outcome (DeLOS-I-trial). Eur Arch Otorhinolaryngol. 2009;266:1291-300.
76. Lefebvre JL, Chevalier D, Luboinski B, Kirkpatrick A, Collette L, Sahmoud T. Larynx Preservation in Pyriform Sinus Cancer: Preliminary Results of a European Organization for Research and Treatment of Cancer Phase III Trial. J Natl Cancer Inst. 1996;88:890-9.
77. Beauvillain C, Mahé M, Bourdin S, Peuvrel P, Bergerot P, Rivière A, et al. Final results of a randomized trial comparing chemotherapy plus radiotherapy with chemotherapy plus surgery plus radiotherapy in locally advanced resectable hypopharyngeal carcinomas. Laryngoscope. 1997;107:648-53.
78. Gupta T, Chopra S, Agarwal JP, Laskar SG, D'cruz AK, Shrivastava SK, et al. Squamous cell carcinoma of the hypopharynx: Single-institution outcome analysis of a large cohort of patients treated with primary non-surgical approaches. Acta Oncol. 2009;48:541-8.
79. Varghese BT, Babu S, Desai KP, Bava AS, George P, Iype EM, et al. Prospective study of outcomes of surgically treated larynx and hypopharyngeal cancers. Indian J Cancer. 2014;51: 104-8.
80. National Institutes of Health (NIH). (2020). SEER Cancer Statistics Review (CSR) 1975-2016. [online] Available from https://seer.cancer.gov/csr/1975_2016/. [Last accessed July, 2020].
81. Varghese BT, Sebastian P, Mathew A. Treatment outcome in patients undergoing surgery for carcinoma larynx and hypopharynx: a follow-up study. Acta Otolaryngol. 2009;129:1480-5.
82. Dedivitis RA, Ribeiro KC, Castro MA, Nascimento PC. Pharyngocutaneous fistula following total laryngectomy. Acta Otorhinolaryngol Ital. 2007;27:2-5.
83. Murray DJ, Gilbert RW, Vesely MJ, Novak CB, Zaitlin-Gencher S, Clark JR, et al. Functional outcomes and donor site morbidity following circumferential pharyngoesophageal reconstruction using an anterolateral thigh flap and salivary bypass tube. Head Neck. 2007;29: 147-54.
84. Varghese BT, Paul S, Elizabeth MI, Somanathan T, Elizabeth KA. Late postradiation laryngeal chondronecrosis with pharyngooesophageal fibrosis. Indian J Cancer. 2004; 41:81-4.
85. Rodriguez J, Point D, Brunin F, Jaulerry C, Brugère J. Surgery of the hypopharynx after radiotherapy. Bull Cancer Radiother. 1996;83:17-23.
86. Davidson J, Keane T, Brown D, Freeman J, Gullane P, Irish J, et al. Surgical salvage after radiotherapy for advanced laryngopharyngeal carcinoma. Arch Otolaryngol Head Neck Surg. 1997;123:420-4.
87. Clark JR, Gilbert R, Irish J, Brown D, Neligan P, Gullane P. Morbidity after flap reconstruction of hypopharyngeal defects. Laryngoscope. 2006;116:173-81.
88. Taki S, Homma A, Oridate N, Suzuki S, Suzuki F, Sakashita T, et al. Salvage surgery for local recurrence after chemoradiotherapy or radiotherapy in hypopharyngeal cancer patients. Eur Arch Otorhinolaryngol. 2010;267:1765-9.
89. Patel RS, Goldstein DP, Brown D, Irish J, Gullane PJ, Gilbert RW. Circumferential pharyngeal reconstruction: history, critical analysis of techniques, and current therapeutic recommendations. Head Neck. 2010;32:109-20.
90. Kadota H, Fukushima J, Nakashima T, Kumamoto Y, Yoshida S, Yasumatsu R, et al. Comparison of salvage and planned pharyngolaryngectomy with jejunal transfer for hypopharyngeal carcinoma after chemoradiotherapy. Laryngoscope. 2010;120:1103-8.
91. Fakhry N, Chamorey E, Michel J, Collet C, Santini L, Poissonnet G, et al. Salvage circular laryngopharyngectomy and radial forearm free flap for recurrent hypopharyngeal cancer. Laryngoscope. 2013;123:910-5.
92. Wookey H. The surgical treatment of carcinoma of the hypopharynx and the oesophagus. Br J Surg. 1948;35:249-66.

CHAPTER

15 Cancers of the Nasal Cavity and Vestibule

Adharsh Anand, Sivakumar Vidhyadharan, Narayana Subramaniam, Samskruthi P Murthy

INTRODUCTION

Sinonasal malignancies are rare when compared to other head and neck sites and comprises only 3% of head and neck cancers.[1] Owing to its intricate anatomy and late presentations the outcomes are also poor when compared to other sites in the head and neck region. The nasal cavity and paranasal sinuses are intimately associated with each other and as well as with orbit, pterygopalatine fossa, infratemporal fossa and as well as anterior and lateral skull base. There are numerous foraminas, canals and fissures that allow communication of these spaces and hence critical structure involvement often occurs. Of these only 20–30% of these cancers have their root of origin from nasal cavity and vestibule. Since malignancies affecting maxilla and ethmoid sinus are discussed elsewhere this chapter is focused on tumors affecting nasal cavity and vestibule.

ANATOMY

The nasal vestibule is the entrance to the nasal cavity and is lined by skin with numerous hair follicles and sebaceous glands. The vestibule is a three sided, pear-shaped cavity, about 1.5 cm in diameter, which ends posteriorly at the limen nasi. The alar cartilages form the anterolateral wall. The medial wall is the columella, formed by the medial wing of the alar cartilage and the anterior portion of the cartilaginous septum. The floor is the maxilla. The lymphatic drainage is to level IB nodes, though occasionally there is risk of the involvement of perifacial nodes at the level of facial neurovascular bundles behind the commissural area.

The nasal cavity begins at the limen nasi and ends at the posterior nares, where it communicates with the nasopharynx. The lateral walls are composed of thin bony folds that project into the nasal cavity, the inferior, medial and superior turbinates. The nasolacrimal duct enters the nasal cavity beneath the inferior turbinate. The ethmoidal bullae and the frontal sinus connect to the nasal cavity with openings in the middle meatus. The sphenoid sinus opens into the nasal cavity via an opening in the anterior wall of the sinus. Approximately 20 branches of the olfactory nerve enter the nasal cavity through the cribriform plate, with nerve fibers distributed over the upper third of septum and the superior nasal turbinate. The epithelium here is nonciliated columnar whereas the inferior portion of the nasal cavity which is the respiratory portion is lined by ciliated columnar. There are numerous collections of lymphoid tissue and mucous glands beneath the epithelium. The lymphatics of the nasal cavity are separated into the olfactory group and respiratory group. The lymphatics of the olfactory region drain posteriorly and terminate in the lateral pharyngeal space in the jugular chain at the skull-base region, while the respiratory lymphatics drain into to the lateral retropharyngeal nodes or even directly to the level II lymph nodes.

EPIDEMIOLOGY

Sinonasal malignancies are twice as common in males and are most commonly seen in the 5th–7th decades of life. This is more often true in carcinomas, though some group of malignancies also present early in life especially lymphoreticular tumors and rhabdomyosarcoma. Squamous cell carcinoma (SCC) and adenocarcinomas are the most common tumors of this region.[2]

Industrial exposure to nickel, leather, textile dust, wood dust, chromium, formaldehyde and asbestos has been implicated as causative factors in sinonasal oncogenesis. Nasal snuff usage also has been associated with sinonasal malignancies; this is a type of powdered tobacco that is sniffed into the nose and is commonly use in South East Asia and some South American countries.

Nasal smoking is another practice that has been associated with sinonasal malignancies.[3-9]

CLINICAL PRESENTATION

Patients can present at any age; carcinomas are common between 5th and 7th decades while sarcomas can present in childhood or adolescence. Malignant lesions of the basal vestibule often present with symptoms of a slow growing mass with attendant crusting and occasional minor bleeding episodes. Pain out of proportion to the accompanying examination findings is uncommon. Patients may also present with nasal obstruction and blood stained discharge.

In case of nasal cavity lesions, nasal obstruction may be the first symptom that is often missed by the patient. The presentation of these patients is usually in advanced stages when symptoms of local spread appear. Some symptoms of early stage diseases are a low-grade chronic infection with discharge, obstruction and minor intermittent bleeding. Depending upon the focus of origin, symptoms vary. An early lateral wall lesion can cause obstruction of the nasolacrimal duct and cause epiphora, while olfactory area lesions can cause anosmia, nasal obstruction and widening of the nasal bridge. Loosening of teeth, radiating pain, ulceration into the oral cavity, trismus, and a bulge in the cheek may all be symptoms and signs of advanced disease.

INVESTIGATIONS

Investigations include an office endoscopy and biopsy that may be a punch or a wedge biopsy depending on the area and access. Further evaluation is based on the histology, which may include cross-sectional imaging in the form of contrast-enhanced computerized tomography (CECT) or magnetic resonance imaging (MRI) in case of epithelial and nonepithelial malignant neoplasms of this region. Cross-sectional imaging should encompass the entire head and neck region. Metastatic evaluation may either be a CT thorax with bone scan and abdominal ultrasound or a positron emission tomography fused with CECT (PET-CT). Histology suggestive of a lymphoproliferative disorder warrants additional staging investigations such as immunohistochemistry, blood biochemistry, and bone marrow aspiration or biopsy. If the histology is mucosal melanoma, sentinel lymph node biopsy may be valuable for the assessment of nodal metastasis. Even metastasis from an unknown primary may present in this region, most commonly renal cell carcinoma. These investigations assist staging and further treatment planning. Basal cell carcinomas (BCC) are often superficial and since lymphatic metastasis are rare, they can be considered for treatment without any further evaluation.

PATHOLOGY

Malignant lesions of the nasal cavity and vestibule exhibit a wide range of pathology mainly due to the diversity of cells in this area. The common tumors are epithelial (SCC), salivary gland (adenocarcinoma, adenoid cystic carcinoma), cutaneous (basal cell carcinoma), neuroendocrine (sinonasal undifferentiated carcinoma, esthesioneuroblastoma), lymphoproliferative (lymphoma) or metastatic (renal cell carcinoma). Further details are discussed in the chapter on tumors of the paranasal sinuses and anterior skull base.

STAGING

There is no universal staging for tumors of the nasal vestibule. Staging does not seem to affect the prognosis as these tumors, as staging often is dependent on the site of origin while survival is dependent on tumor biology. Wang et al. in their series of 36 patients described a staging system for tumors of the nasal vestibule **(Table 1)**.[10]

The nodal staging that they used was similar to the American Joint Committee on Cancer staging for nasal cavity and ethmoid sinus tumors[11] (refer Chapter 16). Only one other report by Patel et al.[12] has used this TNM staging with similar results. For cutaneous malignancies and mucosal melanomas, the staging is as per corresponding histology.

ROUTES OF TUMOR SPREAD

Cancers of the vestibule often spreads locally, with the pattern of invasion depending on the type of cancer; SCC and melanoma are known for early lymphatic metastasis while BCC is locally infiltrative. Cancers of the vestibule spread locally to the adjacent septum and bone that may be the maxillary bone, nasal bone or the hard palate. It may also extend to nearby facial regions such as ala, cheek, upper lip and labial mucosa.

In case of nasal cavity lesions, the most common location of origin is lateral wall of nasal cavity in SCC

Table 1: A staging system for tumors of the nasal vestibule (Wang et al.).[11]

T1	Tumor limited to nasal vestibule involving one or more sites with only superficial invasion
T2	Tumor extending locally to septum, upper lip and philtrum but not fixed to the underlying bone
T3	More invasive/larger lesions

and ethmoidal sinuses in adenocarcinoma. Olfactory neuroblastoma most commonly arises in the anterior skull-base vault and later extends into the nasal cavity and adjacent sinuses. They may have intracranial extension as well. Superior extension may occur to the skull base, dura and intracranial compartment, as well as frontal sinuses. Lateral extension directly involves the ethmoidal and maxillary sinuses, infratemporal fossa and anterolateral cheek. The peculiarity of the midface skeletal framework is the presence of various foramina through which the neurovascular bundles travel. Spread can occur through these foramina also since these are areas of less resistance. Perineural spread can also occur through these areas. The orbital floor and medial orbital walls are at risk; erosion of these walls can result in direct infiltration of the orbital components. Medially the nasal space allows an easy growth anteriorly and posteriorly. More medial growth results in infiltration of the septum and opposite nasal cavity. Inferiorly direct erosion of the nasal floor can result in an oral communication and a fistula. Posterior extension into the nasopharynx and soft palate is also not uncommon. Presentation at late stages often makes it difficult to identify the epicenter of the disease; this is the why the outcomes of nasal cavity and paranasal sinus malignancies are often described together.

RADIOLOGY

Computerized tomography excels at evaluating fine bone details. Because cortical bone and air have no signal on MRI sequences, an analysis of the normal sinus cavity anatomy is difficult with MRI. CT, however, excels at assessing cortical bone. MRI uses varied pulse sequences to interrogate different aspects of the tissues. This is particularly useful for the evaluation of soft tissues, as the different pulse sequences provide a more detailed evaluation of different tissues. With CT, it is often difficult to distinguish proteinaceous fluid from solid material, but MRI sequences allow the assessment of various fluid compositions. MRI often allows scar tissue to be more readily distinguished from surgical material and recurrent tumors.

When locally aggressive lesions are encountered in the nasal cavity or sinuses, the extent of the lesion is an important diagnostic consideration. Although CT can depict bone erosion and distinguish it from expanded or remodeled bone, this distinction is less important in the setting of aggressive pathology, when bone is presumed to have undergone invasion. MRI is preferred because it can more precisely define the extent of disease invasion into soft tissue structures; an example of this is extension across the cribriform plate. MRI is excellent at distinguishing dural involvement from parenchymal involvement by assessing parenchymal edema and the relationship of the tumor to the dura and to gray and white matter. Postcontrast coronal images of the cribriform plate, as well as axial fluid-attenuation inversion recovery (FLAIR) images, are helpful in this evaluation.

Squamous cell carcinoma of the nasal cavity usually has no specific imaging characteristics that distinguish it from other malignancies. Heterogeneous enhancement with central areas of necrosis, are usually present.[13] Melanoma of the nasal cavity may appear as a well-defined nonaggressive mass, similar to a polyp, or it may be aggressive with extensive invasion of surrounding structures. There are usually no specific imaging clues to this diagnosis, but melanotic melanomas may show intrinsically high T1 signal, without gadolinium enhancement, from melanin content.[14]

Melanomas are often vascular, so extensive enhancement is expected when gadolinium agents are administered. Sinonasal undifferentiated carcinoma (SNUC) also has an aggressive, destructive appearance that may be indistinguishable radiographically from other nasal malignancies.

The diagnosis of esthesioneuroblastoma can usually be suggested by its characteristic pattern of spread; this diagnosis should be considered for any mass that crosses the cribriform plate.[15] Extension across the cribriform plate may be seen with other aggressive tumors, and esthesioneuroblastomas may be confined to the nasal cavity or cranial vault, but there is nonetheless a close association between esthesioneuroblastoma and erosion of the cribriform plate. Also characteristic is the presence of cysts along the intracranial margin of the tumor.[16] Involvement of surrounding structures, such as the orbit, is often noted. Esthesioneuroblastoma enhances briskly, but may show areas of central necrosis when large. Involvement of dura, brain, and orbital contents is better assessed with MRI than with CECT, making MRI the preferred modality for staging and follow-up. CECT and MRI are frequently employed together as complementary examinations during diagnostic evaluation.[17]

The inverted papilloma, a benign neoplasm, may have an aggressive radiographic appearance. These lesions usually extend from the lateral nasal wall into the antrum and the nasal cavity and remodel or erode the surrounding bony septations.[18] A characteristic calcification pattern within the tumor is suggestive of this lesion, but is seen in only 10% of cases.[19] On MRI there may be a distinctive pattern of curvilinear enhancement.[20] Because these tumors are prone to recur, and because they are often associated with SCC, imaging plays an important role in the surveillance of patients after treatment of inverted papilloma.

Chondrosarcoma of the sinuses and nasal cavity has a distinctive CT appearance. The chondroid matrix of the tumor demonstrates an irregular array of fine, curvilinear calcifications. It is usually possible to establish a site of origin radiographically. A midline location, arising from the septum, is most characteristic of chondrosarcoma. Surrounding bone structures may be remodeled or invaded. MRI shows heterogeneous high T2 signal, but the calcification pattern makes CT the preferred modality for diagnostic imaging and follow-up. This is the one aggressive lesion that is best imaged with CT, both for staging and for surveillance after treatment.

Concepts helpful in tailoring an imaging approach to sinonasal disease:

- CECT excels at evaluating fine bone detail
- MRI excels at evaluating soft tissues
- Conventional radiographs are of limited diagnostic use
- Aggressive lesions are best imaged with MRI
- Fibro-osseous lesions are usually better assessed with CECT
- MRI is better than CECT for distinguishing neoplasm from entrapped secretions
- MRI is better than CECT for identifying perineural spread
- Desiccated secretions and fungal infections are a potential pitfall on MRI
- Mucosal thickening may be assessed with either modality, but CECT is less costly
- High-resolution CECT is more flexible for post-hoc analyses.

MANAGEMENT

Surgery

Surgery is the mainstay of treatment and offers the best chance of cure in most histologies when disease can be completely resected. The available approaches are as follows:

- *Endoscopic approach:* The advent of rigid nasal endoscopes and powered endonasal instruments has revolutionized the management of sinonasal disorders, especially in chronic inflammatory disease management. The use of these technologies in the management of sinonasal malignancy was looked at with some skepticism especially because of the need to disobey the standard principle of cancer surgery, en-bloc resection. However, many studies that have looked at endonasal approaches in sinonasal malignancy have shown survival and control rates similar to open approaches, which include open craniofacial resections. Hence, minimally invasive endoscopic resection (MIER) has emerged as an alternative to craniofacial resection (CFR) or other open approaches.

Appropriate surgical instrumentation is a requisite for endoscopic tumor resection. Because adequate visualization is critical, a three-chip endoscopic camera with digital enhancement, a high quality, medical-grade monitor, and an assortment of 0, 30, 45, and 70° telescopes should be available. Powered instrumentation, including soft-tissue shavers and surgical drills, facilitate rapid removal of soft-tissue and bone respectively. Soft-tissue shaver tips are available in 40, 60, 90, and 120° angles that facilitate tumor removal in maxillary and frontal sinuses. Bipolar cautery devices allow for hemostasis and minimize bloody contamination of the surgical field.

Another revolution that has happened is the advent of computer-assisted surgery (CAS). Surgical navigation allows the preoperative imaging data and surgical plan to be directly correlated with the operative field, providing a better safety profile and thereby decreasing morbidity and increasing the efficacy of surgery. The intranasal carotid Doppler is also a very useful tool during extensive anterior and lateral skull-base surgery.[21,22]

Preoperative lumbar drain placement is an option that has been contentious, often left to the surgeon. If there is a skull-base defect anticipated, some surgeons practice a prophylactic tracheostomy to divert the airway to avoid postoperative pneumocephalus. Broadly, MIER encompasses two seemingly divergent surgical strategies. The first strategy may be termed the outside-in approach, in which the surgeon chooses to outflank the tumor by dissecting around the tumor, typically in a submucoperiosteal plane. The second alternative is the inside-out approach, in which the core of large-bulky tumors is removed first and then the peripheral margins of the tumor are collapsed inward for removal. In a few instances, the surgeon may choose only one of these strategies, but in most instances both strategies are used selectively in the same case.

Tumor removal for MIER requires the compulsive tracking of points of tumor attachment, which must be completely dissected to achieve sound surgical margins. The surgeon must develop a three-dimensional tumor map as the tumor is removed. Intraoperative frozen sections are frequently used to guide the resection; 20 or more frozen sections during MIER are not unusual. Complete unilateral or, if clinically indicated, bilateral sphenoethmoidectomy and maxillary antrostomy are performed in most cases. Endoscopic septectomy may be required if the tumor involves the septum or to increase exposure within the paranasal sinus confines. Frontal sinusotomy or endoscopic frontal sinus drill-out may be necessary to obtain the anterior margin for the tumor resection. Unilateral or bilateral endoscopic orbital decompression for removal of the orbital wall may be used to clear the lateral margins. Of course, direct extension into the orbit with invasion of the orbital soft tissue contents may necessitate orbital exenteration. This procedure previously required open approaches, whereas more recently the minimally invasive approach using endoscopic power-assisted orbital exenteration has also been successful.[23]

The skull base is usually addressed after the other parts of the tumor have been removed. Whether to resect the cribriform plate or ethmoid roof is generally decided intraoperatively. If the tumor extends to or frankly erodes this boundary, then resection of the cribriform plate or bony ethmoid roof is appropriate. Angled diamond burr tips can be instrumental in achieving precise and atraumatic resection of this bony margin. Cutting burrs should be avoided on the skull base because they may cause inadvertent tearing of the dura and even intracranial injury. After bone removal, the dura may be sampled for frozen section. If the frozen section shows neoplasm, then dural resection is required. If the tumor has no evidence of extensive transdural violation, endoscopic dural resection should be considered; however, intraoperative consultation with neurosurgery should be obtained. Extensive dural or direct intraparenchymal involvement cannot be cleared strictly through the MIER technique. In these cases, bifrontal craniotomy is required for clearing the superior margin of the tumor. Skull-base defects are appropriately reconstructed.

The extent of surgery depends on the extent of involvement. Postoperative care includes nasal pack removal after 2–3 days. The patient can be discharged with saline nasal spray to keep the cavity clean and wet. Nasal toileting is started 2 weeks postsurgery where the debris and crusts are removed endoscopically without disturbing the reconstructed skull base. Contraindications for endoscopic approach is only for those tumors where accessibility is an issue like lateral part of frontal sinus, extensive intracranial involvement and also when there is extensive maxillary sinus, nasal bone or orbital involvement, where an open approach is a necessity.

- *Open approaches:* These have been discussed in detail in the chapter on paranasal sinuses and anterior skull base.

  In general, the surgical approach based on tumor location and extent is as follows:
  - *Purely intranasal:* Septectomy or medial maxillectomy based on lateral nasal wall involvement
  - *Related to nasal cavity and maxilla:* Limited maxillectomy (medial or infrastructure), subtotal or total maxillectomy
  - *Related to nasal cavity and ethmoid:* Ethmoidectomy or ethmoidosphenoidectomy
  - *Related to anterior skull base:* Anterior craniofacial resection

Depending on the extent of lesion, the above procedures are done in combination and extended procedures like orbital exenteration and infratemporal clearance may have to be added. In case of endoscopic surgery, Draf procedures have to be done if frontoethmoidal recess involvement is present.

Management of the Neck

In the case of nasal vestibule lesions, the nodal metastasis rate reported at presentation is under 10%.[24-27] Even in nasal cavity lesions, the nodal metastasis rate at presentation is low, hence the neck is not electively managed as for oral cavity carcinoma. However this decision also rests on the histology of tumor; mucosal melanomas are known to metastasize early to regional lymph nodes and sentinel node biopsy may be attempted in N0 cases in this scenario. In the node positive neck, selective neck dissection or modified radical neck dissection is performed as per institutional practice. Elective neck irradiation is a practice in T3 and T4 tumors.

Radiotherapy

Upfront radiotherapy is preferred for thin superficial lesions with SCC or BCC histology especially those at critical areas of the nose where reconstruction after excision is a challenge. In cases of BCC, electron radiotherapy can be used to reduce toxicity to the surrounding tissues. Brachytherapy has been reported to be of use in small lesions of the septum and columella with good locoregional outcomes. The median dose usually delivered is 65 Gy.

Adjuvant radiotherapy is planned for all stage III/IV tumors after surgery. The median dose differs for specific areas. In case of positive margins, the dose delivered is usually 66–70 Gy and for high-risk areas where there is high chance for micrometastasis or tumor seeding the dose delivered is 60 Gy. For low-risk areas, the dose delivered is usually 54 Gy. Orbit and optic nerve are critical structures to be shielded while designing the radiotherapy treatment plan.

Chemotherapy

Chemotherapy is the mainstay of treatment in lymphomas and metastases from other sites. Induction chemotherapy is practiced in some cases of Kadish C olfactory neuroblastomas, where the chemotherapy used is etoposide or platinum based. Depending upon the response, further treatment is planned. Adjuvant cisplatin chemotherapy is given concurrently with radiotherapy in SCC where there are positive margins or if there is extranodal extension.

OUTCOMES

Outcomes depend on the histology, extent of the disease and the initial treatment plan and expertise. Cancers of the nasal vestibule have good oncological outcomes with 5-year survival outcomes close to 80% even in large lesions (Wang T3 stage). The same may not hold true for nasal cavity tumors as they have a variety of histologies, ranging from low-grade SCC to high-grade mucosal melanoma. Histology-based outcomes are described elsewhere in this book as they are common to the nasal cavity, paranasal sinuses and anterior skull base.

CONCLUSION

Tumors of the nasal cavity and vestibule are a rare and diverse spectrum of disorders. With the exception of cutaneous malignancies, very few institutions or practitioners have extensive experience in their management. Multidisciplinary care and tailor-made treatment plans can offer good oncological outcomes with modest treatment-related morbidity.

REFERENCES

1. Silverberg E. Cancer statistics, 1980. CA Cancer J Clin. 1981; 31(1):13-28.
2. Carrau RL, Myers EM, Johnson JT. Paranasal sinus carcinoma—diagnosis, treatment, and prognosis. Oncology (Williston Park, NY). 1992;6(1):43-50.
3. Bussi M, Gervasio CF, Riontino E, Valente G, Ferrari L, Pira E, et al. Study of ethmoidal mucosa in a population at occupational high risk of sinonasal adenocarcinoma. Acta otolaryngologica. 2002;122(2):197-201.
4. Gordon I, Boffetta P, Demers PA. A case study comparing a meta-analysis and a pooled analysis of studies of sinonasal cancer among wood workers. Epidemiology; 1998. pp. 518-24.
5. Sunderman FW. Nasal toxicity, carcinogenicity, and olfactory uptake of metals. Ann Clin Lab Sci. 2001;31(1):3-24.
6. De Flora S. Threshold mechanisms and site specificity in chromium (VI) carcinogenesis. Carcinogenesis. 2000;21(4): 533-41.
7. Luce D, Leclerc A, Bégin D, Demers PA, Gérin M, Orlowski E, et al. Sinonasal cancer and occupational exposures: a pooled analysis of 12 case-control studies. Can Cause Cont. 2002;13(2):147-57.
8. Mastrangelo G, Fedeli U, Fadda E, Milan G, Lange JH. Epidemiologic evidence of cancer risk in textile industry workers: a review and update. Toxicol Indust Health. 2002;18(4):171-81.
9. Kraus DH, Maghami E. Cancer of the nasal cavity and paranasal sinuses. Expert Rev Antican Ther. 2004;4(3):411-24.
10. Gress DM, Edge SB, Greene FL, Washington MK, Asare EA, Brierley JD, et al. Principles of cancer staging. AJCC Cancer Staging Manual, 8th edition. New York: Springer-Verlag; 2017. p. 30.
11. Wang CC. Treatment of carcinoma of the nasal vestibule by irradiation. Cancer. 1976;38(1):100-6.
12. Patel P, Tiwari R, Karim AB, Nauta JJ, Snow GB. Squamous cell carcinoma of the nasal vestibule. J Laryngol Otol. 1992; 106(4):332-6.
13. Loevner LA, Sonners AI. Imaging of neoplasms of the paranasal sinuses. Neuroimaging Clinics. 2004;14(4):625-46.
14. Kim SS, Han MH, Kim JE, Lee CH, Chung HW, Lee JS, et al. Malignant melanoma of the sinonasal cavity: explanation of magnetic resonance signal intensities with histopathologic characteristics. Am J Otolaryngol. 2000;21(6):366-78.
15. Pickuth D, Öbrunner SY, Spielmann RP. Computed tomography and magnetic resonance imaging features of olfactory neuroblastoma: an analysis of 22 cases. Clin Otolaryngol Allied Sci. 1999;24(5):457-61.
16. Som PM, Lidov M, Brandwein M, Catalano P, Biller HF. Sinonasal esthesioneuroblastoma with intracranial extension: marginal tumor cysts as a diagnostic MR finding. Am J Neuroradiol. 1994;15(7):1259-62.
17. Bradley PJ, Jones NS, Robertson I. Diagnosis and management of esthesioneuroblastoma. Curr Opin Otolaryngol Head Neck Surg. 2003;11(2):112-8.
18. Dammann F, Pereira P, Laniado M, Plinkert P, Löwenheim H, Claussen CD. Inverted papilloma of the nasal cavity and the paranasal sinuses: using CT for primary diagnosis and follow-up. Am J Roentgenol. 1999;172(2):543-8.
19. Savy L, Lloyd G, Lund V, Howard D. Optimum imaging for inverted papilloma. J Laryngol Otol. 2000;114(11):891-3.
20. Ojiri H, Ujita M, Tada S, Fukuda K. Potentially distinctive features of sinonasal inverted papilloma on MR imaging. Am J Roentgenol. 2000;175(2):465-8.
21. Olson G, Citardi MJ. Image-guided functional endoscopic sinus surgery. Otolaryngol Head Neck Surg. 2000;123(3):188-94.
22. Citardi MJ, Batra PS. Image-guided sinus surgery: current concepts and technology. Otolaryngol Clin North Am. 2005; 38(3):439-52.
23. Batra PS, Lanza DC. Endoscopic power-assisted orbital exenteration. Am J Rhinol. 2005;19(3):297-301.
24. Wong CS, Cummings BJ. The place of radiation therapy in the treatment of squamous cell carcinoma of the nasal vestibule. Acta Oncologica. 1988;27(3):203-8.
25. Pantelakos ST, McGuirt WF, Nussear DW. Squamous cell carcinoma of the nasal vestibule and anterior nasal passages. Am J Otolaryngol. 1994;15(1):33-6.
26. Schaefer SD, Hill GC. Epidermoid carcinoma of the nasal vestibule: current treatment evaluation. Laryngoscope. 1980; 90(10):1631-5.
27. Samaha M, Yoskovitch A, Hier MP, Black MJ. Squamous cell carcinoma of the nasal vestibule. J Otolaryngol Head Neck Surg. 2000;29(2):98.

CHAPTER 16

Cancers of the Paranasal Sinuses and Anterior Skull Base

Narayana Subramaniam, Sivakumar Vidhyadharan, Samskruthi P Murthy

INTRODUCTION

Tumors of the paranasal sinuses and anterior skull base are relatively rare, accounting for an estimated 2–3% of head and neck malignancies.[1] Additionally, the histology is diverse, resulting in a lack of high-level evidence for treatment. Given the anatomical complexity of the location, access constraints and the abundance of critical structures requiring preservation to prevent treatment-related morbidity, there is no better example of tumors requiring multidisciplinary treatment.

Although rare, identifying these lesions early is of utmost importance as they are potentially curable and the morbidity associated with treatment of early lesions is low. Additionally, they have nonspecific symptoms, such as unilateral epistaxis, nasal discharge, anosmia and nasal block, which are often mistaken for benign conditions such as rhinosinusitis, and either neglected or resected incompletely. By the time the patient presents with unequivocal symptoms of an invasive sinonasal lesion such as headache or abnormal vision, the lesion is advanced and may not be curable, and even if curable treatment may be extremely morbid.

However recent advances in surgical technique and instrumentation, and radiotherapy delivery, supplemented by improvement in imaging and diagnostic pathology have resulted in excellent outcomes for patients being treated for these tumors. Additionally there are extensive treatment options for advanced lesions, which are no longer relegated to palliative care. Thorough knowledge and expertise along with multidisciplinary care are vital to offer these patients good oncological outcomes and quality of life.

EPIDEMIOLOGY

Given that the term "sinonasal malignancies" refers to a group of heterogeneous cancers, there are no distinct epidemiological features. Incidence is generally higher in males, and epithelial malignancies present in the fifth or sixth decade,[2] however tumors like esthesioneuroblastoma have no sex predilection[3] and rhabdomyosarcoma are common in patients under 10 years old.[4] Given the significant variability in patient demographics and mode of presentation, the index of suspicion must be high to make an early diagnosis.

RISK FACTORS

In a significant proportion of cases, the exact etiology of these tumors is unknown. The strongest linked etiological factors have been inhalants, especially in industrial workers. First described at the turn of the 19th century, it was postulated that a patient developed maxillary sinus cancer due to chromium exposure.[5] Other agents associated with a higher risk of sinonasal cancers are formaldehyde and nickel. Intestinal type adenocarcinoma (ITAC) arguably has the strongest occupational link, especially in those chronically exposed to wood and leather dust.[6,7] A recent systematic review and meta-analysis showed that occupational exposure was most common in adenocarcinomas and that in addition to wood and leather dust and formaldehyde, there was a significantly increased risk of sinonasal cancer in those with in the textile and construction industries.[8] Industrial exposure is likely to be responsible for the geographical heterogeneity in these tumors; adenocarcinoma is more common in Europe than the US as hardwoods found in Europe are more carcinogenic and European factories adopted safety measure later.[9] It is expected that the histology distribution will be altered in the coming decades again due to more awareness and safer working environments. Squamous cell carcinoma has been linked to heavy tobacco and alcohol exposure.[5]

CLINICAL EXAMINATION

The clinical presentation of these patients varies greatly based on the extent of the lesion. Early disease can present with innocuous symptoms indistinguishable from inflammatory rhinosinusitis while advanced disease can present with unequivocal symptoms like visual disturbances and cranial palsy, which are highly suspicious for malignancy. Hence the clinical suspicion while evaluating these patients needs to be high; clinical features that do not fit the pattern of benign sinonasal disease (new onset at later age, unilateral polyps or masses, unexplained epistaxis, proptosis and diplopia) should prompt detailed investigation.

Nasal symptoms include ipsilateral nasal obstruction, rhinorrhea, epistaxis, nasal pain or headache or anosmia. These may be associated with orbital symptoms such as diplopia, decreased visual acuity, proptosis, and epiphora. Advanced lesions involving the soft tissue may be associated with infraorbital hypoesthesia, skin changes or cranial nerve palsies. Maxillary cancers, due to their unique location, can present with a wide variety of symptoms: involvement of the cribriform plate and ethmoid sinus causes anosmia, involvement of the floor of the orbit causes diplopia and chemosis, infraorbital nerve involvement causes facial hypoesthesia, medial extension into the nasal cavity causes nasolacrimal duct obstruction and epiphora, posterolateral extension into the infratemporal fossa causes trismus, involvement of the anterior soft tissue causes skin changes, and involvement of the floor can cause loosening of upper alveolar teeth and ulceration of the palate.

Lesions may or may not be visible in the nasal cavity. Tumors are very rarely seen on anterior rhinoscopy; diagnostic nasal endoscopy is required for thorough evaluation. Findings suspicious for malignancy are a unilateral polypoidal lesion that appears friable with heterogenous mucosa arising from the lateral wall of the nose. The exact point of attachment of the lesion is crucial to arrive a diagnosis—packing the nose with decongestants and adrenaline to allow a clearer, detailed evaluation is invaluable. Evaluation of the extent of the lesion is crucial for surgical planning.

Examination of the eye is a vital part of clinical examination; one should assess for proptosis, extraocular movement, and visual acuity. Detailed examination of individual cranial nerves is vital, as these tumors can involve the cranial nerve either be direct extension or by perineural spread. Direct involvement of III, IV, and VI cranial nerve can occur at the orbital apex **(Fig. 1)**, while cavernous sinus **(Fig. 2)** involvement can affect III, IV, VI, and V (V_1 and V_2). Jugular foramen and leptomeningeal involvement is not unheard of; this can be involvement of IX, X and XI. Examination of the neck is required to detect lymph node spread; although the incidence of nodal spread is low, lymphadenopathy is not unheard of. In certain histologies such as esthesioneuroblastoma and rhabdomyosarcoma, lymphadenopathy may be an indication for induction chemotherapy and hence should not be missed.

APPLIED ANATOMY AND ROUTES OF TUMOR SPREAD

The maxillary sinus is the largest of the paranasal sinuses and is located below the eye, within the maxillary bone. It is in the shape of an inverted pyramid; the roof is the floor of the orbit and infraorbital canal, medially is the lateral nasal wall, anteriorly is the maxillary bone and soft tissue of the face, inferiorly is the maxillary alveolar process, posteromedially is the pterygopalatine fossa and posterolaterally is the infratemporal fossa. The drainage occurs through the semilunar hiatus into the middle meatus of the nose.

The ethmoid sinus is termed as a labyrinth as it is a pattern of multiple interconnected air sinuses rather than a large individual cavity. There is significant variation in size, shape and pneumatization, and cross sectional imaging needs to be studied to determine this preoperatively. The sinus is located between the lateral wall of nose (superior and middle turbinate) medially, the medial wall of the orbit (lamina papyracea) laterally, the sphenoid sinus posteriorly and the anterior skull base (fovea ethmoidalis) superiorly. The sinus is divided by the basal lamella (which connects the middle turbinate to the lamina papyracea) into the anterior and posterior cells, which are anatomically and functionally distinct. The posterior cells drain into the superior meatus, while the anterior cells drain into the middle meatus of the nasal cavity.

The frontal sinus is bounded anteriorly by the anterior table of the frontal bone, posteriorly by the thinner posterior table (that separates the sinus from the frontal lobes), and inferiorly by the roof of the orbit. Pneumatization is highly variable, and this can affect the surgical approach. The sinus drains into the middle meatus in a varied manner.

The sphenoid sinus is a result of pneumatization of the sphenoid bone and is located behind the ethmoid sinus. They are paired and develop separately from the nasal capsule of the embryonic nose, often with a single intervening septum of varying thickness. The sinuses themselves may have varying incomplete septations. They are bounded anteriorly by the posterior ethmoid cells and the sphenoethmoid recess, posteriorly by the tuberculum sellae and clivus, laterally by the

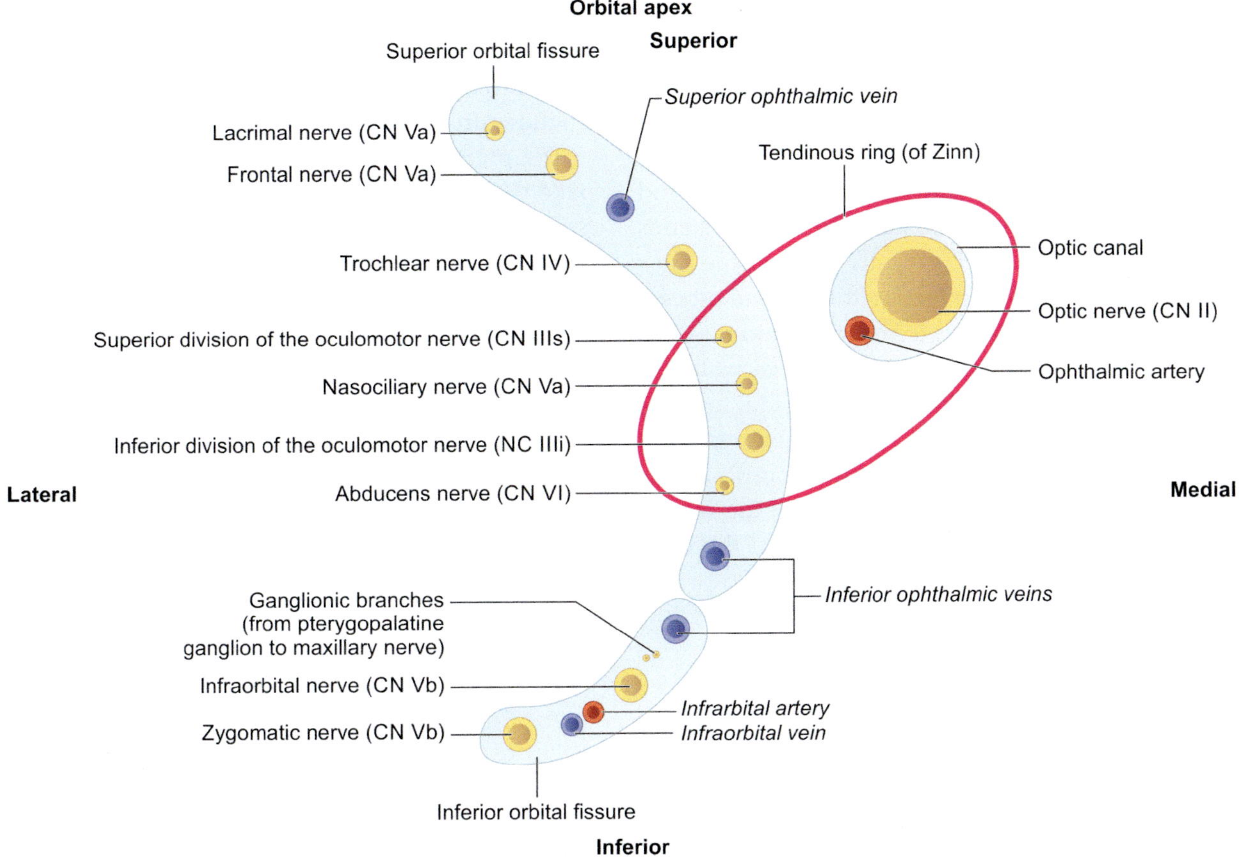

Fig. 1: Schematic diagram of orbital apex.

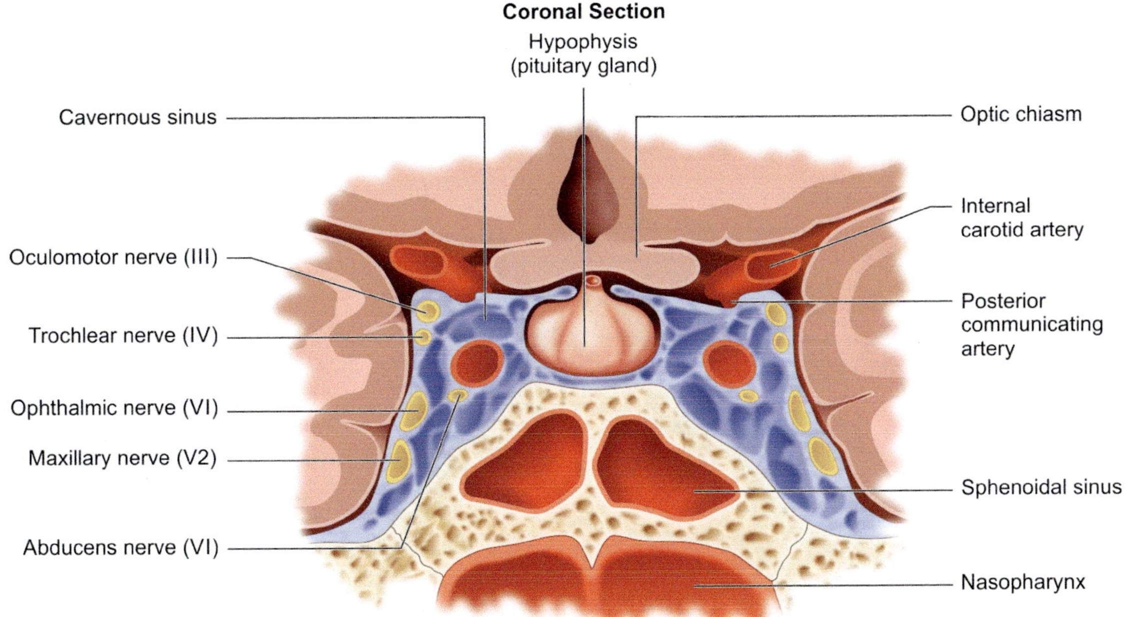

Fig. 2: Coronal section of cavernous sinus.

internal carotid artery and cavernous sinus and the planum sphenoidale (bony roof of the sphenoid sinus) superiorly. A very important surgical relation is the cavernous sinus, which receives blood via the superior and inferior ophthalmic veins through the superior orbital fissure anteriorly from the basilar plexus of veins posteriorly, draining into the internal jugular vein via the superior and inferior petrosal veins. The internal carotid and cranial nerves III, IV, V (V_1 and V_2), and VI pass through the lateral part of the sinus **(Fig. 3)**.

The orbit, although technically not a part of the skull base, due to its anatomical proximity to it and the paranasal sinuses, requires special mention. The bony orbit is pyramidal in shape with the base anteriorly and the apex posteriorly. The medial wall of the orbit extends from the anterior lacrimal crest anteriorly to the apex posteriorly; the lamina papyracea is a thin-walled process of ethmoid bone that separates it from the ethmoid sinus anteriorly. The superior aspect of the medial wall also transmits the superior and inferior ethmoidal arteries through their respective foramina. The zygoma in front and the greater wing of sphenoid behind contribute the lateral wall of the orbit. The orbital plate of the frontal bone forms the roof of the orbit. The apex of the orbit is an important route of spread of tumors intracranially, and contains structures that traverse the superior and inferior orbital fissure and the optic foramen. The structures are illustrated in **Figure 4**.

The pterygopalatine fossa (PPF) is small but critical space that allows tumor spread between the sinonasal cavity, orbit, infratemporal fossa, and the cranial cavity. The PPF is an inverted pyramid in shape **(Fig. 5)** and is bounded by the posterior surface of the maxilla and maxillary sinus cavity anteriorly, the base of medial and lateral pterygoid plates and greater wing of sphenoid posteriorly, the greater wing of sphenoid and the middle cranial fossa superiorly, the sphenoid bone and perpendicular of the palatine bone medially and the pyramidal process of the palatine bone inferiorly. The contents of the PPF can be divided into an anterior

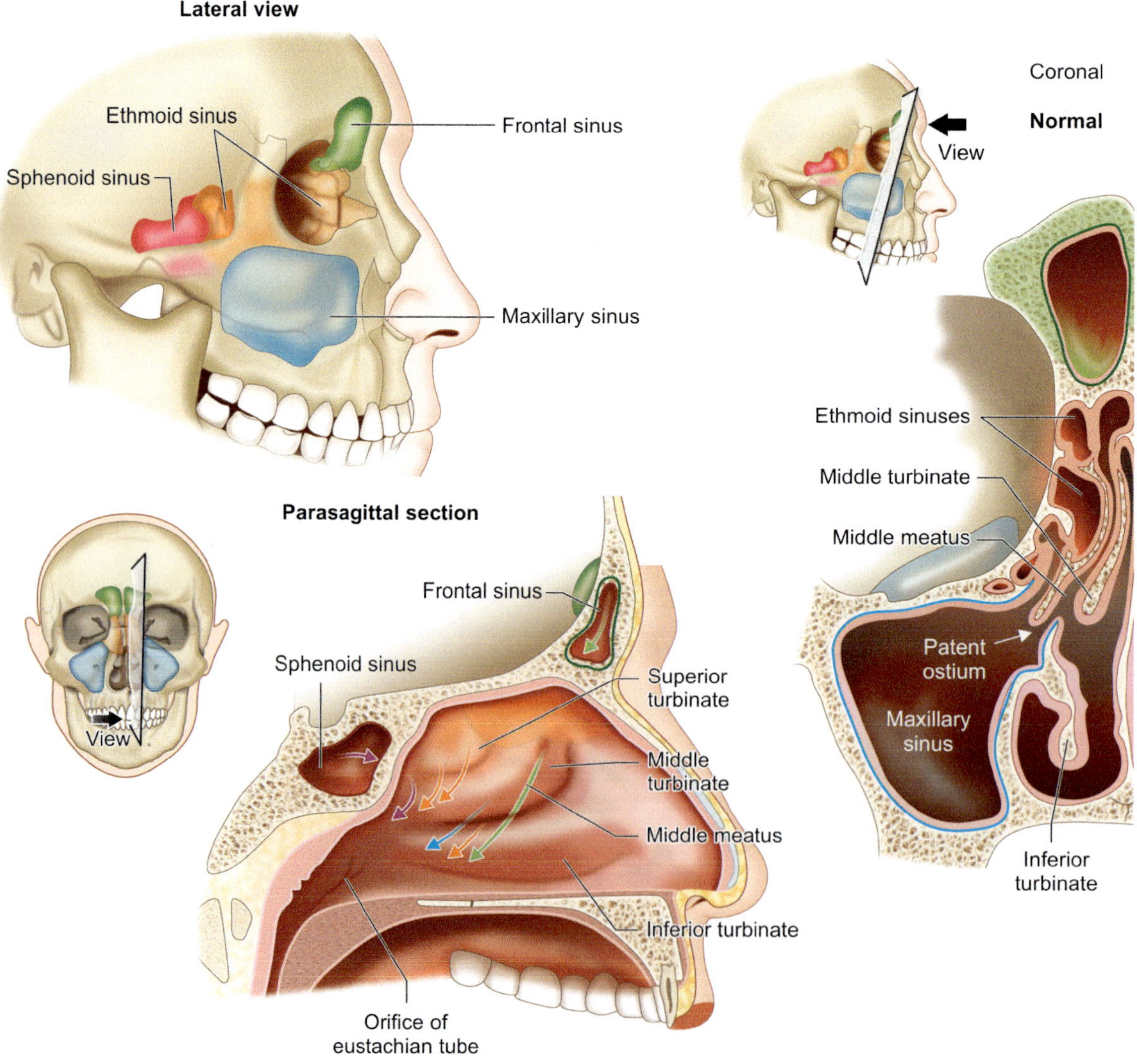

Fig. 3: Cross-sectional view of paranasal sinuses.

vascular space, which contains the termination of the internal maxillary artery, and a posterior neural space that contains the maxillary division of the trigeminal nerve and the pterygopalatine ganglion. The PPF communicates anteriorly with the orbit through the inferior orbital fissure (infraorbital nerve), medially with the nasal cavity through the sphenopalatine foramen (sphenopalatine artery and nerve), laterally with the infraorbital through the pterygomaxillary fissure (posterior superior alveolar nerve), posterosuperiorly with the skull base through the Vidian canal (Vidian nerve), foramen rotundum (maxillary nerve) and palatovaginal canal (pharyngeal branch of the maxillary nerve and pharyngeal artery) and inferiorly with the oral cavity through the greater palatine canal (greater and lesser palatine nerves and descending palatine artery and vein).

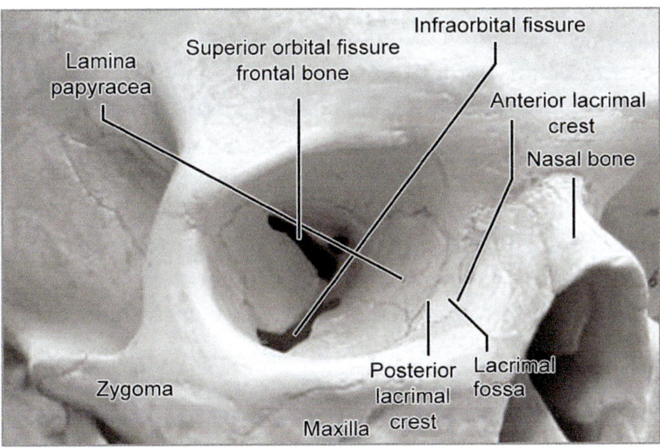

Fig. 4: Bony anatomy of orbit.

The anterior skull base divides the anterior cranial fossa (ACF) and the sinonasal cavity. The anterior skull base spans anteriorly from the posterior table of the frontal sinus till the planum sphenoidale and anterior clinoid process posteriorly. The frontal bone encloses the ACF anterolaterally, forming the lateral boundary of the anterior skull base. The frontal crest is a ridge in the midline of the anterior cranial fossa that forms the attachment of the falx cerebri. The floor of the ACF comprises the orbital process of the frontal bone, with the central deeper portion formed by the ethmoid bone. The ethmoid bone bears the cribriform plate medially and the lamina papyracea laterally. The cribriform plate has multiple perforations through which olfactory rootlets traverse with their dural attachments, while the lamina papyracea is a thin sheet of bone that can be involved by tumors of the ethmoid sinus, to involve the orbit. Posteriorly, the floor of the ACF is formed by the planum sphenoidale, which is an important landmark for sphenoid sinus and optic nerve surgery. Medially the lesser wing of the sphenoid bone forms the anterior clinoid process, which is another important landmark, for identification of the optic nerve and supracavernous internal carotid artery.

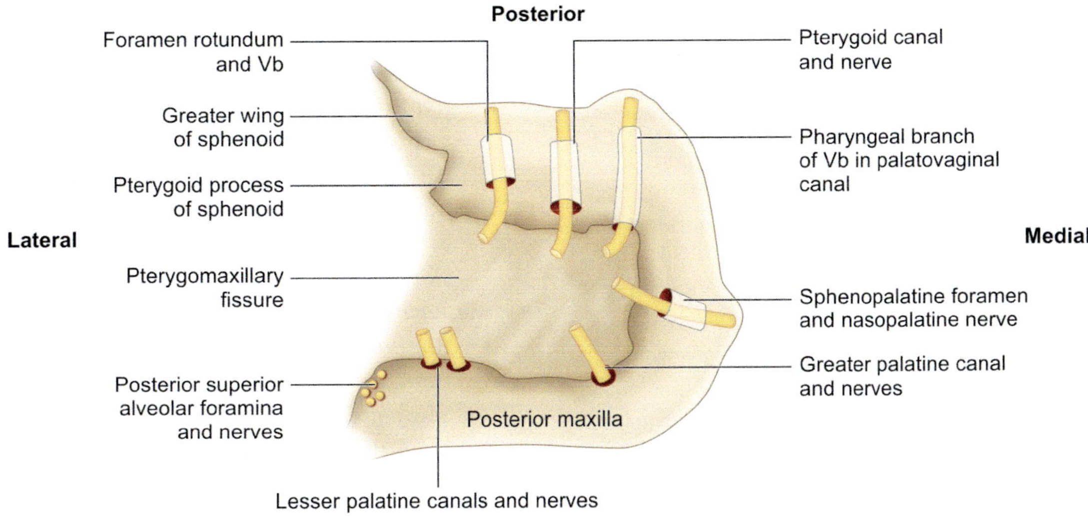

Fig. 5: Right pterygopalatine fossa as viewed from below.

PATHOLOGY

Lesions of this region are a challenge for not only the surgeon, but for the pathologist as well, as the histology of these tumors is diverse with often overlapping morphology. Additionally, due to access constraints, the tissue available for sampling is often scanty. Modern techniques like in situ hybridization (ISH) and polymerase chain reaction (PCR) have revolutionized the treatment of these tumors, however for optimal patient care it is crucial that clinicians and pathologists work together, as rarely do either have enough information individually to make definitive treatment recommendations.

Techniques available for tissue characterization:

- *Histology:* Several diverse tissue types exist in the sinonasal cavity and skull base, including but not limited to squamous epithelium, respiratory epithelium, olfactory epithelium, submucosal salivary glands, blood and lymphatic vessels, peripheral nerve, bone, cartilage, and fat. Identifying the tissue of origin helps determine the nature of the tumor. Additional criteria such as cellular architecture, cytomorphology, nuclear atypia, and presence of mitoses help further characterize these lesions.
- *Immunohistochemistry:* In tumors with indistinct morphology, especially those with poorer differentiation, immunohistochemistry (IHC) is a vital tool to detect the type of tumor being dealt with. Some of the common antibodies used are as shown below **(Table 1)**.[10]

Table 1: Antibodies used for different target tissues in immunohistochemistry.

Antibody used	*Target tissue*
Cytokeratins (CK)	Epithelial tissue such as squamous and mucosal cells (e.g., squamous cell carcinoma)
Vimentin	Mesenchymal tissue such as muscle, connective tissue (e.g., sarcomas)
Epithelial membrane antigen (EMA)	Epithelial tissue (e.g., salivary gland tumors and poorly differentiated carcinomas)
Leukocyte common antigen (LCA)	Lymphocytes and plasma cells (lymphoma)
S-100	Neural crest derivatives (malignant melanoma)
CD-68	Macrophages and histiocytes (malignant fibrous histiocytoma)
Factor VIII and CD 31	Endothelial cells (hemangioma and angiofibroma)
Neuron specific enolase (NSE)	Neuroendocrine tissue (olfactory neuroblastoma)

- *Advanced techniques:* Molecular probes (which includes ISH and PCR) can identify specific nucleic acid sequences which aid in diagnosis; this can be done by identifying the presence of infections (Epstein Barr virus in nasopharyngeal carcinoma) or specific translocations that help identify (PLAG1 identification in pleomorphic adenoma) or determine behavior of certain tumors (MECT1-MAML2 translocation shows favorable outcomes in mucoepidermoid carcinoma). Techniques such as flow cytometry can be used for DNA ploidy analysis, which aids in the identification of rare tumors such as chordoma.[11]

Pathological classification of tumors occurring in the sinonasal tract and anterior skull base:

- *Epithelial tumors:*
  - *Squamous cell carcinoma:* This arises in the squamous epithelial of the sinonasal tract and upper respiratory tract. It has a high propensity of invasion through soft tissue and bone, with high rates of lymphatic and perineural spread. Grossly, tumors can be proliferative, infiltrative or combinations of both. They vary significantly in differentiation, further characterized by cytomorphology, presence of keratin pearls and intercellular bridges; however tumors involving the skull base are more commonly moderately or poorly differentiated.[12]
  - *Adenoid cystic carcinoma:* These arise from the intercalated duct cells of the mucous secreting minor salivary glands arising in the sinonasal tract and skull base. Grossly they appear circumscribed and well or partially capsulated and rubbery to firm in consistency. On histology, they have uniform cells with basophilic mucinous substance and a hyalinized eosinophilic material and small hyperchromatic round to oval nuclei. They are graded based on whether the histology has a tubular, cribriform or solid appearance.[13] They have a lower propensity for lymphatic spread but are notorious for perineural invasion, often with skip metastases along the course of nerves.
- *Mesenchymal tumors:*
  - *Rhabdomyosarcoma:* They originate in the skeletal muscle and have a varying degree of maturation. They are the most common histology occurring in children or young adults, and are classified into orbital, parameningeal, and nonorbital/parameningeal. They may be associated with lymph node or distant metastases. Grossly these tumors are irregular and infiltrative with no

characteristic gross findings. On histology they are characteristically small, round, blue-cell tumors with prominent hyperchromatic nuclei that stain darkly. They are further subdivided into embryonal, alveolar, and pleomorphic subtypes.[14] Categorization and staging are crucial to decide on primary modality of management.

- *Chondrosarcoma:* They originate in cartilage, affecting either the bones or soft tissue. They are relatively rare but have no particular gender or age distribution. Grossly they are osteolytic, causing destruction of bone or soft tissue with extensive local infiltration occurring before they cause symptoms. Histologically, they are classified as conventional, mesenchymal, myxoid, clear cell, and anaplastic variants. They are hypercellular with cells present within lacunae and stroma has a hyaline matrix that may be spindled.[15]
- *Chordoma:* These are slow-growing but locally aggressive malignant neoplasms that originate in notochord remnants of the axial skeleton. They occur in the midline and are irregular in shape with osteolytic bone destruction and calcification. Histologically they have a variety of growth patterns, with cells having a physaliferous (bubble-shaped or vacuolated) appearance due to the presence of cells with round nuclei and abundant vacuolated cytoplasm. These vacuoles contain glycogen, with or without mucous. They can be of classic, chondroid or dedifferentiated types.[16]

- *Lymphoproliferative tumors:*
  - *Lymphoma:* These are malignant proliferations of lymphoid cells having a B- or T-cell origin. In the head and neck, they can arise within the lymph nodes or extranodally. They are more commonly associated with immunosuppressed states, such as HIV or after solid organ transplant.[17] They can involve the skull base either through contiguous spread from the sinonasal tract, lymph nodes or as a de-novo primary lymphoma of the skull base.[18] Grossly they have no characteristic appearance and histology is variable depending on whether they are B- or T-cell, Hodgkin's or non-Hodgkin's lymphoma; immunohistochemistry is invariably required to establish a diagnosis. Treatment is predominantly nonsurgical.
- *Tumors arising from melanocytes:*
  - *Malignant melanoma:* These are malignant tumors arising from the melanocytes in the mucosa of the sinonasal tract or skull base. Majority of these arise in the nasal septum, lateral wall or turbinates of the nasal cavity. They are usually polypoidal or sessile in appearance with variable color (pink, brown or black), with or without ulceration of the mucosal surface. The histological characterization requires special staining and cells are large and pleomorphic with an epithelioid or spindle-shaped morphology with a variable distribution of cells. They have prominent nucleoli with the presence of mitoses and necrosis (which contribute to staging). They are aggressive tumors that are associated with higher locoregional failure rates (unlike cutaneous melanomas, which are associated with distant metastases).[19]
- *Neuroendocrine tumors:*
  - *Olfactory neuroblastoma:* This is an uncommon neoplasm that is believed to arise from olfactory stem cells in the olfactory mucosa of the nasal vault, in the region of the cribriform plate of ethmoid.[20] Grossly they appear reddish or grayish in appearance, polypoidal and may be vascular. Low-grade tumors have well-circumscribed cell nests and intervening fibrillary stroma; however, this structure is lost in high-grade tumors. True rosettes (Flexner-Wintersteiner rosettes) indicate an olfactory differentiation while pseudorosettes (Homer-Wright rosettes) are not specific for olfactory differentiation and may also be seen in other neuroendocrine tumors; both are considered characteristic but are not present in a majority of cases. Tumors are divided into four Hyam's grades (I-IV) based on the architecture, fibrillary matrix, mitosis, necrosis, nuclear pleomorphic, and the presence of rosettes; this has prognostic significance. Nodal spread has a poor prognosis, as does distant metastases.[21]
  - *Neuroendocrine carcinoma:* These are a spectrum of tumors, ranging from well-differentiated carcinoid tumors to poorly differentiated small cell carcinomas. Tumors are categorized as neuroendocrine when histology shows neuroendocrine differentiation, epithelial differentiation (either by virtue of arising in an epithelial- or mucosal-lined passage or positive immunohistochemical staining for cytokeratin), and immunohistochemical positivity for neuroendocrine markers (CD56/N-CAM, synaptophysin or chromogranin).[22] Symptoms are associated with local invasion, however in small cell tumors, paraneoplastic syndromes (commonly syndrome of inappropriate secretion of antidiuretic hormone) have

been reported.[23] Their gross appearance and histology are similar to olfactory neuroblastoma; however, these tumors lie on a spectrum of differentiation. Number of mitoses and Ki-67 can help determine prognosticate patients.[24]

- *Tumors of unknown origin:*
  - *Sinonasal undifferentiated carcinoma:* These are aggressive tumors believed to be of Schneiderian epithelial origin but having no squamous or glandular differentiation.[25] It progresses rapidly and is destructive with early involvement of the orbit and cranial cavity. Histologically, they appear as small, round, blue cell tumors but immunohistochemistry is distinct from other sinonasal malignancies; they stain positive for cytokeratin and may have variable positivity for chromogranin and synaptophysin. They are associated with mitoses and necrosis.[26] They require aggressive multimodal therapy but are often associated with poor survival.
- *Metastases to the skull base:* Primary tumors of the prostate, lung, pancreas, kidney, thyroid, and breast have metastasized to the skull base.[27,29] These are identified by immunohistochemistry and organ-directed therapies are administered. Palliative resection or radiotherapy may be considered for symptomatic relief.
- Tumor-like conditions of the sinonasal tract and anterior skull base:
  - *Inflammatory pseudotumors:* These are quasineoplastic lesions that involve multiple systems in the body, most commonly the lung and orbit. Although not technically malignant, these lesions are destructive and clinically and radiologically mimic malignant lesions.[30,31] These are lesions comprised of inflammatory and myofibroblastic spindle cells, in view of which more recent literature has suggested that they should be referred to "inflammatory myofibroblastic tumors" as it is a more specific term.[32] Clinically they present with nonspecific symptoms of involvement of the nasal cavity and paranasal sinuses, through local invasion.[33] Grossly polypoidal lesions with mucosal edema and bony destruction may be seen. Histological manifestations are complex; the main components are myofibroblasts and inflammatory cells (lymphocytes, plasma cells, macrophages, and eosinophils). There may be areas with vasculitis and stromal fibrosis as well.[34] Immunohistochemical staining typically shows three patterns—only positive vimentin expression, positive expression of myogenic proteins such as desmin, smooth muscle actin and muscle specific actin, and positive expression of cytokeratin. These tumors may also stain positive for anaplastic lymphoma kinase (ALK) aberrant expression. Treatment is by complete surgical excision, however for patients unfit for radical treatment or unresectable lesions, long-term steroid or immunosuppressant use has been shown to be effective.[35]
  - *Fibrous dysplasia:* This is a benign, fibro-osseous disorder that results from the replacement of healthy bone with fibrous tissue that is weak. It can involve one bone (monostic) or several (polyostotic).[36] Symptoms are mainly compressive and lesions can rarely undergo malignant transformation to osteosarcoma, particularly after radiotherapy.[37] Histology shows the presence of irregular and immature fibrillary bony trabeculae with peripheral arrangement of fibroblastic spindle cells. These trabeculae are arranged in "Chinese-letter" pattern. These need to differentiated from other similar lesions such as ossifying fibroma, osteomyelitis, and osteosarcoma.
  - *Angiofibroma:* These are also benign tumors that are locally aggressive and infiltrative. They occur almost exclusively in males; occurrence in females is doubtful. They occur commonly in the adolescent age group and arise from the posterolateral nasal wall or sphenopalatine foramen.[38] Symptoms are due to local extension causing epistaxis, nasal blockage, and visual disturbances, with up to a fifth of patients having intracranial involvement. Although there is no malignant potential, sarcomatous transformation has been shown to occur after massive doses of radiation.[39] Grossly these tumors are rubbery to firm in consistency, with smooth surface and extremely vascular. The histology shows a combination of vascular channels ("staghorn" pattern) having a single layer of endothelial cells and interspersed fibrous stroma. Treatment is surgical but these surgeries are complicated in view of the extreme vascularity and extensive local infiltration; preoperative hormonal therapy and embolization have been described. Palliative radiotherapy has also been described for unresectable lesion and unfit patients.[40,41]
  - *Inverted papilloma:* This is a benign growth arising from the Schneiderian epithelium of the

nasal cavity and paranasal sinus that is known to be locally invasive with a high local recurrence rate, and the possibility of focal malignant transformation within the lesion.[42] It may be associated with human papilloma virus infection but this has not been established definitively. Grossly these have a granular mulberry-like appearance and arise from the lateral nasal wall, are unilateral, and may have a grayish hue.[43] Histologically, they have endophytic or inverted growth pattern with proliferation of squamous epithelium into the underlying stromal tissue as clefts or islands. These epithelial cells may have clear cell features, suggestive of glycogen content. Foci of invasive malignancy are common (around 10%). Treatment required complete excision, which includes subperiosteal resection of the bony nests. Some may respond well to radiotherapy.[44]

AJCC 8th edition staging for cancers of nasal cavity and paranasal sinuses.

Maxillary sinus	
T1	Tumor limited to mucosa of maxillary sinus mucosa without erosion of destruction of bone
T2	Tumor causing bone erosion or destruction including extension into hard palate and/or middle meatus, not including extension to posterior maxillary wall or pterygoid plates
T3	Tumor invades the bony posterior wall of maxillary sinus, subcutaneous tissues, floor or the medial wall of the orbit, pterygoid fossa or ethmoid sinuses
T4a	Tumor involves the anterior orbital contents, skin of the cheek, pterygoid plates, sphenoid or frontal sinuses
T4b	Tumor invades the orbital apex, dura, brain, middle cranial fossa, cranial nerves other than maxillary division of trigeminal nerve, nasopharynx or clivus
Nasal cavity or ethmoid sinus	
T1	Tumor restricted to any one subsite, with or without bony invasion
T2	Tumor invading two subsites in a single region or extending to involve an adjacent region within the nasoethmoidal complex, with or without bony invasion
T3	Tumor extends to invade the medial wall or floor of the orbit, maxillary sinus, palate, or cribriform plate
T4a	Tumor invades any of the following: anterior orbital contents, skin of the nose or cheek, minimal extension to the anterior cranial fossa, pterygoid plates, sphenoid or frontal sinuses
T4b	Tumor invades any of the following: orbital apex, dura, brain, middle cranial fossa, cranial nerves other than maxillary division of trigeminal nerve (V2), nasopharynx, or clivus

Contd...

Contd...

Nasal cavity or ethmoid sinus	
N1	Metastases to single lymph node, 3 cm or less in greatest diameter
N2a	Metastases to single ipsilateral node 3–6 cm in size or metastases to a single lymph node <3 cm in size with ENE
N2b	Metastases to multiple ipsilateral node 3–6 cm in size
N2c	Metastases to bilateral nodes 3–6 cm in size
N3a	Metastases to nodes >6 cm in size without ENE
N3b	Metastases to any node >3 cm in size with ENE
M0	No metastases
M1	Metastatic disease
Kadish staging for olfactory neuroblastoma:[45]	
Stage A	Tumor confined to the nasal cavity
Stage B	Tumor involving the nasal cavity and paranasal sinuses
Stage C	Tumor spread beyond the nasal cavity and paranasal sinuses
Modified Kadish staging for olfactory neuroblastoma[46]	
Stage A	Tumor confined to the nasal cavity
Stage B	Tumor involving the nasal cavity and paranasal sinuses
Stage C	Tumor spread beyond the nasal cavity and paranasal sinuses, including cribriform plate, skull base, orbit or intracranial spread
Stage D	Nodal or distant metastases

RADIOLOGY

For tumors of the sinonasal tract and anterior skull base, imaging is crucial for staging and treatment planning. The local extent of the disease requires special assessment of involvement of the orbit, dura and brain parenchyma and perineural invasion, which can determine the intent and modality of treatment. Nodal assessment is also important even though nodal spread is rare in these tumors, as it prognosticates patients and can alter the management protocol. In this setting, CT and MRI with intravenous contrast are often used in a complementary fashion; both have their advantages and disadvantages.[47] PET-CT is used in advanced lesions for assessing distant metastasis and can also be used for radiotherapy planning,[48] especially in tumors where the exact extent is poorly delineated on clinical examination or conventional cross sectional imaging.

CT Imaging of Sinonasal and Anterior Skull Base Tumors

Axial CT images should be acquired using multidetector CT with a slice thickness of 0.5–0.625 mm to assess subtle changes in osseous anatomy, with reconstruction to coronal and sagittal planes. Intravenous contrast is necessary to assess soft tissue extent; the plain CT of the paranasal sinuses used for assessment of benign pathologies is likely to miss information crucial to diagnosis and staging. Neoplastic lesions usually appear as solid with moderate enhancement on contrast administration. Bone erosion is well appreciated on CT, and is more likely to be sign of malignancy (although benign lesions such as inflammatory pseudotumors and inverted papilloma are capable of causing bone erosion as well). Intralesional calcification can also be seen in squamous cell carcinoma, inverted papilloma, adenocarcinoma, and olfactory neuroblastoma.[49] For patients undergoing endoscopic surgery, a crucial determination is the point of attachment of the tumor: often the tumor grows to encompass the whole nasal cavity and the origin of the tumor needs to be identified so the subperiosteal bony nests or digitations are adequately resected.

MRI Imaging of Sinonasal and Anterior Skull Base Tumors

MRI has the advantage over CT of having better soft tissue resolution and better detection of perineural invasion; however, it tends to overestimate bony involvement. Neoplasms on MRI usually have an intermediate signal-intensity on T1- and T2-weighted sequences. T2-weighted sequences help differentiate the intermediate-signal intensity of the tumor and the high signal-intensity of the surrounding inflamed tissue and reactionary edema. High signal-intensity on T2-weighted images is rare in malignancies, except in salivary gland malignancies and neural-origin tumors.[50] Necrosis can also alter the signal-intensity of T2-weighted images, hence correlation of T1- and T2-weighted images are crucial for accurate assessment. Contrast-enhanced fat saturated images are also important to acquire.

Additional imaging considerations:

- *Perineural invasion:* Thin axial and coronal T1 sequences are helpful to identify asymmetry and fat infiltration of the juxtaforaminal fat pads at the skull base (inferior alveolar foramen, superior orbital fissure, pterygopalatine fossa, and stylomastoid foramen). Coronal T2 fat-suppressed images identify sequelae of perineural invasion such as denervation of the muscle of mastication and facial expression (initially T2 hyperintensity with increased bulk and enhancement post contrast enhancement and later on atrophic changes result in T1 hyperintensity, atrophy and no enhancement on contrast films).[51] Other features include thickening or enhancement of nerve branches, "skip" lesions in the pterygopalatine fossa or Meckel's cave or widening of skull base foramina.
- *Anterior cranial fossa involvement:* As the tumor extends beyond the nasoethmoid roof, intracranial spread may occur via the floor of the anterior cranial fossa. A combination of sagittal and coronal imaging best demonstrates this spread. Early erosion of the cribriform plate is well detected on coronal CT, while spread beyond this into the extradural space, dura, and parenchyma is better seen on MRI. Dural invasion needs to be differentiated from dural inflammation (appearing as linear enhancement) that can be seen with extradural spread; the specific features for dural involvement are focal nodularity, thickening over 5 mm and pial enhancement.[52] Parenchymal invasion can be seen along with perilesional edema.
- *Orbital involvement:* Coronal sections are useful as this usually occurs through the inferior or medial wall. Like involvement of the anterior cranial fossa, the first sign is subtle bone erosion through the orbital floor or lamina papyracea, then involving the extraconal fat and then the extraocular muscles and globe. The periorbita is a resilient barrier to tumor invasion and is initially displaced before it is invaded. T1-weighted fat-suppressed images can help identify invasion into the periorbita but it is not reliable; gross involvement is readily identified preoperatively but subtle involvement needs to be determined by periorbital stripping intraoperatively, aided by frozen section assessment. The reliable signs of orbital involvement that can be identified on cross-sectional imaging are a nodular interface with the orbit, altered signal intensities, and edema of the extraocular muscles and nasolacrimal canal involvement.[53,54]
- *Infratemporal fossa and middle cranial fossa involvement:* This usually occurs through the posterolateral wall of the maxilla or the pterygomaxillary fissure. Bony erosion is seen well on CT, while early soft tissue infiltration into the muscles of mastication, retromaxillary fat involvements are better appreciated on MRI. Perineural invasion assessment is crucial here as it is a common route of spread in this region. From the infratemporal fossa, the tumor can spread to the orbit and to the middle cranial fossa.[55,56]

- *Specific radiological findings in nonepithelial tumors:*
    - *Olfactory neuroblastoma:* These present as enhancing unilateral nasal cavity soft tissue masses. The point of attachment, the cribriform plate of ethmoid, may or may not be demonstrable. As they expand they may cause bowing and destruction of bone. They gradually expand to involve the paranasal sinuses and cranial cavity. Reactionary hyperostosis or new bone formation is usually absent.
    - *Juvenile angiofibroma:* On both CT and MRI they appear as lesions of the posterior nasal cavity or nasopharynx that strongly enhance on contrast films. The epicenter is the sphenopalatine foramen. As they grow they involve the surrounding sinuses, orbit or cranial cavity. "Holman-Miller sign" refers to the anterior bowing of the posterior maxillary wall that occurs due to thinning and pressure atrophy of the bone due to tumor growth in juvenile angiofibromas.
    - *Solitary fibrous tumor:* Formerly referred to as hemangiopericytomas, these arise from endothelial cells and commonly occur in the nasal cavity or paranasal sinuses. They are expansile, bone remodeling lesions with variable enhancement.
    - *Osteosarcoma:* These are lesions that appear as irregular masses with osteolysis or combined lytic-sclerotic bone lesions with intralesional reactive new bone formation.
    - *Chondrosarcoma:* These appear as an irregular mass with scattered intralesional calcifications, with low and high signals on T1- and T2-weighted images respectively. They have a "ring and arc pattern" due to enhancement of the margins and intervening fibrinous septae.[57,58]
    - *Fibrous dysplasia:* These lesions appear as enlarged bone with a dense ground-glass appearance. Although osteolytic, they may have interspersed areas of calcification. On MRI, they may have low to intermediate signal intensity on all sequences but enhance on contrast administration.

TREATMENT PRINCIPLES

Generally, surgery with or without adjuvant therapy is the mainstay of treatment for tumors of the paranasal sinus. These tumors are suspected to have a lower radio-sensitivity than other subsites due to the uneven transmission of ionizing radiation through a complex soft tissue-bone-air interface.[59] Administration of radiotherapy using conventional techniques to these areas is also associated with significant morbidity due to the anatomical proximity of several organs at risk (OARs) such as the eye, brain parenchyma, and pituitary gland. Additionally, surgical treatment has progressed significantly, allowing resection of significant tumors in a safe manner with limited morbidity.

As per the National Comprehensive Cancer Network guidelines, early stage disease (I/II) is usually adequately treated with a single modality of treatment while advanced stage disease (III/IV) requires multimodality treatment.[60]

- For T1-2 disease, surgery is the first choice of treatment, with radiotherapy being a less-favored alternative
- For T3/4 disease, surgery is also the primary choice of treatment with therapy as guided by the final histology. Chemoradiotherapy is acceptable as a primary treatment in select conditions
- Unresectable disease is treated as per the patient's performance status
- Partially or inadequately resected disease (which is a commonly encountered situation in sinonasal tumors due to mistaking them for benign disorders) ideally needs a multidisciplinary evaluation followed by either re-resection or adjuvant therapy.

EARLY STAGE DISEASE (T1-2)

Surgery: As with other subsites of the head and neck, the goal of surgery for malignant sinonasal tumors is an en-bloc circumferential resection; however given the anatomical constraints of the region, this is more often than not impossible. Not unlike microlaryngeal surgery, surgery has evolved to encompass piecemeal resection, which when performed adequately with circumferential margins negative for malignancy, are oncologically sound, especially in the context of endoscopic surgery. Even early stage tumors require a clear operative plan after multidisciplinary discussion; surgeons need to well aware of the natural history of disease and biological behavior of these tumors to avoid incomplete and suboptimal treatment.

Endoscopic surgery is an attractive option, however it needs to be kept in mind that a compromise in oncological principles results in very poor survival outcomes and significant patient morbidity. If endoscopic surgery is not feasible due to the tumor itself, technical limitations of instrument or the surgeon, open surgery affords excellent outcomes in early stage disease. In endoscopic surgery the morbidity spared is a facial incision, which needs to be considered in the context of the patient's general condition and fitness for prolonged anesthesia and tumor biology; a quick open surgery with meticulous skin closure often affords good cosmetic outcomes. However incidence of early stage disease is still low due to the paucity of symptoms associated with these diseases; they are not amenable for unaided clinical examination and are evaluated when they are symptomatic, which is usually in advanced cases. The approaches to these tumors are discussed subsequently.

The neck is not routinely addressed electively in early sinonasal tumors due to the very low risk of occult metastases. If the patient requires radiotherapy for the primary tumor, elective irradiation of the neck is an option that can be considered. A decision to surgically address the neck needs to be taken based on the histology and the stage of the tumor; however nodal metastasis is rare both at presentation (12%) or following treatment (13%).[60] Tumors involving the maxillary alveolus, cheek skin may have a higher incidence of nodal recurrence and consequently poorer survival.[61,62] Additionally, a cervicotomy is being performed for microvascular reconstruction of the defects following sinonasal resections, an elective neck dissection of levels I-II may be prudent; a nodal recurrence in this setting may be difficult to salvage.

Radiotherapy: Radical radiotherapy for early tumors of the ethmoid and maxilla has been described in several centers, however several studies have shown that treatment with radical radiotherapy results in worse survival outcomes and morbidity.[60,63-67] Given the rarity of these tumors, the results in literature were not segregated stage-wise, hence these recommendations are likely to have been made considering individual subsites in entirety. Radiotherapy is the first choice of treatment in certain histologies (lymphoma and plasmacytoma) and in patients unfit for or not desirous of surgery. Adjuvant radiotherapy is administered after surgery in the presence of risk features, such as high-risk histologies (such as sinonasal undifferentiated carcinomas), margin positivity, nodal disease, poor differentiation, high grade, and perineural invasion.

LOCALLY ADVANCED DISEASE (T3-4)

Surgery: Surgery is the mainstay for locally advanced disease of the paranasal sinuses. Adequate surgical clearance is the goal, which can be performed endoscopically or via an open approach depending on the experience of the surgical team. Disease restricted to the paranasal sinuses can be performed using transfacial approaches, while resection of the anterior skull base, dura or brain parenchyma requires a combined approach known as "craniofacial resection" where the resection of the sinonasal disease is performed through an endoscopic or transfacial approach combined with a craniotomy, to ensure adequate exposure to resect the tumor, control bleeding, and repair the dural defect. Technical details are described subsequently.

The neck may be addressed electively with surgery for certain histologies such as squamous cell carcinoma, while irradiation is preferred for other histologies like esthesioneuroblastoma. Clinically or radiologically suspicious cervical lymphadenopathy requires neck dissection. As in early disease, cervicotomy for microvascular anastomosis provides an opportunity to address the neck in a limited manner (levels I-II).

Radiotherapy: Radical radiotherapy is preferred only in patients unfit or not desirous of surgery or unresectable (T4b) disease. Due to the potential morbidity of dose delivery to the OARs, more precise radiotherapy delivery techniques (like intensity modulated radiotherapy and proton therapy) are preferred. Addition of concurrent chemotherapy is suggested in aggressive histologies for incremental benefit, however evidence is scanty. Individual regimens are discussed subsequently.

Adjuvant radiotherapy is indicated in virtually all locally advanced sinonasal tumors, even in the absence of positive margins and risk features, in order to consolidate local control. As a majority of these tumors are associated with local failure, this is of paramount importance to improve survival and preserve quality of life.

Chemotherapy: The role of chemotherapy is clearest in squamous cell carcinoma, where the NCCN recommends the use of concurrent cisplatin for curative intent chemoradiotherapy and induction chemotherapy with docetaxel, cisplatin, and 5-fluorouracil for unresectable disease, based on extrapolation of results from other trials.[68,69]

The role of induction chemotherapy in sinonasal tumors is primarily in T4b disease to determine intent of treatment, or in early orbit involvement to avoid orbital exenteration.[70,71] Newer data is now emerging that response to induction chemotherapy in certain histologies, such as SNUC, may predict favorable responses and outcomes with chemoradiotherapy,[72] however nonrandomized and retrospective data require careful consideration before application to practice.

SURGICAL APPROACHES

Endoscopic approaches: Surgeons undertaking endoscopic resection need to be experienced in endoscopic tumor resection, with the ability to convert to open surgery for safety or oncological reasons. The instrumentation required for resection of these lesions includes high-powered instruments such as a microdebrider, high-speed drills, diamond-tipped drills, and bipolar cautery. Two-member teams commonly perform surgery using the three or fourhanded technique on either side of the nasal septum. Although the tumor is removed piecemeal, the point of attachment of tumor needs to be identified, marked out and removed in entirety, with negative margins on frozen section circumferentially. Normal structures may need to be removed for access to the tumor; the corridors most commonly used for access are transnasal (via the nasal cavity), transantral (through the maxillary antrum), and transsphenoidal (through the roof of the sphenoid sinus).

Depending on the histology, the extent of resection varies; for an olfactory neuroblastoma the olfactory bulbs and tracts require excision along with the point of attachment of the tumor to the cribriform plate of ethmoid, while for a squamous cell carcinoma arising in an inverted papilloma a subperiosteal resection needs to be performed to remove nests of cells within the maxillary bone. A preoperative biopsy allows the resection to be tailored to the patient. Experienced surgeons have pushed the boundaries of endoscopic surgery, so contraindications to endoscopic approaches may be more relevant than indications. The absolute contraindications to endoscopic surgery with curative intent are requirement of orbital exenteration, maxillectomy (except for medial wall resection), tumors involving skin, anterior or lateral involvement of the frontal sinus, involvement of the dura or the brain parenchyma and involvement of the internal carotid artery, cavernous sinus or the optic chiasma.[73] Relative contraindications are orbital apex involvement and pterygomaxillary space or infratemporal fossa involvement.

Open approaches: Complete surgical excision of tumors of the paranasal sinuses and skull base is a challenging prospect, even today. The first description of a complete excision of the superior maxillary bone was given by Lizars in 1829,[74] however he was unable to completely clear the pterygoid process completely. This issue was not solved for over a century, when in the 1960s Conley and Dingman pioneered techniques that allowed adequate access to the infratemporal fossa and pterygomaxillary fissure to clear the posterior maxilla.[75] Similarly, paranasal sinus tumors involving the anterior or middle cranial fossa were deemed unresectable until in 1963 Ketcham described a series of patients treated with a combined craniofacial approach, which continues to be the standard of care to this day.[76]

The approach to open surgical extirpation of these tumors is two-fold; the skin incision which allows access to the paranasal sinuses and skull base, and the extent of bony resection. The ideal approach should allow adequate access to remove the tumor with margins, exposure of the surrounding vital structures and sufficient exposure for reconstruction as and when required. The incisions are shown in **(Table 2)**.

The extent of resection depends on the extent of the tumor. The aim of surgical excision is complete monobloc removal of the tumor, however this is difficult especially in certain areas where the bone is thin and brittle, such as the cribriform plates. In these cases, precise anatomical mapping of the tumor with complete removal aided by frozen section and the "layer concept" (surgical removal of the subsequent uninvolved anatomical layer) aid in adequate clearance—margin adequacy measured in mm as with other subsites is not practical or feasible. In certain locations (such as dura) even a 1 mm margin is accepted as free, while in others (infrastructural maxilla) larger margins are advisable. Margin adequacy also depends on the grade of the tumor—high-grade tumors require more aggressive clearance wherever feasible. This is what makes multidisciplinary management in these patients crucial—the decision to operate, the feasibility and extent of surgery, and the role of adjuvant therapy need to be decided on a case-by-case basis.

Table 2: Incisions and indications for various approaches (shown in **Figure 6**).

Incision	*Indications*
Lynch's incision	Access to the ethmoid sinus and floor of the frontal sinus
Moure's lateral rhinotomy incision	Access to the nasal cavity, ethmoid sinus or anterior skull base
Weber Ferguson incision	Access to tumor involving the maxilla extending superiorly to the infraorbital nerve
Dieffenbach's modification of Weber Ferguson incision	Allows better access to the floor of the orbit
Borle's extension of Weber Ferguson incision	Allows access to the temporal fossa to harvest the temporalis flap for reconstruction of maxillary defect
Weber Ferguson Longmire incision	Additional palatal incision allows for maxillary swing as an approach, (e.g., recurrent nasopharyngeal tumors)
Facial degloving approach	Vestibular incision allows good access to the anterior maxilla avoiding scars on the face, however can be used in very selected malignant tumors

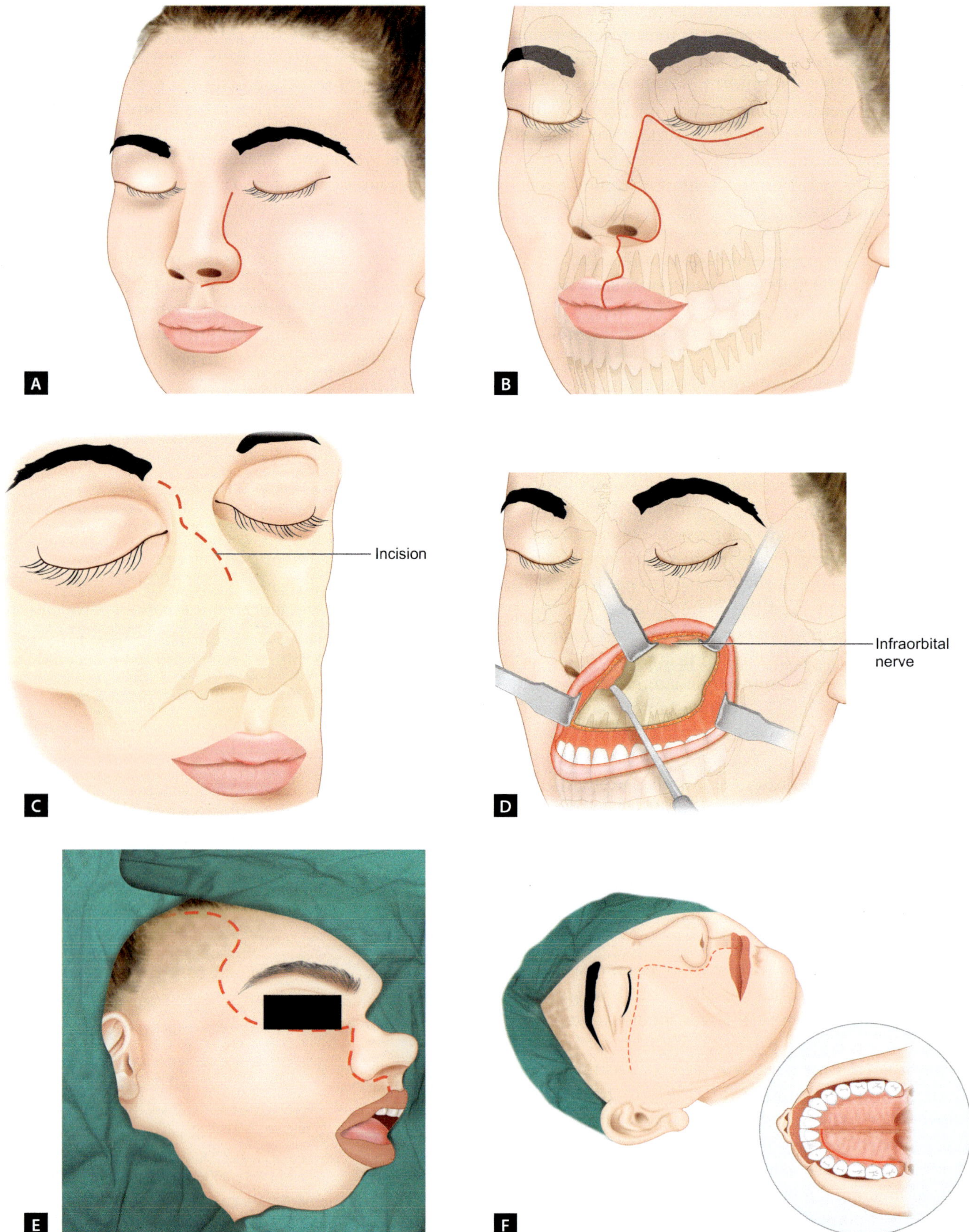

Figs. 6A to F: Maxillectomy incisions. (A) Moure's lateral rhinotomy incision; (B) Dieffenbach's modification of Weber Ferguson incision; (C) Lynch's incision; (D) Facial degloving approach; (E) Borle's extension; (F) Weber Ferguson Longmire incision.

Maxillectomy: Resection of the maxilla can be performed for tumors arising from or adjacent to the maxillary sinus. Circumferential resection of the tumor is performed to ensure margins in all directions. Access may be endoscopic (for medial maxillectomy), transoral, transfacial or extended. For malignant tumors, the principle employed is that the approach should allow excellent access to even the most difficult to reach parts of the tumor; functional and cosmetic considerations are second to oncological ones. Skin planes are raised in the subperiosteal plan to allow the resection to remain bloodless while preserving blood supply to the face. Infiltration near the greater palatine foramen with 2% xylocaine and adrenaline allows the intraoral cuts to remain relatively bloodless. The infraorbital nerve is usually sacrificed unless the vertical extent of resection is low. A high-speed drill is preferred for resection to prevent excess bone loss and immediate packing after osteotomies helps prevent excessive blood loss. Bleeding from the internal maxillary artery is best managed with ligation while bleeding from the pterygoid plexus if the infratemporal fossa is being resected in continuity is prevented by division of the muscle and loose areolar tissue with bipolar forceps or a harmonic scalpel; veins here retract after resection and can be difficult to coagulate subsequently. The most common defect classification is the Liverpool Classification, proposed by Brown in 2000[77] **(Fig. 7)**. It divides the extent of maxillectomy into a vertical component (class I involves removal of alveolar bone without creation of an oroantra fistula, class II involves removal of alveolus and antral wall causing oronasal or oroantral fistula, class III involves resection of maxilla with floor of orbit with or without periorbital tissue and class IV involves maxillectomy and orbital contents with or without anterior skull base) and a horizontal component (resection of hard palate without removal of teeth bearing alveolus, resection of up to half of the hard palate, resection of over half of the hard palate with preservation of part of one side and complete resection of the hard palate). **Figure 8** shows a compartmental resection of a T4 maxilla tumour reconstructed with a soft tissue flap.

Ethmoidectomy: Endoscopic approaches are used for very early tumors limited to the ethmoid sinus that the surgeon is comfortably clearing completely. The external approach to the ethmoid sinus is via the Lynch incision, subperiosteal dissection of the medial orbital contents and piecemeal removal of the lamina papyracea. This is not a reasonable approach for most malignant tumors. Also majority of ethmoidal tumors are advanced at presentation;[78] they often involve the maxillary sinus and anterior cranial fossa **(Fig. 9)** that require maxillectomy and craniofacial resection respectively.

Sphenoidectomy: Like ethmoid sinuses, sphenoid sinus tumors are rare and often advanced at presentation.[79] Few of these patients are candidates for radical surgery as a result, requiring combined transfacial and cranial approaches. Surgical considerations include resectability, prognosis (based on grade and stage of tumor), cure/control rates with non-surgical therapies, and post-operative morbidity (especially in cases requiring cavernous sinus and brain parenchymal resections).

Craniofacial resection: Craniofacial resection is considered the standard treatment for tumors involving the anterior skull base. It involves a combined approach to excise the sinonasal and cranial components of the

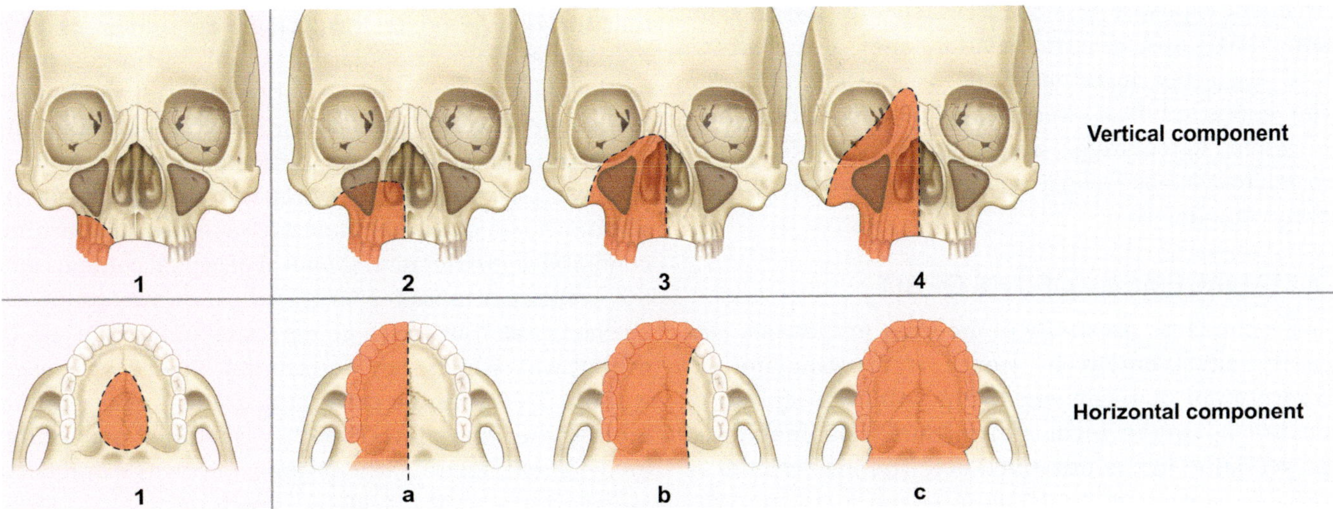

Fig. 7: Brown's classification of maxillectomy defects.

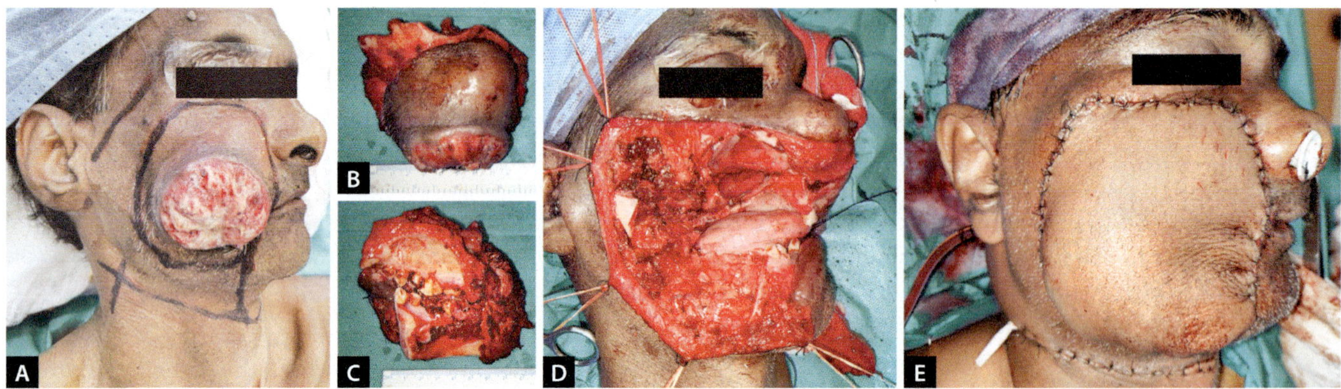

Figs. 8A to E: (A) Clinical appearance of an advanced maxillary cancer; (B) Anterior view of compartment resection; (C) Posterior view showing upper and lower alveoli and gingivobuccal sulcus; (D) Final defect showing the skull base; (E) Defect reconstructed with bipaddled anterolateral thigh flap.

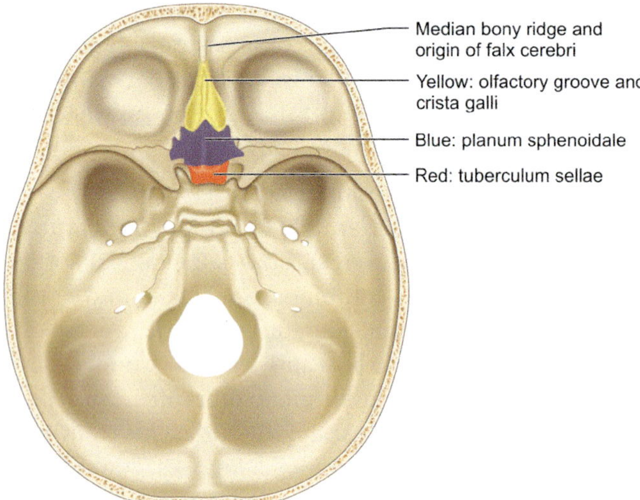

Fig. 9: Parts of the anterior cranial fossa.

tumor en-bloc. Most commonly the wide bifrontal craniotomy with a lateral rhinotomy approach affords excellent exposure to most areas, such as the anterior sphenoid sinus, cavernous sinus, apex of the orbital and even the infratemporal fossa. Depending on the extent of bony resection, reconstruction may be limited to requiring a watertight seal of the dura alone or microvascular reconstruction with soft tissue and/or bony components.

MANAGEMENT OF THE ORBIT

Given the close proximity of the orbit to the sinonasal cavity, involvement by tumor is not uncommon. Appropriate management of the orbit is required to ensure adequate local control and also functional preservation in the preserved eye. The involvement of the orbit varies by the location of the tumor and the histology, and these factors also influence the ability of the surgeon to preserve the eye during resection. It is also to be noted that patients with gross orbital involvement may or may not have symptoms, which makes detailed imaging and clinical evaluation of vision in all patients mandatory. Symptoms, such as proptosis, diplopia, epiphora may occur in about half of patients with sinonasal tumors, but not all symptoms relate to orbital involvement; they may be associated with blockage of the lacrimal drainage system or bony remodeling of the orbital floor.[80] Tumors of the ethmoid often involve the orbit via erosion of the cribriform plate while those of the maxilla most often involve the orbit through destruction of the medial wall and floor of the orbit. However, they have also been known to spread via natural foramina and perineural invasion.

Following violation of the bone by tumor, the periorbita also acts as a barrier to tumor spread due to its dense connective tissue component.[81] Importantly, once this is breached, the tumor has access to the orbital contents without any further barriers or checks to spread. Classifications of orbital involvement are numerous, with arguably the most popular by Ianetti,[82] who described grade I as destruction of medial orbital wall, grade II as extraconal invasion of the periorbital fat and grade III as invasion of medial rectus, optic nerve, ocular bulb or skin overlying the eyelid. He proposed that only grade III tumors needed orbital clearance (removal of orbital contents) or exenteration (removal of orbital contents and the eyelids). A more recent classification was proposed by Neel et al.,[83] in which grade 1 was tumor adjacent to orbital wall which may be thinned, bowed or eroded without breach of the periorbita, grade 2 where tumor erodes the orbital wall with resectable periorbital involvement, grade 3 where tumor involves extraocular muscle intraconal fat, globe or orbital apex, grade 4 where the tumor invades the nasolacrimal system, eyelids or lacrimal sac and grade 5 where there is cavernous sinus or optic canal involvement or massive intracranial involvement. Here as well, grades 1–2 can be managed with conservative surgical procedures while grades 3 and above require orbital sacrifice (except for selected patients of grade 4). In patients receiving conservative surgical approaches with limited involvement or extraconal fat, frozen section has been shown to be useful to establish adequate surgical clearance.[83,84] Several studies have shown that when combined with adjuvant radiotherapy, less aggressive resections (open or endoscopic) have good 5-year local control rates in the range of 60–65%.[85-87]

Another strategy in patients with orbital involvement is induction chemotherapy; the rationale here is to reduce tumor volume allowing less aggressive local resection and better treatment of micrometastatic disease; however patients may progress on the treatment leading to disease no longer being eligible for curative treatment strategies.[88] A major challenge in interpreting the data is that it is retrospective (and hence potentially affected by selection bias), involves multiple histologies and stages, and utilizes multiple chemotherapy regimens. The histologies that showed a good response to induction chemotherapy were squamous cell carcinoma treated with platinum, fluorouracil, and taxane combinations showing a response rate of 67–80%[89-92] and esthesioneuroblastoma/sinonasal endocrine carcinoma treated with platinum and etoposide showing a response rate of 60–80%.[93-95] It is essential to realize that offering patients induction chemotherapy is predicated on their ability to tolerate these regimens, and puts them at the risk of worsening performance status and ineligibility for curative intent therapy and disease progression, and needs to be made in a multidisciplinary setting.

Outcomes following eye preservation in conservative procedures are acceptable; Imola and Schramm reported results in the preserved eye as functional without impairment in 54%, functional with impairment in 37%, and nonfunctional in 9%.[96] Most common complaint was globe malposition due to improper orbital floor reconstruction. Radiotherapy also increases the likelihood of ophthalmic symptoms such as pain, redness, ectropion, and dryness. From this data it is clear that if the eye is preserved, it is crucial to ensure proper position and integrity of the orbital floor. Minimal bony resections of the walls or floor may not merit reconstruction however subtotal or total floor defects (>75% surface area) and multi-segmental defects (resection of the orbital floor and one or more wall) require rigid fixation.[97] This can be achieved with vascularized flaps or titanium mesh, however the latter has the risk of extrusion following adjuvant radiotherapy; the ideal is a microvascular composite free flap with bone and soft tissue.[98]

CAROTID SACRIFICE

As with any tumor in the head the neck, sacrifice of the common/internal carotid artery for paranasal sinus or anterior skull base neoplasms requires careful consideration of the anatomy **(Fig. 10)**. The following section is devoted to carotid sacrifice for head and neck tumors in general, however this decision needs to be taken on an individualized basis, often with input from neuroradiology, neurosurgery, and vascular surgery as and where required.

Background

In most cases, involvement or encasement of the common carotid artery has been considered a contraindication to primary surgical therapy for head and neck neoplasms (deemed as stage T4b on AJCC/NCCN staging systems) due to the high risk of stroke associated with carotid resection.[99] However with better imaging, perioperative care, and surgical technique, patients having carotid involvement are more often becoming surgical candidates with acceptable morbidity. Often cross-sectional imaging has poor specificity to determine actual invasion as opposed to peri-tumor inflammation (especially in irradiated patients), meaning that patients require thorough evaluation and preparation for a carotid resection, even if the tumor can ultimately be dissected off the carotid without sacrifice.[100] Given the potential morbidity of carotid resection, carotid resection needs to be oncologically and functionally worthwhile for the patient. These patients must be potentially curable; patients should have completely resectable disease with a reasonable prognosis, good performance status and willingness to undergo surgery in spite of the potentially devastating neurological sequelae.

Preoperative Evaluation

Preoperative evaluation of carotid involvement using CT or MRI has been shown to have varying levels of accuracy with high inter-observer variation; however, the criterion of involvement of 270 or more of the carotid circumference has been shown to be accurate to determine ability to dissect the tumor off an intact carotid artery.[101] However once it is decided that the carotid may need to be sacrificed, carotid artery balloon test occlusion (BTO) is considered the gold standard evaluation to determine the effect of internal carotid occlusion on

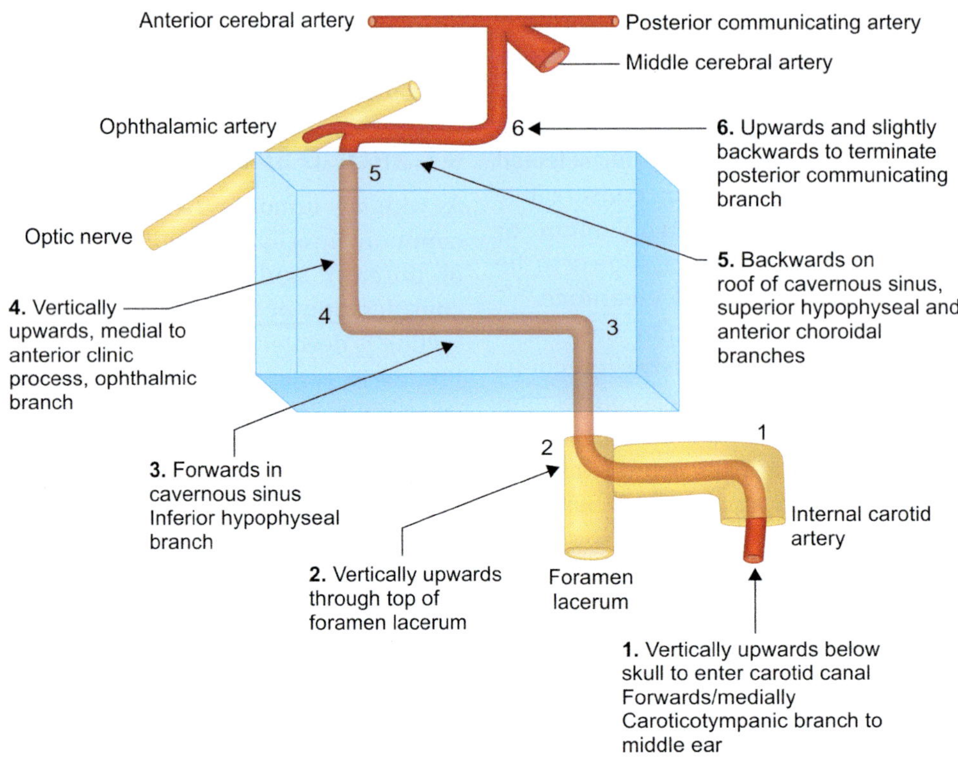

Fig. 10: Anatomy of right internal carotid artery.

cerebrovascular circulation. Without any temporary test occlusion, it is estimated that the incidence of stroke after permanent carotid artery occlusion (such as ligation) is 17–30%.[102,103] This is a modified four-vessel digital subtraction angiography of the cerebral circulation where a balloon is used to occlude the internal carotid artery (usually for 15–30 mins) to determine if the contralateral supply through the circle of Willis is adequate to maintain cerebral perfusion. If the patient has no signs of symptoms of ischemia, they are said to have "passed" and are likely to tolerate carotid sacrifice without reconstruction, while those who have not "passed" require reconstruction either as a single stage or two stage (carotid bypass first followed by resection) procedure. However, there is a caveat here; up to 30% of patients who have passed the BTO still have a risk of stroke following carotid sacrifice due to embolic showers from the distal carotid stump following ligation or the stress of intraoperative hypotension further compromising cerebral blood flow.[104] This has led to patients being grouped as *low risk* (passed BTO with adequate cerebral flow), *moderate risk* (passed BTO with inadequate cerebral blood flow), and *high risk* (failed BTO with no cerebral blood flow). Several techniques have been used to better assess cerebral blood flow after carotid occlusion when compared to clinical evaluation, such as Tc99m SPECT scanning, xenon-enhanced contrast CT and arterial stump measurement, however this is challenging and may not be available in all centers.[105]

Surgical approaches:
- With focal involvement of the carotid wall, peeling or subadventitial may be attempted; however, this may lead to weakening of the wall and subsequent rupture, especially in patients previously receiving radiotherapy
- Ligation of the involved segment is feasible only in low-risk patients, however even they have a risk of stroke postoperatively
- Carotid substitution can be performed with autografts (such as greater saphenous vein or superficial femoral artery grafts) or synthetic grafts (such as Dacron) used as conduits or patches to replace or bridge the resected area.
- Extracranial-intracranial bypass is used when the upper internal carotid artery (petrous or cavernous) is involved, with a surgical bypass created between the external carotid artery and the middle cerebral artery. They are further classified as:
    - *Low flow bypass:* The frontal or parietal branch of the superficial temporal artery is anastomosed to a cortical branch of the middle cerebral artery with a blood flow of 20–70 mL/min

- *Intermediate flow bypass:* Radial artery interposition graft is used between the external carotid and middle cerebral arteries with a blood flow of 60–100 mL/min
- *High flow bypass:* Saphenous vein graft interposition is used between external carotid and middle cerebral arteries with a blood flow of 100–200 mL/min

OUTCOMES

Reporting survival outcomes of paranasal sinus and anterior skull base cancers as a whole is misleading as survival and treatment response varies significantly with histology and stage at presentation. One of the largest studies, showing SEER data for over 6,000 patients, reported 5-year relative survival as 55%.[106] The survival varied significantly with the biological aggression of the histological subtype; low-risk subtypes such as esthesioneuroblastoma and adenoid cystic carcinoma had 5-year survival of around 70%, intermediate-risk subtypes such as squamous cell and adenocarcinoma had survival rates of 50–60% while high-risk subtypes such as melanoma and sinonasal undifferentiated carcinoma had survival rates of around 35%. With newer treatment modalities, such as targeted therapies, this may improve.

COMPLICATIONS

The surgical complication rates are highest with craniofacial resection. An international study of 334 patients published in 2005 showed that postoperative mortality was 4.5%, and complications occurred in 32.9%,[107] even though these were specialized centers with significant technical expertise. The common complications are wound and healing related, CSF leak and meningitis, orbital complications and systemic complications following major surgery. Adjuvant radiotherapy is also not without risk. Surgical wound dehiscence, sinonasal cutaneous fistula, ocular complications (optic atrophy, cataract, xerophthalmia and ectropion), and skull base osteoradionecrosis are known to occur. However their incidence may be minimized with good surgical technique, use of vascularized tissue for wound closure, and more modern radiotherapy delivery techniques.[108]

RECURRENCE AND FOLLOW-UP

Recurrence is common in this group of malignancies, with patients developing recurrences years after initial treatment. For this reason, regular follow-up is advised life-long. Regular endoscopic evaluation is recommended for patients whose tumor bed is accessible for examination, and also to evaluate and treat sequelae of treatment (such as crusting, epiphora). MRI within 3 months following surgery may act as a baseline for further assessment. The UK guidelines advise MRI evaluation every 3–4 months for the first year, every 6 months from the second to fifth year and then every 6–9 months subsequently;[73] however this decision needs to be made based on the patient and disease characteristics.

REFERENCES

1. Muir CS, Nectoux J. Descriptive epidemiology of malignant neoplasms of nose, nasal cavities, middle ear and accessory sinuses. Clin Otolaryngol Allied Sci. 1980;5:195-211.
2. Caplan LS, Hall I, Levine RS, Zhu K. Preventable risk factors for nasal cancer. Ann Epidemiol. 2000;10:186-91.
3. Carey RM, Godovchik J, Workman AD, Kuan EC, Parasher AK, Chen J, et al. Patient, disease, and treatment factors associated with overall survival in esthesioneuroblastoma. Int Forum Allergy Rhinol. 2017;12:1186-94.
4. Ognjanovic S, Linabery AM, Charbonneau B, Ross JA. Trends in childhood rhabdomyosarcoma incidence and survival in the United States, 1975-2005. Cancer. 2009;18:4218-26.
5. 't Mannetje A, Kogevinas M, Luce D, Demers PA, Bégin D, Bolm-Audorff U, et al. Sinonasal cancer, occupation, and tobacco smoking in European women and men. Am J Ind Med. 1999;36(1):101-7.
6. Hadfield EH. A study of adenocarcinoma of the paranasal sinuses in woodworkers in the furniture industry. Ann R Coll Surg Engl. 1970;46(6):301-19.
7. Klintenberg C, Olofsson J, Hellquist H, Sökjer H. Adenocarcinoma of the ethmoid sinuses. A review of 28 cases with special reference to wood dust exposure. Cancer. 1984;54(3):482-8.
8. Binazzi A, Ferrante P, Marinaccio A. Occupational exposure and sinonasal cancer: a systematic review and meta-analysis. BMC Cancer. 2015;15(1):49.
9. Blot WJ, Chow WH, McLaughlin JK. Wood dust and nasal cancer risk. A review of the evidence from North America. J Occup Environ Med. 1997;39(2):148-56.
10. Surgery of the skull base. In: Donald PJ (Ed). Pathology of Skull Base Tumors. Philadelphia: Lippincott-Raven; 1998.
11. Diaz RJ, Guduk M, Romagnuolo R, Smith CA, Northcott P, Shih D, et al. High-resolution whole-genome analysis of skull base chordomas implicates FHIT loss in chordoma pathogenesis. Neoplasia. 2012;14(9):788.
12. Harbo G, Grau C, Bundgaard T, Overgaard M, Elbrønd O, Søgaard H, et al. Cancer of the nasal cavity and paranasal sinuses: a clinico-pathological study of 277 patients. Acta Oncologica. 1997;36(1):45-50.
13. Nascimento AG, Amaral AL, Prado LA, Kligerman J, Silveira TR. Adenoid cystic carcinoma of salivary glands. A study of 61 cases with clinicopathologic correlation. Cancer. 1986;57(2):312-9.
14. Hicks J, Flaitz C. Rhabdomyosarcoma of the head and neck in children. Oral Oncol. 2002;38(5):450-9.

15. Sen CN, Sekhar LN, Schramm VL, Janecka IP. Chordoma and chondrosarcoma of the cranial base: an 8-year experience. Neurosurgery. 1989;25(6):931-41.
16. O'Connell JX, Rosenberg AE, Renard LG, Liebsch NJ, Efird JT, Munzenrider JE. Base of skull chordoma. A correlative study of histologic and clinical features of 62 cases. Cancer. 1994;74(8):2261-7.
17. Han MH, Chang KH, Kim IO, Kim DK, Han MC. Non-Hodgkin lymphoma of the central skull base: MR manifestations. J Comput Assist Tomogr. 1993;17(4):567-71.
18. Oyama H, Nagane M, Shibui S, Nomura K, Mukae K. Skull base malignant lymphoma: a case report and review of the literature. Jpn J Clin Onco. 1992;22:131.
19. Narasimhan K, Kucuk O, Lin HS, Heilbrun LK, Carron M, Venkatramanamoorthy R, et al. Sinonasal mucosal melanoma: a 13-year experience at a single institution. Skull Base. 2009; 19(4):255.
20. Kadish S, Goodman M, Wang CC. Olfactory neuroblastoma—a clinical analysis of 17 cases. Cancer. 1976;37(3):1571-6.
21. Lund VJ, Howard D, Wei W, Spittle M. Olfactory neuroblastoma: past, present, and future? Laryngoscope. 2003;113(3):502-7.
22. Bell D, Hanna EY, Weber RS, DeMonte F, Triantafyllou A, Lewis JS Jr, et al. Neuroendocrine neoplasms of the sinonasal region. Head Neck. 2016;38(Suppl 1):E2259-66.
23. Ma ATW, Lei KIK. Small cell neuroendocrine carcinoma of the ethmoid sinuses presenting with generalized seizure and syndrome of inappropriate antidiuretic hormone secretion: a case report and review of the literature. Am J Otolaryngol. 2009;30:54-7.
24. Kao HL, Chang WC, Li WY, Li A C-H, Li A F-Y. Head and neck large cell neuroendocrine carcinoma should be separated from atypical carcinoid on the basis of different clinical features, overall survival, and pathogenesis. Am J Surg Pathol. 2012;36:185-92.
25. Hafezi S, Seethala RR, Stelow EB, Mills SE, Leong IT, MacDuff E, et al. Ewing's family of tumors of the sinonasal tract and maxillary bone. Head Neck Pathol. 2011;5:8-16.
26. Shah K, Perez-Ordóñez B. Neuroendocrine neoplasms of the sinonasal tract: neuroendocrine carcinomas and olfactory neuroblastoma. Head Neck Pathology. 2016;10(1): 85-94.
27. Mickel RA, Zimmerman MC. The sphenoid sinus: a site for metastasis. Otolaryngol Head Neck Surg. 1990;102:709.
28. Hirai O, Kikuchi H, Hashimoto N. Skull base metastasis. Head Neck. 1991;13:89.
29. Merimsky O, Inbar M, Grosswasser-Reider I, Neudorfer M, Chaitchik S. Sphenoid and cavernous sinuses involvement as first site of metastasis from a fallopian tube carcinoma. Tumori. 1993;79:444.
30. Ong HS, Ji T, Zhang CP, Li J, Wang LZ, Li RR, et al. Head and neck inflammatory myofibroblastic tumor (IMT): evaluation of clinicopathologic and prognostic features. Oral Oncol. 2012;48:141-8.
31. Lazaridou M, Dimitrakopoulos I, Tilaveridis I, Iordanidis F, Kontos K. Inflammatory myofibroblastic tumor of the maxillary sinus and the oral cavity. Oral Maxillofac Surg. 2014;18:111-4.
32. Gleason BC, Hornick JL. Inflammatory myofibroblastic tumors: where are we now? J Clin Pathol. 2008;61:428-37.
33. Chen YF, Zhang WD, Wu MW, Ou-Yang D, Zhang Q. Inflammatory myofibroblastic tumor of the head and neck. Med Oncol. 2011;28(1):349-53.
34. Fujii H, Fujisada H, Kondo T, Takahashi T, Okada S. Orbital pseudotumor: histopathological classification and treatment. Ophthalmologica. 1985;190: 230-42.
35. Segawa Y, Yasumatsu R, Shiratsuchi H, Tamae A, Noda T, Yamamoto H, Komune S. Inflammatory pseudotumor in head and neck. Auris Nasus Larynx. 2014;41(3):321-4.
36. Yagoda MR, Selesnick SH. Temporal bone fibrous dysplasia and cholesteatoma leading to the development of a parapharyngeal abscess. J Laryngol Otol. 1994;108:51.
37. Ruggieri P, Sim FH, Bond JR, Unni KK. Malignancies in fibrous dysplasia. Cancer. 1994;73:1411.
38. Kapadia SB, Popek EJ, Barnes L. Pediatric otorhinolaryngic pathology: diagnosis of selected lesions. Pathol Annu. 1994;29:159.
39. Barnes L, Weber PC, Krause JR, Contis L, Janecka I. Angiofibroma: a flow cytomet-ric evaluation of 31 cases. Skull Base Surg. 1992;2:195.
40. Tang IP, Shashinder S, Gopala Krishnan G, Narayanan P. Juvenile nasopharyngeal angiofibroma in a tertiary centre: ten-year experience. Singapore Med J. 2009;50(3):261-4.
41. Overdevest JB, Amans MR, Zaki P, Pletcher SD, El-Sayed IH. Patterns of vascularization and surgical morbidity in juvenile nasopharyngeal angiofibroma: a case series, systematic review, and meta-analysis. Head Neck. 2018;40(2):428-43.
42. Melroy CT, Senior BA. Benign sinonasal neoplasms: A focus on inverting papilloma. Otolaryngol Clin North Am. 2006;39:601-17.
43. Krouse JH. Endoscopic treatment of inverted papilloma: Safety and efficacy. Am J Otolaryngol. 2001;22:87-99.
44. Strojan P, Jereb S, Borsos I, But-Hadzic J, Zidar N. Radiotherapy for inverted papilloma: a case report and review of the literature. Radiol Oncol. 2013;47(1):71-6.
45. Kadish S, Goodman M, Wang CC. Olfactory neuroblastoma: a clinical analysis of 17 cases. Cancer. 1976;37:1571-6.
46. Dulguerov P, Calcaterra T. Esthesioneuroblastoma: the UCLA experience 1970–1990. Laryngoscope. 1992;102:843-49.
47. Eggesbø HB. Imaging of sinonasal tumors. Cancer Imaging; 2012. p. 136.
48. Kapoor V, Fukui MB, McCook BM. Role of 18FFDG PET/CT in the treatment of head and neck cancers: posttherapy evaluation and pitfalls. Am J Roentgenol. 2005;184(2):589-97.
49. Lloyd GAS. Epithelial tumors. In: Diagnostic imaging of the nose and paranasal sinuses. London: Springer Verlag; 1988. pp. 95-110.
50. Som PM, Shapiro MD, Biller HF, Sasaki C, Lawson, W. Sinonasal tumors and inflammatory tissues: differentiation with MR imaging. Radiology. 1988;167:803-8.
51. Gandhi M, Sommerville J. The imaging of large nerve perineural spread. J Neurol Surg B Skull Base. 2016;77(02):113-23.
52. Eisen MD, Yousem DM, Montone KT, Kotapka MJ, Bigelow DC, Bilker WB, et al. Use of preoperative MR to predict dural, perineural, and venous sinus invasion of skull base tumors. Am J Neurorad. 1996;17:1937-45.
53. Graamans K, Slootweg PJ Orbital exenteration in surgery of malignant neoplasms of the paranasal sinuses. Arch Otolaryngol Head Neck Surg. 1989;115:977-80.
54. Suarez C, Llorente JL, Fernandez De Leon R, Maseda E, Lopez A. Prognostic factors in sinonasal tumors involving the anterior skull base. Head Neck. 2004;26:136-44.
55. Ginsberg LE, DeMonte F. Imaging of perineural tumor spread from palatal carcinoma. AJNR Am J Neuroradiol. 1998;19: 1417-22.

56. Mancuso AA, Harnsberger HR, Dillon WP. Paranasal sinuses, nasal cavity, and facial bones. In: Workbook for MRI and CT of the head and neck, 2nd edition. Baltimore: Williams & Wilkins; 1988. pp. 56-76.
57. Aoki J, Sone S, Fujioka F, Terayama K, Ishii K, Karakida O, Imai S, et al. MR of enchondroma and chondrosarcoma: rings and arcs of Gd-DTPA enhancement. J Comput Assist Tomogr. 1991;15:1011-6.
58. De Beuckeleer LH, De Schepper AM, Ramon F, Somville J. Magnetic resonance imaging of cartilaginous tumors: a retrospective study of 79 patients. Eur J Radiol. 1995;21:34-40.
59. Pfister DG, Ang KK, Brizel DM, Burtness BA, Busse PM, Caudell JJ, et al. Head and neck cancers, version 2.2013. Featured updates to the NCCN guidelines. J Natl Compr Canc Netw. 2013;11(8):917-23.
60. Dulguerov P, Jacobsen MS, Allal AS, Lehmann W, Calcaterra T. Nasal and paranasal sinus carcinoma: are we making progress? A series of 220 patients and a systematic review. Cancer. 2001;92:3012-29.
61. Lavertu P, Roberts JK, Kraus DH, et al. Squamous cell carcinoma of the paranasal sinuses: the Cleveland Clinic experience 1977-1986. Laryngoscope. 1989;99:1130-6.
62. Paulino AC, Fisher SG, Marks JE. Is prophylactic neck irradiation indicated in patients with squamous cell carcinoma of the maxillary sinus? Int J Radiat Oncol Biol Phys. 1997;39:283-9.
63. Magrini SM, Nicolai P, Somensari A, Scheda A, Bignardi M, Bonetti B, et al. Which role for radiation therapy in ethmoid cancer? A retrospective analysis of 84 cases from a single institution. Tumori Journal. 2004;90(6):573-8.
64. Parsons JT, Mendenhall WM, Mancuso AA, Cassisi NJ, Million RR. Malignant tumors of the nasal cavity and ethmoid and sphenoid sinuses. Inter J Rad Oncol Biol Phy. 1988;14(1):11-22.
65. Baker R, Cherry J, Lott S, Bischofberger WB. Carcinoma of the maxillary sinus. Arch Otolaryngol. 1966;84:201-4.
66. Knegt PP, De Jong PC, Van Andel JG, de Boer MF, Eykenboom W, van der Schans E. Carcinoma of the paranasal sinuses. Results of a prospective pilot study. Cancer. 1985;56:57-62.
67. Lindeman P, Eklund U, Petruson B. Survival after surgical treatment in maxillary neoplasms of epithelial origin. J Laryngol Otol. 1987;101:564-8.
68. Vermorken JB, Remenar E, Van Herpen C, Gorlia T, Mesia R, Degardin M, et al. Cisplatin, fluorouracil, and docetaxel in unresectable head and neck cancer. New Engl J Med. 2007;357(17):1695-704.
69. Adelstein DJ, Li Y, Adams GL, Wagner Jr H, Kish JA, Ensley JF, et al. An intergroup phase III comparison of standard radiation therapy and two schedules of concurrent chemoradiotherapy in patients with unresectable squamous cell head and neck cancer. J Clin Oncol. 2003;21(1):92-8.
70. Brasnu D, Laccourreye O, Bassot V, Laccourreye L, Naudo P, Roux FX. Cisplatin-based neoadjuvant chemotherapy and combined resection for ethmoid sinus adenocarcinoma reaching and/or invading the skull base. Arch Otolaryngol Head Neck Surg. 1996;122:765-68.
71. Hanna EY, Cardenas AD, DeMonte F, Roberts D, Kupferman M, Weber R, et al. Induction chemotherapy for advanced squamous cell carcinoma of the paranasal sinuses. Arch Otolaryngol Head Neck Surg. 2011;137(1):78-81.
72. Amit M, Abdelmeguid AS, Watcherporn T, Takahashi H, Tam S, Bell D, et al. Induction chemotherapy response as a guide for treatment optimization in sinonasal undifferentiated carcinoma. J Clin Oncol. 2019;37(6):504.
73. Lund VJ, Clarke PM, Swift AC, McGarry GW, Kerawala C, Carnell D. Nose and paranasal sinus tumors: United Kingdom national multidisciplinary guidelines. J Laryngol Otol. 2016;130(S2):S111-8.
74. Sisson Sr GA, Toriumi DM, Atiyah RA. Paranasal sinus malignancy: a comprehensive update. Laryngoscope. 1989;99(2):143-50.
75. Dingman DL, Conley JJ. Lateral approach to the pterygomaxillary region. Ann Otol Rhinol Laryngol. 1970;79(5):967-9.
76. Ketcham AS, Wilkins RH, Van Buren JM, Smith RR. A combined intracranial facial approach to the paranasal sinuses. Am J Surg. 1963;106:698-703.
77. Brown JS, Rogers SN, McNally DN, Boyle M. A modified classification for the maxillectomy defects. Head Neck. 2000;22:17-26.
78. Lin CY, Chen HH, Chen HH, Fang SY, Tsai ST. Ethmoid sinus cancer: results of treatment with surgery and combined therapy. Acta Otolaryngol. 2004;124(10):1220-5.
79. DeMonte F, Ginsberg LE, Clayman GL. Primary malignant tumors of the sphenoidal sinus. Neurosurgery. 2000;46(5):1084-92.
80. Lund VJ. Malignant tumors of the nasal cavity and paranasal sinuses. ORL J Otorhinolaryngol Relat Spec. 1983;45:1-12.
81. Converse JM. Periorbita or periorbitum? Plast Reconstr Surg. 1977;60(1):106.
82. Iannetti G, Valentini V, Rinna C, Ventucci E, Marianetti TM. Ethmoido-orbital tumors: our experience. J Craniofac Surg. 2005;16:1085-91.
83. Neel GS, Nagel TH, Hoxworth JM, Lal D. Management of orbital involvement in sinonasal and ventral skull base malignancies. Otolaryngol Clin North Am. 2017;50:347-64.
84. Christianson B, Perez C, Harrow B, Batra PS. Management of the orbit during endoscopic sinonasal tumor surgery. Int Forum Allergy Rhinol. 2015;5:967-73.
85. Itami J, Uno T, Aruga M, Ode S. Squamous cell carcinoma of the maxillary sinus treated with radiation therapy and conservative surgery. Cancer. 1998;82:104-7.
86. Nishino H, Ichimura K, Tanaka H, Ishikawa K, Abe K, Fujisawa Y, et al. Results of orbital preservation for advanced malignant maxillary sinus tumors. Laryngoscope. 2003;113:1064-9.
87. Jansen EP, Keus RB, Hilgers FJ, Haas RL, Tan IB, Bartelink H. Does the combination of radiotherapy and debulking surgery favor survival in paranasal sinus carcinoma? Int J Radiat Oncol Biol Phys. 2000;48:27-35.
88. Bossi P, Saba NF, Vermorken JB, Stojan P, Pala L, de Bree R, et al. The role of systemic therapy in the management of sinonasal cancer: a critical review. Cancer Treat Rev. 2015;41:836-43.
89. Bjork-Eriksson T, Mercke C, Petruson B, Ekholm S. Potential impact on tumor control and organ preservation with cisplatin and 5-fluorouracil for patients with advanced tumors of the paranasal sinuses and nasal fossa. A prospective pilot study. Cancer. 1992;70:2615-20.
90. Hanna EY, Cardenas AD, DeMonte F, et al. Induction chemotherapy for advanced squamous cell carcinoma of the paranasal sinuses. Arch Otolaryngol Head Neck Surg. 2011;137:78-81.

91. Ock CY, Keam B, Kim TM, Doo Hee Han, Tae-Bin Won, Se-Hoon Lee et al. Induction chemotherapy in head and neck squamous cell carcinoma of the paranasal sinus and nasal cavity: a role in organ preservation. Korean J Intern Med. 2016;31:570-8.
92. McCary WS, Levine PA, Cantrell RW. Preservation of the eye in the treatment of sinonasal malignant neoplasms with orbital involvement. A confirmation of the original treatise. Arch Otolaryngol Head Neck Surg. 1996;122:657-9.
93. Mitchell EH, Diaz A, Yilmaz T, Roberts D, Nicholas L, DeMonte F, et al. Multimodality treatment for sinonasal neuroendocrine carcinoma. Head Neck. 2012;34:1372-6.
94. Su SY, Bell D, Ferrarotto R, Phan J, Roberts D, Kupferman ME, et al. Outcomes for olfactory neuroblastoma treated with induction chemotherapy. Head Neck. 2017; 39:1671-9.
95. Patil VM, Joshi A, Noronha V, Sharma V, Zanwar S, Dhumal S, et al. Neoadjuvant chemotherapy in locallyadvanced and borderline resectable nonsquamous sinonasal tumors (esthesioneuroblastoma and sinonasal tumor with neuroendocrine differentiation). Int J Surg Oncol. 2016;2016: 6923730.
96. Imola MJ, Schramm VL Jr. Orbital preservation in surgical management of sinonasal malignancy. Laryngoscope. 2002;112:1357-65.
97. Cordeiro PG, Santamaria E, Kraus DH, Strong EW, Shah JP. Reconstruction of total maxillectomy defects with preservation of the orbital contents. Plast Reconst Surg. 1998;102(6): 1874-84.
98. Rajapurkar M, Thankappan K, Sampathirao LM, Kuriakose MA, Iyer S. Oncologic and functional outcome of the preserved eye in malignant sinonasal tumors. Head Neck. 2013;35(10):1379-84.
99. Freeman SB, Hamaker RC, Borrowdale RB, Huntley TC. Management of neck metastasis with carotid artery involvement. Laryngoscope. 2004;114(1):20-4.
100. Mourad M, Saman M, Stroman D, Lee T, Ducic Y. Carotid artery sacrifice and reconstructon in the setting of advanced head and neck cancer. Otolaryngol Head Neck Surg. 2015; 153:225-30.
101. Yousem DM, Hatabu H, Hurst RW, Seigerman HM, Montone KT, Weinstein GS, et al. Carotid artery invasion by head and neck masses: prediction with MR imaging. Radiology. 1995;195(3):715-20.
102. Schorstein J. Carotid ligation in saccular intracranial aneurysms. Br J Surg. 1994;28:50-70
103. Norlen G. The pathology diagnosis and treatment of intracranial saccular aneurysms. Proc R Soc Med. 1952;45:291-302.
104. Standard SC, Ahuja A, Guterman LR. Balloon test occlusion of the internal carotid artery with hypotensive challenge. Am J Neuroradiol. 1995;16(7):1453-8.
105. Andersen AR, Friberg HH, Schmidt JF, Hasselbalch SG. Quantitative measurements of cerebral blood flow using SPECT and [99mTc]-d,l-HM-PAO compared to xenon-133. J Cereb Blood Flow Metab. 1988;8(6):S69-81.
106. Turner JH, Reh DD. Incidence and survival in patients with sinonasal cancer: a historical analysis of population-based data. Head Neck. 2012;34(6):877-85.
107. Ganly I, Patel SG, Singh B, Kraus DH, Bridger PG, Cantu G, et al. Craniofacial resection for malignant paranasal sinus tumors: report of an International Collaborative Study. Head Neck. 2005;27(7):575-84.
108. Jang JW, Chan AW. Prevention and Management of Complications after Radiotherapy for Skull Base Tumors: A Multidisciplinary Approach. Advances in Oto-Rhino-Laryngology; 2012. pp. 163-73.

CHAPTER 17

Cancers of the Nasopharynx

Vivek Shetty, Saurabha Kumar, Narayana Subramaniam

INTRODUCTION

The nasopharynx is the superior-most part of the pharynx that lies behind the posterior nares and communicates with the nasal cavity anteriorly and the oropharynx inferiorly. A roof, a posterior wall, two lateral walls, and a floor bound the nasopharynx. The roof is made up of mucosa overlying the posterior part of the sphenoid bone, which slopes posteriorly to form the posterior wall. Further below is the arch of the atlas over which lie the pharyngobasilar fascia and the superior-most fibers of the superior constrictor. The mucosa in the upper roof contains lymphoid tissue, called adenoids, in the midline.

The Eustachian tube communicates with the lateral pharyngeal wall. The cartilaginous component of the Eustachian tube enters the lateral wall of the pharynx through the sinus of Morgagni, which represents a gap in the musculature and a potential route of spread of tumors. The posterior lip of the Eustachian tube opening is the torus tubarius, behind which is the mucosal fold known as the "fossa of Rosenmüller".

The nasal surface of the soft palate forms the floor of the nasopharynx. The isthmus is the gap between the soft palate and the posterior pharyngeal wall, through which the nasopharynx communicates with the oropharynx below. Adjacent foramina facilitate the spread of malignancy, such as the foramen lacerum that communicates with the middle cranial fossa, jugular foramen, foramen ovale, foramen spinosum, the carotid, and hypoglossal canals.

The epithelial lining of the nasopharynx has three cell types: pseudostratified columnar epithelium which predominates at birth, squamous cell type common in adulthood and an intermediate pseudostratified cuboidal type which represents a transition between the two. In the adult, most commonly the anterior nasopharynx is lined by pseudostratified ciliated respiratory epithelium while nonkeratinized squamous epithelium lines the posterior aspect. There is a transition zone between the two, lined by columnar epithelium with microvilli. Innervation of the mucosa is by the pharyngeal branch of the pterygopalatine ganglion. The most common sites of origin of nasopharyngeal cancer are the fossa of Rosenmüller, posterior wall, and anterior walls.[1]

EPIDEMIOLOGY

Nasopharyngeal carcinoma (NPC) is a rare disease in most populations, except in a few endemic regions. It is 2.3 times more common in males.[2] The risk of NPC rises with age, peaking at around 50–60 years in high-risk populations. Worldwide incidence is 87,000 new cases per annum, and the estimated deaths due to the disease is 51,000 per annum, which is 0.6% of all cancers.[1] Age standardized rate is 1.2 per 100,000 person-years.[1] It is, however, endemic to Southern China, while high incidences are also found in South-east Asia, North-east India, North Africa and the Arctic.[3,4] According to Wei et al., the age-standardized incidence in China is around 2.31 per 100,000 person years.[5] In India, it is uncommon in most region, reporting an incidence of <1 per 100,000 person-years, except in north-eastern states where incidence as high as 4.3 has been reported.[6]

PATHOLOGY

Nasopharyngeal carcinoma is widely believed to be of squamous origin. There are three main pathological types as per the WHO classification—keratinizing squamous cell carcinoma (SCC), non-keratinizing carcinoma, and basaloid squamous cell carcinoma[7] **(Fig. 1)**.

- Keratinizing SCCs exhibit conventional features such as keratinization with intercellular bridges and squamous pearls. They are graded as well, moderately or poorly differentiated tumors. They are not associated with Epstein–Barr virus (EBV) and form a small proportion of NPCs worldwide, especially in endemic areas.

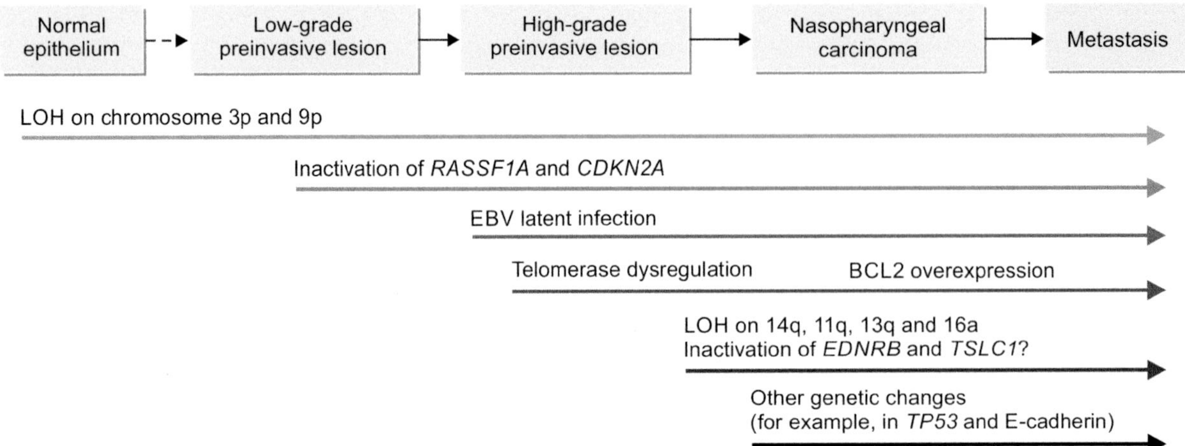

Fig. 1: Pathogenesis of nasopharyngeal carcinoma. (BCL2: B-cell lymphoma 2; *CDKN2A*: cyclin-dependent kinase inhibitor 2A; EBV: Epstein–Barr virus; EBER: Epstein-Barr virus-encoded RNAs; *EDNRB*: endothelin receptor type B; LOH: loss of heterozygosity; *RASSF1A*: Ras-association domain family 1 isoform A; *TSLC1*: tumor suppressor in lung cancer 1)

- Nonkeratinizing carcinomas are strongly associated with EBV. They are the most common histology type in endemic areas.[3] They can be undifferentiated or differentiated. The differentiated type shows either papillary or plexiform growth pattern with stratified cells delineated from the surrounding stroma. The undifferentiated variety, on the other hand, exhibits a syncitial growth pattern. This may be either cohesive (Regaud type) or dyscohesive (Schmincke type), although that has no bearing on clinical behavior, prognosis or management. In contrast to SCCs which have desmoplastic stromal reaction, nonkeratinizing carcinomas exhibit a prominent lymphoid stroma, leading to them being labeled lymphoepitheliomas.
- Basaloid SCC is a high-grade variant of SCC. They consist of mitotically active basaloid cells with pale-staining nuclei in a variety of growth patterns. Conventional squamous pattern is either absent or seen as a minor component of the tumor. Of the three, nonkeratinizing carcinomas have the best prognosis.

RISK FACTORS

The epidemiological data suggests multifactorial causation involving a complex interplay between genetic and environmental factors.[8]

Environmental Factors

- Epstein–Barr virus is a human pathogenic herpes virus that infects over 90% of the global population.[9] It was first isolated in Burkitt's lymphoma cell lines and was the first human oncogenic virus discovered.[10] EBV infection can be either lytic or latent. Latent infection involves only one viral genome replication with each cell cycle whereas in lytic infection, a high number of genomes are produced for transmission.[11] Establishment of latent EBV infection in nasopharyngeal epithelial cells is believed to be a critical event in the development of nonkeratinizing NPC.[12,13] EBV has been found in most tumor cells in almost all cases of nonkeratinized NPC, but not in normal nasopharyngeal epithelial cells, even those adjacent to the tumor **(Flowchart 1)**. It is even found in in-situ carcinomas suggesting that it is an important step in the pathogenesis of NPC and happening even before invasive malignancy develops. It is thought to require an undifferentiated phenotype of epithelial cell for stable EBV infection to set in. In normal nasopharyngeal epithelium, EBV infected cells generally arrest or become senescent due to increased expression of p16 and p21. Hence, stable infection is only possible when there is inactivation of tumor suppressor genes such as *p16* and *RASSF1A* (Ras-association domain family 1 isoform A) and an overactivation of cyclin D1.[12,14] Epstein–Barr virus in nasopharyngeal epithelium displays type II latency, i.e., there is expression of EBV-encoded small RNAs (EBER1/2), Epstein–Barr nuclear antigens-1 (EBNA-1), latent membrane proteins (LMP)-2A/B, LMP-1, and BamH1-A rightward transcripts (BARTs) in the viral genome.[12,15] Further events such as programmed death ligand-1 (PDL1) and PDL2 upregulation help these infected cells evade host immune response. Nuclear factor kappa-light-chain-enhancer of activated B cells (NF-κB) pathway activating mutations have also been reported in up to 41% of tumors.[16] Whole exome sequencing studies have shown few additional acquired mutations, strongly suggesting a prominent role of the EBV-encoded products in tumorigenesis.

Flowchart 1: Pathogenesis of malignant transformation of the nasopharyngeal epithelium.

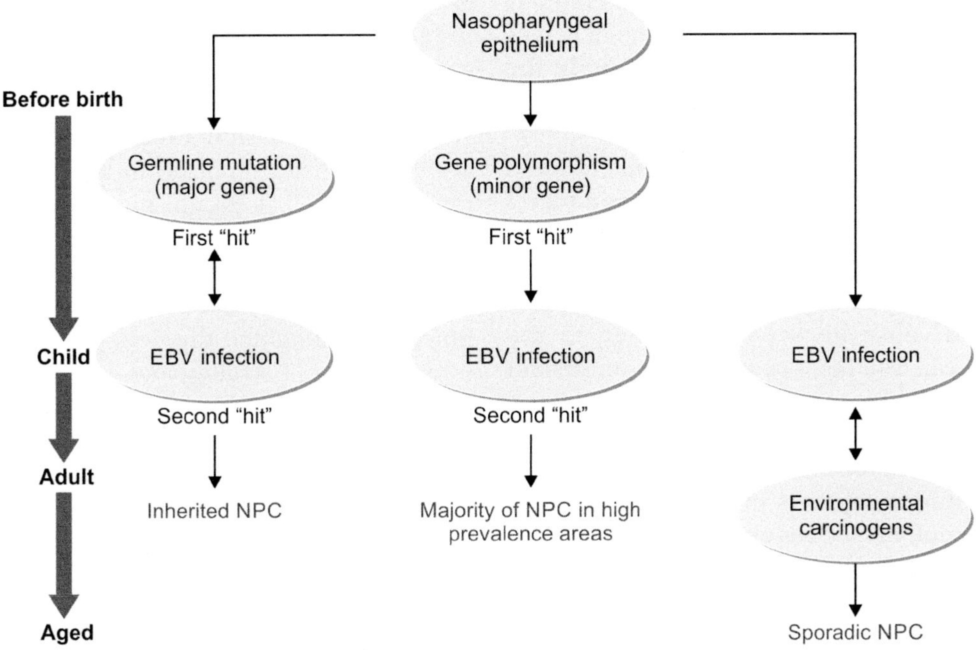

(EBV: Epstein–Barr virus; NPC: nasopharyngeal carcinoma)

These products, especially of those of LMP1 expression, dysregulate various cancer-related genes and enhance NPC tumor heterogeneity. Additional acquired mutations such as p53, RAS, etc. lead to development of subclones that cause local recurrence or distant metastasis.[12,14]

- Human papilloma virus (HPV) has also been reported as a possible etiological factor in NPC, especially in nonendemic regions.[17-19] It has been reported in both keratinizing as well as nonkeratinizing types. HPV-associated NPCs have been reported to have better survival compared to non-virus-associated NPC, with comparable prognosis to EBV-associated NPC.[20]
- Lifestyle factors such as smoking and diet are also known as etiological factors of NPC. Smoking has been reported to significantly increase the risk of the disease.[21,15-34] Any history of smoking is said to carry a moderate risk, which is reported to be dose-dependent. Tobacco usage is associated with keratinizing type of NPC, especially in the western population.
- Dietary factors have been linked to nasopharyngeal cancer, especially in endemic areas. Cooking of salt-cured food exposes the nasopharyngeal mucosa to carcinogenic volatile nitrosamines. Consumption of salted fish rich in nitrosamines (often used as a weaning food in early childhood) and preserved vegetables is also an established risk factor for NPC.[22,23] Consumption of fresh fruits and vegetables, on the other hand, has been reported to have a protective effect.[23,26]

Genetic Factors

Genetic factors play an equally important role in NPC pathogenesis. Their role in EBV-related disease is already discussed. A recent review reported evidence for etiological association of NPC with immune-related human leukocyte antigen (HLA) class I genes, deoxyribonucleic acid (DNA) repair gene *RAD51L1*, cell-cycle control genes *MDM2* and *TP53*, and cell adhesion/migration gene *MMP2*.[27] Chinese studies have reported HLA loci in *6p21* and *CLPTM1L/TERT* loci in 5p15 as having the strongest association with endemic nonkeratinizing NPC.[28,29] Once case-control study showed that having a first-degree relative with NPC could increase risk by seven times;[30] based on evidence of clustering within families, some have called for screening of first-degree relatives of those with NPC.[31]

CLINICAL PRESENTATION

Symptoms at the time of presentation depend on the stage and structures involved. The most common epicenter for primary tumor is the fossa of Rosenmüller. The tumor can extend anteriorly to involve the nasal cavity, paranasal sinuses, pterygoid fossa and even the orbit; laterally to the parapharyngeal and infratemporal spaces; inferiorly into the oropharynx; and posteriorly and superiorly into the sphenoid sinus, clivus, skull base and intracranial structures. Superiorly, invasion of the fibrocartilaginous structure of the foramen lacerum can lead to involvement of the cavernous sinus, causing neuropathy of the nerves present there. The first nerve to be involved is usually the abducens, followed by branches of the trigeminal. Involvement of cranial nerves III and IV indicates more extensive disease within the sinus. In parapharyngeal spread, nerves IX, X, and XI can be affected.

Lymph node involvement is very common. The first echelon nodes are the retropharyngeal nodes and level II lateral neck nodes. Skip metastasis in the absence of first echelon involvement is uncommon. Bilateral nodal involvement is also common. Extensive retropharyngeal involvement can cause neck pain radiating to the head, orbit, and ear. The most common site for distant metastasis is bone followed by lung and liver. Bone involvement can present with severe bone pain, but the others are usually asymptomatic.

Initial presenting symptoms include painless neck swelling; nasal symptoms such as epistaxis or nasal block; ear discharge or hearing loss; or deficits of one or more of the above-mentioned cranial nerves. Trotter's triad is the term given to the cluster of symptoms associated with advanced nasopharyngeal cancer at the fossa of Rosenmüller: unilateral deafness due to secretory otitis media, ipsilateral facial pain due to involvement of the trigeminal nerve at the foramen ovale and soft palate immobility due to vagal involvement.

Direct visualization of the lesion is through a nasal endoscopy. Lesions are most commonly proliferative or polypoidal or submucosal. Although lesions may appear well delineated and discrete, imaging is always required to determine extent. Clinically evident lesions can be biopsied using topical anesthetic administered nasally; however, bleeding may be brisk, requiring nasal packing. NPC has distinctive microscopic features, as described earlier. Sometimes, however, the undifferentiated type may be difficult to distinguish from lymphoma. In case of any doubt, immunohistochemistry can be used to confirm the diagnosis, using leukocyte common antigen (LCA) and a pancytokeratin (CK) marker to differentiate the two. EBER in situ hybridization (ISH) is also useful in confirming nonkeratinized NPC. Squamous secondaries in the neck with unknown primary can often be of nasopharyngeal origin; a core biopsy with EBER ISH can confirm the origin of the disease in such a setting.

RADIOLOGY

Imaging is essential for staging. The primary and nodal disease can be assessed with a CT or MRI. While CT is good for detecting early cortical erosion of bone, MRI is better at delineation of the soft tissue extent, especially in the parapharyngeal space, infratemporal fossa and bone marrow as well as in assessing intracranial extension. It is also useful in imaging perineurial spread.

Positron emission tomography-computed tomography (PET-CT) has been reported to be useful in prognosticating the primary disease.[30] Increased heterogeneity of uptake of ^{18}F-fluorodeoxyglucose (FDG) on PET has been reported to portend a poorer prognosis.

Positron emission tomography-computed tomography has been reported to be superior in detecting regional as well as distant metastasis.[31-33] The common sites for distant metastases are bone, lungs, and liver; and PET has been found to be more sensitive than conventional modalities for detection of these lesions. A recent review, however, highlighted the deficiency of PET in primary tumor staging (T staging) and, hence, recommends both MRI and PET-CT for accurate staging of NPC.[32]

STAGING

The American Joint Committee on Cancer (AJCC) 8th edition staging **(Table 1)**, represented a few deviations from the previous staging systems: T4 criteria "masticator space" and "infratemporal fossa" which were often used synonymously were replaced by specific soft tissue description to avoid ambiguity, adjacent muscle involvement (including pterygoids and prevertebral muscle) was downstaged from T4 to T2 based on recent data showing a good response to treatment in this group, and nodal staging replaced supraclavicular involvement with more contemporary definitions such as nodal disease below and above the cricoid cartilage.[34,35] For endemic nasopharyngeal cancer, competing staging systems exist, such as the Hong Kong, Guangzhou and Guangxi systems, which follow the same principles but have different definitions based on local extent of disease. It has been shown that these systems may outperform AJCC 8th edition in the context of endemic NPC.[36]

ROUTES OF TUMOR SPREAD

Nasopharyngeal cancer can spread locoregionally with involvement of the adjacent structures, lymphatic spread and hematogenous spread is also common. NPCs commonly originate in the fossa of Rosenmüller and spread along well-defined routes. Locoregionally, there is commonly bilateral involvement with local extension to the tensor veli palatine muscle (TVPM) and nasal cavity.

The anatomic sites were classified as based on rate of locoregional involvement or spread:

- *High-risk sites:* TVPM, nasal cavity, sphenoid bone, pterygoids, clivus, petrous apex, prevertebral muscle, and foramen lacerum
- *Medium-risk sites:* Foramen ovale, great wing of the sphenoid bone, oropharynx, medial pterygoid muscle, cavernous sinus, pterygopalatine fossa, sphenoidal sinus, hypoglossal canal, lateral pterygoid muscle, ethmoid sinus, and jugular foramen

Table 1: The American Joint Committee on Cancer (AJCC), 8th edition/Union for International Cancer Control (UICC) staging for nasopharyngeal cancer.

Stages	*Descriptions*
T0	No tumor identified, but EBV-positive cervical node(s) involvement
T1	Tumor confined to nasopharynx, or extension to oropharynx and/or nasal cavity without parapharyngeal involvement
T2	Tumor with extension to parapharyngeal space, and/or adjacent soft tissue involvement (medial pterygoid, lateral pterygoid, prevertebral muscles)
T3	Tumor with infiltration of bony structures at skull base, cervical vertebra, pterygoid structures, and/or paranasal sinuses
T4	Tumor with intracranial extension, involvement of cranial nerves, hypopharynx, orbit, parotid gland, and/or extensive soft tissue infiltration beyond the lateral surface of the lateral pterygoid muscle
N1	Unilateral metastasis in cervical lymph node(s) and/or unilateral or bilateral metastasis in retropharyngeal lymph node(s), 6 cm or smaller in greatest dimension, above the caudal border of cricoid cartilage
N2	Bilateral metastasis in cervical lymph node(s), 6 cm or smaller in greatest dimension, above the caudal border of cricoid cartilage
N3	Unilateral or bilateral metastasis in cervical lymph node(s), >6 cm in greatest dimension; and/or extension beyond the caudal border of cricoid cartilage
M0	No metastases
M1	Metastatic disease
Stage I	T1 N0 M0
Stage II	T0/1 N1 M0, T2 N0/1 M0
Stage III	T0/1/2 N2 M0, T3 N0/1/2 M0
Stage IVA	T4 N0/1/2, Any T N3 M0
Stage IVB	Any T Any N M1

(EBV: Epstein–Barr virus)

- *Low-risk sites*: Orbit, infratemporal fossa, cervical vertebrae, maxillary sinus, hypopharynx, and frontal sinus

There was higher involvement of the high-risk sites and the medium and low risk would be involved following the involvement of the high-risk sites. Bilateral nasopharyngeal extension was common but local extension bilaterally was not very frequent.

Nodal metastasis occurs commonly in retropharyngeal nodes and cervical nodes from level II, III, and IV. In NPC there is a high-level V and supraclavicular nodal involvement (27% and 22%, respectively). Skip metastasis is uncommon at 7.9% and distant nodal involvement was also seen in around 3–5% of the patients.

Nasopharyngeal cancers have higher frequency of distant metastasis when compared with other head and neck tumors. Distant metastases commonly involve bone (75%), lung (46%), and liver (13%).[37]

NONSQUAMOUS CELL CARCINOMA PATHOLOGY

Nasopharyngeal masses are most commonly benign in etiology even in adults, with lymphoid hyperplasia being a common entity. Nasopharyngeal cancers are the most common malignant lesion followed by lymphomas, plasmacytoma, and rhabdomyosarcomas.[38]

TREATMENT

Radiotherapy has remained the treatment of choice for all the stages of NPC as it is a radiosensitive tumor and the anatomic location of the disease limits surgical exposure and approaches. With technological advancements in radiotherapy delivery, cure rates have further improved with reduction in treatment-related morbidity. Although EBV testing is important for prognostic information, there is no evidence to suggest differential treatment for patients based on their EBV status.

The dose recommended for curative treatment of NPC is 66–70 Gy to the gross tumor and positive nodes. The dose to the high-risk areas can be of the range of 60–66 Gy, with low-risk volumes receiving a minimum of 54 Gy in 30–35 fractions with conventional fractionation. Bilateral prophylactic nodal radiation is recommended in NPC in view of high incidence of nodal recurrences even in node-negative cases with subsequent poor survival and distant metastasis even after salvage therapy.[39]

Radiotherapy was previously delivered after two-dimensional (2D) planning, resulting in more acute toxicity and poorer quality of life outcomes. With technological advancements in the field of radiotherapy, there has been better tumor control with improved sparing of the normal surrounding structures from radiotherapy-related toxicity. Various studies have shown that there has been a clear disease-free survival advantage of using newer techniques such as intensity modulated radiation therapy (IMRT) and three-dimensional conformal radiation therapy (3DCRT) over 2D techniques. IMRT was clearly superior to 3DCRT in parotid-sparing radiotherapy delivery, resulting in lower rates of long-term xerostomia **(Table 2)**.[40-44]

Intensity modulated radiation therapy can be considered the standard of care for NPC as meta-analyses have failed to find a significant improvement in survival with proton therapy.[45] However, proton therapy has better sparing of normal tissues such as oral cavity and dysphagia and aspiration-related structures (DARS), resulting less feeding tube placement.[46] Studies comparing various advanced IMRT techniques failed to demonstrate significant advantage of helical tomotherapy or volumetric arc therapy over conventional IMRT.[47]

Table 2: Landmark trials in nasopharyngeal carcinoma.

Study	*Number of subjects*	*Trial design*	*Results*
Al Sarraf et al.[40]	147	70 Gy with 3 weekly CDDP—adjuvant chemotherapy vs. 70 Gy	3 years OS—47% vs. 78%
Chan et al.[42,43]	350	70 Gy with weekly CCDP vs. 70 Gy	5 years OS—59% vs. 70%
Wee et al.[44]	221	70 Gy with 3 weekly CDDP—adjuvant chemotherapy vs. 70 Gy	2 years OS—78% vs. 85%

(CDDP: cisplatinum or cis-diamminedichloroplatinum)

Brachytherapy is used in various centers to attempt deliver higher dose to the primary site. Brachytherapy is delivered as an additional boost. The American Brachytherapy Society has recommended the use of high dose rate (HDR) of brachytherapy for the treatment of early stage NPC. Brachytherapy is delivered using a plastic flexible tube that will fit into the nasopharyngeal space or with a customized applicator. Doses of 6 Gy in two fractions after 70 Gy with external therapy have shown good results while other trials have reported higher side effects such as increased crusting leading to halitosis and pain without any survival advantage.[43,48]

Altered fractionation has been studied in comparison with conventional fraction but the Hong Kong nasopharyngeal carcinoma study group studied convention fractionation with accelerated fractions of 6 days a week treatment with concurrent chemotherapy in both the arms and without. The study showed a positive outcome of accelerated fraction with concurrent chemotherapy in comparison to conventional fractionation, event free survival of 94% versus 70%, but with additional acute and late toxicity.[49]

Radiotherapy with Concurrent Chemotherapy

Intergroup trial 0099 is credited to be the trial that introduced chemotherapy to NPC. In the trial patients were enrolled to radiotherapy alone or concurrent cisplatin-based concurrent chemoradiotherapy (CRT), followed by adjuvant 5-fluorouracil and cisplatin-based adjuvant chemotherapy. There was 78% versus 54% survival benefit at 3 years that was later translated to 5 years survival in the update.[20]

Adjuvant therapy following CRT has been in debate since INT0099 trial due to poor tolerance and high dropout from adjuvant chemotherapy. The MACH-NPC meta-analysis studied the various options of chemotherapy with radiotherapy or radiotherapy alone and concluded that there is a significant advantage of adding chemotherapy to the radiotherapy schedule especially with CRT; this translated into an absolute survival benefit of 6.3% at 5 years. The benefit of adjuvant chemotherapy following completion of CRT was not significant.[50] Yan et al., in another meta-analysis induction, adjuvant, and concurrent chemoradiotherapy which all showed a similar advantage over radiotherapy alone. There was no advantage of adding adjuvant chemotherapy to concurrent chemoradiotherapy.[51,52]

Induction chemotherapy has also been used, predominantly in locally advanced cases. The rationale is that induction chemotherapy can reduce the tumor burden and allow for smaller definitive radiation fields to limit toxicity. Induction chemotherapy with platinum, docetaxel, and 5-fluorouracil followed by CRT was shown to improve 3-year failure free survival to 80% (from 72% when treated with CRT alone.[53] Another meta-analysis by Song et al. showed that adding induction chemotherapy to CRT reduced progression and metastases.[54,55] Compared to earlier meta-analyses like that by Liang ZG et al., which showed no benefit of induction chemotherapy, these were more specific in their selection of chemotherapy protocols.[56,57] Although it is tempting to generalize these results, it is important to understand the context of these clinical trials: only patients who are fit enough to tolerate induction chemotherapy are included. Data showing that these regimens are well-tolerated, are from trial data, and not population-based data and if patients are unlikely to tolerate these regimens, they should not be administered at the cost of defaulting on CRT, which is without the mainstay of their treatment.

Recurrent/Metastatic Nasopharyngeal Carcinoma

Nasopharyngeal carcinoma have a 5–7% chance of presenting with metastatic disease. Based on the size of the tumor and nodal involvement, there is a 25–30% chance of metastatic recurrence within 3 years of post-treatment. Chemotherapy remains the mainstay of treatment for metastatic disease, however, there is no consensus on the monochemotherapy versus multi-agent chemotherapy. Cisplatin combinations with paclitaxel, docetaxel, and gemcitabine are the most commonly used regimens with similar response rates as cisplatin and 5-fluourouracil regimens of 25–75%, and median survival of 9.5–15 months. Targeted agents gefitinib, sorafenib, and cetuximab have been tried but with no significant benefit.[58]

Locoregional recurrence can be managed with re-irradiation, depending on the extent of disease and the previous field of irradiation. IMRT for re-irradiation has shown good response rates with the added advantage of limiting toxicity, which can be significant in this setting. Doses up to 70 Gy have been delivered in re-irradiation setting with acceptable toxicity. In selected patients, 5-year local control rates up to 86% and overall survival of up to 38% have been achieved. Brachytherapy and stereotactic radiotherapy are other modalities that have been used commonly for salvage therapy, both as single modality and as boost to IMRT.[56]

Treatment-related Complications

Radiotherapy for NPC is associated with significant post-therapy complications. Due to proximity of multiple critical structures the rates of complications have been higher than in irradiation of other head and neck subsites. Mucositis is the predominant acute toxicity, which is worse when radiotherapy is combined with chemotherapy. The reported toxicity is hearing loss, endocrine dysfunction, temporal lobe necrosis, and cranial neuropathies. Trismus can develop as a late complication and needs to be differentiated from a recurrence. Xerostomia is common and can be severe. Temporal lobe necrosis, although rare today, is a dreaded complication. It can be asymptomatic and identified on MRI imaging but in a few it can translate into clinical picture of headache, memory loss, and neurological deficits. Skull base osteoradionecrosis with internal carotid artery bleeding is rare but potentially fatal. Delayed bulbar palsy can develop up to 2 decades after treatment in up to 20% of patients and can result in significant functional disability; it can result in deafness, dysarthria, dysphagia, and shoulder dysfunction. Radiation-induced second cancers are usually EBV-negative and are not uncommon. The incidences of toxicity are lesser with better conformal techniques such IMRT being used.[57,58]

SURGICAL APPROACHES

While surgery is not a primary modality for treatment of NPC, it has a role to play in a salvage setting.[59-61] Patients with recurrent cT1–3 have been reported to have very good salvage rates with surgery, while select rT4 patients may also achieve locoregional control. Intracranial extension has been reported to be a poor prognostic feature.[61] A recent meta-analysis reported a 5-year overall survival of 58% and disease specific survival of 63% in selected recurrent cases treated with surgery, demonstrating good salvage rates with the modality. They further reported adjuvant radiotherapy offering significant survival advantage in this cohort.

Surgery for the nasopharynx has traditionally been considered challenging due to the deep anatomical location and difficult access. Proper access is paramount to successful salvage since margin status is an important determinant of outcome, and a positive or close margin has been associated with poor disease control as well as overall survival.[62] A number of open surgical approaches have been described for nasopharyngectomy.[63] Details given below are in brief, for further details please refer to the chapter on anterior skull base tumors.

- *Lateral approach:* The Fisch approach.
  - *Approach:* A postauricular incision followed by total parotidectomy and mastoidectomy with translocation of facial nerve. The zygomatic arch and temporalis attachment is then divided to approach the parapharyngeal space along the middle cranial fossa. The pterygoid muscles are detached from the plate and the internal carotid artery is isolated medially and retracted.
  - *Accessible areas:* Ipsilateral nasopharynx, infratemporal fossa, and parapharyngeal space.
  - *Disadvantages:* Limited access to contralateral wall of nasopharynx, multiple cranial nerves palsies (V, VII, IX, and X), and disruption of masticatory function and trismus.
  - *Use:* This is preferred only when complete exposure of the internal carotid artery is required for vascular control with other approaches being preferred in view of reduced morbidity.
- *Inferior approach:* Transpalatal approach.
  - *Approach:* A hard palate mucosal incision is placed and a submucosal flap is raised. The soft palate is then detached from the hard palate. The posterior part of the hard palate bone as well as the inferior turbinates can be removed to improve access.
  - *Accessible areas:* Nasopharynx.
  - *Disadvantages:* No access to parapharyngeal space or infratemporal fossa, postoperative dysphagia, nasal regurgitation and palatal fistula (especially in the irradiated patient).
  - *Use:* This approach is used for small lesions located in the middle of the nasopharynx with almost no lateral extension.
- *Inferolateral approach:* Transcervico-mandibulo-palatal approach.
  - *Approach:* A lower lip-split and transverse cervical incision is combined with a paramedian mandibulotomy. The mucosal lip incision extended

along the floor of the mouth to the anterior tonsillar pillar, followed by detachment of the soft palate from the hard palate. The internal carotid access is traced from the neck for access.
    - *Accessible areas:* Nasopharynx, ipsilateral parapharyngeal space, and infratemporal fossa.
    - *Disadvantages:* Palatal defect, dysphagia, velopharyngeal incompetence, trismus, mandibular malunion with malocclusion.
    - *Use:* Less common with the advent of anterolateral approach and advances in endoscopic surgery. It was used when the inferior approach was adequate but internal carotid artery vascular control was required.
- *Anterolateral approach:* Facial translocation/maxillary swing approach.
    - *Approach:* A Weber–Ferguson incision with upper lip split and lateral extension to the zygoma is placed. Osteotomies are performed at the anterior maxillary wall below the orbital floor, over the hard palate lateral to the nasal septum, the anterior zygoma, and between the posterior maxillary wall and the pterygoid plates to allow the maxilla to swing forward, preserving its anterior soft tissue attachments; this is crucial to retain vascularity of the bone.
    - *Accessible areas:* Nasopharynx and parapharyngeal space. Complete facial translocation also provides access to the infratemporal fossa.
    - *Disadvantages:* Known complications include avascular necrosis of parts of the maxilla, palatal fistula, lower lid ectropion, epiphora, medial canthus misalignment, nasolacrimal duct obstruction, frontal muscle palsy, and visible facial scars.
    - *Use:* This is the approach of choice for open surgery, but is used sparingly with the advent of endoscopic surgery.
- *Anterior approach:* Mid-face degloving approach.
    - *Approach:* Mucosal incision is placed along the whole upper gingivolabial sulcus. Separate intercartilage incisions along the nasal ala, extended to a transfixation incision of the nasal columella, followed by separation of the nasal tip and ala from nasal bone. The intraoral incision is then connected to the nasal incision through the premaxilla. Bilateral medial maxillectomy can be performed to increase exposure.
    - *Accessible area:* Nasopharynx
    - *Disadvantages:* No access to parapharyngeal space, infratemporal fossa, limited access to inferior part of nasopharynx due to floor of nose and no vascular control of the internal carotid artery.
    - *Use:* This approach can only be used for small tumors close to the midline. It is sparingly used in the endoscopic era.

Endoscopic Surgery

The endonasal endoscopic approach has drastically improved outcomes in nasopharyngectomy. It provides better visualization of the surgical field while avoiding many of the above-mentioned complications of open surgeries. A transpterygoid approach, achieved by removing the medial and posterior maxillary wall, followed by the drilling of the vidian canal and removal of the medial pterygoid wall, provides a wide access to the parapharyngeal space as well as the infratemporal fossa. A recent pooled analysis of 300 patients undergoing endoscopic salvage surgery for NPC has reported promising results, especially in recurrent cT1–3 patients, with negative margins achieved in up to 91.1% of the patients, and local control of up to 80%.[60] The key to good outcome in this cohort is early detection and complete resection.

RECURRENCE AND FOLLOW-UP

Post-treatment clinical and radiological evaluation is crucial to confirm cure. Clinical examination is by endoscopy and imaging can be in the form of CT, MRI or PET-CT. Usually performed 12 weeks after completion of treatment.[64] Imaging earlier than this can result in false positive results. In addition to evaluation of recurrence, it is also important to evaluate post-treatment sequelae such as lymphedema and cranial nerve dysfunction, and arrange appropriate referrals for management. NPC has a propensity for delayed recurrence and often involves the bones, liver, and lungs.[65] Follow-up is usually once in 3 months for the first 2 years, then every 4–6 months till the fifth year and annual visits subsequently. Post-treatment plasma EBV DNA levels can also be used to monitor for recurrence and levels at diagnosis have also been shown to correlate with prognosis.[64]

The prognosis in appropriately treated NPC is good; a contemporary series showed that 5-year OS in those treated with IMRT ± chemotherapy for stage I, II, III, and IVA/B were 100%, 94.3%, 83.6%, and 70.5%, respectively.[44] However, the challenge in this cohort remains balancing cure rates with long-term morbidity, especially in younger patients who present with the disease, and this is where further efforts are required.

REFERENCES

1. Ferlay J, Soerjomataram I, Dikshit R, Eser S, Mathers C, Rebelo M, et al. Cancer incidence and mortality worldwide: sources, methods and major patterns in GLOBOCAN 2012. Int J Cancer. 2015;136(5):E359-86.
2. Yu MC, Yuan JM. Epidemiology of nasopharyngeal carcinoma. Semin Cancer Biol. 2002;12(6):421-9.
3. Chang ET, Adami HO. The enigmatic epidemiology of nasopharyngeal carcinoma. Cancer Epidemiol Biomarkers Prev. 2006;15(10):1765-77.
4. Wee JT, Ha TC, Loong SL, Qian CN. Is nasopharyngeal cancer really a "Cantonese cancer"? Chin J Cancer. 2010;29:517-26.
5. Wei KR, Zheng RS, Zhang SW, Liang ZH, Li ZM, Chen WQ. Nasopharyngeal carcinoma incidence and mortality in China, 2013. Chin J Cancer. 2017;36(1):90.
6. Kataki AC, Simons MJ, Das AK, Sharma K, Mehra NK. Nasopharyngeal carcinoma in the Northeastern states of India. Chin J Cancer. 2011;30(2):106-13.
7. Chan JKC, Bray F, McCarron P. Nasopharyngeal carcinoma. In: Barnes L, Eveson JW, Sidransky D, Reichart P (Eds). WHO classification of tumours. Pathology and genetics of head and neck tumours. Lyon: International Agency for Research on Cancer (IARC) Press; 2005. pp. 85-97.
8. Jia WH, Collins A, Zeng YX, Feng BJ, Yu XJ, Huang LX, et al. Complex segregation analysis of nasopharyngeal carcinoma in Guangdong, China: evidence for a multifactorial mode of inheritance (complex segregation analysis of NPC in China). Eur J Hum Genet. 2005;13:248-52.
9. Cohen JI, Fauci AS, Varmus H, Nabel GJ. Epstein-Barr virus: an important vaccine target for cancer prevention. Sci Transl Med. 2011;3(107):107-7.
10. Epstein MA, Achong BG, Barr YM. Virus particles in cultured lymphoblasts from Burkitt's lymphoma. Lancet. 1964;1(7335):702-3.
11. McKenzie J, El-Guindy A. Epstein-Barr virus lytic cycle reactivation. Curr Top Microbiol Immunol. 2015;391:237-61.
12. Tsao SW, Tsang CM, To KF, Lo KW. The role of Epstein-Barr virus in epithelial malignancies. J Pathol. 2015;235(2): 323-33.
13. Niedobitek G. Epstein-Barr virus infection in the pathogenesis of nasopharyngeal carcinoma. Mol Pathol. 2000;53(5): 248-54.
14. Tsao SW, Tsang CM, Lo KW. Epstein–Barr virus infection and nasopharyngeal carcinoma. Phil Trans R Soc B. 2017;372 (1732).
15. Kang MS, Kieff E. Epstein-Barr virus latent genes. Exp Mol Med. 2015;47(1):e131.
16. Li YY, Chung GT, Lui VW, To KF, Ma BBY, Chow C, et al. Exome and genome sequencing of nasopharynx cancer identifies NF-κB pathway activating mutations. Nat Commun. 2017;8:14121.
17. Lin Z, Khong B, Kwok S, Cao H, West RB, Le QT, et al. Human papillomavirus 16 detected in nasopharyngeal carcinomas in white Americans but not in endemic Southern Chinese patients. Head Neck. 2014;36(5):709-14.
18. Chan YH, Lo CM, Lau HY, Lam TH. Vertically transmitted nasopharyngeal infection of the human papillomavirus: Does it play an aetiological role in nasopharyngeal cancer? Oral Oncol. 2014;50(5):326-9.
19. Dogan S, Hedberg ML, Ferris RL, Rath TJ, Assaad AM, Chiosea SI. Human papillomavirus and Epstein-Barr virus in nasopharyngeal carcinoma in a low-incidence population. Head Neck. 2014;36(4):511-6.
20. Chua MLK, Wee JTS, Hui EP, Chan ATC. Nasopharyngeal carcinoma. Lancet. 2016;387(1022):1012-24.
21. Yong SK, Ha TC, Yeo MC, Gaborieau V, McKay JD, Wee J. Associations of lifestyle and diet with the risk of nasopharyngeal carcinoma in Singapore: a case-control study. Chin J Cancer. 2017;36(1):3.
22. Jia WH, Luo XY, Feng BJ, Ruan HL, Bei JX, Liu WS, et al. Traditional Cantonese diet and nasopharyngeal carcinoma risk: a large-scale case-control study in Guangdong, China. BMC Cancer. 2010;10:446.
23. Jia WH, Qin HD. Non-viral environmental risk factors for nasopharyngeal carcinoma: A systematic review. Semin Cancer Biol. 2012;22(2):117-26.
24. Xue WQ, Qin HD, Ruan HL, Shugart YY, Jia WH. Quantitative association of tobacco smoking with the risk of nasopharyngeal carcinoma: a comprehensive meta-analysis of studies conducted between 1979 and 2011. Am J Epidemiol. 2013;178(3):325-38.
25. Chang ET, Liu Z, Hildesheim A, Liu Q, Cai Y, Zhang Z, et al. Active and Passive Smoking and Risk of Nasopharyngeal Carcinoma: A Population-Based Case-Control Study in Southern China. Am J Epidemiol. 2017;185(12):1272-80.
26. Polesel J, Serraino D, Negri E, Barzan L, Vaccher E, Montella M, et al. Consumption of fruit, vegetables, and other food groups and the risk of nasopharyngeal carcinoma. Cancer Causes Control. 2013;24(6):1157-65.
27. Hildesheim A, Wang CP. Genetic predisposition factors and nasopharyngeal carcinoma risk: a review of epidemiological association studies, 2000-2011: Rosetta Stone for NPC: genetics, viral infection, and other environmental factors. Semin Cancer Biol. 2012;22(2):107-16.
28. Bei JX, Zuo XY, Liu WS, Guo YM, Zeng YX. Genetic susceptibility to the endemic form of NPC. Chin Clin Oncol. 2016; 5(2):15.
29. Bei JX, Su WH, Ng CC, Yu K, Chin YM, Lou PJ, et al. A GWAS Meta-analysis and Replication Study Identifies a Novel Locus within CLPTM1L/TERT Associated with Nasopharyngeal Carcinoma in Individuals of Chinese Ancestry. Cancer Epidemiol Biomarkers Prev. 2016;25:188-92.
30. Huang B, Chan T, Kwong D, Chan WKS, Khong PL. Nasopharyngeal carcinoma: investigation of intratumoral heterogeneity with FDG PET/CT. AJR Am J Roentgenol. 2012;199(1):169-74.
31. Chang MC, Chen JH, Liang JA, Yang KT, Cheng KY, Kao CH, et al. Accuracy of whole-body FDG-PET and FDG-PET/CT in M staging of nasopharyngeal carcinoma: a systematic review and meta-analysis. Eur J Radiol. 2013;82:366-73.
32. Vellayappan BA, Soon YY, Earnest A, Zhang Q, Koh WY, Keong Tham IW, et al. Accuracy of ^{18}F-fluorodeoxyglucopositron emission tomography/computed tomography in the staging of newly diagnosed nasopharyngeal carcinoma: a systematic review and meta-analysis. Radiol Oncol. 2014; 48:331-8.
33. Chua ML, Ong SC, Wee JT, Ng DC, Gao F, Tan TW, et al. Comparison of 4 modalities for distant metastasis staging in endemic nasopharyngeal carcinoma. Head Neck. 2009;31:346-54.
34. Chang JT, See LC, Tang SG, Lee SP, Wang CC, Hong JH. The role of brachytherapy in early-stage nasopharyngeal carcinoma. Int J Radiat Oncol Bio Phys. 1996;36(5):1019-24.
35. Huang CJ, Leung SW, Lian SL, Wang CJ, Fang FM, Ho YH, et al. Patterns of distant metastases in nasopharyngeal carcinoma. Kaohsiung J Med Sci. 1996;12(4):229-34.

36. Cheng JC, Chao KS, Low D. Comparison of intensity modulated radiation therapy (IMRT) treatment techniques for nasopharyngeal carcinoma. Int J Cancer. 2001;92(2): 126-32.
37. Ramaekers BL, Pijls-Johannesma M, Joore MA, van den Ende P, Langendijk JA, Lambin P, et al. Systematic review and meta-analysis of radiotherapy in various head and neck cancers: comparing photons, carbon-ions and protons. Cancer Treat Rev. 2011;37(3):185-201.
38. Pan XB, Chen KH, Huang ST, Jiang YM, Ma JL, Liang ZG, et al. Comparison of the efficacy between intensity-modulated radiotherapy and two-dimensional conventional radiotherapy in stage II nasopharyngeal carcinoma. Oncotarget. 2017;8(44):78096-104.
39. Li WF, Sun Y, Chen M, Tang LL, Liu LZ, Mao YP, et al. Locoregional extension patterns of nasopharyngeal carcinoma and suggestions for clinical target volume delineation. Chin J Cancer. 2012;31(12):579-87.
40. Al-Sarraf M, LeBlanc M, Giri PG, Fu KK, Cooper J, Vuong T, et al. Chemoradiotherapy versus radiotherapy in patients with advanced nasopharyngeal cancer: phase III randomized Intergroup study 0099. J Clin Oncol. 1998;16:1310-7.
41. Lee AWM, Lau WH, Tung SY, Chua DT, Chappell R, Xu L, et al. Preliminary Results of a Randomized Study on therapeutic gain by concurrent chemotherapy for regionally-advanced nasopharyngeal carcinoma: NPC-9901 trial by the Hong Kong Nasopharyngeal Cancer Study Group. J Clin Oncol. 2005;23:6966-75.
42. Chan AT, Leung SF, Ngan RKC, Teo PML, Lau WH, Kwan WH, et al. Overall survival after concurrent cisplatin-radiotherapy compared with radiotherapy alone in locoregionally advanced nasopharyngeal carcinoma. J Natl Cancer Inst. 2005;97:536-9.
43. Chao HL, Liu SC, Tsao CC, Lin KT, Lee SP, Lo CH, et al. Dose escalation via brachytherapy boost for nasopharyngeal carcinoma in the era of intensity-modulated radiation therapy and combined chemotherapy. J Radiat Res. 2017; 58(5):654-60.
44. Wee J, Tan EH, Tai BC, Wong HB, Leong SS, Tan T, et al. Randomized trial of radiotherapy versus concurrent chemoradiotherapy followed by adjuvant chemotherapy in patients with American Joint Committee on Cancer/ International Union against cancer stage III and IV nasopharyngeal cancer of endemic variety. J Clin Oncol. 2005; 23:6730-8.
45. Kong L, Lu JJ. Reirradiation of locally recurrent nasopharyngeal cancer: history. Chin Clin Oncol. 2016;5(2):26.
46. Lee AW, Law SC, Ng SH, Chan DK, Poon YF, Foo W, et al. Retrospective analysis of nasopharyngeal carcinoma treated during 1976-1985: late complications following megavoltage irradiation. Br J Radiol. 1992;65(778):918-92.
47. Lee AW, Poon YF, Foo W, Law SC, Cheung FK, Chan DK, et al. Retrospective analysis of 5037 patients with nasopharyngeal carcinoma treated during 1976-1985: overall survival and patterns of failure. Int J Radiat Oncol Biol Phys. 1992;23(2):261-70.
48. Lee AW, Tung SY, Chan ATC, Chappell R, Fu YT, Lu TX, et al. Preliminary results of a randomized study (NPC9902 Trial) on therapeutic gain by concurrent chemotherapy and/or accelerated fractionation for locally advanced nasopharyngeal carcinoma. Int J Radiat Oncol Biol Phys. 2006;66(1):142-51.
49. Liao SH, Ng SH, Chang JTC, Chan SC, Ko SF, Wang HM, et al. Nodal metastases of nasopharyngeal carcinoma: patterns of disease on MRI and FDG PET. Eur J Nucl Med Mol Imag. 2004;31(8):1073-80.
50. El-Taher M, Ali K, Aref Z. Histopathological Pattern of Nasopharyngeal Masses in Adults. Otolaryngol (Sunnyvale). 2017;7(3):1000311.
51. Blanchard P, Lee A, Marguet S, Leclercq J, Ng WT, Ma J, Chan ATC, et al. Chemotherapy and radiotherapy in nasopharyngeal carcinoma: an update of the MAC-NPC meta-analysis. Lancet Oncol. 2015;16:645-55.
52. Yan M, Kumachev A, Siu LL, Chan KKW. Chemoradiotherapy regimens for locoregionally advanced nasopharyngeal carcinoma: A Bayesian network meta-analysis. Eur J Cancer. 2015;51(12):1570-9.
53. Sanguineti G, Geara FB, Garden AS, Tucker SL, Ang KK, Morrison WH, et al. Carcinoma of the nasopharynx treated by radiotherapy alone: determinants of local and regional control. Int J Radiat Oncol Biol Phys.1997;37(5):985-99.
54. Bensoudaa Y, Kaikania W, Ahbeddoua N, Rahhalia R, Jabrib M, Mrabtia H, et al. Treatment for metastatic nasopharyngeal carcinoma. Eur Ann Otorhinolaryngol Head Neck Dis. 2011;128:79-85.
55. Song Y, Wang W, Tao G, Zhou X. Survival benefit of induction chemotherapy in treatment for locally advanced nasopharyngeal carcinoma—A time-to-event meta-analysis. Oral Oncol. 2015;51:764-9.
56. Sun Y, Li WF, Chen NY, Zhang N, Hu GQ, Xie FY, et al. Induction chemotherapy plus concurrent chemoradiotherapy versus concurrent chemoradiotherapy alone in locoregionally advanced nasopharyngeal carcinoma: A phase 3, multicentre, randomised controlled trial. Lancet Oncol. 2016;17(11):1509-20.
57. Liang ZG, Zhu XD, Tan AH, Jiang YM, Qu S, Su F, et al. Induction Chemotherapy Followed by Concurrent Chemoradiotherapy Versus Concurrent Chemoradiotherapy with or without Adjuvant Chemotherapy for Locoregionally Advanced Nasopharyngeal Carcinoma: Meta-analysis of 1,096 Patients from 11 Randomized Controlled T. Asian Pacific J Cancer Prev. 2013;14(1):515-21.
58. Na'ara S, Amit M, Billan S, Cohen JT, Gil Z. Outcome of patients undergoing salvage surgery for recurrent nasopharyngeal carcinoma: a meta-analysis. Ann Surg Oncol. 2014;21(9):3056-62.
59. Vlantis AC, Lee DLY, Wong EWY, Chow SMW, Ng SK, Chan JYK. Endoscopic nasopharyngectomy in recurrent nasopharyngeal carcinoma: a case series, literature review, and pooled analysis. Int Forum Allergy Rhinol. 2016;XX:1-8.
60. Suárez C, Rodrigo JP, Rinaldo A, Langendijk JA, Shaha AR, Ferlito A. Current treatment options for recurrent nasopharyngeal cancer. Eur Arch Otorhinolaryngol. 2010;267(12): 1811-24.
61. Chan JY, To VS, Chow VL. Multivariate analysis of prognostic factors for salvage nasopharyngectomy via the maxillary swing approach. Head Neck. 2014;36:1013-7.
62. Tsang RK, Wei WI. Salvage surgery for nasopharyngeal cancer. World J Otorhinolaryngol Head Neck Surg. 2015;1(1): 34-43.
63. Chao SS, Loh KS, Tan LK. Modalities of surveillance in treated nasopharyngeal cancer. Otolaryngology—Head Neck Surg. 2003;129(1):61-4.
64. Hui EP, Ma BB, Chan KA, Chan CM, Wong CS, To KF, et al. Clinical utility of plasma Epstein-Barr virus DNA and ERCC1 single nucleotide polymorphism in nasopharyngeal carcinoma. Cancer. 2015;121(16):2720-9.
65. Sun X, Su S, Chen C, Han F, Zhao C, Xiao W, et al. Long-term outcomes of intensity-modulated radiotherapy for 868 patients with nasopharyngeal carcinoma: an analysis of survival and treatment toxicities. Radiother Oncol. 2014;110(3):398-403.

CHAPTER 18

Cancers of the Temporal Bone

Vidya Bhushan R, Narayana Subramaniam, Samskruthi P Murthy, Sivakumar Vidhyadharan

INTRODUCTION

Primary cancers of the temporal bone and lateral skull base are comparatively rare, accounting for 0.2% of all head and neck cancers. They constitute a heterogeneous group of cancers with numerous sites of origin. About 60–80% of temporal bone tumors arise in the external auditory canal.[1]

The rarity of temporal bone cancers and the complexity of the region's anatomy make treating temporal bone malignancies difficult. Although several treatment modalities have been described in the literature, there is a lack of consensus regarding best treatment, mainly due to the absence of prospective randomized studies.[2] The most frequently reported treatment involves surgical resection with or without adjuvant radiotherapy. Chemotherapy, brachytherapy or alternative treatment methods such as superselective intra-arterial chemotherapy injection have been described in the literature. However, their exact role remains to be determined. 5-year locoregional control rates range from 70% in early disease to 20% in advanced disease.[3]

APPLIED ANATOMY

- The temporal bone consists of the following parts: squamous, petrous, mastoid, tympanic, and styloid process.
- The anterior portion of the petrous pyramid forms the posterior aspect of the middle cranial fossa. The caudal or inferior portion contains the exiting jugular vein and the entry of the carotid artery. Finally, the posterior portion forms the lateral portion of the posterior cranial fossa and contains internal auditory canal for the seventh and eighth cranial nerves.
- The internal carotid artery has a thick sheath protecting it. This sheath is thicker proximally and becomes progressively thinner toward the horizontal segment. Beneath the sheath, the artery is surrounded by a plexus of veins, more prominent at its horizontal segment. Bleeding occurring from these veins can be controlled easily by Surgicel® packing. The horizontal segment of the internal carotid artery runs in an anteromedial direction along a line from the spine of the sphenoid, foramen spinosum, foramen ovale, and ending at the pterygoid process.[4]
- The genu of the internal carotid artery is closely related to the cochlea. The distance between the two varies from 1 to 5 mm. The geniculate ganglion is again closely related to the genu of the horizontal internal carotid artery.
- The mandibular condyle, middle meningeal artery, maxillary nerve, and eustachian tube—all lie lateral to the transverse portion of the internal carotid artery. Sacrificing these structures or displacing them is mandatory to control this segment of the artery from the lateral aspect.[4]
- The facial nerve is supplied through three main arterial systems: (1) labyrinthine, (2) the middle meningeal, and (3) the stylomastoid arteries.

ETIOLOGY

For most patients, the cause is unknown. Sun exposure is linked with skin cancers of the temporal region. Radiotherapy has been linked with squamous cell cancer of the middle ear and ear canal. Some investigators have linked chronic otitis media and cholesteatoma to the ear canal and middle ear cancer, but this cause probably accounts for only a few tumors in most modern studies.[5]

HISTOLOGY

Squamous cell carcinoma (SCC) has been the most studied and reported of malignant tumors of the ear and temporal bone, but most of the other tumors behave similarly and share the generally poor outcome

Table 1: Malignant tumor types involving the temporal bone.

Epithelial tumors	• Squamous cell carcinoma • Basal cell carcinoma • Basosquamous carcinoma • Hidradenocarcinoma • Melanoma • Sarcomatoid carcinoma • Sebaceous cell carcinoma
Mesenchymal tumors	• Chondrosarcoma • Osteosarcoma • Rhabdomyosarcoma • Pleomorphic sarcoma • Spindle-cell sarcoma
Salivary gland tumors	• Adenoid cystic carcinoma • Acinic cell carcinoma • Adenocarcinoma • Carcinoma ex pleomorphic adenoma • Mucoepidermoid carcinoma • Malignant mixed carcinoma
Others	• Clivus chondroma • Hemangiopericytoma • Neuroendocrine carcinoma • Peripheral nerve sheath tumor

of this disease. Various malignant tumor types that involve the temporal bone are represented in **Table 1**.

CLINICAL PRESENTATION

It is not uncommon for patients with temporal bone tumor to present late. SCC of the temporal bone has a slightly higher prevalence in men than women. The median age at presentation of SCC of the temporal bone is in the seventh decade. The clinical features of SCC of the temporal bone are nonspecific; therefore, most of the cases are misdiagnosed, especially in the early stages.

Suspicious features are chronic otalgia, bloody otorrhea, bleeding, facial swelling, facial palsy, swelling along the mastoid region, unusual asymmetrical conductive or sensory neural hearing loss, giddiness, neurological deficits, and ulceration and granulation tissue in the canal. Otorrhea, otalgia, and hearing loss make a classic triad for temporal bone cancer symptomatology, but this is seen in only 10% of patients who have temporal bone cancer. Other symptoms such as trismus, dysphagia, and hoarseness are seen less commonly and are usually associated with advanced-stage disease.

The physical examination of these patients demands scrutiny of the external ear, ear canal, tympanic membranes, parotid gland, periauricular skin, cervical lymph nodes, and cranial nerves. Microscopic examination of the ear canal is vital to determine the extent of disease into the ear canal.

PATTERNS OF INVASION

These tumors spread mainly by direct invasion into the temporal bone and neighboring structures (parotid, infratemporal fossa, dura, and brain). Leonetti and colleagues looked at different paths of invasion of temporal bone tumors. They identified that tumors grow superiorly through the tegmen, anteriorly through the glenoid fossa and infratemporal space, inferiorly through the hypotympanum and jugular foramen, posteriorly into the mastoid, and medially through the carotid canal and inner ear.[5] The reason for aggressiveness cannot only be attributed to the disease biology, but also due to the various potential routes of diffusion to the surrounding structures (**Figs. 1A and B**). Microscopic invasion seems to be frequent through the intraosseous vessels and Haversian canals.[6]

The skin of the ear canal is 0.5–1 mm thick in the cartilaginous part and only 0.2 mm thick in the bony part of the external ear canal. Lesions of the bony canal, therefore, have greater propensity to invade the bone.[7]

Growths occurring in the anterior canal wall have a higher predisposition for lymphatic spread. The breach in the continuity of the cartilaginous portion of the ear canal provides swift passage for tumor extension. Tumors originating in or extending to the middle ear have ready access to natural passages such as the eustachian tube and air cells above, below, and behind the labyrinth. When the primary tumor is discovered during surgery for middle ear disease, the chances of tumor spread via the jugular foramen and metastases to retropharyngeal lymph nodes of Rouviere are known.[8]

EVALUATION

Diagnostic imaging is imperative for understanding the three-dimensional anatomy of these tumors. Contrast-enhanced high-resolution computed tomography (CT) and magnetic resonance imaging (MRI) provide complementary details. A CT scan is generally obtained as an initial study. It gives excellent details of bony anatomy. Because surgery is the mainstay of temporal bone cancer treatment, the bony anatomy is especially crucial for temporal bone surgeons. MRI lacks bony detail; its use is reserved as an adjunct, especially in cases in which dural involvement or perineural invasion is suspected. Dural involvement is an important factor for preoperative decision-making and also as a prognosticator. Inflammed dura may mimic tumor involvement, hence enhancement beyond 5 mm thickness, discontinuity of nodular enhancement and pial invasion are indicators of dural involvement by the tumor.[9,10]

Internal carotid artery proximity of involvement to the tumor must mandate further studies.

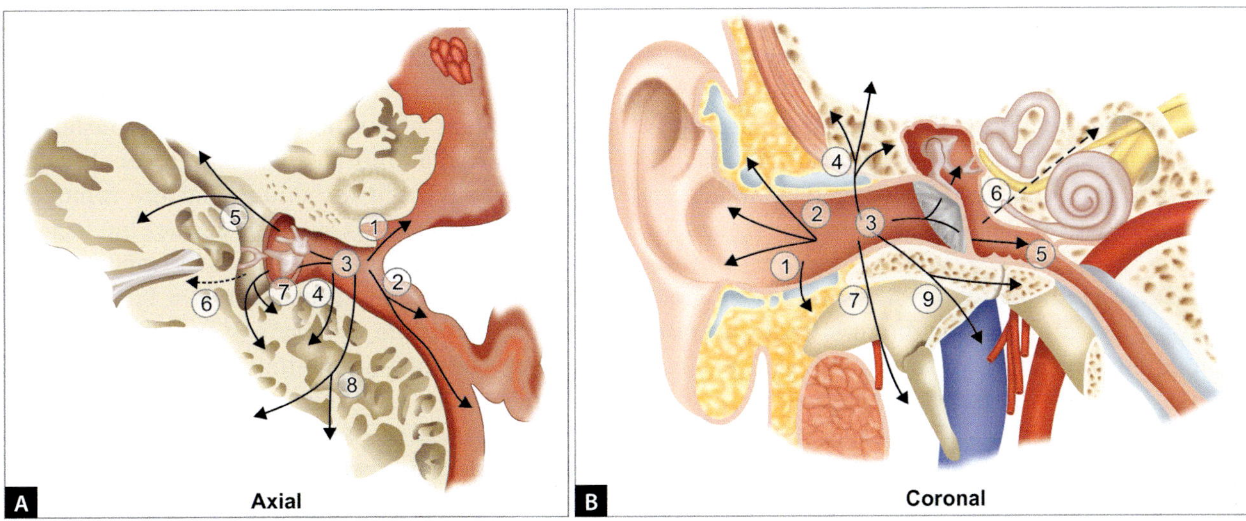

1. Anteriorly: Cartilaginous ear canal → parotid gland
2. Concha → postauricular sulcus
3. Tympanic membrane → middle ear
4. Posteriorly → mastoid
5. Anterior mesotympanum → carotid artery and eustachian tube
6. Inner ear → round window or otic capsule
7. Along the facial nerve → infratemporal fossa
8. Through the mastoid, posterior fossa dura, and sigmoid sinus
9. Beneath the skull base → jugular fossa, carotid artery and lower cranial nerves

Figs. 1A and B: Routes of spread of temporal bone cancer.

Balloon test occlusion (BTO) has been proposed by itself as a preoperative evaluation but has also been paired with additional testing such as hypotensive challenge, xenon-enhanced CT, ^{99m}Tc-HMPAO SPECT and transcranial Doppler ultrasonography.[11] BTO decreases the risk of postoperative ischemic stroke from up to 30% in unselected patients to <13% in patients passing this test. Temporal bone tumors can involve cerebral venous sinus, which may further assessment with cerebral venous drainage by MR venogram. Electrophysiological evaluation of the motor branches and assessment of facial nerve secretory/sensory function (e.g., tear production, taste) should be considered as well.[12] Pure tone audiogram for hearing evaluation should be done preoperatively.

STAGING

The University of Pittsburgh staging system is one of the most widely accepted and used criteria for staging tumors of the temporal bone.[13,14] The staging system is depicted in **Table 2**.

Table 2: Modified Pittsburgh staging system for temporal bone malignancy.[13,14]

T1	Tumor limited to the external auditory canal (EAC) without bony erosion or evidence of soft tissue involvement
T2	Tumor limited to the EAC with bone erosion (not full thickness) or limited soft tissue involvement (<0.5 mm)
T3	Tumor eroding the osseous EAC (full thickness) with limited soft tissue involvement (<5 mm) or tumor involving the middle ear and/or mastoid
T4	Tumor eroding the cochlea, petrous apex, medial wall of the middle ear, carotid canal, jugular foramen, or dura; or tumor with extensive soft tissue involvement (>5 mm), such as involvement of temporomandibular joint or styloid process; or with evidence of facial paresis
N1	Single ipsilateral regional node <3 cm in size
N2a	Single ipsilateral regional node 3–6 cm in size
N2b	Multiple ipsilateral nodes
N2c	Bilateral or contralateral nodes
N3	Nodal deposit >6 cm
M0	No metastases
M1	Metastatic disease

SURGICAL APPROACH

The complex anatomy of the region presents a great challenge to the surgeon in achieving oncological clearance while limiting postoperative morbidity. Clinical research on surgical approaches, after the reports from Parson and Lewis,[15] Conley and Novack[16] and Lewis,[17] has focused mainly on two options: en bloc or piecemeal resection. The latter removes the tumor bit by bit up until normal tissue is encountered, whereas en bloc resections follow an anatomical plane of dissection through normal tissue.

The radicality achieved with extensive surgery is the most important independent factor influencing prognosis though it is not clear how surgical margins can be considered "free" in the bone. The en bloc resections with lateral or subtotal temporal bone resections (LTBR and STBR), though more likely to ensure gross radicality, encounter the problem of microscopic diffusion in the bone and may explain the relatively high recurrence rate after surgery with pathologically free margins (**Figs. 2A and B**).[6]

En bloc resection (advocated by Parsons and Lewis, Conley and Novac, and Lewis et al.) is considered to be a useful method of controlling the local recurrence because of the low possibilities of residual tumor and tumor dispersion. The en bloc resection of the temporal bone by the lateral approach with safety margins is useful for resecting tumors that have infiltrated the petrous apex and the cranial base.[18,19] The internal carotid artery can be resected if the cerebral blood flow volume is 30 mL/100 mg/min or more on the preoperative test.[18]

A surgical approach must be tailored to the site and the extent of the lesion. When the posterior wall of the external auditory canal (as in a canal-wall down tympanoplasty) and the middle ear are removed, the overlying skin is closed in a "cul-de-sac", the facial nerve is left in place, and the labyrinth is the medial boundary of bone removal, the procedure is a lateral petrosectomy or, according to Fisch, subtotal petrosectomy. The term "lateral" is a better term that describes the concept where bone removal stops at the labyrinth, remaining lateral to it. If the extension of bone removal includes the labyrinth and internal auditory canal (independently if the procedure becomes extra- or transdural), a "subtotal petrosectomy" is then performed, or as Fisch described, total petrosectomy. In the subtotal petrosectomy, the inner boundary of the block resection extends from the carotid canal to the jugular fossa, and includes transection of the petrous bone medial to the labyrinth and through

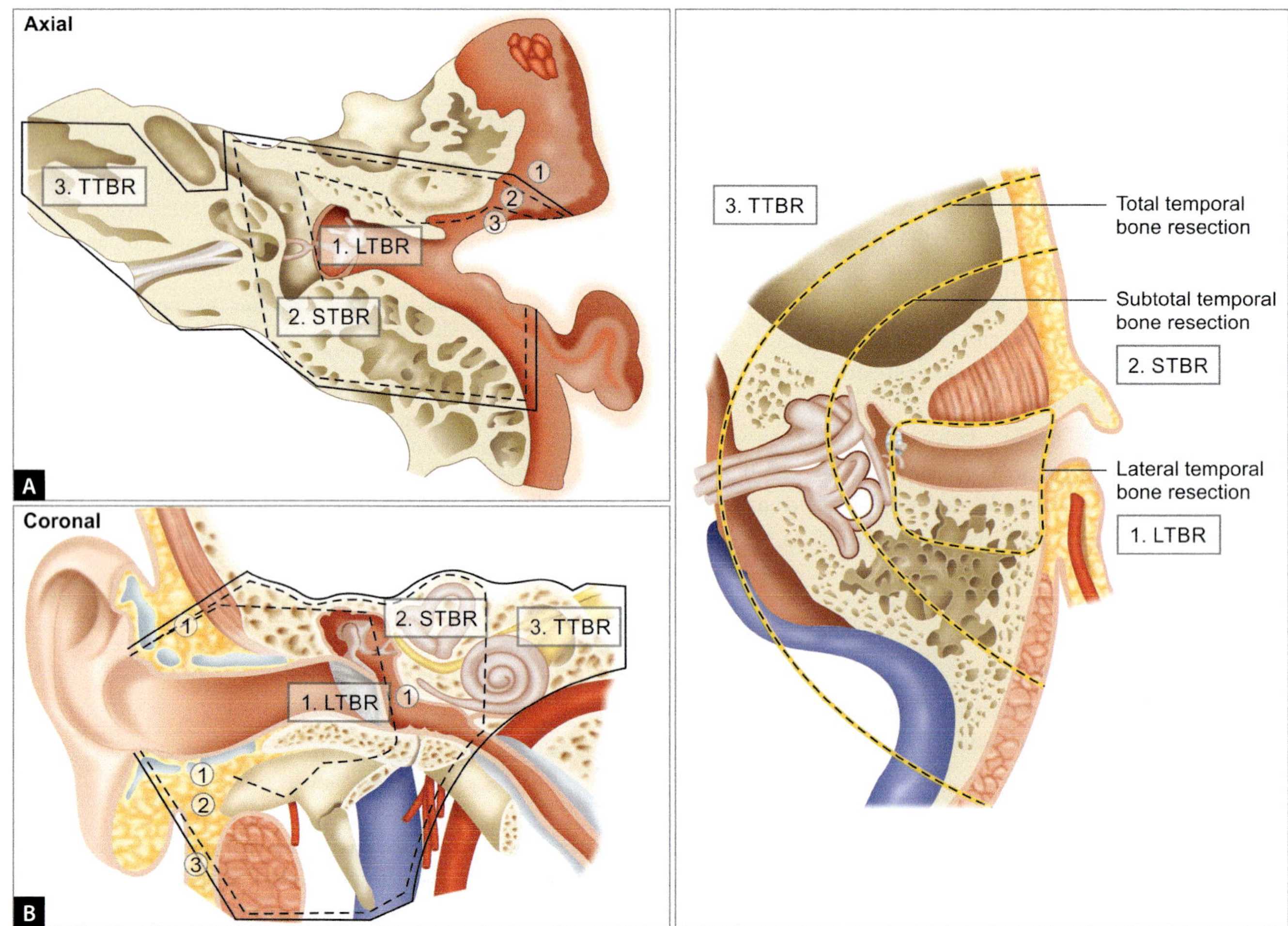

Figs. 2A and B: Margins of temporal bone resection.

the internal auditory canal. The auditory canal and the facial nerve are sacrificed.

Total petrosectomy extends further to include the petrous apex. In both subtotal and total petrosectomy, the dura is preserved or, if resected, repaired. Lateral temporal bone resection (LTBR) should be regarded as the minimum oncological operation for T1 and T2 lesions.[20] Essential elements of LTBR are (1) excision lateral to facial nerve (2) conchal bowl resection, and (3) bony cuts involve mastoid to middle fossa dura (or leaving a thin layer of bone), anteriorly into zygomatic air cells and temporomandibular joints (TMJ), inferiorly to stylomastoid foramen, hypotympanum to the TMJ.[15,16] Extended temporal bone resection (ETBR) is required for more extensive tumors involving the middle ear. The essential elements of ETBR are: (1) facial nerve sacrifice, (2) posterior and middle craniotomy, (3) labyrinthectomy, (4) transection of internal auditory canal, (5) resection of petrous tip, (6) exposure of intrapetrous portion of the carotid, and (7) total parotidectomy.

The subtotal temporal bone resection (STBR) involves temporal and occipital craniotomies, freeing the carotid and four osteotomies to deliver the specimen. There is a subtemporal osteotomy from the carotid canal to the posterior side of the petrous bone, with transection of the proximal third of the internal auditory canal, a second osteotomy through the occipital craniotomy, from the petrous bone to the jugular foramen (preserving its medial wall), a third osteotomy from the jugular fossa to the carotid canal, and a fourth from the carotid canal to the glenoid fossa through the temporal craniotomy.

Kollert et al.[21] recommends stage-dependent LTBR or STBR combined with parotidectomy and neck dissection. Prasad et al.[22] noted that STBR appears to be more beneficial than LTBR or mastoidectomy, with 5-year survivals of 42%, 29%, and 17%, respectively. A review of 26 publications including 144 patients showed that patients with tumor confined to the external auditory canal (EAC) had similar survival, regardless of the type of surgery performed (e.g., mastoidectomy, lateral TBR, and STBR).[1] Patients with an extension of the disease into the middle ear had longer survival times if they underwent an STBR.[23]

Management of the Parotid Gland

The incidence of parotid involvement in temporal bone SCC is reportedly in the range of 10–62%.[24] Superficial parotidectomy should be a part of en bloc resection as a standard treatment for SCC, even if a patient shows no clinical or radiological evidence of salivary gland involvement or close margins.[25-27] Hosokawa et al. used CT to study focal defects in the anterior–inferior canal wall of the tympanic bone in search of indicators of an anterior spread in SCC, and recommended superficial parotidectomy as necessary in all resections, noting that deep lobe was rarely involved.[27] Total parotidectomy is recommended in T4 SCC with virtually all cases revealing direct parotid involvement.

Management of the Facial Nerve

Irrespective of the approach, a central problem in extirpating lesions of the lateral skull base is the location of the facial nerve. Because of its long and irregular route through the temporal bone, any attempt at petrous resection often forces the surgeon either to sacrifice the facial nerve or, more commonly, to reroute it.[28,29] Historically, management of the facial nerve required either anterior or posterior mobilization as described by Fisch[30] and House and Hitselberger,[31] respectively.

Higgins and Antonio[32] conducted a systematic review and meta-analysis of studies on temporal bone SCC published between 1976 and 2008 to ascertain the impact of facial palsy on survival outcomes. They concluded that facial nerve involvement is associated with a poor outcome, and that survival outcomes for those with facial palsy more closely resembled the survival curves for advanced-stage T4 disease. Transposition requires skeletonization of the facial nerve in the Fallopian canal, resection of attachments to the canal, and displacement of the facial nerve in an anterior or posterior direction. Extrinsic and intrinsic blood supply is placed in jeopardy, especially with first genu rerouting. However, rerouting of the facial nerve provides maximal jugular bulb and tumor exposure and facilitates tumor resection. Anterior rerouting of the facial nerve is a maneuver designed to enhance exposure of the jugular foramen and carotid canal during resection of cranial base tumors.

Role of Neck Dissection

In the literature, there are reported rates of 4.5–31.8% nodal positivity after neck dissection, with a cumulative involvement of 17.7%.[33] The rate of micrometastases in the clinically negative neck was 17%. The prevalence of lymph node involvement in temporal bone cancers at presentation varies from 10 to 23% but is connected with a grave prognosis.[34,35] A planned dissection of levels Ib–III enables en bloc resection of the tumor, parotid, and lymph nodes. The risk of metastases at level IV should be considered in cases with positive nodes at higher levels, or in tumors recurring after surgery and/or radiotherapy. Extending the dissection to include level V is generally recommended in cases of therapeutic neck dissection and intraoperative positive nodes.[36]

Role of Adjuvant Therapy

Postoperative radiotherapy (PORT) is commonly indicated for advanced temporal bone SCC (T3/T4), in cases with intracranial invasion, adverse pathological features (as perineural/vascular invasion, close or positive surgical margins), and lymph node metastases or extranodal extension. Although the matter is still debated, a significant number of authors have advocated the use of PORT in T2 disease in view of it being an aggressive disease. Adjuvant external-beam radiotherapy should cover a target volume that includes at least the petrosal bone, the parotid fossa, and the retroauricular region. Intensity-modulated techniques may well reduce dose to the ipsilateral cochlea (if this is separate from the tumor volume) and oral cavity. Chronic otomastoiditis and temporal bone necrosis following radiotherapy can be reduced by restricting the volume of bone treated to high dose as far as possible.

In a recent meta-analysis by Oya et al., the 5-year overall survival rate of early-stage external canal SCC was 77%. PORT was administered in 45% of stage I patients and 68% of stage II patients. Survival analysis of all patients showed no differences between the surgery-only and surgery with PORT groups; however, PORT exhibited a better prognosis than surgery alone among patients with stage I disease ($p = 0.003$). This result indicated that PORT can be considered the standard therapy for stages I/II external auditory canal SCC.[37]

Ogawa et al. suggest that radiation therapy does not affect disease-free survival (DFS) in T1.[38] Authors of that study found the 5-year DFS rate in T1, T2 and T3 patients to be 83, 45 and 0% in the group treated with radiotherapy alone ($p < 0.0001$) and 75, 75 and 46% in the group that underwent surgery with PORT ($p = 0.13$). A multi-institutional review by Yin et al.[39] has suggested increased survival with chemotherapy in stage III/IV disease, if combined with surgery and PORT (surgery with PORT and surgery with chemoradiotherapy had a 5-year survival of 28.7% and 52.5%, respectively).

Prasad et al. did not find improved survival with the addition of PORT to temporal bone resection (TBR); (TBR and PORT vs. TBR alone had a 5-year survival of 48% and 44.4%, respectively).[22]

There is conflicting data in the literature regarding the benefits of chemotherapy with or without radiation. Takenaka et al. recently performed a meta-analysis on case series published between 2006 and 2013 to assess the efficacy of chemoradiotherapy (CRT) for advanced disease. The 5-year overall survival rate of 752 patients was 57%. In the individual patient data meta-analysis, the 5-year overall survival rates of patients who received surgery ± PORT, preoperative CRT, definitive CRT, and surgery with postoperative CRT were 53.5%, 85.7%, 43.6%, and 0%, respectively.[40] The value of this meta-analysis is limited by the different chemotherapeutic protocols used in the studies considered, the very small size of the samples and the inclusion of only eight patients treated preoperatively with CRT.

Role of Reconstructive Surgery

Reliable and robust reconstruction of the lateral skull base is needed to prevent complications. The type of reconstruction depends on several factors: the size of the defect, history of preoperative radiotherapy, vascular and dural coverage, and cosmesis. The considerations in reconstruction are protection of the brain when dura mater is breached, the size of the skin defect, the auricular defect, tissue volume, mandible defect and facial nerve deficits. Cervicofacial, temporalis, and other local flaps have been utilized for small superficial periauricular cutaneous defects for decades; however, the small tissue volume they provide limits their use. Regional flaps provide considerable volume but are limited by length and the amount of tension that can be placed on the vascular pedicle. Free-flap reconstruction has become the standard-of-care for definitive management of large cutaneous and skull-base defects.

REHABILITATION

Facial Nerve

A cable graft from intratemporal facial nerve to intra-parotid branches can be performed if there is enough proven tumor-free proximal facial nerve (otherwise other options can be considered, see chapter on facial nerve disorders in head and neck cancer) and if the peripheral branches can be identified. Useful donor nerves include greater auricular nerve, sural nerve, or lateral cutaneous nerve of thigh (easily available if harvesting an anterolateral thigh free flap).[1] Gold weights, tarsorrhaphy, canthoplasty, brow lifts, and static slings each have a role to play.

Hearing and Vestibular Rehabilitation

Osseointegrated implants offer patients an option for hearing restoration and for prosthesis fixation. Implants can be placed either at the time of primary surgery or at a time after completion of therapy. Loading can begin in 3 months in patients if the patient is not treated with radiotherapy. However, 6 months are allowed to pass before using an implant in an irradiated field.[41] Total conductive hearing loss can be rehabilitated through an osseointegrated bone anchored hearing aid (BAHA). Total hearing loss can be rehabilitated through either a BAHA or a bilateral contralateral routing of signals (BI-CROS) aid. Postoperative vertigo is expected if there is resection of a functioning labyrinth. If vestibular compensation is protracted and incomplete, referral for vestibular rehabilitation services should be considered.

RECURRENCE

Although complete excision with free margins is the main goal of temporal bone oncological surgery, relatively high local recurrence rates have been reported, even in patients whose final pathology report confirmed free margins. Even though histopathological accuracy has improved over the years, it is still not easy to analyze margins in bone and at the interface between tumor and bone. Numerous sections of the specimen are probably needed and further analyzes are mandatory to investigate hidden microscopic pathways of tumor diffusion. Furthermore, perineural involvement might also account for the rapid recurrence rate in addition to bony involvement/invasion.

The clinical behavior of SCC recurring in temporal bone makes it necessary to question the selection criteria for curative or palliative surgery for recurrent lesions. Salvage surgery might be considered for early recurrences. Recurrences tend to occur within the first 2 years after completion of therapy. A large study of 157 patients with temporal bone tumors showed a mean time to recurrence of 13 months. In this study, recurrences were 12.7% local, 6.4% regional, and 13.4% distant. The most common sites for distant spread are lung, brain, and dermal metastases.[42] Morris et al.[43] showed recurrence rates of 20.5% for local disease, 5.5% for regional disease, and 22.9% for distant disease.

PROGNOSIS

The pathological status of surgical margins is reported as the main factor influencing the outcome and the recurrence rate, although how reliable "free margins" are defined in the bone is still a matter of discussion. The difference in outcomes for those with and without anterior extension of T4 tumors was recently investigated,[44] showing a significantly better prognosis in those with anterior extension. Extensive erosion of the bone was also a negative prognostic factor. The pathological grading of the tumor was reported as a factor related to worse prognosis only in a limited number of series. In part, facial nerve involvement continues to be controversial with a significant adverse prognostic role. Dura mater infiltration evidence (both radiological and/or pathological) was reported in most of the series as the strongest negative prognostic factor affecting survival.[19,42]

PALLIATION

The local issues that affect patients when tumors are inoperable or recur are generally pain (particularly through dural involvement) and fungation. Therefore, a comprehensive analgesic regimen is required to manage pain. Fungation can be a particular problem, made worse by the prominent site of the cancer. Radiotherapy can be given for palliative intent, if not already given, and can be useful for both pain and fungation. Short fractionation schedules may well be appropriate in these situations. If RT has previously been given and there is a reasonable interval (>12 months), then reirradiation is sometimes beneficial.[45]

CONCLUSION

Management of temporal bone tumors is challenging due to rarity of disease, complexity of anatomy and absence of universal consensus on treatment modalities. Most of the management principles are derived from retrospective case series to provide the best possible treatment.

REFERENCES

1. Homer JJ, Lesser T, Moffat D, Slevin N, Price R, Blackburn T. Management of lateral skull base cancer: United Kingdom national multidisciplinary guidelines. J Laryngol Otol. 2016;130(S2):S119-24.
2. Nakagawa T, Kumamoto Y, Natori Y, Shiratsuchi H, Toh S, Kakazu Y, et al. Squamous cell carcinoma of the external auditory canal and middle ear: an operation combined with preoperative chemoradiotherapy and a free surgical margin. Otol Neurotol. 2006;27(2):242-9.
3. Chen WY, Kuo SH, Chen YH, Lu SH, Tsai CL, Cheng JC, et al. Postoperative intensity-modulated radiotherapy for squamous cell carcinoma of the external auditory canal and middle ear: treatment outcomes, marginal misses, and perspective on target delineation. Int J Radiation Oncol Biol Physics. 2012;82(4):1485-93.
4. Sanna M, De Donato G, Taibah A, Russo A, Falcioni M, Mancini F. Infratemporal fossa approaches to the lateral skull base. The Keio J Med. 1999;48(4):189-200.
5. Gidley PW, DeMonte F. Temporal bone malignancies. Neurosurg Clin. 2013;24(1):97-110.
6. Zanoletti E, Marioni G, Franchella S, Munari S, Pareschi R, Mazzoni A, et al. Temporal bone carcinoma: classical prognostic variables revisited and modern clinico-pathological evidence. Rep Pract Oncol Radiother. 2016;21(4):386-90.
7. Tiwari R, Brouwer J, Quak J, Tobi H, Winters H, Mehta D. Squamous cell carcinoma of the external auditory canal and middle ear results of treatment with subtotal temporal bone resection and postoperative radiotherapy. Indian J Otolaryngol Head Neck Surg. 2002;54(3):179-83.

8. Stell PM, McCormick MS. Carcinoma of the external auditory meatus and middle ear: prognostic factors and a suggested staging system. Journal Laryngol Otol. 1985;99(9):847-50.
9. Feiz-Erfan I, Suki D, Hanna E, DeMonte F. Prognostic significance of transdural invasion of cranial base malignancies in patients undergoing craniofacial resection. Neurosurgery. 2007;61(6):1178-85.
10. Ahmadi J, Hinton DR, Segall HD, Couldwell WT. Surgical implications of magnetic resonance-enhanced dura. Neurosurgery. 1994;35(3):370-7.
11. Tansavatdi K, Dublin AB, Donald PJ, Dahlin B. Combined Balloon Test Occlusion and SPECT Analysis for Carotid Sacrifice: Angiographic Predictors for Success or Failure? J Neurol Surg Part B: Skull Base. 2015;76(04):249-51.
12. Schick B, Dlugaiczyk J. Surgery of the ear and the lateral skull base: pitfalls and complications. GMS Curr Top Otorhinolaryngol, Head Neck Surg. 2013;12.
13. Moody SA, Hirsch BE, Myers EN. Squamous cell carcinoma of the external auditory canal: an evaluation of a staging system. Otol Neurotol. 2000;21(4):582-8.
14. Arriaga M, Curtin H, Hirsch BE, Takahashi H, Kamerer DB. Staging proposal for external auditory meatus carcinoma based on preoperative clinical examination and computed tomography findings. Ann Otol, Rhinol Laryngol. 1990;99(9):714-21.
15. Parsons H, Lewis JS. Subtotal resection of the temporal bone for cancer of the ear. Cancer. 1954;7(5):995-1001.
16. Conley JJ, Novack AJ. The surgical treatment of malignant tumors of the ear and temporal bone: Part I. AMA arch otolaryngol. 1960;71(4):635-52.
17. Lewis JS. Temporal bone resection: review of 100 cases. Arch Otolaryngol. 1975;101(1):23-5.
18. Asano K, Somekawa Y, Yoshioka I, Ikeda H. En bloc resection of the temporal bone by the lateral approach in carcinoma of the middle ear associated with skull base infiltration with reference to the resection of the petrous apex. Skull Base Surg. 1998;8(04):195-204.
19. Masterson L, Rouhani M, Donnelly NP, Tysome JR, Patel P, Jefferies SJ, et al. Squamous cell carcinoma of the temporal bone: clinical outcomes from radical surgery and postoperative radiotherapy. Otol Neurotol. 2014;35(3):501-8.
20. Zhang T, Li W, Dai C, Chi F, Wang S, Wang Z. Evidence-based surgical management of T1 or T2 temporal bone malignancies. Laryngoscope. 2013;123(1):244-8.
21. Kollert M, Draf W, Minovi A, Hofmann E, Bockmühl U. Carcinoma of the external auditory canal and middle ear: therapeutic strategy and follow up. Laryngo-rhino-otologie. 2004;83(12):818-23.
22. Prasad S, Janecka IP. Efficacy of surgical treatments for squamous cell carcinoma of the temporal bone: a literature review. Otolaryngol Head Neck Surg. 1994;110(3):270-80.
23. Chang CH, Shu MT, Lee JC, Leu YS, Chen YC, Lee KS. Treatments and outcomes of malignant tumors of external auditory canal. Am J Otolaryngol. 2009;30(1):44-8.
24. Choi JY, Choi EC, Lee HK, Yoo JB, Kim SG, Lee WS. Mode of parotid involvement in external auditory canal carcinoma. J Laryngol Otol. 2003;117(12):951-4.
25. Okada T, Saito K, Takahashi M, Hasegawa Y, Fujimoto Y, Terada A, et al. En bloc petrosectomy for malignant tumors involving the external auditory canal and middle ear: surgical methods and long-term outcome. J Neurosurg. 2008;108(1):97-104.
26. Bibas AG, Ward V, Gleeson MJ. Squamous cell carcinoma of the temporal bone. J Laryngol Otol. 2008;122(11):1156-61.
27. Hosokawa S, Mizuta K, Takahashi G, Okamura J, Takizawa Y, Hosokawa K, et al. Surgical approach for treatment of carcinoma of the anterior wall of the external auditory canal. Otol Neurotol. 2012;33(3):450-4.
28. Haijin Y, Shiming Y. Otolaryngology: Open Access; 2017.
29. Pensak ML, Jackler RK. Removal of jugular foramen tumors: the fallopian bridge technique. Otolaryngol Head Neck Surg. 1997;117(6):586-91.
30. Fisch U. Infratemporal fossa approach for glomus tumors of the temporal bone. Ann Otol, Rhinol Laryngol. 1982;91(5):474-9.
31. House WF, Hitselberger WE. The transcochlear approach to the skull base. Arch Otolaryngol. 1976;102(6):334-42.
32. Higgins TS, Antonio SA. The role of facial palsy in staging squamous cell carcinoma of the temporal bone and external auditory canal: a comparative survival analysis. Otol Neurotol. 2010;31(9):1473-9.
33. Moffat DA, Wagstaff SA, Hardy DG. The outcome of radical surgery and postoperative radiotherapy for squamous carcinoma of the temporal bone. Laryngoscope. 2005;115(2): 341-7.
34. Martinez-Devesa P, Barnes ML, Milford CA. Malignant tumors of the ear and temporal bone: a study of 27 patients and review of their management. Skull Base. 2008;18(1):1-8.
35. Simo R, Homer J. Follow-up of head and neck cancers. In: Roland NJ, Paleri V (Eds). Head and Neck Cancer: Multidisciplinary Management Guidelines. London: ENT-UK; 2011. pp. 362-6.
36. Rinaldo A, Ferlito A, Suárez C, Kowalski LP. Nodal disease in temporal bone squamous carcinoma. Acta Otolaryngologica. 2005;125(1):5-8.
37. Oya R, Takenaka Y, Takemura K, Ashida N, Shimizu K, Kitamura T, et al. Surgery with or without postoperative radiation therapy for early-stage external auditory canal squamous cell carcinoma: a meta-analysis. Otol Neurotol. 2017;38(9):1333-8.
38. Ogawa K, Nakamura K, Hatano K, Uno T, Fuwa N, Itami J, et al. Treatment and prognosis of squamous cell carcinoma of the external auditory canal and middle ear: a multi-institutional retrospective review of 87 patients. Int J Radiation Oncol Biol Physics. 2007;68(5):1326-34.
39. Yin M, Ishikawa K, Honda K, Arakawa T, Harabuchi Y, Nagabashi T, et al. Analysis of 95 cases of squamous cell carcinoma of the external and middle ear. Auris Nasus Larynx. 2006;33(3):251-7.
40. Takenaka Y, Cho H, Nakahara S, Yamamoto Y, Yasui T, Inohara H. Chemoradiation therapy for squamous cell carcinoma of the external auditory canal: A meta-analysis. Head Neck. 2015;37(7):1073-80.
41. Walker DD, Babu S. Temporal Bone Paraganglioma: Hearing Outcomes and Rehabilitation. J Neurol Surg Part B: Skull Base. 2019;80(2):209-13.
42. Gidley PW, Thompson CR, Roberts DB, DeMonte F, Hanna EY. The oncology of otology. Laryngoscope. 2012; 122(2):393-400.
43. Morris LG, Mehra S, Shah JP, Bilsky MH, Selesnick SH, Kraus DH. Predictors of survival and recurrence after temporal bone resection for cancer. Head Neck. 2012;34(9):1231-9.
44. Mazzoni A, Danesi G, Zanoletti E. Primary squamous cell carcinoma of the external auditory canal: surgical treatment and long-term outcomes. Acta Otorhinolaryngologica Italica. 2014;34(2):129.
45. Pemberton LS, Swindell R, Sykes AJ. Primary radical radiotherapy for squamous cell carcinoma of the middle ear and external auditory canal—a historical series. Clinical Oncology. 2006;18(5):390-4.

CHAPTER 19

Tumors of the Salivary Glands

Federico Bolognesi, Narayana Subramaniam, Samskruthi P Murthy, Sivakumar Vidhyadharan

INTRODUCTION

Salivary gland tumors are a heterogeneous group of pathologies that are morphologically, clinically, and histologically diverse, often presenting significant diagnostic and management challenges to both pathologists and surgeons. This group of lesions is considered one of the most interesting and stimulating of the head and neck areas for its diagnostic complexity and its morphological diversity. The classification system proposed by World Health Organization (WHO) in 2005, later modified in 2017, distinguishes benign tumors and primary or secondary malignancies, depending on the tissue of origin **(Table 1)**.[1-3]

As already mentioned, salivary gland tumors are relatively rare, with an annual total incidence between 0.4 and 13.5 per 100,000 patients per year. According to the WHO, salivary gland tumors include about 6% of head and neck neoplasms and about 0.5% of all malignancies.[4,5] About 80% of salivary gland tumors are benign and most of them are localized in the parotid gland (80%) and in the submandibular gland (10–15%), while the sublingual gland and accessory salivary glands are rarely affected (5–10%).[6,7]

About 80% of the salivary gland tumors are benign and most of them are localized to the parotid gland (80%) and in the submandibular gland (10–15%), while the sublingual gland and accessory salivary glands are rarely affected (5–10%). About 85% of parotid tumors, 50–60% of submandibular gland tumors, 50% of the minor salivary gland tumors, and 10–20% of the sublingual gland tumors are benign **(Table 2)**.

Mucoepidermoid carcinoma is the most common malignant tumor of the parotid (21–26%), followed by carcinoma ex pleomorphic adenoma (5–18%), acinic cell carcinoma (9–24%), and adenocarcinoma not otherwise specified (NOS) (11–15%). The parotid is also a common site for metastases coming from squamous cell carcinomas (SCCs) and malignant melanomas of the head and neck, mostly from the skin of the temporal region.[8,9]

Tumors of the submandibular gland are much less than those with the parotid (4–11%) and about half of them are pleomorphic adenomas. The remainders are malignant tumors such as adenoid cystic carcinoma (ACC), mucoepidermoid carcinoma, carcinoma ex pleomorphic adenoma, SCC, and non-Hodgkin's lymphoma. The most common malignant neoplasm of the intraoral salivary gland is mucoepidermoid carcinoma (47–52%), followed by cystic adenoid carcinoma (14–23%) and polymorphous adenocarcinoma (12–19%). Tongue and the retromolar region salivary neoplasms are almost always malignant. Other common intraoral sites are palate (33%), upper lip (20%), and buccal mucosa (17%).[10-13,13a]

The average age of the occurrence of salivary tumors is 45 years, with a peak in incidence between the 5th and 6th decade. The average age of onset is higher for malignancy than benign tumors; for malignant tumors the peak is around the sixth decade of life. The age of onset is also influenced by the histological subtype; mean age at diagnosis of acinic cell carcinoma is 51 years, whereas for the SCC it is 72 years. Most aggressive tumors tend to present at an advanced age, usually in the seventh decade. White patients are affected about 1.4 times more than the black population.

Vascular tumors account for 60% of cases; among these, hemangioma is the tumor most often encountered. Hemangiomas account for 90% of all salivary gland tumors in children <1 year of which one-third are present at birth. Hemangiomas arise most commonly in the parotid glands but can also arise in submandibular and minor salivary glands. Malignant salivary gland tumors in children and adolescents are very rare, with an estimated annual incidence of 0.08 per 100,000 of these.

Mucoepidermoid carcinoma is the most common accounting for >60% with an average age of 13.4 years at diagnosis.[14-17]

RISK FACTORS

There are no specific risk factors for salivary gland tumors and, therefore, the etiology of such neoplasms is largely unknown. In some cases there may be genetic alterations; in others, they may be associated with viral infections such as Epstein–Barr virus (EBV) as in the case of poorly differentiated carcinoma and lymphoepithelial carcinoma of the parotid gland of Asian and Inuit populations.[18]

Also, some of these tumors are linked to exposure to industrial pollutants in silica, nickel, and rubber manufacturing. An increase in salivary gland tumors was also reported after exposure to nuclear radiation at Hiroshima and Nagasaki.[19] The role of smoking has been emphasized by numerous authors, particularly in Warthin's tumors, as chronic irritation from smoking is thought to cause proliferation of embryonic salivary duct remnants in the lymph nodes. Recently, an increase in the frequency of this tumor in women has been reported, which could be explained by an increase in female smoking.[20,21]

Table 1: World Health Organization (WHO) classification of salivary gland tumors.

Salivary gland tumors	
Benign	*Malignant*
Pleomorphic adenoma • Metastasizing pleomorphic adenoma	Acinic cell carcinoma
Myoepithelioma	Mucoepidermoid carcinoma
Basal cell adenoma	Adenoid cystic carcinoma
Warthin's tumor	Polymorphous low-grade adenocarcinoma
Oncocytoma	Epithelial myoepithelial carcinoma
Canalicular adenoma and other ductal adenomas	Clear cell carcinoma
Lymphadenoma • Sebaceous lymphadenoma • Nonsebaceous lymphadenoma • Sebaceous lymph adenocarcinoma	Basal cell adenocarcinoma
Ductal papilloma • Inverted ductal papilloma • Intraductal papilloma • Sialadenoma papilliferum	Sebaceous adenocarcinoma
Cystadenoma	Intraductal carcinoma
Other epithelial lesions • Intercalated duct lesions • Nodular oncocytic hyperplasia • Lymphoepithelial lesions Sclerosing polycystic adenosis	Salivary duct carcinoma
Soft tissue tumors • Hemangioma • Lipoma/sialolipoma • Nodular fasciitis	Oncocytic carcinoma
Borderline tumors • Sialoblastoma	Adenocarcinoma, not otherwise specified (NOS) • Cystadenocarcinoma • Mucinous adenocarcinoma
	Myoepithelial carcinoma
	Carcinoma ex pleomorphic adenoma
	Secretory carcinoma
	Carcinosarcoma
	Squamous cell carcinoma
	Large cell carcinoma
	Lymphoepithelial carcinoma
	Poorly differentiated carcinoma • Neuroendocrine carcinoma • Undifferentiated carcinoma • Large cell neuroendocrine • Small cell neuroendocrine carcinoma
	Hematolymphoid tumors • Hodgkin's lymphoma • Diffuse large B-cell lymphoma • Extranodal marginal zone B-cell lymphoma of MALT
	Secondary tumors that have metastasized to the salivary gland from another location • Cutaneous malignancies • Renal cell carcinoma • Lung cancer

(MALT: mucosa-associated lymphoid tissue)

Table 2: Incidence of malignancy in salivary gland tumors.

	Parotid	*Submandibular*	*Sublingual*	*Minor*
Benign	85%	50–60%	10–20%	50%
Malignant	15%	40–50%	80–90%	50%

ANATOMY

Salivary glands are classified as major salivary glands (parotid, submandibular, and sublingual) and minor salivary glands (located in the oral cavity, in the palatal, labial, and buccal mucosa). The parotid is the largest salivary gland with a weight of approximately 30 g. It is the first major salivary gland to form at the 5th–6th week of intrauterine development; it has an ectodermal origin and is formed in the oral cavity by epithelial buds with salivary canaliculi appearing around the 12th week, surrounded by the myoepithelial cells that contract the canaliculi, and the acini during secretion. The gland is included in a fibrous capsule that generally is formed around the 3rd month of development and follows the contours of the parotid region. The parotid capsule is continuous with the superficial component of the deep cervical fascia. The gland extends from the zygomatic arch superiorly to the posterior belly of the digastric inferiorly, and rests posteriorly on the ramus of the mandible. Anteriorly, the parotid fascia continues with the fascia over the masseter muscle forming the parotidomasseteric fascia. From a surgical point of view it is important to have a detailed knowledge of the topographic anatomy of the parotid region, as described below.

Parotid Region

The parotid region occupies the lateral part of the deep intermediate space of the face that is pyramid-shaped with a lateral base and medial apex, of which three walls are well-delineated: (1) the side, (2) back wall, and (3) front walls. The lateral wall lies between the tragus posteriorly and the posterior edge of the ascending ramus of the mandible anteriorly: it is the anatomical area in which the clinical examination of the gland takes place. Inferiorly, the limit is represented by a line traced from the lower edge of the mandible body. The anterior wall of the parotid region comprises the masseter muscle, the mandibular ramus, the sphenomandibular ligament, the medial pterygoid muscle, and the stylomandibular ligament, which separate the parotid region from the infratemporal fossa on the front. The upper aspect of the parotid region is narrow, lying between the anterior temporomandibular joint and the external acoustic meatus. In contrast, the lower end is broad, formed by a septum which separates the parotid gland from the submandibular gland.

The lower portion of the parotid is called the tail and overlaps the angle of the mandible, extending over the sternocleidomastoid muscle. Many benign tumors are found in this region. The deep extension of parotid gland extends behind the mandible ramus through the stylomandibular tunnel to enter the prestyloid parapharyngeal space. The parotid gland is traversed by the facial nerve that arbitrarily divides the parotid gland into two lobes, superficial and deep. However, this is a theoretical subdivision: the two lobes cannot be anatomically or radiologically individualized.[22]

The facial nerve enters this region after exiting the temporal bone through the stylomastoid foramen, passing between the digastric muscle and the styloid muscle to enter the gland at the level of its posterior surface, immediately dividing into two main branches, the temporofacial branch and the cervicofacial branches. These are divided into five branches: (1) frontal, (2) zygomatic, and (3) upper buccal branches (from the temporofacial branch); (4) lower buccal and (5) marginal mandibular branches (from the cervicofacial branch).

The facial nerve is accompanied by four afferent veins: (1) the maxillary vein, (2) the occipital vein, (3) the superficial temporal vein, and (4) the auricular vein. The superficial temporal vein and the maxillary vein form the retromandibular vein. This passes close to the lower pole of the parotid gland and divides into a posterior branch, which forms the external jugular vein after joining the posterior auricular vein, and an anterior branch which joins the facial vein. The retromandibular vein is an important surgical landmark because the facial nerve divides into its temporofacial and cervicofacial branches just behind the retromandibular vein, lying just superficial to it. Finally, the external carotid artery passes on the medial face of the parotid gland, running from the bottom to the top to divide into two branches at the level of the condyle, the superficial temporal artery and the internal maxillary artery. The parasympathetic innervation of the parotid is given by the glossopharyngeal nerve whereas sympathetic innervation originates from the superior cervical ganglion of the paravertebral chain.

Submandibular Region

The submandibular region is located below the floor of the oral cavity and has a triangular shape, with medial, superolateral wall, and inferolateral walls. It is limited laterally by the medial aspect of the body of the mandible, inferiorly by the portion of the cervical fascia stretched between the inferior margin of the mandible and the hyoid bone and by the concavity of the intermediate tendon of the digastric muscle, medially by the hyoglossus and mylohyoid muscles and posteriorly it is separated from the parotid gland by interglandular septum.

The region contains the submandibular gland, which has an endodermic origin. It weighs 7–8 g and has the shape of a triangular prism; there are faces such as lateral, medial, and lower faces. The lateral face is related anteriorly with the submandibular fossa of the mandible and posteriorly with the medial pterygoid muscle. The medial face is related with the mylohyoid, hyoglossus, stylohyoid muscles, and with the intermediate tendon of the digastric muscle; on the hyoglossus muscle, the submandibular gland covers the hypoglossal nerve. The lower face is related with the superficial cervical fascia and it is crossed by the anterior facial vein. From the medial face of the gland, an anterior extension arises which moves forward between the hyoglossus and mylohyoid muscles, until it reaches the sublingual gland. The facial artery is related to the posterior part of the lateral face, it first runs deep into the superficial lobe and then emerges between the lateral surface of the gland and mandibular insertion of the medial pterygoid muscle, from which it reaches the inferior margin of the mandible. The submental artery and vein run between the surface of the gland and the mandible.

The submandibular duct (of Wharton) has a length of 4–5 cm. It emerges from the medial face of the gland and moves obliquely forward, upward, and medially, together with the anterior extension of the gland, until it reaches the sublingual groove, running on the inner face of the sublingual gland in relation to the sublingual artery and the lingual nerve. It opens in the sublingual groove on the apex of the sublingual caruncle.

Submandibular lymph nodes are located between the salivary gland and the mandible. Sometimes one or more lymph nodes can be incorporated into the salivary gland. The parasympathetic fibers originate from the superior salivary nucleus and through the facial nerve, the chorda tympani nerve (where they run together with the gustatory fibers for the two anterior thirds of the tongue) and the lingual nerve reach the submandibular ganglion; hence, the postganglionic fibers go to the glandular parenchyma. Sympathetic fibers reach the submandibular gland starting from the upper cervical ganglion, following the plexus that forms around the facial artery. The arterial blood supply comes from multiple branches of the facial and lingual arteries. Venous blood drains predominantly into the deep lingual vein.

Sublingual Gland

The sublingual gland is a major salivary gland and is situated in the sublingual region. The gland has an ovoid shape and weighs 2–3 g. It has lateral and medial faces, upper and lower margins, and anterior and posterior poles. The lateral face is related to the sublingual dimple of the mandible. The medial face is related to the genioglossus and longitudinal inferior muscles of the tongue, lingual nerve, sublingual artery, and submandibular duct. The upper margin of the gland raises the mucosa of the sublingual sulcus in the sublingual fold. The lower margin is related to the mylohyoid muscle. The anterior extremity is related to the origin of the genioglossus muscle. The main sublingual duct (Rivinus' duct) emerges from the medial aspect of the gland and runs outside the submandibular duct, opening into the sublingual caruncle, and beside the submandibular duct itself. The innervation is the same as that of the submandibular glands. The arterial supply comes from the sublingual branch of the lingual artery and the submental branch of the facial artery, with venous drainage into the deep lingual vein.

Parapharyngeal Space

The parapharyngeal space is a deep region of the neck placed laterally to the lateral wall of the pharynx and commonly described as an inverted pyramid with apex at the hyoid bone and base at the skull base. This pyramid has four walls: (1) medial, (2) anterior, (3) lateral, and (4) posterior. The medial wall corresponds to the superior constrictor muscle of the pharynx, the anterior wall to the medial pterygoid muscle and to the ramus of the mandibular, and the lateral wall is composed of the deep lobe of the parotid gland covered by the deep parotid fascia and the posterior belly of the digastric muscle. Posteriorly is the prevertebral fascia and cranially the pharyngeal space continues with the masticatory space. On the dorsal side, there is a septum that divides the parapharyngeal space from the retropharyngeal one, referred to as "Charpy's sagittal septum".

The parapharyngeal space is divided into two distinct parts by the styloid process and by the stylomandibular fascia: the prestyloid compartment anteriorly and the retrostyloid compartment posteriorly. The former has the shape of a dihedral angle with an anterior vertex, and contains the branches of the carotid artery such as the ascending pharyngeal artery and the palatine artery, while the second is almost entirely occupied by the vascular-nerve bundle consisting of the internal carotid artery, the internal jugular vein, the sympathetic trunk, and the cranial nerves IX–XII. Parotid masses can involve the parapharyngeal spaces in two distinct ways: tumors can arise within the deep lobe of the parotid gland and, therefore, extend into the parapharyngeal space through the stylomandibular tunnel or they can arise from the parotid tissue presenting itself as an isolated mass within the prestyloid parapharyngeal space.

Anatomical Landmarks for Identification of the Facial Nerve

The facial nerve emerges from the petrous part of the temporal bone through the stylomastoid foramen. The nerve emerges at the level of the posterior belly of the digastric muscle and from its point of emergence is directed forward and outward, almost horizontally along the upper wall of the retrostyloid space. At this level, the facial nerve is accompanied by a venous plexus and the stylomastoid artery, which is a branch of the posterior auricular artery.[23]

In this short retroparotid tract, the nerve passes external to the styloid apophysis. It then enters into the parotid region between the posterior belly of the digastric muscle laterally and the styloid muscle medially. The landmark where the nerve goes into the gland is schematically placed at the same distance from the zygoma and from the angle of the jaw, at about 25 mm depth.

Here we report the main landmarks used for the anterograde dissection of the main trunk of the facial nerve in its extracranial portion.[24-27]

- The triangular process of tragus cartilage represents a very important landmark for the facial nerve identification and is commonly referred to as the "pointer". Recently data shows that the nerve trunk is about 13.6 ± 11.00 mm anterior and deep to the pointer.
- The tympanomastoid suture is one of the main landmarks used because it is easily palpable in the deepest part of the cartilaginous portion of the external auditory canal. The facial nerve emerges a few millimeters (3.79 ± 2.92 mm) deep to its edge.
- The posterior belly of the digastric muscle is a convenient landmark, although it is a muscle and it might be dependent on the force of retraction. The overall average of the distance between the posterior belly of the digastric muscle and the extra-temporal segment of the facial nerve trunk is 8.79 ± 3.99 mm.
- The styloid process represents a less safe and less reliable surgical landmark because it could be absent or poorly developed in 50% of cases, often it is not easily identifiable; it is deeper than the same nerve and sometimes can present elongation or calcification of the stylohyoid ligament (i.e., Eagle syndrome). The average distance reported in literature between the styloid process and the facial nerve trunk is 9.80 ± 0 mm from the nerve trunk.
- The mastoid process is located at an average distance of 10.49 ± 1.42 mm from the facial nerve trunk.
- The external auditory meatus is located at an average distance of 11.77 ± 1.42 mm from the facial nerve trunk.
- The transverse process of C1 is located at an average distance of 14.99 ± 1.68 mm from the facial nerve trunk.

These measurements can be affected by atrophy of the mandible, gender, ethnicity or side, and much of the existing data is based on cadaveric studies and not on live patients. Within the parotid, the nerve takes a superficial course as it moves toward the medial aspect of the face, and it is important to consider that at its origin the nerve may have a transverse and not antero-posterior direction.

In the dissection of the facial nerve, it is important to free the fascial attachments in the pretragal and pretympanic parts of the gland as well as broad inferior dissection to mobilize the gland of the digastric muscle. In difficult cases, the facial nerve must be exposed in retrograde way. The dissection can start from any of the distal branches of the facial nerve, identified at the anterior edge of the gland, where the facial nerve becomes very superficial, running in the subcutaneous space.

The marginal mandibular branch can be identified inferiorly at the level of the superior and posterior portion of the submandibular gland. It is interesting to note that marginal mandibular nerve is divided into two branches in more than half of cases, or can remain unique. Rarely, the chin branches can reach up to six branches.[28] In adults, these branches often are below the mandibular angle and run for about 1.5 cm below the lower edge of the mandible; however, some branches may drop up to 3 cm below the jaw. During this course, the chin branch crosses the facial pedicle on average at 24 mm from the posterior margin of the mandibular angle. The buccal branch is located at the level of the midface and runs along the lower face of the masseter in close relation to the parotid duct. Surgically, the frontal and temporal branches are particularly vulnerable, since they run in a region where the superficial musculoaponeurotic system (SMAS) is very fine and directly subcutaneous.[29] This region can be marked with a triangle formed by the earlobe, the outer edge of the eyebrow, and the upper external corner of the forehead.[30]

The peripheral branches of the facial nerve form the parotid plexus through multiple anastomotic arcades. These anastomoses are important during facial nerve dissection since any accidental damage to one of the smaller branches often does not cause any facial weakness due to the double innervation of adjacent branches. The studies by Davis on 350 cadaveric facial nerves demonstrated these anastomotic relationships between adjacent branches, defining six different anastomotic patterns.[31]

CLINICAL EVALUATION

The diagnosis of a salivary neoplasm is often accidental and in most cases recognized by self-palpation of the patient. In the parotid gland, the superficial lobe is most often affected (90%) and, therefore, it typically appears in the form of a mass located anteriorly and inferiorly to the ear lobule that fills the retromandibular sulcus. These tumors are more often unilateral and when they develop in the deep part of the gland, or in its pharyngeal or cervical extension, the symptoms are represented by swallowing disorders as they extend toward the anterior parapharyngeal or prestyloid space. Deep lobe involvement may be identified on intraoral examination.

For the submandibular gland, neoplasms are often palpable in the submandibular region, below the mandible, with bi-digital palpation the best way to clinically distinguish these from enlarged lymph nodes; as the submandibular gland has a superficial and deep component on either side of the mylohyoid, these can be palpated bi-digitally while lymph nodes cannot. In the case of involvement of the sublingual gland, there is usually a swelling in the anterior floor of the mouth with overlying intact mucosa.

A malignant tumor should be suspected in the event of pain, irregularity of the surface of the swelling, hard consistency, adherence to the skin or deeper layers restricting mobility, rapid growth, suspicious lymphadenopathy, facial nerve paresis or palsy or evidence of distant metastases.

IMAGING

Imaging is a fundamental step in the diagnosis of salivary gland neoplasms, especially for malignancy, both to assess the nature of the lesion and to plan the surgery. In case of malignancy the main objective is to evaluate the extension of the neoplasm in terms of extension, perineural extension, lymphatic spread, lymph node involvement, and distant spread.[32]

Ultrasonography

Ultrasound represents today the examination of choice for the first diagnosis, especially for superficial parotid lesions. It is a noninvasive and low-cost examination, useful for the study of the superficial lobe of the parotid gland, submandibular and sublingual glands. It allows a simultaneous evaluation of the lymph node stations of the neck, particularly during the follow-up; besides it allows to guidance for needle biopsy. Despite being an excellent tool to differentiate solid lesions from cystic lesions and to assess the degree of vascularization of the neoplasm, it is an operator-dependent examination and does not allow accurately visualization of the deep lobe of the parotid gland or the minor salivary glands.[33-35]

Cross-sectional Imaging

Computed tomography (CT) and magnetic resonance imaging (MRI) provide important information regarding the size of the nodule, infiltration into adjacent tissues, macroscopic vascular or perineural invasion, and lymph node status. CT scan is the most widely performed diagnostic test, which often represents the first test to identify, sometimes in a random manner, a neoplasm of the salivary glands. CT scan is extremely rapid to perform and is particularly useful in the identification of bone infiltration, such as temporal bone or mandible, or in case of lesions that present calcifications within. Perineural extension can be evidenced by a dilation of the foramina of the skull base or by a loss of fat on soft tissue images. Furthermore, the accurate assessment of the retropharyngeal space, which cannot be clinically assessed, is well performed with CT. Extranodal extension can also be identified through indistinct fat planes and stranding of soft tissue with invasion of adjacent structures. The use of contrast media (except for allergic cases) is mandatory to have a better definition of the images and, therefore, of the tumor extension. The major pitfall of CT is the presence of image artifacts due to dental filling materials such as amalgam, dental implants or prostheses. CT perfusion imaging is an advanced method of evaluation that can be performed quantitatively to assess tumor vasculature.[36,37]

Magnetic resonance imaging with contrast medium represents the gold standard for the study of salivary gland neoplasms. MRI allows an accurate evaluation of deeper tissues and especially extraglandular or perineural diffusion in the case of malignant neoplasms, as well as the visualization of the interface between neoplasia and surrounding tissues. As far as perineural diffusion is concerned, the evaluation of both the trigeminal nerve and the facial nerve is very important for malignant tumors that have a high propensity for nerve invasion. It has a sensitivity of 87% and a specificity of 94%. A field of view not exceeding 250 mm and a cut thickness of 5 mm or less is desirable. Benign tumors generally have smooth and well-defined margins, a hyperintense signal on T2-weighted images and are often superficially localized. Malignant tumors, on the other hand, especially high-grade tumors, have poorly defined margins, invasion of adjacent tissues, low T2 signal, heterogeneous contrast enhancement, cystic areas and central necrosis. Cystic areas are observed in 50% of benign tumors and in 78% of malignant ones. Central cystic areas are visible only in malignant tumors. The presence of irregular thickening and peripheral nodules within the lesion wall are more commonly observed in malignant tumors.[38,39]

Intraparotid lymph node metastases from malignant neoplasms of the skin of the face, ear, and scalp, mostly SCC and melanoma, are recognized by an increase in size of the ipsilateral intraparotid lymph nodes, in addition to hypointense signal in T1 and intermediate or hyperintense signal in T2. The contrast medium enhancement highlights well the lymph nodes inside the parotid fat and the possible central necrotic areas with no enhancement. Diffusion-weighted MR imaging with the calculation of the apparent diffusion coefficient (ADC) may help differentiate between benign and malignant; tumors with high ADC value are more likely to be benign. Dynamic-enhanced imaging (DCE) technology which uses contrast-enhanced curves to characterize tumor angiogenesis and tissue enhancement; malignant tumors demonstrate rapid enhancement, but washout tends to be slower than in benign lesions. Protonic MR spectroscopy of the salivary glands can also aid in this distinction; tumors with choline/creatine ratios >2.4 are likely to be benign.[40] The disadvantages of MR imaging include possible contraindications to magnetic field exposure, such as pacemakers or neural stimulators, presence in the patient's body of nonmagnetic metals and relatively long scan times, which can increase the likelihood of movement or require use of sedation in claustrophobic patients.

Positron emission tomography-computed tomography (PET-CT) is used above all in locally advanced malignant neoplasms in stage to evaluate for distant metastases. Although high-grade salivary neoplasms tend to show higher maximum standardized uptake values than low-grade and benign ones, it is not reliable to differentiate a malignant salivary gland neoplasm from a benign one **(Table 3)**.[41]

Table 3: Key imaging characteristics of salivary gland neoplasms.[41]

Neoplasms	*Imaging characteristics*
Pleomorphic adenoma	Bright T2 signal, sharp margins, heterogeneous nodular enhancement, lobulated contours and dark T2 rims
Carcinoma ex pleomorphic adenoma	Newly infiltrative margins and rapid increase in size of a previous well-circumscribed mass
Warthin's tumor	Hypercellular microcysts, multifocal in 20%
Mucoepidermoid carcinoma	Partially cystic mass with ill-defined margins
Adenoid cystic carcinoma	Perineural spread and local invasion
Oncocytoma	Vanishing mass on T2-weighted images and T1 with contrast, FDG avid on PET
Lipoma	Fat attenuation on CT, fat suppression on MRI
Intraparotid metastases	Parotid tail or pretragal mass with primary malignancy that may be identifiable
Hemangioma	T2 hyperintense, homogeneous enhancement
Tumor-like lesions	
Ranula	T2 hyperintense lesion in sublingual space
Venous malformation	T2 hyperintense, gradual enhancement, may have phleboliths
Lymphatic malformation	Trans-spatial, hemorrhage-fluid levels
Arteriovenous malformation	Clustered nidus, arterial feeder, and draining vein

(CT: computed tomography; FDG: fluorodeoxyglucose; PET: positron emission tomography)

CYTOLOGY AND FROZEN SECTION

Preoperative differentiation between a benign and malignant neoplasm is very important in determining the timing and type of surgical intervention.[42,42a] Cytological examination using fine-needle aspiration cytology (FNAC) is an economic diagnostic procedure, widely accessible, minimally invasive, and oncologically safe; the risk of neoplastic dissemination appears irrelevant. The best accuracy is obtained by performing the procedure under ultrasound control. Sometimes in the diagnosis of cystic tumors, such as mucoepidermoid carcinomas, may require a repetition of the examination. The percentage to correctly establish a diagnosis between benign or malignant neoplasm of the salivary glands by the FNAC varies from 81 to 98%.[1,43]

In response to the limits of FNAC in the diagnosis of salivary gland neoplasms, to increase its reproducibility and promote its clinical relevance, a group of international pathologists has proposed a classification scheme for the reporting of FNAC samples of the salivary glands known as the "Milan System for Reporting Salivary Gland Cytopathology (MSRSGC)". The MSRSGC classifies the FNAC results of the salivary glands in the following diagnostic categories: nondiagnostic, non-neoplastic, atypia of undetermined significance, benign neoplasia, neoplasm of the salivary glands of uncertain malignant potential, and suspicious for malignancy and malignant. This is based on risk stratification rather than specific histological subtypes.[44]

Despite the fact that FNAC may not be able to effectively distinguish between a cellular inflammatory lesion and a neoplasm or a benign neoplasm and a well-differentiated malignant neoplasm due to overlapping cytological and architectural features, in most cases it is effective in distinguishing between a non-neoplastic and neoplastic process and identifying the most common neoplasms and metastases from other sites in the body. FNAC has a sensitivity of 87–100% and specificity of 90–100% when used to distinguish benign and malignant salivary gland tumors. Recent reviews have shown that the specificity is high for the diagnosis of neoplasm (95–98%) and malignancy (85–96%). Sensitivity is lower and more variable for the diagnosis of neoplasm (95–96%) and for malignancy (79–87%). As far as benign neoplasms are concerned, sensitivity and specificity of FNAC are 95% and 93%, respectively. For neoplasm of the salivary glands of uncertain malignant potential or suspected malignancy, the sensitivity and specificity of FNAC are 88% and 74%, respectively. Therefore, although a positive FNAC diagnosis is quite reliable, the false-negative rate associated with FNAC is still quite high (up to 20%).[45,46] For inconclusive or equivocal cytology in spite of adequate sampling, immunohistochemistry and identification of genomic alterations represent the next step in diagnostic testing **(Table 4)**.

For parapharyngeal neoplasms, it is easy to access lesions located in the prestyloid space that medialize the lateral wall of the pharynx through the transoral route for FNAC. However, for retrostyloid lesions, a blind approach may put neurovascular structures at risk. Yousem et al. described a novel image-guided method in which the needle is introduced through the soft tissues anterior to the mandibular ramus to reach the parapharyngeal space through the masticatory space.[47]

Frozen section allows a refinement of the diagnosis, especially in the case of malignant neoplasms; it is often used to confirm the presence of a neoplasm if the cytology is not diagnostic or if the cytopathological diagnosis is in contrast with the clinical features or intraoperative findings, and to determine the local and lymph node extension of the disease. It may also be used to confirm the presence of a high-grade neoplasm of the deep lobe and the need for neck dissection. The overall accuracy of frozen section is clinically acceptable (sensitivity of 90% and specificity of 99%), with a precision slightly higher than that of FNAC. It can be used to confirm the diagnosis in those patients undergoing surgery with a negative FNAC.

HISTOLOGY

- *Benign epithelial tumors*[2,5,48-50]
    - *Monomorphic adenoma:* Fairly frequent tumors, relatively small, well-delineated, encapsulated, and unifocal. They consist of epithelial elements in a fairly poor stroma and lack mesenchymal tissue.
    - *Warthin's tumor:* Composed of oncocytic cells and a lymphoid stroma. On histology there are vegetations covered with epithelial cells and immersed in cavities with an acidophilic content. The stroma contains a variable proportion of lymphoid tissue with follicles. Malignant transformation is exceptional (1%) to non-Hodgkin lymphoma. It can occur bilaterally and multifocally and in the latter case the risk of recurrence is greater. It is usually a rounded tumor, smooth on the surface, fluctuating and chamois yellow-colored. Sectioned, a viscous, brownish liquid emerges from this nodule. It consists of tubular or cystic structures with papillary formations bordered by a double eosinophilic cellular layer, in a stroma rich in lymphocytes. The inner cellular layer is formed by tall cylindrical cells, with abundant, acidophilic and finely granular cytoplasm.
    - *Oncocytoma:* Benign, solid, rounded, and well-delineated tumor characterized by the proliferation of oxyphil cells. It is a tumor organized in cords of large cells with eosinophilic, granular, and regular cytoplasm in a poor stroma. The oncocyte cell is an epithelial cell derived from metaplasia of the cells that form the epithelium of the acinar or tubular structures. It has an abundant and finely granular eosinophilic cytoplasm with a central pyknotic nucleus. There are three types of oncocytic lesions: (1) the disseminated and non-encapsulated form (diffuse oncocyte hyperplasia) which invades large portions of the parotid gland, until it completely occupies it; (2) the nodular form (multifocal nodular oncocytic hyperplasia) which presents several nodules without capsules inside a normal parenchyma; and (3) the third form, the oncocytoma, is a unique and encapsulated tumor, sometimes within a multinodular form.
    - *Pleomorphic adenoma:* Round or fusiform, hard, slow-growing, and indolent tumor. Macroscopically, this tumor generally appears as a rounded lesion, surrounded by a pseudocapsule.

Table 4: Genomic alterations and immunohistochemistry in salivary gland tumors.[2,59-64]

Tumor	*Chromosomal rearrangement*	*Gene and mechanism (FISH probes)*	*Prevalence*	*Immunostains*
Pleomorphic adenoma	8q12 translocations 12q13-15 translocations	*PLAG1* fusions/amplification *HMGA2* fusions/amplification	>50% ~15%	AE1/AE3, CK5/6, S100, p63
Carcinoma ex pleomorphic adenoma	8q12 translocations 12q13-15 translocations 17p13.1 12q15 amplification	*PLAG1* fusions/amplification *HMGA2* fusions/amplification *TP53* mutation HRAS mutation *MDM2*	72.7% 13.6% ~25–50% 25% ~50%	No data available
Myoepithelial carcinoma	8q12 t(12,22) (q21;q12)	*PLAG1* fusions *EWSR1-ATF1*	37.5% 12.5%	No data available
Clear cell carcinoma (hyalinizing)	t(12;22) (q21;q12)	*EWSR1-ATF1* *EWSR1-CREM*	80–93% <5%	CK5/6, p63+
Tubulotrabecular basal cell adenoma	3p22.1	*CTNNB1* hotspot mutation	37.5–80%	No data available
Membranous basal cell adenoma	16q12.13 deletion	*CYLD/LOH* mutation	36–80%	No data available
Basal cell adenocarcinoma	16q12.1	*CYLD* mutation	29%	No data available
Mucoepidermoid carcinoma	t(11;19) (q21;p13) t(11;15) (q21;q26) 9p21.3	*CRTC1-MAML2* *CRTC3-MAML2* *CDKN2A* deletion	40–80% 5–6% 25–35%	CK5/6+, p63–
Secretory carcinoma (mammary analog)	t(12;15) (p13;q25) t(12;10) (p13;q11) t(12;7) (p13;q31)	ETV6-NTRK3 ETV6-RET ETV6-MET	~95–98% ~2–5% <1%	GATA3+, S100+ MUC4+ Mammoglobin+
Intraductal carcinoma, intercalated duct type	10q11.21	*RET* fusions	46.7%	No data available
Intraductal carcinoma, apocrine type	3q26.32 11p15.5	*PIK3CA* mutations (apocrine type) *HRAS* mutations (apocrine type)	High High	No data available
Epithelial-myoepithelial carcinoma	11p15.5	*HRAS* hotspot mutation	25–77.8%	No data available
Salivary duct carcinoma	17q21.1 8p11.23 17p13.1 3q26.32 11p15.5 Xq12 10q23.31	*HER2* amplification *FGFR1* amplification *TP53* mutation *PIK3CA* mutation *HRAS* mutation *AR* copy gain *PTEN* loss *CDKN2A* loss	31% 10.3% 55–56% 20–33.3% 33.3% 35% 38% 10%	GATA3+, AR+, CK7+
Adenoid cystic carcinoma	6q22-23 translocations 8q13 translocations 9q34.3	*MYB* fusion/activation/amplification *MYBL1* fusion/activation *NOTCH* mutations (solid type)	~80% ~10% 13.7%	CD117+ S100 + CK5/6+, p63+
Polymorphous adeno-carcinoma, classic type	14q12	*PRKD1* hotspot mutation	73–75%	No data available
Polymorphous adenocarcinoma cribriform type	14q12 19q13.2 2p22.2	*PRKD1* fusions *PRKD2* fusions *PRKD3* fusions	38% 14.3% 19%	No data available
Acinic cell carcinoma	19q31.1 9q31	*MSANTD3* fusion/amplification *NR4A3* fusion/activation	4.4% 86%	No data available

(FISH: fluorescence in situ hybridization)

The pleomorphic adenoma consists of an epithelial component, formed by cylindrocubic cells, and a myoepithelial part, appearing as hyaline cells; the two components are interspersed with a stroma which is myxoid, mucoid, or chondroid. Three subtypes have been isolated: (1) the hypocellular (rich stroma, the most frequent and most likely to relapse), (2) the hypercellular, and (3) the classic form (equal distribution of epithelial, myoepithelial, and stroma cells). An important feature of pleomorphic adenomas is the presence of pseudopods and satellite nodules, which frequency varies according to the cellular subtype (23–75% in hypercellular adenomas, 33–62% in hypocellular adenomas, and 21–80% in classic adenomas). The pseudocapsule can have a variable thickness or be locally deficient. Exceptionally, an apparently typical pleomorphic adenoma can give metastases that have a histological appearance similar to the primitive tumor, probably following multiple recurrences or repeated surgical operations that allow some tumors to gain vascular access and metastasize, mainly to bone, lungs, and lymph nodes.

- *Myoepithelial adenoma:* Composed exclusively of myoepithelial cells. Can have different possible structures: solid, reticular, or myxoid. There is a similarity to pleomorphic adenoma due to the presence of myoepithelial cells, however, the myoepithelial adenoma does not present in ductal differentiation; it demonstrates a frank demarcation between cellular elements and the stroma. This distinction is important because myoepitheliomas have a more aggressive course compared to pleomorphic adenomas with a higher malignant transformation risk.

- *Malignant epithelial tumors*[51-64]
  - *Mucoepidermoid carcinoma:* Macroscopically appears hard, grayish-white or gray-red, noncapsulated and more or less circumscribed according to the tumor grading: high-grade tumors tend to have less defined limits. There may be cystic areas, especially in low-grade forms. The macroscopic appearance varies according to the degree of the tumor; this tumor develops starting from the salivary channels and it is characterized by the presence of epidermoid cells, mucous cells and intermediate cells. This neoplasm is divided into low-grade, intermediate, and high-grade tumors, depending on their histological differentiation. The proportion of various cell types varies from one tumor to another, and even within the same tumor. Low-grade tumors are well-differentiated, circumscribed but not capsulated and with a cystic prevalence, most often <4 cm in diameter, formed by well-differentiated epithelial cells and mucous-producing cells. High-grade tumors are poorly differentiated, generally with a diameter >4 cm, solid and with hemorrhagic and necrotic areas; mucous-producing cells are rare and the epidermoid component prevails. Several systems have been proposed for the determination of the grading of this neoplasm, although none has been universally accepted. A recent system that takes into account five histopathological features (cystic component, neural invasion, necrosis, mitotic index, and cellular anaplasia) appears to be reproducible in defining these tumors with low, intermediate, and high degree of malignancy.
  - *ACC:* It consists of two cell types: (1) canal type ductal cells and (2) myoepithelial cells. The tumor develops from the intercalated duct, and is formed by small, dark canalicular cells and myoepithelial cells, which are arranged in trabeculae interspersed by hyaline or mucoid stroma insulas. Three structural types are described: (1) cribriform, (2) tubular, or (3) solid pattern. The tumor was graded by Szanto et al. as grade I (cribriform or tubular), grade II (<30% solid) or grade III (>30% solid).[53] Perineural or perivascular invasion is very characteristic as these are biologically aggressive tumors with a high propensity for metastasis, even years after the surgical excision of the primary tumor. Tumors with a predominantly tubular and cribriform component are less aggressive course than those with a solid component >30%. Lymph node spread is rare (except for oral cavity primaries) and metastasis is the most common to the lung.
  - *Acinic cell carcinoma:* Macroscopically, the tumor is not capsulated, but usually well-circumscribed. Its surface is crumbly, fragile, and gray-white colored. It can take on a solid or cystic appearance. It is a malignant epithelial tumor, which presents with some cellular differentiations toward acinar cells. It is considered as a low-grade tumor. These tumors are formed by cells similar to the serous cells of the salivary glands, rounded or polyhedral, arranged in sheets or in acini, with cytoplasm having characteristic of basophilic granulations. Many authors believe that this tumor

originates from the neoplastic transformation of intercalated ductal cell into serous acinar cells. Calcifications may be present.

- *Salivary duct carcinoma:* This is a particularly aggressive malignant tumor similar to intraductal and ductal infiltrating high-grade breast carcinoma. It is usually poorly circumscribed, rapidly infiltrating the adjacent soft tissues with frequent perineural and vascular invasion. Two subtypes are distinguished based on grading: high- and low-grade. It shows a variety of growth patterns, both solid and cystic, ranging from cribriform to solid to micropapillary, which resembles low-grade ductal carcinoma in situ or atypical ductal breast hyperplasia. The tumor cells are monomorphic and ovoid and uniformly spaced with round nuclei and scanty eosinophilic cytoplasm.
- *Carcinoma ex pleomorphic adenoma:* These patients have a typical history of a long-standing pleomorphic adenoma (at least 3 years), with rapid growth in recent months. The risk and rapidity of malignant transformation are proportional to the length of time elapsed and the number of relapses that preceded it. The malignant component is more frequently represented by a poorly differentiated adenocarcinoma (ductal or NOS type) or by an undifferentiated carcinoma. While most carcinoma ex pleomorphic adenoma is now recognized as salivary duct carcinoma, there are also other morphological subtypes including myoepithelial carcinoma and epithelial-myoepithelial carcinoma that are less aggressive. Nuclear polymorphism and hyperchromasia are frequent. The nuclear atypia characterizes the tumor grading and correlates directly with the prognosis. The diagnosis is based on the simultaneous presence of vestiges of the pleomorphic adenoma and more or less differentiated carcinomatous cells. It is a tumor usually poorly circumscribed and, for the most part, largely infiltrating. Three subtypes have been described: (1) noninvasive-intracapsular carcinoma within a pleomorphic adenoma, (2) minimally invasive carcinoma within a pleomorphic adenoma, and (3) highly invasive carcinoma (>1.5 mm infiltration from tumor capsule in to adjacent tissues). Features that determine malignant transformation are areas of necrosis, hemorrhage, calcification, or excessive hyalinization.
- *Mammary analog secretory carcinoma:* This was described for the first time in 2010 and is a salivary glandular neoplasm very similar to the secretory carcinoma of the breast. It is positive for the fusion of the *ETV6-NTRK3* genes [t (12;15) (p13;q25)]. It has an equal sex predilection and commonly occurs in minor salivary sites. It shows a multivacuolated eosinophilic cytoplasm and a papillary cystic architecture. It is periodic acid-Schiff positive with a globular pattern. It is S100 and mammaglobin positive, and DOG1 negative. Despite being typically indolent, it has a 25% of risk of lymph node metastasis.
- *Carcinosarcoma:* This is an extremely rare tumor consisting of a mixture of carcinomatous and sarcomatous elements. The carcinomatous component is usually represented by moderately- or poorly-differentiated ductal carcinoma or undifferentiated carcinoma, while the sarcomatous component consists mainly of chondrosarcoma or osteosarcoma. It often arises in recurrences of polymorphic adenoma, or within a polymorphic adenoma. It is a locally aggressive tumor.
- *Epithelial-myoepithelial carcinoma:* It is a characteristically multinodular lesion, sometimes with cystic spaces, poorly circumscribed, with variously mixed tubular and solid architecture. It is composed of a variable percentage of the two cell types (ductal and myoepithelial-epithelial), which form typical duct-like structures. The biphasic morphology is represented by an inner layer of ductal lining (epithelial-type cells) and an outer layer of clear cells (myoepithelial-type cells). It is a rare epithelial tumor whose atypical myoepithelial cells present an index of high mitotic activity, aggressive growth and frequent vascular and perineural invasion.
- *Oncocytic carcinoma:* It consists of oncocytes (cells with finely granular eosinophilic cytoplasm and round vesicular nucleus, often with prominent nucleoli) and often represents the malignant transformation of its benign counterpart. It is a high-grade, noncapsulated tumor that often infiltrates adjacent soft tissues, lymphatic vessels and nerves. The evaluation of the MIB1 proliferation index to discriminate malignant from benign oncocytoma is useful.
- *Lymphoepithelial carcinoma:* This is an undifferentiated carcinoma accompanied by an abundant non-neoplastic lymphoid infiltrate. It shows a particular racial predilection for the Inuit populations of the Arctic regions, Chinese of Southeast Asia and for the Japanese. In the endemic areas, the association between

EBV and lymphoepithelial carcinoma is almost 100%, a fact that suggests an important role for EBV in the genesis of these tumors. It must be distinguished above all from metastatic undifferentiated carcinoma, in particular from nasopharyngeal carcinoma, from which it is morphologically indistinguishable.
- *Small cell carcinoma:* It is a rare malignant tumor of the salivary glands characterized by a proliferation of small anaplastic cells with poor cytoplasm, finely granular nuclear chromatin, and modest or absent nucleoli. There are usually a high number of mitoses. It is a tumor similar to small cell lung cancer and it is, hence, necessary to exclude a primary lung cancer. It is a poorly circumscribed tumor that often infiltrates the salivary parenchyma and adjacent soft tissues with extensive areas of necrosis and hemorrhage, vascular, and perineural invasion. Most small cell carcinomas express neuroendocrine markers, such as chromogranin A or synaptophysin.

- *Other epithelial lesions*
  - *Sclerosing polycystic adenosis:* It is an inflammatory and reactive slow-growing lesion characterized by fibrocystic changes and adenosis of the salivary glands, especially the parotid. It is well-defined and nonencapsulated. The main feature of this lesion is focal cystic spaces within fibrotic stoma.
  - *Intercalated duct hyperplasia:* It is a proliferation of intercalated tubules of the intercalated duct caliber. It presents as nonencapsulated expanded proliferations that preserve the lobular architecture of the acinar duct unit.
  - *Nodular oncocytic hyperplasia:* It presents in most cases as a lesion of the parotid gland and has a peak in the fifth–sixth decade of life. It is formed by multiple nonencapsulated solid to tubulotrabecular nodules of oncocytes.
  - *Lymphoepithelial lesions:* These are characterized by metaplastic ducts infiltrated by lymphocytes. Malignant transformation usually affects the lymphoid component, resulting in mucosa-associated lymphoid tissue (MALT) lymphoma.
- *Soft tissue lesions*
  - *Hemangioma:* This is the most common nonepithelial tumor with an incidence of 30% in the major salivary glands. It is the most common parotid tumor in infancy. It is a vascular lesion occurring due to an abnormal proliferation of endothelial cells. It consists of both vascular proliferation and the salivary gland structures with entrapped ducts and effaced acini amid proliferating thin-walled endothelium-lined cavernous type of blood vessels.
  - *Nodular fasciitis:* It has a peak in the third–fourth decade of life and it is usually characterized by rapid growth. It consists of a well-defined but focally permeable myofibroblastic proliferation, with little cellular atypia. It is positive for *USP6* gene fusion. The cells can be spindles or stellate-like.

STAGING

The American Joint Committee on Cancer 8th edition/Union for International Cancer Control staging for salivary gland cancers is as described in **Table 5**. Like oral cancer, it has incorporated extranodal extension (ENE) into the newest edition of the staging system.

OUTCOMES

The 5-year survival of salivary gland cancers is highly variable, dependent on histology, stage, grading, lymph node metastases, and performance status. Arguably, histology is the single most prognostic determinant; high-grade tumors such as salivary duct carcinomas are

Table 5: The American Joint Committee on Cancer (AJCC), 8th edition/the Union for International Cancer Control (UICC) staging for salivary gland cancers.

AJCC 8th edition/UICC staging for salivary gland cancer	
T1	Tumor ≤2 cm in the greatest dimension without extraparenchymal extension
T2	Tumor >2 cm but ≤4 cm in greatest dimension without extraparenchymal extension
T3	Tumor >4 cm or tumor having extraparenchymal extension
T4a	Moderately advanced local disease: skin, mandible, ear canal and/or facial nerve
T4b	*Very advanced local disease*: Skull base and/or pterygoid plates and/or encasing common carotid artery
N1	Metastases to single lymph node, 3 cm or less in the greatest diameter
N2a	Metastases to single ipsilateral node 3–6 cm in size or metastases to a single lymph node <3 cm in size with ENE
N2b	Metastases to multiple ipsilateral node 3–6 cm in size
N2c	Metastases to bilateral nodes 3–6 cm in size
N3a	Metastases to nodes >6 cm in size without ENE
N3b	Metastases to any node >3 cm in size with ENE
M0	No metastases
M1	Metastatic disease

(ENE: extranodal extension)

Table 6: 5-year overall survival of salivary gland cancers based on histology.

Histology	*5-year overall survival*
Polymorphous adenocarcinoma	90–100%
Acinic cell carcinoma	75–96%
Low-grade mucoepidermoid carcinoma	75–100%
Intermediate grade mucoepidermoid carcinoma	70–95%
High-grade mucoepidermoid carcinoma	22–51%
Adenoid cystic carcinoma	35–92%
Salivary duct carcinoma	20–35%
Carcinoma ex pleomorphic adenoma	30–96%
Myoepithelial carcinoma	67%
Squamous cell carcinoma	25–30%
Sebaceous carcinoma	62%
Lymphoepithelial carcinoma	75–86%

associated with a short disease-free interval and a high propensity for distant metastases, while ACC has a high propensity for local recurrence and distant metastases which can occur over a decade after treatment. **Table 6** shows the reported 5-year survival in salivary gland cancers related to tumor histology.[65-78]

TREATMENT PRINCIPLES

As per the National Comprehensive Cancer Network guidelines, early stage disease (I/II) is usually sufficiently treated with single modality treatment while advanced stage disease (III/IV) requires multimodality treatment.[79]

For T1–2 disease, surgery is the first choice of treatment, with adjuvant radiotherapy reserved for situations such as:
- Low-grade tumor with suspected spillage
- Gross perineural invasion
- High-grade tumors
- ACC

For T3/T4a disease, surgery is also the choice of treatment with indications for adjuvant radiotherapy being:
- Intermediate or high-grade tumor
- Positive margins
- Perineural invasion
- >1 node involvement
- Lymphovascular invasion
- Extranodal extension

For T4b (unresectable disease), treatment is dependent on the patient's performance status and likelihood of cure.
- Curative intent radiotherapy or concurrent chemoradiotherapy offers the best chance of cure.
- Palliative radiotherapy offers locoregional control and symptom relief without survival benefit.
- Best supportive care is used when the patient is unlikely to withstand any therapy and has a very low life expectancy.

For N0 disease, selective neck dissection is indicated in:
- High-grade tumors
- Advanced disease (T3/4)
- High-risk angioinvasive subtype

In cases with a low likelihood of occult nodal spread, if the primary tumor requires adjuvant radiotherapy, elective neck irradiation is a reasonable approach with limited morbidity.

For N+ disease, selective or comprehensive neck dissection is indicated, based on the nodal burden. Adjuvant radiotherapy is indicated for patients having >1 node positive. In selected high-risk patients, adjuvant concurrent chemoradiotherapy may be considered:
- High-grade histology
- Positive margins
- Perineural invasion
- Extranodal extension
- Lymphovascular invasion

In these patients, the role of concurrent chemotherapy is to increase locoregional control, but there is a paucity of evidence that shows that addition of chemotherapy to adjuvant radiotherapy offers a discernable improvement in survival. Often these decisions need to be made in a multidisciplinary tumor board setting.

SURGICAL CONSIDERATIONS

Both benign and malignant tumors can often be approached with the similar techniques and surgical strategies; in all cases a resection is recommended that involves the removal of the tumor with an adequate margin of healthy tissue surrounding it. In any case, the tumor site, extent and the histology influence the treatment plan.[79-81]

Parotid Gland

With regard to the malignant tumors of the parotid gland, at any stage and low grade, a superficial or total parotidectomy with preservation of the facial nerve is indicated; in high-grade or deep tumors a total parotidectomy with preservation of the facial nerve is indicated. Usually, for benign tumors, a complete or partial superficial parotidectomy or an extracapsular dissection is chosen. The main objective is the preservation of the facial nerve and its branches, except in cases where it is infiltrated with consequent preoperative facial paralysis or if the dissection attempts to preserve the

Table 7: Comparison of parotid surgical techniques and complication risk.

Surgery	*Transient facial nerve dysfunction**	*Permanent facial nerve dysfunction*	*Frey's syndrome*	*Salivary fistula*	*Bleeding*
Enucleation	0–11%	0–3.5%	0%	–	–
Extracapsular dissection	3.9–16%	0–8%	0–16%	0.3–<10%	0.8–3.5%
Partial superficial parotidectomy	1.9–56.3%	0–10%	2.2–32.3%	0–13.8%	0.7–6.3%
Superficial parotidectomy	8–45%	0–44.4%	5.3–54.5%	0–9.9%	3.8–16%
Total parotidectomy	0–64.6%	0–10%	8–69.7%	<1–10%	1.7–13%

Key: *: 6–8 months

nerve leads to tumor spills and grossly positive margins. The different surgical approaches are mentioned below **(Table 7)**.

- *Enucleation:* Simple removal of a circumscribed, encapsulated, and easily clearable formation from the surrounding tissues, interrupting the capsule and its content removed in block or by piecemeal resection, thus leaving residual tumor tissue, without the simultaneous removal of perilesional cuff of healthy parotid gland tissue. The dissection of the facial nerve is not required. Recurrences after simple enucleation are frequent (20–40%) and require the use of radiotherapy to reduce the risk of local recurrence. Enucleation was widely used in the past since the first described by Senn[82] in but for the aforementioned reasons, this technique is no longer recommended.[83,84]
- *Extracapsular dissection:* It corresponds to a partial exeresis of the preneural portion of the parotid gland due to a clinically benign, superficial, hardly clearable formation, of a size not exceeding 2.5–4 cm without pseudocapsule rupture if it is a pleomorphic adenoma. It is performed by contextually removing a cuff of perilesional healthy parotid tissue, remaining in the compartment of loose areolar tissue at least 2–3 mm from the tumor.[85]
- *Superficial parotidectomy:* It consists of the removal of the superficial lobe of the parotid gland and the whole parenchyma superficial to the facial nerve; it is the common choice for low- and intermediate-grade malignant tumors located in the superficial lobe, which do not involve the facial nerve, in addition to benign tumors of diameter more than 3–4 cm. It can be performed through two modalities of facial nerve dissection:[86-91]
  - *Retrograde:* This starts from one of the peripheral branches and following their course backward until the main bifurcation of the facial nerve and the common trunk. The Stensen's duct is identified, at the level of the anterior border of the gland, as landmarks for the search of the buccal branch of the facial nerve that is located superficially to the duct. The retromandibular vein is used as a landmark for the identification of the marginal mandibular branch of the facial nerve and the zygomatic arch for the zygomatic branch of the facial nerve. Once reaching the bifurcation and the common trunk of the facial nerve, the gland is removed starting from its posterior margin.
  - *Anterograde:* This is a more widely used technique and comprises dissection of the flap below the superficial musculoaponeurotic system superficial to the parotid capsule, identification of the greater auricular nerve and sternocleidomastoid, tragal pointer and posterior belly of digastric in order to locate the facial nerve trunk, which is then dissected bluntly from proximal to distal, removing the parotid tissue superficial to the nerve.
- *Partial superficial parotidectomy:* It consists in the same approach of superficial parotidectomy with removal of the tumor with only a surrounding cuff of noninvolved glandular parenchyma (aims for a 1-cm circumferential margin); the remaining portion of superficial parotid gland is preserved. It is especially indicated for benign mobile tumors <3–4 cm located in the superficial lobe or at the level of the tail of the parotid. It requires the dissection of the only branches of the facial nerve next to the neoplasm.[92-94] **Figures 1A to D** show a partial superficial parotidectomy for a malignant neoplasm.
- *Total parotidectomy:* It consists of the total removal of the parotid parenchyma (superficial and deep to the facial nerve). Total parotidectomy is indicated in cases of tumors involving the deep lobe, even without involvement of the facial nerve, high-grade malignant tumors with high risk of metastasis, malignant tumors with the presence of intraparenchymal or

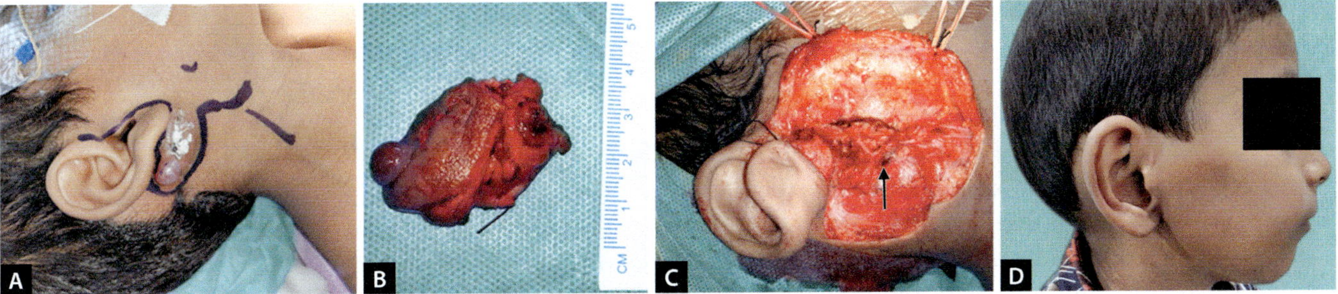

Figs. 1A to D: (A) Recurrent high-grade mucoepidermoid carcinoma parotid in a 5-year-old child with skin involvement; (B) Resected tumor specimen; (C) Intact facial nerve showing typical anatomy in children (arrow); (D) Follow-up at 18 months.

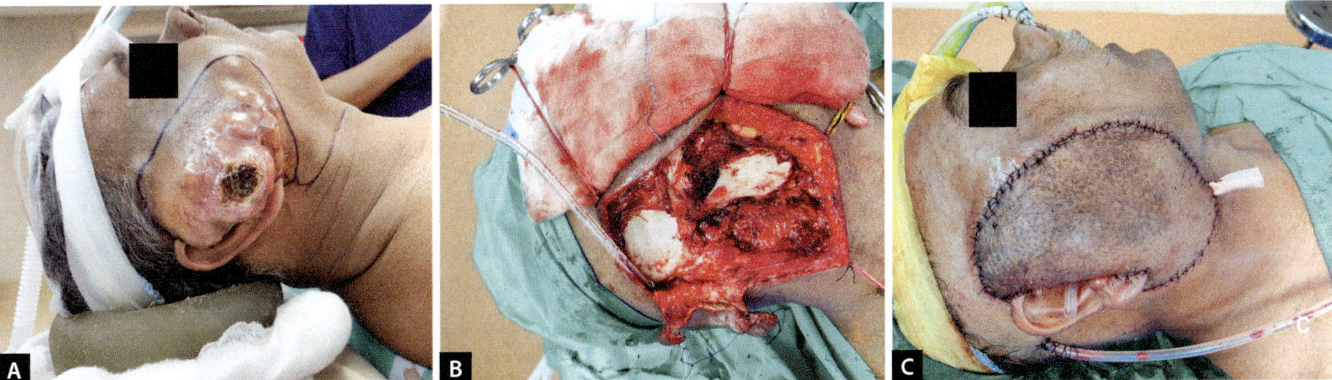

Figs. 2A to C: Re-recurrent pleomorphic adenoma following spillage during surgery. (A) Clinical image; (B) Defect postradical parotidectomy; (C) Defect reconstructed with fasciocutaneous anterolateral thigh flap.

nodal metastases (N+), and patients having macroscopically positive margins after superficial parotidectomy. It requires the dissection of the facial nerve conducted with the same approach as superficial parotidectomy.[95-97]

- *Radical parotidectomy:* It is a total parotidectomy with sacrifice of the facial nerve and its branches. It has the same indications of the total parotidectomy, with the addition of completely or partially removing of the facial nerve due to macroscopic involvement of it by the tumor. **Figures 2A to C** show a radical parotidectomy for a re-recurrent pleomorphic adenoma.
- *Extensive radical parotidectomy:* Radical parotidectomy extended to at least one of the surrounding structures (skin, mastoid, mandible, temporomandibular joint, masticatory muscles, infratemporal fossa, and petrosal bone).

Parapharyngeal Space Involvement

Tumors located in the parapharyngeal space are quite rare and often due to the absence of precise symptoms, they are diagnosed late and randomly. Pleomorphic adenoma is the most common benign salivary tumor in the parapharyngeal space while ACC is the most common malignant tumor. The surgical approaches to the parapharyngeal space are divided into:[98-100]

- *Transoral:* For a long time reserved to the small-sized neoplasms (<3 cm) of the prestyloid space, it avoids skin incisions with excellent esthetic results but this approach has poor surgical exposure, less neurovascular control and high risk of rupture. Transoral robotic surgery (TORS) also allows direct access with excellent visualization and instrumentation. The disadvantage of using the transoral approach is the necessity to divide the pharyngeal mucosa and the upper constrictor muscle, often causing prolonged postoperative pain. Furthermore, the inability to grasp and handle the tumor capsule safely with blunt instruments during TORS, the working angle and the lack of carotid artery protection mean that there is a high rate of pseudocapsule rupture in pleomorphic adenomas by the robot gripper. Therefore, O'Malley recommended the combined use of TORS and blunt tools or finger dissection for the posterior portion of the tumor leaving a small layer of facial tissue overlying the internal carotid artery.[101,102]

- *Transcervical-transparotid:* Mostly used for the lesions that involve the facial nerve, starting from the deep lobe of the parotid and invading the parapharyngeal space, of diameter <4–5 cm; it can also be used for poststyloid space injuries. This technique consists of the extension in the parotid region of the cervical access, the completion of the superficial parotidectomy and the subsequent access to the deep lobe and the parapharyngeal space. The division of the styloid process, as proposed by Olsen, is useful to increase surgical exposure.[103] Through this access, it is possible to identify and preserve the facial nerve and the cranial nerves IX–XII and the sympathetic chain, carotid arteries, and the internal jugular vein.
- *Transcervical:* It represents the most common surgical approach to remove poststyloid styloid and is characterized by a curvilinear incision at the level of the hyoid bone. The submandibular gland can be maintained and retracted anteriorly or removed. Through an incision of the deep fascia at the submandibular space, the parapharyngeal space is exposed. To increase surgical exposure, the stylohyoid and styloglossus muscles, posterior belly of the digastric muscle, and the stylomandibular ligament can be divided. This approach allows a good view of the parapharyngeal space, cranial nerves, and large vessels. It is generally used for benign tumors with a diameter <4–5 cm which can also be removed by blunt dissection with the fingers (blind finger dissection); although inadequate surgical exposure in case of malignant tumors or very large benign tumors with cranial extension can result in rupture or bleeding.
- *Transcervical-transmandibular:* For more complex cases, malignant tumors or large benign tumors (diameter >4–5 cm), an osteotomy of the mandible is indicated: it can be performed in median or paramedian position, preserving the mental nerve. This technique allows "mandibular swing" and is used mostly for malignant or invasive tumors involving the mucosa of the pharyngeal wall or invasion of the skull base or the masticator space. It often requires tracheostomy and nasogastric tube. Alternatively, a double osteotomy of the mandible can be performed (parasymphysis and condyle) as proposed by Seward[104] thus avoiding a lip incision, mental nerve damage, and an intraoral incision. For those malignant lesions of the parapharyngeal space that involve the skull base or the jugular foramen or with intracranial extension the infratemporal approach combined with the transcervical or transcervical-transparotid approach as required.[105,106]

Submandibular Gland

- Benign and small tumors of the submandibular gland can be treated with complete removal of the gland through a curvilinear lateral cervical incision made approximately two fingers below the angle of the jaw.
- For low-grade early-stage tumors malignant tumors stage I–II, with no clinical and radiographic signs of lymph node involvement and extraglandular extension, the treatment of choice is exclusively surgical based on complete excision of the gland and complete removal of the adjacent soft tissues of the submandibular triangle (IB lymph node level). Weber et al. demonstrated that submandibular neoplasms are managed significantly better when they are treated as a neck dissection rather than a gland removal performed mostly for benign inflammatory processes.[107]
- For high-grade malignant tumors, it is better to include also the II and III nodal level in the dissection, thus removing also the lymph node stations with greater risk of metastatic localization.[108-112]

Sublingual Gland

- Regarding the malignant tumors, for early-stage (I–II) tumors, low-grade, with diameter <2 cm, without clinical and radiographic signs of lymph node involvement and extraglandular extension, the treatment of choice is exclusively surgical based on complete excision of the sublingual gland and the ipsilateral submandibular gland due to the fact that the ductal system is often infiltrated or damaged during surgery.
- For advanced stage (III–IV) tumors with a diameter >2 cm, en-bloc excision of the neoplasm by pull-through is indicated and, if the primary tumor is represented by ACC, it also provides, in most of the cases, the sacrifice of the lingual nerve with frozen section on the distal stump. Through the preoperative CT scan it is possible to define the exact extension of the neoplasm and involvement of the mandibular bone (in case of periosteal involvement, a marginal resection is recommended while in the case of gross bone erosion, a segmental resection of the mandible is mandatory). The lymph node dissection of levels I–III is recommended in case of N0 disease, or a therapeutic neck dissection in case of N+ disease.

The indication for radiotherapy follows the principles expressed for neoplasms of the other salivary glands: stage III–IV, high-grade tumors, with perineural infiltration, positive resection margins, N+, and extranodal disease. In case of locoregional recurrences, if the neoplasm is resectable, a wide resection with the sacrifice of involved structures is required.[113-117]

Neck Dissection

If the Blair incision is extended to the neck, a lymphadenectomy can be easily performed; however, the treatment of the neck in patients with parotid gland cancers is still controversial. The incidence of lymph node metastases from malignant parotid tumors range from 10 to 46%, and the incidence of occult metastases was 2 to 50%.[118,119] Evidence suggests that a therapeutic neck dissection is indicated in all cases of clinically positive nodal disease (N+). Parotid tumors often metastasize to level IIB and therefore the risk of involving the level V is high; hence, a therapeutic neck dissection must also include the VA and VB levels. Another high-risk feature for occult lymph node metastases (especially mucoepidermoid carcinoma and adenocarcinoma, and more rarely for ACC) in addition to a diameter >4 cm is macroscopic extraglandular extension, the tumor type, facial pain, and paralysis; with these conditions neck dissection is mandatory even in patients with a negative neck (N0). Another risk factor is represented by the histology that represents an independent predictor factor for occult cervical lymph node metastases (35% for adenocarcinoma, 35% for high-grade mucoepidermoid carcinoma, 33% for salivary duct carcinoma, 29% for undifferentiated carcinoma, and 17% for mixed malignant carcinoma) with a 33% of risk in T1-2 and 38% in T3-4 patients. Finally, the localization of the primary tumor also represents an independent risk factor for the presence of lymph node metastases, as shown by Terhaard et al. (submandibular gland, parotid gland, oral cavity, and other localizations had a nodal metastasis in 42%, 25%, 9%, and 36%, respectively) **(Table 8)**.[65,66,69,76,120-130]

Table 8: Incidence of cervical lymph node metastases associated with salivary gland tumors based on histology.

Histology	*Incidence of cervical lymph node metastases*
Polymorphous adenocarcinoma	9–15%
Adenocarcinoma	20–25%
Acinic cell carcinoma	1–47%
Low-grade mucoepidermoid carcinoma	3–8%
Intermediate-grade mucoepidermoid carcinoma	20%
High-grade mucoepidermoid carcinoma	50–85%
Adenoid cystic carcinoma	4–38%
Salivary duct carcinoma	43–60%

RADIOTHERAPY

The role of postoperative radiotherapy (PORT) is essentially complementary to the surgery and is used as adjuvant therapy in patients with high-risk factors. Scientific evidence shows that PORT is correlated with improved overall survival and local control especially in patients with high-grade neoplasms. Target RT volumes must be adapted based on the extent of the disease prior to surgery. The clinical target volume (CTV) must be based on the extent of the disease including the parapharyngeal space and the temporal fossa in parotid tumors and the tissues surrounding the gland in the submandibular ones. In case of skin involvement and/or very superficial tumors of the parotid or submandibular gland, a bolus should be given on the scar region. In the case of perineural invasion, frequent in ACC, the field must cover the entire course of the nerve up to the skull base. The common indications for PORT are:[131-133]

- High-risk histology (high-grade adenocarcinoma NOS, salivary duct carcinoma, high-grade mucoepidermoid carcinoma, solid ACC, carcinoma ex pleomorphic adenoma, and other high-grade tumors)
- Advance local disease (T3/T4)
- Margin status (macroscopically positive margins clearly indicated, microscopically positive margins more controversial)
- High-grade tumors (G3/4)
- Perineural invasion
- Extranodal extension
- Capsule rupture (controversial)
- Recurrence (controversial)

For early lesions (T1/T2) with favorable histotype, if tumor resection is macroscopically and microscopically complete there is no indication for complementary treatment with radiotherapy. ACC and salivary ductal carcinoma are generally exceptions because of the high risk of recurrence and perineural diffusion of these tumors; however, even this is controversial and needs to be decided in a multidisciplinary setting in a case-by-case basis. Although tempting to use adjuvant radiotherapy to improve locoregional control, it may counter intuitively preclude future use. In case of incomplete or inadequate resection, PORT is often indicated. For the early stage tumors with clear margins and no risk factors such as PNI or LVI, PORT is unlikely to offer any benefit.

For locally advanced tumors (T3/T4) there is a consensus in literature to consider adjuvant PORT unless there is particular reason not to. In N0 cases where the neck is not being addressed surgically there is a definite role for elective neck irradiation in those histologies with a potential for nodal spread. Elective neck irradiation includes at least ipsilateral levels Ib, II, and III. If adjuvant PORT is being administered for nodal disease after neck dissection, levels I–V should be irradiated. For malignant submandibular gland tumors receiving elective neck irradiation levels I–III are addressed; for bulky tumors or tumors approaching the midline contralateral neck irradiation (either level I or levels I–III) should be considered.

Pleomorphic adenoma represents a peculiar scenario because although it is a benign tumor, PORT may be recommended after surgical clearance of recurrent tumors. Retrospective studies have shown the benefit of PORT in reducing the risk recurrence in these patients.

In a setting of adjuvant PORT for patients who have undergone a curative intent resection with clear margins, CTV should receive 60 Gy. The operated field should receive at least 60 Gy while the adjacent undissected regions with a risk of relapse are to receive 54–56 Gy. The undissected N0 neck is to receive 46–50 Gy. In a patient with high-risk features such as gross residual disease, positive margins, extensive nodal disease, and extranodal extension, 66–70 Gy is the indicated dose. When there is extensive perineural invasion, the entire course of the involved nerve needs to be targeted up to the skull base (most often with 56–63 Gy).

Exclusive radiotherapy alone or in combination with chemotherapy is indicated treatment for patients with unresectable neoplasms and those unfit for or refusing surgery (recommended dose 66–70 Gy). A therapeutic option in patients with macroscopic disease not eligible for surgical resection is particle therapy. There are several reports on the results of radical neutron therapy that have shown the possibility of achieving a long-term local control rate between 50 and 80%.

Currently, the most used types of hadron therapy are proton therapy (PT) and carbon ion radiotherapy (CIRT) for the treatment of deep tumors; in fact, the dose-depth profile of these ions is characterized by a low dose in the entry canal and a very high dose (Bragg peak) next to their target.[134-137] In this way and thanks to the electric charge of these particles, it is possible to direct the beam on the target with remarkable precision, saving the healthy tissues and the noble structures of the body. Recent studies have shown satisfactory results in terms of OS in patients suffering from locally advanced parotid tumors, especially ACC, subjected to exclusive therapy with carbon ions (64 Gy in 16 fractions for 4 weeks) in order to avoid dysfunctions to facial nerve: 5-year OS and progression-free survival were 70.1% and 49.2% respectively, with poor performance status and skull base invasion as significant risk factors for OS. Proton therapy can instead be used to save toxicity (mucositis, dysphagia, and weight loss) in selected subpopulations, as demonstrated by a recent retrospective comparison conducted by MD Anderson. Studies on fast neutron-based radiotherapy in patients with salivary gland carcinoma have shown a 5-year locoregional control and OS rates of 57–58% and 51–72%, respectively.[138-140] So far, hadron therapy, especially carbon ions radiotherapy, is indicated for unresectable neoplasms or in patients who are not candidates for surgery or as adjuvant therapy, especially in cases of tumor residue R1 or R2; in fact, for tumors considered radio-resistant, such as salivary gland tumors like ACC, the treatment with carbon ions seems to be more advantageous in terms of better dose of energy distribution, compared to photons and neutrons radiotherapy, which have more late toxicity.

CHEMOTHERAPY AND TARGETED THERAPY

Although most patients with salivary gland cancer have a potentially curable disease at the time of presentation, a significant percentage of patients will experience recurrent or metastatic disease, particularly those with stage III/IV disease. Distant metastases are more common than locoregional recurrence and the most frequent sites are lung, bone, and liver. Metastases in low-grade tumors are rare, while ACC (solid type), salivary duct carcinoma, high-grade mucoepidermoid carcinoma, adenocarcinoma and carcinoma ex pleomorphic adenoma are not uncommon. Advanced stage, close or involved margins, vascular invasion, and histological grade represent risk factors predictive of distant metastases. In case of isolated lung metastases, metastasectomy may be considered, particularly in ACC. Surgery for lung metastases can be considered in oligometastatic lesions, minimal or no pleural involvement and reasonable disease-free interval.[141-143]

The addition of chemotherapy to radiotherapy remains controversial and is generally prescribed for palliative treatment of symptomatic relapsed disease (which is not resectable due to extent of disease or patient factors).[144] There are no National Comprehensive Cancer Network recommendations about specific chemotherapy regimens and so far there are no randomized trials determining standard of care. Conventional chemotherapy with cisplatin and 5-fluorouracil or cisplatin, doxorubicin, and cyclophosphamide are used as a first-line of treatment. However, no chemotherapy regimens have been shown to reliably prolong or improve overall or disease-free survival in these tumors; no improvement of survival was observed in patients who had objective responses compared to those who did not.[145-148] This is the study of an ongoing Radiation Therapy Oncology Group (RTOG) trial that is yet to postresults (NCT01220583).

In ACC, chemotherapy should be used for symptomatic cases or those with rapid neoplastic growth. In this setting, chemotherapy may have a palliative in recurrent, progressive, and symptomatic ACC after having considered other therapeutic options such as palliative radiotherapy, metastasectomy of solitary lesions or embolization/radiofrequency ablation of liver lesions. First-line therapy should be dictated by patient characteristics and comorbidities, toxicity problems, patient costs and preferences. Two options can be identified as first-line therapies: chemotherapy with a single drug and combined chemotherapy. For single drug chemotherapy, mitoxantrone alone and vinorelbine or epirubicin (anthracycline) are reasonable options based on prospective clinical trial data that showed good objective responses in addition to stabilizing the disease and maintaining a profile of favorable toxicity; neither paclitaxel nor cisplatin is recommended due to the lack of proven activity for paclitaxel and the availability of less toxic choices for cisplatin. In a setting of polychemotherapy, cisplatin, anthracycline, 5-fluorouracil, cyclophosphamide, vincristine, and bleomycin are active and safe agents. A combination of cisplatin and anthracycline is the most used combination in clinical practice although unfortunately the results obtained with chemotherapy in ACC are still unsatisfactory. Combination therapy appears to be superior to monotherapy, although the toxicities are consistently higher, emphasizing the importance of applying these therapies only in selected patients with good clinical conditions (performance status of 0–1) and without comorbidity. Monotherapy regimens in ACC achieved a response rate of 13% with a duration of response of 5–20 months, while the cisplatin, doxorubicin, and cyclophosphamide (CAP regimen) was associated with a response rate of 25% with a duration of response variable from 6 to 77 months.[149]

Most studies have been conducted on ACC and there is limited evidence on other histologies. For mucoepidermoid carcinoma, systemic treatment based on cisplatin is administered more frequently in high-grade disease. For adenocarcinoma NOS and salivary duct carcinoma, regimens that have been used include cisplatin or paclitaxel monotherapy and combinations with vinorelbine or capecitabine (CAP). A meta-analysis by Rizk et al. in a cohort of salivary gland tumors showed that the median survival increased by 2.5 and 4.9 months for platinum and anthracycline-treated patients respectively.[150] It also showed that there was no significant difference in survival between patients treated with cisplatin or carboplatin-based monochemotherapy and polychemotherapy, only increased toxicity in the latter **(Table 9)**.[148,151-156]

Numerous targeted therapies are currently being studied: these therapies target specific tumor receptors and are used in patients with advanced disease. The most investigated targeted therapies are those targeting androgen receptors and receptors with tyrosine kinase activity such as the c-kit, epidermal growth factor receptors (EGFR) 1 and 2 (HER2). Unfortunately, our current knowledge on targeted therapy is mainly based on clinical cases and small cohorts of patients suffering from salivary gland carcinomas. All these receptors can be overexpressed in different types of salivary gland carcinomas. Overexpression of the HER2 protein is more frequent in salivary duct carcinomas (SDC) while EGFR mutations are rarely found (<5%) in salivary gland carcinomas. Unfortunately, 20–25% of carcinomas have a *RAS* mutation (mainly *H-RAS*), which may explain the resistance to this type of therapy.

Salivary glands carcinomas that overexpress HER2 can be treated with the anti-HER2 antibody, trastuzumab. HER2 and EGFR overexpression carcinomas without EGFR/*RAS* mutations could be treated by lapatinib, an anti-HER2/EGFR inhibitor. In EGFR mutated carcinomas (without RAS activation), inhibition could be obtained with gefitinib, while for those overexpressing EGFR (EGFR and RAS-not mutated), anti-EGFR monoclonal

Table 9: Overall response rate of various chemotherapeutic regimens in salivary gland tumors in prospective studies.

Drug	*Overall response rates*	*Median overall survival*
Cisplatin	18%	14 months
Vinorelbine	20%	9 months
Vinorelbine and cisplatin	44%	19 months
Paclitaxel	26%	13 months
Gemcitabine and cisplatin	24%	14 months
Mitoxantrone	6–12%	18 months
Epirubicin	10%	15 months
Gemcitabine	No response	N/A

Table 10: Hormone receptor status in salivary gland carcinomas.

Tumor	*VEGF*	*c-kit*	*HER2*	*EGFR*	*ER*	*PR*	*ADR*
Mucoepidermoid carcinoma	↑	↓↓	↑	↑	↓↓	↓↓	↓↓
Adenocarcinoma	↑	↓↓	↑	↑	↓↓	↓↓	↓↓
Adenoid cystic carcinoma	↑↑↑	↑↑↑	↓↓	↓	↓↓	↓↓	↓↓
Salivary duct carcinoma	↑↑	↓↓	↑↑	↑	↓↓	↓↓	↑↑↑

(ADR: androgen receptor; c-kit: CD-117; EGFR: epidermal growth factor receptor, ER: estrogen receptor; HER2: human epidermal growth factor receptor 2; PR: progesterone receptor; VEGF: vascular endothelial growth factor)

antibody therapy with cetuximab, could be beneficial **(Table 10)**.[131,157,158] Estrogen receptor (ER) tamoxifen and toremifene antagonists and antiandrogen receptor (AR) therapy with bicalutamide may be additional options. Favorable responses to androgenetic deprivation therapy (ADT) have been reported, although it is limited only to tumors that express androgen receptors and almost exclusively for male patients. Antiangiogenic agents have also been evaluated in advanced salivary gland tumors; partial remission was described in a phase I study after three cycles with axitinib, a potent inhibitor of VEGF 1–3 receptors.

PEDIATRIC SALIVARY GLAND TUMORS

About 5% of salivary gland tumors occur in the pediatric population, of which half (40–60%) are malignant. They are mainly localized at the parotid and more common after 10 years of age with a slight female preponderance. Mucoepidermoid carcinoma and acinic cell carcinoma are the most common histologies.[159-162] Rhabdomyosarcoma is common nonepithelial malignancy[163,164] while pleomorphic adenoma and hemangioma are common benign histologies in this population. The main risk factors for the development of salivary gland carcinomas in pediatric patients are the EBV, especially in cases of undifferentiated carcinomas of the Inuit population, and previous radiotherapy to the region. As in adults, CT or MRI is indicated for diagnosis and in younger patients, they may require a sedation or general anesthesia of the patient. MRI is preferable to CT as it avoids radiation exposure.

Most salivary gland tumors that occur in the pediatric patient are low grade and presented at an early stage, therefore survival is better than tumors in adult patients.[164-166] The histological grade and the clinical stage represent the two most critical prognostic factors. As in adults, the gold standard for the treatment of salivary glands neoplasms in the pediatric patient is surgery. Some studies report a risk of facial nerve dysfunction function higher than adult patients, especially for those patients who receive a total parotidectomy. As above mentioned, most salivary gland tumors that occur in the pediatric patient are low grade and presented at an early stage and therefore the incidence of nodal spread or occult metastases is rather low (about 11–17%). The indications to address the neck are the same as in adults, but the surgeon needs to consider lymph node hyperplasia, especially in younger children, which can be mistaken for metastatic disease.

The indications for radiotherapy are the same of the adult patients, although in pediatric patients a higher risk of postradiation therapy complications such as delayed facial growth and facial dysmorphism, dental complications, endocrine dysfunction, cataract, hearing loss, and secondary malignant neoplasms (especially sarcomas, skin, and thyroid neoplasms) must be taken into account.[167] Therefore, it is recommended, when possible, to use intensity modulated radiotherapy or proton beam therapy, limited to the primary area and a long-term follow-up in order to evaluate late side effects and secondary malignant neoplasms. Like adult patients, chemotherapy is usually reserved for cases with unresectable progressive disease, which is not amenable to surgery or radiation therapy.[137]

REFERENCES

1. Barnes L, Eveson JW, Reichart P, Sidransky D. Pathology and Genetics of Head and Neck Tumours. Lyon, France: IARC Press; 2005.
2. Seethala RR, Stenman G. Update from the 4th Edition of the World Health Organization Classification of Head and Neck Tumours: Tumors of the Salivary Gland. Head Neck Pathol. 2017;11(1):55-67.
3. Sowa P, Goroszkiewicz K, Szydelko J, Chechlinska J, Pluta K, Domka W, et al. A Review of Selected Factors of Salivary Gland Tumour Formation and Malignant Transformation. Biomed Res Int. 2018;2018:2897827.
4. Eveson JW, Cawson RA. Salivary gland tumors. A review of 2410 cases with particular reference to histological types, site, age, and sex distribution. J Pathol. 1985;146:51-8.
5. Spiro RH. Salivary neoplasms: overview of a 35-year experience with 2,807 patients. Head Neck Surg. 1986;8: 177-84.

6. Califano J, Eisele DW. Benign salivary gland neoplasms. Otolaryngol Clin North Am. 1999;32:861-73.
7. Gaillard J, Gandon J, Laudenbach P, Jezequel J, Beauvillain de Montreuil C, Fontanel JP, et al. Pathologie médicale et chirurgicale de la région parotidienne. Société française d'ORL et pathologie cervicofaciale. Paris: Arnette; 1981. p. 261.
8. Koul R, Dubey A, Butler J Cooke AL, Abdoh A, Nason R. Prognostic factors depicting disease specific survival in parotid-gland tumors. Int J Radiat Oncol Biol Phys. 2007; 68:714-8.
9. Bron LP, Traynor SJ, McNeil EB, O'Brien CJ. Primary and metastatic cancer of the parotid: comparison of clinical behaviour in 232 cases. Laryngoscope. 2003;113:1070-5.
10. Pinkston JA, Cole P. Incidence rates of salivary gland tumors: results from a population-based study. Otolmyngol Head Neck Surg. 1999;120:834-40.
11. Wahiber P, Anderson H, Biorldund A, Möller T, Perfekt R. Carcinoma of the parotid and submandibular glands—a study of survival in 2465 patients. Oral Oncol. 2002;38:706-13.
12. Guzzo M, Ferrari A, Marcon I, Collini P, Gandola L, Pizzi N, et al. Salivary gland neoplasms in children: the experience of the Istituto Nazionale Tumori of Milan. Pediatr Blood Cancer. 2006;47(6):806-10.
13. Luna MA, Batsakis JG, el-Naggar AK. Salivary gland tumors in children. Ann Otol Rhinol Laryngol. 1991;100(10):869-71.
13a. Skolnik EM, Friedman M, Becker S, Sisson GA, Keyes GR. Tumors of the major salivary glands. Laryngoscope. 1977; 87:843-51.
14. Woods Je, Chong GC, Beahrs OJ. Experience with 1,360 primary parotid tumors. Amer J Surg. 1975;130:460-2.
15. Mehta D, Willging JP. Pediatric salivary gland lesions. Semin Pediatr Surg. 2006;15(2):76-84.
16. Shapiro NL, Bhattacharyya N. Clinical characteristics and survival for major salivary gland malignancies in children. Otolaryngol Head Neck Surg. 2006;134(4):631-4.
17. Lennon P, Silvera VM, Perez-Atayde A, Cunningham MJ, Rahbar R. Salivary gland tumors in children: a retrospective clinical review. Pediatr Hematol Oncol. 2014;31(8):681-6.
18. Anantharajan N, Ravindranathan N, Rajadurai P. Lympho-epithelial carcinoma of the parotid gland, a very unusual tumor: a case report and review. Ear Nose Throat J. 2013; 92(9):E7-E9.
19. Saku T, Hayashi Y, Takahara O, Matsuura H, Tokunaga M, Tokunaga M, et al. Salivary tumors among atom bomb survivors, 1950-1987. Cancer. 1997;79(8):1465-775.
20. Chung YK, Khoo ML, Heng MK, Hong GS, Soo KC. Epidemiology of Warthin's tumour of the parotid gland in an Asian population. Br J Surg. 1999;86:661-4.
21. Lamelas J, Terry JH, Alfonso AE. Warthin's tumor: Multi-centricity and increasing incidence in women. Am J Surg. 1987;154:347-51.
22. Thibault F, Halimi P, Bely N, Chevallier JM, Bonfils P, Lellouch-Tubiana A, et al. Internal architecture of the parotid gland at MR imaging: facial nerve or ductal system? Radiology. 1993;188:701-5.
23. Ji YD, Donoff RB, Peacock ZS, Carlson ER. Surgical Landmarks to Locating the Main Trunk of the Facial Nerve in Parotid Surgery: A Systematic Review. J Oral Maxillofac Surg. 2018; 76(2):438-43.
24. Witt RL, Weinstein GS, Rejto LK. Tympanomastoid suture and digastric muscle in cadaver and live parotidectomy. Laryngoscope. 2005;115(4):574-7.
25. Rea PM, McGarry G, Shaw-Dunn J. The precision of four commonly used surgical landmarks for locating the facial nerve in anterograde parotidectomy in humans. Ann Anat. 2010;192(1):27-32.
26. Greyling LM, Glanvill R, Boon JM, Schabort D, Meiring JH, Pretorius JP, et al. Bony landmarks as an aid for intra-operative facial nerve identification. Clin Anat. 2007;20:739.
27. Cannon CR, Replogle WH, Schenk MP. Facial nerve in parotidectomy: a topographical analysis. Laryngoscope. 2004;114:2034.
28. Toure S, Vacher C, Bertrand JC. Étude anatomique du rameau marginal. de la mandibule du nerf facial. Rev Stomatol Chir Maxillofac. 2004;105(3):149-52.
29. Correia Pde C, Zani R. Surgical anatomy of the facial nerve as related to ancillary operations in rhytidoplasty. Plast Reconstr Surg. 1973;52(5):549-52.
30. May M. The facial nerve. Stuttgart: Thieme Thieme Medical Publishers; 1986.
31. Davis RA, Anson BJ, Budinger JM, Kurth LR. Surgical anatomy of the facial nerve and parotid gland based upon a study of 350 cervicofacial halves. Surg Gynecol Obstet. 1956;102(4): 385-412.
32. Lobo R, Hawk J, Srinivasan A. A Review of Salivary Gland Malignancies: Common Histologic Types, Anatomic Considerations, and Imaging Strategies. Neuroimaging Clin North Am. 2018;28(2):171-82.
33. Bialek EJ, Jakubowski W, Zajkowski P, Szopinski KT, Osmolski A. US of the major salivary glands: anatomy and spatial relationships, pathologic conditions, and pitfalls. Radiographics. 2006;26(3):745-63.
34. Scholbach T, Scholbach J, Krombach GA, Gagel B. New method of dynamic color Doppler signal quantification in metastatic lymph nodes compared to direct polarographic measurements of tissue oxygenation. Int J Cancer. 2005; 114(6):957-62.
35. Zengel P, Schrotzlmair F, Reichel C, Paprottka P, Clevert DA. Sonography: the leading diagnostic tool for diseases of the salivary glands. Semin Ultrasound CT MR. 2013;34(3): 196-203.
36. Razek AA, Tawfik AM, Elsorogy LG, Soliman NY. Perfusion CT of head and neck cancer. Eur J Radiol. 2014;83(3):537-44.
37. Atkinson C, Fuller J 3rd, Huang B. Cross-Sectional Imaging Techniques and Normal Anatomy of the Salivary Glands. Neuroimaging Clin North Am. 2018;28(2):137-58.
38. Christe A, Waldherr C, Hallett R, Zbaeren P, Thoeny H. MR imaging of parotid tumors: typical lesion characteristics in MR imaging improve discrimination between benign and malignant disease. Am J Neuroradiol. 2011;32:1202-7.
39. Abdel Razek AAK, Mukherji SK. State-of-the-Art Imaging of Salivary Gland Tumors. Neuroimaging Clin N Am. 2018; 28(2):303-17.
40. King A, Yeung D, Ahuja A, Tse GMK. Salivary gland tumors at in vivo proton MR spectroscopy. Radiology. 2005;237:563-9.
41. Kessler AT, Bhatt AA. Review of the Major and Minor Salivary Glands, Part 2: Neoplasms and Tumor-like Lesions. J Clin Imaging Sci. 2018;8:48.
42. Bussu F, Parrilla C, Rizzo D, Almadori G, Paludetti G, Galli J. Clinical approach and treatment of benign and malignant parotid masses, personal experience. Acta Otorhinolaryngol Ital. 2011;31(3):135-43.
42a. Sood S, McGurk M, Vaz F. Management of salivary gland tumours: United Kingdom national multidisciplinary guide-lines. J Laryngol Otol. 2016;130(S2):S142-S149.

43. Colella G, Cannavale R, Flamminio F, Foschini MP. Fine-needle aspiration cytology of salivary gland lesions: A systematic review. J Oral Maxillofac Surg. 2010;68:2146-53.
44. Baloch ZW, Faquin WC, Layfield LJ. Is it time to develop a tiered classification scheme for salivary gland fine-needle aspiration specimens? Diagn Cytopathol. 2017;45:285-6.
45. Rajendra Santosh AB, Bakki SR, Manthapuri S. A review of research on cytological approach in salivary gland masses. Indian J Dent Res. 2018;29(1):93-106.
46. Schmidt RL, Hall BJ, Wilson AR, Layfield LJ. A systematic review and meta-analysis of the diagnostic accuracy of fine-needle aspiration cytology for parotid gland lesions. Am J Clin Pathol. 2011;136(1):45-59.
47. Yousem DM, Sack MJ, Scanlan KA. Biopsy of parapharyngeal space lesions. Radiology. 1994;193(3):619-22.
48. Seifert G, Langrock I, Donath K. A pathological classification of pleomorphic adenoma of the salivary glands (author's transl). Hno. 1976;24(12):415-26.
49. Alshagroud R, Kamoh A, Popat SR, Brandwein-Weber M, Aguirre A. Metastasizing pleomorphic adenoma case report and review of the literature. Head Neck Pathol. 2017;11(4):487-93.
50. Ponniah I, Suresh Kumar P, Karunakaran K, Shankar KA, Kumaran MG, Preeti LN. Hemangioma in minor salivary glands: real or illusion. Diagn Pathol. 2006;1(1):21.
51. Monoo K, Sageshima M, Ito E, Nishihira S, Ishikawa K. Histopathological grading and clinical features of patients with mucoepidermoid carcinoma of the salivary glands. Nippon Jibiinkoka Gakkai Kaiho. 2003;106(3):192-8.
52. Goode RK, Auclair PL, Ellis GL. Mucoepidermoid carcinoma of the major salivary glands: clinical and histopathologic analysis of 234 cases with evaluation of grading criteria. Cancer: Interdiscipl Int J Am Cancer Soc. 1998;82(7):1217-24.
53. Szanto PA, Luna MA, Tortoledo ME, White RA. Histologic grading of adenoid cystic carcinoma of the salivary glands. Cancer. 1984;54(6):1062-9.
54. Ito K, Tsukuda M, Kawabe R, Nakagawa C, Matsushita K, Kubota A, et al. Benign and malignant oncocytoma of the salivary glands with an immunohistochemical evaluation of Ki-67. ORL. 2000;62(6):338-41.
55. Savera AT, Sloman A, Huvos AG, Klimstra DS. Myoepithelial carcinoma of the salivary glands: a clinicopathologic study of 25 patients. Am J Surg Pathol. 2000;24(6):761-74.
56. Katabi N, Gomez D, Klimstra DS, Carlson DL, Lee N, Ghossein R. Prognostic factors of recurrence in salivary carcinoma ex pleomorphic adenoma, with emphasis on the carcinoma histologic subtype: a clinicopathologic study of 43 cases. Hum Pathol. 2010;41(7):927-34.
57. Di Palma S. Carcinoma ex pleomorphic adenoma, with particular emphasis on early lesions. Head Neck Pathol. 2013;7(1):68-76.
58. Leung SY, Chung LP, Yuen ST, Ho CM, Wong MP, Chan SY. Lymphoepithelial carcinoma of the salivary gland: in situ detection of Epstein-Barr virus. J Clin Pathol. 1995; 48(11):1022-7.
59. Andersson MK, Stenman G. The landscape of gene fusions and somatic mutations in salivary gland neoplasms-Implications for diagnosis and therapy. Oral Oncol. 2016; 57:63-9.
60. Andreasen S, Kiss K, Mikkelsen LH, Channir HI, Plaschke CC, Melchior LC, et al. An update on head and neck cancer: new entities and their histopathology, molecular background, treatment, and outcome. Apmis. 2019;127(5):240-64.
61. Badlani J, Gupta R, Balasubramanian D, Smith J, Luk P, Clark J. Primary salivary gland malignancies: a review of clinicopathological evolution, molecular mechanisms and management. ANZ J Surg. 2018;88(3):152-7.
62. Weinreb I, Zhang L, Tirunagari LM, Sung YS, Chen CL, Perez-Ordonez B, et al. Novel *PRKD* gene rearrangements and variant fusions in cribriform adenocarcinoma of salivary gland origin. Genes Chromosomes Cancer. 2014;53(10):845-56.
63. Skálová A, Vanecek T, Sima R, Laco J, Weinreb I, Perez-Ordonez B, et al. Mammary analogue secretory carcinoma of salivary glands, containing the *ETV6-NTRK3* fusion gene: a hitherto undescribed salivary gland tumor entity. Am J Surg Pathol. 2010;34(5):599-608.
64. Persson M, Andrén Y, Mark J, Horlings HM, Persson F, Stenman G. Recurrent fusion of MYB and NFIB transcription factor genes in carcinomas of the breast and head and neck. Proceed Nat Acad Sci. 2009;106(44):18740-4.
65. Castle JT, Thompson LD, Frommelt RA, Wenig BM, Kessler HP. Polymorphous low grade adenocarcinoma: a clinicopathologic study of 164 cases. Cancer: Interdiscipl Int J Am Cancer Soc. 1999;86(2):207-19.
66. Evans HL, Luna MA. Polymorphous low-grade adenocarcinoma: a study of 40 cases with long-term follow up and an evaluation of the importance of papillary areas. Am J Surg Pathol. 2000;24(10):1319-28.
67. Hickman RE, Cawson RA, Duffy SW. The prognosis of specific types of salivary gland tumors. Cancer. 1984;54(8):1620-4.
68. Witt RL. Major salivary gland cancer. Surg Oncol Clin North Am. 2004;13(1):113-27.
69. Guzzo M, Andreola S, Sirizzotti G, Cantu G. Mucoepidermoid carcinoma of the salivary glands: clinicopathologic review of 108 patients treated at the National Cancer Institute of Milan. Ann Surg Oncol. 2002;9(7):688-95.
70. Clode AL, Fonseca I, Santos JR, Soares J. Mucoepidermoid carcinoma of the salivary glands: a reappraisal of the influence of tumor differentiation on prognosis. J Surg Oncol. 1991;46(2):100-6.
71. Hamper K, Lazar F, Dietel M, Caselitz J, Berger J, Arps H, et al. Prognostic factors for adenoid cystic carcinoma of the head and neck: a retrospective evaluation of 96 cases. J Oral Pathol Med. 1990;19(3):101-7.
72. Perzin KH, Gullane P, Clairmont AC. Adenoid cystic carcinomas arising in salivary glands. A correlation of histologic features and clinical course. Cancer. 1978;42(1):265-82.
73. Guzzo M, Palma SD, Grandi C, Molinari R. Salivary duct carcinoma: clinical characteristics and treatment strategies. Head Neck: J Sci Spec Head Neck. 1997;19(2):126-33.
74. Barnes L, Rao U, Krause J, Contis L, Schwartz A, Scalamogna P. Salivary duct carcinoma: Part I. A clinicopathologic evaluation and DNA image analysis of 13 cases with review of the literature. Oral Surg Oral Med Oral Pathol. 1994;78(1):64-73.
75. Tortoledo ME, Luna MA, Batsakis JG. Carcinomas ex pleomorphic adenoma and malignant mixed tumors: histomorphologic indexes. Arch Otolaryngol. 1984;110(3):172-6.
76. Fonseca I, Soares J. Epithelial-myoepithelial carcinoma of the salivary glands. A study of 22 cases. Virchows Archiv A. 1993;422(5):389-96.
77. Shemen LJ, Huvos AG, Spiro RH. Squamous cell carcinoma of salivary gland origin. Head Neck Surg. 1987;9(4):235-40.
78. Sheen TS, Tsai CC, Ko JY, Chang YL, Hsu MM. Undifferentiated carcinoma of the major salivary glands. Cancer: Interdiscipl Int J Am Cancer Soc. 1997;80(3):357-63.

79. Colevas AD, Yom SS, Pfister DG, Spencer S, Adelstein D, Adkins D, et al. NCCN guidelines insights: head and neck cancers, version 1.2018. J Nat Comp Cancer Network. 2018; 16(5):479-90.
80. Bradley PJ. Pleomorphic salivary adenoma of the parotid gland: which operation to perform? Curr Opin Otolaryngol Head Neck Surg. 2004;12:69-70.
81. Touquet R, Mackenzie IJ, Carruth JA. Management of the parotid pleomorphic adenoma, the problem of exposing tumour tissue at operation. The logical pursuit of treatment policies. Br J Oral Maxillofacial Surg. 1990;28(6):404-8.
82. Senn N. The pathology and surgical treatment of tumors. Philadelphia, PA: WB Saunders; 1900.
83. Anderson R. Benign mixed tumours of the parotid gland. Cancer Head Neck Proc Int Symposium. 1975;37:1555-8.
84. Gleave EN, Whittaker JS, Nicholson A. Salivary tumours—experience over thirty years. Clin Otolaryngol Allied Sci. 1979;4(4):247-57.
85. McGurk M, Thomas BL, Renehan AG. Extracapsular dissection for clinically benign parotid lumps: reduced morbidity without oncological compromise. Br J Cancer. 2003; 89(9):1610-3.
86. Xu ZJ, Chen LS, Zhan JD, Xu MM, Zhang B, Huang SL, et al. Modified rhytidectomy incision and modified Blair incision contrast research in superficial parotid gland tumor resection. J Clin Otorhinolaryngol Head Neck Surg. 2017;31(21):1684-7.
87. Terris DJ, Tuffo KM, Fee WE. Modified facelift incision for parotidectomy. JLaryngol Otol. 1994;108(7):574-8.
88. Stankovic P, Wittlinger J, Timmesfeld N, Stephan SH, Georgiew R, Guenzel T, et al. Antero- vs. retrograde nerve dissection in parotidectomy: a systematic review and meta-analysis. Eur Arch Otorhinolaryngol. 2018;275(6):1623-30.
89. Furusaka T, Tanaka A, Matsuda H, Hasegawa H, Asakawa T, Shigihara S. Cervical branch of the facial nerve approach for retrograde parotidectomy compared with anterograde parotidectomy. Acta Otolaryngol. 2014;134(11):1192-7.
90. Emodi O, El-Naaj IA, Gordin A, Akrish S, Peled M. Superficial parotidectomy versus retrograde partial superficial parotidectomy in treating benign salivary gland tumor (pleomorphic adenoma). J Oral Maxillofacial Surg. 2010; 68(9):2092-8.
91. Zhang SS, Ma DQ, Guo CB, Huang MX, Peng X, Yu GY. Conservation of salivary secretion and facial nerve function in partial superficial parotidectomy. Int J Oral Maxillofacial Surg. 2013;42(7):868-73.
92. Zbären P, Vander Poorten V, Witt RL, Woolgar JA, Shaha AR, Triantafyllou A, et al. Pleomorphic adenoma of the parotid: formal parotidectomy or limited surgery. Am J Surg. 2013; 205(1):109-18.
93. Li C, Xu Y, Zhang C, Sun C, Chen Y, Zhao H, et al. Modified partial superficial parotidectomy versus conventional superficial parotidectomy improves treatment of pleomorphic adenoma of the parotid gland. Am J Surg. 2014;208(1): 112-8.
94. Larian B. Parotidectomy for benign parotid tumors. Otolaryngol Clin North Am. 2016;49(2):395-413.
95. Blair VP. Surgery and Diseases of the Mouth and Jaws. St. Louis: CV Mosby; 1917.
96. Casani AP, Cerchiai N, Dallan I, Seccia V, Sellari Franceschini S. Benign tumours affecting the deep lobe of the parotid gland: how to select the optimal surgical approach. Acta Otorhinolaryngol Ital. 2015;35:80-7.
97. Johnson JT, Ferlito A, Fagan JJ, Bradley PJ, Rinaldo A. Role of limited parotidectomy in management of pleomorphic adenoma. J Laryngol Otol. 2007;121(12):1126-8.
98. Riffat F, Dwivedi RC, Palme C, Fish B, Jani P. A systematic review of 1143 parapharyngeal space tumors reported over 20 years. Oral Oncol. 2014;50(5):421-30.
99. Carrau RL, Myers EN, Johnson JT. Management of tumors arising in the parapharyngeal space. Laryngoscope. 1990; 100(6):583-9.
100. Datarkar AN, Deshpande A. Giant parapharyngeal space pleomorphic adenoma of the deep lobe of parotid presenting as obstructive sleep apnoea: a case report and review of the diagnostic and therapeutic approaches. J Maxillofacial Oral Surg. 2015;14(3):532-7.
101. Goodwin Jr WJ, Chandler JR. Transoral excision of lateral parapharyngeal space tumors presenting intraorally. Laryngoscope. 1988;98(3):266-9.
102. O'Malley Jr BW, Quon H, Leonhardt FD, Chalian AA, Weinstein GS. Transoral robotic surgery for parapharyngeal space tumors. ORL. 2010;72(6):332-6.
103. Olsen KD. Tumors and surgery of the parapharyngeal space. Laryngoscope. 1994;104:1-28.
104. Lazaridis N, Antoniades K. Double mandibular osteotomy with coronoidectomy for tumours in the parapharyngeal space. Br J Oral Maxillofacial Surg. 2003;41(3):142-6.
105. Bozza F, Vigili MG, Ruscito P, Marzetti A, Marzetti F. Surgical management of parapharyngeal space tumours: results of 10-year follow-up. Acta Otorhinolaryngologica Italica. 2009;29(1):10.
106. Bradley PJ, Eisele DW. Salivary Gland Neoplasms. Adv Otorhinolaryngol. Basel, Karger. 2016;78:120-31.
107. Weber RS, Byers RM, Petit B, Wolf P, Ang K, Luna M. Submandibular gland tumors: Adverse histologic factors and therapeutic implications. Arch Otolaryngol Head Neck Surg. 1990;116(9):1055-60.
108. Roh JL, Choi SH, Lee SW, Cho KJ, Nam SY, Kim SY. Carcinomas arising in the submandibular gland: high propensity for systemic failure. J Surg Oncol. 2008;97(6):533-7.
109. Storey MR, Garden AS, Morrison WH, Eicher SA, Schechter NR, Ang KK. Postoperative radiotherapy for malignant tumors of the submandibular gland. Int J Radiat Oncol Biol Phys. 2001;51(4):952-8.
110. Lee RJ, Tan AP, Tong EL, Satyadev N, Christensen RE. Epidemiology, prognostic factors, and treatment of malignant submandibular gland tumors: a population-based cohort analysis. JAMA Otolaryngol Head Neck Surg. 2015;141(10):905-12.
111. Huang TT, Chou YF, Wen YH, Chen PR. Resected tumours of the sublingual gland: 15 years' experience. Br J Oral Maxillofacial Surg. 2016;54(6):625-8.
112. Rinaldo A, Ferlito A, Pellitteri PK, Robbins KT, Shaha AR, Bradley PJ, et al. Management of malignant submandibular gland tumors. Acta Otolaryngol. 2003;123(8):896-904.
113. Zdanowski R, Dias FL, Barbosa MM, Lima RA, Faria PA, Loyola AM, et al. Sublingual gland tumors: clinical, pathologic, and therapeutic analysis of 13 patients treated in a single institution. Head Neck. 2011;33(4):476-81.
114. de Brito Santos IR, Kowalski LP, de Araujo VC, Logullo AF, Magrin J. Multivariate analysis of risk factors for neck metastases in surgically treated parotid carcinomas. Arch Otolaryngol Head Neck Surg. 2001;127(1):56-60.
115. Armstrong JG, Harrison LB, Thaler HT, Friedlander-Klar H, Fass DE, Zelefsky MJ, et al. The indications for elective

treatment of the neck in cancer of the major salivary glands. Cancer. 1992;69(3):615-9.
116. Lombardi D, McGurk M, Vander Poorten V, Guzzo M, Accorona R, Rampinelli V, et al. Surgical treatment of salivary malignant tumors. Oral Oncol. 2017;65:102-13.
117. Carlson ER, Schlieve T. Salivary gland malignancies. Oral Maxillofacial Surg Clin. 2019;31(1):125-44.
118. Klussmann JP, Ponert T, Mueller RP, Dienes HP, Guntinas-Lichius O. Patterns of lymph node spread and its influence on outcome in resectable parotid cancer. Eur J Surg Oncol (EJSO). 2008;34(8):932-7.
119. Ali S, Palmer FL, DiLorenzo M, Shah JP, Patel SG, Ganly I. Treatment of the neck in carcinoma of the parotid gland. Ann Surg Oncol. 2014;21(9):3042-8.
120. Yoo SH, Roh JL, Kim SO, Cho KJ, Choi SH, Nam SY, et al. Patterns and treatment of neck metastases in patients with salivary gland cancers. J Surg Oncol. 2015;111(8):1000-6.
121. Lau VH, Aouad R, Farwell DG, Donald PJ, Chen AM. Patterns of nodal involvement for clinically N0 salivary gland carcinoma: refining the role of elective neck irradiation. Head Neck. 2014;36:1435-9.
122. Greig SR, Chaplin JM, McIvor NP, Izzard ME, Taylor G, Wee D. Acinic cell carcinoma of the parotid gland: Auckland experience and literature review. ANZ J Surg. 2008;78(9):754-8.
123. Gomez DR, Katabi N, Zhung J, Wolden SL, Zelefsky MJ, Kraus DH, et al. Clinical and pathologic prognostic features in acinic cell carcinoma of the parotid gland. Cancer. 2009;115(10):2128-37.
124. Hoffman HT, Karnell LH, Funk JF, Robinson RA, Menck HR. National Cancer Data Base report on cancer of the head and neck: acinic cell carcinoma. Head Neck. 1999;21: 297-309.
125. Stennert E, Kisner D, Jungehuelsing M, Guntinas-Lichius O, Schröder U, Eckel HE, et al. High incidence of lymph node metastasis in major salivary gland cancer. Arch Otolaryngol Head Neck Surg. 2003;129(7):720-3.
126. Spiro RH, Huvos AG, Berk R, Strong EW. Mucoepidermoid carcinoma of salivary gland origin: a clinicopathologic study of 367 cases. Am J Surg. 1978;136(4):461-8.
127. Spiro RH, Huvos AG, Strong EW. Adenoid cystic carcinoma of salivary origin: a clinicopathologic study of 242 cases. Am J Surg. 1974;128(4):512-20.
128. Sur RK, Donde B, Levin V, Pacella J, Kotzen J, Cooper K, et al. Adenoid cystic carcinoma of the salivary glands: a review of 10 years. Laryngoscope. 1997;107(9):1276-80.
129. Brandwein MS, Jagirdarmd J, Patil J, Biller H, Kaneko M. Salivary duct carcinoma (cribriform salivary carcinoma of excretory ducts) a clinicopathologic and immunohisto-chemical study of 12 cases. Cancer. 1990;65(10):2307-14.
130. Brandwein-Gensler M, Hille J, Wang BY, Urken M, Gordon R, Wang LJ, et al. Low-grade salivary duct carcinoma: description of 16 cases. Am J Surg Pathol. 2004;28(8):1040-4.
131. Terhaard CH, Lubsen H, Van der Tweel I, Hilgers FJ, Eijkenboom WM, Marres HA, et al. Salivary gland carcinoma: independent prognostic factors for locoregional control, distant metastases, and overall survival: results of the Dutch head and neck oncology cooperative group. Head Neck: J Sci Special Head Neck. 2004;26(8):681-93.
132. Mahmood U, Koshy M, Goloubeva O, Suntharalingam M. Adjuvant radiation therapy for high-grade and/or locally advanced major salivary gland tumors. Arch Otolaryngol Head Neck Surg. 2011;137(10):1025-30.
133. Lewis AG, Tong T, Maghami E. Diagnosis and management of malignant salivary gland tumors of the parotid gland. Otolaryngol Clin North Am. 2016;49(2):343-80.
134. Griffin TW, Pajak TF, Laramore GE, Duncan W, Richter MP, Hendrickson FR, et al. Neutron vs photon irradiation of inoperable salivary gland tumors: results of an RTOG-MRC cooperative randomized study. Int J Radiation Oncol Biol Phys. 1988;15(5):1085-90.
135. Douglas JG, Laramore GE, Austin-Seymour M, Koh WJ, Stelzer K, Griffin TW. Treatment of locally advanced adenoid cystic carcinoma of the head and neck with neutron radiotherapy. Int J Radiation Oncol Biol Phys. 2000;46(3):551-7.
136. Orlandi E, Iacovelli NA, Bonora M, Cavallo A, Fossati P. Salivary gland. Photon beam and particle radiotherapy: present and future. Oral Oncol. 2016;60:146-56.
137. Grant SR, Grosshans DR, Bilton SD, Garcia JA, Amin M, Chambers MS, et al. Proton versus conventional radio-therapy for pediatric salivary gland tumors: acute toxicity and dosimetric characteristics. Radiother Oncol. 2015;116(2): 309-15.
138. Castello A, Olivari L, Lopci E. Adenoid cystic carcinoma: focus on heavy ion therapy and molecular imaging. Am J Nucl Med Mole Imag. 2018;8(1):1.
139. Locati LD, Guzzo M, Bossi P, Massone PP, Conti B, Fumagalli E, et al. Lung metastasectomy in adenoid cystic carcinoma (ACC) of salivary gland. Oral Oncol. 2005;41(9): 890-4.
140. Budd GT, Groppe CW. Adenoid cystic carcinoma of the salivary gland: Sustained complete response to chemotherapy. Cancer. 1983;51(4):589-90.
141. Venook AP, Tseng Jr A, Meyers FJ, Silverberg I, Boles R, Fu KK, et al. Cisplatin, doxorubicin, and 5-fluorouracil chemotherapy for salivary gland malignancies: a pilot study of the Northern California Oncology Group. J Clin Oncol. 1987;5(6):951-5.
142. Dreyfuss AI, Clark JR, Fallon BG, Posner MR, Norris Jr CM, Miller D. Cyclophosphamide, doxorubicin, and cisplatin combination chemotherapy for advanced carcinomas of salivary gland origin. Cancer. 1987;60(12):2869-72.
143. Creagan ET, Woods JE, Rubin J, Schaid DJ. Cisplatin-based chemotherapy for neoplasms arising from salivary glands and contiguous structures in the head and neck. Cancer. 1988;62(11):2313-9.
144. Wang X, Luo Y, Li M, Yan H, Sun M, Fan T. Management of salivary gland carcinomas: a review. Oncotarget. 2017;8(3): 3946.
145. Laurie SA, Ho AL, Fury MG, Sherman E, Pfister DG. Systemic therapy in the management of metastatic or locally recurrent adenoid cystic carcinoma of the salivary glands: a systematic review. Lancet Oncol. 2011;12(8):815-24.
146. Hill ME, Constenla DO, A'hern RP, Henk JM, Rhys-Evans P, Breach N, et al. Cisplatin and 5-fluorouracil for symptom control in advanced salivary adenoid cystic carcinoma. Oral Oncol. 1997;33(4):275-8.
147. Ross PJ, Teoh EM, A'hern RP, Rhys-Evans PH, Harrington KJ, Nutting CM, et al. Epirubicin, cisplatin and protracted venous infusion 5-Fluorouracil chemotherapy for advanced salivary adenoid cystic carcinoma. Clin Oncol. 2009;21(4): 311-4.
148. Gilbert J, Li Y, Pinto HA, Jennings T, Kies MS, Silverman P, et al. Phase II trial of taxol in salivary gland malignancies (E1394): a trial of the Eastern Cooperative Oncology Group. Head Neck: J Sci Spec Head Neck. 2006;28(3):197-204.

149. Airoldi M, Garzaro M, Pedani F, Ostellino O, Succo G, Riva G, et al. Cisplatin + Vinorelbine Treatment of Recurrent or Metastatic Salivary Gland Malignancies (RMSGM). Am J Clin Oncol. 2017;40(1):86-90.
150. Rizk S, Robert A, Vandenhooft A, Airoldi M, Kornek G, Machiels JP. Activity of chemotherapy in the palliative treatment of salivary gland tumors: review of the literature. Eur Arch Otorhinolaryngol. 2007;264(6):587-94.
151. Licitra L, Marchini S, Spinazzè S, Rossi A, Rocca A, Grandi C, et al. Cisplatin in advanced salivary gland carcinoma. A phase II study of 25 patients. Cancer. 1991;68(9):1874-7.
152. Airoldi M, Pedani F, Succo G, Gabriele AM, Ragona R, Marchionatti S, et al. Phase II randomized trial comparing vinorelbine versus vinorelbine plus cisplatin in patients with recurrent salivary gland malignancies. Cancer. 2001; 91(3):541-7.
153. Mattox DE, Von Hoff DD, Balcerzak SP. Southwest Oncology Group study of mitoxantrone for treatment of patients with advanced adenoid cystic carcinoma of the head and neck. Invest New Drugs. 1990;8(1):105-7.
154. Verweij J, De Mulder PH, De Graeff A, Vermorken JB, Wildier J, Kerger J, et al. Phase II study on mitoxantrone in adenoid cystic carcinomas of the head and neck. Ann Oncol. 1996;7(8):867-9.
155. Vermorken JB, Verweij J, De Mulder PH, Cognetti F, Clavel M, Rodenhuis S, et al. Epirubicin in patients with advanced or recurrent adenoid cystic carcinoma of the head and neck: a phase II study of the EORTC Head and Neck Cancer Cooperative Group. Ann Oncol. 1993;4(9): 785-8.
156. van Herpen CM, Locati LD, Buter J, Thomas J, Bogaerts J, Lacombe D, et al. Phase II study on gemcitabine in recurrent and/or metastatic adenoid cystic carcinoma of the head and neck (EORTC 24982)/ . Eur J Cancer. 2008;44: 2542-5.
157. Laurie SA, Licitra L. Systemic therapy in the palliative management of advanced salivary gland cancers. J Clin Oncol. 2006;24(17):2673-8.
158. Sen M, Prestwich R. Chemotherapy and Targeted Therapy. In: Bradley PJ, Eisele DW (Eds). Salivary Gland Neoplasms. Adv Otorhinolaryngol. Basel: Karger Publishers; 2016. pp. 148-56.
159. Bradley PJ, Eisele DW. Salivary gland neoplasms in children and adolescents. In: Bradley PJ, Eisele DW (Eds). Salivary Gland Neoplasms. Basel: Karger Publishers; 2016. pp. 175-81.
160. Ord RA, Carlson ER. Pediatric salivary gland malignancies. Oral Maxillofacial Surg Clin. 2016;28(1):83-9.
161. Verma J, Teh BS, Paulino AC. Characteristics and outcome of radiation and chemotherapy-related mucoepidermoid carcinoma of the salivary glands. Pediatr Blood Cancer. 2011;57(7):1137-41.
162. Loy TS, McLaughlin R, Odom LF, Dehner LP. Mucoepidermoid carcinoma of the parotid as a second malignant neoplasm in children. Cancer. 1989;64(10):2174-7.
163. Sultan I, Rodriguez-Galindo C, Al-Sharabati S, Guzzo M, Casanova M, Ferrari A. Salivary gland carcinomas in children and adolescents: a population-based study, with comparison to adult cases. Head Neck. 2011;33(10):1476-81.
164. Galer C, Santillan AA, Chelius D, Huh W, El-Naggar A, Hanna E, et al. Minor salivary gland malignancies in the pediatric population. Head Neck. 2012;34(11):1648-51.
165. Deng R, Huang X, Hao J, Ding J, Hu Q. Salivary gland neoplasms in children. J Craniofac Surg. 2013;24(2):511-3.
166. Kessler A, Handler SD. Salivary gland neoplasms in children: a 10-year survey at the Children's Hospital of Philadelphia. Int J Pediatr Otorhinolaryngol. 1994;29(3):195-202.
167. Denys D, Kaste SC, Kun LE, Chaudhary MA, Bowman LC, Robbins KT. The effects of radiation on craniofacial skeletal growth: a quantitative study. Int J Pediatr Otorhinolaryngol. 1998;45(1):7-13.

CHAPTER

20

Paragangliomas and Neurogenic Tumors of the Head and Neck

Athira Ramakrishnan, Sivakumar Vidhyadharan, Samskruthi P Murthy, Narayana Subramaniam

INTRODUCTION

Paragangliomas are rare and typically benign tumors of the paraganglia, clusters of neuroendocrine cells that are associated with the peripheral nervous system. Broadly, they can be divided into two categories: (1) adrenal paragangliomas, where they are known as pheochromocytomas and (2) extra-adrenal paragangliomas. Within the extra-adrenal category, 70% can be found within the head and neck, where they are also known as chemodectomas, nonchromaffin tumors, and glomus tumors.[1] Pheochromocytomas and sympathetic paragangliomas are almost clinically active most of the time, while parasympathetic paraganglioma are usually not clinically active, with 1–3% of head and neck paraganglioma showing elevated catecholamines.

The bulk of the paragangliomas of the head and neck originate from the parasympathetic nervous system. In the head and neck, they are described in relation to their site of origin and the adjacent major neurovascular structures **(Fig. 1)**.[2,3] Additionally they have a low likelihood of physiological activity and may have a familial or genetic component to their etiology.

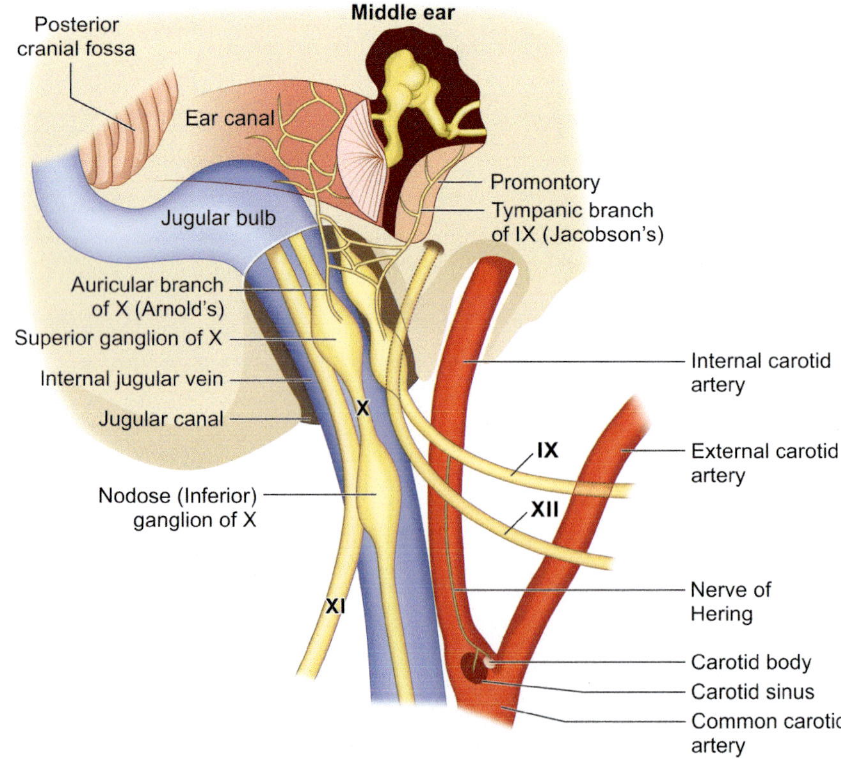

Fig. 1: Common sites of head and neck paragangliomas and relationship to the lower cranial nerves.

Paraganglia refer to a group of cell clusters that are responsible for vasoactive peptides that influence the baroreceptor and chemoreceptor reflexes that maintain blood pressure. Extra-adrenal paragangliomas are either branchiomeric or vagal.[4-6] Carotid body tumors occur at the carotid bifurcation, jugular paragangliomas occur at the jugular bulb, tympanic paragangliomas occur in the middle ear mucosa while vagal and laryngeal paragangliomas occur in the vagus nerve and larynx, respectively.[7] They have a variable rate of growth and often present as an asymptomatic lesion detected on clinical examination or on routine imaging. Rare sites of occurrence are orbital, sinonasal tract, thyroid, nasopharynx, facial skeleton, and cavernous sinus.[8,9] The most common lesions are carotid body tumors and jugular tumors, with vagal paragangliomas accounting for <5%.

EPIDEMIOLOGY AND RISK FACTORS

These are rare tumors, accounting for around 0.5% of all head and neck tumors. The majority of head and neck paragangliomas (HNPG) are benign; however, it is suspected that up to 20% may be malignant due to their unique histology malignancy is diagnosed based on the presence or absence of metastases to nonendocrine tissues.[10,11] Malignancy rates are higher in sporadic lesions than in familial lesions, except in succinate dehydrogenase complex subunit B (SDHB) mutations where over two-thirds of patients develop malignant paragangliomas. Another feature that dictates malignancy risk; about a quarter of orbital and laryngeal paragangliomas are malignant, which is higher than lesions in other sites.[12]

The sex distribution varies; carotid body tumors are more common in men, while vagal paragangliomas are more common in women.[8] The median age at diagnosis is the fifth decade of life, with these lesions very rarely seen in children.[13] As these lesions can be hereditary in up to a quarter of patients, genetic investigation is mandated.[14] The succinate dehydrogenase (SDH) group of genes has been demonstrated to be associated with familial cases of paraganglioma.[15] When familial, a thorough evaluation for multiple tumors is indicated (reported as high as 78–87%). Genetic syndromes such as MEN IIA/B (multiple endocrine neoplasia type IIA and IIB), von Hippel–Lindau syndrome can also be associated with paragangliomas.[15-18]

The only factors seen to predispose to development of paragangliomas is chronic hypoxia resulting from living in high-altitude areas. These have been shown to be distinct from familial cases by a lower risk of bilaterality and no identifiable genetic mutations.[19-23]

GENETIC MUTATIONS

The genes that have been shown to be associated with paragangliomas are SDH subunits D, B, and C. The inheritance of these mutations may be autosomal dominant with development of paragangliomas only when the inheritance is from the father.[6] Patients with SDH mutations are likely to be younger males (<40 years) with a family history, multiple lesions, and a previous pheochromocytoma. Risk of malignancy is low except with SDHB **(Table 1)**.[24]

HISTOLOGY

These tumors have two major components, the chief cells (type I) and the sustentacular cells (type II). The chief cells stain positively for chromogranin, synaptophysin, neuron-specific enolase and other neurofilament stains, while the sustentacular cells are fibrovascular supportive elements that stain positive for S100. Clusters of these two cell types appear as nests of cells, or "Zellballen" on low power microscopy.[25]

CAROTID BODY TUMORS

The carotid body is a chemoreceptor organ made of glomus cells that have the primary function of sensing the chemical make-up of the blood, specifically sampling levels of pH, oxygen, and carbon dioxide. The primary stimulators of the carotid body include acidemia, hypercarbia, and hypoxia. These stimulators result in downstream sympathetic nervous system effects,

Table 1: Familial head and neck paraganglioma syndromes.[2]

Paraganglioma type	*Mutation*	*Risk of multifocality*	*Risk of malignancy*	*Risk of pheochromocytoma*
1	SDHD	High	Low	Intermediate
2	Unknown	Unknown	Unknown	Unknown
3	SDHC	Low	Low	No
4	SDHB	Intermediate	Intermediate	High

(SDHB: succinate dehydrogenase complex subunit B; SDHC: succinate dehydrogenase complex subunit C; SDHD: succinate dehydrogenase complex subunit D)

in turn causing increased heart rate, blood pressure, respiratory rate, and pulmonary tidal volumes. Low partial pressures of oxygen are thought to be the most potent stimulant of the carotid body. Grossly, the carotid body is a small reddish brown-tan ovoid structure only 3–5 mm in diameter. It is located within the adventitia of the common carotid posterior and medially to the carotid bifurcation. Blood supply comes primarily from small feeder blood vessels from the ascending pharyngeal artery, a branch of the external carotid artery. Afferent innervation leaves via Hering's nerve that is a branch of the glossopharyngeal nerve. In regard to the pharyngeal space, carotid body tumors are considered to be the most common tumor of the poststyloid pharyngeal space.

The classical carotid body tumors grow at the bifurcation of the carotid artery and present as a painless, mobile, slow-growing neck mass that may be pulsatile and transmit bruits. If these tumors extend into the parapharyngeal space, they can be associated with cranial nerve palsies (typically X/XII) and can damage the sympathetic chain through further progression. A classic sign of a tumor of the carotid body (known as "Fontaine's sign") is seen when the tumor is palpated and it is laterally mobile but is fixed in the cranial-caudal direction. Less than 10% of these patients present with symptoms related to cranial nerve dysfunction. Given its location within the carotid sheath, the vagus nerve (X) is the most common cranial nerve affected; however, palsies may be routinely seen in cranial nerves IX, X, XI, and XII as well as the sympathetic chain, depending on the size and erosive qualities of the mass. Involvement of these nerves can result in many deficits including hoarseness, dysphagia, shoulder dysfunction, neck, and tongue weakness.[25-27]

Shamblin Classification

The Shamblin classification system was initially developed based on intraoperative findings in order to help predict postoperative morbidity in carotid body tumors. The classification was then subsequently extrapolated to imaging findings to determine operative course and morbidity.

- *Type I:* The least invasive tumor type which correlates to splaying the main carotid branches but not encasing them. These tumors are minimally attached to blood vessels and are removed by complete resection with minimal risk to the patient.
- *Type II:* More adherent to the vessels and partially encasing the external and internal carotids. Resection of these lesions carries higher risk of complication but is still possible without disruption of the carotid vessels.
- *Type III:* These are the most invasive lesions and indicate that the external and internal carotids are completely encased by the tumor. Often these tumors are considered unresectable. If resection is undertaken, it is highly risky and often requires interruption of blood flow to the brain with vascular reconstruction.

Additional risks associated with surgery of these lesions are injury to X (leading to aspiration and vocal issues), XI (leading to shoulder pain and weakness), and XII (leading to speech and swallowing issues). It is important to note that there is a significantly high rate of aspiration and dysphagia with concurrent X and XII injuries. Disruption of the adjacent sympathetic cervical chain which lies posterior to the carotid sheath may lead to an ipsilateral Horner's syndrome (ptosis, miosis, and anhydrosis), and blood flow interruption to the carotid arteries or associated embolism even without injury or transection may both cause stroke.[27]

JUGULOTYMPANIC TUMORS

Glomus tympanicum and glomus jugulare tumors have now been grouped together. Glomus tympanicum tumors are specifically confined to the middle ear space. Similar to jugulare tumors, they arise from the paraganglia tissue on the tympanic branch of IX (Jacobson's nerve) and are the most common tumor of the middle ear. The classical features are pulsatile tinnitus and hearing loss. Computed tomography (CT) of the temporal bone may show a rounded mass adjacent to the cochlear promontory. Glomus jugulare tumors arise from the paraganglia tissue around the jugular bulb. They arise either along Jacobson's nerve or Arnold's nerve (X). Classical symptoms are similar to those associated with glomus tympanicum. Due to their location, glomus jugulare tumors have a higher risk of cranial nerve injury during surgery (up to one-third of patients experience this). Also glomus jugulare tumors can be multiple.[27] In advanced lesions, the temporal bone may undergo enlargement, expansion and destruction, resulting in a "moth-eaten" appearance; this does not occur in tympanic paragangliomas that are smaller, less aggressive, and spares the jugular bulb and ossicles.[26]

The Fisch classification is the primary system used to categorize these tumors **(Figs. 2 to 7)**:[28]

- *Type A:* Tumors limited to the middle ear cleft (which designates glomus tympanicum).
- *Type B:* Tumors are limited to the tympanomastoid area but jugular bulb and carotid artery are both intact.

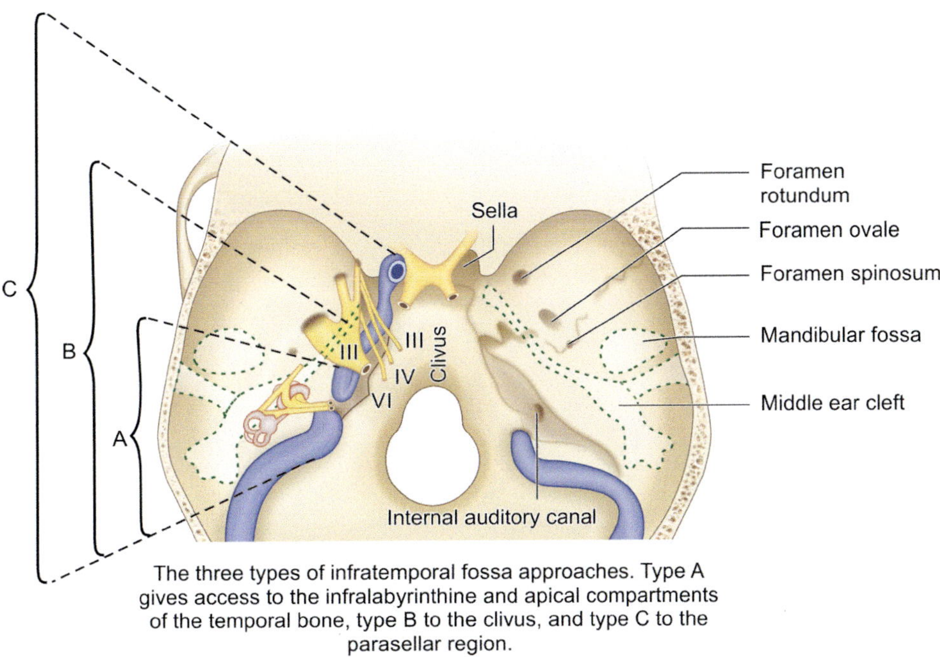

Fig. 2: Overview of exposure with Fisch approaches.

- *Type C:* Tumors involving the infralabyrinthine compartment of the temporal bone are considered type C and subdivided into C1–4 based on their degree of extension into the petrous and subsequent portions of the carotid canal.
  - *C1:* Tumor eroding carotid canal but not involving carotid artery
  - *C2:* Tumors involving vertical petrous carotid artery
  - *C3:* Tumors involving the horizontal carotid canal, but not foramen lacerum
  - *C4:* Tumors involving foramen lacerum and cavernous sinus
- *Type D:* Tumors with intracranial extension
  - *De1:* Extradural extension of <2 cm medial dural displacement
  - *De2:* Extradural extension of >2 cm medial dural displacement
  - *Di1:* Intradural extension of <2 cm
  - *Di2:* Intradural extension of >2 cm
  - *Di3:* Neurosurgically unresectable tumors

Another system known as the Glasscock/Jackson criteria has been used to characterize these tumors **(Table 2)**.[28]

On examination of these tumors, the tympanic membrane has bluish appearance which blanches on positive pressure with pneumatic otoscopy (Brown's sign). Extension through tympanic membrane can present as a polypoidal mass in ear canal. Middle ear tumors can extend along facial nerve, spread posteriorly into mastoid cavity, anteriorly along prelabyrinthine cells to involve petrous carotid. Rarely otic capsule involvement can present with vertigo. Due to proximity to the skull base, there is a high risk of invasion of cranial nerves IX to XII. Involvement of facial nerve in mastoid can result in facial paralysis as a presenting sign. Erosion of jugulocarotid spine leads to involvement of vertical petrous carotid artery and further anterior extension will lead to involvement of the horizontal segment. Further medial extension will lead to involvement of clivus and cavernous sinus. Occasionally, they can extend to infratemporal fossa and parapharyngeal space.[25,27] An osseous erosion around the jugular bulb is believed to be indicative of either a jugular or jugulotympanic paraganglioma rather than a tympanic paraganglioma.[26]

GLOMUS VAGALE

The last and possibly most ominous paraganglioma of the head and neck is the glomus vagale tumor. These tumors arise from one of the three ganglia situated along the vagus nerve as it approaches and enters the skull base. There is an inferior, middle, and superior ganglion. These tumors are the most likely of the head and neck paragangliomas to become malignant but the rarest, representing only approximately 5% of the head and

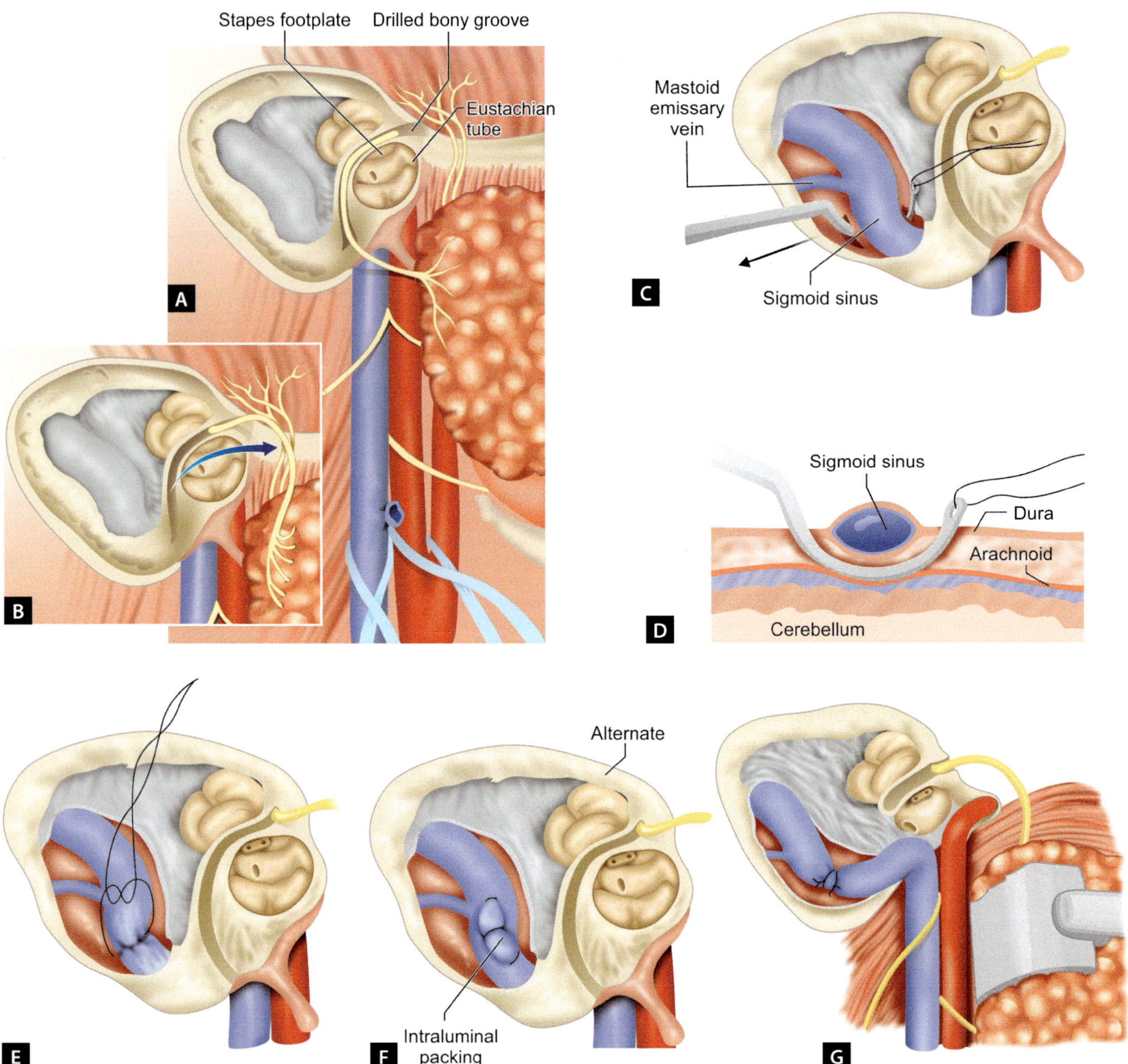

Figs. 3A to G: Fisch type A approach. (A and B) Type A dissection; (C) Mastoidectomy with exposure of sigmoid sinus and facial nerve; (D) Transfixation ligature with aneurysm needle; (E) Proximal and distal ligation; (F) Intraluminal packing as an alternative approach; (G) Exposure of jugular bulb and internal carotid artery after facial translocation.

neck paragangliomas. Grossly these tumors are situated more superiorly than carotid body tumors would be and can also be distinguished by the fact that they reside between the internal carotid and internal jugular vein instead of between the carotid branches. This tumor shows a female preponderance of 3:1. Lesions that originate superiorly may have a dumbbell appearance while lesions originating inferiorly often involve the poststyloid parapharyngeal space. Nearly 22% of vagal tumors already have intracranial extension at the time of diagnosis and this is the primary cause of death in these patients. Up to 50% exhibit cranial nerve deficits at time of presentation, primarily affecting X, IX, XI, and XII.

The staging system for glomus vagale tumors was developed in 1993 by Browne et al.[29]

- *Type I* tumors lie in the parapharyngeal space without evidence of jugular foramen invasion.
- *Type II* tumors have jugular foramen invasion but do not violate the skull base.
- *Type III* tumors present with deep invasion of the jugular foramen and/or middle ear with extension into the skull base (Classic "dumbbell" appearance).

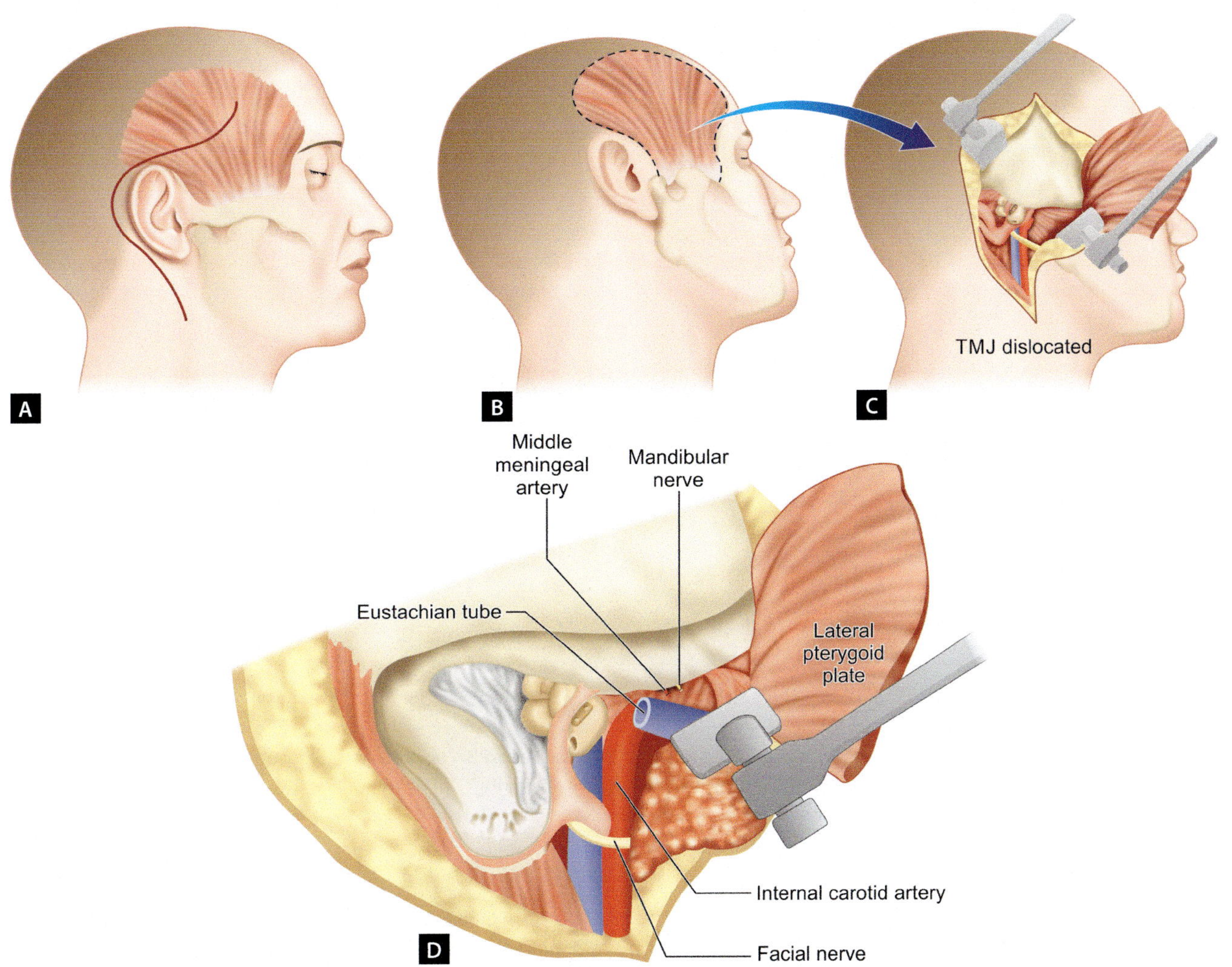

Figs. 4A to D: Fisch type B dissection exposes the petrous apex, clivus and superior infratemporal fossa. (A) Incision; (B) Downward reflection of temporalis; (C) Additional exposure after TMJ dislocation; (D) V3 can be transected and ICA exposed. (TMJ: temporomandibular joint)

DIAGNOSTIC EVALUATION

A detailed history and clinical examination are mandatory, with a special emphasis on cranial nerve evaluation and identifying symptoms and signs of catecholamine excess or malignant transformation. Family history of associated syndromes should be sought. The advantage of detecting SDH mutations is that patients may be screened and paragangliomas diagnosed while they are limited to reduce treatment-related morbidity. Additionally, siblings and children of SDH mutation carriers should be considered for genetic testing and, if found to harbor a mutation, screened via a 24-hour urine screening. Normal serum catecholamine levels effectively rule out a functioning tumor.

IMAGING

Ultrasound: Sonographic imaging may be utilized for initially evaluating a neck lump identified on clinical examination. It usually would reveal a well-defined heterogeneously hypoechoic mass with pronounced internal vascularity on color Doppler. By evaluating the internal and external carotid arteries and their patterns of displacement in detail along with cross-sectional assessment, a diagnosis of carotid body and vagal paragangliomas may be suggested.[26]

CT scan: CT with contrast is essential to evaluate the extent of lesion along with adjacent bony destruction. These lesions have early and robust enhancement with contrast administration. Delineation of pattern of invasion and skull base destruction is essential for surgical planning. Erosion of jugulotympanic spine, expansion of jugular foramen, involvement of mastoid, and middle ear are some signs to look for in glomus tympanicojugular lesions.

For primary imaging assessment of possible carotid body paragangliomas, either CT or magnetic resonance imaging (MRI) may be used to show an enhancing and

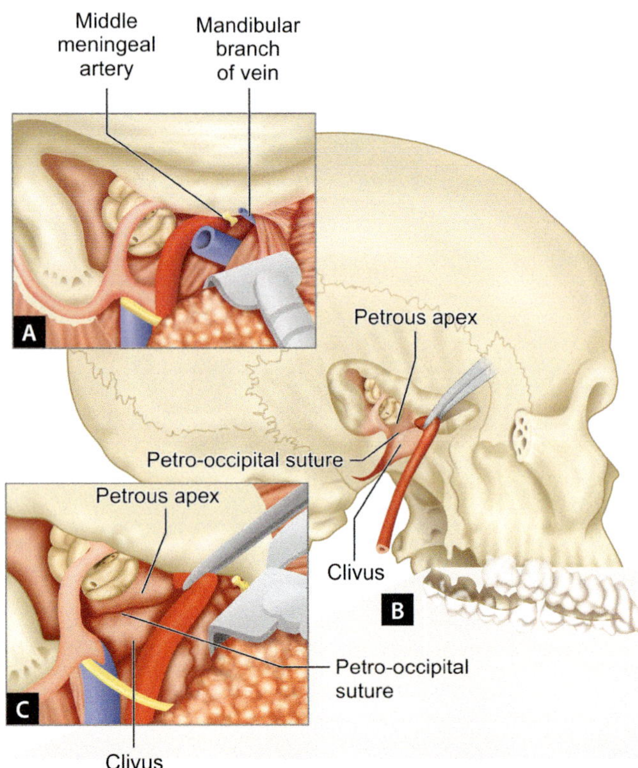

Figs. 5A to C: Fisch type C dissection exposes rostral clivus, cavernous sinus, sphenoid sinus and nasopharynx through removal of pterygoid base.

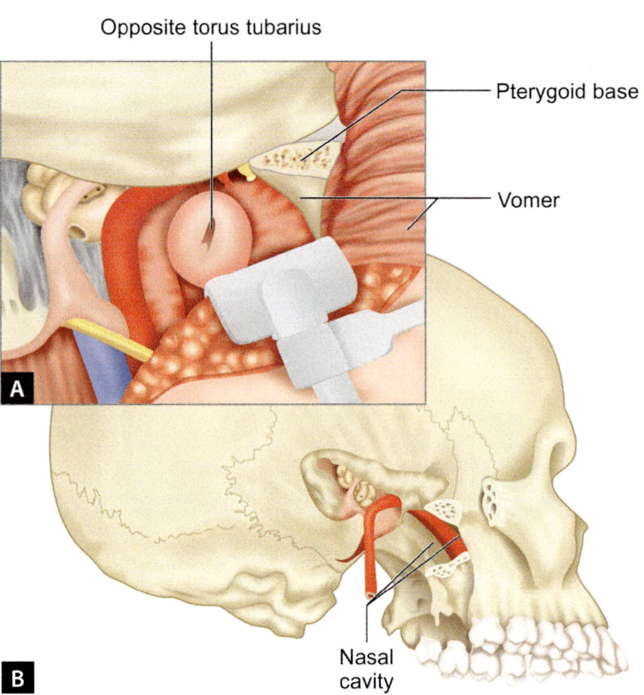

Figs. 7A and B: Nasopharynx exposure through removal of pterygoid processes and muscles.

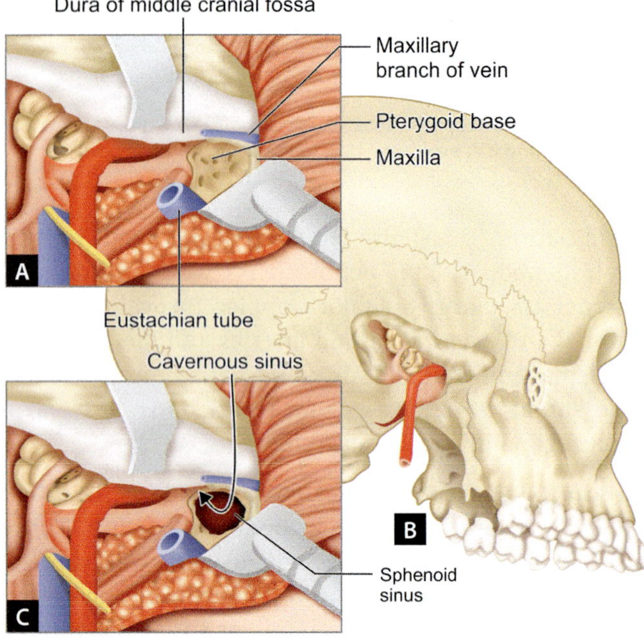

Figs. 6A to C: Exposure of cavernous sinus.

attenuating soft tissue mass located within the carotid space placed at the bifurcation of the carotids. Accompanying mass effect causes splaying of the internal and external carotid arteries and the pathognomonic

Table 2: Classification of glomus tympanicum and glomus jugulare.

Glomus tympanicum	*Glomus jugulare*
I: Small mass limited to promontory	*I:* Small tumor involving jugular bulb, middle ear, and mastoid
II: Tumor completely filling middle ear space	*II:* Tumor extending under internal auditory canal; may have intracranial canal extension
III: Tumor filling middle ear and extending into mastoid	*III:* Tumor extending into petrous apex; may have intracranial canal extension
IV: Tumor filling middle ear, extending into the mastoid or through tympanic membrane to fill the external auditory canal; may extend anterior to carotid	*IV:* Tumor extending beyond petrous apex into clivus or infratemporal fossa; may have intracranial canal extension

"Lyre sign". In vagal paragangliomas, the carotid vessels are likely to be displaced anteromedially. In cases of high-vagal paragangliomas, CT is also helpful in evaluation of osseous involvement of the anterior skull base.[26]

MRI: It is complementary to CT and can provide delineation of lesion, surveillance, and detection of concurrent paraganglioma in head and neck and confirmation of the diagnosis of paraganglioma. "Salt and pepper"

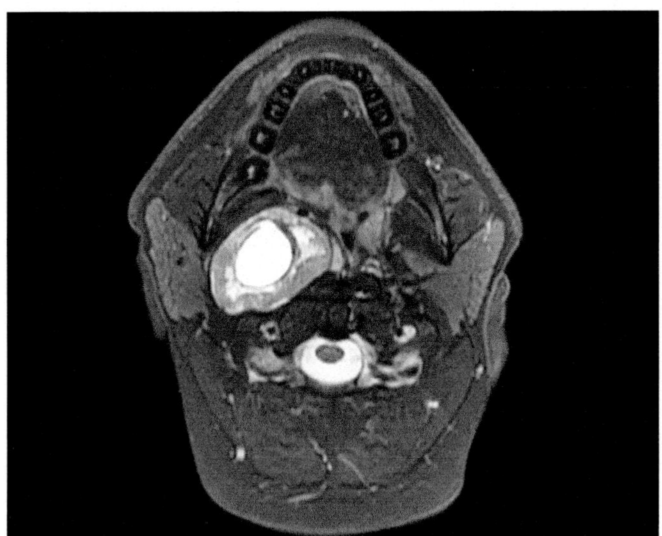

Fig. 8: Schwannoma of the right vagus showing intense enhancement on T2W MR.

appearance on T2-weighted images due to high flow of vascular voids is essentially pathognomonic of paraganglioma and is the most apparent in tumors >1 cm. Vascular displacement and extent of intracranial involvement are accurately determined. Normally, tumors such as schwannomas and neurofibromas are less vascular and do not reveal the characteristic flow voids as observed in paragangliomas **(Fig. 8)**.[26]

Dihydroxyphenylalanine-positron emission tomography (DOPA-PET): DOPA-PET is the diagnostic imaging method of choice, demonstrates the highest sensitivity and specificity for the detection of paragangliomas, and identifies possible lesions <1 cm with certainty. This imaging should be used to confirm suspicious findings in familial cases and/or as a screening method at the time of diagnosis of genetic predisposition and as a follow-up procedure every 2–3 years. With DOPA-PET, possible paragangliomas or metastatic lymph nodes even <1 cm can be identified with certainty, in contrast to MRI or CT scan.[23] This means that an absence of DOPA uptake would practically rule out any metastatic lymph nodes, but for evaluation of structural detail and extent of spread CT and MRI are unavoidable. A minority of paragangliomas (1–3%) demonstrate clinical or biochemical evidence of hormonal activity. The evaluation of the 24-hour urinary catecholamine excretion (increased two- to threefolds) is a prerequisite to exclude catecholamine excess, especially in the case of a planned operative procedure. The current literature seems to overstate the number of catecholamine secreting tumors. Konstantinos et al. in their analysis of 175 patients showed that the number of hormonal active paragangliomas of the head and neck area, as defined by an increased 24-hour urinary catecholamine excretion, is essentially negligible (1 out of 175 patients).[27]

Angiography: Angiography plays a less significant role in the diagnosis, but plays a crucial role in embolization. Angiography provides a detail map of tumor blood supply and venous drainage, delineates flow dynamics, and also provides information about cerebral circulation. Selective preoperative embolization can be executed to reduce intraoperative blood loss. Angiographic balloon occlusion test in cases that may require internal carotid artery resection is paramount to anticipate perioperative morbidity. Temporarily occluding the carotid siphon within the cavernous sinus and monitoring neurologic dysfunction by means of clinical examination, electroencephalogram (EEG) and/or Xenon CT can be performed. MR angiogram can map feeder vessels and also confirms the diagnosis. Both, MRA and CTA permit assessment of perfusion of the mass, identification of feeding vessels and revealing the presence of multicentric disease, and aiding in performing either embolization or surgical resection. Head and neck paragangliomas classically have many enhancing, feeding peritumoral arteries and veins.[26]

TREATMENT

The treatment options for paragangliomas of the head and neck are most commonly observation, surgery or radiotherapy (RT). The choice of treatment depends on the histology, tumor size, symptomatology, patient demographics, anticipated treatment-related morbidity, and physician preference and expertise. To allow a systematic approach, multidisciplinary algorithms have been proposed that simplify decision-making.[3]

Surgical excision was considered the standard approach to paragangliomas of the head and neck for decades. It is still preferred for carotid body tumors that are limited in size (<5 cm) and lack carotid encasement. This allows for complete excision with low risk of bleeding and disruption of cerebral blood flow. In cases of bilateral carotid body tumor, surgical excision may lead to baroreflex failure syndrome, characterized by wide fluctuations in blood pressure with episodes of severe hypertension and tachycardia in response to stress, pain or exertion. In these cases, resection of the smaller tumors and radical radiotherapy to the larger tumor is indicated. In cases of malignancy or in biochemically active tumors, adjuvant radiotherapy may be indicated.[1] Approaches to carotid body tumor and jugular/vagal paragangliomas are illustrated in **Flowcharts 1 and 2**.[3]

With improvement in microsurgical technique and perioperative care including embolization techniques, the

Flowchart 1: Approach to carotid body tumors (CBT).

Presence of CBT

Single CBT

Jugular or vagal tumor + CBT

Bilateral CBT

Magnetic resonance angiography

Surgery for CBT

RT for jugular/ vagal tumor

Surgery for smaller-sized CBT

RT for larger-sized CBT

Surgery

Salvage surgery if regrowth

Salvage reirradiation or observation

Salvage RT if growth

(CBT: carotid body tumor; RT: radiotherapy)

Flowchart 2: Approach to jugular/vagal paragangliomas.

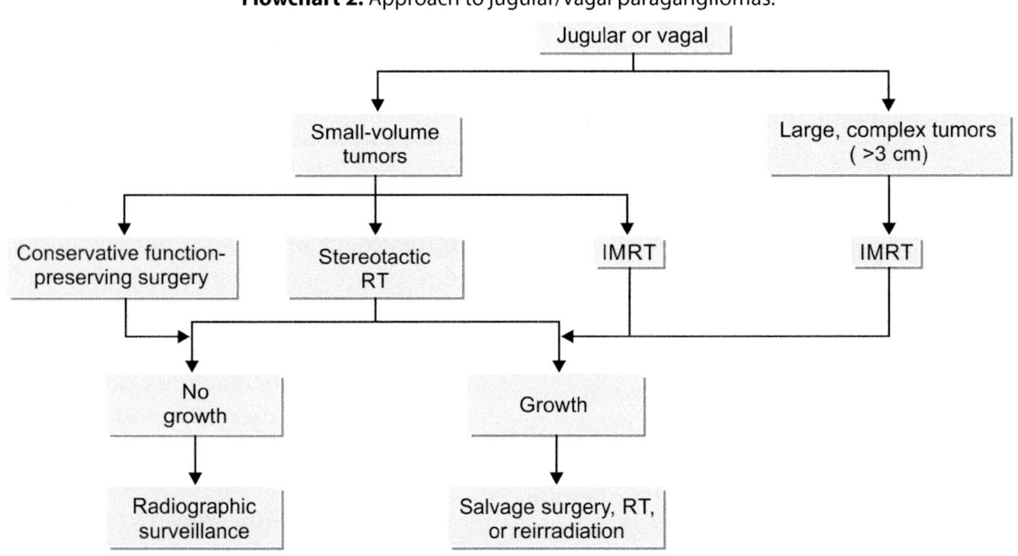

(IMRT: intensity-modulated radiotherapy; RT: radiotherapy)

surgical morbidity associated with these resections has reduced considerably over time.[30] However, it is crucial for the surgeon to anticipate the extent of postoperative morbidity, since surgery and RT have comparable local control rates in most series.[31] In elderly patients, especially those with comorbid illness that preclude anesthesia, radiotherapy should be considered the initial treatment choice. This is also the choice for patients with tumors that have expanded to extensively involve the skull base or the intracranial compartment. A systematic review by Suárez of jugular and vagal paragangliomas showed that RT had better local control and lower incidence of major morbidity.[31] Stereotactic radiosurgery (SRS) is also an attractive treatment option in those with skull-base tumors and lesions <3 cm. Local control rates are excellent and it allows for shorter treatment duration but the risk of hearing loss following treatment of tympanojugular paragangliomas is around 50%. When compared with RT for other histologies in the head and neck, the advantage of RT for paragangliomas is the dosage required is lower; the standard dose of external beam of RT is 45 Gy at 1.8 Gy per daily fraction. Higher doses do not improve control rates but are associated with higher complication rates. For SRS, the optimal dose described is 12–15 Gy.[32]

Intensity-modulated RT (IMRT) allows for smaller treatment volumes and resultant improved morbidity profiles. Use of MRI for treatment planning may improve precision. However, very small treatment volumes may result in geographical miss and reduced local control rates.

For patients with slow-growing benign lesions and modest life expectancy, observation of these lesions may be the best approach. It is to be considered, however, that once cranial nerve deficits begin to appear, they may be irreversible; the relatively low morbidity of profile of RT requires to be weighed against cranial nerve deficits.[33,34]

SURGICAL APPROACHES

- *Carotid body tumors:* Depending on the vertical extent of the tumor either a transverse or vertical incision can be utilized. The sternocleidomastoid muscle is dissected off the carotid sheath to expose the tumor. The X and XI cranial nerves are isolated to avoid injury. The common carotid artery is dissected out proximally and distally and vessels loops are placed on it. Subadventitial dissection is performed in Shamblin types I/II to dissect between the tumor and the carotid artery wall. Gentle handling prevents intimal injury. The principles of carotid sacrifice are detailed in the chapter on tumors of the paranasal sinuses and anterior skull base.
- *Fisch approaches:*[35] These approaches to the infratemporal fossa were described to access tumors of the temporal bone and skull base. Detailed figures explaining them have been shown.
  - *Type A:* This allows access to the jugular bulb, vertical petrous carotid, and posterior infratemporal fossa. It involves radical mastoidectomy, anterior translocation of the facial nerve, and dissection of the posterior infratemporal fossa.
  - *Type B:* This allows access to the petrous apex, clivus, and superior infratemporal fossa by reflection of the temporalis on to the coronoid process and zygoma.
  - *Type C:* This allows access to the nasopharynx, peritubal space, rostral clivus, parasellar area, pterygopalatine fossa, and anterosuperior infratemporal fossa by removal of the base of pterygoid process and removal of the floor of the middle cranial fossa and pterygoid muscles.

FOLLOW-UP

For patients on observation with no active management, regular imaging is important to determine when intervention is required. For patients who have undergone complete resection or RT, follow-up may be indicated with ultrasound or cross-sectional imaging. Sporadic cases require an annual MRI of the head and neck, especially in jugulotympanic paragangliomas for the first 2 years. In carotid body or vagal tumors, ultrasound may be adequate. In familial cases, evaluation of the abdomen may also be indicated. The follow-up for each patient needs to be tailor-made based on completeness of treatment, likelihood of recurrence, presence of malignancy, and other factors.

REFERENCES

1. Kumar V, Abbas A, Fausto N, Aster J. Robbins and Cotran: Pathological Basis of Disease, 8th edition. Philadelphia, PA: Saunders; 2010.
2. Pellitteri PK, Rinaldo A, Myssiorek D, Gary Jackson C, Bradley PJ, Devaney KO, et al. Paragangliomas of the head and neck. Oral Oncol. 2004;40:563-75.
3. Hu K, Persky MS. Treatment of head and neck paragangliomas. Cancer Control. 2016;23(3):228-41.
4. Pearse AG. The diffuse neuroendocrine system: peptides, amines, placodes and the APUD theory. Prog Brain Res. 1986; 68:25-31.
5. Pearse AG. The diffuse neuroendocrine system and the implications of the APUD concept. Int surg. 1979;64: 5-7.
6. Schwaber MK, Glasscock ME, Nissen AJ, Jackson CJ, Smith PG. Diagnosis and management of catecholamine secreting glomus tumors. Laryngoscope. 1984;94:1008-15.
7. Yuan Y, Shi H, Tao X. Head and neck paragangliomas: diffusion weighted and dynamic contrast enhanced magnetic resonance imaging characteristics. BMC Med Imaging. 2016; 16:12.
8. Martin TP, Irving RM, Maher ER. The genetics of paragangliomas: a review. Clin Otolaryngol. 2007;32:7-11.
9. Kollert M, Minovi AA, Draf W, Bockmuhl U. Cervical paragangliomas-tumor control and long-term functional results after surgery. Skull Base. 2006;16:185-91.
10. Offergeld C, Brase C, Yaremchuk S, Mader I, Christian Rischke H, Gläsker S, et al. Head and neck paragangliomas: clinical and molecular genetic classification. Clinics (Sao Paulo). 2012;67(Suppl 1):19-28.
11. McCrary HC, Babajanian E, Calquin M, Carpenter P, Casazza G, Naumer A, et al. Characterization of malignant head and neck paragangliomas at a single institution across multiple decades. JAMA Otolaryngol Head Neck Surg. 2019; 145(7):641-6.
12. Chino JP, Sampson JH, Tucci DL, Brizel DM, Kirkpatrick JP. Paraganglioma of the head and neck: long-term local control with radiotherapy. Am J Clin Oncol. 2009;32:304-7.
13. Papaspyrou K, Mann WJ, Amedee RG. Management of head and neck paragangliomas: review of 120 patients. Head Neck. 2009;31:381-7.
14. Cadiñanos J, Llorente JL, de la Rosa J, Villameytide JA, Illán R, Durán NS, et al. Novel germline SDHD deletion associated with an unusual sympathetic head and neck paraganglioma. Head Neck. 2011;33(8):1233-40.
15. Burnichon N, Rohmer V, Amar L, Herman P, Leboulleux S, Darrouzet V, et al. The succinate dehydrogenase genetic testing in a large prospective series of patients with paragangliomas.J Clin Endocrinol Metab. 2009;94:2817-27.
16. Boedeker CC, Hensen EF, Neumann HP, Maier W, van Nederveen FH, Suárez C, et al. Genetics of hereditary head and neck paragangliomas. Head Neck. 2014;36:907-16.
17. Bayley JP, Kunst HP, Cascon A, Lourdes Sampietro M, Gaal J, Korpershoek E, et al. SDHAF2 mutations in familial and

sporadic paraganglioma and phaeochromocytoma. Lancet Oncol. 2010;11:366-72.

18. Kirmani S, Young WF. Hereditary Paraganglioma-Pheochromocytoma Syndromes. 2008 May 21 [updated 2012 Aug 30]. In: Pagon RA, Adam MP, Ardinger HH, Bird TD, Dolan CR, Fong CT, Smith RJH, Stephens K (Eds). Gene Reviews VR [Internet]. Seattle (WA): University of Washington, Seattle; 1993-2014.
19. Cerecer-Gil NY, Figuera LE, Llamas FJ, Lara M, Escamilla JG, Ramos R, et al. Mutation of SDHB is a cause of hypoxia related high altitude paraganglioma. Clin Cancer Res. 2010; 16:4148-54.
20. Astrom K, Chen JE Willet-Brozick, Aston CE, Baysal BE. Altitude is a phenotypic modifier in hereditary paraganglioma type 1 evidence for oxygen sensing defect. Hum Genet. 2003;113:228-37.
21. Hinerman RW, Amdur RJ, Morris CG, Kirwan J, Mendenhall WM. Definitive radiotherapy in the management of paragangliomas arising in the head and neck: a 35-year experience. Head Neck. 2008;30:1431-8.
22. Lee JH, Barich F, Karnell LH, Robinson RA, Zhen WK, Gantz BJ, et al. National Cancer Data Base report on malignant paragangliomas of the head and neck. Cancer. 2002;94:730-7.
23. Williams MD. Paragangliomas of the head and neck: an overview from diagnosis to genetics. Head Neck Pathol. 2017;11:278-87.
24. Neumann HP, Erlic Z, Boedeker CC, Rybicki LA, Robledo M, Hermsen M, et al. Clinical predictors for germline mutations in head and neck paraganglioma patients: cost reduction strategy in genetic diagnostic process as fall-out. Cancer Res. 2009;69:3650-6.
25. Papaspyrou K, Mewes T, Rossman H, Fottner C, Schneider-Raetzke B, Bartsch O, et al. Head and neck paragangliomas: report of 175 patients (1989-2010). Head Neck. 2012;34(5): 632-7.
26. Thelen J, Bhatt AA. Multimodality imaging of paragangliomas of the head and neck. Insights Imaging. 2019;10(1): 2-9.
27. Manolidis S, Hu KS, Persky MS. Paragangliomas of the head and neck. In: Harrison LB, Sessions RB, Kies MS (Eds). Head and Neck Cancer: A Multidisciplinary Approach Hardcover, 4th edition. Philadelphia: Lippincott Williams & Wilkins (LWW); 2013. pp. 745-76.
28. Woolen S, Gemmete JJ. Paragangliomas of the head and neck. Neuroimaging Clin N Am. 2016;26(2):259-78.
29. Browne JD, Fisch U, Valavanis A. Surgical therapy of glomus vagale tumors. Skull Base Surg. 1993;3(4):182-92.
30. Brink I, Hoegerle S, Klisch J, Bley TA. Imaging of pheochromocytoma and paraganglioma—review. Fam Cancer. 2005;4(1): 61-8.
31. Suárez C, Rodrigo JP, Bodeker CC, Llorente JL, Silver CE, Jansen JC, et al. Jugular and vagal paragangliomas: systematic study of management with surgery and radiotherapy. Head Neck. 2013;35(8):1195-204.
32. Jacob JT, Link MJ, Foote RL. Stereotactic radiosurgery for glomus tumors. In: Lunsford LD, Sheehan J (Eds). Intracranial Stereotactic Radiosurgery. New York, NY: Thieme Medical Publishers; 2009. pp. 84-9.
33. Van der Mey AG, Frijns JH, Cornelisse CJ, Brons EN, van Dulken H, Terpstra HL, et al. Does intervention improve the natural course of glomus tumors? A series of 108 patients seen in a 32-year period. Ann Otol Rhinol Laryngol. 1992;101:635-42.
34. Smith J, Harvey R, Owen D, Prince M, Carol B, Gregory W, et al. Head and neck paragangliomas: a two-decade institutional experience and algorithm for management: paragangliomas of the head and neck. Laryng Invest Otolaryngol. 2017;2(6):380-9.
35. Fisch U. Infratemporal fossa approach to tumours of the temporal bone and base of the skull. J Laryngol Otol. 1978;92(11):949-67.

CHAPTER 21

Melanomas of the Head and Neck

Samskruthi P Murthy, Sivakumar Vidhyadharan, Narayana Subramaniam

INTRODUCTION

Melanomas arise from the malignant transformation of melanocytes. Melanocytes are neural crest in origin and, hence, melanomas can arise in skin and other sites as well. In head and neck, cutaneous melanomas are common, while primary mucosal melanomas are quite rare. The following chapter is divided into cutaneous and noncutaneous melanoma.

CUTANEOUS MELANOMA

Introduction

Cutaneous melanoma of the head and neck region constitutes 25–30% of all melanomas. Sun exposed areas are commonly affected with face (40–60%), scalp (14–49%), neck (20–29%), and ear (8–11%) involved in decreasing order of occurrence.[1-3] Melanoma incidence is gradually rising at the rate of 5% increase in incidence per year and mortality has increased at 2% per year.[4,5] The estimated loss of years due melanoma mortality is 20.4 years (when compared to 16.6 years in other malignancies),[6] which reflects how melanoma often affects the young, healthy population, and has a high mortality.

Etiology

- *Ultraviolet (UV) radiation:* Frequent exposure to UV radiation is a major etiologic factor in causation of cutaneous melanoma. UVB light (290–310 nanometers) and UVA (320–400 nanometers) are both known to be risk factors, UVB more than UVA.[7] UVB causes pyrimidine dimers and UVA causes oxidative DNA damage. Frequent use of tanning beds is also associated with increased risk. The risk of melanoma with UV exposure is dose and duration dependent.
- *Personal characteristics:* Skin type (Fitzpatrick type I and II), blonde or red hair, and blue eyes is associated with increased risk of melanoma.[8]
- *Atypical mole syndrome:* Atypical mole syndrome associated with a defect in *CDKN2A* gene, that encodes for p16, is associated with risk of melanoma. This mutation has high penetrance and carries a 100% risk of melanoma among relatives.[9]
- *Xeroderma pigmentosa:* Xeroderma pigmentosa, characterized by defective nucleotide excision repair, especially thymine dimers, is associated with increased risk of all cutaneous cancers.[10]
- *Pre-existing lesions:* About 80% of melanoma arises from pre-existing lesions. Congenital nevi that measure >20 cm has a 10% increased lifetime risk of developing melanoma.[11] Dysplastic nevi, which are characterized by indistinct borders, carry the highest risk of malignant transformation than other types of nevi.

Molecular Pathogenesis

Various molecular and chromosomal aberrations are identified in melanoma that helps in differentiating melanoma from benign nevi. These aberrations are evolutionary changes that result in progression from nevi to melanoma. Mutations of p53, *Rb* gene, and *PTEN* that are commonly associated with other cancers are rarely seen in melanoma and occur only in advanced stages. In the early stages, mutations in the RAS-RAF-MEK-extracellular-signal-regulated kinase (ERK) pathway, *PI3K/PTEN*, and c-*KIT* pathways have been recognized in cutaneous melanoma.[12] Mutations of *CD2KA* locus (*p16INK/p14ARF*) flag the malignant transformation of nevi to melanoma and is found in 25% of familial melanoma.[12] Various other pathways such as the Wnt signaling pathway, melanocortin signaling pathway (a-MSH/melanocortin-1 receptor/cAMP), and loss of the *p16INK4a* cyclin-dependent kinase also play an essential role in melanoma carcinogenesis. Of all these, the mitogen-activated protein kinase (MPAK) pathway plays a significant role and is utilized as diagnostic and prognostic marker and also as a potential therapeutic target.

The clinical subtypes based on etiology can be divided into chronic and nonchronic sun damage (non-CSD) melanoma. Each one is associated with distinct molecular signature. Non-CSD subtype is associated with B-type Raf (BRAF) mutations (56%) while *KIT* aberrations are seen in 28% of chronic sun damage (CSD) subtype; non-CSD subtype does not express *KIT* aberrations.[13]

Biomarkers and Treatment Implications

- *B-Raf protooncogene mutation: BRAF* is a serine-threonine kinase that activates the MAPK pathway. It is commonly seen in younger age, trunk melanoma, and intermittent sun exposure. Most common mutation is at V600E (80%) and V600K (15%) at 600th codon.[13] *BRAF V600E* is associated with good response to BRAF/MEK inhibitors. Other codon mutations are associated with reduced response. BRAFVE1 immunohistochemistry (IHC) can be used as a rapid screening test for BRAF mutations. BRAF inhibitors recommended in cutaneous melanoma are vemurafenib and dabrafenib.
- *KIT protooncogene mutation (c-KIT): KIT* is a tyrosine kinase receptor. Mutations of c-*KIT* are associated commonly with mucosal and non-CSD melanoma. Mutations are associated with good response to *KIT* inhibitors.[12] c-*KIT* inhibitor indicated in cutaneous melanoma is imatinib.
- *NRAS proto-oncogene: NRAS* mutations are GTPase dependent and activate the MAPK pathway. *NRAS* is strongly associated with poor survival and commonly seen in advanced cases. *NRAS* mutations are rarely associated with *BRAF* or *KIT* mutations.[12] The presence of *NRAS* mutation is an indication to stop further molecular profiling. MEK inhibitors may show a partial response, but is negligible. MEK inhibitor approved for use in cutaneous melanoma is trametinib.
- *Programmed death-ligand-1 (PD-L1):* PD-L1 is a co-regulatory molecule that inhibits T cell-mediated antitumor response. PD-L1 is expressed on tumor cells and tumor-infiltrating macrophages. PD-L1 IHC staining is considered positive when there is tumor cell membranous staining at any level. PD-L1 expression >5% is considered high and associated with good response to nivolumab or nivolumab + iplimumab therapy.[14] Low PD-L1 expression predicts inadequate response with nivolumab. Routine PD-L1 testing is not recommended for treatment decisions.

Molecular Testing

Biopsy with IHC is the gold standard to diagnose melanoma. Few dysplastic nevi may be difficult to be distinguished from melanoma by histopathology and use of molecular testing to differentiate benign from malignant has been studied. Molecular markers are also extensively studied in prognostication of disease. Their efficacy in prognostication in comparison with known pathological factors is variable, but most studies have shown that they are inferior to tumor thickness and nodal status as prognosticators. Various tests are available commercially and their use is represented in **Table 1**.[15]

Table 1: Adjunctive molecular profiling tests available for melanocytic neoplasm.

Technique	*Clinical use*	*Accuracy*	
		Sensitivity	*Specificity*
Chromosomal analysis			
Fluorescence in situ hybridization	• Diagnosis in histologically ambiguous melanocytic neoplasms • Distinguishing benign melanocytic nevi from malignant melanoma	43–100%	29–80%
Comparative genomic hybridization	Distinguishing benign melanocytic nevi from malignant melanoma	92–96%	87–100%
Gene expression profiling			
Decision Dx-Melanoma (Castle Biosciences, Friendswood, Texas)	Assessing metastasis risk in malignant melanoma, with negative sentinel lymph node biopsy	85–100%	54–78%
myPath Melanoma (Myriad Genetics, Salt Lake City, Utah)	Distinguishing benign melanocytic nevi from malignant melanoma	55–90%	88–93%
Pigmented Lesion Assay (DermTech, Inc, La Jolla, California)	Clinical decision tool (prebiopsy) for malignant melanocytic neoplasms	91%	53–69%

Indications for Molecular Testing

The National Comprehensive Cancer Network (NCCN) recommendation for molecular testing in cutaneous melanoma are:

- Stage III patients with high risk for recurrence
- Stage IV patients

In these patients, *BRAF*, *NRAS* and *c-KIT* mutations need to tested.[16] Broader gene profiling is recommended if feasible in stage IV disease.

Clinical Presentation

Cutaneous melanoma commonly involves men more than women with a median age of presentation of 59 years. The major subtypes of clinical presentation of melanoma are superficial spreading melanoma (SSM), nodular melanoma (NM), acral-lentiginous melanoma (ALM), and lentigo maligna melanoma (LMM).[17] SSM is the most prevalent type comprising 65% of clinical presentation. Variegated patches of gray brown or black characterize SSM. In early stages, lesions show a radial growth pattern, which at a later stage grows vertically to involve deeper structures. Nodular melanoma (NM) comprises 20% of all presentation and is an aggressive variant characterized by numerous mitotic figures, invasive growth pattern and ulceration. Lentigo maligna melanoma (LMM) is seen in 5% of cases. Histologically melanocytes are placed at the level of reticular dermis hence appears as insignificant lesions clinically and are most often misdiagnosed. Other rarer types such as desmoplastic melanoma are seen in the head and neck region, which is associated with higher local recurrence and increased perineural spread. These are most often amelanotic.[17]

Pathology and Pathological Prognosticators

Histology of melanoma is characterized by presence of atypical melanocytes along the epidermo-dermal junction with variable growth pattern beyond papillary dermis depending on the invasiveness of tumor. The diagnosis of melanoma can sometimes be challenging as they mimic various other malignancies. IHC plays a vital role in diagnosis. S-100 antigen has high sensitivity but lacks specificity.[18] HMB-45 melanosomal antigen is highly specific for pigmented cells. The melanosomal protein MART-1/Melan-Ais also recommended. Enzymatic proteins such as tyrosinase, TRP-1 and TRP-2, and structural melanosomal proteins, collectively called melanogenesis-related proteins (MRPs), which are highly specific and sensitive for cells of melanocyte origin can also be used as IHC marker.[18] Various histological subtypes are defined by World Health Organization (WHO), they are superficial spreading melanoma, nodular melanoma, lentigo maligna melanoma, acral lentiginous melanoma, mucosal-lentiginous melanoma, desmoplastic/neurotropic melanoma, melanoma arising from a blue nevus, melanoma arising from a giant congenital nevus, melanoma of childhood, nevoid melanoma, persistent melanoma, and melanoma, not otherwise classified. The pathological prognosticators and their definition are described below:[19]

- *Tumor thickness:* It is defined as the upper edge of the granular layer of the epidermis of the overlying skin. If the lesion is ulcerated, the base of the ulcer to the deepest point of tumor invasion in millimeter is measured. Depth is measured perpendicular to the skin using an ocular micrometer. Breslow's thickness and Clark levels are also known prognosticators of melanoma.
- *Tumor ulceration:* It is considered as an independent prognostic factor and also affects the staging. Ulceration is defined as full-thickness epidermal defect with evidence of reactive changes and thinning or effacement, in the absence of recent surgical procedure. Whenever a biopsy is taken, a full-thickness biopsy must be performed so that depth can be measured. The point of biopsy must be documented so that when the final excision specimen is examined, the biopsy site can be made out and not confused as ulceration.
- *Mitotic rate:* It is also a strong predictor of outcome. The mitotic rate is expressed as the number of mitosis per mm^2. The figures are counted in invasive melanoma cells. The mm^2 with maximum mitosis (hotspot) is counted.
- *Lymphovascular invasion:* It is defined as melanoma cells within the lamina of blood vessels, or lymphatic must be documented.
- *Perineural invasion:* It must also be described in the report with the same definition as perineural invasion in mucosal SCC.
- *Microsatellite tumor deposit:* Like microscopic cutaneous metastasis, it is found adjacent or deep to primary tumor. The microsatellite is tumor nest >0.05 mm in diameter and is separated from the tumor by at least 0.3 mm of normal tissue.
- *In-transit metastasis:* These occur >2 cm from the primary tumor but not beyond closest lymph nodal basin. The impact of in-transit metastasis on survival is higher than nodal burden.

Evaluation

In the history, a presence of pre-existing lesions, sun exposure, and family history must be documented.

The location of the lesion is important as scalp, ear, cheek, and neck in a descending order portend worst prognosis.

The acronym ABCDE describes features of melanoma in a pre-existing nevi. Asymmetry, irregular border, color variation, diameter >6 mm, and evolution of the mole are considered signs of malignant transformation of a mole.[17] The diagnosis is made by incision biopsy. If the lesion is small, then excisional biopsy with a 2-mm margin can be done. Shave biopsy is avoided as it affects assessment of depth.[16]

The staging workup is based on the clinical stage of the disease where the biopsy report is utilized for microstaging the tumor.[16] **Table 2** shows the American Joint Committee on Cancer (AJCC), 8th edition, classification. In stage I/II disease, imaging for distant metastasis is not advocated while a preliminary ultrasound to assess regional lymph nodes can be done. In stage III, likelihood of distant metastasis is 0.5–3.7%. In patients with palpable nodes, the rate increases to 16% and hence metastatic workup must include computed tomography (CT) of neck, abdomen, pelvis, and magnetic resonance imaging (MRI) of brain or whole-body positron emission tomography (PET) CT.[16] All stage III/IV patients must be evaluated for distant metastasis. PET-CT has a sensitivity of 68–87% and specificity of 92–98%.[20] Use of PET-CT in stage I/II melanoma is not advocated due to very low specificity of PET-CT in this group. Serum LDH level is of prognostic value but not a marker to detect distant metastasis. Serum LDH is an independent prognostic factor, predicting response, progression-free survival, and overall survival.[16]

The American Joint Committee on Cancer, 8th edition, was modified based on collaborative data from International Melanoma Database and Discovery Platform (IMDDP) which included melanoma patients from 10 institutions treated after 1998 and comprised of >46,000 patients.[21]

Treatment

Surgery forms the primary treatment modality for resectable melanoma. The recommendations for adequate margins have been depicted in the table as per NCCN recommendations **(Table 3)**.[16] Assessment and evaluation of the margins is based on the principles

Table 2: Cutaneous melanoma TNM staging—the American Joint Committee on Cancer (AJCC), 8th edition.

T stage	*N stage*	*M stage*
TX: Primary tumor thickness cannot be assessed.	*NX:* Regional nodes not assessed [e.g., sentinel lymph node (SLN) biopsy not performed, regional nodes previously removed for another reason]	*M0:* No evidence of distant metastasis
T0: No evidence of primary tumor (e.g., unknown primary or completely regressed melanoma)	*N0:* No regional metastases detected	*M1:* Evidence of distant metastasis *M1a:* Distant metastasis to skin, soft tissue including muscle, and/or nonregional lymph node
Tis (melanoma in situ)	*N1* *N1a:* One clinically occult (i.e., detected by SLN biopsy) *N1b:* One clinically detected *N1c:* No regional lymph node disease with IT/MM	*M1b:* Distant metastasis to lung with or without M1a sites of disease
T1: ≤1.0 mm *T1a:* <0.8 mm without ulceration *T1b:* <0.8 mm with ulceration or 0.8–1 mm with or without ulceration	*N2* *N2a:* 2 or 3 clinically occult (i.e., detected by SLN biopsy) *N2b:* 2 or 3, at least one of which was clinically detected *N2c:* One clinically occult or clinically detected with IT/MM	*M1c:* Distant metastasis to non-CNS visceral sites with or without M1a or M1b sites of disease
T2: >1.0–2.0 mm *T2a:* >1.0–2.0 mm without ulceration *T2b:* >1.0–2.0 mm with ulceration	*N3* *N3a:* Four or more clinically occult (i.e., detected by SLN biopsy) *N3b:* Four or more, at least one of which was clinically detected, or the presence of any number of matted nodes *N3c:* Two or more clinically occult or clinically detected and/or presence of any number of matted nodes with IT/MM	*M1d:* Distant metastasis to CNS with or without M1a, M1b, or M1c sites of disease
T3: >2.0–4.0 mm *T3a:* >2.0–4.0 mm without ulceration *T3b:* >2.0–4.0 mm with ulceration		No LDH elevation LDH elevation
T4: >4.0 mm *T4a:* >4.0 mm without ulceration *T4b:* >4.0 mm with ulceration		

(IT: in-transit metastases: MM: microsatellite metastases; LDH: lactate dehydrogenase)

Table 3: National Comprehensive Cancer Network (NCCN) margin recommendation in cutaneous melanoma.[16]

Tumor thickness	*Recommended clinical margin*
In situ	0.5–1 cm
≤1.0 mm	1 cm
>1–2 mm	1–2 cm
>2–4 mm	2 cm
>4 mm	2 cm

already described in the chapter on nonmelanoma skin cancers. In large lesions, a 2-cm margin may be difficult to achieve in complex anatomical areas of head and neck, and hence 1–2 cm margin with complete circumferential assessment of margins must be the goal. Various earlier trials have shown equivocal outcomes with wider margins.[22-26] A recent UK-based prospective trial has shown that a wider margin in tumors >2 mm thick significantly improves melanoma-specific survival. The follow-up period of the trial was 8.8 years. Although this is the only prospective trial in melanoma proving better control with wider margins, it failed to show benefit of a 3-cm margin over a 2-cm one.[27]

Management of the Neck

Sentinel lymph node biopsy (SLNB) must be performed in cases with tumor thickness >1 mm. SLNB is a procedure to identify subclinical nodal metastasis in stage one and stage two melanoma.[16] The utility of SLNB is based on technical aspects of the procedure and method of pathological examination. A positive SLNB is associated with high risk of recurrence and these patients must be subjected to a complete neck dissection and adjuvant therapy.[16] The technique consists of four stages namely preoperative dynamic lymphoscintigraphy or single positron emission tomography (SPECT) scan which has better anatomical accuracy, intraoperative identification by isosulfan blue or methylene blue, and gamma probe identification of radio-labeled lymph nodes. Pathological examination must include routine hematoxylin and eosin staining, serial step sectioning and IHC with HMB-45 and Melan-A. About 5–40% are upstaged by SLNB. The utility of SLNB in melanoma with tumor thickness <1 mm is controversial.[16]

The MSLT-1 trial initiated in 1994 proved the utility of SLNB in melanoma.[28] The trial proved the prognostic value of SLNB in patients with tumors >1.2 mm thick and demonstrated SLNB status as the strongest predictor of disease-free survival. In this trial false negative rate was 20%.

^{99m}Tc tilmanocept (lymphoseek) is a CD206 receptor-targeted agent, which has shown an increased identification of melanoma containing lymph node,[29] however, its use is still limited. The identified nodes must be excised with cervical incision. When SLN is detected in the parotid, modified Blair incision is placed, and nodal clearance is done after finding the facial nerve. SLNB localized nodes can be intraparotid (51.4%) and extraparotid (26.4%).[30] A completion of comprehensive neck dissection is indicated after positive SLNB. 11.5% of the patients had additional positive nonsentinel lymph node, which was an independent prognostic factor for recurrence (HR: 1.78). All at-risk nodal stations must be cleared. An imaginary plane that passes through the external auditory canal has been used to divide primary melanomas into anterior and posterior lesions. The lesions anterior to this line neck dissection must include level I–V with superficial parotidectomy. The lesions posterior to this line will require posterolateral neck dissection.

Role of Radiation Therapy

The role of radiation as a primary modality treatment in a curative setting is limited. Various retrospective studies have shown efficacy of definitive primary radiation but with a higher relapse rate.[31,32] This could be due to the limitation in defining clinical and true (pathological) tumor borders.

Radiation plays an important role in reducing the risk of recurrence, especially in the nodal basin. Studies have shown that adjuvant RT was helpful in patients with positive excision margin, Breslow's thickness >4 mm and also lesions of head and neck, as achieving adequate margin in this region may be difficult due to complexity of the anatomy.[33-35] The only prospective phase III trial aimed at studying the benefit of adjuvant RT in patients with higher risk for nodal recurrence reported significantly lower nodal recurrence in the adjuvant RT group.[36] The trial included patients with ≥1 parotid node, ≥2 cervical nodes, ≥3 cm node in the neck and extranodal extension to be significant factors that affect the risk of nodal recurrence.

Adjuvant Systemic Therapy

Traditionally, high-dose interferon-α has been used as an adjuvant systemic treatment in melanoma patients to reduce risk of recurrence and has been widely studied and used over many years. Various trials are available that have shown improvement in recurrence-free survival and overall survival, but the meta-analysis from these trials has shown that the improvement in event-free and overall survival is <4%.[37] With the advent of targeted therapy and immune checkpoint inhibitors and various prospective randomized trials supporting their benefit in the adjuvant setting has almost replaced interferon-α as an adjuvant agent. The current NCCN recommendations do not support the use of interferon-α for adjuvant therapy in cutaneous melanoma. The SWOGS0008 phase III trial has shown the efficacy of a biochemotherapy regimen using cisplatin, vinblastine, dacarbazine, interleukin, and interferon-α with improved recurrence-free survival of 4 years versus 1.9 years in the high-dose interferon-α group.[38] Due to increased toxicity in high-dose interferon-α and biochemotherapy regimen, the current evidence recommends targeted therapy or immune checkpoint inhibitors in the adjuvant setting. The recommendations and evidence supporting their use have been described in **Table 4**.

Most of the trials that have studied the efficacy have not included in-transit disease in their inclusion criteria. In-transit disease can be managed with local therapy, regional therapy (that may not be useful in head and neck) and systemic therapy. Talimogene laherparepvec (T-VEC), a modified herpes virus, delivers localized expression of granulocyte-macrophage colony-stimulating factor inducing tumor cell lysis has shown durable response rate, overall response rate, and complete response in 16.3%, 26.4%, and 11.1%, which was significantly better than subcutaneous injection of GM-CSF in patients with in-transit metastasis.[44] Other modalities such as interleukin-2, Bacillus Calmette-Guérin, and Rose Bengal (a photosensitizing dye) have shown promising results but are not recommended in clinical use setting. Molecular targeted therapies/immune checkpoint inhibitors are not indicated in the induction setting.

Management of Distant Metastases

Rate of distant metastases in cutaneous melanoma is quite high. Molecular characterization of the metastatic tumor must be done to guide the planning of systemic therapy. Radiation therapy for painful bone metastasis can be advocated. BRAF inhibitors have shown radiosensitive property, hence, it can be used concurrently with RT. BRAF inhibitors are started >3 days before RT and >1 day before stereotactic radiosurgery (SRS) for brain metastasis. Limited oligometastases, if resectable, can be excised with negative margins. The NCCN recommendations and Food and Drug Administration (FDA) approved targeted therapy in metastatic and adjuvant therapy is described in **Table 5**.

Follow-up Strategy

Stage I/II patients should be examined every 6–12 months for the first 5 years then yearly for the next 5 years. Stage III/IV patients need closer follow-up with 3–6 monthly follow-up for the first 2 years, then 6–12 months next 3 years and annually for the next 5 years. Imaging with CT scan/MRI brain or PET-CT is recommended within the first 3 years of follow-up.[16] Ultrasound neck for patients with high-risk of regional recurrence can be advised. Sun protection strategies, as described in the chapter of nonmelanoma skin cancer, must be followed.

Table 4: Evidence supporting the use of targeted therapy and immune checkpoint inhibitors in the adjuvant setting of cutaneous melanoma.[16]

Trial	*Inclusion criteria (stage) (AJCC 7th Edition)*	*Treatment arms*	*Median follow-up (in years)*	*RFS/DFS*
Immune checkpoint inhibitors				
Eggermont et al.[39]	IIIA > 1 mm, IIIB/C	HD-Ipi Pbo	5.3	41 vs. 30% (5 years)
Weber et al.[40]	IIIB/C, IV	Nivo + Pbo HD-Ipi + Pbo	1.6	71 vs. 61% (1 year)
Eggermont et al.[41]	IIIA > 1 mm, IIIB/C	Pembro Pbo	1.2	75 vs. 61% (1 year)
BRAF targeted therapy				
Long et al.[42]	IIIA > 1 mm, IIIB/C	Dab + Tram Pbo	2.8	58 vs. 39% (3 years)
Maio et al.[43]	IIC, IIIA > 1 mm, IIIB/C	Vem Pbo	2.8	62 vs. 53% (2 years)

(DFS: disease-free survival; Ipi: ipilimumab; nivo: nivolumab; Pbo: placebo; pembro: pembrolizumab; RFS: recurrence-free survival; tram: trametinib; vem: vemurafenib)

Table 5: Indications and Food and Drug Administration (FDA) approval for molecular therapy in cutaneous melanoma in adjuvant and unresectable/metastatic setting.[16]

Agent	*Indication in unresectable/ metastatic melanoma*	*Indication in adjuvant therapy*
Immune checkpoint inhibitors		
Ipilimumab	Yes	Positive regional nodes postcomplete nodal dissection
Nivolumab	Yes	Positive regional nodes, adjuvant postsurgical excision of metastasis
Pembrolizumab	Yes	Positive regional nodes postcomplete nodal dissection
Ipilimumab/Nivolumab	Yes	Not approved
BRAF targeted therapy		
Dabrafenib	Yes with BRAF V600E +	Not approved
Vemurafenib	Yes with BRAFV600E +	Not approved
BRAF/MEK combinations		
Dabrafenib/Trametinib	Yes with BRAFV600E/K+	Positive regional nodes postcomplete nodal dissection with BRAFV600E +
Vemurafenib/Cobimetinib	Yes with BRAFV600E +	Not approved
Encorafenib/Binimetinib	Yes with BRAFV600E/K+	Not approved

Prognosis

Five years survival in Stages I, II, and III is >90%, 45–77% and 27–70%, respectively. For metastatic disease, the 5-year survival rate is <20%.[45]

MUCOSAL MELANOMA

Introduction

Primary mucosal melanoma (PMM) of the head and neck is one of the rare cancers. Head and neck region comprises more than half of all PMM in the body with the sinonasal tract being the most frequent followed by oral cavity, larynx, and pharynx. PMM accounts for 0.03% of all cancers and 1.3% of all melanoma.[46,47] 55% of PMM arise in head and neck region.[47] The prognosis of PMM of head and neck is worse than cutaneous melanomas. Due to rarity of the disease, most of the management strategies are derived from retrospective studies or extrapolated from cutaneous melanoma trials.

Etiology

The causative factor for PMM is unknown.[48] Even though most patients with sinonasal or laryngeal PMM are associated with smoking, its influence on causing melanoma is unknown. Racial pigmentation has seen no preponderance of PMM in one race over the other. PMM is mostly linked to embryology. Melanocytes migrate as neurocristic derivatives in endodermal or ectodermal mucosa, which could give rise to PMM.[49] Melanocytes are detected in oral cavity mucosa at 20 weeks of gestation and nonmigration of these melanocytes could result in PMM at a later stage.[50]

Like cutaneous malignancy, various genetic changes in the intracellular signaling pathway have been associated with PMM. C-*KIT* (CD117) is overexpressed in 80% of cases and somatic mutations of *KIT* are seen in 10–30% of cases.[50] *CD117* forms a potential target for therapy in PMM.

B-type Raf mutations are commonly seen in cutaneous melanoma, but is uncommon in PMM, seen only in <10% of cases.[51] RAS-MAPK pathway mutations are seen in 20% and overexpressed in >90% of PMM.[50] *CDKN2A* mutations are observed in 50% of PMM.[52]

Presentation and Evaluation

Commonly present in fifth to eighth decade of life with equal gender preponderance.[48] PMM of sinonasal region comprises <5% of all sinonasal malignancies.[53] They commonly affect the lateral wall of the nose and nasal septum. Most sinonasal PMM present at a late-stage, by which time discerning the anatomical origin of the tumor becomes difficult.[54] Among the paranasal sinuses, PMM most commonly affects the maxillary sinus, followed by ethmoid and sphenoid sinuses. Presenting symptoms are like any other tumors of the sinonasal region. Nasal PMM have a better prognosis than those involving sinuses, probably due to a higher rate of skull base, orbit and/or facial soft tissue involvement in sinuses. Evaluation of PMM in the sinonasal area must include CT scan and MRI to assess the extent of locoregional disease and determine resectability. In PMM of sinonasal region, nodal metastasis occurs in 10–20% and distant metastases in <10% distant metastases.[55] During the course of the disease, 40–50% develop distant metastases to lung, brain, bone, and liver.[56] Based on clinical observation, PMM of genitourinary tract were classified as unilocular or multilocular; the same was evaluated in the sinonasal region, and tumors that was multilocular (defined by the presence of multiple lesions in different location at diagnosis, with a margin of tumor-free cells) was associated with unfavorable disease-specific survival.[57]

Other Sites

Oral cavity of PMM is the next most common site and comprises 40% of all PMM in the head and neck region. Most of the lesions are situated in the upper maxillary ridge and hard palate.[48] Rate of lymph nodal metastasis is higher (25%) and the risk increases exponentially beyond the thickness of 5 mm.[58,59] Melanoma of the larynx and pharynx are less common. PMM of the nasopharynx is associated with regional and distant metastasis rates of 65% and 60%, respectively.[48]

Pathological evaluation is similar to cutaneous melanoma reporting.[60] Radiological imaging is based on the site involved. Distant metastasis workup is recommended in advanced cases, clinically palpable node and recurrent tumors.

Staging System

Primary mucosal melanoma of head and neck can be staged based on Ballantyne,[61] modified Prasad,[62] AJCC (7th edition) for mucosal melanoma of head and neck region[63] or carcinoma of the sinonasal region as per AJCC 8th edition, as shown in **Table 6**. The staging system proposed by Ballantyne is simple to use but is limited as no other prognostic factors such as size, local extension of tumor is taken into consideration. The AJCC, 7th edition, mucosal melanoma staging is not updated in the 8th edition. Michel et al. compared Ballantyne, modified Prasad, AJCC (7th edition) for mucosal melanoma of head and neck region and carcinoma of sinonasal region as per AJCC, 7th edition, staging system, and showed that carcinoma of sinonasal region as per AJCC, 7th edition, staging system proved to be the best predictor of disease-free and overall survival.[64]

Treatment

Locoregional Management

Surgery with adequate margins forms the mainstay of treatment. The important prognosticator of survival outcome in PMM is complete excision. Positive surgical margins are associated with a 21% increased risk of dying due to the disease.[65] Hence, local control must be achieved. Intraoperative frozen section assessment of margins is advocated as they correlate well with final histopathology report.[66] In most cases, there is a discrepancy in gross visible tumor and final histopathologically assessed tumor extent. Failure to achieve local control increases the risk of distant metastasis to 71%, as opposed to 14% in patients with good local control.[67] Local recurrence is difficult to salvage, as only 25% can be salvaged. Studies have shown the safety of endoscopic excision in nasal PMM with comparable outcomes as open surgery at 10 years follow-up.[68,69] Advanced cases of sinonasal region will require craniofacial resection to achieve adequate local control. Diseases of oral cavity, larynx, and pharynx are surgically treated based on resection principles of squamous cell carcinoma of the respective sites. Role of neck dissection in sinonasal PMM may be conservative due to the lower rate of nodal metastases. However, oral cavity is associated with higher rate of nodal metastases and hence the neck must be addressed electively. Role of SLNB is sinonasal tumors has been studied, but their routine clinical use is difficult to define.[70,71]

Radiotherapy

Melanoma is traditionally regarded as radioresistant tumor. The proximity of vital structures, especially in sinonasal region, may limit the use of radiation in this region. Newer technologies such as intensity-modulated radiation therapy, volumetric-modulated arc therapy, tomotherapy, carbon-ion therapy, neutrons, and proton therapy have allowed improved dose gradient and dose painting within the RT field. Indication for adjuvant RT is in sinonasal PMM where margin assessment is difficult, extensive tumor and positive margins.[72] RT in the

Table 6: Staging systems for primary mucosal melanoma of the head and neck.

Ballantyne 1970[61]	*Prasad 2004*[62]	*Mucosal melanoma TNM 2009*[63]		
Stage I: Any T N0 M0 *Stage II*: Any T N+ M0 *Stage III*: Any T Any N0 M+	*Level I:* In situ *Level II:* Invasion to lamina propria *Level III:* Deep tissue invasion	*T3:* Epithelial/submucosal (limited to mucosa) *T4a:* Deep soft tissue, cartilage, bone *T4b:* Involvement of brain, dura, skull base	*N0:* No regional nodes *N1:* Regional nodes positive *M0:* No distant metastasis *M1:* Presence of distant metastasis	*Stage III:* T3N0 *Stage IVa:* T4aN0, T3/T4aN1 *Stage IVb:* T4b Stage IVc M1

adjuvant setting has shown improvement in local control in doses >54 Gy. Various studies have proven improved locoregional control with no benefit on survival, as the rate of distant metastases is not affected by postoperative radiation.[48,72]

Definitive RT can be administered in advanced, recurrent tumors, unresectable tumors where photons, neutrons, or carbon ions therapy has shown local control of 61–85%.[73]

Systemic Therapy

Role of systemic therapy in PMM is extrapolated from cutaneous melanoma evidence. Molecular profiling in PMM is recommended to include identification of alterations in *KIT, BRAF*, and *N-RAS*. Biochemotherapy has shown promising results in unresectable, metastatic PMM tumors.[74] The role of targeted therapy in unresectable PMM is limited with most studies showing a low response rate. Imatinib has shown response of 26% and ipilimumab a response rate of 6–12%.[75] Further studies are required to optimize targeted therapy in PMM.

Prognosis

Most studies have shown 5-year overall survival of <30%.[76] The prognosticators of outcome in PMM are surgical margin status, tumor thickness >5 mm, clinical-stage, >10 mitotic figures per high power field, lymphovascular invasion, age >70 years and amelanotic subtype.[48,54,77]

Follow-up Strategy

No defined recommendations for follow-up of PMM exist. The follow-up recommendation similar to that of squamous cell carcinoma counterparts in their respective subsite may be followed.

CONCLUSION

Cutaneous melanomas are aggressive tumors. Tumor resection with adequate margins forms the cornerstone of management in this group of patents. Molecular characterization of the tumor in melanoma is essential. With the recent trend of targeted therapies and immunotherapy, the survival of cutaneous melanoma patients has significantly improved. PMM of the head and neck are rare and carry worse prognosis than their cutaneous counterparts. Use of targeted therapy in the adjuvant setting for PMM is yet to be defined.

REFERENCES

1. Bodenham DC. Malignant melanoma of the head and neck. Excerpta Medica; 1975. pp. 85-91.
2. Conley J, Hamaker RC. Melanoma of the head and neck. The Laryngoscope. 1977;87(5):760-4.
3. Franklin JD, Reynolds VH, Bowers JD, Lynch JB. Cutaneous melanoma of the head and neck. Clin Plast Surg. 1976;3(3): 413-27.
4. Kosary CL, Altekruse SF, Ruhl J, Lee R, Dickie L. Clinical and prognostic factors for melanoma of the skin using SEER registries: collaborative stage data collection system, version 1 and version 2. Cancer. 2014;120:3807-14.
5. Nikolaou V, Stratigos AJ. Emerging trends in the epidemiology of melanoma. Br J Dermatol. 2014;170(1):11-9.
6. Ekwueme DU, Guy Jr GP, Li C, Rim SH, Parelkar P, Chen SC. The health burden and economic costs of cutaneous melanoma mortality by race/ethnicity-United States, 2000 to 2006. J Am Acad Dermatol. 2011;65(5):S133-e1.
7. Jhappan C, Noonan FP, Merlino G. Ultraviolet radiation and cutaneous malignant melanoma. Oncogene. 2003;22(20): 3099-112.
8. Bataille V, Bishop JA, Sasieni P, Swerdlow AJ, Pinney E, Griffiths K, et al. Risk of cutaneous melanoma in relation to the numbers, types and sites of naevi: a case-control study. Br J Cancer. 1996;73(12):1605-11.
9. Nelson AA, Tsao H. Melanoma and genetics. Clin Dermatol. 2009;27(1):46-52.
10. Cleaver JE. Cancer in xeroderma pigmentosum and related disorders of DNA repair. Nat Rev Cancer. 2005;5(7):564-73.
11. Watt AJ, Kotsis SV, Chung KC. Risk of melanoma arising in large congenital melanocytic nevi: a systematic review. Plast Reconstruct Surg. 2004;113(7):1968-74.
12. Russo AE, Torrisi E, Bevelacqua Y, Perrotta R, Libra M, McCubrey JA, et al. Melanoma: molecular pathogenesis and emerging target therapies. Int J Oncol. 2009;34(6):1481-9.
13. Kibbi N, Kluger H, Choi JN. Melanoma: clinical presentations. In: Kaufman HL, Mehnert JM (Eds). Melanoma: Cancer Treatment and Research. Cham: Springer; 2016. pp. 107-29.
14. Mahoney KM, Freeman GJ, McDermott DF. The next immune-checkpoint inhibitors: PD-1/PD-L1 blockade in melanoma. Clinical therapeutics. 2015;37(4):764-82.
15. Lee JJ, Lian CG. Molecular testing for cutaneous melanoma: an update and review. Arch Pathol Lab Med. 2019;143(7): 811-20.
16. National Comprehensive Cancer Network. (2020). NCCN Clinical Practice Guidelines in Oncology (NCCN Guidelines VR) cutaneous melanoma 2.2020. National Comprehensive Cancer Network, Inc.; 2020. [online] Available from NCCN.org. [Last accessed July, 2020].
17. Ward WH, Lambreton F, Goel N, Jian QY, Farma JM. Clinical presentation and staging of melanoma. In: Ward WH, Farma JM (Eds). Cutaneous Melanoma: Etiology and Therapy [Internet]. Brisbane (AU): Codon Publications; 2017.
18. Ohsie SJ, Sarantopoulos GP, Cochran AJ, Binder SW. Immunohistochemical characteristics of melanoma. J Cutan Pathol. 2008;35(5):433-44.
19. Frishberg DP, Balch C, Balzer BL, Crowson AN, Didolkar M, McNiff JM, et al. Protocol for the examination of specimens from patients with melanoma of the skin. Arch Pathol Lab Med. 2009;133(10):1560-7.
20. Jiménez-Requena F, Delgado-Bolton RC, Fernández-Pérez C, Gambhir SS, Schwimmer J, Pérez-Vázquez JM, et al. Meta-analysis of the performance of ^{18}F-FDG PET in cutaneous melanoma. Eur J Nucl Med Mole Imag. 2010;37(2):284-300.
21. Gershenwald JE, Scolyer RA, Hess KR, Sondak VK, Long GV, Ross MI, et al. Melanoma staging: evidence-based changes in the American Joint Committee on Cancer eighth edition

cancer staging manual. CA: A Cancer J Clin. 2017;67(6): 472-92.
22. Veronesi U, Cascinelli N. Narrow excision (1-cm margin): a safe procedure for thin cutaneous melanoma. Arch Surg. 1991;126(4):438-41.
23. Veronesi U, Cascinelli N, Adamus J, Balch C, Bandiera D, Barchuk A, et al. Thin stage I primary cutaneous malignant melanoma. N Engl J Med. 1988;318(18):1159-62.
24. Cohn-Cedermark G, Rutqvist LE, Andersson R, Breivald M, Ingvar C, Johansson H, et al. Long-term results of a randomized study by the Swedish Melanoma Study Group on 2-cm versus 5-cm resection margins for patients with cutaneous melanoma with a tumor thickness of 0.8–2.0 mm. Cancer: Interdiscipl Int J Am Cancer Soc. 2000;89(7):1495-501.
25. Khayat D, Rixe O, Martin G, Soubrane C, Banzet M, Bazex JA, et al. Surgical margins in cutaneous melanoma (2 cm versus 5 cm for lesions measuring less than 2.1-mm thick) Long-term results of a large European multicentric phase III study. Cancer: Interdiscipl Int J Am Cancer Soc. 2003;97(8):1941-6.
26. Gillgren P, Drzewiecki KT, Niin M, Gullestad HP, Hellborg H, Månsson-Brahme E, et al. 2-cm versus 4-cm surgical excision margins for primary cutaneous melanoma thicker than 2 mm: a randomised, multicentre trial. The Lancet. 2011;378(9803):1635-42.
27. Hayes AJ, Maynard L, Coombes G, Newton-Bishop J, Timmons M, Cook M, et al. Wide versus narrow excision margins for high-risk, primary cutaneous melanomas: long-term follow-up of survival in a randomised trial. The Lancet Oncol. 2016;17(2):184-92.
28. Morton DL, Cochran AJ, Thompson JF, Elashoff R, Essner R, Glass EC, et al. Sentinel node biopsy for early-stage melanoma: accuracy and morbidity in MSLT-I, an international multicenter trial. Ann Surg. 2005;242(3):302.
29. Sondak VK, King DW, Zager JS, Schneebaum S, Kim J, Leong SP, et al. Combined analysis of phase III trials evaluating [99m Tc] tilmanocept and vital blue dye for identification of sentinel lymph nodes in clinically node-negative cutaneous melanoma. Ann Surg Oncol. 2013;20(2):680-8.
30. Loree TR, Tomljanovich PI, Cheney RT, Hicks Jr WL, Rigual NR. Intraparotid sentinel lymph node biopsy for head and neck melanoma. The Laryngoscope. 2006;116(8):1461-4.
31. Hedblad MA, Mallbris L. Grenz ray treatment of lentigo maligna and early lentigo maligna melanoma. J Am Acad Dermatol. 2012;67(1):60-8.
32. Fogarty GB, Hong A, Scolyer RA, Lin E, Haydu L, Guitera P, et al. Radiotherapy for lentigo maligna: a literature review and recommendations for treatment. Br J Dermatol. 2014; 170(1):52-8.
33. Agrawal S, Kane III JM, Guadagnolo BA, Kraybill WG, Ballo MT. The benefits of adjuvant radiation therapy after therapeutic lymphadenectomy for clinically advanced, high-risk, lymph node-metastatic melanoma. Cancer: Interdiscipl Int J Am Cancer Soc. 2009;115(24):5836-44.
34. Pinkham MB, Foote MC, Burmeister E, Thomas J, Meakin J, Smithers BM, et al. Stage III melanoma in the axilla: patterns of regional recurrence after surgery with and without adjuvant radiation therapy. Int J Radiat Oncol Biol Phys. 2013; 86(4):702-8.
35. Strojan P, Jančar B, Čemažar M, Perme MP, Hočevar M. Melanoma metastases to the neck nodes: role of adjuvant irradiation. Int J Radiat Oncol Biol Phys. 2010;77(4):1039-45.
36. Henderson MA, Burmeister BH, Ainslie J, Fisher R, Di Iulio J, Smithers BM, et al. Adjuvant lymph-node field radiotherapy versus observation only in patients with melanoma at high risk of further lymph-node field relapse after lymphadenectomy (ANZMTG 01.02/TROG 02.01): 6-year follow-up of a phase 3, randomised controlled trial. The Lancet Oncol. 2015; 16(9):1049-60.
37. Ives NJ, Suciu S, Eggermont AM, Kirkwood J, Lorigan P, Markovic SN, et al. Adjuvant interferon-α for the treatment of high-risk melanoma: an individual patient data meta-analysis. Eur J Cancer. 2017;82:171-83.
38. Flaherty LE, Moon J, Atkins MB, Tuthill R, Thompson JA, Vetto JT, et al. Phase III trial of high-dose interferon alpha-2b versus cisplatin, vinblastine, DTIC plus IL-2 and interferon in patients with high-risk melanoma (SWOG S0008): An intergroup study of cancer and leukemia Group B, Children's Oncology Group, Eastern Cooperative Oncology Group, and Southwest Oncology Group. J Clin Oncol: Official J Am Soc Clin Oncol. 2014;32(33):3771-8.
39. Eggermont AM, Chiarion-Sileni V, Grob JJ, Dummer R, Wolchok JD, Schmidt H, et al. Prolonged survival in stage III melanoma with ipilimumab adjuvant therapy. N Engl J Med. 2016;375(19):1845-55.
40. Weber J, Mandala M, Del Vecchio M, Gogas HJ, Arance AM, Cowey CL, et al. Adjuvant nivolumab versus ipilimumab in resected stage III or IV melanoma. N Engl J Med. 2017;377(19):1824-35.
41. Eggermont AM, Blank CU, Mandala M, Long GV, Atkinson V, Dalle S, et al. Adjuvant pembrolizumab versus placebo in resected stage III melanoma. N Engl J Med. 2018;378(19):1789-801.
42. Long GV, Hauschild A, Santinami M, Atkinson V, Mandalà M, Chiarion-Sileni V, et al. Adjuvant dabrafenib plus trametinib in stage III BRAF-mutated melanoma. N Engl J Med. 2017; 377(19):1813-23.
43. Maio M, Lewis K, Demidov L, Mandalà M, Bondarenko I, Ascierto PA, et al. Adjuvant vemurafenib in resected, BRAFV600 mutation-positive melanoma (BRIM8): a randomised, double-blind, placebo-controlled, multicentre, phase 3 trial. The Lancet Oncol. 2018;19(4):510-20.
44. Andtbacka RH, Kaufman HL, Collichio F, Amatruda T, Senzer N, Chesney J, et al. Talimogene laherparepvec improves durable response rate in patients with advanced melanoma. J Clin Oncol. 2015;33(25):2780-8.
45. Tas F. Metastatic behavior in melanoma: timing, pattern, survival, and influencing factors. J Oncol. 2012;2012.
46. Jangard M, Hansson J, Ragnarsson-Olding B. Primary sinonasal malignant melanoma: a nationwide study of the Swedish population, 1960-2000. Rhinology. 2013;51(1):22-30.
47. Chang AE, Karnell LH, Menck HR. The National Cancer Data Base report on cutaneous and noncutaneous melanoma: a summary of 84,836 cases from the past decade. Cancer: Interdiscipl Int J Am Cancer Soc. 1998;83(8):1664-78.
48. López F, Rodrigo JP, Cardesa A, Triantafyllou A, Devaney KO, Mendenhall WM, et al. Update on primary head and neck mucosal melanoma. Head Neck. 2016;38(1):147-55.
49. Gorsky M, Epstein JB. Melanoma arising from the mucosal surfaces of the head and neck. Oral Surg Oral Med Oral Pathol Oral Radiol Endodontol. 1998;86(6):715-9.
50. Lourenço SV, Fernandes JD, Hsieh R, Coutinho-Camillo CM, Bologna S, Sangueza M, et al. Head and neck mucosal melanoma: a review. Am J Dermatopathol. 2014;36(7):578-87.
51. Chraybi M, Alsamad IA, Copie-Bergman C, Baia M, André J, Dumaz N, et al. Oncogene abnormalities in a series of primary melanomas of the sinonasal tract: NRAS mutations and

cyclin D1 amplification are more frequent than KIT or BRAF mutations. Human Pathol. 2013;44(9):1902-11.
52. Turri-Zanoni M, Medicina D, Lombardi D, Ungari M, Balzarini P, Rossini C, et al. Sinonasal mucosal melanoma: molecular profile and therapeutic implications from a series of 32 cases. Head Neck. 2013;35(8):1066-77.
53. Mendenhall WM, Amdur RJ, Hinerman RW, Werning JW, Villaret DB, Mendenhall NP. Head and neck mucosal melanoma. Am J Clin Oncol. 2005;28(6):626-30.
54. Moreno MA, Roberts DB, Kupferman ME, DeMonte F, El-Naggar AK, Williams M, et al. Mucosal melanoma of the nose and paranasal sinuses, a contemporary experience from the MD Anderson Cancer Center. Cancer. 2010;116(9):2215-23.
55. Rinaldo A, Shaha AR, Patel SG, Ferlito A. Primary mucosal melanoma of the nasal cavity and paranasal sinuses. Acta Otolaryngol. 2001;121(8):979-82.
56. Medhi P, Biswas M, Das D, Amed S. Cytodiagnosis of mucosal malignant melanoma of nasal cavity: A case report with review of literature. J Cytol/Indian Acad Cytol. 2012;29(3):208-13.
57. Rossi OS, Vital D, Soyka MB, Roth TN, Huber GF, Holzmann D. Multilocular sinonasal malignant melanoma: a poor prognostic subgroup. Eur Arch Otorhinolaryngol. 2015;272(1):123-9.
58. Umeda M, Shimada K. Primary malignant melanoma of the oral cavity—its histological classification and treatment. Br J Oral Maxillofacial Surg. 1994;32(1):39-47.
59. Patel SG, Prasad ML, Escrig M, Singh B, Shaha AR, Kraus DH, et al. Primary mucosal malignant melanoma of the head and neck. Head Neck: J Sci Specialt Head Neck. 2002;24(3):247-57.
60. Prasad ML, Jungbluth AA, Iversen K, Huvos AG, Busam KJ. Expression of melanocytic differentiation markers in malignant melanomas of the oral and sinonasal mucosa. Am J Surg Pathol. 2001;25(6):782-7.
61. Ballantyne AJ. Malignant melanoma of the skin of the head and neck: an analysis of 405 cases. American J Surg. 1970; 120(4):425-31.
62. Prasad ML, Patel SG, Huvos AG, Shah JP, Busam KJ. Primary mucosal melanoma of the head and neck: a proposal for microstaging localized, stage I (lymph node-negative) tumors. Cancer: Interdiscipl Int J Am Cancer Soc. 2004;100(8): 1657-64.
63. Edge SB, Compton CC. The American Joint Committee on Cancer: the 7th edition of the AJCC cancer staging manual and the future of TNM. Ann Surg Oncol. 2010;17(6):1471-4.
64. Michel J, Perret-Court A, Fakhry N, Braustein D, Monestier S, Richard MA, et al. Sinonasal mucosal melanomas: the prognostic value of tumor classifications. Head Neck. 2014; 36(3):311-6.
65. Penel N, Mallet Y, Mirabel X, Van JT, Lefebvre JL. Primary mucosal melanoma of head and neck: prognostic value of clear margins. Laryngoscope. 2006;116(6):993-5.
66. Tajudeen BA, Vorasubin N, Sanaiha Y, Palma-Diaz MF, Suh JD, Wang MB. Sinonasal mucosal melanoma: 20-year experience at a tertiary referral center. Int Forum Allergy Rhinol. 2014; 4(7):592-7.
67. Lee SP, Shimizu KT, Tran LM, Juillard G, Calcaterra TC. Mucosal melanoma of the head and neck: the impact of local control on survival. Laryngoscope. 1994;104(2):121-6.
68. Lund VJ, Stammberger H, Nicolai P, Castelnuovo P, Beal T, Beham A, et al. European position paper on endoscopic management of tumours of the nose, paranasal sinuses and skull base. Rhinol Suppl. 2010;22:1-43.
69. Nicolai P, Battaglia P, Bignami M, Villaret AB, Delu G, Khrais T, et al. Endoscopic surgery for malignant tumors of the sinonasal tract and adjacent skull base: a 10-year experience. Am J Rhinol. 2008;22(3):308-16.
70. Sta I, Koranda P, Beneš P. Sentinel lymph node biopsy: a new perspective in head and neck mucosal melanoma. Melanoma Res. 2006;16(5):423-7.
71. Baptista P, Velloso MJ, Salvinelli F, Casale M. Radioguided surgical strategy in mucosal melanoma of the nasal cavity. Clin Nucl Med. 2008;33(1):14-8.
72. Liao JJ, Parvathaneni U, Laramore GE, Thompson JA, Bhatia S, Futran ND, et al. Fast neutron radiotherapy for primary mucosal melanomas of the head and neck. Head Neck. 2014;36(8):1162-7.
73. Krengli M, Masini L, Kaanders JH, Maingon P, Oei SB, Zouhair A, et al. Radiotherapy in the treatment of mucosal melanoma of the upper aerodigestive tract: analysis of 74 cases. A Rare Cancer Network study. Int J Radiat Oncol Biol Phys. 2006;65(3):751-9.
74. Bartell HL, Bedikian AY, Papadopoulos NE, Dett TK, Ballo MT, Myers JN, et al. Biochemotherapy in patients with advanced head and neck mucosal melanoma. Head Neck: J Sci Spec Head Neck. 2008;30(12):1592-8.
75. Guo J, Si L, Kong Y, Flaherty KT, Xu X, Zhu Y, et al. Phase II, open-label, single-arm trial of imatinib mesylate in patients with metastatic melanoma harboring c-Kit mutation or amplification. J Clin Oncol. 2011;29(21):2904-9.
76. Jethanamest D, Vila PM, Sikora AG, Morris LG. Predictors of survival in mucosal melanoma of the head and neck. Ann Surg Oncol. 2011;18(10):2748-56.
77. Shuman AG, Light E, Olsen SH, Pynnonen MA, Taylor JM, Johnson TM, et al. Mucosal melanoma of the head and neck: predictors of prognosis. Arch Otolaryngol Head Neck Surg. 2011;137(4):331-7.

CHAPTER 22

Nonmelanoma Skin Cancers of the Head and Neck

Samskruthi P Murthy, Sivakumar Vidhyadharan, Narayana Subramaniam

INTRODUCTION

Skin cancers are among the most frequent cancers worldwide, especially in the Caucasian population. Skin cancers comprise 20–30% of all cancers in Caucasians and 1–2% of all cancers in Black and Asian populations.[1] The skin is the largest organ and is primarily composed of two layers, the epidermis and dermis. Different cell-types result in a range of diverse tumors. Basal and squamous cell carcinomas arise from keratinocytes, melanoma arises from melanocytes, sebaceous cyst carcinoma arises from sebaceous glands in dermis and Merkel cell carcinoma (MCC) is hypothesized to arise from Merkel cells. Based on the cell of origin, skin cancers can be broadly classified into melanoma and nonmelanoma skin cancers (NMSC). NMSC can be further classified as epithelial and nonepithelial skin cancers **(Flowchart 1)**.

ANATOMY OF THE SKIN

The epidermis consists of keratinocytes, melanocytes, Merkel cells, and Langerhans cells. The epidermis is subdivided into strata basale, spinosum, granulosum, and corneum (from deep to superficial). Stratum basale is connected to the dermis by the basement membrane. Dermis contains the neurovascular component of the skin and consists of papillary deeper reticular layers. The dermis is primarily composed of collagen and elastin, which is formed by fibroblasts. This layer also mounts sweat glands (sebaceous glands). The dermis overlies subcutaneous tissue also called as hypodermis. The subcutaneous tissue consists of fat, perforating blood vessels, superficial fascia and nerves. Subcutaneous tissue anchors skin to deeper muscles and bone.

Flowchart 1: Classification of skin cancers.

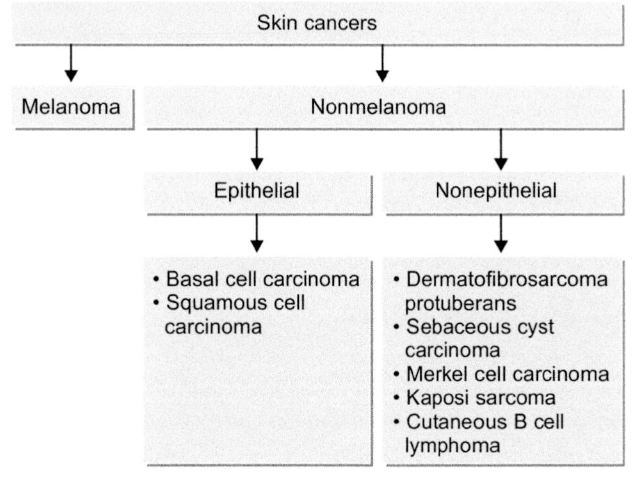

NONMELANOMA SKIN CANCERS

Epithelial Skin Cancers

Nonmelanoma skin cancers are more common than melanoma in the head and neck region. Majority of NMSC consists of epithelial skin cancers [basal cell carcinoma (BCC) and cutaneous squamous cell carcinoma (cSCC)]. There has been 65% increase in the incidence of NMSC since 1980, but the incidence has plateaued since 2000. The exact incidence of NMSC in India is uncertain.[2]

Epidemiology and Carcinogenesis

Cutaneous squamous cell carcinoma and BCC arise from keratinocytes. Ultraviolet radiation (UVR) exposure is the primary etiologic factor in causation of NMSC with ultraviolet B (UVB-wavelength is 290–320 nm) playing a pivotal role in the induction of skin cancer. Depletion of ozone layer further accentuates UV exposure with a 2–4% increase in incidence for every 1% reduction in the ozone layer.[3] The low incidence of NMSC among dark skinned people is attributed to the protective nature of epidermal melanin, with a protection factor of up to 13.4% in Black populations. The epidermis in

Table 1: List of genetic disorders linked to nonmelanoma skin cancers (NMSC).

Condition	*Transmission*	*Gene involved*	*Function*
Conditions increasing risk of basal cell carcinoma:			
Basal cell nevus syndrome	AD	*PTCH1, PTCH2,* and *SUFU*	Hedgehog signaling pathway
Bazex–Dupré–Christol syndrome	XLD	Unknown	DNA repair and regulation of cell cycle
Conditions increasing risk of cutaneous squamous cell carcinoma:			
Xeroderma pigmentosum	AR	*XPA-XPG* and *XPV*	Nucleotide excision repair
Multiple self-healing squamous epithelioma	AD	*TGFBR1*	TGF-β signal transduction
Oculocutaneous albinism	AR	*TYR, OCA2, TYRP1, SLC45A2*	Melanin synthesis
Epidermodysplasia verruciformis	AR	*EVER1* and *EVER2*	Signal transduction in endoplasmic reticulum
Dyskeratosis congenita	AD	*TERC, TINF2, TERT, RTEL1*	Telomere maintenance and trafficking
Huriez syndrome	AD	Unknown	Unknown
Rothmund–Thomson syndrome	AR	*RECQL4* and *C16Orf57*	Chromosomal stability, telomere maintenance and trafficking
Bloom syndrome	AR	*BLM/RECQL3*	Chromosomal stability
Werner syndrome	AR	*WRN/RECQL2*	Chromosomal stability

(AD: autosomal dominant; AR: autosomal recessive; BLM: Bloom syndrome; DNA: deoxyribonucleic acid; *EVER1*: epidermodysplasia verruciformis 1; *EVER2*: epidermodysplasia verruciformis 2; *OCA2*: oculocutaneous albinism type II; *PTCH1*: protein patched homolog 1; *PTCH2*: protein patched homolog 2; *RECQL2*: RecQ Protein-Like 2; *RECQL3*: RecQ Protein-Like 3; *RTEL1*: regulator of telomere elongation helicase 1; *SUFU*: suppressor of fused protein; *TERC*: telomerase RNA component; *TINF2*: TERF1 interacting nuclear factor 2; *TERT*: telomerase reverse transcriptase; TGF-β: transforming growth factor-β; *TYR*: tyrosinase; *TYRP1*: tyrosinase-related protein 1; XLD: X-linked dominant)

dark-skinned subjects transmits only 7.4% of UVB and 17.4% of UVA while that of white-skinned individuals transmit 24% and 55%, respectively.[4] Dark-skinned individuals have larger and more melanized melanosomes, which is protective. A 6–33 times greater dose of UVR is required to cause perceptible erythema among dark-skinned than fair-skinned people.[4]

Ultraviolet B radiation causes pyridine adducts by inducing covalent bonding between pyrimidine and results in photomutagenic substances (pyrimidine—pyrimidine and cyclopyrimidine dimers), while UVB causes reactive oxygen radicals by photo-oxidative stress-mediated mechanisms. The effect of UVA is indirect DNA damage. About 90% of cSCC and 50% BCC have shown a mutated variant of p53 positivity.[5] Inactivation of p53 as a consequence of UVR results in clonal expansion of keratinocytes due to resistance to apoptosis.

Association of human papillomavirus (HPV) with skin cancers has been studied and has shown that DNA from HPV subtypes has been identified in 90% of NMSC among immunocompromised and 50% of immunocompetent patients.[6] However, no specific type of HPV has shown any strong association with skin cancers, unlike in cervical or oropharyngeal cancers.

The sonic hedgehog pathway plays a vital role in the causation of BCC and has been studied extensively as a critical target for chemotherapy. Patched 1 gene on chromosome 9q encodes for the sonic hedgehog receptor, which is mutated in approximately 30–90% of sporadic BCC.[7]

Indoor tanning is being increasingly used in the White population, with an estimated incidence of exposure of 35% of the general population in the US, with the incidence higher among university students. A large meta-analysis has shown that indoor tanning is associated with cSCC with a 67% higher risk when compared to those nonexposed.[8] Various genetic disorders associated with NMSC are listed in **Table 1**.

Various other etiologic factors such as arsenic, coal tar, and radiation therapy also play a role in carcinogenesis of NMSC. BCC commonly occurs in areas of previous radiation therapy.[5] Immune deficient patients are prone to skin cancers. Renal transplant patients have 18 times higher risk of developing skin cancer than controls. Patients with NMSC have increased risk of developing synchronous or metachronous NMSC, with an incidence as high as 39% in one of the studies.[2]

PRESENTATION AND EVALUATION

Basal Cell Carcinoma

Basal cell carcinoma commonly described as rodent ulcer presents with indurated borders and a deep ulcerated center. Various forms are described namely nodular, cystic, morphoeic or infiltrative, micronodular, superficial and pigmented each with a characteristic appearance. Approximately 30–40% of BCC are mixed type.[9] Even though clinical presentation is almost diagnostic, superficial lesion may be difficult to identify and are commonly misdiagnosed as other skin disorders such as psoriasis, which can mimic superficial BCC. Morphoeic or infiltrative type has ill-defined margins are also hard to notice and most often present late. BCC are proposed to occur along with embryonic fusion lines in the head and neck region, but this notion has been challenged.

Deep biopsy to include deep reticular dermis is the gold standard for diagnosis of BCC; superficial biopsies are not advisable. On histopathology, BCC is characterized by basaloid cells that proliferate parallel to epidermis arranged in strands or nodules.[10] Morpheaform or infiltrative BCC is characterized by poorly circumscribed deeply infiltrative borders, with infiltration commonly seen into the reticular dermis.[10]

BerEP4 is a monoclonal antibody that binds to glycoproteins expressed in human epithelial cells. Immunohistochemistry (IHC) stain for BerEp4 can be used to distinguish BCC from cSCC as all subtypes of BCC stain strongly positive for BerEp4 while cSCC does not.[11]

Cutaneous Squamous Cell Carcinoma

Cutaneous squamous cell carcinoma presents in sun-exposed areas of the body and are commonly associated with precancerous lesions such as actinic keratitis or Bowen's disease. Appearance of induration is usually the first sign of malignant transformation in a pre-existing skin lesion. cSCC usually presents with ill-defined edges and adhered crusts. Deep biopsy to include deep reticular dermis is the gold standard for diagnosis of cSCC. Histologically, cSCC is an epithelial tumor with dermal infiltration and signs of cornification. Degree of differentiation is based on level of keratinization and can be classified as well—moderate—poorly differentiated tumors. The Broder's classification of four-tier grading system into grade I–IV can also be used.[12] The common variants of cSCC are adenosquamous, verrucous, and spindle-cell carcinoma.[13] Spindle-cell carcinoma is associated with occurrence of spindle-shaped cells with minimal differentiation and may sometimes be difficult to distinguish from sarcomas. In such situation, IHC stains with cytokeratin (CK) and epithelial membrane antigen (EMA) will be strongly positive in cSCC. Spindle-cell carcinoma is commonly seen in immuno-compromised and irradiated skin. Verrucous SCC is very rare and classically presents with endo-exophytic growth, hyperkeratosis, acanthosis, mild atypia, and good differentiation. The borders are pushing than infiltrating. *Adenosquamous SCC* is also a rare variant, which presents with true mucin secreting glandular differentiation within foci of SCC. The probable origin of cell could be pluripotent epithelial cells near or within sacral segments of sweat glands. These tumors are highly aggressive with high rate of recurrence and metastasis.

IMAGING

The American Association of Dermatologists has detailed the indications for imaging in NMSC.[14] The indications are as follows:

- *Probable bone involvement:* Bone invasion especially in tumors (both cSCC and BCC) involving scalp, periorbital region has a tendency to involve bone. Clinical fixation of the tumor is an obvious sign, but in suspected recurrent cases, there is a higher chance of subclinical erosion of the bone CT scan is recommended. High resolution of CT scan with detailed bone cuts helps in evaluating the extent of bone involvement.
- *Probable orbital involvement:* Tumors involving medial canthus of the eye have a higher predilection for orbital involvement. Clinical signs such as restriction in movement of the eyeball are obvious, but early invasion is difficult to define clinically. MRI with contrast enhancement is ideal for studying changes in the intraorbital fat which T1-weighted contrast-enhanced fat-suppressed images giving the best delineation of early tumor involvement.
- *Assessment of deep soft tissue extension:* The depth of extension in infiltrating tumors may be difficult to assess in areas with complex anatomy such as perioral, periorbital, and periaural region. Contrast-enhanced MRI gives a better soft tissue delineation than CT scan.
- *Evaluation of regional nodes and distant metastasis:* Basal cell carcinomas are rarely metastatic. Nodal involvement and distant metastatic involvement needs to be assessed in high-risk cSCC. The imaging that gives best delineation of primary can be used to assess draining lymph nodes as well. The diagnostic criteria are same as mucosal head and neck SCC.
- *Suspected cases of perineural spread:* Involvement of second and third division of trigeminal nerve and facial nerve is common. PNI is rarely reported in BCC but is more common in cSCC. Clinical evidence of PNI may be evident and must be suspected when tumors are present in areas of close proximity to major nerves.

- *Postoperative surveillance for recurrent disease:* When tumors are resected and reconstructed with either local or distant flap or large surrounding tissue re-arrangement, assessment of recurrent disease becomes difficult. In such cases, imaging may be required for surveillance.

Noninvasive Imaging Tools

With rising incidence of skin cancers, noninvasive imaging tools have emerged to screen, diagnose, and monitor patients with cutaneous malignancy.[15] Dermatoscopy is a noninvasive microscopic technique, which uses incident light with reduction specular reflectance either with interface fluid or polarized light. It helps to differentiate between pigmented BCC and melanoma. Confocal microscopy (CM) is a noninvasive method, which provided cellular level resolution with serial optical sections up to a depth of papillary dermis. Optical coherence tomography (OCT) uses low coherence light source to image nontransparent tissues. Unlike CM, OCT provides structural resolution up to a depth of reticular dermis. Use of these techniques needs training and cannot be used routinely by everyone. However, biopsy with histopathology evaluation remains the gold standard in diagnosing skin cancer; the role of noninvasive imaging is only in high-risk condition when lesions to be biopsied are to be triaged based on noninvasive techniques. A combination of CM or OCT along with dermascope helps in better refinement of dermatoscopic findings with better depth evaluation capacity.

STAGING AND RISK STRATIFICATION

The American Joint Committee on Cancer (AJCC) 8th edition, which is classically used to stage cancers, has made the following changes from previous staging system **(Table 2)**.

- Primary tumor size cut-off of 4 cm was introduced to distinguish T2 and T3.
- Depth of invasion (DOI) of >6 mm and perineural invasion (PNI) ≥ 1 mm is now considered as T3.

The AJCC has grouped both cSCC and BCC for staging and thus may not represent all the risk factors important for prognostication. The National Comprehensive Cancer Network (NCCN) recommends the following features as high risk in BCC.[16]

- *Location:* Presence of tumor in area which constitutes central face, eyelids, eyebrows, periorbital skin, nose, lips, chin, mandible, preauricular and postauricular skin/sulci, temple, and ear.

Table 2: The American Joint Committee on Cancer (AJCC), 8th edition, T-staging in nonmelanoma skin cancers (NMSC).

Category	*Definition*
Tx	Primary tumor cannot be assessed
Tis	Carcinoma in situ
T1	Tumor ≤2 cm in the greatest dimension
T2	Tumor >2 cm, but ≤4 cm in the greatest dimension
T3	Tumor >4 cm in maximum dimension or minor bone erosion or perineural invasion or deep invasion
T4	*T4a:* Tumor with gross cortical bone/marrow invasion
	T4b: Tumor with skull base invasion and/or skull-base foramen involvement

Deep invasion defined as invasion beyond the subcutaneous fat or >6 mm as measured from the granular layer of adjacent normal epidermis to the base of tumor.
Perineural invasion defined as tumor cells within the nerve sheath of a nerve lying deeper than the dermis or measuring 0.1 mm or larger in caliber or presenting with clinical or radiological involvement of named nerves without skull base invasion or transgression.

- *Size:* Tumors more than 2 cm is considered as high risk while the presence of tumor in high-risk area immaterial of the size is considered high risk.
- Ill-defined borders
- Presence of a lesion in previously irradiated area and immunosuppressed individual
- Perineural invasion—even though rare, its presence is considered high risk.
- Aggressive growth pattern on histology (micronodular, infiltrative or morpheaform). Low risks are tumors with well-defined borders and with histological subtype such as superficial or nodular type.
- *Age: Not* considered as a risk factor as the literature shows conflicting results.

In cSCC the risk stratification is similar to BCC with the following additions:[17]

- *Depth:* Defined by College of American Pathologists (CAP) as the distance in millimeters from the deepest point of invasion to the granular layer excluding parakeratosis and scale crust. A depth of ≥2 mm is considered as high-risk tumor.
- *Degree of differentiation*: Well- or moderately-differentiated are low-risk tumors and poorly-differentiated are high-risk tumors.
- *Histologic subtype:* Acanatholytic, adenosquamous, and metaplastic types are considered as high-risk tumors.
- Presence of lymphovascular involvement is high-risk tumor.

Risk of regional disease is higher in cSCC. The risk stratification based on regional involvement is varied.

Table 3: The American Joint Committee on Cancer (AJCC), 8th edition, N-staging in nonmelanoma skin cancers (NMSC).

Category	*Definition*
NX	Regional lymph nodes cannot be assessed
N0	No regional lymph node metastasis
N1	Metastases to single ipsilateral lymph node, 3 cm or less in the greatest diameter and without ENE
N2a	Metastases to single ipsilateral node >3 cm but not >6 cm in the greatest dimension and no ENE *or* metastases to single ipsilateral lymph node 3 cm or less with ENE
N2b	Metastases to multiple ipsilateral node none >6 cm in the greatest dimension and no ENE
N2c	Metastases to bilateral or contralateral lymph nodes, none >6 cm in the greatest dimension and no ENE
N3a	Metastases to nodes >6 cm in the greatest dimension without ENE
N3b	Metastases to node measuring >3 cm with ENE

(ENE: extranodal extension)

O'Brien et al. proposed risk stratification for regional disease based on parotid involvement and other cervical nodal involvement.[18] The reproducibility of this staging system was not uniform in all studies, hence it is not commonly used. NCCN has stratified regional disease into low, medium, and high risk.[17]

- *Low-risk:* One lymph node ≤3 cm positive, no extranodal extension (ENE)
- *Medium-risk:* One lymph node >3 cm positive with no ENE or ≥2 lymph nodes positive with no ENE
- *High-risk:* One or more lymph nodes positive with ENE or incompletely excised disease

Retrospective studies have shown that number of nodes, ENE, involvement of parotid, LN size to be good prognosticators.[19-21] While with the addition of ENE in the recent AJCC staging system, it also provides good risk stratification **(Table 3)**.

TREATMENT

Resectable Disease

Surgery is the mainstay of treatment in BCC. Wide excision with adequate margins is essential and achieves a disease-free survival of 96% at 5 years.[22] Even though various nonsurgical modalities exist, surgical excision achieves the best outcome. Surgical excision with margin assessment either with Mohs micrographic surgery (MMS) or complete circumferential peripheral and deep margin assessment under intraoperative frozen section is recommended. Standard excision without evaluation of complete margins is not advisable. Randomized trial data from the Netherlands has shown better control with MMS with 10-year recurrence rates in primary and recurrent tumors of 4.4% and 3.9% when compared to standard excision, which showed recurrence rates of 12.2% and 13.5%, respectively.[23] Low-risk tumors are resected with a margin of 3–4 mm and depth of resection up to mid-subcutaneous tissue in superficial tumors. High-risk tumors need resection margin of >4 mm and a depth of resection as mandated by the deep extent of tumor.[16]

Like BCC, cSCC is also managed by surgery. Evaluation of the margin either with MMS or complete circumferential peripheral and deep margin assessment under intraoperative frozen section is recommended. The recommended margins for cSCC are 4 mm for low risk and 6 mm or more for high-risk cases with a depth of mid-subcutaneous tissue in superficial tumors and deeper plane in high-risk tumors.[17] The NCCN recommendations in high-risk tumor mention wider margins with no cut-off, as high-risk tumors have variable clinical characteristics and extension.[17] A meta-analysis that has evaluated MMS and standard excision for cSCC recommends MMS, as it is associated with lower recurrence rates than standard excision.[24] The 5-year recurrence rate with MMS was 3.1% and 10% for primary and recurrent tumors, respectively. The meta-analysis also mentions variability in cure rates with MMS based on size and differentiation of tumor, but the cure rates are uniformly improved with MMS when compared with standard excision. The NCCN recommends circumferential peripheral and deep margin assessment under intraoperative frozen section as an alternative to MMS; however, it is to be noted that the discrepancy between paraffin section and intraoperative frozen section can be as high as 10–20% in NMSC.[25] The only way to reduce the discrepancy is by perfect orientation of the specimen and better communication with pathologist for sectioning of representative margin.

MANAGEMENT OF THE NECK

Studies have shown that recurrence and metastasis in sentinel lymph node biopsy (SLNB) positive tumor is as high as 33–45% and is associated with lower 3-year disease specific survival.[26] The NCCN does not recommend SLNB for cSCC, as the use of SLNB in improving outcomes and selection criteria is unclear in literature.[17] The risk factors for lymph node metastasis are:[27]

- Tumors measuring >4 cm
- Tumors infiltrating deeper than subcutaneous fat
- Tumors with poor differentiation
- Peritumoral inflammation
- Lymphovascular invasion
- Perineural invasion
- Recurrent lesion

Cases with these risk features must be evaluated thoroughly preoperatively for nodal involvement. NCCN recommends selective neck dissection (SND) when single node is involved and comprehensive neck dissection when more than one nodes are involved.[17] Superficial parotidectomy is advocated when parotid nodes are involved, as almost all the nodes in parotid are present in a plane anterior to retromandibular vein. Radiation therapy (RT) to the neck is not recommended as a primary modality of treatment. Studies have shown better outcomes in terms of both survival and recurrence when nodal disease is addressed with surgery and adjuvant RT than either surgery or RT alone. The indication for chemoradiotherapy for ENE positive nodes is extrapolated from mucosal head and neck squamous cell carcinomas (HNSCC), as there are no comparative trials available for cSCC.[17] Nodal recurrence is usually seen within 10–19 months of treatment of primary disease. Nodal metastasis is associated with a distant metastasis rate of 4–27%.[27] When parotid nodes are involved, especially in anterolateral skin tumors, elective neck dissection can be considered as rate of occult neck metastasis to deep cervical chain can be as high as 42%.[28]

RADIOTHERAPY IN NONMELANOMA SKIN CANCERS

Definitive Radiotherapy

Surgery forms the mainstay of treatment in NMSC. Definitive RT as the primary treatment modality is considered based on various tumors and patient factors.

Tumor Factors

There is only one randomized controlled trial that has compared RT with surgery in 347 patients with facial BCC with tumors measuring <4 cm. Even though tumor control of 92.5% was achieved with RT, it was still inferior to surgery, which had a control rate of 99.3%.[29] Various studies have achieved high-control rate of 90% with RT but is still inferior to surgery.[30-32] Even the long-term cosmesis and patient reported outcomes were inferior in RT group.

There are no RCTs comparing RT and surgery for cSCC. Various studies have reported good control rates with RT, especially in superficial tumors.[33,34] The role of definitive RT in NMSC is restricted to very superficial tumors and early preinvasive tumors involving large areas of head and neck wherein surgical resection may lead to more significant morbidity.[33]

Use of RT as definitive treatment for advanced cases for both BCC and cSCC is associated with high failure rate and locoregional control of 58–68% at 5 years.[35-37] Therefore, even in advanced cases, surgery with margin-controlled excision followed by adjuvant radiation when indicated gives the best possible oncologic and functional outcome.

Patient Factors

An unfit patient with poor performance status and multiple comorbidities may not be able to undergo surgery and can be treated with definitive RT. Elderly patients are often treated with hypofractionated dose (5–7 Gy in 5–6 fractions) for convenience and when long-term outcomes with hypopigmentation and skin atrophy is not an issue. Younger patients with longer life expectancy can be treated with 2–2.5 Gy over 4–5 weeks with use of modern inverse planning techniques for the best cosmetic and oncologic outcomes.[17]

Adjuvant Radiotherapy

Clear-cut indications for adjuvant therapy do not exist due to the lack of randomized trials supporting their use. The NCCN recommends adjuvant RT for all high-risk (mentioned in section of risk stratification) cases of BCC and cSCC, margin positivity and presence of nodal disease.[17] Adjuvant RT has shown to improve locoregional control without benefit on survival. Dose and fractionation of RT in the adjuvant setting is similar to mucosal head and neck SCC.

Role of Superficial Therapies

The best oncologic and cosmetic outcome is achieved by surgery. Superficial therapies are inferior and the NCCN recommends superficial therapies only in following indications:[16,17]

- Anatomically complex areas with superficial BCC
- Cutaneous squamous cell carcinoma with in situ changes

The following therapies are recommended:

- *Cryotherapy:* It is a procedure where tumor lysis is achieved by freeze thaw cycles applied repeatedly. It achieves poorer cosmetic outcome in nonsuperficial lesions.
- *Cytotoxic creams such as imiquimod and 5-fluorouracil:* Cosmetic outcome is reported better than surgery, but clearance and efficacy is poorer than surgery.
- *Photodynamic therapy (PDT):* It is a procedure wherein photosensitizing agent such as aminolevulinate or 5-aminovulinic acid (ALA) is locally applied on the lesion and exposed to the light source. PDT was associated with good cosmetic outcome while the oncologic outcome was inferior to surgery.

Various studies have compared different modalities with variable outcomes, but the choice of superficial therapy must be based on patient preference.

MANAGEMENT OF MARGINS IN NONMELANOMA SKIN CANCERS

A 360-degree margin evaluation with complete assessment of peripheral and deep margin is paramount in skin cancer. MMS or complete circumferential peripheral with deep margin assessment, with techniques as described below:

- *Mohs micrographic surgery:* MMS is a specialized technique for margin assessment, which was first proposed by Dr Frederick Mohs in 1930s.[38] It was first described with fixed tissue technique with prefixation of surrounding skin with zinc chloride. This aspect has fallen out of vogue and presently no tissue fixation technique is recommended. Curettage of the proliferative component of tumor can be done but this is left to surgeon's preference. The margins are delineated and oriented with hash marks (superficial scalpel marks) on both the tumor and patient margin edge for orientation. Then a No. 15 or 10 scalpel is used to cut with a 45° angle to the skin in such a way that the cutting edge is beveled inwards. This is extremely important, as flattening of the margin tissue on the slide is possible only if the edge is beveled. After excision, the specimen is re-oriented with color. Then the tissue is frozen with epidermis/superficial edge in direct contact with optimum cutting temperature compound. The tissue is laid with epidermis down, so that superficial epidermis and the deepest resection margin are in the same plane for pathological evaluation. Layer-by-layer margin excision is continued until negative margins are achieved.[39] MMS needs specialized training by the surgeon and can be time-consuming.
- *Complete circumferential peripheral and deep margin assessment:* It varies from MMS wherein the margins are rendered by pathologist (not by the surgeon as in MMS).[40] The margins are analyzed by en face tangential analysis where the specimen is placed epidermis down and margins are sectioned circumferentially.

A few principles relating to management of margin that are of significance are:

- Until all margins are clear pathologically, no reconstruction must be planned.
- Gross undermining and tissue de-arrangement of surrounding skin is avoided as much as possible.
- Surrounding inflammatory changes, if present, must be considered as tumor.
- For patients with surrounding large areas of precancerous lesion, no tissue de-arrangement must be done and surrounding areas, if not amenable for resection, can be managed with superficial therapies.

SYSTEMIC THERAPY

Basal Cell Carcinoma

Hedgehog pathway inhibitor is recommended in cases of unresectable local disease and BCC with distant metastasis. The recommended drugs are vismodegib and sonidegib.[31-41] The time to response ranges from 2.6 to 4 months. The duration of sustained response ranges from 9.5 to 22 months. Adverse reactions occurred in 25–32% of cases with first onset of adverse reactions at approximately 6 months. Side effects include muscle spasm, alopecia, taste loss, fatigue, weight loss, nausea, and diarrhea. Sonidegib is also associated with elevated creatinine kinase. The dose of vismodegib is 150 mg and sonidegib is 200 mg, both once daily. Even though trial tested a higher dose of sonidegib (300 mg) both doses showed similar efficacy rates and higher dose was associated with higher rates of adverse reactions.[42]

CUTANEOUS SQUAMOUS CELL CARCINOMA

Locally Advanced Squamous Cell Carcinoma

Only small retrospective studies exist that have studied responses of locally advanced SCC that are unlikely to be cured by surgery. These studies have included patients with operable disease that have refused surgery or those with residual disease after resection. However, due to absence of any comparable randomized trial, systemic therapy is not routinely recommended. Its use concomitant with RT for nonmetastatic locally advanced disease that may not be amenable for surgery can be considered, and dosage and protocol are same as mucosal HNSCC.[17]

Induction chemotherapy with cytotoxic therapy and EGFR inhibitor has shown to reduce tumor burden and has made large invasive lesions amenable for surgery or RT; however, their routine use is not recommended. The response rates with cytotoxic drugs such as cisplatin, cisplatin + 5 FU or vindesine is limited and the supporting evidence is sparse. Multiple studies including phase 2 trials have shown response to EGFR inhibitors with limited response in distant metastasis.[43-45] Cetuximab is preferred over cytotoxic therapy due to low-toxicity profile in a distant metastasis setting.

Recently approved anti-PD-1 agents nivolumab and pembrolizumab have been used for metastatic HNSCC with platinum resistance which has shown promising results.[46,47] While the trials did not include cases of cSCC, their use can be recommended in a trial setting for unresectable or metastatic disease. Few early feasibility trials have tested immunotherapy in cSCC.[48,49]

Follow-up

The NCCN recommendations are as follows:[16,17]

- In a case of BCC the risk of developing another BCC is 30–50% in the next 5 years and patient is also at an increased risk of developing SCC or melanoma. The first 2 years are crucial and full body evaluation must be done at follow-up. High-risk patients may need long-term follow-up beyond 5 years.
- Like BCC, patients with cSCC are also prone for development of another cSCC with a rate of 30–40% over 5 years. The recurrence rates are as high as 70–80% in 2 years. Therefore, a long-term close monitoring is recommended.
- Follow-up recommendations are based on risk stratification. Low-risk patient can be followed up once every 3 months for the first 2 years then 6-monthly for next 3 years. Patients with regional disease or high risk need follow-up every 1–3 months for 1st year, 2–4 months next year, 4–6 months for the next 3 years and yearly for a lifetime. Patient's self-education and strict sun protection are essential along with close follow-up.

MANAGEMENT OF HIGH-RISK DISEASE

Patients with actinic keratosis and Bowen's disease are more prone to developing multiple tumors at once. The presence of field cancerization and multiple adjacent tumors in close proximity may make surgical excision difficult. Superficial therapies in a single setting or upfront radiation therapy can be recommended in actinic keratosis or Bowen's disease with low-risk tumors. A prior biopsy to prove the lesion is pathologically low-risk before application of superficial therapy is essential. In cases with extensive lesions in the high-risk area can be surgical excised and surrounding in situ changes can be managed by superficial therapy with minimal rearrangement of the surrounding tissue. In patients on immunosuppression following strategies can be tried.

- Dose reduction of immunosuppressant
- Switch over to mammalian target of rapamycin (mTOR) inhibitors for immunosuppression
- When NMSC is surgically not amenable, oral capecitabine can be suggested.[17]

PREVENTION OF NONMELANOMA SKIN CANCERS

Patient Education[17]

Patient education is paramount in both patients with high-risk condition and all patients with diagnosed skin cancer. At the time of diagnosis of high-risk condition and after treatment of newly diagnosed skin cancer patient, education regarding self-examination and regular use of sun protection is mandatory.

Sun Protection Strategy[50]

- Refrain from sun exposure between 10 AM and 4 PM
- Sun protective clothing such as round hat with a rim all around, wraparound sunglasses, and hand gloves up to sleeves should be used.
- Application of sunscreen of at least SPF 15 which block both UVA and B. Application must be repeated every 2 hours when outside, even on cloudy days.
- Routine vitamin D supplementation is not recommended despite the common belief that sun protection strategies may reduce vitamin D levels; studies have shown that dietary vitamin D absorption compensates for this.

Self-examination[17]

- Patient and patient's family members must be educated regarding identifying new lesions and also to look for lymph nodes.
- Monthly self-examination results in early identification and better cure rates in high-risk patients.

Chemoprevention

- Oral retinoids and synthetic retinoids (e.g., isotretinoin) have been tested and have shown efficacy in preventing new SCC in very high-risk conditions such as transplant recipients, psoriasis on psoralen and ultraviolet A (PUVA) therapy, and xeroderma pigmentosum. Their use beyond very high-risk conditions is not recommended, as trials have shown no benefit out of these indications. Topical retinoid is not recommended. The toxicity profile of oral retinoid namely cheilitis, excessive peeling of skin, hair disorders, and headaches are commonly reported.[51]
- Oral nicotinamide has emerged as an alternative to retinoid with lower toxicity profile. Recent trial has shown a benefit of 30% reduction in cSCC and 20% reduction in BCC with oral 500 mg BID dose for 12 months.[52] Even though the trial has compared it with placebo and not with oral retinoids, due to the better safety profile, oral nicotinamide is recommended.
- Oral celecoxib (cyclo-oxygenase 2 inhibitor) has not shown any benefit in risk reduction of development of newer lesions. Its association with severe and fatal toxicity such as cardiovascular thrombotic events and gastrointestinal (GI) adverse events make the use of celecoxib detrimental.[51]

NONMELANOMA NONEPITHELIAL SKIN CANCERS

Dermatofibrosarcoma Protuberans

Introduction

Dermatofibrosarcoma protuberans (DFSP) is a rare mesenchymal tumor arising from the dermis that is characterized by indolent growth, high local recurrence rate and an extremely low metastatic rate. Diagnosis of DFSP has always been challenging with its pathological features and biological behavior ranging between those of dermatofibroma and malignant fibrous histioma. Given the slow growth of DFSP, most lesions present late in advanced stage. Head and neck are the second most common sites for DFSP to occur.

Presentation

The incidence is as low as 4.5 cases per million cases per year in the US and it affects more than women.[53] It can occur at any age, but most commonly presents between second and fifth decades of life. The slow infiltrative growth pattern of the tumor commonly mimics benign skin lesions in early stages. The lesion is adherent to dermis but is freely mobile over structures at depth. The pattern of growth can be flat, elevated, and subcutaneous nodule or multinodular.[51] Peripheral satellite lesions are common which at a later stage coalesce to form large tumors that involve the skin and can cause ulceration.[52] In scalp, adherence to periosteum is earlier than adherence to deeper structures elsewhere in the body. DFSP are shown to have frequent irregular finger projections that represent growth of the tumor along the reticular dermis.[51] The tumor in early stages grows radially and then reaches a rapid growth period during which the tumor grows vertically down to adhere to deeper structures.[52]

Adenosine deaminase severe combined immunodeficiency is a rare disorder caused by mutation of adenosine deaminase 1 gene that codes for the enzyme required for purine metabolism and is characterized by dysfunctional T, B, and natural killer cells. In its severe form, it is fatal in 1–2 years, while milder forms exist. Its association with DFSP cannot be explained, but patients with this disorder have an incidence of DFSP of up to 67% and often present at a very early age (first decade of life).[54-56] Patients diagnosed with this disorder must be closely monitored for DFSP throughout their life.

Pathology

Dermatofibrosarcoma protuberans is characterized by rearrangement of chromosome 17 and 22, which results in fusion of *collagen type I α-1* gene and platelet derived growth factor beta *(PDGF-β)* gene, which as a consequence results in overexpression of PDGF-β receptor.[57,58] This tyrosine kinase receptor forms a potential for targeted therapy in DFSP. Almost 90% of tumors manifest this chromosomal rearrangement.[59] Darier and Ferrand first described the clinicopathologic features of DFSP in 1924.[60] Pathologically, it is a spindle-cell neoplasm with high cellularity and low collagen content. DFSP is characterized by storiform arrangement with fat entrapment, which appears as honeycomb. Various histologic variants include myxoid, granular cell, and pigmented type.[61] Of particular interest, there are fibromatosis, sarcomatoid variants with high mitotic index (median of 7 mitoses per high power field), high recurrence and metastatic potential, lower CD-34 expression, and positivity for p53 mutations. They represent a dedifferentiation variant and account for 10–15% of DFSP.[62]

Biopsy remains the gold standard for diagnosis. Differential diagnoses are dermatofibroma, benign fibrous histioma, malignant fibrous histioma, atypical fibroxanthoma, giant cell fibroblastoma, and diffuse neurofibroma. Immunohistochemistry plays a vital role in differentiating DFSP from others. IHC strongly stains for CD34, CD44, and vimentin.[63,64] DFSP stains negative for factor XIIIa that is positive for dermatofibroma.[63]

Imaging

Dermatofibrosarcoma protuberans must be evaluated with MRI. Tumors are commonly associated with finger-like projections and satellite lesions, which are better visualized with MRI. CT scan is advocated only when bone involvement is suspected. MRI helps in accurate mapping of the tumor essential for complete removal and better local control. Tumor has low-signal intensity on T1-weighted (T1W) and high-signal intensity (higher than fat) on T2-weighted (T2W).[65] Fast spin echo sequences can be of additional value. These tumors rarely metastasize and no metastatic workup is done except in cases with fibrosarcomatous changes, where evaluation of chest for lung metastasis may be warranted.

Treatment

Surgical excision with radial margins of 2–4 cm and depth up to deep investing fascia or periosteum (in scalp lesions) is the standard of treatment.[17] Excision with adequate margins is essential during the first excision as it gives the best outcome. If there is margin positivity then re-excision must be planned. In the head and neck region, achieving 2–4 cm may be difficult; in these cases, MMS has been advocated.[66] Margin control with

CD34 IHC assessment can help in better clearance.[67] Tissue rearrangement and reconstruction must be delayed if margin clearance is suspect, as undermining surrounding tissue may result in tumor seeding. Radiotherapy is indicated in the postoperative setting with positive margins not amenable for further resection and as a primary modality in unresectable tumors.[68,69]

Chromosome 17 and 22 translocation results in overexpression of PDGF-β receptor, which is a potential target for tyrosine kinase inhibitor imatinib mesylate.[70] It is indicated in adult patients with unresectable disease, metastatic disease, and recurrence after multiple excisions and not amenable for further resection.[17] Local recurrence rates are varied between 10 and 60% and low regional recurrence rate of 1% and distant metastasis rate of 4–5%.[71,72] Follow-up once in 6 months with a primary focus on local recurrence is recommended.

Sebaceous Carcinoma

Sebaceous carcinoma is rare but aggressive tumor arising from sebaceous glands. In the head and neck region, they are broadly classified as periocular and extraocular;[73] both have different clinicopathologic behavior. Sebaceous carcinoma is exceedingly rare in the general population but is associated with Muir–Torre syndrome, which is characterized by mutations of mismatch repair genes namely *MLH1, MSH2, MSH6,* and *PMS2.* This syndrome is also associated with visceral malignancy of genitourinary and colorectal. It is also strongly associated with sebaceous carcinoma that many experts recommend genetic testing for Muir–Torre syndrome in all patients with sebaceous carcinoma.[73,74]

Presentation

Sebaceous carcinoma commonly occurs among men in their fifth decade of life. Extraocular is in the Caucasian population while periocular is common in the Asia Pacific population. Atypical chalazion, chronic unilateral blepharitis in an adult male must raise suspicion for sebaceous carcinoma.[73]

Diagnosis

Deep biopsy is mandated for extraocular while a superficial shave biopsy may suffice for periocular tumors. Histologically, tumors show variable growth patterns with extraocular tumors showing lobular, vacuolated, infiltrative growth patterns while periocular tumors show lobular mixed papillary variations.[73] Pagetoid spread is characterized by subclinical growth pattern, increased risk of local recurrence, and metastasis. Extraocular tumors are mostly well or moderately differentiated while periocular show moderate-to-poor differentiation.[75] IHC shows positivity for nuclear factor XIIIa, EMA, and adipophilin. Androgen receptor positivity (>50% staining) is considered as a poor prognostic sign and is more common in periocular tumors.[76,77]

Imaging

Periocular tumors need imaging when:
- Lesion involves full thickness of the eyelid.
- Pagetoid growth pattern is seen.
- Tumor is poorly differentiated, which has higher rate of occult nodal metastasis.[73]

Larger tumors in the periocular region may have deeper infiltration to orbital contents, paranasal sinus, skull base which mandates thorough assessment with MRI. Palpable lymph nodes must be evaluated with imaging. Recurrent tumors also need imaging for primary assessment and nodal evaluation. Staging for periocular tumors is as per the American Joint Committee on Cancer (AJCC), 8th edition, eyelid tumors and for extraocular tumors, as per skin carcinoma staging **(Table 4)**.

Table 4: The American Joint Committee on Cancer (AJCC), 8th edition, staging of eyelid tumors.

Category	*Definition*
T1	Tumor ≤10 mm in the greatest dimension
T1a	Does not involve tarsal plate or eyelid margin
T1b	Invades tarsal plate or eyelid margin
T1c	Involves full thickness of eyelid
T2	Tumor >10 mm but ≤20 mm in the greatest dimension
T2a	Does not involve tarsal plate or eyelid margin
T2b	Invades tarsal plate or eyelid margin
T2c	Involves full thickness of eyelid
T3	Tumor >20 mm but ≤30 mm in the greatest dimension
T3a	Does not involve tarsal plate or eyelid margin
T3b	Invades tarsal plate or eyelid margin
T3c	Involves full thickness of eyelid
T4	Any eyelid tumor involving adjacent ocular, orbital or facial structure
T4a	Invades ocular or intraorbital structures
T4b	Invades or erodes bony walls of the orbit or extends to paranasal sinuses or invades the lacrimal sac, nasolacrimal duct or brain
N1	Metastasis in a single ipsilateral regional node ≤ 3 cm in dimension
N1a	Based on clinical evaluation or imaging findings
N1b	Based on lymph node biopsy
N2	Metastasis in a single ipsilateral regional lymph node, >3 cm in the greatest dimension or bilateral/contralateral lymph nodes
N2a	Based on clinical evaluation or imaging findings
N2b	Based on microscopic findings
M1	Distant metastasis

Treatment

Surgical excision with 1 cm margin is considered adequate. Margin control with MMS or complete circumferential peripheral and deep margin assessment recommended, especially in periocular lesions, as 1 cm margins may be difficult to achieve.[73] Periocular tumors with pagetoid growth pattern and mapping biopsies to assess subclinical growth pattern of the tumor is necessary. Mapping biopsies in the form of circumferential biopsies around the tumor over palpebral and bulbar conjunctiva can be performed.[78] Orbital exenteration may be required in cases with retrobulbar extension, orbital fat, extraocular muscles, and sclera.[73]

Elective neck dissection or parotidectomy is not recommended.[73] Parotidectomy and neck dissection based on the location of primary tumor must be performed when nodes are involved on imaging.

Adjuvant radiotherapy is not routinely advocated. Margin positivity, large primary tumors, and LN involvement are indications for adjuvant RT.[79] PNI as a sole indication for adjuvant RT in sebaceous carcinoma is questionable as supporting data is insufficient.[73]

Definitive RT (55 Gy) in sebaceous carcinoma has shown good local control, with a 5-year disease-free survival of 54%.[80,81]

Evidence to support systemic therapy for management of metastatic disease is sparse. Platinum-based chemotherapy, targeted therapy with agents, targeting androgen receptors, and anti-EGFR therapies have been studied with variable response rates.[73]

Prognosis and Follow-up

Disease-free survival at 3 years is 18% and 25.6% for extraocular and periocular tumors, respectively. The rate of distant metastasis during the course of the disease is 1.8% for extraocular and 12.5% for periocular tumors.[73] Follow-up visits are once in 6 months for the first 3 years and then annually.

Merkel Cell Carcinoma

Merkel cell carcinoma is an extremely rare tumor of the skin with epithelial and neuroendocrine differentiation. It is a highly aggressive tumor with a high rate of regional and distant metastasis. The incidence is 0.13 per 100,000 in Europe and 1.6 per 100,000 in Australia.[82,83] It commonly occurs in white populations with only 1% of the dark-skinned population affected by it. MCC commonly occurs in the head and neck region, especially the lips. MCC is a rapidly growing tumor with 63% showing rapid growth of primary at 3 months, 26–36% with lymph node involvement and 6–16% with distant metastasis at presentation.[84-86]

Pathogenesis

Various etiologies have been proposed. The initial hypothesis that it arises from Merkel cells that are tactile epithelial cells at the epidermal-dermal junction has been challenged. Merkel cells play a key role in afferent sensory impulse from the skin. A multifactorial process has been proposed with various factors such as viral pathogen, immunosuppression, and UV exposure, all playing a role in the carcinogenesis. Nonviral tumors are associated with mutation of p53, NOTCH, phosphoinositide 3-kinase/AKT serine/threonine kinase (PI3K/AKT) which could be attributed to UV exposure.[87,88] Merkel cell polymyxovirus (MCPyV) that is a nonenveloped double-stranded DNA virus is a common dermal commensal.[89] It was first described in 2008 by Feng et al., with integrated viral, DNA is seen in 66–80% of cases and is now considered pathognomonic of MCC.[90] It affects codependent translation regulator and retinoblastoma protein family, which in turn activate survivin, which downregulates apoptosis. MCPyV oncoprotein antigen can be quantified, which helps in prognostication and recurrence surveillance. A prospective study with 219 newly diagnosed MCC patients has shown that MCPyV oncoprotein antigen negative patients have shorter recurrence period and raising titers signify early recurrence.[91]

Pathology

Merkel cell carcinoma consists of small round basophilic monomorphous cells at reticular dermis extending into subcutaneous tissue. These cells contain large nuclei with inconspicuous cytoplasm. MCC often gets misdiagnosed clinically and are diagnosed pathologically.[92] Various small round cell tumors need to be differentiated from other tumors such as small cell lung cancer, neuroblastoma, rhabdomyosarcoma, metastatic carcinoid, desmoplastic small cell tumor, amelanocytic melanoma, mesenchymal chondrosarcoma, Ewing sarcoma, lymphoma, and osteosarcoma. It is difficult to differentiate between small cell lung cancer and MCC. 75–100% of MCC express positivity for CK20, which appears as a paranuclear dot on microscopy. Small cell lung cancers express thyroid transcription factor 1 (TTF-1) but never CK20. Other neuroendocrine markers such as chromogranin, synaptophysin, neuron specific enolase; neurofilament can be used when CK20 is negative.[92,93] The College of American Pathologists (CAP) recommends the following pathological features to be included in the final report for adequate staging of the tumor.[17]

- Maximum tumor diameter and extension
- Extracutaneous spread

- Lymphovascular invasion
- Mitotic rate
- Infiltrative growth pattern
- Lymphocyte infiltration
- Presence of second malignancy

Evaluation

In early stages, they clinically present as subcutaneous nodules with reddish-purple hue. The acronym "AEIOU" consisting of *a*symptomatic, rapid *e*xpansion, *i*mmunosuppression, *o*lder than 50, and *U*V exposure of light skin describes characteristics of MCC well. However, most MCC is misdiagnosed clinically and the diagnosis is established on histology. There is no consensus regarding imaging modality of choice.[94] CT or MRI, whichever gives better delineation of the primary, can be chosen to evaluate regional nodal basin.[95] Rate of distant metastasis is high at presentation and hence evaluation with PET-CT with MRI brain or CT neck/chest/abdomen/pelvis with MRI brain may be required in recurrent cases, high nodal disease, and unresectable cases.[95,96] There is no consensus on appropriate imaging modality. All clinically significant node disease must be evaluated with ultrasound-guided fine-needle aspiration, as presence of concomitant lymphoma or metastatic small cell lung cancer is a possibility.

The AJCC, 8th edition, has based its staging system on a National Cancer Data Base (NCDB) analysis of 9,387 cases with a median follow-up of 28.2 months **(Table 5)**.[97]

Treatment

Due to rarity of disease and rapid progression, prospective trials in management of MCC are rare. Primary tumor, when resectable, must be resected with 1–2 cm margins with thorough margin assessment as described earlier.[17] Before excision, sentinel node biopsy is recommended by NCCN in all clinically negative nodal disease. The SLNB positivity in clinically negative disease ranges from 30 to 38%.[98] SLNB with thorough serial step sectioning and addition of IHC for CK20 is recommended. The head and neck region is associated with technical challenges with SLNB.[98] In a node positive disease, comprehensive nodal dissection is recommended. Postoperative radiation is recommended for positive margins, positive nodal disease.[17]

Routine use of adjuvant RT in early stages with negative margins and negative nodal disease on SLNB is not recommended. Unresectable disease and metastatic disease are managed with chemotherapy.[17]

Unlike other subsites, the first line of therapy is immunotherapy. The JAVELIN Merkel 200 trial included stage IV MCC with distant metastases treated with avelumab (anti-PD-L1 inhibitor)[99,100] showed as progression-free survival of 9.1 months on interim analysis. When response rate in resistant cases (resistant to one or more lines of cytotoxic chemotherapy) was evaluated, an overall response of 33% was documented. Results from this trial led to the Food and Drug Administration (FDA) approval of the use of avelumab in metastatic MCC. Anti-PD-1 inhibitors such as pembrolizumab and nivolumab have also been tested. In cases not responding to immunotherapy, cytotoxic therapies such as cisplatin, carboplatin with or without etoposide, or the CAV [cyclophosphamide-Adriamycin® (doxorubicin)-vincristine] regimen are recommended.[17]

Table 5: The American Joint Committee on Cancer (AJCC), 8th edition, staging of Merkel cell carcinoma.

Category	Definition
T1	Tumor ≤20 mm in the greatest dimension
T2	Tumor >20 mm but ≤50 mm in the greatest dimension
T2a	Does not involve tarsal plate or eyelid margin
T3	Tumor >50 mm in the greatest dimension
T4	Primary tumor invades fascia, muscle, cartilage or bone
N1a	Microscopic regional lymph node metastasis following dissection, clinically occult
N1b	Microscopic confirmation of clinically detected regional lymph node metastasis
N2	In transit metastasis without lymph node metastasis
N3	In transit metastasis with lymph node metastasis
M1	Distant metastasis

Surveillance

About 90% of recurrence occurs in the first 2 years (median 8 months); hence, surveillance during the first 2 years must be rigorous. Imaging modalities may be required. These patients are at an increased risk of second primary MCC and other cutaneous and non-cutaneous malignancy. Especially in risk individuals, annual PET-CT may be recommended to detect distant metastasis.[17]

CONCLUSION

Skin cancers have a varied presentation and outcome based on the cell of origin. Locally infiltrative basal cell carcinoma, DFSP to highly aggressive Merkel cell carcinoma forms the wide spectrum of skin tumors. Surgical excision forms the primary treatment modality in all skin cancers. The role of other modalities in skin cancers is limited; however, recent advances in targeted therapy have the potential to improve longevity and quality of life in metastatic disease.

REFERENCES

1. Gloster HM Jr, Neal K. Skin cancer in skin of color. J Am Acad Dermatol. 2006;55(5):741-60.
2. Panda S. Nonmelanoma skin cancer in India: Current scenario. Indian J Dermatol. 2010;55(4):373.
3. Bais AF, Lucas RM, Bornman JF, Williamson CE, Sulzberger B, Austin AT, et al. Environmental effects of ozone depletion, UV radiation and interactions with climate change: UNEP Environmental Effects Assessment Panel, update 2017. Photochem Photobiol Sci. 2018;17(2):127-79.
4. Brenner M, Hearing VJ. The protective role of melanin against UV damage in human skin. Photochem Photobiol. 2008;84(3):539-49.
5. Didona D, Paolino G, Bottoni U, Cantisani C. Non-melanoma skin cancer pathogenesis overview. Biomedicines. 2018;6(1):6.
6. Rangwala S, Tsai KY. Roles of the immune system in skin cancer. Br J Dermatol. 2011;165(5):953-65.
7. Skoda AM, Simovic D, Karin V, Kardum V, Vranic S, Serman L. The role of the Hedgehog signaling pathway in cancer: a comprehensive review. Bosnian J Basic Med Sci. 2018;18(1):8-20.
8. Wehner MR, Shive ML, Chren MM, Han J, Qureshi AA, Linos E. Indoor tanning and non-melanoma skin cancer: systematic review and meta-analysis. BMJ. 2012;345:e5909.
9. Buljan M, Bulat V, Šitum M, Lugović Mihić L, Stanić-Duktaj S. Variations in clinical presentation of basal cell carcinoma. Acta Clinica Croatica. 2008;47(1):25-30.
10. Crowson AN. Basal cell carcinoma: biology, morphology and clinical implications. Modern Pathol. 2006;19(2):S127-47.
11. Tellechea O, Reis JP, Domingues JC, Baptista AP. Monoclonal antibody Ber EP4 distinguishes basal-cell carcinoma from squamous-cell carcinoma of the skin. Am J Dermatopathol. 1993;15(5):452-5.
12. Gee HE, Veness MJ. High-risk cutaneous squamous cell carcinoma. Curr Otorhinolaryngol Reports. 2018;6(2):120-8.
13. Yanofsky VR, Mercer SE, Phelps RG. Histopathological variants of cutaneous squamous cell carcinoma: a review. J Skin Cancer. 2011;2011.
14. Humphreys TR, Shah K, Wysong A, Lexa F, MacFarlane D. The role of imaging in the management of patients with nonmelanoma skin cancer: when is imaging necessary? J Am Acad Dermatol. 2017;76(4):591-607.
15. Bakos RM, Blumetti TP, Roldán-Marín R, Salerni G. Noninvasive imaging tools in the diagnosis and treatment of skin cancers. Am J Clin Dermatol. 2018;19(1):3-14.
16. Bichakjian CK, Olencki T, Aasi SZ, Alam M, Andersen JS, Berg D, et al. Basal cell skin cancer, version 1.2016, NCCN clinical practice guidelines in oncology. J Nat Comp Cancer Network. 2016;14(5):574-97.
17. National Comprehensive Cancer Network (2020). NCCN Clinical Practice Guidelines in Oncology (NCCN Guidelines VR) Squamous Cell Skin Cancer 1.2020. National Comprehensive Cancer Network, Inc.; 2020. [online] Available from NCCN.org. [Last accessed July, 2020].
18. O'Brien CJ, McNeil EB, McMahon JD, Pathak I, Lauer CS, Jackson MA. Significance of clinical stage, extent of surgery, and pathologic findings in metastatic cutaneous squamous carcinoma of the parotid gland. Head Neck: J Sci Spec Head Neck. 2002;24(5):417-22.
19. Vauterin TJ, Veness MJ, Morgan GJ, Poulsen MG, O'Brien CJ. Patterns of lymph node spread of cutaneous squamous cell carcinoma of the head and neck. Head Neck. 2006;28(9):785-91.
20. Andruchow JL, Veness MJ, Morgan GJ, Gao K, Clifford A, Shannon KF, et al. Implications for clinical staging of metastatic cutaneous squamous carcinoma of the head and neck based on a multicenter study of treatment outcomes. Cancer. 2006;106(5):1078-83.
21. Hinerman RW, Indelicato DJ, Amdur RJ, Morris CG, Werning JW, Vaysberg M, et al. Cutaneous squamous cell carcinoma metastatic to parotid-area lymph nodes. Laryngoscope. 2008;118(11):1989-96.
22. Fahradyan A, Howell AC, Wolfswinkel EM, Tsuha M, Sheth P, Wong AK. Updates on the management of non-melanoma skin cancer (NMSC). Healthcare (Basel). 2017;5(4):82.
23. Mosterd K, Krekels GA, Nieman FH, Ostertag JU, Essers BA, Dirksen CD, et al. Surgical excision versus Mohs' micrographic surgery for primary and recurrent basal-cell carcinoma of the face: a prospective randomised controlled trial with 5-years' follow-up. Lancet Oncol. 2008;9(12):1149-56.
24. Rowe DE, Carroll RJ, Day CL Jr. Prognostic factors for local recurrence, metastasis, and survival rates in squamous cell carcinoma of the skin, ear, and lip: implications for treatment modality selection. J Am Acad Dermatol. 1992;26(6):976-90.
25. Nicoletti G, Brenta F, Malovini A, Musumarra G, Scevola S, Faga A. Study to determine whether intraoperative frozen section biopsy improves surgical treatment of non-melanoma skin cancer. Mole Clin Oncol. 2013;1(2):390-4.
26. Matthey-Giè ML, Boubaker A, Letovanec I, Demartines N, Matter M. Sentinel lymph node biopsy in nonmelanoma skin cancer patients. J Skin Cancer. 2013;2013:267474.
27. Jennings L, Schmults CD. Management of high-risk cutaneous squamous cell carcinoma. J Clin Aesthetic Dermatol. 2010; 3(4):39-48.
28. Haksever M, Akduman D, Demir M, Aslan S, Yanılmaz M, Solmaz F. The treatment of neck and parotid gland in cutaneous squamous cell carcinoma of face and forehead and the review of literature. Ann Med Surg. 2015;4(1):48-52.
29. Avril MF, Auperin A, Margulis A, Gerbaulet A, Duvillard P, Benhamou E, et al. Basal cell carcinoma of the face: surgery or radiotherapy: Results of a randomized study. Br J Cancer. 1997;76(1):100-6.
30. Wilder RB, Kittelson JM, Shimm DS. Basal cell carcinoma treated with radiation therapy. Cancer. 1991;68(10):2134-7.
31. Wilder RB, Shimm DS, Kittelson JM, Rogoff EE, Cassady JR. Recurrent basal cell carcinoma treated with radiation therapy. Arch Dermatol. 1991;127(11):1668-34.
32. Childers BJ, Goldwyn RM, Ramos D, Chaffey J, Harris JR. Long-term results of irradiation for basal cell carcinoma of the skin of the nose. Plast Reconstr Surg. 1994;93(6):1169-73.
33. Veness MJ. The important role of radiotherapy in patients with non-melanoma skin cancer and other cutaneous entities. J Med Imag Radiat Oncol. 2008;52(3):278-86.
34. Veness MJ, Ong C, Cakir B, Morgan G. Squamous cell carcinoma of the lip. Patterns of relapse and outcome: reporting the Westmead Hospital experience, 1980–1997. Australasian Radiol. 2001;45(2):195-9.
35. Lee WR, Mendenhall WM, Parsons JT, Million RR. Radical radiotherapy for T4 carcinoma of the skin of the head and neck: a multivariate analysis. Head Neck. 1993;15(4):320-4.
36. Al-Othman MO, Mendenhall WM, Amdur RJ. Radiotherapy alone for clinical T4 skin carcinoma of the head and neck with surgery reserved for salvage. Am J Otolaryngol. 2001; 22(6):387-90.
37. Kwan W, Wilson D, Moravan V. Radiotherapy for locally advanced basal cell and squamous cell carcinomas of the skin. Int J Radiat Oncol Biol Phys. 2004;60(2):406-11.

38. Mohs FE. Origin and progress of Mohs micrographic surgery. In: Snow SN, Mikhail G. Wisconsin Mohs Micrographic Surgery, 2nd edition. United States: Wiley; 2006.
39. Chen EL, Srivastava D, Nijhawan RI. Mohs micrographic surgery: development, technique, and applications in cutaneous malignancies. Semin Plast Surg. 2018;32(2):60-8.
40. Kimyai-Asadi AR, Katz T, Goldberg LH, Ayala GB, Wang SQ, Vujevich JJ, et al. Margin involvement after the excision of melanoma in situ: the need for complete en face examination of the surgical margins. Dermatol Surg. 2007;33(12):1434-41.
41. Sekulic A, Migden MR, Oro AE, Dirix L, Lewis KD, Hainsworth JD, et al. Efficacy and safety of vismodegib in advanced basal-cell carcinoma. N Engl J Med. 2012;366(23):2171-9.
42. Migden MR, Guminski A, Gutzmer R, Dirix L, Lewis KD, Combemale P, et al. Treatment with two different doses of sonidegib in patients with locally advanced or metastatic basal cell carcinoma (BOLT): a multicentre, randomised, double-blind phase 2 trial. Lancet Oncol. 2015;16(6):716-28.
43. Picard A, Pedeutour F, Peyrade F, Saudes L, Duranton-Tanneur V, Chamorey E, et al. Association of oncogenic mutations in patients with advanced cutaneous squamous cell carcinomas treated with cetuximab. JAMA Dermatol. 2017;153(4):291-8.
44. Preneau S, Rio E, Brocard A, Peuvrel L, Nguyen JM, Quéreux G, et al. Efficacy of cetuximab in the treatment of squamous cell carcinoma. J Dermatol Treat. 2014;25(5):424-7.
45. Trodello C, Pepper JP, Wong M, Wysong A. Cisplatin and cetuximab treatment for metastatic cutaneous squamous cell carcinoma: a systematic review. Dermatol Surg. 2017; 43(1):40-9.
46. Ferris RL, Blumenschein Jr G, Fayette J, Guigay J, Colevas AD, Licitra L, et al. Nivolumab for recurrent squamous-cell carcinoma of the head and neck. N Engl J Med. 2016; 375(19):1856-67.
47. Seiwert TY, Burtness B, Mehra R, Weiss J, Berger R, Eder JP, et al. Safety and clinical activity of pembrolizumab for treatment of recurrent or metastatic squamous cell carcinoma of the head and neck (KEYNOTE-012): an open-label, multicentre, phase 1b trial. Lancet Oncol. 2016;17(7):956-65.
48. Maubec E, Boubaya M, Petrow P, Basset-Seguin N, Grob JJ, Dréno B, et al. Pembrolizumab as first-line therapy in patients with unresectable cutaneous squamous cell carcinoma (cSCC): Phase 2 results from CARSKIN. J Clin Oncol. 2019;37(15):9547.
49. Papadopoulos KP, Owonikoko TK, Johnson ML, Brana I, Gil-Martin M, Perez RP, et al. REGN2810: A fully human anti-PD-1 monoclonal antibody, for patients with unresectable locally advanced or metastatic cutaneous squamous cell carcinoma (CSCC)—Initial safety and efficacy from expansion cohorts (ECs) of phase I study. J Clin Oncol. 2017;35(15): 9503.
50. Sanchez G, Nova J, Rodriguez-Hernandez AE, Medina RD, Solorzano-Restrepo C, Gonzalez J, et al. Sun protection for preventing basal cell and squamous cell skin cancers. Cochrane Database Syst Rev. 2016;7(7):CD011161.
51. Wright TI, Spencer JM, Flowers FP. Chemoprevention of nonmelanoma skin cancer. J Am Acad Dermatol. 2006; 54(6):933-46.
52. Chen AC, Martin AJ, Choy B, Fernández-Peñas P, Dalziell RA, McKenzie CA, et al. A phase 3 randomized trial of nicotinamide for skin-cancer chemoprevention. N Engl J Med. 2015;373(17):1618-26.
53. Stivala A, Lombardo GA, Pompili G, Tarico MS, Fraggetta F, Perrotta RE. Dermatofibrosarcoma protuberans: our experience of 59 cases. Oncol Letters. 2012;4(5):1047-55.
54. Pack GT, Tabah EJ. Dermatofibrosarcoma protuberans: a report of thirty-nine cases. AMA Arch Surg. 1951;62(3): 391-411.
55. Burkhardt BR, Soule EH, Winkelmann RK, Ivins JC. Dermatofibrosarcoma protuberans: study of fifty-six cases. Am J Surg. 1966;111(5):638-44.
56. Kesserwan C, Sokolic R, Cowen EW, Garabedian E, Heselmeyer-Haddad K, Lee CC, et al. Multicentric dermatofibrosarcoma protuberans in patients with adenosine deaminase-deficient severe combined immune deficiency. J Allerg Clin Immunol. 2012;129(3):762-9.
57. Bridge JA, Neff JR, Sandberg AA. Cytogenetic analysis of dermatofibrosarcoma protuberans. Cancer Genet Cytogen. 1990;49(2):199-202.
58. Patel KU, Szabo SS, Hernandez VS, Prieto VG, Abruzzo LV, Lazar AJ, et al. Dermatofibrosarcoma protuberans COL1A1-PDGFB fusion is identified in virtually all dermatofibrosarcoma protuberans cases when investigated by newly developed multiplex reverse transcription polymerase chain reaction and fluorescence in situ hybridization assays. Hum Pathol. 2008;39(2):184-93.
59. Noujaim J, Thway K, Fisher C, Jones RL. Dermatofibrosarcoma protuberans: from translocation to targeted therapy. Cancer Biol Med. 2015;12(4):375-84.
60. Darier J. Dermatofibromes progressifs et recidivants ou fibrosarcomes de la peau. Ann Dermatol Venereol. 1924;5: 545-62.
61. Gloster JH, Harris KR, Roenigk RK. A comparison between Mohs micrographic surgery and wide surgical excision for the treatment of dermatofibrosarcoma protuberans. J Am Acad Dermatol. 1996;35(1):82-7.
62. Szollosi Z, Nemes Z. Transformed dermatofibrosarcoma protuberans: a clinicopathological study of eight cases. J Clin Pathol. 2005;58(7):751-6.
63. Zelger B, Sidoroff A, Stanzl U, Fritsch PO, Ofner D, Jasani B, et al. Deep penetrating dermatofibroma versus dermatofibrosarcoma protuberans: a clinicopathologic comparison. Am J Surg Pathol. 1994;18(7):677-86.
64. Mentzel T, Beham A, Katenkamp D, Dei Tos AP, Fletcher CD. Fibrosarcomatous ("high-grade") dermatofibrosarcoma protuberans: clinicopathologic and immunohistochemical study of a series of 41 cases with emphasis on prognostic significance. Am J Surg Pathol. 1998;22(5):576-87.
65. Torreggiani WC, Al-Ismail K, Munk PL, Nicolaou S, O'Connell JX, Knowling MA. Dermatofibrosarcoma protuberans: MR imaging features. Am J Roentgenol. 2002; 178(4):989-93.
66. Serra-Guillén C, Llombart B, Nagore E, Guillén C, Requena C, Traves V, et al. Mohs micrographic surgery in dermatofibrosarcoma protuberans allows tumour clearance with smaller margins and greater preservation of healthy tissue compared with conventional surgery: a study of 74 primary cases. Br J Dermatol. 2015;172(5):1303-7.
67. Jimenez FJ, Grichnik JM, Buchanan MD, Clark RE. Immunohistochemical margin control applied to Mohs micrographic surgical excision of dermatofibrosarcoma protuberans. J Dermatol Surg Oncol. 1994;20(10):687-9.
68. Du K, Li J, Tang L, Lin X, Kong X, Liao X, et al. Role of postoperative radiotherapy in dermatofibrosarcoma protuberans: a propensity score-matched analysis. Radiat Oncol. 2019; 14(1):20.
69. Ballo MT, Zagars GK, Pisters P, Alan Pollack MD. The role of radiation therapy in the management of dermatofibrosarcoma protuberans. Int J Radiat Oncol Biol Phys. 1998;40(4): 823-7.

70. Labropoulos SV, Razis ED. Imatinib in the treatment of dermatofibrosarcoma protuberans. Biol Targets Ther. 2007; 1(4):347-52.
71. Ruiz-Tovar J, Guarino MF, Callejas ME, Velardo AA, Bermejo JA, Navarro LC. Dermatofibrosarcoma protuberans: Review of 20-years experience. Clin Translat Oncol. 2006; 8(8):606-10.
72. Hayakawa K, Matsumoto S, Ae K, Tanizawa T, Gokita T, Funauchi Y, et al. Risk factors for distant metastasis of dermatofibrosarcoma protuberans. J Orthopaed Traumatol. 2016;17(3):261-6.
73. Owen JL, Kibbi N, Worley B, Kelm RC, Wang JV, Barker CA, et al. Sebaceous carcinoma: evidence-based clinical practice guidelines. Lancet Oncol. 2019;20(12):e699-714.
74. Shalin SC, Lyle S, Calonje E, Lazar AJ. Sebaceous neoplasia and the Muir–Torre syndrome: important connections with clinical implications. Histopathology. 2010;56(1):133-47.
75. Misago N, Toda S, Narisawa Y. Two histopathologic patterns of well-differentiated extraocular sebaceous carcinoma. J Cutan Pathol. 2011;38(10):767-74.
76. Jakobiec FA, Mendoza PR. Eyelid sebaceous carcinoma: clinicopathologic and multiparametric immunohistochemical analysis that includes adipophilin. Am J Ophthalmol. 2014; 157(1):186-208.
77. Mulay K, Shah SJ, Aggarwal E, White VA, Honavar SG. Periocular sebaceous gland carcinoma: do androgen receptor (NR3C4) and nuclear survivin (BIRC5) have a prognostic significance? Acta Ophthalmol. 2014;92(8):e681-7.
78. Kaliki S, Ayyar A, Dave TV, Ali MJ, Mishra DK, Naik MN. Sebaceous gland carcinoma of the eyelid: clinicopathological features and outcome in Asian Indians. Eye. 2015;29(7): 958-63.
79. Shields JA, Saktanasate J, Lally SE, Carrasco JR, Shields CL. Sebaceous carcinoma of the ocular region: the 2014 Professor Winifred Mao Lecture. Asia-Pacific J Ophthalmol. 2015;4(4):221-7.
80. Yen MT, David TT, Wu X, Wolfson AH. Radiation therapy for local control of eyelid sebaceous cell carcinoma: report of two cases and review of the literature. Ophthal Plast Reconstruct Surg. 2000;16(3):211-5.
81. Takagawa Y, Tamaki W, Suzuki S, Inaba K, Murakami N, Takahashi K, et al. Radiotherapy for localized sebaceous carcinoma of the eyelid: a retrospective analysis of 83 patients. J Radiat Res. 2019;60(5):622-9.
82. Youlden DR, Soyer HP, Youl PH, Fritschi L, Baade PD. Incidence and survival for Merkel cell carcinoma in Queensland, Australia, 1993-2010. JAMA Dermatol. 2014; 150(8):864-72.
83. van der Zwan JM, Trama A, Otter R, Larrañaga N, Tavilla A, Marcos-Gragera R, et al. Rare neuroendocrine tumours: results of the surveillance of rare cancers in Europe project. Eur J Cancer. 2013;49(11):2565-78.
84. Santamaria-Barria JA, Boland GM, Yeap BY, Nardi V, Dias-Santagata D, Cusack JC. Merkel cell carcinoma: 30-year experience from a single institution. Ann Surg Oncol. 2013; 20(4):1365-73.
85. Tarantola TI, Vallow LA, Halyard MY, Weenig RH, Warschaw KE, Grotz TE, et al. Prognostic factors in Merkel cell carcinoma: analysis of 240 cases. J Am Acad Dermatol. 2013;68(3):425-32.
86. Lemos BD, Storer BE, Iyer JG, Phillips JL, Bichakjian CK, Fang LC, et al. Pathologic nodal evaluation improves prognostic accuracy in Merkel cell carcinoma: analysis of 5823 cases as the basis of the first consensus staging system. J Am Acad Dermatol. 2010;63(5):751-61.
87. Harms PW, Collie AM, Hovelson DH, Cani AK, Verhaegen ME, Patel RM, et al. Next generation sequencing of Cytokeratin 20-negative Merkel cell carcinoma reveals ultraviolet-signature mutations and recurrent TP53 and RB1 inactivation. Modern Pathol. 2016;29(3):240-8.
88. Harms PW, Vats P, Verhaegen ME, Robinson DR, Wu YM, Dhanasekaran SM, et al. The distinctive mutational spectra of polyomavirus-negative Merkel cell carcinoma. Cancer Res. 2015;75(18):3720-7.
89. Coursaget P, Samimi M, Nicol JT, Gardair C, Touzé A. Human Merkel cell polyomavirus: virological background and clinical implications. APMIS. 2013;121(8):755-69.
90. Feng H, Shuda M, Chang Y, Moore PS. Clonal integration of a polyomavirus in human Merkel cell carcinoma. Science. 2008;319(5866):1096-100.
91. Paulson KG, Lewis CW, Redman MW, Simonson WT, Lisberg A, Ritter D, et al. Viral oncoprotein antibodies as a marker for recurrence of Merkel cell carcinoma: a prospective validation study. Cancer. 2017;123(8):1464-74.
92. Gollard R, Weber R, Kosty MP, Greenway HT, Massullo V, Humberson C. Merkel cell carcinoma: review of 22 cases with surgical, pathologic, and therapeutic considerations. Cancer: Interdiscipl Int J Am Cancer Soc. 2000;88(8):1842-51.
93. Andea AA, Coit DG, Amin B, Busam KJ. Merkel cell carcinoma: histologic features and prognosis. Cancer. 2008; 113(9):2549-58.
94. Müller-Richter UD, Gesierich A, Kübler AC, Hartmann S, Brands RC. Merkel cell carcinoma of the head and neck: Recommendations for diagnostics and treatment. Ann Surg Oncol. 2017;24(11):3430-7.
95. Siva S, Byrne K, Seel M, Bressel M, Jacobs D, Callahan J, et al. 18F-FDG PET provides high-impact and powerful prognostic stratification in the staging of Merkel cell carcinoma: a 15-year institutional experience. J Nucl Med. 2013;54(8):1223-9.
96. Hawryluk EB, O'Regan KN, Sheehy N, Guo Y, Dorosario A, Sakellis CG, et al. Positron emission tomography/computed tomography imaging in Merkel cell carcinoma: a study of 270 scans in 97 patients at the Dana-Farber/Brigham and Women's Cancer Center. J Am Acad Dermatol. 2013;68(4): 592-9.
97. Harms KL, Healy MA, Nghiem P, Sober AJ, Johnson TM, Bichakjian CK, et al. Analysis of prognostic factors from 9387 Merkel cell carcinoma cases forms the basis for the new 8th edition AJCC staging system. Ann Surg Oncol. 2016;23(11):3564-102.
98. Grotz TE, Joseph RW, Pockaj BA, Foote RL, Otley CC, Bagaria SP, et al. Negative sentinel lymph node biopsy in Merkel cell carcinoma is associated with a low risk of same-nodal-basin recurrences. Ann Surg Oncol. 2015;22(12):4060-6.
99. Kaufman HL, Russell J, Hamid O, Bhatia S, Terheyden P, D'Angelo SP, et al. Avelumab in patients with chemotherapy-refractory metastatic Merkel cell carcinoma: a multicentre, single-group, open-label, phase 2 trial. Lancet Oncol. 2016; 17(10):1374-85.
100. Kaufman HL, Russell JS, Hamid O, Bhatia S, Terheyden P, D'Angelo SP, et al. Updated efficacy of avelumab in patients with previously treated metastatic Merkel cell carcinoma after ≥1 year of follow-up: JAVELIN Merkel 200, a phase 2 clinical trial. J Immunother Cancer. 2018;6(1):7.

CHAPTER 23

Thyroid Malignancies

Samskruthi P Murthy, Sivakumar Vidhyadharan, Narayana Subramaniam

INTRODUCTION

Thyroid cancer is the most common endocrine malignancies with an increasing incidence over the last few decades. It is broadly classified into differentiated and undifferentiated tumors. Differentiated thyroid cancer (DTC) arises from either thyroid follicular cells or parafollicular C cells. DTC carries an excellent prognosis with a 10-year survival rate of 90–95%.[1] On the other end of the spectrum, undifferentiated tumor-like anaplastic thyroid cancer is almost always fatal with 1-year survival of <20%.[2] The following chapter includes management strategies in DTC and anaplastic thyroid cancer.

ANATOMY AND PHYSIOLOGY OF THYROID GLAND

The thyroid is an endocrine gland situated in the anterior compartment of the neck. It is mainly composed of follicular cells and parafollicular cells that give rise to differentiated thyroid cancer. The surgical anatomy of the thyroid gland is intricate and complex and is explained under the section on thyroidectomy. The primary function of the gland is secretion of thyroxine (3, 5, 3', 5' iodothyronine or T4) and tri-iodothyronine (3, 5, 3' iodothyronine or T3). Iodine plays an important role in thyroid hormone production. The required minimum daily intake of iodine is 59 μg.[3] Sodium iodide symporters situated at the basolateral membrane of follicular cells facilitate iodine transmembrane transport against an electrochemical gradient.[3] Sodium iodide symporter is also expressed in differentiated thyroid cancer and hence can take up the iodine-131 isotope. Thyroglobulin (Tg) is a homodimeric glycol protein (660 kDa) that is stored in thyroid follicles as colloid, which forms a substrate for thyroid hormone synthesis.[4] Tg is cleaved to T3 and T4 by the follicular apical enzymes (thyroid peroxidase). Thyroid peroxidase catalyzes, iodination of tyrosine residues of Tg, which in turn get absorbed into follicular cells and are secreted into blood across the basement membrane.[4] Both normal thyroid tissue and differentiated thyroid cancers secrete thyroglobulin.

EPIDEMIOLOGY

There has been an exponential increase in papillary thyroid carcinoma (PTC). This increase is believed to be due to an increase in detection methods by the usage of routine scan that identifies otherwise indolent tumors.[5] The incidence of PTC in autopsies has not grown proportionally with incidence in the population, favoring over diagnosis as one of the reasons for the increase in incidence.[6] Nevertheless, the increase is seen even in the large tumors that can be attributed to environmental and lifestyle changes. Despite the rise in incidence, the mortality rate has been stable over decades (0.5 cases per 100,000 persons).[7] This finding makes the rising incidence more relevant as early detection must translate to improved survival. When overdiagnosis is the only cause, then there must be a corresponding decline in the incidence of large, aggressive tumors due to early detection but there has been an increase in numbers of advanced tumors.[8] Similarly overdetection would imply an increase in incidence across all histologies of thyroid cancer, but this has been seen only in PTC.[8] Bernier et al. studied age-standardized incidence rates from 39 US cancer registries and found an increase in pediatric thyroid cancers (10–19 years of age) from 4.77/million in 1998 to 8.82/million in 2013; the increased rates were for both papillary and follicular carcinoma and both early and advanced stages of thyroid cancer.[9]

RISK FACTORS

Various risk factors for thyroid cancer have been proposed and studied.

- *Radiation:* Radiation is a well-known cause of thyroid cancer. The superficial situation of the thyroid gland in the neck exposes the gland to higher doses of radiation than other subsites. The Chernobyl incidence released a massive dose of ^{131}I which resulted in reporting of over 4,000 cases from the area.[10] With a recent increase in the use of CT scans, the routine radiation exposure of a person has increased from an average of 3 mSv/year in 1980 to 6 mSv/year in 2006 in the US.[11] The iodinated contrast medium also concentrates in the thyroid, which further increases the radiation absorption by the gland. While the direct evidence of thyroid cancer and CT scans has not been evaluated, but there is a documented increased exposure. The use of radioactive iodine/radioiodine ablation (RAI) for hyperthyroidism has seen a gradual fall over decades. Meta-analysis has shown a relative risk (RR) for thyroid, kidney stomach cancer in these patients to be 1.99, 1.7, and 1.1 respectively.[12] Radiotherapy in the head and neck region among children results in second malignancy among which thyroid comprises 7.5%.[13]
- *Iodine deficiency:* Iodine deficiency results in an increase in thyroid-stimulating hormone (TSH) levels, which acts as a tumor growth factor. Rodent models have shown an increased risk of thyroid cancer among iodine deficient rodents with prolonged TSH elevation.[14] Iodine deficiency is associated with an increased incidence of follicular carcinoma than PTC.
- *Elevated TSH:* Various studies have shown a positive correlation between increased risk of thyroid cancer and elevated TSH.[15,16] Even though no direct correlation is proven, the incidence of Hashimoto's thyroiditis and thyroid cancer have increased in parallel. Periods of elevated TSH levels and oxidative stress associated with the autoimmune process could be the cause.
- *Nonthyroid hormones:* Studies have shown an increased risk of thyroid cancer among obese patients. The insulin resistance and hyperinsulinemia associated with obesity could be the causative factor. Insulin stimulates thymocyte proliferation, differentiation, and also transformation.[17] The exact mechanism is unknown. A recent meta-analysis assessed the relation of thyroid cancer risk and reproductive factors.[18] They have reported that women of reproductive age and during pregnancy are more prone to thyroid cancer than women at ends of the reproductive age.

THYROID CANCER IN INDIA

Epidemiological studies about thyroid cancer in India are limited. The incidence of thyroid cancer has drastically increased in Thiruvananthapuram from 6.9 per 100,000 females in 2006 to 13.3 in 2012.[19] While the incidence in Delhi, Mumbai, Bengaluru, and Chennai have remained stable at 2–4.1 per 100,000 females between 2006 and 2012. While, on the other hand, the cancer mortality has been stable at 0.4–0.5 per 100,000 females in all five cities. The peak rise was among <40 years.

EVALUATION OF THE THYROID NODULE

Thyroid nodules are common and need evaluation to differentiate between benign and malignant nodules. Fine-needle aspiration cytology (FNAC) remains the gold standard in the diagnosis of malignant thyroid nodules. Before subjecting the patient to invasive FNAC, ultrasound (US) features are used to guide suspicious nodules that require FNAC.

Ultrasound

Various US risk stratifications are available which have been modified over the years. American College of Radiology–Thyroid Imaging, Reporting and Data System (ACR TI-RADS),[20] American Thyroid Association US stratification,[21] Korean Society of Thyroid Radiology (KSThR),[22] and American Association of Clinical Endocrinologists (AACE)/American College of Endocrinology (ACE)/Associazione Medici Endocrinology (AME) risk stratifications are a few.[23]

The American Thyroid Association (ATA) and the American College of Radiology (ACR) thyroid imaging reporting and data system (TI-RADS) are the most common US staging systems used. ATA has a pattern-oriented approach. Unlike the ATA US stratification system, ACR TI-RADS is a point-based system in which the sonologist evaluates all visible nodules and awards points for each feature. These points are then added up and the TI-RAD level is assigned. When compared to other US systems, ACR TI-RADS size cut-off is higher, which is based on the fact that the US tends to overestimate the size of the nodule. Bachar et al. showed a discrepancy between pathological and sonological size, which showed the US mean diameter of 2.65 ± 1.07 cm correlating with a pathological mean diameter of 1.97 ± 1.17 cm.[24] ACR TI-RADS has explained assigning points when US features cannot be determined, which is most often seen when calcifications overshadow the rest of the nodule for evaluation. Yoon et al. have shown that the ATA US system led to noncategorization of 3.4% of nodules, of which 18.2% were malignant.[25] Due to the point-based system, interobserver variability is reduced with ACR TI-RADS and leads to lesser invasive procedures in nonsignificant nodules. The percentage of benign nodules biopsied is least with ACR TI-RADS (47.1%) when compared to ATA US and KSThR TI-RADS.

Ultrasound-guided FNAC is indicated when thyroid nodule is not palpable, posteriorly placed, small nodules, previously failed unguided FNAC and cystic nodules with solid component. US-guided FNAC of the lymph nodes is indicated when nodes are nonpalpable, cystic, and small nodes.[21]

Fine-needle Aspiration Cytology

Fine-needle aspiration cytology of thyroid nodule remains the gold standard in diagnosing malignancy. The Bethesda system for reporting thyroid cytology was proposed to facilitate uniform terminology for reporting FNAC reports of thyroid nodules.[26] The Bethesda system is one of the most widely accepted reporting systems that aids in better communication between cytologist and treating endocrinologist/surgeon concerning understanding and interpretation of the report. It consists of five categories with a defined rate of malignancy of each category. Newer pathological entities and changing terminology in thyroid cancer has led to a change in the rate of malignancy for each category. The presence of nuclear pseudoinclusions, psammoma bodies, and true papillae are characteristic of PTC cytology.

Fine-needle aspiration cytology is considered adequate when at least six groups of follicular cells with each containing at least 10 cells are present.[27] Cytology slide is considered benign when abundant colloid is present even though the cells are sparse. Atypia of undetermined significance (AUS) could be cellular or architectural atypia or both. The rate of AUS reported by a cytologist must be limited to <10%, for laboratory reports to be considered of adequate quality.[28] Follicular neoplasm or suspicious for follicular neoplasm (FN/SFN) is defined as "follicular-patterned cells with mild nuclear changes (increased nuclear size, nuclear contour irregularity, and/or chromatin clearing) can be classified as FN/SFN as long as true papillae and intranuclear pseudoinclusions are absent".[27] The earlier noninvasive follicular variant of papillary carcinoma thyroid is now termed "noninvasive follicular thyroid neoplasm with papillary-like nuclear features" (NIFTP). It significantly affects risk of malignancy in category 3 and above.[29] NIFTP is a pathological diagnosis and treatment consists of lobectomy, which is in line with category recommendation. Hence, from a management point of view, NIFTP does not affect the management recommendation. The earlier belief that a 3-month gap between FNAC is warranted to avoid cellular atypia is not recommended. ATA recommends no such delay in repeat FNAC, as the presence of malignancy affects the final prognosis.[21]

Molecular Genetics in Thyroid Cancer

Thyroid cancer initiation and progression is a consequence of the accumulation of genetic and epigenetic changes. Two main pathways mediate the carcinogenesis. Mitogen-activated protein kinase (MAPK) activation is essential for tumor initiation, which occurs as a result of chromosomal rearrangements such as *RET/PTC* and tropomyosin receptor kinase (TRK) and point mutations that involve *RAS, BRAF*.[30] RET and neurospecific receptor kinase (NRK) encode cell membrane tyrosine kinases and *BRAF/RAS* are intracellular signal transducers. Point mutations are a consequence of sporadic and dietary mutagenesis, while chromosomal rearrangement and chromosomal fragility are a consequence of radiation-induced carcinogenesis. *RET* gene fuses with an active promoter that drives ligand-independent RET/PTC protein, which results in stimulation of MAPK signaling and initiates tumorigenesis.[30] The fusion between *PAX8* and *PPARγ* gene results in *PAX8/PPARγ* protein overexpression, the mechanism of which is not fully defined. BRAF is a serine-threonine kinase that is activated by RAS, results in inactivation of the MAPK signaling pathway. The most common point mutation is adenine substitution at 1,799 nucleotide position resulting in replacement of valine by glutamate at residue 600 (Val 600 Glu). RAS encode G-proteins that transmit signal from tyrosine kinase inhibitors (TIKs), activate both MAPK and *PI3-AKT* pathway. *NRAS* codon 61 and *HRAS* codon 61 are the most common point mutations in thyroid cancer. *TP53* and *CTNNB1* genes mutation is commonly associated only with poorly differentiated carcinoma (PDC) and anaplastic carcinoma.[31] They drive tumorigenesis by encoding for effectors that activate the *PI3-AK* pathway. The role of identification of molecular markers is essential as they play a role in diagnosis, prognostication, and targeted therapy.

Molecular Markers for Diagnosis

The prevalence of mutations specific to tumors along with their prevalence of occurrence is summarized in **Table 1**.[30]

Table 1: Thyroid cancer and mutation profiles.

Characteristics	*Papillary carcinoma*	*Follicular carcinoma*	*Poorly differentiated carcinoma*	*Anaplastic carcinoma*	*Medullary carcinoma*
Prevalence %	80–85	10–15	<2	1–2	3–5
Pattern of spread	Nodal metastasis	Hematogenous spread to bones, lungs	Invasive local tumor, nodal and hematogenous metastasis	Invasive local tumor, nodal and hematogenous metastasis	LN and hematogenous metastasis
10-year survival %	95–98	90–95	50	<10	60–80
Common mutations with prevalence in percentage	*BRAF*: 40–45	*RAS*: 40–50	*RAS*: 20–40	*TP53*: 50–80	Familial forms: *RET* > 95
	RAS: 10–20	*PAX8/PPAR-γ*: 30–35	*TP53*: 20–30	*TP53*: 50–80 *CTNNB1*: 5–60	Sporadic: *RET*: 40–50
	RET/PTC: 10–20	*PIK3CA*: <10	*BRAF*: 10–20	*RAS*: 20–40 *BRAF*: 20–40	Sporadic: *RAS*: 25
	TRK: <5	*PTEN*: <10	*CTNNB1*: 10–20	*PIK3CA*: 10–20 *PTEN*: 5–15	
			PIK3CA: 5–10	*AKT1*: 5–10	
			AKT1: 5–10		

Table 2: Commercially available molecular testing kit and their interpretation.

	Afirma gene expression classifier	*ThyroMIR + ThyGenX*	*Thyroseq*
Method	*mRNA* gene expression	Multiplex PCR + MicroRNA expression	Next-generation sequencing
Test characteristics	mRNA expression of 167 genes	100 genetic alterations in 8 genes + 10 mRNA expression	56 genes V2 112 genes V3
Sensitivity %	92	89	86
Specificity %	27	85	79
NPV %	91	96	94
PPV %	30	66	58
Rule in/rule out/ combined	Rule out test	Combined	Combined
Duration of result	<2 weeks	10–14 days	<2 weeks
Pattern of report	• Cytopathology resulted then GSC is evaluated on BIII/IV only • GSC resulted as benign or suspicious • Additional analysis for *BRAF*^{V600E}, MTC, *RET/PTC1* and *3*	• *ThyGenX* oncogene reported • If *ThyGenX* negative, then ThyraMIR assessed and reported as high or low risk	Positive or negative with detailed results for each type of molecular marker tested
Interpretation	• *Benign:* Consider surveillance • *Suspicious:* Consider surgery	• *7GP positive:* Consider surgery • *ThyraMIR high:* Consider surgery • *ThyraMIR low:* Consider surveillance	• *Negative:* Consider surveillance • *Positive:* Consider surgery

(MTC: medullary thyroid cancer; NPV: negative predictive value; PCR: polymerase chain reaction; PPV: positive predictive value; PTC: papillary thyroid carcinoma; RNA: ribonucleic acid)

The use of molecular markers in the diagnosis of thyroid malignancy is restricted to Bethesda 3 and 4 cytology reports. The use of molecular markers is being explored to avoid excessive surgery and also to avoid completion surgery if the report indicates high-risk pathology. Various test panels are tested and available commercially. **Table 2** shows various commercially available molecular testing kit and their interpretation.[32,33]

The interpretation of these test panels is based on the concept of "ruling in" and "ruling out". A "rule in" test is a highly specific test that when positive points toward malignancy and active intervention has to be planned. While a "rule out" test is a highly sensitive test that is when negative rules out the possibility of malignancy in the nodule. The interpretation of molecular markers cannot solely aid the management decision, but must always be made in conjunction with cytology report. The FNAC aspirate is sent for molecular marker test panel.

The recent meta-analysis reported that postvalidation studies available for Afirma-GEC and Thyroseq V2 are intermediate to good quality of evidence.[34] Afrima has the maximum evidence available with consistent high sensitivity of 90%. Thyroseq V2 has shown high overall diagnostic accuracy with an expected rate of avoided surgery of 79%. The cost-effectiveness of these tests versus surgery hinders the use of these tests. Molecular testing is set with limitations and merits, and hence when used, patients must be counseled. ATA does not recommend routine use of molecular tests.[21]

Prognostic Implications of Molecular Markers

BRAF is associated with aggressive variant of PTCs such as tall cell variant. It is commonly associated with extrathyroidal extension, higher rates of recurrence, presents with larger tumors, and has a propensity for dedifferentiation.[30] *RET*/PTC chromosomal rearrangements associated with younger patients and propensity for nodal metastasis. *RAS* mutations are commonly associated with follicular tumors. They have a greater propensity for distant metastasis. Telomerase reverse transcriptase (*TERT*) mutations are rare in thyroid malignancies with an incidence of 4.2% alone and combined with *BRAF* in 6.2% of cases.[30] *TERT* mutations are an independent predictor of recurrence and mortality and are associated with poor survival.

MANAGEMENT OF THYROID CANCER

Imaging in Thyroid Cancer

Residual disease is common in DTC and the only way to reduce resurgeries is by adequate preoperative imaging and planning. Various modalities such as US, computed tomography (CT), magnetic resonance imaging (MRI) scans, and positron-emission tomography (PET)-CT are used in preoperative assessment.[35]

Ultrasound

The objectives of preoperative imaging are to assess the extent of primary tumor and rest of the thyroid gland and to assess neck lymph nodes in the lateral compartment and central compartment. In US, the presence of the thyroid gland between trachea and carotid affects the assessment of central compartment nodes.

Ultrasound assessment of primary tumor: Assessment of location, extent, focality, and invasion of surrounding structures must be assessed. Invasion to carotid artery, trachea, and esophagus needs further evaluation with cross-sectional imaging such as CT.

Ultrasound assessment of lymph nodes: The sensitivity of the US to identify metastatic nodes ranges from 25 to 60%, while specificity ranges from 80 to 90%.[36,37]

- *Location of nodes:* The involvement of nodes is progressive from level VI to level III/IV to level II. Involvement of contralateral nodes in the absence of contralateral thyroid lobe involvement is less with contralateral level VI involvement in 5–25% and contralateral lateral nodes in 5–14%. The involvement of level V and IIb is rare with <5% involvement.[35]
- *Size:* Nodes measuring >1 cm is considered metastatic with a sensitivity of 68% and sensitivity of 75%.
- *Shape:* Rounded nodes are considered malignant.[38] Solbiati index is a valuable tool to objectively assess the shape of the node. It is calculated by the ratio of long and short axes of the node. A ratio of <2.0 is considered suspicious of malignancy and value of >2.0 as benign.[39] The sensitivity is 46% and specificity of 64%.
- *Calcifications:* Microcalcifications are seen in lymph nodes with metastasis and are 100% specific.[38]
- *Echogenicity:* Benign nodes are uniformly hypoechoic with central hilar enhancement. While malignant nodes typically exhibit mixed echogenicity, hyperechoic, and sometimes can be cystic.[40] Cystic nodes represent increased tumor aggressiveness and are common in younger patients.
- *Hypervascularity:* Normal/benign nodes express hypervascularity along hilum. While malignant nodes express a disordered vascularity throughout the node with peripheral vascularity. Peripheral vascularity has the highest sensitivity and specificity of 86% and 82%, respectively.[40]

Additional considerations: Fine-needle aspiration cytology is not mandatory when US features are specific to metastasis and does not change the extent of surgery.[41-43] FNAC must be performed with 27-gauge needle to acquire adequate cells. Tg assessment of the FNA needle washout can be used to improve the sensitivity of the cytology report; a cutoff of 1 ng/mL for washouts prepared with up to 1 mL of solvent is suggested. Tg washout may especially be helpful in cases with cystic nodes. US-guided FNAC is suggested for nodes >0.8 cm.[42,43]

Ultrasound after previous surgery is tricky due to postoperative inflammation, fibrosis, and scarring and reactive adenopathy. The rate of false positivity is also high. Hence, re-evaluation after 6 months is suggested, if the initial tumor is nonaggressive.[35]

Ultrasound is the first line of imaging modality in DTC; cross-sectional imaging is advised only in select cases. However, the US is limited in the evaluation of deep neck structures that are shielded by air or bone.

The indications for cross-sectional imaging are:[35]

- Invasive primary tumor with suspicious involvement of carotid artery, esophagus, trachea, and larynx
- Large primary/nodal disease which cannot be evaluated by US
- Extranodal extension with involvement of carotid, artery or deep neck spaces such as retropharyngeal space
- Extension of primary/nodal disease into mediastinum
- Posteromedial located tumors that are not well visualized with US.

Figures 1 to 3 show various presentations of DTC on CT.

A combination of US and cross-sectional imaging can be used to gain 15% sensitivity in the evaluation of lymph nodes.[35] MRI imaging is associated with motion artifacts with benefit of noniodinated gadolinium contrast.

Functional Imaging in Differentiated Thyroid Cancer

Positron-emission tomography with computed tomography (PET-CT) imaging at present has a limited role in papillary and follicular carcinoma of thyroid except in postoperative setting when Tg is elevated with negative iodine scan. DTC has low fluorodeoxyglucose (FDG) avidity that results in false-negative findings reducing the diagnostic accuracy of FDG. About 0–50% of DTC express glucose transporter.[44] The correlations between glucose transporter (GLUT)-3, GLUT-4, and standardized uptake values (SUV) are significant in DTC. The sensitivity and specificity of FDG-PET with US, CT with contrast is comparable with respect to identification of lymph nodes.[45] Hence, US or cross-sectional imaging will suffice. Less than 4% of patients present with distant metastasis and hence a routine metastatic preoperative workup is not advisable.[46] As the tumor dedifferentiates, it loses its property of iodine avidity and glucose metabolism increases. The use of FDG-PET CT in the evaluation of distant metastasis in aggressive histologies such as anaplastic thyroid carcinoma might be justifiable.[47] Increased FDG-uptake in either primary or recurrent tumor signifies aggressive disease or dedifferentiated tumor; the SUV value is of prognostic significance.

Incidentalomas: These are thyroid nodules that are not palpable but are identified on imaging. Incidentalomas detected by PET-CT has a rate of malignancy of 10–63.3%.[35,48] Hence, all FDG avid incidentalomas must be evaluated to rule out malignancies even if they measure <1 cm. FDG incidentalomas are most often associated with aggressive histology. PET-CT in AUS has shown varied results with sensitivity ranging from 57 to 100%.[49]

Preoperative Thyroglobulin

The specificity and sensitivity of Tg with intact thyroid is of limited value. Preoperative measurement of serum Tg

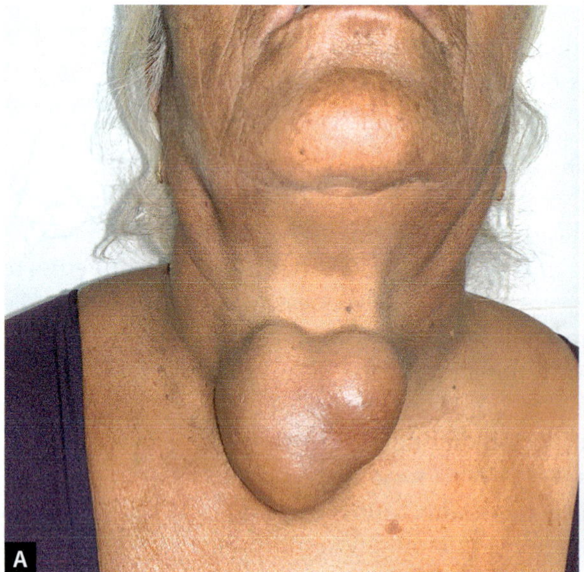

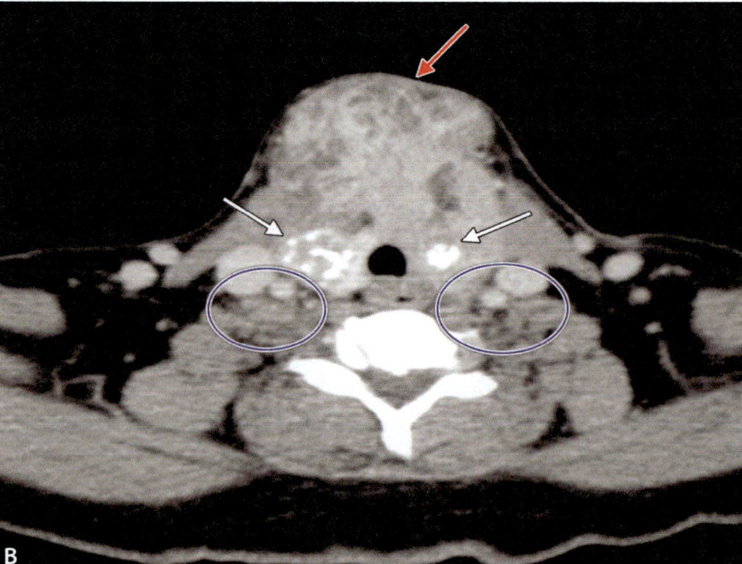

Figs. 1A and B: (A) Clinical photo of a 60-year-old female patient with long standing history of thyroid swelling (>15 years) and proven papillary carcinoma thyroid; (B) Contrast enhanced CT of the same patient showing invasive tumor involving whole thyroid gland (red arrow), strap muscles and skin anteriorly macrocalcification (white arrows), lymph nodal metastasis in level VI compartment (purple circles).

is futile as various nonmalignant thyroid disorders such as autoimmune thyroiditis, benign adenoma, subacute thyroiditis, and Graves' disease can raise serum Tg. ATA 2015 does not recommend routine preoperative assessment of Tg.[21]

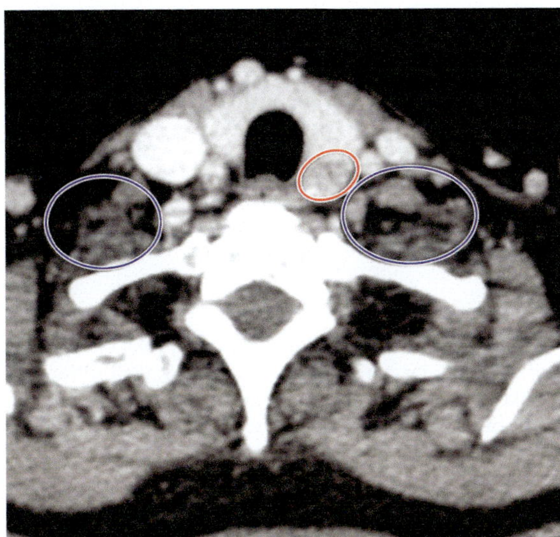

Fig. 2: Axial sections of contrast enhanced CT depicting incidentally detected thyroid nodule (proven papillary carcinoma thyroid in left lobe of thyroid (red circle) with bilateral level VI and IV lymph nodal metastasis (blue circles).

Pathology

The pathology of thyroid cancers is confusing and ever-changing. To simplify pathology of tumors arising from follicular cells, pathologic features can be defined by following characteristics.[50] **Table 3** describes various pathological characteristics that define the variant.

- *Papillae:* The architecture of tumor consists of papillae that are composed of a central fibrovascular core, lined by single or multiple layers of cells.
- *Nuclear features of papillary carcinoma:* The characteristic nuclear changes consists pseudonuclear inclusions, nuclear grooving, and distinct nucleoli. The classical orphan Annie eye is formed due to the clearing of chromatin in the nuclei.
- *Capsular invasion:* There is no definite consensus. Transgression of tumor capsule either through the whole thickness or incomplete transgression is considered as capsular invasion.
- *Angioinvasion:* Defined as the invasion of vascular space by the invasion of tumor cells through the vessel with accompanying thrombus. Vascular invasion can be differentiated by lymphatic invasion as vascular invasion stain positive for CD31. Greater than 4 foci of angioinvasion increase the risk of recurrence.
- *Encapsulation:* Intact tumor capsule.

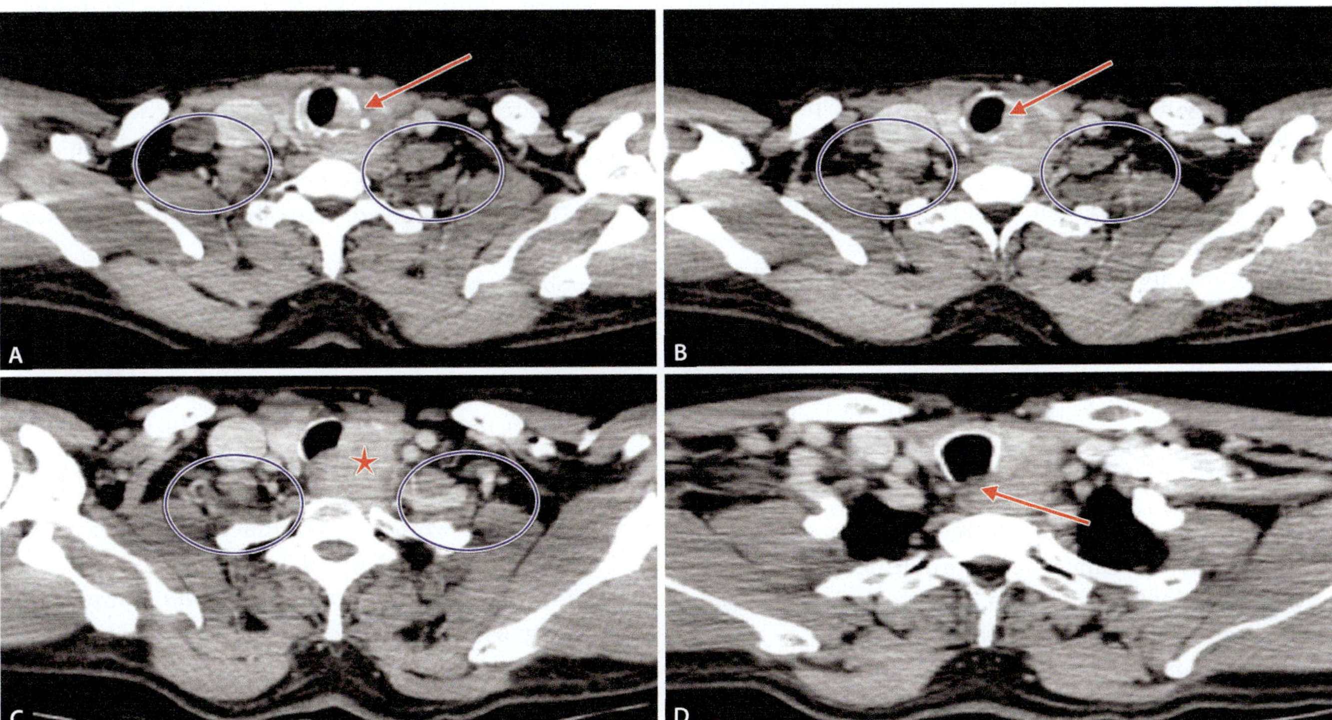

Figs. 3A to D: Axial sections of contrast enhanced CT of a 52-year-old patient with proven papillary carcinoma thyroid. (A and B) Red arrow showing tumor invasion through the cricoid cartilage and blue circles depicting lateral cervical lymph nodal metastasis; (C) Red star showing thyroid tumor involving left thyroid lobe, left tracheo-esophageal grove, tracheal cartilage and esophageal involvement and blue circles depicting lateral cervical lymph nodal metastasis; (D) Red arrow showing thyroid tumor invading esophagus and posterior tracheal wall.

Table 3: Pathological features of follicular cell-derived tumors.

Type	*Papillae*	*Nuclear features of PTC*	*Capsular invasion*	*Angioinvasion*	*Follicular architecture*	*Encapsulated*
Malignant tumors						
PTC: Classical	+	+	-	-	-	-
FV-PTC	–	+	–	–	+	
MI-FC	–	–	+	– #	+	
EA-FC			–	+	+	+
WI-FC	–	–	+	+	+	
WDCa-NOS	–	–	+	+	–	
Borderline malignant tumors						
NIFTP	–	+	–	–	–	
WDT-UMP	?	+ or ?	?	?		+
FT-UMP	–	–	?	?	+	+

(PTC: papillary thyroid carcinoma; FV-PTC: follicular variant-papillary thyroid carcinoma; MI-FC: minimally invasive follicular carcinoma; EA-FC: encapsulated angioinvasive follicular carcinoma; WI-FC: widely invasive follicular carcinoma; WDCa–NOS: well-differentiated carcinoma—not otherwise specified; NIFTP: noninvasive follicular thyroid neoplasm with papillary-like nuclear features; WDT-UMP: well-differentiated tumor of uncertain malignant potential; FT-UMP: follicular tumor of uncertain malignant potential; +: present; –: absent; ?: variable)

as per College of American Pathologists (CAP)

- *Extrathyroidal extension:* Microscopic extrathyroidal extension is difficult to identify, as an extension to surrounding fatty tissue can be misleading. The current staging considers extension to strap muscles as significant.
- *Psammoma bodies:* Laminated calcification of the central core of papillae can result in psammoma bodies. While calcification of colloid is seen in Hurthle cell neoplasm.
- *Margin:* The margin in the thyroid gland is difficult to assess, as the capsule of the thyroid gland is deficient in various areas. The outer surface of the thyroid gland is considered as margin.
- *Microscopic and macroscopic nodal metastasis:* No consensus. Even though metastasis <2 mm is defined as microscopic, 2–10 mm as small and >10 mm as large (as proposed by Randolph et al.), this has not been prospectively validated.

The characteristic features that help in diagnosing common thyroid cancer and borderline tumors of the thyroid are detailed in **Table 3**. Further characteristics of uncommon tumors are as follows:

- *Variants of papillary thyroid carcinoma*
  - *Tall cell variant:* Tall cell is twice as tall as wide. More than 50% of cells must be tall cells to diagnose a tall cell variant. Occurs in older patients, presents as large tumors, and extrathyroidal extension is common. Dedifferentiation has been described. 10-year OS is 79%, which is much lower than classical papillary carcinoma.[51]
  - *Diffuse sclerosing variant:* Incidence is very rare, comprising 3% of papillary carcinoma.[52] Characterized by areas of squamous metaplasia, extensive calcification, and extensive lymphocytic infiltrates. The tumor commonly involves the whole gland and is grossly very hard on palpation. Commonly occurs in children and young adults. Often associated with regional and distant metastasis.
  - *Solid variant*: One of the variants with a high mortality rate of 10–12% at 10 years of follow-up.[53] While solid variant associated with children of the post-Chernobyl incident, it is associated with a better prognosis.[54] This needs to be differentiated from poorly differentiated carcinoma. The solid variant still presents with nuclear features of papillary while the papillary growth pattern is replaced by solid growth.
- *Poorly differentiated thyroid carcinoma:* Turin criteria for diagnosis consists of:[55]
  - Insular/solid/trabecular growth pattern
  - Absence of conventional nuclear features of PTC and presence of one of the following:
    - Tumor necrosis
    - Convoluted nuclei
    - Mitosis >3 × 10 high power fields (HPF)

Even the foci consisting of 10% of PDC can affect the survival outcome. PDC forms a bridge in clinical behavior between DTC and anaplastic thyroid carcinoma.

- *Primary squamous cell carcinoma (SCC) of the thyroid*: Similar to SCC of other areas. Stain positive for *PAX8* which is negative if it is metastatic to the thyroid.[56]
- *Primary thyroid lymphoma:* It is rare comprising 1–5% of all thyroid malignancies. The most common are non-Hodgkin's lymphoma such as diffuse large β-cell lymphoma (DLBCL), mucosal-associated lymphoid tissue lymphoma (MALT), or mixed variants.[56]
- *Primary thyroid sarcoma:* Comprises <1.5% of all thyroid malignancies. Includes angiosarcoma, fibrosarcoma, leiomyosarcoma, and malignant fibrous histiocytoma. In all cases, the possibility of distant metastasis to thyroid must be ruled out.[56]

The intraoperative frozen section for confirmatory diagnosis in tumors with nonspecific FNAC reports is not advocated, because of low sensitivity and high false-negative rate.[57] Frozen section is not advisable as it is associated with various limitations such as sampling error in capsule examination, freeze artifact and distortion, blood vessel collapse, difficulty in distinguishing between iatrogenic capsular rupture, difficulty in distinguishing capsular entrapment, and true capsular invasion. The final histopathological evaluation becomes difficult due to sampling during the frozen section. Capsule sampling to rule out capsular invasion is difficult as the capsule cannot be accurately sampled on frozen section.

Extent of Surgery

The extent of thyroidectomy has been debated for decades. The guidelines and recommendations for the extent of surgery, especially in low-risk group, have been ever changing. Due to the absence of prospective trials, most of the recommendations are based on retrospective studies that are either institutional data or large population-based data.[58] The current ATA recommends hemithyroidectomy for unifocal tumors measuring <4 cm without evidence of any adverse features (such as extrathyroidal extension and lymph node metastasis) preoperatively.[21] The studies of significance favoring less than total thyroidectomy and total thyroidectomy are listed in **Table 4.**[58-66]

The risk stratification of low risk and intermediate-high risk is based on histopathology report. Hence, emergence of adverse features in postoperative histopathology report may mandate total thyroidectomy to facilitate RAI. The rate of occurrence of adverse features that may mandate completion of thyroidectomy ranges from 43 to 59.1%.[67,68] Hence, estimation of one's own regional or institutional data is crucial to counsel patients.

Table 4: Studies that have assessed efficacy extent of thyroidectomy in differentiated thyroid cancer (DTC).[58]

Study	*Number of patients*	*Source of data*	*Follow-up in years*	*Conclusion*
In favor of total thyroidectomy				
Mazzaferri et al.[59]	1,355	Institution	15.7	Tumors >1.5 cm near total thyroidectomy with radioiodine therapy offers better outcome
Hay et al.[60]	1,656	Institution	18	No survival benefit with more aggressive surgery but associated with significant lower risk of recurrence
Bilimoria et al.[61]	52,173	Population-based data	5.8	Total thyroidectomy is associated with lower recurrence rate and improved survival compared with lobectomy
In favor of lobectomy				
Cady et al.[62]	631	Institution	15	Patients at low-risk or with small carcinomas can be treated satisfactorily by lobectomy
Shah et al.[63]	146	Institution	20	Lobectomy in low-risk patients is as safe as total thyroidectomy
Mandelsohn et al.[64]	22,724	Population database	9.1	Extent of surgical resection does not significantly impact overall or disease-specific survival
Nixon et al.[65]	889	Institution	8.25	No significant difference between the two surgical groups in overall survival/disease-specific survival/local recurrence/distant recurrence rate
Adam et al.[66]	61,775	Population database	6.8	Overall survival was similar in patients undergoing total thyroidectomy versus lobectomy for tumors 1.0–4.0 cm

TOTAL THYROIDECTOMY AND APPLIED ANATOMY

Total or hemithyroidectomy is the current standard of treatment in patients with differentiated thyroid cancer when indicated. Theodor Billroth introduced modern thyroid surgery, and Theodor Kocher refined it, by introducing the concept of capsular dissection. Kocher's procedures were completed with a mortality of 1% and a minimal morbidity that was reported from 900 thyroid procedures; it was for his work on physiology, pathology, and surgery of the thyroid that he received a Nobel Prize in 1909. The procedure of total thyroidectomy is broken down into the following headings:[69]

- *Management of external branch of superior laryngeal nerve (EBSLN):* EBSLN is a neglected nerve during thyroid surgery but injury to it can cause significant impairment for those who use their voices professionally. The nerve can be identified successfully in 60–90% of the cases.[70] Various classifications describing the relation of EBSLN with upper pole of thyroid and constrictor muscle are presented in **Table 5.**[71,72]

  The key step in identifying the nerve during thyroidectomy is by developing a medial avascular plane before ligation of superior thyroid vessels between the cricothyroid muscle and the medial border of the superior pole of thyroid. This can be achieved by lateral traction of the superior pole of the thyroid. The classical teaching of ligating the superior thyroid vessels blindly in a bunch must be avoided as superior laryngeal nerve lies in close proximity to per Cernea type 2A and 2B classifications.[69] Hence, after creating the medial avascular plane, superior thyroid vessels must be identified individually and ligated separately.
- *Capsular dissection:* In earlier years, the recurrent laryngeal nerve (RLN) was identified lateral to the thyroid gland and was dissected throughout its entire length in the neck. This resulted in an increased risk of devascularization of the parathyroid gland and also neural injury. Capsular dissection avoids this and is commenced high on the surface of the thyroid gland, dividing only the terminal branches of the inferior thyroid artery.[69] The dissection is commenced from the lower pole and progressed toward the upper pole. During the dissection, inferior parathyroid glands can be identified and successfully preserved. This method of dissection preserves vascular supply to parathyroid glands and minimum dissection and manipulation of the recurrent laryngeal nerve.
- *Recurrent laryngeal nerve dissection:* The RLN arises from vagus at the level of the subclavian artery on the right and arch of the aorta on the left. The term "recurrent" is used as the nerve loops around the respective artery to run along the tracheoesophageal groove and enter larynx by piercing the inferior border of inferior constrictor muscle. The nerve runs behind common carotid arteries at the mediastinal inlet and above the nerve is bounded medially by the trachea and laterally by carotid artery. On the right, the nerve runs more laterally, while it almost runs a vertical course on the left. The left nerve is longer, measuring 12 cm, while on the right it measures 7 cm with a mean diameter of 1.3 mm. The nerve crosses branches of inferior thyroid artery, which is subject to anatomical variations. In most of the cases the nerve runs anterior

Table 5: Classifications of external branch of superior laryngeal nerve (EBSLN) anatomy.

Type	Description	Incidence	Remark
Cernea et al.[71]			
Type I	Nerve crosses superior thyroid vessels 1 cm above upper pole edge of superior pole	68% small/normal gland 23% in enlarged gland	
Type IIA	Nerve crosses superior thyroid vessels <1 cm from upper pole edge of superior pole	18% in small/normal gland 15% in enlarged gland	Asians most often have either of type II SLNB
Type IIB	Nerve crosses below upper border of superior pole	14% in small/normal gland 54% in enlarged gland	
Friedman et al.[72]			
Type I	Nerve runs superficial to inferior constrictor muscle		
Type II	Nerve penetrates muscle (inferior constrictor) in lower portion of muscle		
Type III	Nerve penetrates muscle (inferior constrictor) superiorly and remains protected the whole length	20%	As the nerve stays hidden, it is difficult to identify SLNB in type III

(SLNB: sentinel lymph node biopsy)

to the artery. The distal segment of the nerve runs underneath the inferior constrictor muscle to enter the larynx at the inferior edge of the thyroid cartilage. The most constant landmark of the nerve is the point of entry into the inferior constrictor muscle and this is not subject to distortion in any kind of thyroid pathology. The nerve may occasionally branch along its cervical course in the last 2 cm, usually above the intersection of the inferior thyroid artery and the nerve. The anterior branch is the motor branch while the posterior branch most often is sensory. The relationship of the nerve with tubercle of Zuckerkandl (ToZ) and ligament of Berry is extremely important. ToZ is closely associated with the nerve and is described as an arrow pointing to the nerve. The nerve runs medial to ToZ and the likelihood it running lateral to tubercle is extremely low with an incidence of 0.8–7%.[73]

Tubercle of Zuckerkandl being a component of the thyroid gland is also affected by pathologies of the thyroid gland. When enlarged, it may grow around the RLN giving a false impression of the nerve piercing the ToZ. The superior parathyroid gland is situated posterior and superior to ToZ. During the lateral approach to finding the RLN, ToZ is a useful landmark for the identification of the distal RLN. Transection of TZ during thyroidectomy is not advocated and it must be resected completely.

The ligament of Berry is posterior condensation of the pretracheal fascia that suspends it to the cricotracheal complex. The middle thyroid vein, when present (30%), must be ligated before starting the capsular dissection along the lateral surface of the thyroid. This enables a 120° arc of rotation of the thyroid lobe achieved by anteromedial traction of the lobe, which results in straightening RLN and its displacement from the trachea-esophageal groove. The ligament of Berry has a superficial vascular plane, which consists of terminal branches and tributaries of inferior thyroid artery and vein, and this layer runs lateral to the nerve. On division of this layer, the distal part of the nerve is exposed and the nerve is seen lying over the deep fibrous layer. The deep fibrous layer is relatively avascular and extends from cricoid to first or third tracheal ring.

Sympathetic inferior laryngeal nerve anastomotic branch (SILAB) can be confused with a non-RLN. In 2% of cases, SILAB is larger than RLN. Whenever there is a doubt, the nerve must be traced laterally; a nonrecurrent laryngeal nerve (NRLN) will arise from the vagus while SILAB most often arise from middle cervical ganglia.[74]

Table 6: Course of nonrecurrent laryngeal nerve.

Nonrecurrent internal laryngeal nerve (NRLN)	*Course*
Type I	The NRLN arises from cervical vagus directly and descends into the larynx at the level of the superior thyroid pole along with vessels of the superior thyroid pedicle
Type IIA	The NRLN arises from the cervical vagus directly and follows a transverse path parallel to and over the trunk of the inferior thyroid artery (ITA), at the level of the isthmus
Type IIB	The NRLN follows a transverse path parallel to and under the trunk of ITA, marking a downward curve

Nonrecurrent laryngeal nerve has an incidence on the right side of around 0.61%. This occurs as a consequence of abnormal absorption of the fourth right branchial arch, which results in a retroesophageal right subclavian artery. Nonrecurrence on the left side is extremely rare with incidents of 0.04% and is known to occur only in situs inversus.[75] The points of entry of a nonrecurrent nerve are described in **Table 6**.

Approaches to Recurrent Laryngeal Nerve

Various surgical approaches have been described:[73]

- *Lateral approach:* It is the most common approach that is performed in routine open thyroidectomy, where the nerve is identified at the level of the middle of the thyroid lobe. In this approach, the superior and inferior thyroid poles are detected first and then the middle of the thyroid vein is ligated for maximum retraction of the thyroid lobe, anteromedially to expose the paratracheal region. This approach utilizes the inferior thyroid artery, ligament of Berry and ToZ as markers of nerve. The nerve is identified and detected in the distal 2 cm near its entry into the inferior constrictor muscle.
- *Superior approach:* It is one of the most challenging approaches that should be used as a last resort in large thyroids with retrosternal extension. The superior pole of thyroid is retracted laterally to locate RLN at the inferior margin of inferior constrictor muscle. The laryngeal entry point being the most constant anatomical site makes this approach most accurate.
- *Inferior approach:* It is usually considered in cases of revision surgery. The nerve is identified between

the retracted strap muscles and the carotid artery. The nerve lies in an area which is previously undissected and hence is easier to identify. The nerve runs as a single trunk and hence its identification in this area is beneficial. This approach is associated with a higher possibility of compromising inferior parathyroid gland vascularity.

The vascularity of the parathyroid gland must always be checked by capsular prick with a needle to look for capillary bleed. If absent, transplantation of the parathyroid gland is recommended.[76] In theory, autotransplantation can cause short-term hypocalcemia but has the potential to avoid permanent hypocalcemia.

Intraoperative nerve monitoring of RLN: The gold standard to identify RLN is by intraoperative visualization and detailed knowledge regarding its normal and variant anatomy. Use of intraoperative nerve monitoring (IONM) to identify the nerve is always used as an adjuvant to visualization.[77] IONM is not used as a proxy to poor knowledge and experience concerning nerve visualization. Various studies have proven the safety of using IONM in thyroidectomy. A review has shown no benefit when compared with IONM and RLN visualization.[78] The rate of transient and permanent RLN palsy was the same among the two groups. The cost-effectiveness was better in the visualization only group. Currently, there is no recommendation of routine use of IONM during every total thyroidectomy.[32]

The clinical situations where IONM benefit over visualization are reoperation, resection of large thyroid with substernal extension, preoperative vocal cord palsy, locally infiltrative thyroid disease with functioning RLN, and prognostication of the nerve.[79] IONM is associated with a steep learning curve especially regarding the management of machinery, circuit, and also the interpretation of signals.

Intraoperative nerve monitoring setup: When IONM is planned, a preoperative thorough laryngeal examination to document vocal cord mobility is mandatory. No muscle relaxant must be used. The circuit consists of stimulator and response circuit each with efferent electrode, afferent electrode and ground electrode. Both circuits are connected to interface connector and electromyography (EMG) monitor. The stimulator electrode can be a probe used to stimulate the nerve or an electrode cuff (cuff around the vagus nerve). The response electrode is embedded within the intubation tube at a length corresponding to the level of the vocal cord. The relation of electrode and vocal cord is variable, based on patient height and extend of cervical extension intraoperatively. The length variability can be up to 6 cm and hence position must be checked after positioning the patient.

A strength of 2 mA is used to identify and 1 mA to monitor the nerve.[79] Loss of signal (LOS) is defined as a decrease in signal strength to <50% and increase in latency by 10%. When there is loss of signal the algorithm to further manage has been well-defined. The point at loss of signal, the nerve distal to that point is involved. An EMG amplitude of 250 microvolt is considered as a normal postoperative nerve. During nerve stimulation, laryngeal twitch can be elicited at the posterior aspect of cricoid. Whenever there is a loss of signal with loss of laryngeal twitch, the contralateral nerve is stimulated.[80] When the contralateral nerve stimulation results in laryngeal twitch, ipsilateral loss of function must be suspected. When laryngeal twitch is present on the ipsilateral side and contralateral stimulation is absent then the response circuit may need to be rechecked. During LOS, the site must be recorded along with the differences between global and segmental loss. Intermittent monitoring is most often performed but it has a low positive predictive value due to circuit problems. Continuous monitoring has better positive predictive value but is associated with adverse events such as hemodynamic instability due to continuous vagal stimulation.

Prognostication of the nerve: Prognostication of the nerve function is important when the nerve is involved by the tumor. In thyroid cancer, 50% of patients with preoperative vocal cord palsy and 60% with infiltrated nerve showed EMG activity. When there is detectable EMG activity in the nerve, the continuity of the nerve must be maintained.[81]

Recurrent laryngeal nerve involvement is associated with high recurrence rate but does not affect survival. Hence, a remnant of the disease up to 5–8 mm can be left behind in cases with positive EMG.

When there is identified LOS, reversible causes such as ligature close to the nerve and traction on the nerve can be corrected.

- *Completeness of thyroidectomy:* This is the most vital. The common areas where remnants of thyroid tissue are left behind are superior pole of the thyroid, ToZ, and the area around ligament of Berry. The embryonal rests of thyroid such as pyramidal remnant and thyrothymic tract must also be excised.

- *Identifying parathyroids:* The inferior parathyroid gland is located within a radius of 1 cm either inferior or lateral to the inferior pole of the thyroid. The position of inferior parathyroid is variable. Superior parathyroid gland is more constant and lies within a 1 cm radius of cricothyroid articulation, 1 cm cranial to the junction of inferior thyroid artery, and the RLN. The parathyroid gland is soft elliptical and flat in shape have a discrete sliding moment and is colored tan brown. The plane of superior parathyroid gland is dorsal to RLN while the inferior parathyroid gland is ventral to RLN.[76]

REMOTE ACCESS THYROID SURGERY

Thyroid surgeries have evolved over centuries from major surgery with increased mortality and morbidity to a daycare procedure where the patient is discharged in a day without a drain, largely due to improved instruments for better hemostasis. Innovations in surgical technology have paved way to remote access thyroid surgery, which utilizes incisions which are hidden and aided by endoscopic or robotic instruments to access the thyroid bed. Various approaches have been described and can be broadly classified into extracervical approaches and cervical approaches.

Extracervical Approaches

These are the breast approach, transaxillary approach, and bilateral axilla breast approach. Breast approach was developed in 2000 and utilizes an incision along anterior axillary line. The major disadvantage is excessive dissection plane to reach thyroid bed. The transaxillary approach involves a 3-cm incision along the anterior fold of axilla through which 5–10 mm trocars are inserted. An additional trocar can be inserted adjacent to the incision to gain access for an additional instrument center neck is approached by raising subcutaneous flap up to clavicle and subplatysmal flap in the supraclavicular region. In the gasless approach, the incision can be 5–6 cm and the elevated flap is held in place by a self-retaining retractor. The access to the central compartment is gained between sternal and clavicular heads of sternocleidomastoid (SCM). The thyroid gland is exposed by separating and elevating the lateral border of the strap muscles. This approach can utilize three or four working ports. The major drawback is that the contralateral side is difficult to access and this can be addressed using a 30° scope and rotation of the operative bed. The position of the arm in extension has led to injuries of the brachial plexus due to prolonged traction on the brachial plexus during the surgery.[82,83]

Bilateral axilla breast approach is a modification of the above-described approaches where 5/10 mm ports are placed in the periareolar on both sides.[84] The main advantage of this approach is that it closely resembles conventional open thyroid surgery, gives wider access for the free maneuvering of instruments, prevents clashing of instruments, and provides maximum working ports. However, the extent of dissection is more. The cervical approaches have their scar hidden in the upper chest area which may not be acceptable in the western population. The main advantages are: it gives easier access to the central compartment and the trajectory is caudocranial and hence the orientation of anatomy is easier, multiple ports can be used and both robotic and endoscopic instruments can be used with any of the extracervical procedures.

Cervical Approaches

The facelift retroauricular approach utilizes a postauricular incision that is hidden along the hairline. This approach has reduced area of dissection and relies on familiar dissection planes. The thyroid bed is closer to the central compartment than the transaxillary approach.[84] The subplatysmal plane is maintained by preserving the greater auricular nerve and external jugular vein. A critical triangle bounded by the anterior border of SCM and posterior border of sternohyoid and inferiorly superior border of omohyoid forms the doorway to the central compartment.[85] This approach can only accommodate three instruments and the trajectory of dissection is craniocaudal. Even patients with high BMI can undergo this approach.

The transoral approach was first described in 2008 where the sublingual approach was used.[86] The access is gained by a 1.5-cm incision along the floor of the mouth, just anterior to the frenulum of tongue, and two separate 1.5 cm is placed in the oral vestibule lateral to mental nerve. Once submental pocket is reached, the midline and the lateral pockets are connected in the submental area and furthered into the thyroid compartment. Due to the increased risk of neuropathy this procedure has become unpopular. The transoral endoscopic thyroidectomy vestibular approach (TOETVA) has emerged as a modification to transoral approach.[87,88] It utilizes a midline incision in the oral vestibule along with gingivolabial sulcus, staying medially between the mental nerves. The surgical axis in this approach involves the least tissue dissection along the familiar tissue planes. This approach technically should give better access to the entire central compartment. Dentition and cervical spine instability may be roadblocks to this approach.

Indications: These are thin body habitus, absence of excessive body fat, a well-circumscribed nodule measuring <3 cm, a thyroid lobe measuring <6 cm, no evidence of thyroiditis or extrathyroid extension.[89] The contraindications are extrathyroidal extension, Graves' disease, previous substernal extension, and previous neck surgery.[89] Drawbacks of remote access thyroid surgery is the long learning curve; surgeons with experience of over 40 cases are considered safe.

Safety Profile

The contraindications mentioned earlier have been superseded by advances in technology and attainment of improved surgical skills. Studies have shown that minimal extrathyroidal extension to strap muscles can be effectively resected. Lateral lymph node metastases are also cleared by robotic lateral neck dissection. The operative morbidities such as hematoma, pain, RLN palsy, and hypocalcemia are all shown to be comparable between remote access and open surgery.[90] However, oncologic outcomes are not the same. Studies have shown that lateral compartment even in the presence of multiple nodes can be cleared effectively, but central compartment lymph nodal clearance is shown to be inferior in remote access thyroidectomy.[91,92] The completeness of resection as evaluated with post-total thyroidectomy serum Tg has significantly higher Tg in the remote access thyroidectomy group.[92] Assessment of thyroid tissue on radioiodine scans has shown no significant difference[93,94] implying low remnant volume. The survival rates and recurrence between remote access thyroidectomy and open surgery have been the same but with follow-up of only <2–5 years.[91]

MANAGEMENT OF NECK NODES

The thyroid gland is composed of rich intrathyroidal lymphatic channels that form dense networks around the thyroid follicle and exit the gland along the vascular network. The first echelon lymph nodes are located in level VI that in turn drain to level IV and VII. Prelaryngeal nodes are the most common group involved. The upper pole can drain to level II/III without involving level VI. The lymphatic channels that run along the inferior thyroid artery follow the paratracheal route, continue posteriorly behind the carotid artery, and drain at the junction of the internal and subclavian vein. A few lymphatics run anterior to carotid sheath to involve lateral nodes. The rate of nodal metastasis is represented in **Table 7**.[32]

Table 7: Nodal metastasis rate in differentiated thyroid cancer (DTC).[32]

Level of cervical lymph node	*Rate of lymph node metastasis in DTC*
I	5–9%
II	IIA: 47–60%; IIB: 8–27%
III	67–71%
IV	61–71%
V	Va: 3–20%; Vb: 8–48%
VI	40–60%

Therapeutic central compartment dissection is indicated when nodes are involved in preoperative assessment or on clinical palpation during surgery. The prophylactic central compartment is done when lateral nodes are involved, in T3/T4 disease or if dissection is likely to alter management.[21] Therapeutic lateral neck dissection is indicated when nodes in the lateral compartment are involved, while prophylactic lateral neck dissection is not recommended. Overall survival at 14 years is 82% without lymph-node metastasis that drops to 7.9% when extensive nodal metastasis is present.[95] The risk of recurrence further increases with multiple metastases, large nodes, and extracapsular extension than those with microscopic disease. The extent of neck dissection for palpable lateral neck nodes must involve levels IIA–VB.[21]

The role of prophylactic central compartment dissection is a controversial issue where proponents of prophylactic level VI dissection argue that identification of disease in the central compartment can be helpful in staging and planning of adjuvant therapy. However, prophylactic level VI dissection has shown no benefits to long-term outcome.[96,97] The risk of recurrence in macroscopic nodal disease is significantly higher than microscopic nodal positivity. Central compartment dissection must include prelaryngeal, pretracheal, and paratrachea nodes on the ipsilateral side. The nodal yield to efficiently identify occult metastasis is 6,9,18 in lateral neck dissection and 3,4,8 in central neck dissection in T1b, T2, and T3 tumors, respectively.[98]

Central Neck Dissection Technique[97]

The central compartment is composed of levels VI and VII, which is bounded superiorly by hyoid bone, inferiorly by the sternal notch in level VI and crossing of the innominate artery to define level VII. The compartment is further bound laterally by the carotid artery and posteriorly by prevertebral fascia. The central compartment is further divided into prelaryngeal, pretracheal, and paratracheal regions. Central neck dissection must include clearance of all three regions. Berry picking of the nodes must not be performed, as it is associated with higher rates of recurrence and revision surgery. The prelaryngeal region extends from the upper margin of hyoid up to the lower border of the thyroid cartilage. Pretracheal dissection extends from lower margin of thyroid cartilage up to suprasternal notch. All the fibrofatty tissue from the anterior wall of trachea must be cleared. The paratracheal region is technically difficult to dissect due to the presence of RLN and the inferior parathyroid gland. Dissection must extend from the lower border of cricoid cartilage up to innominate artery and laterally the carotid artery. The dissection is begun laterally by exposing the carotid artery dividing the carotid sheath and freeing all the tissue along the medial aspect of the carotid artery. The course of the RLN is delineated from the point of entry at the inferior constrictor muscle up to the thoracic inlet. On the right side, the nerve forms a superior lateral triangle and inferior medial triangle. After the identification of the inferior parathyroid gland and its blood supply from the inferior thyroid artery, all the nodal tissues are dissected off the prevertebral fascia. Even in extensive paratracheal dissection, the superior parathyroid glands that are dorsal to RLN can be preserved with good vascularity. In revision central compartment dissection, excessive scarring in the area can make dissection extremely challenging. The anterior arch of cricoid is identified, from which the entry point of the RLN can be identified. The carotid artery dissection is completed and the strap muscles are divided inferiorly to expose the paratracheal region completely. An inferior approach to identify the RLN must be employed.

Radioiodine Therapy

Radioiodine therapy (RIT) plays a pivotal role in the management of differentiated thyroid cancer. RIT treatment is defined as administration of iodine 131—sodium or potassium iodide for irradiation of thyroid remnant or differentiated thyroid cancer tumor. The treatment with RIT can be broadly classified into RAI, radioiodine remnant ablation, and radioiodine treatment.

- Radioiodine remnant ablation is defined as a modality that is directed to ablate thyroid and its remnants so that the follow-up surveillance can be effectively done with serum Tg and diagnostic whole-body scintigraphy.
- Radioiodine ablation is directed to treat microscopic remnants of the thyroid gland or differentiated thyroid cancer as an adjuvant in the postoperative setting.
- Radioiodine treatment consists of radioiodine administration that is targeted against recurrent or metastatic thyroid cancer that is not amenable for surgery.

Fundamentals of Radioiodine Therapy

Iodine-131 is the most common isotope that is used for radioiodine treatment. The half-life of an isotope is defined as the time it takes to decrease in activity by 50%. The half-life is divided into biological and effective half-life. Biological half-life is defined as the time radioiodine takes to decrease in quantity in a person's body as a result of excretion by urine, sweat, saliva by 50%, which takes approximately 80 days when normal thyroid is present and 12 days for extrathyroidal tissue.[99] The effective half-life, on the other hand, is a reduction in the activity by 50% as a result of radioactive decay, which takes approximately 7 days for thyroid compartment and 8 hours for extrathyroidal tissue.[99] The radioactive decay of iodine-131 is by β-decay. Iodine-131 undergoes mechanical transformation where a neutron emits a proton and an electron. The emission product releases energy in the range of 250–800 KeV,[99] which is extremely useful in directed ablation of the tissue of interest, as the energy range travels less than a millimeter before depositing their energy. This decay occurs in the cells that highly concentrate iodine-131.

The common terminology used in RIT is Becquerel (Bq), Curie (Ci), and Gray (Gy). The terms "Becquerel" and "Curie" are used while expressing the amount of radioiodine administered during the procedure, while the term "Gray" is used when expressing the amount of radiation absorbed by the organ or tissue.

Dosimetry is the amount of radioiodine that has to be administered to the patient to achieve the required ablation. It can be calculated by three methods: (1) fixed-dose, (2) remnant-based dosimetry, and (3) bone marrow/blood dosimetry.

1. *Fixed dose* of radioiodine administration is the most often adopted method in most centers across the world due to ease of administration and to lessen the technical and logistic problems that are associated with other methods of dosimetric calculation.[81] In the fixed-dose approach, all patients based on their risk stratification and the indication for radioiodine are administered a fixed-dose of radioiodine. The empirical or fixed-dose varies among different centers but the most common doses are as follows:
   - For low-risk patients (stage I/II disease) are commonly treated with 30–50 mCi of radioiodine.
   - High-risk patients are treated with a dose range of 100–200 mCi.
   - Intermediate-risk group the dose can vary between 30 and 150 mCi based on institutional protocol.
   - In bone and diffuse lung metastasis high doses of radioiodine may have to be administered (200 mCi)

but potential complications such as bone marrow depression and lung fibrosis must be borne in mind.

2. *Dosimetric method* by estimation of maximum tolerable blood radioactivity is another method. This method involves measuring radiation activity in the patient's blood sample over 4 or more days after administration of iodine-131. The whole body retention must be <80 mCi at 48 hours of iodine-131 administration.[99] This method is protective against myelosuppression and lung fibrosis that can occur with high doses, but the main limitation is that the absorbed dose to the tumor is not known.
3. *Remnant or lesion-based dosimetry* is calculated by measuring the uptake and clearance of iodine-131 by the lesion of interest. The areas of remnant thyroid and metastatic disease that need to be treated are calculated by serial gamma camera images that are acquired up to 96 hours after administration of radioiodine.[99] This approach is also called a Maxon approach to honor the key developer. The mass of lesion to be treated has to be precalculated by the means of imaging modalities like CT and/or ultrasound. Lesion-based dosimetry with iodine-124 can also be used to calculate the radioiodine concentration in differentiated thyroid cancer, but its complex decay activity complicates the process.

Dosimetric calculations are not standardized in children and are challenging in children who are below adult size and in stages of development. The dose of iodine-131 that needs to be administered is calculated by the child's total body surface area. For children, the dose can be adjusted as per the body weight with the range of 1.85–7.4 MBq/kg or by fixed-dose as one-third of adult activity at 5 years, half the adult activity at 10 years or 5/6th of adult activity at 15 years.[100] The use of recombinant TSH (rTSH) in children is debated.

In conclusion, even though the use of an empirical fixed dose is easier, there is a chance of undertreating or overtreating a patient. While other methods are cumbersome to use and the calculation method may be subjected to the effect of stunning, other dosimetric methods allow the individualization of the radioiodine treatment.

Patient Preparation for Radioiodine Treatment

- *Low iodine diet:* Low iodine diet must be advised 2 weeks before treatment up to 2 days after the administration.[101] The purpose is to deplete body iodine stores and to maximize uptake of radioiodine by the target tissue. A dietary allowance of ≤50 µg/day is recommended. The dietary recommendation varies from region to region due to different food practices in different areas within the country. The use of iodinated contrast during a CT scan can expose the patient to large amounts of iodine. Every 100 mL of IV contrast contains 150 mg of iodine per mL that corresponds to >15 g of iodine in a single dose of IV contrast for imaging. Hence, use of iodinated contrast must be avoided and even if used must be a month before RIT.[102] A 24-hour urinary iodine of ≤100 µg is considered acceptable for use while planning RIT.
- *Lithium:* It is known to increase the biological half-life of iodine-131 by 50% in tumor deposits and 90% in normal thyroid.[103] Lithium in the dose of 300 mg is given three times a day, 5 days before iodine-131 administration. The use of lithium is contraindicated in patients with cardiac arrhythmia, renal insufficiency, seizures, and patients on calcium channel blockers. Most centers do not use lithium as a routine pre-application protocol.
- *Hypothyroidism:* Recommended before RIT. Hypothyroidism or elevated TSH can be achieved by various approaches the most common approach employed is stopping LT4 for a period of 3–4 weeks before RIT. A second approach is to switch from levothyroxine to tri-iodothyronine (T3) for some 3 weeks, which is topped 2 weeks before RIT. The two randomized noninferiority trials have shown the oncologic safety and efficacy of using recombinant TSH in the low-risk group of patients.[104,105] Recombinant TSH is administered as an intramuscular injection of dose 0.9 mg on day 1 and day 2. Following the injection, the mean peak TSH concentration reached is 116 mIU/L at 24 hours after the injection and starts to decline on day 4, and reaches the baseline in 6–7 days. Radioiodine therapy or scan is conducted on day 3. Post-therapy scan and/or serum Tg measurement is done between days 7 and 10 depending on the intent of RIT. Empirically serum, TSH levels of >30 mIU/L are considered imperative for radioiodine administration, although there are no studies that have documented the same. The administration of recombinant TSH is not indicated in high-risk differentiated thyroid cancer. An absolute advantage of recombinant TSH is in patients with ischemic heart disease who cannot tolerate prolonged hypothyroidism. The ESTIMABL phase III trial was reassessed in terms of quality of life and cost-effectiveness of using recombinant TSH.[10] The study showed that recombinant TSH

could be cost-effective if the price was lowered by 30%. Studies have shown that health-related quality of life was significantly better in patients who received recombinant TSH especially during the periablation period, while the quality of life later on (approximately 3 months from administration) was equal in those receiving recombinant TSH and those on thyroxine withdrawal. The improvement was seen in physical health-related and vitality domains during the evaluation.[106]

Stunning

Stunning is defined as reduced radioiodine uptake and efficacy due to suboptimal therapeutic and/or biological effects of radioiodine administration. Stunning is commonly induced due to a higher dose administered during a preablation scan or during dosimetric calculations.[107] This can be avoided by restricting the administration of radioiodine to 3–10 MBQ. Iodine-124 PET-CT is emerging as an alternative to preablation scan and for dosimetric evaluation but the extent of stunning with iodine-124 is yet unknown.

PRINCIPLES OF THYROID REMNANT ABLATION

The term "thyroid remnant ablation" is restricted to cases where the indication of RIT is remnant normal thyroid or tumor tissue due to incomplete surgery. Thyroid or disease remnant that is <2 g is considered as small and remnant >2 g is considered as large. When thyroid remnant is <2 g, ablation is successful in 94% of patients this falls to 68% when the remnant is large.[108] Routine use of remnant ablation is controversial, especially in large remnants. A randomized prospective clinical trial by Bal et al. has shown that increase in doses of iodine-131 beyond 50 mCi resulted in a plateau in the dose-response curve[109] and the following study by the same author in 2004 showed that patients receiving <25 mCi had a worse response rate.[110]

As a general rule, large remnants must be resected and must not be considered for RAI. The current ATA guidelines recommend lobectomy in patients with unifocal tumor measuring <4 cm. The follow-up rationale using radioiodine scan and serum Tg in low-risk tumors with remnant thyroid lobe is still undefined and debatable. The normal thyroid tissue concentrates iodine more than the tumor thyroid tissue and hence in the presence of large normal thyroid remnant, multiple RAI doses need to be administered to reach biochemical cure.

Radioiodine Ablation

The indications of RAI are based on risk stratification as per ATA.[21] ATA recommends 30 mCi in low-risk group when indicated and 100–150 mCi for patients with increased risk of recurrence.[21] The contraindications of RAI are pregnancy, breastfeeding, patients with bone marrow depression, pulmonary function restriction, and patients with neurological symptoms or neural damage caused by the metastasis from thyroid cancer.

American Thyroid Association Low-risk Patients

Among the lower risk patients, the principle of ablation is meant to enhance sensitivity and specificity of serum Tg during the follow-up period. Two randomized noninferiority prospective trials have shown the efficacy of using a low dose of radioiodine 30 mCi is as effective as the high dose.[104,105] The Hi-Lo trial showed a response rate of 85% in those receiving low dose radioiodine and response rate of 88.9% in those receiving high dose that shows that the low dose was noninferior. The other trial showed a response of 91.1% and 93.5% in high dose at 95% confidence intervals. Low-dose therapy was also associated with shorter hospital stay than those receiving high dose (1 vs. 3 days). The adverse effect rates in the high-dose group are also higher (33%) than those of the low-dose group (21%). Low-risk differentiated thyroid cancer has a 5-year regional and distant recurrence-free survival of 98% and 100% without RAI. ATA does not recommend RAI for low-risk patients.[21]

American Thyroid Association Intermediate-risk Category

There is limited data to support the use of radioiodine and its efficacy in the intermediate-risk group of patients. RAI in patients with stage III disease which mainly includes those with >45 years, with tumors >4 cm, microscopic invasion and also lymph-node metastasis has shown benefit.[111] The efficacy of RAI in younger patients has been uncertain. Aggressive histological variants of PTC have shown inferior survival, especially in diffuse sclerosing variant and tall cell variant, even in patients who received RAI. Studies have shown that microscopic lymph-node metastasis and a larger number of nodal metastasis is associated with reduced survival.[112] While the risk of recurrence increases even for $BRAF^{V600E}$ they are most often associated with aggressive histology, nodal metastasis, and extrathyroidal extension-making risk attributed to *BRAF* alone difficult to interpret.[113] In conclusion in an intermediate-risk group, there is limited data examining the efficacy of RIT. Both HiLo and ESTIMBL1 trials have included intermediate-risk factors namely extrathyroidal extension and lymph node metastasis and have shown efficacy with low-dose RAI and this is the only prospective evidence available for intermediate-risk group.

American Thyroid Association High-risk Category

Radioiodine ablation is routinely recommended in high-risk patients. Radioiodine treatment in high-risk patients is usually administered a high dose ranging from 100 to 150 mCi.[21] The use of rTSH usage in high-risk groups is not recommended.

Precautions to Minimize Radioiodine Uptake and Retention

Liberal oral hydration, use of lemon juice, and sour candy to increase the salivary flow and use of laxatives to decrease the time contact with intestines and urinary bladder can help in reducing radiation exposure. Patients with renal failure should undergo dialysis within 24 hours following RAI for faster iodine-131 clearance.[99]

Fertility after Iodine-131 Treatment

Most women have temporary amenorrhea that recovers within 6 months. The temporary amenorrhea represents temporary ovarian failure characterized by high serum FSH level. For each millicurie of radioiodine administration, the ovary receives a radiation dose of 0.14 Cu. Studies have shown that after the initial menstrual irregularity the outcome on subsequent pregnancy or offspring is not altered. However, one of the studies has shown an increased risk of miscarriage of 20% during the first year of radioiodine administration. Hence, after RIT, patient is advised for contraception during the first year.[114] During pregnancy, suppressive doses of thyroxine must be continued with close monitoring of TSH levels. The radiation dose to the testis is 0.085 Cu for every mCi of RAI administered. Men are asked to avoid fathering a child for a period of 4–6 months, especially if a single ablation dose is given.[115] Gonadal damage may be cumulated in patients who received multiple high doses. The radiation dose to testis and ovary is by radioactivity in the blood and retention of radioiodine in the intestine and bladder. Hence, adequate hydration and use of laxatives must be considered. Sperm banking may need to be considered in patients who are planned for multiple high doses of RAI.

Pre- and Post-therapy Radioiodine Scan

Preablative radioiodine scan is avoided in many centers but the combination of stimulated serum Tg along with the preablation scan helps in the modification in management decision in 31% of cases and can also change the risk stratification in 15% of patients.[116] The post-therapy scan is highly sensitive and hence is usually performed no sooner than 72 hours. The ablation success rate is evaluated 6–12 months after the RIT in intermediate- and high-risk group patients. The definition of success is a negative follow-up diagnostic whole-body scan or thyroid update below 0.1% along with no detectable serum Tg and no evidence of structural disease in the neck by ultrasonography.[117]

FOLLOW-UP STRATEGY IN DIFFERENTIATED THYROID CANCER

Risk Stratification

Differentiated thyroid cancer is associated with extremely good outcomes with a 10-year overall survival of 93% and 85% in papillary and follicular carcinomas, respectively.[1] It has been shown that after the initial treatment, 78% of the treatment cost is borne by the patient during the follow-up period.[118] Hence, it is extremely important to risk stratify the patient for early detection and appropriate treatment of recurrent disease. The TNM staging, MACES, AGES, and various other stratification systems have been proposed that help in risk stratifying patients based on clinical and pathological features. Most of the staging systems assess survival, while DTC is characterized by long survival and higher recurrence. Hence, risk stratification must be aimed at assessing rate of recurrence rather than survival. The risk of recurrence and the biological behavior of tumor changes over time, hence a patient who was initially a low-risk can become a high-risk patient later on.[119] The current ATA guidelines recommend a dynamic risk stratification which is a continuous process from initial therapy (based on histopathological features) to treatment response.[21] The risk estimates continue to be modified during follow-up and disease-specific mortality can change over time as a function of the clinical course of the disease and response to the therapy. Dynamic risk stratification is assessed at various time points, described below:

- *Post surgery:* Based on histopathology report, patient is classified as low-/intermediate-, and high-risk group. Adjuvant therapy is planned based on this risk level.

- *Response to therapy:* Response is accessed after completion of treatment. The stratification consists of excellent response, biochemical incomplete response, structural incomplete response, and intermediate response. Further follow-up and management of the patient are based on response to the therapy.

The initial stage after the surgery is vital in deciding immediate adjuvant treatment for the patient. The validation and concept of response to therapy was initially described by Tuttle et al,[119] based on response to therapy during the first 2 years of follow-up.

The risk of recurrence is considered as a continuum as patients cannot be strictly classified into low, intermediate, and high risk. Individualized management recommendations can be done using ATA recommended risk levels. Various retrospective studies have shown that a substantial portion of intermediate- and high-risk patients who show excellent response to therapy have a very low risk of recurrence and can be appropriately stratified based on their response to treatment.[120-122]

The basis of ATA recommended dynamic risk stratification is based on retrospective data. This can be applied only to patients who have undergone total thyroidectomy and RAI. Momesso et al.[123] and Park et al.[107] have proposed stratifications for patients undergoing lobectomy or total thyroidectomy without RAI. However, the proposed Tg cutoff value proposed in the study has not been validated. ATA risk stratification does not include PDTC and Hurthle cell carcinoma, which are known to have increased risk of recurrence and a poorer survival than other DTC.[122]

Thyroid-stimulating Hormone Suppression

The level of TSH suppression is based on the response to treatment. Thyroid cancer cells also express TSH receptors which when stimulated increase iodine uptake and Tg release. This forms the basis of stimulated Tg and elevated TSH before RIT. After lobectomy, TSH must be maintained within normal limits. A high-dose of T4 commonly used to suppress disease can cause bone mineral loss, which is extremely problematic in children and postmenopausal woman. The increased levels of LT4 can also lead to increased atrial contraction, increased cardiac contractility, ventricular hypertrophy and systolic/diastolic dysfunction.[124] While prescribing high doses of T4 the potential adverse effects must be borne in mind. The levels of TSH suppression are:[21]

- No TSH suppression inpatient with excellent response treatment.
- Mild suppression (TSH 0.1–0.5 mU/L) in cases with intermediate and biochemical incomplete response with high-risk comorbidity.
- Moderate/complete suppression (TSH < 0.1 mU/L) in cases with structural incomplete response and biochemical incomplete response with no comorbidities.

Serum Thyroglobulin

Thyroglobulin is a thyroid-specific marker, as no other tissues secrete Tg, but its sensitivity depends on various factors. DTC has good prognosis and patients have long survival and use of Tg as a tumor marker plays a key role.[108] Levels of serum Tg correlate well with the volume of thyroid tissue with 1 ng/mL corresponding to 1 g of thyroid tissue, reducing to 0.5 ng/mL when TSH is <0.1 mU/L. Tg ranges between 20 and 25 ng/mL with an intact normal thyroid gland. The half-life of Tg is variable between 1 and 3 days.[108] The time-lapse between total thyroidectomy and Tg measurement as per ATA recommendation is 3–4 weeks[21] and NCCN recommendation is 6–12 weeks.[125] Postoperative Tg is also depended on various factors such as completion of the surgery, level of TSH, presence of regional/distant metastasis, and functional sensitivity of the assay used. Grade of tumor does not affect Tg levels; PDTC can produce high levels of Tg and well-differentiated thyroid tumors can produce low levels. Tg gives us information on recurrence and metastatic disease, estimate of disease load, response to treatment, and also in risk stratification.

Thyroglobulin Assay

Thyroglobulin measurement is done by two methods namely radioimmunoassay (RIA) and immunometric assay (IMA). IMA has largely replaced RIA, as IMA has an automated process, forms a stable labeled antibody reagent, and also requires a short incubation period to achieve maximum test sensitivity. RIA uses rabbit polyclonal antibody and IMA uses isotopic immunoradiometric and nonisotopic primary chemiluminescence.

Immune assay factors that affect the levels of Tg are:[126]

- *Between the method bias:* The methods express a threefold difference in Tg level when Tg Ab is absent. Hence, during the long-term follow-up of patient, changing method of Tg assessment can affect the identification of recurrent disease. As changes as small as 1.5 µg/L is considered significant, a threefold increase can affect the specificity of the test.
- *Between run precision:* All biochemical test machines are subject to change in reagent lots and machine instrument calibration, which can affect Tg level even affecting tests done in the same laboratory over the years. To avoid both errors, the calibration of

immunoassay must meet the criteria recommended by the Community Bureau of Reference of the Commission of the European Communities (CRM-457, BCR Brussels) recommended in 1994.

- *High-dose hook effect:* When Tg level is high, it exceeds the capture and signal capacity of the reagent antibody and results in underestimation of Tg. This can happen in metastatic disease that may have Tg levels > 1,000 ng/mL.
- *Antibody interference:* Thyroglobulin antibodies (TgAb) are IgG antibodies, which are detected is approximately 25% of DTC patients. Tg molecules bind with TgAb and affect serum assessment by both methods. IMA tends to underestimate the Tg level in the presence of TgAb. Underestimation occurs when reagent lacks species specificity and reagent gets precipitated by TgAb, thus preventing binding of reagent to Tg. Tg complexes with TgAb and also circulates as free Tg, which is not recognized by the IMA method. Epitome masking is necessary for monoclonal antibodies used in IMA to recognize Tg, where noncompetitive reagents of IMA do not recognize large Tg-TgAb complexes. TgAb interference can be significant when the IMA method is used as even very low or undetectable TgAb can affect Tg estimation. While overestimation can occur in RIA method when TgAb sequester Tg-I-125 tracer used in RIA. RIA reagents are polyclonal and competitive reagents, which can recognize both free and TgAb complexes. Heterophilic antibody in the circulation can cause overestimation of Tg by forming a false bridge between capture and signal monoclonal antibodies. Heterophilic antibody interference is not seen in the RIA method. As TgAb inference is more in IMA, many centers prefer to measure TgAb by RIA method of assessment. Underestimation is more problematic as it defeats the purpose of Tg as a tumor marker.
- *Nonassay related factors that influence Tg secretion:* These are amount of thyroid/tumor tissue present, tissues capability to secrete Tg, injury to thyroid tissue releases Tg, (e.g., postsurgery, repeat FNAC), duration of TSH stimulation and increased metabolic clearance of Tg-TgAb complexes.

Stimulated versus Nonstimulated Thyroglobulin

0.5 ng/mL of Tg is secreted per gram of thyroid tissue when TSH is <0.1 mU/L.[108] When nonstimulated Tg is to be assessed, the TSH level must be stable across all readings and the functional sensitivity of the method used to assess must be high. In cases when thyroid suppression cannot be stopped, rTSH can be used. Under thyroid suppression, Tg level is undetectable in 98% of cases. IMA methodology has evolved; first-generation of IMA methods had a sensitivity of 1.0 µg/L, while the second generation had a functional sensitivity of 0.1 µg/L. When IMA second-generation methodology is used, Tg can be assessed under thyroid suppression,[21] but TgAb must be absent as they interfere with Tg estimation. A meta-analysis has shown that unstimulated Tg has a high negative predictive value but poor positive predictive value; hence, elevated unstimulated Tg must be followed by stimulated Tg assessment.[127] Tg determination is most sensitive when TSH is elevated and thyroid hormone suppressive doses are stopped. Tg is measured after two doses of 0.9 mg dose of rTSH and is most sensitive at 4 days after the first dose of rTSH with sensitivity as high as 100% (Tg cut-off is 2 ng/mL).[21,108] The level of Tg cutoff value based on response to treatment is represented in **Table 8.**[21] Tg doubling time of <1 year is considered as progressive recurrent disease.

Table 8: Significant Tg cutoff values.[21]

Status	*Level of thyroglobulin (Tg)*
Post-thyroidectomy without RAI	No universal consensus Suppressed Tg < 0.1 ng/mL
Excellent response	Suppressed Tg < 0.2 ng/mL or TSH stimulated Tg < 1 ng/mL
Biochemical incomplete response	Suppressed Tg > 1 ng/mL or stimulated Tg > 10 ng/mL
Intermediate response	Nonstimulated Tg detectable, but <1 ng/mL Stimulated Tg detectable, but <10 ng/mL

(TSH: thyroid-stimulating hormone)

MANAGEMENT OF RECURRENT TUMORS

The rate of recurrence is dependent on various factors. The disease status after initial treatment must be recorded before defining recurrence to differentiate between recurrent and persistent disease. Disease recurrence is defined as the identification of biochemical or structural disease in a patient with a period of disease-free interval. Persistent disease is when a patient does not have a disease-free interval after initial therapy.

Recurrent Primary Tumor

The recurrent tumor is defined by level of Tg elevation and/or structural disease identified on ultrasound or cross-sectional imaging. The management principles of recurrent thyroid disease is based on various factors:[128]

- All thyroid bed recurrences must be differentiated into nodal and primary recurrence which may be the best identified by cross-sectional imaging.

- Previous surgery morbidity such as RLN paralysis, hypoparathyroidism must be documented. Active surveillance or no treatment to the recurrent primary is an option when there is small volume disease in the thyroid bed in previously operated area with contralateral RLN palsy.
- The volume of recurrent disease must be determined by imaging, RAI scan or PET CT.
- Patience factors such as age and comorbidity must also be taken into consideration while planning further management.
- The extent of the site and progression or stability of distant metastasis if present must also be documented.

The extent of surgery during revision must be aimed to remove any remaining normal thyroid tissue and clear all the recurrent primary tumor with detailed mapping done preoperatively with imaging if previously not addressed the nodal basin with increased risk of metastasis must also be cleared as a future surgery might be difficult.

Principles of Revision Thyroidectomy[129]

- During revision surgery, microvascular clips and silk sutures placed in previous surgery may mimic a hard tumor.
- Strap muscles must be cut inferiorly to expose the entire central compartment.
- Invasion to surrounding structures in recurrent tumors is managed as per the extent.

Recurrent Nodal Disease

While treating recurrent nodal disease, the potential benefit from the intervention must be weighed against the oncologic benefit and the resultant morbidity from the surgery. After surgical removal of recurrent nodes, Tg level becomes undetectable only in 50% of cases and has no benefit on overall survival.

The management principles are based on the following factors:[128]

- Primary tumor factors such as adverse histology of the primary tumor, inability of the primary tumor to concentrate radioiodine, rapid elevation or doubling time of Tg, presence of *BRAF/RAS* mutations, *RET/PTC* rearrangements may mandate aggressive management.
- Nodal factors such as presence of invasive features (extranodal extension) and change in the size of lymph nodes are factors pointing toward active intervention.
- Patience factors such as age, significant comorbidity, and vocal cord paralysis on the contralateral side are important factors.

The nodal size cut-off of <0.8 cm and <1 cm for the central and lateral compartment is considered non-significant and must not be further evaluated.[21] During active surveillance, if the node increases to >3–5 mm/year, then the node must be evaluated. Parapharyngeal and retropharyngeal nodal disease are rarely seen in the recurrent disease. CT-guided FNAC must be used to diagnose the recurrence before any active intervention is planned.

The extent of neck dissection is based on nodal level involvement. Superselective neck dissection is performed in the previously operated neck and formal neck dissection (levels II–V) in patients who have not undergone neck dissection previously. Berry-picking of nodes is not advisable even in a recurrent disease.[21] Nonsurgical modality such as ethanol injection (where 95% ethanol is injected directly into the node), laser ablation (in which heat energy induces necrosis), and radiofrequency ablation can also be used where surgery is not advisable.[21]

Distant Metastasis in Recurrence

The status of distant metastasis must always be determined while treating recurrent disease. Extensive progressive distant metastasis receives priority over nodal or primary disease and the treatment is guided by distant metastasis. Management of distant metastasis is described later in the chapter.

LOCALLY ADVANCED THYROID CANCER

Invasive thyroid cancer is defined as a disease that extends outside the thyroid gland/capsule of metastatic nodes to involve adjacent structures. The incidence of invasive thyroid cancer is variable in the literature ranging from 1 to 23%.[130] The variability is attributed to differences in the histology. The presentation of invasive thyroid cancer is most commonly a palpable neck mass, hoarseness dysphagia, hemoptysis, and dyspnea.[131]

Biology of Invasive Thyroid Cancer

The progress of thyroid cancer from well-differentiated tumors to poorly differentiated thyroid carcinoma is a continuum.[30] Histological sybtypes such as tall cell, Hurthle cell, poorly differentiated, and solid variant of PTC are commonly locally aggressive. The incidence of extrathyroidal extension (ETE) also increases with an increase in the size of primary and duration of the disease. Microscopic ETE is seen even in micropapillary thyroid cancer (21%).[132] The thyroid capsule is a discontinuous fibroadipose tissue and the isthmus lies in direct contact with subcutaneous fat and strap muscles. Hence, interpretation of extrathyroid and extension in this area must be documented carefully. The paratracheal lymph nodes can exhibit extracapsular extension, which may involve the RLN, trachea, or esophagus.

Infiltrated Recurrent Laryngeal Nerve

The suspicion of RLN starts from history of hoarseness of voice and a preoperative vocal cord palsy. Occult infiltration of the RLN can be found. When the vocal cords are mobile, the RLN must be carefully dissected and preserved. Shaving of the tumor from the nerve can be done as the microscopic disease does not affect survival or further recurrence. Partial layer resection where <50% of nerve thickness is preserved can be done with intact nerve function.[131] Understanding of RLN microanatomy is essential. 2 cm below the level of cricoid 55% of nerve fibers are motor and 45% are sensory, while at the entry point motor fibers consist of 80% as sensory branches to trachea and esophagus is given before entry point. The adductor and abductor fibers are not spatially segregated and consist two to four times more adductor fibers than the abductor. If the nerve is transected with no loss of nerve length, primary anastomosis with epineural reanastomosis (9-0 sutures) must be planned. Vocal cord medicalization with fat for temporary but immediate voice relief can be planned. Division of posterior branch of RLN can be transected to prevent cross-connection. When there is segmental loss, nerve graft repair is required where adjoining ansa cervicalis can be used. Nerve anastomosis must not be under tension. Permanent changes in laryngeal framework must not be attempted during immediate surgery, but can be planned after a latent period of at least 6 months.

Invasion of the Muscle

Extension of the thyroid disease to strap muscles (sternohyoid and sternothyroid) can be easily resected without significant morbidity. Involvement of the muscle is one of the earliest signs of aggressive disease.

Invasion of Laryngotracheal–esophageal Complex

Tumor involving larynx or trachea can also involve lateral wall of pharynx, esophagus, and almost always RLN. Hence, the evaluation of infiltrative thyroid disease must consist of cross-sectional imaging with CT scan or MRI along with laryngoscopy, bronchoscopy, and esophagoscopy to evaluate the involvement of any of these structures due to their proximity. Imaging along with endoscopic findings, a perfect tumor mapping must be done so that all conservative approaches with negative margins are explored.

Decision making:[131] Invasive tumor involving central compartment of the neck involves structures that are vital in maintaining functions such as breathing, feeding, and speech. Hence, the extent of resection and the resultant morbidity must be preplanned and the patient must be adequately counseled. The histology of the tumor, grade of differentiation, age of the patient, and the ability of the disease to concentrate radioiodine must be taken into consideration as the outcome is dependent on these factors. A patient with resistant radioiodine tumor and those with aggressive histology must be resected aggressively with adequate margins. Even in a patient with metastatic disease with a tumor that is radioiodine avid, resection with adequate margin must be planned. Presence of distant metastasis is not a contraindication for local management of aggressive disease which can uptake radioiodine.

Invasion of Airway

Airway invasion is challenging to manage and must be considered as an emergency even in the absence of acute respiratory distress. Performing a tracheostomy upfront without disease evaluation may result in inadvertent entry into trachea at the level of tumor invasion or tracheostomy may be made above the level of tumor block. Most importantly, tracheostomy makes further resection—anastomosis challenging as it hinders in tracheal mobilization and results in additional loss of tracheal rings. Patients with suspected airway invasion must be taken up for surgery with adequate evaluation at the earliest. The combined classification of laryngo-tracheal complex invasion proposed by Dralle et al. guides in choosing the appropriate resection and reconstruction option based on the extent of involvement.[133]

Mechanism or route of entry: The common entry points of the laryngotracheal complex are direct extension through thyroid ala and paraglottic space by the tumor situated in superior pole, extension into the trachea by paratracheal metastatic lymph node, direct invasion of the trachea by thyroid isthmus or lower pole of the thyroid.[131]

Laryngeal cartilage involvement: In early stages when only thyroid ala is involved, the involved cartilage can be resected without reconstruction as long as the inner perichondrium is preserved. When cricoid cartilage is involved, the extent of resection is vital. No more than one-third of anterior cartilage can be resected without affecting the stability of the larynx. When more than one-third is resected then reconstruction must be planned. The fundamental principle of reconstruction is to provide vascularized lining to maintain luminal dimension and avoid the development of granulation tissue. Involvement of the cricoarytenoid joint is rare, but when disrupted, the position must be re-established above the reconstructed cricoid.[130]

Laryngeal intraluminal involvement: When the tumor involves beyond the cartilage, aggressive resection must be planned. Lateral invasion of the larynx with unilateral paraglottic space involvement is amenable for vertical front lateral hemilaryngectomy which can be reconstructed with local, regional, or free flaps. Sensate radial artery forearm flap can be used to accommodate the sensory loss.[131]

When there is an anterior extension to involve cricoid-trachea then resection can be done with laryngofissure access. Total laryngectomy with or without pharyngectomy is indicated when >50% of the laryngeal framework is involved or adjacent involvement of pharynx and esophagus. Pharyngectomy defect can be managed with patch pharyngoplasty flap or gastric pull up when esophageal involvement is significant. The resection and reconstruction principles are the same as in SCC of respective sites.

Invasion of Trachea

Trachea is most often invaded by paratracheal lymph nodes and also by thyroid directly. The posterior capsule of the thyroid is thin and comes directly in contact with the anterolateral wall of the trachea. Shin and Grillo staging system defined tracheal invasion into **(Fig. 4)**:[134]

- *Stage 0:* Disease confined to the thyroid gland.
- *Stage I:* Disease extends beyond thyroid gland and involves external perichondrium of tracheal cartilage.
- *Stage II:* Tumor invades between tracheal cartilage and/or minimal erosion of tracheal cartilage.

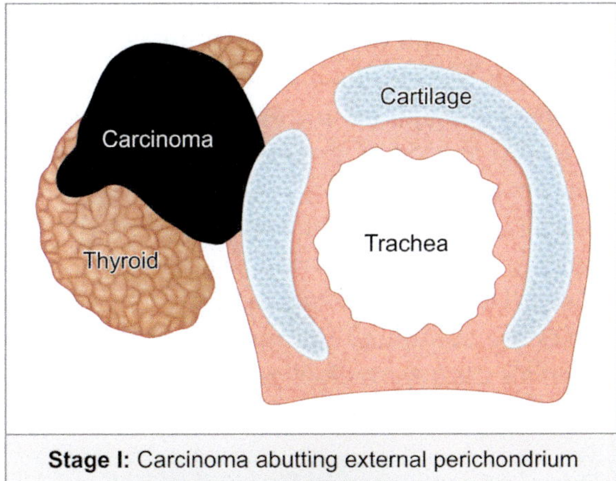

Stage I: Carcinoma abutting external perichondrium

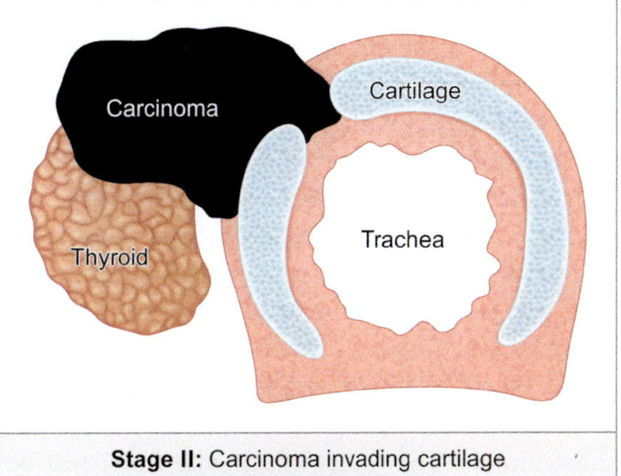

Stage II: Carcinoma invading cartilage

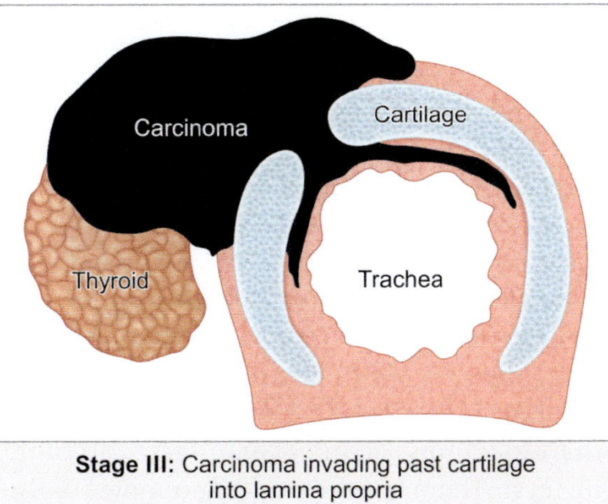

Stage III: Carcinoma invading past cartilage into lamina propria

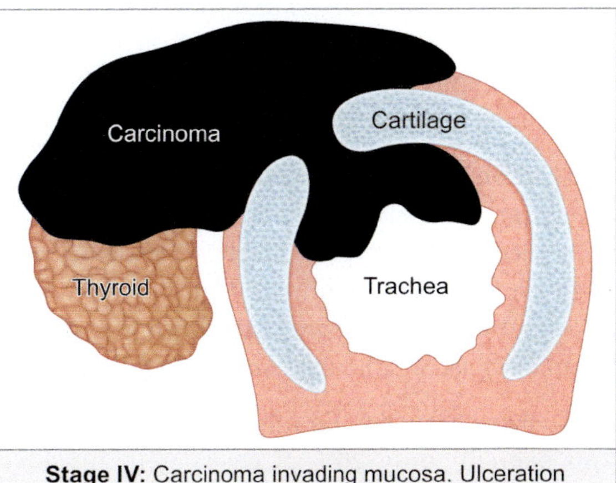

Stage IV: Carcinoma invading mucosa. Ulceration or mass visible within lumen

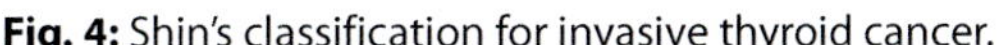

Fig. 4: Shin's classification for invasive thyroid cancer.

- *Stage III:* Tumor invasion between the tracheal cartilages and/or through the tracheal cartilage into lamina propria of tracheal mucosa. The lesion appears as a submucosal bulge on bronchoscopy.
- *Stage IV:* Tumor invades full thickness of the tracheal wall with involvement of tracheal mucosa.

Resection:[131] In stage I disease, shave resection along subperichondrial plane can be achieved. Intraoperatively, the assessment must be thorough, as tumor between the cartilages may be missed by shave resection. When all gross tumors are removed, either by shave excision or cartilage excision, the outcome is the same; however, survival significantly reduces when the gross tumor is left behind. In stages II–IV, when there is inner/partial cartilage invasion or full-thickness tracheal cartilage involvement, then either window resection or segmental resection can be done. Window resection is resecting the involved portion of the trachea, when disease extent is restricted to the anterior or lateral wall of the trachea. The defect can be reconstructed with SCM muscle flap with clavicular periosteum, mesh repair, or sliding tracheoplasty. The window defect created on the tracheal wall can be exteriorized as tracheostomy stoma. The defect can be closed secondarily by titanium mesh embedded in the adjoining skin, which can be raised as a flap to cover the defect with the epidermal layer facing inward into the lumen. The external surface can be closed by local advancement of the skin or deltopectoral flap. Sliding tracheoplasty involves refashioning the resection margins is such a way that the inferior and superior border of resection can be approximated like a jigsaw puzzle. Segmental resection involves resecting whole segment of trachea that is involved with adequate margins. Up to 4–5 rings can be resected. The defect can be closed by end-to-end anastomosis. The anastomotic site must not be under tension. Suprahyoid release and hilar mobilization to gain additional length may be required. Principles of tracheal resection and reconstruction is detailed in the chapter on tracheal malignancy.

Vascular involvement: Carotid artery involvement is rare and can be managed with subadventitial dissection. Segmental resection with bypass surgery can be done, if indicated. Internal jugular vein involvement is common with large lateral nodes. Intravascular tumor emboli are also common in cases of follicular carcinoma thyroid.

Esophageal management: Esophageal involvement is rare and seen in only 20% of cases with invasive disease.[135] Passing a nasogastric tube before resection aids in identification of the esophagus. Disease must be resected with the cuff of muscularis when tumor abuts the esophagus. When there is through-the-wall invasion, either patch or circumferential resection and reconstruction as appropriate must be planned. When the lower end of resection extends into the thoracic esophagus, gastric pull-up procedure can be indicated.

Prognosis of invasive differentiated thyroid cancer: The overall survival in the Mayo clinic series at 5, 10, and 15 years were 79%, 63%, and 54%, respectively.[136] The factors associated with poor prognosis were metastatic to other sites than lung, metastasis >2 cm, cervical metastasis >3 cm and poorly differentiated thyroid carcinoma. About 60% of patient who recur after resection of invasive thyroid disease succumb to the disease.[131]

Special Clinical Scenarios in Differentiated Thyroid Cancer

Pregnancy and Thyroid Cancer

If thyroid cancer is detected in early pregnancy, then the tumor is serially followed up with US. Surgery is recommended when there is an increase in 50% volume and 20% in diameter of disease, the appearance of lymph node metastasis. Surgery is performed at 24 weeks of gestation. If diagnosed later, thyroid cancer is managed after the delivery of the child.[137] There is no difference in final oncologic outcomes when compared between pregnancy and nonpregnancy detected DTC or on the timing of surgery.[137] Hence, when the tumor appears low risk, surgery must be deferred until delivery. In a diagnosis of medullary or anaplastic carcinoma, surgery must be performed as early as possible. In a known DTC patient who conceives, thyroid suppressive doses are continued but monitored closely at 4 weekly intervals till 20th week of gestation and weekly after that until end of pregnancy.

Thyroid Carcinoma in Thyroglossal Cyst

Differentiated thyroid cancer may develop within the thyroglossal cyst. All follicular origin tumors can arise with thyroglossal cyst, with 90% of them are PTC.[138] The treatment consists of the Sistrunk operation (excision of thyroglossal cyst tract and body of hyoid bone) with total thyroidectomy with or without neck dissection depending on the extent of disease. The thyroidectomy specimen is known to harbor a second primary in 11–40% of cases and hence routine of total thyroidectomy with Sistrunk operation is essential. The only indication for Sistrunk operation without total thyroidectomy is micropapillary carcinoma within the cyst. There is evidence that removal of the cyst may be adequate treatment when there is no evidence of disease in the thyroid or the neck; however, this is controversial.

Hurthle Cell Tumors

Hurthle cell tumors (HCTs) are rare thyroid tumors, comprising 10% of all thyroid cancers. The available literature and evidence concerning prognosis, natural history, and management strategies are varied and limited due to low incidence rates. A Hurthle cell is a terminology that describes a thyroid follicular cell with oncocytic changes. They are also found in other organs such as kidney, salivary glands, and parathyroid gland. Hurthle cell is characterized by large polygonal cells with acidophilic granular cytoplasm (due to abundant mitochondria in the cytoplasm), reduced cytoplasm: nuclear ratio and prominent nucleolus.[139] The diagnosis of Hurthle cell variant is made when 75% of a cellular component in the tumor is Hurthle cells. Sippel et al. have shown that HCT with size >6 cm has 50% of the rate of malignancy and <2 cm tumors are rarely malignant.[140] FNAC sensitivity is only 23.8% for HCT.[141]

Hurthle cell carcinoma (HCC) presents in patients aged 50–60 years with a female preponderance. The outcomes of HCC are variable, with earlier studies reporting worse outcomes while more recent studies showing better outcomes.[141] Analysis from the SEER database has shown 5-year and 10-year survival of 85% and 71%, respectively in nonmetastatic disease.[142] They reported age and tumor size as a major prognosticator.

The variation in outcomes of HCC is due to tumor classification: HCTs are classified as Hurthle cell adenoma, HCC, and papillary variant of HCC. Hurthle cell carcinoma is an encapsulated benign tumor, while HCC is considered as a type of a follicular carcinoma charted by follicular architecture, capsular invasion, and angioinvasion. Papillary variant of HCC consists of papillary architecture while papillary nuclear features are typically absent. *RET/PTC* rearrangement positivity in HCC is characteristic of papillary variant HCC.[143] Presence of *RET/PTC* rearrangement is pathognomonic and is recommended to be tested in every case. The papillary variant of HCC behaves like papillary carcinoma with favorable diagnosis and increased LN metastasis than distant metastasis while HCC is more angioinvasive and present with distant metastases more often.[143]

Hurthle cell carcinoma is further classified as minimally invasive and widely invasive. Widely invasive is associated with poorer outcomes. The management, postoperative surveillance is similar to DTC. The belief that radioiodine uptake by HCTs does not occur is not true. They show RAI uptake in the range of 40–70% and must be used as an adjuvant therapy.[143] The role of external beam radiotherapy (EBRT) is the same as in other invasive DTC. Large tumors >6.5 cm, local structure invasion, multiple metastatic nodes, and soft tissue nodules can be recommended for EBRT.[144]

Radiation-induced Thyroid Cancer

Radiation exposure in the early years of life leads to an increase in thyroid cancer risk. The Chernobyl incident showed a 75% increase in risk of developing thyroid cancer.[10] Most cancers were PTC associated with extrathyroidal extension and nodal metastasis, with distant metastasis rates similar to sporadic cases. The solid variant of PTC is the most common variant forming approximately 30% of cases while comprising only <1–3% of sporadic cases. Chromosomal rearrangements are seen in 50–85% of cases, especially RET/PTC rearrangement.[145] The mechanism of chromosomal rearrangement is attributed to spatial contiguity. Radiation exposure causes rejoining of free DNA ends that are nearby. The latency period between exposure and time of presentation is important, as longer latency is associated with less aggressive tumors.[145] There was also a threefold increased risk of thyroid cancer among breast cancer patients with the possibility of radiation exposure to the neck; but even among nonirradiated patients, there was a slight increase incidence, making implications of these findings unclear.

Microcarcinoma

Management of microcarcinoma defers based on presentation. Microcarcinoma is defined as thyroid carcinoma measuring <1 cm. Microcarcinoma that presents with lymph node metastasis, distant metastasis is rare but when present, the management controversy does not exist. When microcarcinoma is incidentally detected, the controversy revolves around active management versus observation. The outcome of micropapillary carcinoma is excellent with locoregional recurrence rates of 2–6% and distant recurrence rates of 1–2%. The management of microcarcinoma thyroid came from two prospective studies by Ito et al.[146] and Sugitani et al.[147] Based on conclusions from the trial, indications for thyroidectomy in microthyroid carcinoma are:

- Tumor located posteriorly adjacent to the trachea or close to the RLN
- Fine-needle aspiration findings suggestive of the high-grade tumor
- Presence of regional lymph node/distant metastases
- Signs of progression during follow-up, defined by 5% growth over 5 years follow-up and 8% growth over 10 years follow-up

Use of molecular studies and their implication in microthyroid carcinoma is not well-defined.[21]

Familial Nonmedullary Thyroid Cancer

Familial nonmedullary thyroid cancer (FNMTC) is defined as the presence of follicular origin thyroid cancer in two or more first-degree family members. The rate of sporadic is 62–69% while this rate drops to 6% if three or more family members are affected.[21] **Table 9** summarizes syndromes associated with FNMTC.

Familial nonmedullary thyroid cancers are mostly PTC followed by Hurthle cell and follicular carcinoma. They are characterized by multifocality, nodal metastasis, and extrathyroidal extension. The overall survival of sporadic and familial cases is similar but disease-free survival is shorter with familial cases as the rate of recurrence is as high as 50%.[32]

Pediatric Thyroid Carcinoma

Thyroid nodules are uncommon in children and is seen in 1–2% of the pediatric population, but compared to adults, the rate of malignancy in thyroid nodules is higher at 20–26%;[1] hence, all pediatric thyroid nodule must be evaluated to rule out malignancy. DTC comprises 1% of all cancers in the prepubertal age and 7% of all adolescent malignancies.[147,148] The most common pediatric thyroid malignancies are PTC, follicular carcinoma, and medullary thyroid carcinoma. The association of malignancy with radiation exposure and familial syndromes must always be ruled out before a management strategy is formed. Most of these tumors are multicentric and nodal involvement and distant metastasis at presentation are seen in 70% and 19–25%, respectively.[149] In spite of this, the overall survival is greater, with a 30-year overall survival rate of 92–99%.[150] Use of the Bethesda system to evaluate thyroid nodule has been studied and has shown the rate of malignancy of 0, 0, 18%, 100%, 100%, and 100% in Bethesda classification type I–VI, respectively.[151]

The extent of surgical resection is debatable but the current ATA guidelines favor total thyroidectomy as the initial resection choice due to higher incidence of multifocality. Thyroid surgery in pediatric group must be performed in a center with high volumes of thyroid surgery.[152] Neck dissection must be done only in patients with involved nodal disease. There is no role of prophylactic lateral or central compartment neck dissection in children with nonmedullary thyroid cancer. The rate of nerve injury is higher (30–40%) and the risk of hypercalcemia is 22% in <6 year age group and 15% in the 7–12 years age group.[153]

Postsurgery risk stratification as per ATA guidelines includes low-, intermediate-, and high-risk group based on clinical presentation, tumor size, regional invasion, and distant metastasis.[150] Postoperative staging to assess complete surgical clearance of disease utilizes serum Tg, TgAb, and whole body iodine scan. Irrespective of the risk stratification, if there is no structural/biochemical disease diagnosed with negative whole body iodine scan and Tg of <2 ng/mL within 12 weeks of surgery, adjuvant radioiodine treatment is not recommended.[150] The indications for RAI are patients with elevating

Table 9: Familial nonmedullary thyroid cancer syndromes.[32]

Syndrome	*Inheritance*	*Gene mutation*	*Subtype of thyroid cancer*	*Extrathyroidal manifestations*
Familial adenomatous polyposis	AD	Inactivating mutation of APC	PTC	Multiple adenomatous polyps in the colon
Gardner's syndrome	AD	Inactivating mutation of APC	PTC	Fibrous dysplasia, fibroma, desmoid tumors, hepatoblastoma, GI tract hamartomas
Cowden's syndrome	AD	PTEN	FTC	Hamartomas
Werner's syndrome	AR	WRN	PTC, FTC, ATC	Premature aging, scleroderma-like changes, muscular atrophy
McCune–Albright syndrome	M	GNAS1	PTC	Café-au-lait spots, polyostotic fibrous dysplasia, endocrinopathies
Carney's complex	AD	PRKAR1	PTC, FTC	Myxoma, schwannomas, tumors of adrenal, pituitary and testicle
DICER1 syndrome	AD	DICER1	PTC, FTC	Pleuropulmonary blastoma (PPB), ovarian Sertoli–Leydig tumors, multicystic nephroma, pineoblastoma
CHEK2 gene mutation		*CHEK2* (tumor suppressor gene)	PTC	

(AD: autosomal dominant: AR: autosomal recessive; ATC: anaplastic thyroid carcinoma; FTC: follicular thyroid carcinoma; M: Mosaicism; PTC: papillary thyroid carcinoma)

Tg level in postoperative period, structural disease that is unresectable and distant metastasis.[150] The preparation for radioiodine treatment is same as adults but the use of recombinant TSH is extrapolated from adult trials. The dosing of radioiodine is as discussed in the section of radioiodine dosimetry. The surveillance is performed with ultrasound and serial Tg based on postoperative risk stratified group. Children with distant metastasis do better than adults with the same load of disease.

Patients must be followed up to 40 years of age or lifelong with reducing frequency if there is no evidence of recurrence. TSH suppressive therapy of 0.5–1.0 mIU/L, 0.1–0.5 mIU/L and <0.1 mIU/L is recommended for low-, intermediate-, and high-risk group, respectively.[150] Even in patients with distant metastasis or unresectable recurrence, TSH suppressive therapy must be continued. The chronic nonphysiological hyperthyroid state can result in accelerated bone maturation with a reduced final height of the patient. The cumulative dose of radioiodine must be balanced against the potential risk of developing long-term complications, including second primary tumors versus benefit of RIT in controlling disease and improved survival. The role of PET-CT in radioiodine resistant cases in pediatric age group is not well-defined; hence, such cases must be evaluated with cross-sectional imaging like CT scan.

Poorly Differentiated Thyroid Cancer

Poorly differentiated thyroid cancer (PDTC) is a distinct entity with an intermediate prognosis between well-differentiated thyroid cancer and anaplastic thyroid cancer. The incidence is rare and it is a biologically aggressive tumor. The existing literature is limited with most of the guidelines based on a few retrospective series. Poorly differentiated thyroid carcinoma has an incidence rate of 0.23–2.6% of thyroid cancers, and they show a female preponderance, presenting most commonly in the sixth decade of life.[154] The pathological criteria to diagnose this cancer was proposed by Turin which can be distinguished on histology; however, establishing a diagnosis on FNAC remains a challenge and the diagnostic FNAC in this is about 6%.[155] The rate of nodal metastasis is 27.8–72.4%, the rate of distant metastasis is 48.5%, and the presence of extranodal extension is 66.6%.[9] The ability of these tumors to concentrated radioiodine has been believed to be modest, however, various studies have shown the ability to be as high as 71%;[156] hence, radioiodine should be used as an adjuvant therapy. PDTC also secrets serum Tg and hence this should be used in their surveillance. This survival outcome is also variable with an overall survival of 62–89.3%.[156] The factors associated with poor prognostication for survival are incomplete resection, age >45 years, and multiple RIT treatments in the past. Presence of gross extranodal extension did not impact survival.

Role of External Beam Radiotherapy in Thyroid Cancer

The role of external beam radiation is not well-defined. Most of the available evidence is largely based on small numbers and retrospective studies. The only trial intended to answer this question started in 2003 was stopped early due to nonacceptance of EBRT in most centers and required accrual was not achieved.[157] Currently, no prospective trial is available and EBRT is restricted to disease that is not amenable for surgery/RAI in the absence of distant metastasis and as an adjuvant setting cases with locally infiltrative disease. Most of the guidelines vary between institutions. In general, the following are accepted as indications of EBRT in thyroid cancer:[158]

- Gross residual disease not amenable to surgery
- Microscopic residual disease at an increased risk of recurrence (such as in an invasive thyroid cancer)
- Recurrent tumors not amenable for surgery

Gross Residual Disease not Amenable for Surgery

One of the largest series with 217 patients of residual disease has shown a benefit with EBRT. The 10-year local relapse-free rate (LRFR) and cause-specific survival (CSS) were 63.4% and 74.1%, respectively.[159] EBRT in residual unresectable disease is recommended after RIA. A dose of 60–70 Gy in 30–35 daily fractions is recommended. EBRT is not indicated in younger patients with radioiodine avid tumors.[160]

Microscopic Residual Disease at an Increased Risk of Recurrence

The definition of microscopic residual disease is difficult, as the surgeon removes all visible gross tumor with adequate margins. In cases that are at high risk for locoregional recurrence are indicated for EBRT. The local recurrence rate is as high as 36% when there is gross extrathyroidal disease and microscopic residual disease. The commonly used indications for EBRT are T4 tumors, multiple positive lymph nodes, gross extranodal extension and gross extrathyroidal extension.[158] The indication for EBRT in extensive nodal disease is limited, as the nodal disease is more easily salvageable than thyroid bed recurrence.

Radiation Technique and Dose

Due to variability in literature, consensus on radiation dose, volumes, and technique is lacking. A dose of 60–70 Gy is advocated by most studies in inoperable disease. For microscopic disease, 50–70 Gy is recommended with an average total dose of 60 Gy is recommended. The tumor volume is also different across the studies. The superior limit was defined as mastoid process, mandible angle, or upper limit of thyroid bed and the inferior margin of field was up to sternal angle or clavicle to include supraclavicular nodes. Significantly better target volume coverage is achieved with intensity modulated radiation therapy (IMRT) than other RT techniques when employed for thyroid cancer.[151] Thyroid bed proximity to spinal cord places it at risk and with dose painting advantage with IMRT as the spinal cord dose can be restricted to <45 Gy.

Combined External Beam Radiotherapy and Radioactive Iodine Therapy/Adjuvant Therapy

The sequence of EBRT and RAI has been debated. In diseases associated with reduced uptake of radioiodine (unfavorable histology, older age, recurrent disease, high FDG uptake, and/or low RAI uptake in known residual disease) EBRT can be considered first.[158]

Thyroglobulin Elevated Negative Iodine Scan

The definition of TENIS includes structural disease that loses ability to concentrate radioiodine, progresses on radioiodine treatment, is partially radioiodine avid, did not ever concentrate radioiodine or elevated thyroglobulin with negative iodine scan with no structurally evident disease. Diagnosis and management of thyroglobulin elevated negative iodine scan (TENIS) is challenging due to rarity of the entity (incidence 2–13%). The diagnosis of TENIS is by exclusion. Some of the features that need to be documented and looked for are:[161,162]

- Significant rise in stimulated serum Tg
- Documentation of initial radioiodine uptake
- Level of TSH may be too low to show an appropriate uptake
- Iodine contamination may have occurred due to improper preparation
- Metastases that are too small to be identifiable on radioiodine scan may have occurred
- There may have been insufficient iodine administration during the scan
- Neck node metastasis deficient in sodium iodide symporter may be present

Evaluation

Initial workup consists of US neck to rule out local and regional recurrence. If the US is negative then PET-CT scan must be performed. This is an absolute indication for use of PET-CT in DTC. The sensitivity of PET-CT increases with elevating TSH levels. A recent meta-analysis in 2019 has proven the diagnostic accuracy of FDG PET-CT in TENIS. If the disease is identifiable and resectable on PET-CT, then resection of the disease is the primary aim. Other modalities are employed only when the disease is not resectable. Elevated Tg with no structural disease on radioiodine scan and PET-CT is a clinical entity that we often encounter, but is associated with good prognosis. The role of empirical I-131 is debated.[161-163]

Treatment Options

- *Surgery:* When the tumor is resectable, surgery achieves best outcome than all other modalities of treatment.
- *External beam radiotherapy:* It is used only when further surgery is not contemplated.[161]
- *Re-differentiation agents:* As the tumor dedifferentiates, it loses its ability to concentrate iodine. Various modalities have been tested to re-differentiate tumor. Retinoids are one of the widely tested agents. In vitro studies, retinoids can upgrade sodium iodine symporter and enhance iodine uptake. Various clinical studies have shown variable response rate from 21.6 to 23%,[166] however, the increased uptake did not transform into a clinical advantage. Thiazolidinedione is a peroxisome proliferator-activated receptor-gamma agonist. Commonly used as an antidiabetic has shown redifferentiation and antiproliferative properties in in vitro studies. A phase II study showed a response of 25% but the same did not translate into a reduction in the size of the disease as per RECIST (response evaluation criteria in solid tumors) criteria.[167] Various other agents are available such as histone deacetylase inhibitor, (e.g., valproic acid, trichostatin, and depsipeptide), DNA demethylating agents, (e.g., 5-azacytidine), and arsenic trioxide, which have shown benefit in in vitro studies but potential clinical use needs to be validated.[168] Selumetinib, a selective MEK inhibitor, was shown in a phase II clinical trial to cause redifferentiation in radiorefractory DTC. The efficacy was higher in patients with an *NRAS* mutation rather than those with *BRAF* mutations.
- *Tyrosinase inhibitors:* Tyrosine kinase inhibitors form one of the main modality of treatment in these patients. They are indicated in iodine refractory cases with proven disease progression. These agents

are tumorostatic and hence of limited value when the disease is stable.[21] TKIs intervene at various levels. They inhibit various pathways, namely mitogen-activated protein kinase (MAPK) pathway, the PI3K-AKT pathway, and vascular endothelial growth factor receptor.[169] The TKIs with proven efficacy and commonly used are sorafenib and lenvatinib. DECISION (stuDy of sorafEnib in loCally advanced or metastatIc patientS with radioactive Iodine-refractory thyrOid caNcer) trial proved the efficacy of sorafenib over placebo in cases with iodine refractory tumors that were locally advanced and metastatic.[170] Progression-free survival was 10.8 months as opposed to 5.8 months in the placebo group. Lenvatinib has also proven efficacy in radioiodine refractory tumors with PFS 18.3 months versus 3.6 months in the placebo arm.[171] TKIs are associated with significant toxicities and adverse events that significantly affect quality of life.[21] Dose reduction due to toxicity was necessary in 78% and discontinuation in 19% with sorafenib. The discontinuation due to adverse effects with lenvatinib was in 14.2%.

Tyrosine kinase inhibitors contraindications:[21]
- Active intestinal disease such as irritable bowel syndrome, diverticulitis
- Liver disease
- Recent tracheal irritation (predisposes to tracheaesophageal fistula)
- Poorly controlled hypertension
- Prolonged QTc interval, arrhythmias
- Untreated brain metastasis

Side effects: Cardiovascular toxicity, predisposes to hypertension, prolonged QTc interval (>480 msec is an indication for stopping TKI), and arrhythmias. Other side effects include ephrotoxicity, hepatotoxicity, cutaneous toxicity such as increased photophobia, sores, photosensitization, and teratogenic potential.

- *177Lu-DOTATATE:* Recent studies have proven an increased expression of somatostatin receptor (SSTR) on the cell surface.[172,173] The expression is higher in patients with PTC. The use of 177Lu-DOTATATE is extrapolated from its utility in neuroendocrine tumors that express SSTR. Patients treated with 177Lu-DOTATATE have shown a longer time to progression and longer survival. The percentage of patients with TENIS expressing SSTR is minimal but in a choice-restricted entity, exploring peptide receptor radionuclide therapy (PRRT) with 177Lu/90Y-DOTATATE therapy can be recommended. The evidence is limited in this regard and lacks standardization.

Prognosis with TENIS where structural disease is identified is worse than patient with elevated Tg with no structural disease, with 3-year overall survival with metastatic disease of <50%.

MANAGEMENT OF DISTANT METASTASIS

Management of distant metastasis in DTC most often needs a multidisciplinary approach. The management guidelines are derived from smaller studies due to the absence of prospective trials.

- *Surgery:* Surgery forms the mainstay of treatment for locoregional disease as well as distant metastasis. When resectable and in oligometastatic patients, surgical resection is accompanied by the best outcome. Surgery also plays a role in palliation especially in bone metastasis with pain, where surgical resection and fixation of pathological fracture is followed by adjuvant therapy may improve pain. Surgery places an important role in brain metastasis and spine metastasis with impending neurological complications. Stopping thyroxine for RAI can result in edema that may further worsen neurological complication.[21] Patients receiving surgery for brain metastasis have shown better survival (6.7 months), when compared to those who did not (3.4 months). In cases with unresectable brain metastasis, radiation and corticosteroids must be the first-line treatment then followed by RAI.
- *Radioiodine therapy:* Distant metastasis occurs most frequently in the lung. RAI forms the mainstay of treatment in RAI avid metastases. The factors associated with favorable outcome are age <40 years, lung-only metastasis, micronodular disease, and PTC.[108] A fixed dose of 100–150 mCi is commonly administered. Most metastatic disease may need multiple therapies usually repeated over 3–12 months. Lung and bone metastasis are the RAI avid disease. The benefits of repeated-dose must be weighed against benefit. The risk of second primary tumors is higher (20 times) with increasing doses of radioiodine. A cumulative dose of 600 mci is associated with increased risk of second primary tumors. Pulmonary fibrosis is also one of the dose-limiting complications for RIA.
- *External beam radiotherapy:* Stereotactic radiosurgery/therapy can be used in large lung and brain metastasis. Bone metastasis irradiation can be recommended to alleviate pain. Hemostatic RT can be planned in cases with symptomatic hemoptysis from lung metastasis. Diffuse lung involvement is best managed by RAI.
- *Cytotoxic therapy:* It has limited use with no survival benefit. Bleomycin, cisplatin, cisplatin or bleomycin with vincristine have been used but with limited benefit.[21] When all other therapies are exhausted, then systemic chemotherapy can be administered.

CONCLUSION

Follicular derived differentiated thyroid cancer is associated with excellent outcomes. Surgery and adjuvant RIT form the primary treatment modalities. The following section includes medullary thyroid carcinoma and anaplastic thyroid carcinoma management.

MEDULLARY THYROID CARCINOMA

Medullary thyroid carcinoma (MTC) is a differentiated thyroid cancer that arises from parafollicular C cell (C cells) of the thyroid which is neuroendocrine in origin. Parafollicular C cells originate from the ultimobranchial bodies that descend inferiorly and get trapped within the junction of upper one-third and lower two-thirds of the thyroid lobe. C cells are more dense in men than in women. MTC form 1–2% of all thyroid cancers. MTC can present in the sporadic form (80%) or as part of inherited tumor syndrome. The behavior of MTC differs from follicular origin DTC in being associated with higher metastasis rate. The 5-year survival in stage I/II/III disease is 93% but falls to 28% in stage IV. Surgery forms the only curative modality of treatment in MTC, while most other modalities play a role in the adjuvant setting or unresectable/metastatic disease.[174,175]

CLINICAL PRESENTATION

Sporadic cases present in the fifth or sixth decade of life while an inherited form of MTC presents at an earlier age. About 50% of MTC present with lymph node spread, 15% present with local invasion and 5–10% present with distant metastasis.[176]

Sporadic MTC presents as single thyroid nodule. Inherited syndromes associated with MTC are usually bilateral and multicentric. Among the inherited forms, the most aggressive and unfavorable outcome is associated with multiple endocrine neoplasia type 2B (MEN2B) and the most indolent course is in familial MTC (MEN2 MTC only). Multiple endocrine neoplasia type 2A (MEN2A) shows a variable degree of aggressiveness. Gene mutation estimates aggressiveness of the tumor. Familial nature is suspected based on positive family history, the presence of multiple endocrine neoplasia and multicentricity of MTC.[177]

These tumors can also secrete adrenocorticotropic hormone (ACTH), calcitonin gene-related peptide (CGRH), which can result in diarrhea, and Cushing's syndrome-like features. Diarrhea can be relieved by somatostatin analog such as octreotide and lanreotide. Cushing's syndrome features are managed with ketoconazole, mifepristone, aminoglutethimide, and metyrapone or mitotane.[178]

Familial Medullary Thyroid Carcinoma

Familial MTC is associated exclusively with *RET* gene mutation. *RET* is a proto-oncogene on chromosome 10q11-2. The gene consists of 21 exons and encodes for the tyrosine kinase transmembrane receptor. *RET* gene is expressed in neural crest cell, urogenital system, and branchial arches. The receptor is divided into three parts based on location. The extracellular domain has a distal cadherin-like region, a juxtamembrane domain with cysteine-rich region and an intracellular domain with tyrosine kinase activity. The RET proto-oncogene mutations are associated with multiple endocrine neoplasia syndrome type 2 (MEN2) and familial medullary thyroid carcinoma (FMTC), which now group under MEN2.[177] MEN2 has an inheritance by autosomal dominance. MEN2 is further classified as:

- *Multiple endocrine neoplasia syndrome type 2A:* It is characterized by MTC (90%), pheochromocytoma (50%), and parathyroid adenoma (20–30%).
- *Multiple endocrine neoplasia syndrome type 2B (also known as MEN3):* It is associated with MTC (90%), pheochromocytoma (40–50%), other features (40–50%) such as mucosal neuroma, marfanoid habitus, medullated corneal nerve fibers, and megacolon.[179]

Almost 98% of MEN2A mutations are located on cadherin-like domain, MEN2B mutations are in relation to tyrosine kinase domain, and FMTC-associated RET mutations affect any of the domains. The domain, codon, risk association, phenotype association of each mutation are represented in **Table 10**. The risk assessment was made based on aggressiveness associated with the respective gene. Aggressiveness was defined based on early age of presentation and frequency of metastatic disease. The American Thyroid Association guidelines described risk stratification is represented in **Table 10**.

GENETIC SCREENING

Genetic screening is advised when there is familial inheritance suspicion in the index case. The index case is subjected to screen *RET* gene mutation and which when positive, blood is taken from all first-degree family members for testing. Adequate counseling and consent must be taken before initiating genetic screening. In sporadic cases, *RET* gene analysis is recommended as 5–7% of clinically apparent sporadic forms on testing. Somatic mutation of *HRAS, KRAS,* and *NRAS* can be in sporadic cases when no *RET* mutation is detected.[180]

A single or multitiered analysis is frequently advocated, which tests commonly known mutations. Sequencing the entire coding region is indicated when

Table 10: Relationship of various *RET* gene mutation with phenotype, pheochromocytoma (PHEO), hyperparathyroidism (HPTH), cutaneous lichen amyloidosis (CLA) and Hirschsprung's disease (HD).

Domain	*Codon*	*Exon*	*Phenotype*	*Risk association**	*PHEO*	*HPTH*	*CLA*	*HD*
Cadherin-like domain	609	10	FMTC MEN2A	Moderate	+/++	+	N	Y
	611	10	FMTC MEN2A	Moderate	+/++	+	N	Y
	618	10	FMTC MEN2A	Moderate	+/++	+	N	Y
	620	10	FMTC MEN2A	Moderate	+/++	+	N	Y
	630	11	FMTC	Moderate	+/++	+	N	N
	634	11	MEN2A	High	+++	++	Y	N
Cysteine-rich domain	768	13	FMTC	Moderate	–	–	N	N
	790–1	13	FMTC	Moderate	+	–	N	N
	804	14	FMTC	Moderate	+	+	Y	N
Tyrosine kinase domain	883	15	MEN2B	High	+++	–	N	N
	891	15	FMTC	Moderate	+	+	N	N
	912	16	FMTC	Moderate	–	–	N	N
	918	16	MEN2B	Highest	+++	–	N	N

(FMTC: familial medullary thyroid carcinoma; MEN2: multiple endocrine neoplasia syndrome type 2)
Notes:
Incidence rate: + = 10%; ++ = 20–30%; +++ = 50%
Y: positive occurrence
N: negative occurrence
**risk stratification as per the American Thyroid Association*

no *RET* mutation is identified on routine single or multi-tiered analysis is done. In suspected MEN2B cases, mutation for 918 codon must be tested first followed by 883, if 918 codon is negative. Exon-10 associated gene mutations followed by exon-11 mutations are tested in MEN2A. Parents whose child has classic MEN2B, patients with cutaneous lichen amyloidosis, and children with Hirschsprung disease are also subjected to genetic testing. Prenatal and preimplantation testing must be suggested when either of parents have MEN2.

DIAGNOSIS

Fine-needle Aspiration Cytology[181]

Cytological evaluation of MTC is characterized by dispersed cell pattern of polygonal cells, azurophilic cytoplasmic granules and eccentrically placed nuclei, and presence of amyloid. The accuracy of FNAC is low with only 50% being diagnosed with MTC based only on FNAC features. Immunohistochemistry (IHC) on the cellblock or FNAC washout for calcitonin (CTN) and chromogranin is advocated in equivocal reports.

Serum Tumor Markers

Serum calcitonin is a polypeptide hormone which is produced exclusively by parafollicular C cells. In normal circumstances, CTN binds to osteoclast and inhibits bone resorption. In an adult, large doses of calcitonin do not bring about changes in the calcium level, but its activity is pronounced during increased bone turn over and inhibits bone resorption. CTN raises even in the presence of microfoci of MTC and hence is the most sensitive marker for MTC. To differentiate CTN released from C cells, the patient can be subjected to calcium 2 mg/kg or pentagastrin 0.5 mg/kg as a challenge test. After the stimulation, there is a 5–10 fold increase in the serum CTN if the origin is from C cells. Procalcitonin is the precursor of CTN which may sometimes interfere with CTN level assessment when immunochemiluminometric analysis is used because patients with inflammatory conditions may present with high procalcitonin, and serum CTN will be reported as high in this situation. Children show a higher level with a cutoff of 40 pg/mL in <6 months and 15 pg/mL in 6 months to 3 years. Children above 3 years have normal adult range of CTN. CTN cutoff value in women and men are 15–25 pg/mL and 70–80 pg/mL, respectively.[182]

Biochemical screening is a method in which patients with a moderate risk of *RET* mutation can be followed up with serial serum CTN and prophylactic thyroidectomy is advised based on the rising level of CTN.[183] Patients with slow-growing tumors have a moderate risk of gene mutation. In them, the rates of tumor growth are 0.4–0.5 mm (N0) and 1.2–1.6 mm (N^+), which gives leeway to perform thyroidectomy only when serum CTN rises.

Carcinoembryonic antigen (CEA) is also a secretory product of C cells, but is not a specific marker.[184] CEA is used as an essential tool in evaluating disease progression. When there is a progressive increase of CEA without elevation in CTN, it represents early epithelial differentiation and a poorly differentiated MTC. Serum CTN and CEA must always be measured concurrently. Calcitonin >20 pg/mL, 50 pg/mL, 200 pg/mL, and 500 pg/mL is associated with lymph nodal metastasis in ipsilateral central, ipsilateral lateral, contralateral central, contralateral lateral, and upper mediastinal nodes, respectively. Preoperative CEA level has also been associated with the presence of >10 nodes and distant metastasis when there has been an incremental increase of serum CEA value. Hence, preoperative assessment of CTN and CEA must be done in all cases; not only does it aid in diagnosis, but also in treatment decision and prognostication.

OTHER PREOPERATIVE EVALUATION

About 5–7% of patients who are clinically apparent sporadic form may have inherited form and hence preoperative evaluation of both adrenal and parathyroid gland must be performed in all cases. Pheochromocytoma can be ruled out by using biochemical tests such as epinephrine to norepinephrine ratio. Measurement of plasma metanephrines is the most sensitive and specific of all the tests. Hypertension is not always associated with pheochromocytoma. Once biochemical suspicion arises a CT scan or an MRI of the abdomen must be performed. If they fail to locate pheochromocytoma, then ^{131}I metaiodobenzylguanidine scan can be performed, which is specific to chromaffin tissue. Parathyroid adenoma or hyperplasia is associated with hyperparathyroidism, hypercalcemia, and hypercalciuria, which can be easily assessed.

IMAGING[185]

Ultrasound of the neck is usually the first and the most frequent preoperative imaging modality. The ultrasound features of MTC are solid hypoechoic nodules with coarse calcification. Further cross-sectional imaging may be required if there are signs of local invasion. Any node that is suspicious on ultrasound must be evaluated with FNAC and CTN assessment of the washout fluid. Distant metastasis must be evaluated in patients with extensive local disease, extensive regional disease, symptoms or signs of distant metastasis and in all patients with calcitonin >500 pg/mL. Distant metastasis evaluation is best done with CT, MRI, and bone scintigraphy. Accurate assessment of local and regional disease is essential, as elevated calcitonin level due to an incomplete surgery will mandate surgery.

The three-phase contrast-enhanced multidetector liver CT and contrast-enhanced MRI are sensitive imaging techniques to assess liver metastases. Lung and mediastinal nodal metastasis can be best evaluated with a CT scan of the chest. Bone metastases can be evaluated with axial MRI and bone scintigraphy which are complementary to each other and combined are most sensitive modality. 12-F-fluoro-2-deoxy-D-glucose (FDG) positron emission tomography/CT (FDG-PET/CT) and 18F-dihydroxyphenyl alanine F-DOPA-PET-CT have limited value in primary setting evaluation. No single imaging modality provides optimal whole-body imaging for MTC.

PATHOLOGY

Microscopic picture of MTC consists of only polyhedral cells with spindle-shaped cells with peripheral palisading in a vascular stroma.[186,187] CTN-IHC staining is diagnostic of MTC, while the differentiated tumor shows stronger positivity to CEA. Cytokeratin-7, cytokeratin-8, TTF1, and chromogranin may also show focal positivity. In all patients, the entire gland must be examined to roll-out multicentricity.

STAGING AND PROGNOSTICATION

The American Joint Committee on Cancer (AJCC) staging is based on the size of the tumor, extrathyroidal extension and nodal and distant metastasis, as depicted in **Table 11**. However, the TNM staging lacks various critical prognostic factors. The 5- and 10-year disease-specific survival in patients who are younger than 40 years and those older are 95/75% and 65/50%, respectively. Immaterial of the age, MEN2B has worse survival than all other variants. The different staging systems for MTC have been evaluated which has shown that EORTC staging system performs better than the AJCC system. Other prognostic factors that affect survival are the paucity of calcitonin staining, increasing CEA and postoperative persistent increased CTN.[188]

MANAGEMENT

Surgery forms the mainstay of treatment in MTC. All other treatment modalities are not curative. Before surgical management, all patients must be assessed for hyperparathyroidism and pheochromocytoma.

Table 11: The American Joint Committee on Cancer (AJCC), 8th edition, TNM staging for medullary thyroid carcinoma.

TX	Primary tumor cannot be assessed
T0	No evidence of primary tumor
T1	Tumor ≤2 cm or less in greatest dimension limited to the thyroid
T1a	Tumor ≤1 cm in greatest dimension limited to the thyroid
T1b	Tumor >1 cm but ≤2 cm in the greatest dimension limited to the thyroid
T2	Tumor >2 cm but ≤4 cm in the greatest dimension limited to the thyroid
T3	Tumor ≥4 cm or with extrathyroidal extension
T3a	Tumor ≥4 cm in the greatest dimension limited to the thyroid
T3b	Tumor of any size with gross extrathyroidal extension invading only strap muscles (sternohyoid, sternothyroid, thyrohyoid, or omohyoid muscles)
T4	Advanced disease
T4a	Moderately advanced disease; tumor of any size with gross extrathyroidal extension into the nearby tissues of the neck, including subcutaneous soft tissue, larynx, trachea, esophagus, or recurrent laryngeal nerve
T4b	Very advanced disease; tumor of any size with extension toward the spine or into nearby large blood vessels, gross extrathyroidal extension invading the prevertebral fascia, or encasing the carotid artery or mediastinal vessels
NX	Regional lymph nodes cannot be assessed
N0	No evidence of locoregional lymph node metastasis
N0a	One or more cytologically or histologically confirmed benign lymph nodes
N0b	No radiologic or clinical evidence of locoregional lymph node metastasis
N1	Metastasis to regional nodes
N1a	Metastasis to level VI or VII (pretracheal, paratracheal, or prelaryngeal/Delphian, or upper mediastinal) lymph nodes. This can be unilateral or bilateral disease
N1b	Metastasis to unilateral, bilateral, or contralateral neck lymph nodes (levels I, II, III, IV, or V) or retropharyngeal lymph node
M0	No distant metastasis
M1	Distant metastasis

Pheochromocytoma must be managed by laparoscopic adrenalectomy under alpha-adrenergic blockade. When the tumor is 1 cm or more, total thyroidectomy with bilateral central nodal clearance is recommended. When one tumor is <1 cm, total thyroidectomy will suffice. The indications for lateral neck dissection are clinically positive lymph nodes, and prophylactic lateral neck dissection is recommended based on the preoperative CTN level and positive level VI nodes.[189]

Management of Inherited Medullary Thyroid Carcinoma

Based on the risk stratification of the gene mutation, prophylactic thyroidectomy is advised.

- *Highest risk gene mutation:* Prophylactic total thyroidectomy with or without level VI dissection with first year of life or when diagnosed. Follow-up with US of the neck, serum CTN, and CEA every 6 months for the first year then annually. Screening for pheochromocytoma at 11 years of age.
- *High-risk gene mutation*: Prophylactic total thyroidectomy within 5 years of life. Follow-up strategy is similar to the highest risk group.
- *Modest risk gene mutation:* Prophylactic total thyroidectomy when serum CTN elevates. Follow-up strategy includes evaluation of serum CTN every 6 months for the first year and then annually. Screen for pheochromocytoma at 16 years of age.
- In adults with detected *RET* gene mutation, biochemical screening with serum CTN must be followed and prophylactic thyroidectomy when serum CTN elevates.

External Beam Radiotherapy

External beam radiotherapy has not been adequately studied in MTC while available evidence has shown slight improvement in disease-free survival in patients who received postoperative RT in the presence of extrathyroidal extension, extensive local and regional involvement. Therapeutic radiation can be considered when the tumor is unresectable without distant metastases.

POST-TREATMENT SURVEILLANCE

Patients are started on thyroid hormone supplementation without TSH suppression. Postoperative surveillance consists of US neck, serum CTN and serum CEA every 3–6 months. When there is undetectable CTN/CEA and no structural evidence of disease on follow-up after the 1st year of therapy, annual follow-up can be planned.

PERSISTENTLY RAISED CALCITONIN LEVELS

Concentration of serum CTN and CEA must be measured every 3 months. About 80% with palpable MTC and 50% with nonpalpable macroscopic disease following curative-intent treatment show persistent elevation of CTN. Complete biochemical cure can be achieved when preoperative CTN is <100 pg/mL. Calcitonin or CEA can be measured over multiple time points to determine the rate at which the value doubles. Calcitonin doubling time is an independent predictor of survival. The doubling time must be calculated at least four-time points over a minimum of 2 years. With a doubling time of 25 months or greater, the risk of progressive disease is 14% and 94% when doubling time was 25 months and less.

If there is no evidence of structural disease in the neck and CTN levels are detectable but <150 pg/mL, then patients can be followed up without any active intervention.

EVALUATION OF RECURRENT OR METASTATIC MEDULLARY THYROID CARCINOMA[190]

Calcitonin >150 pg/mL must be evaluated for metastases and value of >1,000 pg/mL most often represents distant metastasis. Radionuclide imaging plays a vital role in detecting persistent or recurrent MTC. The conventional nuclear imaging techniques such as Technetium-99m pentavalent dimercaptosuccinic acid [^{99m}Tc-(V) DMSA], somatostatin analogs labeled with Indium-111 or Technetium-99m, radioiodinated metaiodobenzylguanidine (MIBG) or radiolabeled anti-CEA antibodies are not sensitive enough to detect MTC relapse when compared to conventional radiological imaging (CT/MRI) and hence have fallen out of vogue.

The three radiopharmaceuticals that are used routinely are FDG, fluorine-18 dihydroxyphenylalanine (FDOPA) and somatostatin analogs labeled with Gallium-68.

- *PET-CT:* FDG PET-CT has shown variable sensitivity (17–95%) and specificity (68–100%). The reason for diversity in these results can be attributed to technical aspects, tumor aspects and also the inclusion criteria of these studies. The detection rate with PET-CT is 59%. Most of MTCs are not very aggressive and may not concentrate FDG, while tumors that are aggressively growing and are characterized by high-serum CTN, high-serum CEA, and steep doubling time increase the diagnostic performance of PET-CT.
- *Fluorine-18 dihydroxyphenylalanine:* The trans-membrane amino acid transporter that is significantly upregulated in neuroendocrine tumors such as MTC takes up FDOPA. The detection rate of MTC with FDOPA is 72%. The detection rate increases to 86% when the CTN doubling time is <24 months. Few researchers have demonstrated an improved detection rate with early image acquisition (15 minutes) when compared to standard acquisition (60 minutes) and suggested a dual-phase FDOPA image acquisition.
- *Somatostatin analogs labeled with Gallium-68:* Somatostatin receptors are commonly expressed on the cell surface of neuroendocrine origin. The diagnostic performance of somatostatin receptor analog is inferior to other nuclear imaging modalities. Nevertheless, they are valuable when therapeutic options are considered. The detection rate is 60%.

The comparative analysis between these imaging modalities has shown that FDOPA performs better than all other nuclear imaging. The roles of FDOPA and FDG-PET are complementary to each other, where FDOPA provides precise diagnostic information in well-differentiated MTC and FDG is superior in dedifferentiated tumors. The main drawback of FDOPA is that it is the most expensive modality for evaluation. No cost-effectiveness studies are available. Due to the wide availability of FDG, it is probably the most frequent imaging modality utilized. The proposed algorithm for the use of radionuclide imaging when the serum CTN is >150 pg/mL is the use of FDOPA PET-CT followed by FDG PET-CT, then followed by somatostatin analog imaging. When CEA level is elevated disproportionately to CTN, then the first preferred modality must be FDG PET-CT.

MANAGEMENT OF RECURRENT OR METASTATIC DISEASE

In case of a recurrence when resectable must be surgically excised. Patients with bone and brain metastasis are managed similar to differentiated thyroid cancer that is radioiodine resistant. Chemoembolization is planned when the disease is disseminated in the liver with <3 cm size and involves less than one-third of the liver.

Targeted Therapy

Mutation of *RET* is virtually present in all patients with familial and inherited MTC. These mutations are also seen in 18–80% of patients in sporadic cases and in *RET* negative MTC, *RAS* mutations are commonly identified. Vascular endothelial growth factor receptors are overexpressed in MTC. Various TKIs have been tested in MTC. Vandetanib and cabozantinib are recommended agents as they have shown increased progression-free survival. Vandetanib is a multitargeted agent which inhibits *RET*, endothelial growth factor, and vascular endothelial growth factor. Vandetanib has shown increased progression-free survival over placebo (HR: 0.46) in a phase III randomized trial, which included 331 patients with unresectable locally advanced or metastatic MTC.[191,192]

Vandetanib (300 mg/day) or cabozantinib (140 mg/day) is used in this setting. Vandetanib has shown a higher progression-free survival of 30.5 months with the median was not reached. Diarrhea, rash, photosensitivity, fatigue, and folliculitis are the common adverse effects with vandetanib. The trial showed that 12% of patient discontinued treatment and 35% had a dose reduction. Cabozantinib is also a multitargeted agent that inhibits *RET*, vascular endothelial growth factor receptor 2 (VEGFR2), and MET. Cabozantinib showed an increased progression-free survival of 11.2 months over placebo (4 months) in a phase III randomized trial (EXAM) in 330 patients with locally advanced or metastatic MTC. The median overall survival achieved was 26.6 months which did not reach statistical significance. Cabozantinib has a higher clinical benefit in *RT918* and *RAS* mutations. It is associated with severe bleeding, gastrointestinal perforation, and fistula. Cabozantinib is associated with discontinuation in 16% and dose reduction in 79%. TKIs must be used as a single agent of first-line systemic therapy agents.

Use of cytotoxic chemotherapy has been studied with doxorubicin, dacarbazine and 5-fluorouracil with low response rates of 15–20% and low durability of the response. Radiolabeled molecules such as 90Y-DOTATOC was evaluated in a phase II trial which included patients with advanced MTC who showed uptake on 111In OctreoScan. The trial reported a 58.1% reduction in CTN doubling time and 29% had a reduction in CTN value. Hematologic toxicity occurred in 13% and 23% developed renal toxicity. Efficacy of pretargeted radionuclide labeled molecules needs further validation for routine use.[193,194]

CONCLUSION

Medullary thyroid carcinoma comprises 1–2% of all thyroid cancers. *RET* gene mutation is commonly associated with MTC. Genetic counseling must be considered in all cases. Serum calcitonin is the most sensitive tumor marker for MTC and plays an essential role in treatment decision and follow-up strategy. Surgery is the only curative treatment available for MTC; hence, preoperative evaluation to accurately assess disease extent is vital to achieve cure. Treatment options in recurrent inoperable tumors are limited to TKIs.

ANAPLASTIC THYROID CARCINOMA

Anaplastic thyroid carcinomas are rare tumors which comprise of 1–2% of all thyroid cancers. These tumors are extremely aggressive and are associated with 100% disease-specific mortality.[195] The median survival in these patients is 3–6 months. There is no consensus on management due to the rarity of the disease and short survival of the patient. Even today, it remains a devastating diagnosis.

EPIDEMIOLOGY

The frequency of anaplastic thyroid carcinoma has shown geographical changes in incidence with higher prevalence in areas of endemic goiter. The incidence is 1–2 cases/million population/year.[196] Recent epidemiological data has shown a decrease in incidence of anaplastic thyroid cancer worldwide.[196]

PATHOPHYSIOLOGY

Nearly half of all ATCs arise in previous or concurrent DTC. These ATC reflect dedifferentiation of DTC. Various genetic alterations that are noticed or expressed in DTC overlap in ATC along with additional alterations. These genetic alterations attained later could be responsible for the aggressive behavior of ATC. The molecular alterations represent a continuum of acquired alterations leading to ATC. The most frequent genetic alterations seen in ATC are *TP53,* combined *BRAF,* and *TERT* mutations most commonly.[197] *TIK3CA, BTEN,* and *RAS* mutations are seen in the rate of 10–20%. These tumors express a higher burden of somatic mutations and are known to acquire *BRAF, RAS* mutations early, and *P53* and *TERT* promoter mutations are acquired later.[197] Mechanisms of immune evasion have also been noted in these tumors and make them an attractive candidate for immunotherapy. They show enriched neutrophils T-cell and tumor-associated macrophages. ATC also has a higher expression of PDL-1.[198] The precipitating event or an etiology factor for transformation into undifferentiated anaplastic cancer is uncertain.

PRESENTATION

These patients typically present with a rapidly enlarging neck mass and associated symptoms of compression and invasion to local structures such as breathing difficulty, stridor, dysphasia, cough, hoarseness of voice, and hemoptysis. Rarely anaplastic thyroid carcinoma can be found incidentally in the surgical specimen of DTC. They present in 5th to 7th decades of life and it is rarely seen in patients <30 years. It affects females more than men in the ratio of 2:1.[2]

DIAGNOSIS

Extensive local invasion to adjoining structures and distant metastasis is seen in 15–50% of patients. The lung is the most common site of distant metastasis (50%)

followed by bone (5–15%) and brain (5%).[199] Diagnosis by FNAC may not always be conclusive of anaplastic thyroid carcinoma. Presence of differentiated thyroid carcinoma in the background may make the reporting more challenging. The presence of biphasic spindle and giant cells, prominent mitotic figures in a background of necrosis, and inflammatory cells are common features on FNAC. The diagnosis of anaplastic thyroid cancer must be a diagnosis of exclusion as various other tumors can mimic features of anaplastic thyroid cancer on cytology and histopathology. Most of these cancers have definitive treatment available while a diagnosis of anaplastic thyroid cancer is devastating due to limited treatment options and poor survival. Differential diagnosis of anaplastic carcinoma is poorly differentiated thyroid carcinoma, primary thyroid SCC, medullary thyroid carcinoma, primary thyroid sarcoma, primary thyroid lymphoma, and metastatic disease to the thyroid. IHC is essential in almost all cases to confirm the diagnosis of anaplastic thyroid cancer. Focal positivity for cytokeratin and vimentin is expressed. They are negative for thyroid transcription factor, Tg and calcitonin. Diffuse expression of *PAX8* and *P53* are common.[200] The microscopic appearances are broadly classified into sarcomatoid, giant cell, and epithelial variants. Sarcomatoid form is characterized by malignant spindle cells similar to pleomorphic sarcoma. Giant cell form is characterized by pleomorphic malignant cells with multiple nuclei. Epithelial form has squamoid tumor nests with abundant eosinophilic cytoplasm.

All cases of anaplastic carcinoma must be evaluated for distant metastasis with CT scan of the neck, chest, abdomen, pelvis, and MRI brain or PET-CT from skull base to mid-thigh level with MRI brain. Cross-sectional imaging of the neck and chest is mandatory to assess the extension of disease, especially to adjacent structures.

TREATMENT

No curative therapy exists. Most patients have an average of 5 months of survival. 1-year survival in ATC is 20%.[125] Half of the patients die of airway complications and others by distant metastasis. The prognostic factors in ATC are age at presentation, dyspnea at presentation, and distant metastases.[201] Patients with disease confined to neck survive 5 months longer than those with extension beyond the neck. At the diagnosis of anaplastic carcinoma, it is critical to counsel patient and patient's family regarding prognosis, management options, and end-of-life care. Most of the clinically apparent ATCs are unresectable. When resectable, total thyroidectomy with nodal region clearance must be attempted.[125] Studies have shown that, even after attempted tumor clearance, there is no significant survival benefit except in cases where the anaplastic carcinoma component is restricted within the thyroid gland.[125]

External beam radiation therapy must be considered after surgery, unresectable tumors and palliation of local symptoms and distant metastases. ATC is considered radio-resistant tumor and primary EBRT rarely achieves local control. Hyperfractionation is considered in ATC. The rationale is to shorten the treatment time and hence reduces the likelihood of tumor repopulation.

Multimodality treatment with surgery, radiation and chemotherapy showed maximum benefit in survival.[125] Surgery (resection of all visible locoregional tumor) followed by doxorubicin 60 mg/m^2 and cisplatin 120 mg/m^2 every 4 weeks. After two cycles of chemotherapy, hyperfractionation of EBRT [1.25 Gy twice daily-6 hours apart for 5 days a week (total dose of 40 Gy)] or addition of boost to the tumor volume to achieve a total dose of (50–55 Gy) is administered. The radiation field includes the region from the mastoid process to the level of carina. 2 weeks after EBRT, chemotherapy is continued, with each cycle 4 weeks apart to a total of six cycles. The regime has shown a response rate of 80% and a median survival of 1 year.[202] The toxicity level in this regime was quite high, with hematologic toxicity as high as 73%. Maximum response was based on the completeness of resection.

In patients with distant metastasis, doxorubicin is the only agent recommended for single-agent therapy. Other recommended systemic therapy regime is carboplatin with paclitaxel or paclitaxel alone.[203,204]

Targeted therapy with dabrafenib and trametinib or larotrectinib are options in the presence of *BRAF*^{V600E} mutation and *NTRK* gene fusion-positive ATC. A phase II trial reported an overall response of 69% with dabrafenib 150 mg twice daily and trametinib 2 mg once daily in patients with *BRAF*^{V600E} mutations.[205] Hence, molecular testing in ATC is recommended to widen the treatment options.

PALLIATION

Palliation of airway obstruction and bleeding is essential. Prophylactic tracheostomies were associated with lower survival, which could be attributed to treatment delay caused by tracheostomy wound-related issues. Tracheostomy, if possible, must be done but tracheostomy-related maintenance and complications such as stomal bleed must be discussed with patient and caretaker.

Various other palliative measures are essential, which are described below:

- *Breathlessness:* Breathlessness is the most challenging symptom to palliate. The sensation of breathlessness can be reduced by morphine 2.5–5 mg hourly + helium 80% and oxygen 20%.
- *Fear and anxiety:* Fear and anxiety can be alleviated with diazepam 2–5 mg 8 hourly or lorazepam 0.5–1 mg 12 hourly.
- *Bleeding:* Active bleeding can be managed with tranexamic acid 500 mg 8 hourly or etamsylate 500 mg 6 hourly.
- *Intractable cough:* Intractable cough can be managed lidocaine 2% nebulization with 4 mL per nebulization.

CONCLUSION

Anaplastic carcinoma thyroid is a rapidly growing tumor and its management must be treated as an oncologic emergency. It is vital to keep the period between diagnosis and end of treatment as short for best for outcome possible. Most tumors present in unresectable or metastatic stage and treatment options are limited.

REFERENCES

1. Sherma SI. Thyroid carcinoma. Lancet. 2003;361(9356):501-11.
2. Nagaiah G, Hossain A, Mooney CJ, Parmentier J, Remick SC. Anaplastic thyroid cancer: a review of epidemiology, pathogenesis, and treatment. J Oncol. 2011;2011.
3. Cavalieri RR. Iodine metabolism and thyroid physiology: current concepts. Thyroid. 1997;7(2):177-81.
4. Dunn JT. Thyroglobulin chemistry, biosynthesis, and proteolysis. Werner and Ingbar's the Thyroid; 2000.
5. Wiltshire JJ, Drake TM, Uttley L, Balasubramanian SP. Systematic review of trends in the incidence rates of thyroid cancer. Thyroid. 2016;26(11):1541-52.
6. Furuya-Kanamori L, Bell KJ, Clark J, Glasziou P, Doi SA. Prevalence of differentiated thyroid cancer in autopsy studies over six decades: a meta-analysis. J Clin Oncol. 2016;34(30):3672-9.
7. Davies L, Welch HG. Current thyroid cancer trends in the United States. JAMA Otolaryngol Head Neck Surg. 2014;140(4):317-22.
8. Morris LG, Myssiorek D. Improved detection does not fully explain the rising incidence of well-differentiated thyroid cancer: a population-based analysis. Am J Surg. 2010;200(4):454-61.
9. Bernier MO, Withrow DR, Berrington de Gonzalez A, Lam CJ, Linet MS, Kitahara CM, et al. Trends in pediatric thyroid cancer incidence in the United States, 1998–2013. Cancer. 2019;125(14):2497-505.
10. Ron E. Thyroid cancer incidence among people living in areas contaminated by radiation from the Chernobyl accident. Health Phys. 2007;93(5):502-11.
11. Sinnott B, Ron E, Schneider AB. Exposing the thyroid to radiation: a review of its current extent, risks, and implications. Endocr Rev. 2010;31(5):756-73.
12. Hieu TT, Russell AW, Cuneo R, Clark J, Kron T, Hall P, et al. Cancer risk after medical exposure to radioactive iodine in benign thyroid diseases: a meta-analysis. Endocr Cancer. 2012;19(5):645-55.
13. Ron E, Lubin JH, Shore RE, Mabuchi K, Modan B, Pottern LM, et al. Thyroid cancer after exposure to external radiation: a pooled analysis of seven studies. Radiat Res. 1995;141(3):259-77.
14. Schaller Jr RT, Stevenson JK. Development of carcinoma of the thyroid in iodine-deficient mice. Cancer. 1966;19(8):1063-80.
15. Boelaert K, Horacek J, Holder RL, Watkinson JC, Sheppard MC, Franklyn JA. Serum thyrotropin concentration as a novel predictor of malignancy in thyroid nodules investigated by fine-needle aspiration. J Clin Endocrinol Metabol. 2006;91(11):4295-301.
16. Kumar H, Daykin J, Holder R, Watkinson JC, Sheppard MC, Franklyn JA. Gender, clinical findings, and serum thyrotropin measurements in the prediction of thyroid neoplasia in 1005 patients presenting with thyroid enlargement and investigated by fine-needle aspiration cytology. Thyroid. 1999;9(11):1105-9.
17. Vella V, Malaguarnera R. The emerging role of insulin receptor isoforms in thyroid cancer: clinical implications and new perspectives. Int J Mol Sci. 2018;19(12):3814.
18. Mannathazhathu AS, George PS, Sudhakaran S, Vasudevan D, Krishna KMJ, Booth C, et al. Reproductive factors and thyroid cancer risk: meta-analysis. Head Neck. 2019;41(12):4199-208.
19. Mathew IE, Mathew A. Rising thyroid cancer incidence in southern India: an epidemic of overdiagnosis. J Endocr Soc. 2017;1(5):480-7.
20. Tessler FN, Middleton WD, Grant EG, Hoang JK, Berland LL, Teefey SA, et al. ACR thyroid imaging, reporting and data system (TI-RADS): white paper of the ACR TI-RADS committee. J Am Coll Radiol. 2017;14(5):587-95.
21. Haugen BR, Alexander EK, Bible KC, Doherty GM, Mandel SJ, Nikiforov YE, et al. 2015 American Thyroid Association management guidelines for adult patients with thyroid nodules and differentiated thyroid cancer: the American Thyroid Association guidelines task force on thyroid nodules and differentiated thyroid cancer. Thyroid. 2016;26(1):1-33.
22. Shin JH, Baek JH, Chung J, Ha EJ, Kim JH, Lee YH, et al. Ultrasonography diagnosis and imaging-based management of thyroid nodules: revised Korean Society of Thyroid Radiology consensus statement and recommendations. Korean J Radiol. 2016;17(3):370-95.
23. Gharib H, Papini E, Garber JR, Duick DS, Harrell RM, Hegedüs L, et al. American Association of Clinical Endocrinologists, American College of Endocrinology, and Associazione Medici Endocrinologi medical guidelines for clinical practice for the diagnosis and management of thyroid nodules–2016 update. Endocr Practice. 2016;22(s1):1-60.
24. Bachar G, Buda I, Cohen M, Hadar T, Hilly O, Schwartz N, et al. Size discrepancy between sonographic and pathological evaluation of solitary papillary thyroid carcinoma. Eur J Radiol. 2013;82(11):1899-903.
25. Yoon JH, Lee HS, Kim EK, Moon HJ, Kwak JY. Malignancy risk stratification of thyroid nodules: comparison between the thyroid imaging reporting and data system and the 2014 American Thyroid Association management guidelines. Radiology. 2016;278(3):917-24.
26. Cibas ES, Ali SZ. The 2017 Bethesda system for reporting thyroid cytopathology. Thyroid. 2017;27(11):1341-6.

27. Misiakos EP, Margari N, Meristoudis C, Machairas N, Schizas D, Petropoulos K, et al. Cytopathologic diagnosis of fine needle aspiration biopsies of thyroid nodules. World J Clin Cases. 2016;4(2):38-48.
28. Ali SZ. Thyroid cytopathology: Bethesda and beyond. Acta Cytol. 2011;55(1):4-12.
29. Zhou H, Baloch ZW, Nayar R, Bizzarro T, Fadda G, Adhikari-Guragain D, et al. Noninvasive follicular thyroid neoplasm with papillary-like nuclear features (NIFTP): implications for the risk of malignancy (ROM) in The Bethesda System for Reporting Thyroid Cytopathology (TBSRTC). Cancer Cytopathol. 2018;126(1):20-6.
30. Nikiforov YE, Nikiforova MN. Molecular genetics and diagnosis of thyroid cancer. Nat Rev Endocrinol. 2011;7(10): 569-80.
31. Donghi R, Longoni A, Pilotti S, Michieli P, Della Porta G, Pierotti MA. Gene p53 mutations are restricted to poorly differentiated and undifferentiated carcinomas of the thyroid gland. J Clin Invest. 1993;91(4):1753-60.
32. Patel KN, Yip L, Lubitz CC, Grubbs EG, Miller BS, Shen W, Angelos P, et al. The American Association of Endocrine Surgeons Guidelines for the definitive surgical management of thyroid disease in adults. Ann Surg. 2020;271(3):e21-93.
33. D'Cruz AK, Vaish R, Vaidya A, Nixon IJ, Williams MD, Vander Poorten V, et al. Molecular markers in well-differentiated thyroid cancer. Eur Arch Otorhinolaryngol. 2018;275(6):1375-84.
34. Vargas-Salas S, Martínez JR, Urra S, Domínguez JM, Mena N, Uslar T, et al. Genetic testing for indeterminate thyroid cytology: review and meta-analysis. Endocr Cancer. 2018; 25(3):R163-77.
35. Yeh MW, Bauer AJ, Bernet VA, Ferris RL, Loevner LA, Mandel SJ, et al. American Thyroid Association statement on preoperative imaging for thyroid cancer surgery. Thyroid. 2015;25(1):3-14.
36. Hwang HS, Orloff LA. Efficacy of preoperative neck ultrasound in the detection of cervical lymph node metastasis from thyroid cancer. Laryngoscope. 2011;121(3):487-91.
37. Choi JS, Kim J, Kwak JY, Kim MJ, Chang HS, Kim EK. Preoperative staging of papillary thyroid carcinoma: comparison of ultrasound imaging and CT. Am J Roentgenol. 2009;193(3):871-8.
38. Leboulleux S, Girard E, Rose M, Travagli JP, Sabbah N, Caillou B, et al. Ultrasound criteria of malignancy for cervical lymph nodes in patients followed up for differentiated thyroid cancer. J Clin Endocrinol Metabol. 2007;92(9): 3590-4.
39. Solbiati L, Osti V, Cova L, Tonolini M. Ultrasound of thyroid, parathyroid glands and neck lymph nodes. Eur Radiol. 2001; 11(12):2411-24.
40. Wunderbaldinger P, Harisinghani MG, Hahn PF, Daniels GH, Turetschek K, Simeone J, et al. Cystic lymph node metastases in papillary thyroid carcinoma. Am J Roentgenol. 2002;178(3):693-7.
41. Boi F, Baghino G, Atzeni F, Lai ML, Faa G, Mariotti S. The diagnostic value for differentiated thyroid carcinoma metastases of thyroglobulin (Tg) measurement in washout fluid from fine-needle aspiration biopsy of neck lymph nodes is maintained in the presence of circulating anti-Tg antibodies. J Clin Endocrinol Metabol. 2006;91(4):1364-9.
42. Snozek CL, Chambers EP, Reading CC, Sebo TJ, Sistrunk JW, Singh RJ, et al. Serum thyroglobulin, high-resolution ultrasound, and lymph node thyroglobulin in diagnosis of differentiated thyroid carcinoma nodal metastases. J Clin Endocrinol Metabol. 2007;92(11):4278-81.
43. Cunha N, Rodrigues F, Curado F, Ilhéu O, Cruz C, Naidenov P, et al. Thyroglobulin detection in fine-needle aspirates of cervical lymph nodes: a technique for the diagnosis of metastatic differentiated thyroid cancer. Eur J Endocrinol. 2007;157(1):101-7.
44. Yasuda M, Ogane N, Hayashi H, Kameda Y, Miyagi Y, Iida T, et al. Glucose transporter-1 expression in the thyroid gland: clinicopathological significance for papillary carcinoma. Oncol Reports. 2005;14(6):1499-504.
45. Adams S, Baum RP, Stuckensen T, Bitter K, Hör G. Prospective comparison of 18-F-FDG PET with conventional imaging modalities (CT, MRI, US) in lymph node staging of head and neck cancer. Eur J Nucl Med. 1998;25(9):1255-60.
46. Martin S, Maurice T, Vathaire FD, Catherine H, Gardet P, Travagli JP, et al. Long-term results of treatment of 283 patients with lung and bone metastases from differentiated thyroid carcinoma. J Clin Endocrinol Metabol. 1986;63(4):960-7.
47. Treglia G, Muoio B, Giovanella L, Salvatori M. The role of positron emission tomography and positron emission tomography/computed tomography in thyroid tumours: an overview. Eur Arch Otorhinolaryngol. 2013;270(6):1783-7.
48. Algin E, Uner A, Akdemir UO, Gumusay O, Kapucu O, Ozet A. The assessment of incidental thyroid lesions on 18F-fluorodeoxyglucose positron emission tomography/computed tomography: A single centre experience. J Oncol Sci. 2017;3(2):57-61.
49. Sciacchitano S, Lavra L, Ulivieri A, Magi F, De Francesco GP, Bellotti C, et al. Comparative analysis of diagnostic performance, feasibility and cost of different test-methods for thyroid nodules with indeterminate cytology. Oncotarget. 2017;8(30):49421.
50. Seethala RR, Asa SL, Carty SE, Hodak SP, McHugh JB, Richardson MS, et al. Protocol for the examination of specimens from patients with carcinomas of the thyroid gland. Coll Am Pathol; 2014.
51. Ghossein R, Livolsi VA. Papillary thyroid carcinoma tall cell variant. Thyroid. 2008;18(11):1179-81.
52. Falvo L, Giacomelli L, D'Andrea V, Marzullo A, Guerriero G, De Antoni E. Prognostic importance of sclerosing variant in papillary thyroid carcinoma. Am Surg. 2006;72(5):438-44.
53. Nath MC, Erickson LA. Aggressive variants of papillary thyroid carcinoma: hobnail, tall cell, columnar, and solid. Adv Anatom Pathol. 2018;25(3):172-9.
54. Fridman M, Lam AK, Krasko O. Characteristics of young adults of Belarus with post-Chernobyl papillary thyroid carcinoma: a long-term follow-up of patients with early exposure to radiation at the 30th anniversary of the accident. Clin Endocrinol. 2016;85(6):971-8.
55. Volante M, Collini P, Nikiforov YE, Sakamoto A, Kakudo K, Katoh R, et al. Poorly differentiated thyroid carcinoma: the Turin proposal for the use of uniform diagnostic criteria and an algorithmic diagnostic approach. Am J Surg Pathol. 2007;31(8):1256-64.
56. Spielman DB, Badhey A, Kadakia S, Inman JC, Ducic Y. Rare thyroid malignancies: an overview for the oncologist. Clin Oncol. 2017;29(5):298-306.
57. McHenry CR, Raeburn C, Strickland T, Marty JJ. The utility of routine frozen section examination for intraoperative diagnosis of thyroid cancer. Am J Surg. 1996;172(6):658-61.
58. Murthy SP, Balasubramanian D, Anand A, Limbachiya SV, Subramaniam N, Nair V, et al. Extent of Thyroidectomy in

Differentiated Thyroid Cancers—Review of Evidence. Indian J Surg Oncol. 2018;9(1):90-6.

59. Mazzaferri EL, Jhiang SM. Long-term impact of initial surgical and medical therapy on papillary and follicular thyroid cancer. Am J Med. 1994;97(5):418-28.
60. Hay ID, Thompson GB, Grant CS, Bergstralh EJ, Dvorak CE, Gorman CA, et al. Papillary thyroid carcinoma managed at the Mayo Clinic during six decades (1940–1999): temporal trends in initial therapy and long-term outcome in 2444 consecutively treated patients. World J Surg. 2002;26(8): 879-85.
61. Bilimoria KY, Bentrem DJ, Ko CY, Stewart AK, Winchester DP, Talamonti MS, et al. Extent of surgery affects survival for papillary thyroid cancer. Ann Surg. 2007;246(3):375-81.
62. Cady BL, Sedgwick CE, Meissner WA, Bookwalter JR, Romagosa VI, Werber JO. Changing clinical, pathologic, therapeutic, and survival patterns in differentiated thyroid carcinoma. Ann Surg. 1976;184(5):541-53.
63. Shah JP, Loree TR, Dharker D, Strong EW. Lobectomy versus total thyroidectomy for differentiated carcinoma of the thyroid: a matched-pair analysis. Am J Surg. 1993;166(4):331-5.
64. Mendelsohn AH, Elashoff DA, Abemayor E, St John MA. Surgery for papillary thyroid carcinoma: is lobectomy enough? Arch Otolaryngol Head Neck Surg. 2010;136(11): 1055-61.
65. Nixon IJ, Ganly I, Patel SG, Palmer FL, Whitcher MM, Tuttle RM, et al. Thyroid lobectomy for treatment of well differentiated intrathyroid malignancy. Surgery. 2012; 151(4):571-9.
66. Adam MA, Pura J, Gu L, Dinan MA, Tyler DS, Reed SD, et al. Extent of surgery for papillary thyroid cancer is not associated with survival: an analysis of 61,775 patients. Ann Surg. 2014;260(4):601-5.
67. Murthy SP, Balasubramanian D, Subramaniam N, Nair G, Babu MJ, Rathod PV, et al. Prevalence of adverse pathological features in 1 to 4 cm low-risk differentiated thyroid carcinoma. Head Neck. 2018;40(6):1214-8.
68. Kluijfhout WP, Pasternak JD, Lim J, Kwon JS, Vriens MR, Clark OH, Shen WT, et al. Frequency of high-risk characteristics requiring total thyroidectomy for 1–4 cm well-differentiated thyroid cancer. Thyroid. 2016;26(6):820-4.
69. Delbridge L. Total thyroidectomy: the evolution of surgical technique. ANZ J Surg. 2003;73(9):761-8.
70. Kochilas X, Bibas A, Xenellis J, Anagnostopoulou S. Surgical anatomy of the external branch of the superior laryngeal nerve and its clinical significance in head and neck surgery. Clin Anatom: Off J Am Assoc Clin Anatom Br Assoc Clin Anatom. 2008;21(2):99-105.
71. Cernea CR, Ferraz AR, Nishio S, Dutra Jr A, Hojaij FC, Dos Santos LR. Surgical anatomy of the external branch of the superior laryngeal nerve. Head Neck. 1992;14(5):380-3.
72. Friedman M, LoSavio P, Ibrahim H. Superior laryngeal nerve identification and preservation in thyroidectomy. Arch Otolaryngol Head Neck Surg. 2002;128(3):296-303.
73. Fundakowski CE, Hales NW, Agrawal N, Barczyński M, Camacho PM, Hartl DM, et al. Surgical management of the recurrent laryngeal nerve in thyroidectomy: American Head and Neck Society Consensus Statement. Head Neck. 2018;40(4):663-75.
74. Raffaelli M, Iacobone M, Henry JF. The "false" nonrecurrent inferior laryngeal nerve. Surgery. 2000;128(6):1082-7.
75. Stewart GR, Mountain JC, Colcock BP. Non-recurrent laryngeal nerve. Br J Surg. 1972;59(5):379-81.
76. Phitayakorn R, McHenry CR. Incidence and location of ectopic abnormal parathyroid glands. Am J Surg. 2006;191(3): 418-23.
77. Randolph GW, Kamani D. Intraoperative neural monitoring in thyroid cancer surgery. Langenbeck's Arch Surg. 2014; 399(2):199-207.
78. Pisanu A, Porceddu G, Podda M, Cois A, Uccheddu A. Systematic review with meta-analysis of studies comparing intraoperative neuromonitoring of recurrent laryngeal nerves versus visualization alone during thyroidectomy. J Surg Res. 2014;188(1):152-61.
79. Poveda MC, Dionigi G, Sitges-Serra A, Barczynski M, Angelos P, Dralle H, et al. Intraoperative monitoring of the recurrent laryngeal nerve during thyroidectomy: a standardized approach (part 2). World J Endocr Surg. 2012;4(1):33-40.
80. Randolph GW, Kobler JB, Wilkins J. Recurrent laryngeal nerve identification and assessment during thyroid surgery: laryngeal palpation. World J Surg. 2004;28(8):755-60.
81. Scharpf J, Randolph G. Intraoperative Nerve Monitoring for Parathyroid Surgery. In Medical and Surgical Treatment of Parathyroid Diseases. Cham: Springer; 2017. pp. 459-68.
82. Ikeda Y, Takami H, Sasaki Y, Kan S, Niimi M. Endoscopic neck surgery by the axillary approach. J Am Coll Surg. 2000;191(3):336-40.
83. Luginbuhl A, Schwartz DM, Sestokas AK, Cognetti D, Pribitkin E. Detection of evolving injury to the brachial plexus during transaxillary robotic thyroidectomy. Laryngoscope. 2012;122(1):110-5.
84. Bhatia P, Mohamed HE, Kadi A, Kandil E, Walvekar RR. Remote access thyroid surgery. Gland Surg. 2015;4(5):376-87.
85. Terris DJ, Singer MC. Robotic facelift thyroidectomy: facilitating remote access surgery. Head Neck. 2012;34(5): 746-7.
86. Witzel K, Von Rahden BH, Kaminski C, Stein HJ. Transoral access for endoscopic thyroid resection. Surg Endoscopy. 2008;22(8):1871-5.
87. Anuwong A. Transoral endoscopic thyroidectomy vestibular approach: a series of the first 60 human cases. World J Surg. 2016;40(3):491-7.
88. Dionigi G, Bacuzzi A, Lavazza M, Inversini D, Pappalardo V, Boni L, et al. Transoral endoscopic thyroidectomy via vestibular approach: operative steps and video. Gland Surg. 2016;5(6):625-7.
89. Berber E, Bernet V, Fahey III TJ, Kebebew E, Shaha A, Stack Jr BC, et al. American Thyroid Association statement on remote-access thyroid surgery. Thyroid. 2016;26(3): 331-7.
90. Liu SY, Ng EK. Robotic versus open thyroidectomy for differentiated thyroid cancer: an evidence-based review. Int J Endocrinol. 2016;2016.
91. Wang YC, Liu K, Xiong JJ, Zhu JQ. Robotic thyroidectomy versus conventional open thyroidectomy for differentiated thyroid cancer: meta-analysis. J Laryngol Otol. 2015;129(6): 558-67.
92. Lang BH, Wong CK, Tsang JS, Wong KP, Wan KY. A systematic review and meta-analysis evaluating completeness and outcomes of robotic thyroidectomy. Laryngoscope. 2015; 125(2):509-18.
93. Lee S, Kim HY, Lee CR, Park S, Son H, Kang SW, et al. A prospective comparison of patient body image after robotic thyroidectomy and conventional open thyroidectomy in patients with papillary thyroid carcinoma. Surgery. 2014; 156(1):117-25.

94. Tae K, Song CM, Ji YB, Kim KR, Kim JY, Choi YY. Comparison of surgical completeness between robotic total thyroidectomy versus open thyroidectomy. Laryngoscope. 2014;124(4): 1042-7.
95. Maksimovic S, Jakovljevic B, Gojkovic Z. Lymph node metastases papillary thyroid carcinoma and their importance in recurrence of disease. Med Arch. 2018;72(2):108-11.
96. Wang TS, Cheung K, Farrokhyar F, Roman SA, Sosa JA. A meta-analysis of the effect of prophylactic central compartment neck dissection on locoregional recurrence rates in patients with papillary thyroid cancer. Ann Surg Oncol. 2013;20(11):3477-83.
97. Pai SI, Tufano RP. Central compartment neck dissection for thyroid cancer. ORL. 2008;70(5):292-7.
98. Robinson TJ, Thomas S, Dinan MA, Roman S, Sosa JA, Hyslop T. How many lymph nodes are enough? Assessing the adequacy of lymph node yield for papillary thyroid cancer. J Clin Oncol. 2016;34(28):3434-9.
99. Luster M, Clarke SE, Dietlein M, Lassmann M, Lind P, Oyen WJ, et al. Guidelines for radioiodine therapy of differentiated thyroid cancer. Eur J Nucl Med Mol Imaging. 2008;35(10): 1941-59.
100. Rivkees SA, Mazzaferri EL, Verburg FA, Reiners C, Luster M, Breuer CK, et al. The treatment of differentiated thyroid cancer in children: emphasis on surgical approach and radioactive iodine therapy. Endocr Rev. 2011;32(6):798-826.
101. Tomoda C, Uruno T, Takamura Y, Ito Y, Miya Y, Kobayashi K, et al. Reevaluation of stringent low iodine diet in outpatient preparation for radioiodine examination and therapy. Endocr J. 2005;52(2):237-40.
102. Amdur RJ, Mazzaferri EL. Intravenous iodinated contrast effects iodine uptake for months. In: Amdur RJ, Mazzaferri EL, Kirwan J (Eds). Essentials of Thyroid Cancer Management. Boston, MA: Springer; 2005. pp. 211-3.
103. Amdur RJ, Mazzaferri EL. Using Lithium Carbonate to Increase the Effectiveness of I-131. In: Amdur RJ, Mazzaferri EL, Kirwan J (Eds). Essentials of Thyroid Cancer Management. Boston, MA: Springer; 2005. pp. 221-7.
104. Schlumberger M, Catargi B, Borget I, Deandreis D, Zerdoud S, Bridji B, et al. Strategies of radioiodine ablation in patients with low-risk thyroid cancer. N Engl J Med. 2012;366(18): 1663-73.
105. Mallick U, Harmer C, Yap B, Wadsley J, Clarke S, Moss L, et al. Ablation with low-dose radioiodine and thyrotropin alfa in thyroid cancer. N Engl J Med. 2012;366(18):1674-85.
106. Borget I, Bonastre J, Catargi B, Déandréis D, Zerdoud S, Rusu D, et al. Quality of life and cost-effectiveness assessment of radioiodine ablation strategies in patients with thyroid cancer: results from the randomized phase III ESTIMABL trial. J Clin Oncol. 2015;33(26):2885-92.
107. Park HM, Gerard SK. Stunning: untoward effect of 131 I thyroid imaging prior to radioablation therapy. In: Park HM, Gerard SK (Eds). Thyroid Cancer. Totowa, NJ: Humana Press; 2006. pp. 337-45.
108. Amdur RJ, Mazzaferri EL. Essentials of thyroid cancer management. New York: Springer; 2005.
109. Bal C, Padhy AK, Jana S, Pant GS, Basu AK. Prospective randomized clinical trial to evaluate the optimal dose of 131I for remnant ablation in patients with differentiated thyroid carcinoma. Cancer: Interdisciplinary Int J Am Cancer Soc. 1996;77(12):2574-80.
110. Bal CS, Kumar A, Pant GS. Radioiodine dose for remnant ablation in differentiated thyroid carcinoma: a randomized clinical trial in 509 patients. J Clin Endocrinol Metabol. 2004;89(4):1666-73.
111. Hay ID, Bergstralh EJ, Grant CS, McIver B, Thompson GB, Van Heerden JA, et al. Impact of primary surgery on outcome in 300 patients with pathologic tumor-node-metastasis stage III papillary thyroid carcinoma treated at one institution from 1940 through 1989. Surgery. 1999;126(6):1173-82.
112. Wang LY, Ganly I. Nodal metastases in thyroid cancer: prognostic implications and management. Future Oncol. 2016;12(7):981-94.
113. Zhu G, Deng Y, Pan L, Ouyang W, Feng H, Wu J, et al. Clinical significance of the BRAFV600E mutation in PTC and its effect on radioiodine therapy. Endocrine connections. 2019;8(6): 754-63.
114. Vini L, Hyer S, Al-Saadi A, Pratt B, Harmer C. Prognosis for fertility and ovarian function after treatment with radioiodine for thyroid cancer. Postgrad Med J. 2002;78(916):92-3.
115. Ceccarelli C, Canale D, Vitti P. Radioactive iodine (131I) effects on male fertility. Curr Opin Urol. 2008;18(6):598-601.
116. Avram AM, Esfandiari NH, Wong KK. Preablation 131-I scans with SPECT/CT contribute to thyroid cancer risk stratification and 131-I therapy planning. J Clin Endocrinol Metabol. 2015;100(5):1895-902.
117. Spencer CA, Fatemi S. Thyroglobulin. In: Mazzaferr EL, Harmer C, Mallick UK, Kendall-Taylor P (Eds). Practical Management of Thyroid Cancer. London: Springer; 2006. pp. 211-28.
118. Lubitz CC, Kong CY, McMahon PM, Daniels GH, Chen Y, Economopoulos KP, et al. Annual financial impact of well-differentiated thyroid cancer care in the United States. Cancer. 2014;120(9):1345-52.
119. Tuttle RM, Tala H, Shah J, Leboeuf R, Ghossein R, Gonen M, det al. Estimating risk of recurrence in differentiated thyroid cancer after total thyroidectomy and radioactive iodine remnant ablation: using response to therapy variables to modify the initial risk estimates predicted by the new American Thyroid Association staging system. Thyroid. 2010; 20(12):1341-9.
120. Hundahl SA, Fleming ID, Fremgen AM, Menck HR. A National Cancer Data Base report on 53,856 cases of thyroid carcinoma treated in the US, 1985-1995. Cancer: Interdiscipl Int J Am Cancer Soc. 1998;83(12):2638-48.
121. Castagna MG, Maino F, Cipri C, Belardini V, Theodoropoulou A, Cevenini G, et al. Delayed risk stratification, to include the response to initial treatment (surgery and radioiodine ablation), has better outcome predictivity in differentiated thyroid cancer patients. Eur J Endocrinol. 2011;165(3):441-6.
122. Krajewska J, Chmielik E, Jarząb B. Dynamic risk stratification in the follow-up of thyroid cancer: what is still to be discovered in 2017. Endocr Cancer. 2017;24(11):R387-402.
123. Momesso DP, Vaisman F, Yang SP, Bulzico DA, Corbo R, Vaisman M, et al. Dynamic risk stratification in patients with differentiated thyroid cancer treated without radioactive iodine. J Clin Endocrinol Metabol. 2016;101(7):2692-700.
124. Spencer CA. Assay of thyroid hormones and related substances. In: Spencer CA (Ed). Endotext [Internet]. MDText.com, Inc; 2017.
125. National Comprehensive Cancer Network. (2020). NCCN Clinical Practice Guidelines in Oncology (NCCN GuidelinesVR) thyroid carcinoma 1.2020. National Comprehensive Cancer Network, Inc.; 2020. [online] Available from NCCN.org. [Last accessed July, 2020].

126. Schlumberger M, Hitzel A, Toubert ME, Corone C, Troalen F, Schlageter MH, et al. Comparison of seven serum thyroglobulin assays in the follow-up of papillary and follicular thyroid cancer patients. J Clin Endocrinol Metabol. 2007; 92(7):2487-95.
127. Giovanella L, Treglia G, Sadeghi R, Trimboli P, Ceriani L, Verburg FA. Unstimulated highly sensitive thyroglobulin in follow-up of differentiated thyroid cancer patients: a meta-analysis. J Clin Endocrinol Metabol. 2014;99(2):440-7.
128. Tufano RP, Clayman G, Heller KS, Inabnet WB, Kebebew E, Shaha A, et al. Management of recurrent/persistent nodal disease in patients with differentiated thyroid cancer: a critical review of the risks and benefits of surgical intervention versus active surveillance. Thyroid. 2015;25(1):15-27.
129. Shaha AR. Revision thyroid surgery–technical considerations. Otolaryngol Clin North Am. 2008;41(6):1169-83.
130. Shindo ML, Caruana SM, Kandil E, McCaffrey JC, Orloff LA, Porterfield JR, et al. Management of invasive well-differentiated thyroid cancer: an American head and neck society consensus statement: AHNS consensus statement. Head Neck. 2014; 36(10):1379-90.
131. Urken ML. Prognosis and management of invasive well-differentiated thyroid cancer. Otolaryngol Clin North Am. 2010;43(2):301-28.
132. Arora N, Turbendian HK, Scognamiglio T, Wagner PL, Goldsmith SJ, Zarnegar R, et al. Extrathyroidal extension is not all equal: implications of macroscopic versus microscopic extent in papillary thyroid carcinoma. Surgery. 2008; 144(6):942-8.
133. Dralle H, Brauckhoff M, Machens A, Gimm O. Surgical management of advanced thyroid cancer invading the aerodigestive tract. In: Clark O, Duh QY, Kebebew E (Eds). Textbook of Endocrine Surgery, 2nd edition. United States: WB Saunders; 2005. pp. 318-33.
134. Shin DH, Mark EJ, Suen HC, Grillo HC. Pathologic staging of papillary carcinoma of the thyroid with airway invasion based on the anatomic manner of extension to the trachea: a clinicopathologic study based on 22 patients who underwent thyroidectomy and airway resection. Hum Pathol. 1993;24(8):866-70.
135. Price DL, Wong RJ, Randolph GW. Invasive thyroid cancer: management of the trachea and esophagus. Otolaryngol Clin North Am. 2008;41(6):1155-68.
136. McCaffrey TV, Bergstralh EJ, Hay ID. Locally invasive papillary thyroid carcinoma: 1940–1990. Head Neck. 1994; 16(2):165-72.
137. Alexander EK, Pearce EN, Brent GA, Brown RS, Chen H, Dosiou C, et al. 2017 Guidelines of the American Thyroid Association for the diagnosis and management of thyroid disease during pregnancy and the postpartum. Thyroid. 2017;27(3):315-89.
138. Patel SG, Escrig M, Shaha AR, Singh B, Shah JP. Management of well-differentiated thyroid carcinoma presenting within a thyroglossal duct cyst. J Surg Oncol. 2002;79(3):134-9.
139. Máximo V, Sobrinho-Simões M. Hürthle cell tumours of the thyroid. A review with emphasis on mitochondrial abnormalities with clinical relevance. Virchows Arch. 2000; 437(2):107-15.
140. Sippel RS, Elaraj DM, Khanafshar E, Zarnegar R, Kebebew E, Duh QY, et al. Tumor size predicts malignant potential in Hürthle cell neoplasms of the thyroid. World J Surg. 2008; 32(5):702-7.
141. Ahmadi S, Stang M. Hürthle cell carcinoma: current perspectives. Onco Targets Ther. 2016;9:6873-84.
142. Goffredo P, Roman SA, Sosa JA. Hurthle cell carcinoma: a population-level analysis of 3311 patients. Cancer. 2013; 119(3):504-11.
143. Ganly I, Ricarte Filho J, Eng S, Ghossein R, Morris LG, Liang Y, et al. Genomic dissection of Hurthle cell carcinoma reveals a unique class of thyroid malignancy. J Clin Endocrinol Metabol. 2013;98(5):E962-72.
144. Zavitsanos P, Amdur RJ, Drew PA, Cusi K, Werning JW, Morris CG. Favorable outcome of Hurthle cell carcinoma of the thyroid treated with total thyroidectomy, radioiodine, and selective use of external-beam radiotherapy. Am J Clin Oncol. 2017;40(4):433-7.
145. Nikiforov YE. Radiation-induced thyroid cancer: what we have learned from Chernobyl. Endocr Pathol. 2006;17(4): 307-18.
146. Ito Y, Uruno T, Nakano K, Takamura Y, Miya A, Kobayashi K, Yokozawa T, et al. An observation trial without surgical treatment in patients with papillary microcarcinoma of the thyroid. Thyroid. 2003;13(4):381-7.
147. Sugitani I, Toda K, Yamada K, Yamamoto N, Ikenaga M, Fujimoto Y. Three distinctly different kinds of papillary thyroid microcarcinoma should be recognized: our treatment strategies and outcomes. World J Surg. 2010;34(6):1222-31.
148. Hogan AR, Zhuge Y, Perez EA, Koniaris LG, Lew JI, Sola JE. Pediatric thyroid carcinoma: incidence and outcomes in 1753 patients. J Surg Res. 2009;156(1):167-72.
149. Sipos JA, Mazzaferri EL. Thyroid cancer epidemiology and prognostic variables. Clin Oncol. 2010;22(6):395-404.
150. Francis GL, Waguespack SG, Bauer AJ, Angelos P, Benvenga S, Cerutti JM, et al. Management guidelines for children with thyroid nodules and differentiated thyroid cancer: the American Thyroid Association guidelines task force on pediatric thyroid cancer. Thyroid. 2015;25(7):716-59.
151. Norlén O, Charlton A, Sarkis LM, Henwood T, Shun A, Gill AJ, et al. Risk of malignancy for each Bethesda class in pediatric thyroid nodules. J Pediatr Surg. 2015;50(7):1147-9.
152. Fahrner R, Übersax L, Mettler A, Berger SM, Seiler CA. Paediatric thyroid surgery is safe-experiences at a tertiary surgical centre. Swiss Med Weekly. 2014;144:w13939.
153. Sosa JA, Tuggle CT, Wang TS, Thomas DC, Boudourakis L, Rivkees S, et al. Clinical and economic outcomes of thyroid and parathyroid surgery in children. J Clin Endocrinol Metabol. 2008;93(8):3058-65.
154. Nishida T, Katayama SI, Tsujimoto M, Nakamura JI, Matsuda H. Clinicopathological significance of poorly differentiated thyroid carcinoma. Am J Surg Pathol. 1999;23(2):205-11.
155. Bongiovanni M, Faquin WC. Poorly differentiated thyroid carcinoma. In: Ali S, Cibas E (Eds). The Bethesda System For Reporting Thyroid Cytopathology. Springer, Boston, MA: Springer; 2010. pp. 129-38.
156. Thiagarajan S, Yousuf A, Shetty R, Dhar H, Mathur Y, Nair D, et al. Poorly differentiated thyroid carcinoma (PDTC) characteristics and the efficacy of radioactive iodine (RAI) therapy as an adjuvant treatment in a tertiary cancer care center. Eur Arch Otorhinolaryngol. 2020;277:1807-14 .
157. Biermann M, Pixberg MK, Riemann B, Schuck A, Heinecke A, Schmid KW, et al. Clinical outcomes of adjuvant external-beam radiotherapy for differentiated thyroid cancer. Nuklearmedizin. 2009;48(3):89-98.
158. Kiess AP, Agrawal N, Brierley JD, Duvvuri U, Ferris RL, Genden E, et al. External-beam radiotherapy for differentiated thyroid cancer locoregional control: A statement of the American Head and Neck Society. Head Neck. 2016;38(4): 493-8.

159. Chow SM, Yau S, Kwan CK, Poon PC, Law SC. Local and regional control in patients with papillary thyroid carcinoma: specific indications of external radiotherapy and radioactive iodine according to T and N categories in AJCC 6th edition. Endocr Cancer. 2006;13(4):1159-72.
160. Schwartz DL, Lobo MJ, Ang KK, Morrison WH, Rosenthal DI, Ahamad A, et al. Postoperative external beam radiotherapy for differentiated thyroid cancer: outcomes and morbidity with conformal treatment. Int J Radiat Oncol Biol Phys. 2009;74(4):1083-91.
161. Basu S, Dandekar M, Joshi A, D'Cruz A. Defining a rational step-care algorithm for managing thyroid carcinoma patients with elevated thyroglobulin and negative on radioiodine scintigraphy (TENIS): considerations and challenges towards developing an appropriate roadmap. Eur J Nucl Med Mol Imag. 2015;42:1167-71.
162. Silberstein EB. The problem of the patient with thyroglobulin elevation but negative iodine scintigraphy: the TENIS syndrome. Semin Nucl Med. 2011;41(2):113-20
163. Altenvoerde G, Lerch H, Kuwert T, Matheja P, Schäfers M, Schober O. Positron emission tomography with F-18-deoxy-glucose in patients with differentiated thyroid carcinoma, elevated thyroglobulin levels, and negative iodine scans. Langenbeck's Arch Surg. 1998;383(2):160-3.
164. Wan Q, Bai L, Zhao G, Zhang Y, Ma Q, Wang R, et al. Diagnostic performance of 18F-FDG-PET/CT in DTC patients with thyroglobulin elevation and negative iodine scintigraphy: a meta-analysis. Eur J Endocrinol. 2019;181(2)(ahead of publishing).
165. Vural GU, Akkas BE, Ercakmak N, Basu S, Alavi A. Prognostic significance of FDG PET/CT on the follow-up of patients of differentiated thyroid carcinoma with negative 131I whole-body scan and elevated thyroglobulin levels: correlation with clinical and histopathologic characteristics and long-term follow-up data. Clin Nucl Med. 2012;37(10):953-9.
166. Coelho SM, Vaisman M, Carvalho DP. Tumour re-differentiation effect of retinoic acid: a novel therapeutic approach for advanced thyroid cancer. Curr Pharm Des. 2005;11(19):2525-31.
167. Kebebew E, Peng M, Reiff E, Treseler P, Woeber KA, Clark OH, et al. A phase II trial of rosiglitazone in patients with thyroglobulin-positive and radioiodine-negative differentiated thyroid cancer. Surgery. 2006;140(6):960-7.
168. Haugen BR. Redifferentiation therapy in advanced thyroid cancer. Curr Drug Targets-Immune, Endocr Metabol Dis. 2004;4(3):175-80.
169. Cabanillas ME, Waguespack SG, Bronstein Y, Williams MD, Feng L, Hernandez M, et al. Treatment with tyrosine kinase inhibitors for patients with differentiated thyroid cancer: the MD Anderson experience. J Clin Endocrinol Metabol. 2010;95(6):2588-95.
170. Brose MS, Nutting CM, Jarzab B, Elisei R, Siena S, Bastholt L, et al. Sorafenib in radioactive iodine-refractory, locally advanced or metastatic differentiated thyroid cancer: a randomised, double-blind, phase 3 trial. Lancet. 2014; 384(9940):319-28.
171. Schlumberger M, Tahara M, Wirth LJ, Robinson B, Brose MS, Elisei R, et al. Lenvatinib versus placebo in radioiodine-refractory thyroid cancer. N Engl J Med. 2015;372(7):621-30.
172. Teunissen JJ, Kwekkeboom DJ, Krenning EP. Staging and treatment of differentiated thyroid carcinoma with radio-labeled somatostatin analogs. Trends Endocrinol Metabol. 2006;17(1):19-25.
173. Jois B, Asopa R, Basu S. Somatostatin Receptor Imaging in Non-131I-Avid Metastatic Differentiated Thyroid Carcinoma for Determining the Feasibility of Peptide Receptor Radionuclide Therapy With 177Lu-DOTATATE: Low Fraction of Patients Suitable for Peptide Receptor Radionuclide Therapy and Evidence of Chromogranin A Level-Positive Neuroendocrine Differentiation. Clin Nucl Med. 2014; 39(6):505-10.
174. Wells Jr SA, Asa SL, Dralle H, Elisei R, Evans DB, Gagel RF, et al. Revised American Thyroid Association guidelines for the management of medullary thyroid carcinoma: the American Thyroid Association Guidelines Task Force on medullary thyroid carcinoma. Thyroid. 2015;25(6): 567-610.
175. Roman S, Lin R, Sosa JA. Prognosis of medullary thyroid carcinoma: demographic, clinical, and pathologic predictors of survival in 1252 cases. Cancer: Interdiscipl Int J Am Cancer Soc. 2006;107(9):2134-42.
176. Williams ED, Brown CL, Doniach I. Pathological and clinical findings in a series of 67 cases of medullary carcinoma of the thyroid. J Clin Pathol. 1966;19(2):103-13.
177. Donis-Keller H, Dou S, Chi D, Carlson KM, Toshima K, Lairmore TC, et al. Mutations in the RET proto-oncogene are associated with MEN 2A and FMTC. Hum Mol Genet. 1993;2(7):851-6.
178. Hijazi YM, Nieman LK, Medeiros LJ. Medullary carcinoma of the thyroid as a cause of Cushing's syndrome: a case with ectopic adrenocorticotropin secretion characterized by double enzyme immunostaining. Hum Pathol. 1992;23(5): 592-6.
179. Quayle FJ, Moley JF. Medullary thyroid carcinoma: including MEN2A and MEN2B syndromes. J Surg Oncol. 2005;89(3): 122-9.
180. Moura MM, Cavaco BM, Leite V. RAS proto-oncogene in medullary thyroid carcinoma. Endocr Relat Cancer. 2015; 22(5):R235-52.
181. Mehdi G, Maheshwari V, Ansari HA, Sadaf L, Khan MA. FNAC diagnosis of medullary carcinoma thyroid: a report of three cases with review of literature. J Cytol/Indian Acad Cytol. 2010;27(2):66-8.
182. Hennessy JF, Gray TK, Cooper CW, Ontjes DA. Stimulation of thyrocalcitonin secretion by pentagastrin and calcium in two patients with medullary carcinoma of the thyroid. J Clin Endocrinol Metabol. 1973;36(1):200-3.
183. Vieira AE, Mello MP, Elias LL, Lau IF, Maciel LM, Moreira AC, et al. Molecular and biochemical screening for the diagnosis and management of medullary thyroid carcinoma in multiple endocrine neoplasia type 2A. Horm Metabol Res. 2002;34(04):202-6.
184. Costante G, Lalami Y, Jungels C, Awada A. Calcitonin and Carcinoembryonic Antigen for the Diagnosis and Management of Medullary Thyroid Carcinoma. In: Giovanella L (Ed). Atlas of Thyroid and Neuroendocrine Tumor Markers. Cham: Springer; 2018. pp. 133-50.
185. Kushchayev SV, Kushchayeva YS, Tella SH, Glushko T, Pacak K, Teytelboym OM. Medullary thyroid carcinoma: an update on imaging. J Thyroid Res. 2019;2019.
186. Haddad RI, Nasr C, Bischoff L, Busaidy NL, Byrd D, Callender G, et al. NCCN guidelines insights: thyroid carcinoma, version 2.2018. J Nat Comp Cancer Network. 2018;16(12):1429-40.
187. Kebebew E, Ituarte PH, Siperstein AE, Duh QY, Clark OH. Medullary thyroid carcinoma: clinical characteristics,

treatment, prognostic factors, and a comparison of staging systems. Cancer: Interdiscipl Int J Am Cancer Soc. 2000;88(5): 1139-48.

188. Terezakis SA, Lee NY. The role of radiation therapy in the treatment of medullary thyroid cancer. J Nat Comp Cancer Net. 2010;8(5):532-41.
189. Kebebew E, Kikuchi S, Duh QY, Clark OH. Long-term results of reoperation and localizing studies in patients with persistent or recurrent medullary thyroid cancer. Arch Surg. 2000;135(8):895-901.
190. Cabanillas ME, Hu MI, Jimenez C. Medullary thyroid cancer in the era of tyrosine kinase inhibitors: to treat or not to treat—and with which drug—those are the questions. J Clin Endocrinol Metabol. 2014;99(12):4390-6.
191. Wells Jr SA, Robinson BG, Gagel RF, Dralle H, Fagin JA, Santoro M, et al. Vandetanib in patients with locally advanced or metastatic medullary thyroid cancer: a randomized, double-blind phase III trial. J Clin Oncol. 2012; 30(2):134-41.
192. Schoffski P, Elisei R, Mueller S, Brose MS, Shah MH, Licitra LF, et al. An international, double-blind, randomized, placebo-controlled phase III trial (EXAM) of cabozantinib (XL184) in medullary thyroid carcinoma (MTC) patients (pts) with documented RECIST progression at baseline. J Clin Oncol. 2012;30(Suppl 15):5508.
193. Bodei L, Cremonesi M, Grana C, Rocca P, Bartolomei M, Chinol M, et al. Receptor radionuclide therapy with 90 Y-[DOTA] 0-Tyr 3-octreotide (90 Y-DOTATOC) in neuroendocrine tumours. Eur J Nucl Med Mol Imaging. 2004; 31(7):1038-46.
194. Bodei L, Handkiewicz-Junak D, Grana C, Mazzetta C, Rocca P, Bartolomei M, et al. Receptor radionuclide therapy with 90Y-DOTATOC in patients with medullary thyroid carcinomas. Cancer Biother Radiopharm. 2004;19(1):65-71.
195. Are C, Shaha AR. Anaplastic thyroid carcinoma: biology, pathogenesis, prognostic factors, and treatment approaches. Ann Surg Oncol. 2006;13(4):453-64.
196. Davies L, Welch HG. Increasing incidence of thyroid cancer in the United States, 1973-2002. JAMA. 2006;295(18):2164-7.
197. Bonhomme B, Godbert Y, Perot G, Al Ghuzlan A, Bardet S, Belleannée G, et al. Molecular pathology of anaplastic thyroid carcinomas: a retrospective study of 144 cases. Thyroid. 2017; 27(5):682-92.
198. Chintakuntlawar AV, Rumilla KM, Smith CY, Jenkins SM, Foote RL, Kasperbauer JL, et al. Expression of PD-1 and PD-L1 in anaplastic thyroid cancer patients treated with multimodal therapy: results from a retrospective study. J Clin Endocrinol Metabol. 2017;102(6):1943-50.
199. Besic N, Gazic B. Sites of metastases of anaplastic thyroid carcinoma: autopsy findings in 45 cases from a single institution. Thyroid. 2013;23(6):709-13.
200. Deeken-Draisey A, Yang GY, Gao J, Alexiev BA. Anaplastic thyroid carcinoma: an epidemiologic, histologic, immunohistochemical, and molecular single-institution study. Hum Pathol. 2018;82:140-8.
201. Sugitani I, Miyauchi A, Sugino K, Okamoto T, Yoshida A, Suzuki S. Prognostic factors and treatment outcomes for anaplastic thyroid carcinoma: ATC Research Consortium of Japan cohort study of 677 patients. World J Surg. 2012; 36(6):1247-54.
202. Lowe NM, Loughran S, Slevin NJ, Yap BK. Anaplastic thyroid cancer: the addition of systemic chemotherapy to radiotherapy led to an observed improvement in survival—a single centre experience and review of the literature. Sci World J. 2014;2014.
203. Higashiyama T, Ito Y, Hirokawa M, Fukushima M, Uruno T, Miya A, et al. Induction chemotherapy with weekly paclitaxel administration for anaplastic thyroid carcinoma. Thyroid. 2010;20(1):7-14.
204. Ain KB, Egorin MJ, DeSimone PA, Collaborative Anaplastic Thyroid Cancer Health Intervention Trials (CATCHIT) Group. Treatment of anaplastic thyroid carcinoma with paclitaxel: phase 2 trial using ninety-six-hour infusion. Thyroid. 2000; 10(7):587-94.
205. Subbiah V, Kreitman RJ, Wainberg ZA, Cho JY, Schellens JH, Soria JC, et al. Dabrafenib and trametinib treatment in patients with locally advanced or metastatic BRAF V600-mutant anaplastic thyroid cancer. J Clin Oncol. 2018;36(1):7.

CHAPTER 24

Disorders of the Parathyroid Gland

Samskruthi P Murthy, Sivakumar Vidhyadharan, Narayana Subramaniam

INTRODUCTION

Abnormalities in parathyroid hormone secretion are common. With the advent of advanced laboratory technology, improved imaging modalities, and better operative techniques, management of parathyroid hormone disorders are more efficient with better cure rates in the recent years. The following chapter describes the management of hyperparathyroidism, hypoparathyroidism, ad parathyroid carcinoma (PC).

CALCIUM HOMEOSTASIS

Calcium homeostasis is critical as various processes in the body are dependent on calcium for normal functioning including contraction of the heart and other muscles, conduction of nerve impulses, clotting of blood, secretion from glandular tissues and intracellular signals. The level of calcium is maintained by a complex interplay between dietary intake, intestinal absorption, skeletal remodeling, and urinary excretion.[1] Parathyroid hormone plays an essential role in monitoring and maintaining extracellular calcium in a precise range.

The level of normal calcium is 8.8–10.5 mg/dL.[2] 50–60% of calcium is bound to a protein-like albumin in the serum. The physiologic property is dependent on the ionized form (free) of calcium. Corrected calcium takes into account the level of albumin. Corrected calcium can be calculated by the formula derived 40 years ago, where corrected calcium in mmol/L = total calcium mmol/L + 0.02 (40-albumin g/L).[3]

Parathyroid hormone (PTH) is secreted by the parathyroid gland. PTH is an 84 amino acid peptide with a plasma half-life of 2–4 minutes.[4] The parathyroid chief cells express the calcium-sensing receptor on the surface of the cell, which continuously monitor extracellular calcium. Drop in calcium level is sensed by the calcium-sensing receptor and triggers a series of intracellular signals and release PTH.[4]

Calcitriol 1,25 dihydroxy vitamin D [1,25-(OH)2D] plays a crucial role in maintaining calcium homeostasis. Cholecalciferol (vitamin D_3) is synthesized in the skin on exposure to ultraviolet (UV) light. It is also supplied by dietary sources. The vitamin D_3 is hydroxylated in the liver to 25-(OH)D. Calcitriol is produced in the kidney by hydroxylation.[4]

Despite variations in the maintenance of calcium homeostasis, the level of ionized calcium is tightly regulated in the normal range (<0.1 mg/dL deviation).[5] PTH increases calcium by bone resorption, which is mediated by interaction with osteoclast to release calcium. Bone remodeling releases and consumes 500 mg of calcium a day and acts as a reservoir of calcium and maintain calcium homeostasis at the expense of bone density.[6] PTH also enhances calcium reabsorption at the distal nephron of the kidney. When the calcium intake increases, there is decreased calcium absorption and increased calcium excretion.

A range of other disorders can also cause hypercalcemia by varied mechanisms. Malignancy-associated hypercalcemia, osteolytic hypercalcemia, sarcoidosis, tuberculosis, endocrinopathies, thiazides, and prolonged immobilization are few causes of nonparathyroid-related hypercalcemia.

HYPERPARATHYROIDISM

Hyperparathyroidism is the increased secretion of PTH by intrinsic abnormalities of the gland (primary/tertiary) or by external stimulus increasing PTH production (secondary).[7] The incidence of primary hyperparathyroidism (pHPT) is approximately 4 per 100,000 people per year.[8] pHPT is one of the most common causes for hypercalcemia and is caused by solitary parathyroid adenoma in 80–85% of cases. PC is exceedingly rare and comprises less than 0.5–5% of cases.[9-11] Secondary hyperparathyroidism occurs when the calcium concentrations decrease, which in turn stimulate secretion of PTH; in these cases, hypercalcemia may not be present. However, some cases do progress to hypercalcemia at later stages. These patients may develop multigland disease (MGD) due to prolonged stimulation, which leads to tertiary hyperparathyroidism.[7] Tertiary hyperparathyroidism is commonly encountered in end-stage renal disease. Lithium therapy stimulates the calcium-sensing receptor and hence increases PTH secretion.

Epidemiology

The prevalence of pHPT is varied in the literature due to criteria used to define pHPT. The prevalence of pHPT has significantly increased from 1970 with the advent of automated calcium testing. More patients with subclinical diseases are being diagnosed, unlike earlier days, when significant target organ manifestations were the presenting features. The estimated prevalence of pHPT is 0.86% in the general population and women, especially in the postmenopausal age group have a higher incidence.[12] Women are affected 2–3 times more often than men.

Pathogenesis

Radiation exposure induces pHPT. The prevalence is directly proportional to radiation dose and also radiation exposure at a younger age group.[7] The incidence of parathyroid tumor was higher in Hiroshima and Chernobyl disaster areas. Even therapeutic external radiation also predisposes to pHPT. The incidence of MGD is similar to the general population; however, they have a higher risk of recurrent disease.

Lithium associated pHPT occurs in 15% of chronic lithium users (>10 years of usage).[7] MGD is reported to be as high as 83.

Signs and Symptoms

Mild hypercalcemia of <11 mg/dL rarely present with any symptoms. Polyuria and dyspepsia are seen in a few cases. Symptoms of hypercalcemia commonly occur with calcium levels >11 mg/dL. At this stage patient may experience fatigue, mild cognitive impairment, and mild neuromuscular symptoms such as muscle weakness. Severe hypercalcemia >13 mg/dL can lead to abdominal pain, vomiting, lethargy, obtundation and even coma. Prolonged hypercalcemia can cause nephrolithiasis, nephrocalcinosis, chondrocalcinosis, and band keratopathy.[7] QT interval is shortened in moderate to severe hypercalcemia.[13] Increased bone resorption, which is out of proportion of osteoclastic bone formation, results in bone loss leading to osteopenia. The bone loss is commonly seen in cortical bone such as distal radius and proximal femur. Cancellous bone involvement is classical to age and menopause-related bone loss.[14] Nephrolithiasis is seen in 15–20% of the patients. Fragility factors are common, which is unrelated to trauma.

History of Clinical Symptoms

Family history of pituitary tumors, hypercalcemia, pancreatic tumors, and kidney stones must be recorded. Radiotherapy exposure is also a risk factor for primary hyperthyroidism. Use of thiazide diuretics and lithium must be ruled out in the personal history.[7]

Laboratory Testing

Before making a diagnosis of hypercalcemia, various other factors that can alter calcium levels must be ruled out. For every 1 mg of albumin or total protein, serum calcium is elevated by 0.8 mg/dL. The first investigation of choice is serum PTH concentration. The evaluation of serum calcium and PTH must be assessed simultaneously. Radioimmunoassay and immunochemiluminometric (ICMA) assay are the two methods commonly employed to assess PTH. Radioimmunoassay has low sensitivity and hence rarely used in present day practice. (1-84) PTH and (7-84) PTH are different fragments in circulation.[15,16] The second generation ICMA measures intact PTH (iPTH) and this is the preferred method. When renal function is compromised, fragments of PTH circulate in the blood at a higher concentration than a patient with normal renal function. Serum phosphorus, electrolytes, BUN, serum creatinine, and 24-hour urine calcium excretion, should also be measured.[7] Hypophosphatemia occurs due to decreased renal threshold for phosphate clearance. Bone specific alkaline phosphatase is a marker to evaluate bone resorption activity and measured when increased bone resorption is suspected.[7]

25-OH vitamin D is inversely related to the level of PTH. Low vitamin D, along with hypercalcemia, can trigger PTH secretion. pHPT with 25-OH vitamin D deficiency is associated with significant hypercalcemia, severe bone disease, and also increased weight of parathyroid adenoma.[17]

Serum creatinine to assess for renal function is mandatory in all cases. Glomerular filtration rate of less than 60 mL/min is associated with increased PTH and bone resorption.[7] 24-hour urinary calcium excretion of more than 400 mg/day is associated with an increased risk of nephrocalcinosis.[7]

Familial hypercalciuria hypercalcemia (FHH) is an autosomal dominant disorder with mutations of renal calcium-sensing receptor. Most of these patients rarely require surgical treatment; hence an unrecognized FHH can lead to unnecessary parathyroid surgery. FHH must always be ruled out in all cases of pHPT. The calcium creatinine clearance ratio is 24-hour urinary calcium/serum calcium ÷ 24-hour urinary creatinine/serum creatinine. When the ratio is <0.01, a diagnosis of FHH is made. When the ratio is >0.02, a diagnosis of pHPT is made.[18] For an intermediate level of 0.01–0.02, other causes such as renal insufficiency vitamin D deficiency and drug-induced hypercalcemia have to be excluded.

Pathology

A normal parathyroid gland weighs 20–50 mg.[19] Hypersecretion of PTH is seen in parathyroid adenoma, hyperplasia or carcinoma. Depending on the number of glands involved, they are further divided into single and MGD. Double adenomas, hyperplastic glands are also part of MGD. Parathyroid adenoma is defined as a well-defined encapsulated neoplasm with rim of normal parathyroid tissue. Parathyroid hyperplasia is characterized by increased cellularity, which involves the whole of the gland.[7] Parathyroid hyperplasia comprises 2–20% of pHPT.

PARATHYROIDECTOMY

Surgical excision of the involved parathyroid gland is the only definitive therapy for pHPT.[7] Conservative management is considered ineffective and less cost-effective than surgery, even in asymptomatic patients.[20-22]

Indications for parathyroidectomy:

- Parathyroidectomy must be indicated in all patients with a confirmed diagnosis of pHPT.[7] An elevated serum calcium level of >1 mg/dL above normal range must be considered for parathyroidectomy immaterial of symptomatology.
- *Target organ manifestations:*
  - *Renal manifestations:* Parathyroidectomy is indicated in nephrolithiasis, nephrocalcinosis, hypercalciuria (urinary calcium >400 mg/dL) and impaired GFR (<60 mL/min).
  - *Bone manifestations:* Presence of osteoporosis, fragility fracture or evidence of vertebral compression fracture mandate parathyroidectomy.
  - *Neurocognitive and neuropsychiatrist manifestations:* Neurocognitive and neuropsychiatrist disturbances as a result of hypercalcemia most often overlaps with various other disorders. When neurocognitive symptoms are the only presenting symptoms, diagnosis of pHPT is often missed. A prospective controlled study has shown that following parathyroidectomy, there was significant improvement of neurological symptoms within 10 days of surgery and significant improvement in overall health status.[23]
  - *Cardiac manifestations:* Mortality from cardiac manifestations of hypercalcemia is most significant in patients with hypertension. Patients with hypertension are at a 50% higher mortality risk than a normotensive patient with pHPT.[24] pHPT patients are associated with increased risk of myocardial infarction/congestive heart failure.[25] The diastolic dysfunction and left ventricular hypertrophy are common in pHPT and are gradually reversed after curative surgery.[26] Valvular calcification, carotid artery stiffness, and increased intima medial thickness are few pathological findings that are not reversed after parathyroidectomy.[27]

Contraindications for minimally invasive parathyroidectomy are:[7]

- Familial primary hyperparathyroidism
- MGD
- High body mass index
- Kyphoscoliosis
- Concurrent thyroid disease
- Gland >4 cm (relative)
- Lithium-induced hyperparathyroidism (relative)
- Suspected PC (relative)

Imaging

The diagnosis and indication for parathyroidectomy is based on history, and biochemical tests of the patient. Imaging modalities are only for localization of the parathyroid gland and not to make a diagnosis of hyperparathyroidism or parathyroid neoplasm. The decision to perform or defer surgery should not be based on imaging characteristics.

Neck Ultrasonography

Ultrasonography (US) is noninvasive inexpensive, and hence US neck must be the first modality of imaging to localize the gland.[7] Normal parathyroid glands are not visible on US. Parathyroid glands are characterized by homogeneity, hypoechogenicity, ovoid shape, and hypervascularity with an extrathyroidal feeding artery entering the parathyroid gland.[28] A recent meta-analysis has demonstrated a positive predictive value of 93.2% (85–100%),[29] and single institutional series have reported sensitivity of 82%[30,31] with US. The sensitivity drops to 35% in MGD.[32]

About 12–67% of patients with pHPT have concomitant thyroid disease and incidence of concomitant thyroid cancer is in the range of 2–17.6%.[33-35] Hence all patients with pHPT must be evaluated for thyroid nodules, and further management must be based on known guidelines of thyroid nodule management.

4D Computed Tomography

The fourth dimension of CT scan (4D CT scan) refers to a differential pattern of contrast enhancement of parathyroid tissue. Parathyroid glands have a rapid uptake and washout time, than adjacent tissue. 4D CT utilizes multiple thin cuts with a spatial resolution of 1 mm that help in better identifying parathyroid glands. 4D CT is the only modality that can also identify normal parathyroid glands. The sensitivity is 89% with a positive predictive value of 93.5%, which is greater than the combined US and sestamibi scan.[29] The sensitivity is sustainably high, even in MGD (62.5–85.7%).[36,37] Availability of 4D CT scan is limited.

Magnetic Resonance Imaging

Magnetic resonance imaging (MRI) is seldom used to localize parathyroid gland. Parathyroid adenoma appears as enhancing lesion with isodensity on T1-weighted image and increased signal intensity on T2-weighted image.[28] The sensitivity of 3T MRI is 97%, and specificity is 97.5%.[38] The sensitivity and specificity of 1.5T MRI is lower than 3T MRI.

Technetium-99m Sestamibi Scintigraphy

Sestamibi (also known as MIBI) is a lipophilic cation ionic complex which is an isonitrile derivative sequesters preferentially into mitochondria rich parathyroid cells. MIBI is bound to radionuclide Technetium-99m (^{99m}Tc). The half-life of ^{99m}Tc-MIBI is 6 hours.[28] Parathyroid scintigraphy needs a small dose of 15–35 m Ci (555–1295 MBq) ^{99m}Tc-MIBI.

Various acquisition protocols are used like digital subtraction and dual-phase acquisition. A larger mitochondrial burden in parathyroid cells than in the thyroid results in uptake and prolonged retention of MIBI within parathyroid cells, while the thyroid uptake washes out earlier due to lower mitochondrial density.[28] Dual-phase acquisition protocol includes image acquisition at 10–15 minutes and 2–3 hours after administration of ^{99m}Tc-MIBI. ^{99m}Tc-pertechnetate or ^{123}iodine are radiotracers specific to thyroid and are used along with ^{99m}Tc-MIBI, which is digitally subtracted to reveal the parathyroid location.[28] While image acquisition can be performed with 2D planar imaging, single positron emission CT (SPECT) or SPECT CT. SPECT CT has the advantage of better spatial configuration and orientation with better anatomical details which is essential, especially while evaluating ectopic glands. ^{99m}Tc-MIBI SPECT sensitivity is 79% and positive-predictive value is 91%.[32] The sensitivity of the test is dependent on the weight of the gland. Sensitivity is 51% with <500 mg gland and 93% when gland weighs >500 mg.[39] The sensitivity of the scan decreases to 44% in MGD. ^{99m}Tc-MIBI is the most common preoperative localization technique used. Combined US and ^{99m}Tc-MIBI scintigraphy has the highest predictive value for parathyroid location, higher than either modality used alone.[40] However, the combination is still limited in MGD.

18F-fluorocholine Positron Emission Tomography

Choline plays a vital role in the synthesis of phospholipids, and 18F-fluorocholine (18FCH) is commonly used to image renal cell carcinoma.[28] Studies have shown that 18FCH is taken up by parathyroid tissue. 3.2 MBq of 18FCH per kg of body weight is injected and the image acquired 60 minutes after administration.[28] The specificity, positive predictive value, negative predictive value and overall accuracy of 18F-fluorocholine positron emission tomography (18FCH-PET) CT are 96%, 90.2%, 97.4%, and 95.3% respectively.[41] Utility of 18FCH-PET MRI has also been studied, which has a sensitivity of 90% and 100% positive predictive value.[42]

Invasive Localization Methods

All invasive methods of localization are used only when the noninvasive methods fail to localize the parathyroid gland or in recurrent/re-operative scenarios.

Ultrasound-guided Fine-needle Aspiration Biopsy with PTH Washout

This method is highly specific (100%) with no false-positive results.[43,44] This procedure is associated with the risk of sampling adjoining thyroid tissue and can also interfere with final histology due to artifacts.[45] Fine-needle aspiration biopsy (FNAB) cannot differentiate between parathyroid adenoma and PC and hence should not be used to differentiate the two.

Selective Parathyroid Venous Sampling

Selective parathyroid venous sampling (SVS) aids in generalized localization of parathyroid into cervical, mediastinal, and laterality based on the PTH output measurements via venous blood sampling from various sites. The exact location of the gland cannot be assessed by this method. This technique needs an experienced interventional radiologist and is not widely available.

The venous return of normally located parathyroid gland is by superior, middle, and inferior thyroid veins. Superior and middle thyroid veins drain into internal jugular vein (IJV) and inferiorly into the brachiocephalic vein. Thoracic glands may drain into the superior thymic vein or internal thoracic veins. The venous sampling is done serially from superior vena cava, right brachiocephalic vein, left brachiocephalic vein, right internal jugular vein, left internal jugular vein, right middle thyroid vein, left superior thyroid vein, right superior thyroid vein, right vertebral vein, left vertebral vein, right subclavian vein, left subclavian vein, left internal thoracic vein, right internal thoracic vein, superior thymic vein, right inferior thyroid vein and left inferior thyroid vein. The PTH values that are 150–200% greater than superior vena cava value are taken as positive. The true positive rate is 71%.[46-48] Prior ligation of vessels in previous surgery may lead to false localization of the gland.

Selective parathyroid venous sampling is used as a last resort to localize parathyroid glands. The first line of localization methods must consist of US-^{99m}Tc-MIBI scintigraphy. Second-line localization can include ultrasound-guided FNAB with PTH washout, 4D CT, 18FCH-PET CT or MRI. The third-line localization modality is SVS.

Embryology of Parathyroid Gland

Inferior and superior parathyroid glands develop from third and fourth branchial pouches respectively during the 5th week of gestation.[49] The third branchial pouch descends inferiorly along thymus and lay inferior to superior parathyroid glands. They can be found anywhere from skull base to mediastinum. Aberrations in descend, accessory tissue, and supernumerary parathyroid glands make parathyroidectomy challenging.

Applied Anatomy of the Parathyroids

Number: Typically four parathyroid glands are present, two on each side of thyroid lobe. About 3–6% of cases may have less than four glands, and 0.6–0.7% may have supernumerary glands (>4).[50] Supernumerary glands are rarely present and are commonly found in thymus. Other sites are laryngeal submucosa, pericardium, aortopulmonary window, lateral to carotid sheath, and also intravagal.

Weight: Normal gland approximately weighs 40 mg while a hyperplastic gland weighs >60 mg.[50]

Appearance: A normal gland is typically light brown or reddish tan. The color of the gland is based on fat content, vascularity, and oxyphil cell concentration. Glandular enlargement replaces surrounding fat and hence appears more gray. The discrete edge of a parathyroid gland glides over the surrounding fat during dissection, which helps in differentiation from other structures. A normal parathyroid gland is flat and leaf-like while enlarged glands are globular.[50]

Symmetry: Superior glands are more constant than inferior glands. 70% of inferior and 80% of superior glands show symmetry.[50]

Relation to recurrent laryngeal nerve (RLN): The relation between the path of RLN and parathyroid glands is the most constant. The identification of which gland is superior or inferior is made based on its relation to RLN and not on location alone. If the RLN path is considered in a coronal plane, then superior parathyroid glands are dorsal and inferior glands are ventral to this plane.[50] Hence the migration path of superior glands are always dorsal to RLN, a plane that is retropharyngeal, retroesophageal, posterior mediastinal, while the migration path of inferior gland is always ventral to RLN plane along with thymus, anterior mediastinum.

Relation to vascular pedicle: Inferior parathyroid gland is supplied by inferior thyroid artery and the superior gland by an anastomotic branch between superior and inferior thyroid arteries. Inferior parathyroid gland in the mediastinum can be supplied by the thymic branch of internal mammary artery.[50]

Gland position:

- *Normal location:* Inferior parathyroid are in close relation to the thymus, and superior parathyroid is in close relation to lateral thyroid anlage with a shorter migration path than the inferior parathyroid gland. Hence, the inferior parathyroid has higher ectopic rates than superior gland. Inferior parathyroid gland rest within 1 cm inferior, posterior or lateral to the inferior pole of thyroid in 50% of cases. Superior parathyroid gland is normally located at cricothyroid articulation or 1 cm cranial to the inferior thyroid artery and RLN intersection.

- *Abnormal location:* Typical variation of the inferior parathyroid gland is commonly along the thyrothymic tract, which represents fat degeneration of uppermost residual thymic gland. Inferior parathyroid glands are present in this location in 25% of cases.[50] Ectopic inferior parathyroid gland can be high in the neck and low in the mediastinum based on rate of descent. Undescended inferior parathyroid glands are located at the carotid bifurcation, 2–3 cm lateral to the superior pole of the thyroid, angle of the mandible or hyoid bone. Overly-descended inferior parathyroid can be found in anterior mediastinum within lower portion of thymus. 1% of inferior parathyroid glands are intrathyroid. Intrathyroidal gland is most challenging to identify and does not include subcapsular parathyroid gland. They can be identified by intraoperative US. Atypical sites of superior parathyroid gland are posterolateral to the superior pole of the thyroid, retrolaryngeal, retro-esophagal or retropharyngeal. Retropharyngeal and retroesophageal sites are most difficult to be identified on US due shadowing from overlying laryngeal cartilage.[50]
- *Acquired migration:* This can occur due to gross enlargement of the gland and regional dynamics secondary to muscular movements of deglutition and respiration. Unlike ectopic gland, the blood supply remains the same, and inferior thyroid artery travels along the migration tract.[50]

Recent meta-analysis on location of the parathyroid gland has shown that 81.5% of cases have four glands.[51] 15.9% of cases have an ectopic location with 11.6% found in the neck and 4.35% in the mediastinum. The most common ectopic location in neck was retro-esophageal or paraesophageal location.

Preoperative management:

- *Calcium supplementation:* Contrary to the belief, even patients with pHPT need calcium supplementation. Low calcium intake, in turn, leads to increased PTH secretion. Natural longitudinal study has shown that dietary intake of calcium does not affect PTH, serum calcium or calcitriol levels.[52] Calcium supplementation has also shown to increase bone density in patients with primary hyperparathyroidism. There is no data to support calcium restriction.[7]
- *Vitamin D supplementation:* A meta-analysis with ten studies has shown that patients with pHPT are associated with reduced levels of vitamin D.[53] A randomized trial compared 2,800 IU daily cholecalciferol (D3) against placebo in pHPT patients for 6 months pre and postoperative period.[54] The patients with vitamin D supplementation showed a significant reduction in the first 25 weeks of treatment. There was no significant difference in serum or urinary calcium at any point of time. However, vitamin D supplementation must be done with caution in cases with significant hypercalciuria. The recommendations of calcium and vitamin D supplementation are controversial, even though guidelines do not recommend against it, there is no regime validated that can be prescribed.
- *Vocal cord status:* All patients undergoing para-thyroidectomy must undergo evaluation for vocal cord mobility.
- *Hypercalcemia:* Severe hypercalcemia is rare in pHPT. Hypercalcemic crisis is defined as albumin corrected serum calcium of >14 mg/dL with signs of multiorgan dysfunction.[7] The management strategy is aimed to correct hypovolemic state, promote renal calcium excretion, and inhibit accelerated bone resorption. Most often, hypercalcemic crisis is precipitated by concurrent precipitating illness, which must be identified and corrected. Euvolemic status can be achieved by infusion of 3–4 L of normal saline over 24 hours, followed by 2–3 L of normal saline infusion until normal urinary output is attained.[55] Urinary excretion is promoted by furosemide (loop diuretic) to block calcium reabsorption at distal nephron and promote calciuresis. Thiazide diuretics are contraindicated. Bone resorption can be prevented by calcitonin, glucocorticosteroids, and bisphosphonates. Cinacalcet is used as a medical management strategy in pHPT patients who cannot undergo surgery. It acts by stimulating calcium sensory receptors on parathyroid chief cells to reduce PTH secretion. Approved dose is 30 mg twice daily.[56] While higher doses are required in hypercalcemic crisis (up to 90 mg twice daily), the safety of such higher doses has not been studied.

Terminology in Parathyroid Surgery

The terminology is based on the number of parathyroid glands excised. Subtotal parathyroidectomy is a term used to define a surgical procedure involving resection of 3.5 glands and the term total parathyroidectomy is used to define a procedure that involves removal of all parathyroid glands. Various studies have also used postoperative serum PTH level to define the extent of parathyroidectomy, but this is variable across studies.[7]

Types of Parathyroidectomy based on Access

Minimally Invasive Parathyroidectomy

Minimally invasive parathyroidectomy (MIP) is defined as a surgical procedure with a restricted field of dissection that is necessary to expose abnormal parathyroid gland. 85% of pHPT is due to single parathyroid adenoma, which can be effectively cured with MIP and operative adjuncts. An absolute prerequisite is preoperative localization of the gland and absence of MGD.

Various procedures have been described.

- *Minimally invasive parathyroidectomy:* This classically utilizes 2–3 cm cervical incisions on the side of the abnormal gland. The procedure can be done under regional anesthesia, or general anesthesia and conventional instruments are used for dissection and access **(Figs. 1A and B)**.
- *Minimally invasive endoscopic parathyroidectomy:* This technique utilizes either a remote access like in remote access thyroidectomy or a lateral cervical route with insufflation.
- *Minimally invasive endoscopic-assisted parathyroidectomy:* This procedure involves access to the area of interest with a 1.5 cm cervical incision where tissue dissection is completed by open access and endoscope is used only to localize parathyroid gland.
- *Minimally invasive image-guided parathyroidectomy:* ^{99m}Tc-MIBI is the only radiotracer used for intraoperative localization of parathyroid glands using a handheld gamma probe. ^{99m}Tc-MIBI is injected intravenously (740MBq) and dual-phase images are acquired. The patient is taken up for image-guided surgery with gamma probe after 2.5–3 hours of injection.

Bilateral Exploration

Bilateral exploration (BE) is a procedure wherein all parathyroid glands are explored and managed as per the indication. BE remains a preferred and time-tested procedure for pHPT.[7] The side with preoperative localized gland is exposed first, and then the contralateral side is explored. The parathyroid glands are first searched for in their expected normal locations. If absent, then the posterior surface of the thyroid gland is explored. If absent in the second location, then ectopic locations are dissected to locate parathyroid glands.

Missing inferior parathyroid glands are first explored in the thyrothymic tract and then the carotid sheath is explored. A missing superior parathyroid is often seen in retropharyngeal or retroesophageal location. During the procedure, the recurrent laryngeal nerve must be dissected throughout its cervical course.

When subtotal parathyroidectomy is planned, then all four glands must be localized and evaluated. The gland chosen for preservation is first preserved and checked for viability. Once the vascularity is confirmed then rest of the glands are resected. When total parathyroidectomy is planned, then least abnormal parathyroid gland is cryopreserved and/or autotransplanted into a vascularized muscular pocket.

Adjuncts to Parathyroid Surgery

Identification of the gland:

- *Visual confirmation of the gland:* Based on size, shape, color, and weight must be assessed, which are a sensitive indicator in the hands of an experienced surgeon.[7]
- *Ex-vivo measurement:* After the gland is excised, ex-vivo measurement of PTH aspirate from the glandular tissue can aid in identification of the gland.

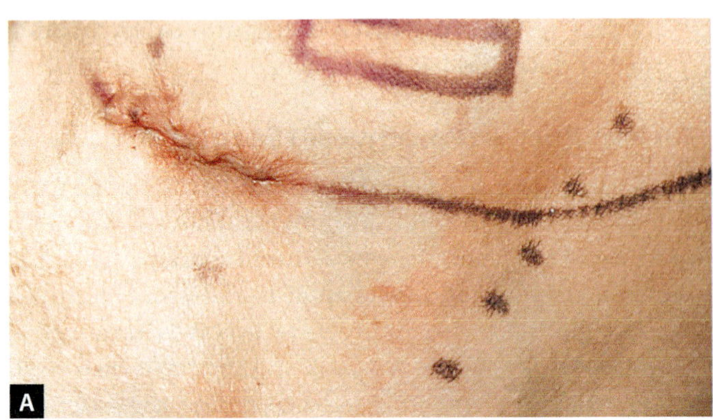

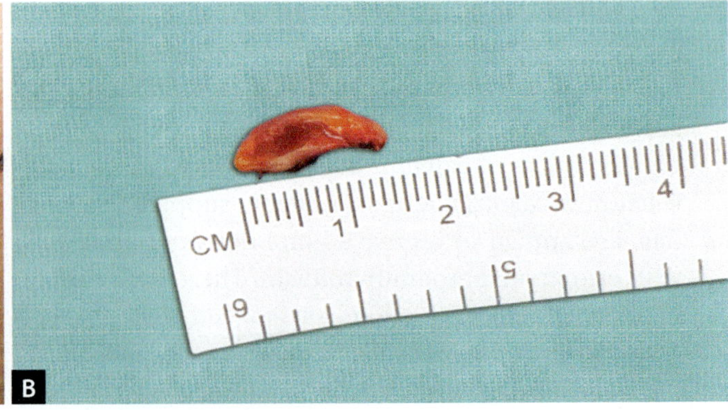

Figs. 1A and B: Minimally invasive parathyroid surgery where a 2 cm neck incision is used (A) to remove a 1.5 cm parathyroid adenoma (B).

The aspirate is sent in 1 mL of normal saline for testing.[7] Frozen section analysis can be used. Freezing artifacts can sometimes affect reporting and hence combining imprint cytology with frozen section analysis can improve the sensitivity of the test. Frozen section is of higher value mainly when imaging modalities cannot localize the gland.[7]

Enhancing visualization and localization of the gland:

- *Methylene blue:* When administered at the rate of 5–7.5 mg/kg body weight diluted in 500 mL of Ringer's lactate and infused over 45–60 minutes can enhance visualization of abnormal glands.[57] However, methylene blue is associated with a high rate of complications and is not widely used. Various other visual aids such as infrared fluorescence and autofluorescence have been studied but not routinely used.
- *Intraoperative ultrasound:* It is a beneficial adjunct in localizing the gland. With the help of smaller footprint probes, intraoperative US can reach areas that are difficult to access. Intraoperative US is precious in identifying intrathyroidal gland.[7]
- *Differential jugular venous sampling:* A differential (>10%) PTH level can help in localizing the side of parathyroid gland.[58] This technique must be used with caution in re-operative cases where vein ligation may affect venous sampling.
- *^{99m}Tc-MIBI radio guidance*: It can be used for localization of the gland. The accuracy of ^{99m}Tc-MIBI drops significantly in MGD and is also associated with high false rate due to uptake in the thyroid. A 20% drop in gamma count from parathyroid bed to ex-vivo count is considered significant.[59] Use of radio-guided technique and intraoperative PTH monitoring in combination is more accurate than radio guidance alone.

Completeness of resection:

- *Intraoperative PTH monitoring (IPM)*: IPM is vital in achieving excellent cure rates. BE is based on comparative size and weight of parathyroid gland, while IPM helps to assess the functionality of the gland. IPM aids in real-time assessment of the success of surgery as 15% of the cases may have MGD.[60] MIP with IPM has achieved cure rates of 97–99%.[61-63] IPM utilizes the short half-life of PTH (3–5 minutes). The rapid analysis can be performed with immunochemiluminescence assay, which can be completed in 8–20 minutes. The level of PTH is depended on the protocol used, the vein blood being drawn, and transport error. Various protocols are described, but most common are Miami and dual criteria protocol:
  - *Miami protocol:*[64-66] Miami protocol is one of the widely used methods of IPM. A preincision and a pre-excision blood sample are drawn. 5 and 10 minutes after the excision is complete, two more blood samples are drawn. When PTH level drops >50% of either preincision or pre-excision sample, the PTH drop is considered as adequate excision, and the procedure is stopped. If the PTH levels are high, then a repeat sample at 15–20 minutes postexcision is drawn for comparison. If >50% drop in the blood sample is not seen after 20 minutes of excision, then BE must be performed. This protocol has shown excellent long-term cure rates of 97–99%.
  - *Dual criteria:*[67,68] Dual criteria is a modification of Miami protocol, in which preincision and 10 minutes postexcision blood sample is drawn. >50% drop in PTH value and return to normal range is considered as significant resection and procedure is abandoned. If the rise in PTH level is persistent, surgery must proceed to BE. The success rate of the procedure when both criteria are met is 97–99%.

Several studies have shown that with either of the protocol, when PTH falls >50% but not <40 pg/mL, the rate of persistence and recurrence is higher.[62,68] A false-positive result is seen in unrecognized MGD, postexcision sample hemodilution or hemolysis.[69] A false-negative result is seen in patients with reduced renal clearance, artificially elevated baseline PTH or hemodilution of the baseline sample.[70]

Autotransplantation and Cryopreservation

Immediate autotransplantation success rate is >90%. Each parathyroid gland must be handled with care, as if it is the last viable gland.[71,72] Glands must be tested for their vascularity by needle prick/surgical blade capsular incision and evaluation of capillary bleed. If the vascularity is compromised, then the gland must be immediately autotransplanted. It is preferable to use a frozen section analysis to confirm parathyroid origin before autotransplant. Extracervical site like forearm is preferable if the likelihood of subsequent development of hyperparathyroidism is high. The site of autotransplantation must be marked with permanent suture or a clip for identification at a later stage.

Autotransplantation includes mincing the parathyroid tissue into 2–3 mm fragments. Two/three fragments are transferred into each vascularized intramuscular pockets (sternocleidomastoid, brachioradialis or pectoralis muscle). An approximate of 6 weeks is required for transplanted fragments to function. Cryopreservation is not routinely used, as the functional preservation of parathyroid tissue is questionable. Here, parathyroid tissue is frozen and thawed before planned autotransplantation. Delayed autotransplantation and cryopreservation is associated with significantly higher rates of nonfunctioning of parathyroid than immediate autotransplantation. In re-operative MGD, cryopreservation has a definite role, as previous resection and vascularity of remaining glands may be difficult to assess. Approximately 60% of preserved glands maintain function after the transfer.[73]

POSTOPERATIVE MANAGEMENT

Hypocalcemia

Immediate hypocalcemia is more common in BE than MIP. Rate of transient hypocalcemia is 5–47%, and the rate of permanent hypocalcaemia is 0–3.6%.[7,74] The calcium levels significantly drop to symptomatic level usually after 24–48 hours. The drop can also occur on the third or fourth day postexcision. Hence, calcium levels need to be monitored and supplemented as required. Long-term calcium supplementation is required in most cases. The standard recommendations for supplementation vary significantly and this is usually performed as per institutional policies. The dose of calcium and vitamin D supplementation requirements are represented in **Table 1**.[75]

Failed Parathyroidectomy

Persistent hyperparathyroidism is defined as raised calcium levels <6 months after parathyroidectomy and recurrent hyperparathyroidism as raised calcium levels >6 months after parathyroidectomy.[7] Causes of failure are commonly a missed MGD, interval development of MGD, residual graft hypertrophy, vascularization of previously devascularized gland and parathyromatosis. Re-surgery is challenging, and the surgeon must utilize all preoperative and intraoperative adjuncts to localize the abnormal gland successfully. The procedure that can be performed with the least morbidity and best cure must be chosen. Before a diagnosis of persistent or recurrent disease is made, all the causes for false-positive results and drug interactions must be ruled out. The threshold for re-surgery must be very high, as the cure rates are lower (82–98%)[76,77] and complication rates are higher than primary parathyroidectomy. All possible preoperative evaluation and surgical adjuncts must be used to achieve the best cure. BE is preferred over a minimal access approach.

Familial Hyperparathyroidism

- *Multiple endocrine neoplasm (MEN) syndromes:* Variants of MEN syndrome are the most common familial forms of hyperparathyroidism.
- *MEN1 syndrome:* MEN1 syndrome is an autosomal dominant hereditary disease with mutations of the *MEN1* gene located on chromosome 11q13, which is a tumor suppressor gene encoding for 610 amino acid—menin protein.[78] The *MEN1* gene mutations are also found in sporadic cases. They almost always arise from the same locus at chromosome 11q13. A mutation of *MEN1* gene is the first hit in MEN1 syndrome, in combination with somatic or postnatal loss of other copy *MEN1* gene (second hit), which results in neoplastic clonal expression. MEN1 syndrome primarily includes hyperparathyroidism, adenoma of the anterior pituitary, and neuroendocrine tumors of gastropancreatic system (insulinoma, gastrinoma and glucagonomas).[79] Presence of two of these neoplasms is defined as MEN1 syndrome. Other manifestations are lipomas, facial angiofibroma, collagenomas, thyroid and adrenal nodules, and foregut carcinoids. The follow-up strategy in a known carrier of MEN1 syndrome is represented in **Table 2**.[78,79] Hyperparathyroidism is the most common and the earliest manifestation with 70% penetrance by 50 years of age. Hyperparathyroidism in MEN1 syndrome is associated with MGD, which is most often asymmetric enlargement. *MEN1* is also

Table 1: Required doses of calcium and vitamin D supplementation.

	Calcium supplementation		*Vitamin D supplementation*	
Gender	*Age in years*	*Dose*	*Age in years*	*Dose*
Women	19–51	1,000 mg/day	≤71	600 IU/day
	≥51	1,200 mg/day	>71	800 IU/day
Men	19–71	1,000 mg/day	≤71	600 IU/day
	>71	1,200 mg/day	>71	800 IU/day

Table 2: Follow-up strategy in a known carrier of MEN1 syndrome.

Tumor	*Penetrance (at 40 years of age)*	*Age to begin evaluation (in years)*	*Biochemical test annually*	*Imaging annually*
Parathyroid adenoma	90%	8	Calcium, PTH	None
Gastrinoma	40%	20	Gastrin, secretin-stimulated gastrin	CT/MRI
Insulinoma	10%	5	Fasting glucose , insulin	CT/MRI
Anterior pituitary	20%	5	PRL, IGF-1	MRI
Foregut carcinoid	2%	20	None	CT
Other enteropancreatic	2–20%	20	Chromogranin A, glucagon, proinsulin	^{111}In-DTPA octreotide scan

(IGF-1: insulin-like growth factor 1; PTH: parathyroid hormone; PRL: prolactin)

associated with higher likelihood of recurrence after parathyroidectomy. Patients with hyperparathyroidism must be treated with total parathyroidectomy and autotransplantation or subtotal parathyroidectomy.[7] A randomized trial compared the efficacy of total parathyroidectomy with autotransplantation versus subtotal parathyroidectomy. There was no significant difference in the outcome. The rate of supernumerary parathyroid glands is higher in MEN1, and hence various studies advocate routine resection of thymus and thymic tract.

- *MEN2:* The hallmark disease of MEN2 with 100% penetrance is medullary thyroid carcinoma. MEN2 syndrome has been described in detail under section medullary carcinoma thyroid. Approximately 10–25% of MEN2 is associated with hyperparathyroidism. The most common mutation associated with hyperparathyroidism is 634 mutation. Prior thyroidectomy makes management of hyperparathyroidism difficult in MEN2. The functionality of the remaining parathyroid glands is difficult to assess, and hence even though MGD is common, a directed approach with removal of only abnormal gland is advocated.[7]
- *MEN4:* About 5–10% of MEN1 syndrome patients do not show mutations of the *MEN1* gene. These patients have mutations of *CDNK1B* gene located on chromosome 12p13. The tumor profile of MEN4 is similar to MEN1.
- *Hyperparathyroidism-jaw tumor syndrome (HPT-JT):* HPT-JT is an autosomal dominant disorder caused by mutation of *CDC73* (previously known as HRPT2) gene.[80,81] *CDC73* encodes the parafibromin protein that plays a role in transcription and post-transcription pathways by forming complexes with RNA polymerase II. The clinical presentation of HPT-JT consists of parathyroid tumors, ossifying jaw tumors, renal abnormalities, and uterine tumors. Hyperparathyroidism has a penetrance of 80–90% by the third decade of life. The risk of malignant transformation of parathyroid glands is higher in HPT-JT (15–38%).[80,81] There is no consensus regarding the extent of parathyroid resection in HPT-JT due to the rarity of the disorder.[7]

HYPOPARATHYROIDISM

Hypoparathyroidism is characterized by low PTH secretion, hypocalcemia, and hyperphosphatemia. Hypoparathyroidism is a common complication after surgery of the central compartment of the neck. Noniatrogenic causes of hypoparathyroidism are rare and are represented in **Table 3**. The manifestations of hypocalcemia as a result of hypoparathyroidism are represented in **Table 4**. The following section focuses on the management of post-thyroidectomy hypoparathyroidism.

Management of Hypoparathyroidism Post-total Thyroidectomy

Assessment

- *Intraoperative period:* The viability of the gland must be assessed based on gross appearance and vascularity of the gland. The appearance can be graded from a scale of 0 (normal color of gland and normal vascularity) to scale of 3 (severely compromised gland with dark brown/pale in appearance and no bleeding on capsular incision). This scale, correlates well with postoperative hypoparathyroidism.[82] Intraoperative measurement of PTH has also been studied to predict hypoparathyroidism postoperatively.[83]
- *Postoperative period:* Calcium level <8.0 mg/dL is considered hypocalcemia in most centers. Various parameters such as serum calcium, a combination of calcium and PTH, ionized calcium, corrected calcium have been reported with good efficacy. In general, PTH level >10 pg/mL signifies returning parathyroid function.[84]

Table 3: Causes of hypoparathyroidism.

Common causes	*Familial causes*
• Surgery of the neck (thyroidectomy 75%) • Radiation-induced • Metastatic infiltration • Hemochromatosis • Wilson's disease	• Digeorge syndrome • Hypoparathyroidism–deafness–renal dysplasia syndrome • Kenny–Caffey syndrome • Sanjad–Sakati syndrome • Mitochondrial trifunctional protein deficiency syndrome • Kearns–Sayre syndrome • Autoimmune polyglandular syndrome • Acquired autoimmune hypoparathyroidism
Pseudohypoparathyroidism (peripheral resistance to PTH)	*Secondary to hypomagnesemia*
• Pseudohypoparathyroidism type 1a/b/c • Blomstrand lethal chondrodysplasia • Pseudopseudohypoparat-hyroidism	• Alcohol intake • Malnutrition • Malabsorption

(PTH: parathyroid hormone)

Table 4: Signs and symptoms of acute and chronic hypoparathyroidism.

Neuromuscular	*Neurological*	*Cardiovascular*
• Fatigue • Generalized muscle weakness • Muscle cramping • Neuromuscular irritability • Laryngospasm and stridor • Bronchospasm and wheezing • Elevated creatinine kinase	• Paresthesia • Seizers • Poor memory • Poor concentration • Depression • Anxiety • Chorea • Parkinsonism	• Arrhythmias • Heart block • Congestive heart failure • Prolonged QT interval
	Gastrointestinal	*Ophthalmic*
	• Constipation • Abdominal cramps • Steatorrhea	• Papilledema • Cataract

Management

Acute hypocalcemia is an emergency and must be treated at the earliest. 1–2 g of calcium gluconate in 50 mL of 5% dextrose is infused over 20 minutes under 12-lead electrocardiogram monitoring.[85] Each vial of calcium gluconate contains 93 mg of elemental calcium. A bolus of intravenous calcium gluconate increases calcium level for 2–3 hours. Hence, continued transfusion along with calcium assessment every 8 hours must be continued until calcium level reaches 7.5 mg/dL.[84]

Oral calcium supplementation is administered at 1–3 g of elemental calcium every 3–4 hours. Calcium carbonate (40% elemental calcium) and calcium citrate (21% of elemental calcium) are commonly used calcium salts. Serum calcium must be maintained at the lower limit of the normal range. Calcitriol administration (0.25–0.5 μg/day) is advocated when calcium levels continue to fall despite oral calcium supplementation.[85] Low magnesium levels impair PTH release and must be assessed in cases that do not respond to oral calcium treatment.[85] Recombinant PTH(1–84) has shown to reduce calcium supplementation in 50% of cases, and 43% were independent of any supplementation with 50–100 μg subcutaneous infection daily.[86]

The management algorithm of hypocalcemia is varied across all institutions. The institutional protocol that is tested for efficacy must be followed, as there are no standard protocols for hypocalcemia management in post-thyroidectomy.

PARATHYROID CARCINOMA

Parathyroid carcinoma are rare, accounting for <1% of hyperparathyroidism.[9] PC are challenging to diagnose preoperatively, as most often, the presentation is similar to other causes of pHPT.

Epidemiology

The incidence of PC is rare and only presents as a part of hyperparathyroidism spectrum. Globally, Japan has reported a high incidence of PC.[87] The variation in incidence between decades is also wide, with most population-based studies showing increasing incidences over time. PC commonly presents in the fifth or fourth decades of life and affects both genders equally.[88]

Molecular Biology

The triggering genetic abnormality in causation of PC is unknown. *CDC73* gene mutation in HPT-JT is associated with higher rates of PC. Various mutations of PRUNE2, FAT3, AKAP9, ZEB1, and ADCK1 are frequently known to occur.[89,90] CCND1 amplification is observed in 29% of tumors.

Clinical Presentation

Most of the patients with PC have serum calcium levels >14 mg/dL and manifest symptoms and signs of target organ disease. Most patients present with renal and skeletal manifestation, unlike in benign parathyroid adenoma. Nonfunctioning PC is exceedingly rare. Few patients can present with local signs and symptoms of local invasion such as change in voice and dysphagia. Most PC measure >3.5 cm and hence are palpable in the neck, while parathyroid adenomas are smaller and are rarely palpable in the neck.[88]

Pathology

Parathyroid adenoma and PC are difficult to differentiate even on pathological evaluation. Schantz and Castleman defined pathological characteristics of PC.[91] The principle histologic features of PC are trabecular pattern, mitotic figures, thick fibrous bands, capsular invasion, and vascular invasion. The key histologic feature of PC is invasion. Capsular invasion either complete or partial transgression, extension to surrounding thyroid and fatty tissue are various spectrum of invasion. Tumor necrosis, prominent nucleoli, and high mitotic figure (5 mitoses/50 hpf) are associated with poor prognosis.[92]

Atypical parathyroid adenoma is a terminology used to denote parathyroid adenomas with all features of PC but without invasion.[88] Immunohistochemistry (IHC) can aid in improving the accuracy of PC.[93] PTH, chromogranin A, GATA 3 positivity helps in identifying the tissue to be of parathyroid origin. Ki-67 proliferation index (>5%) and nuclear loss of parafibromin aid in differentiating PC from benign lesion. Nuclear loss of parafibromin also predicts a higher rate of recurrence.[88]

Imaging

The imaging algorithm is similar to parathyroid adenoma. Invasive features on US must mandate cross-sectional imaging. Nam et al. recommended features such as heterogeneous echotexture, irregular shape, uncircumscribed margin, and intranodular calcification as differentiating features of PC from adenoma.[94] The sensitivity and specificity of differentiating PC from adenoma with these US features is 100% and 96.7% respectively. The depth to width ratio of >1 is also suggestive of malignancy.[95] Often ^{99m}Tc-MIBI cannot differentiate between benign and malignant, but a recent study has shown a higher peak of retention index in PC.[96] The role of PET/CT has been primarily in evaluating regional and distant metastases. 18FCH has shown promising results.

US-guided FNAB has a limited role in suspected PC cases, due to fear of capsular rupture and tumor seeding.[97] However, FNAB can be used to reliably diagnose metastatic disease.

Staging

There is no Union for International Cancer Control (UICC) proposed TNM staging for PC. Two commonly quoted TNM staging systems are represented in **Table 5**.

Treatment

Surgery

En bloc resection of the tumor at initial surgery forms the only curative treatment option for PC. En bloc resection including tumor resection with ipsilateral thyroid lobe and adjacent involved structures with adequate gross margins is considered adequate.[88] Most often, preoperative diagnosis is not available, and intraoperative findings must guide the suspicion of PC and adequate surgery. The best chance of cure is during initial surgery. Some cases may not present with features of invasion, making diagnosis of PC difficult. Re-operation with ipsilateral thyroid lobe excision and central compartment clearance within 1 month of initial surgery is known to reduce recurrence.[99] Care must be taken to preserve the capsule of tumor intact to avoid tumor spillage. The incidence of regional lymph nodal involvement ranges between 6.5 and 32.1% at initial diagnosis.[100] Neck dissection of involved nodal stations must be performed. Role of prophylactic neck dissection in improving locoregional control or survival is controversial. Even though, some authors routinely advocate central compartment dissection in all cases of PC. Hsu et al. reviewed SEER cancer registry for PC patients and reported that the rate of regional metastasis was significantly higher in patients with tumors >3 cm (21 vs. 2.8%) and advocated prophylactic neck dissection

Table 5: TNM staging systems for parathyroid carcinoma.

Shaha et al.[98]	*Schulte et al.*[9]
T1: Tumor <3 cm *T2:* Tumor >3 cm *T3:* Tumor of any size with invasion of surrounding soft tissue *T4:* Massive central compartment disease invading trachea, esophagus, recurrent disease	*T1:* Evidence of capsular invasion *T2:* Invasion of surrounding structures excluding vital organs *T3:* Evidence of vascular invasion *T4:* Invasion of vital organs, i.e., hypopharynx, larynx, recurrent laryngeal nerve, and carotid artery
N0: No regional node metastases *N1:* Regional lymph nodes metastases *M0:* No evidence of distant metastases *M1:* Evidence of distant metastases	*Nx:* Lymph node not assessed *N0:* No regional node metastases *N1:* Regional lymph nodes metastases *M0:* No evidence of distant metastases *M1:* Evidence of distant metastases
TNM stage I: T1N0M0 II: T2N0M0 IIIa: T3N0M0 IIIb: T4N0M0 IIIc: Any T, N1, M0 IV: Any T, any N, M1	*TNM stage* I: T1-2N0M0 II:T3N0M0 III: Any T, N1, M0 or T4 IV: Any N, M1

in tumors measuring >3 cm.[101] However, they showed that the presence of regional metastases did not affect disease-specific survival.

Radiotherapy

Parathyroid carcinoma is a radioresistant tumor. The indication for adjuvant radiotherapy (RT) is not well defined. The principle of adjuvant RT is to reduce locoregional recurrences and hence in tumors with a high risk of recurrence, adjuvant RT must be recommended. Various risk stratification systems have been reported. Schulte has classified the presence of capsular invasion and invasion to surrounding soft tissue as low risk and vascular invasion, lymph nodal metastases, invasion to vital organs as a high-risk group.[9] The MD Anderson risk stratification was based on features of vascular invasion, serum calcium >15 mg/dL and age >65 years as significant predictors of reduced recurrence-free survival.[102] Patients were stratified as low, moderate, and high risk when 0, 1 and >2 features were present. The 2-year recurrence-free survival in the low, moderate, and high-risk group was 97%, 72%, and 27% respectively. Hence patients with these moderate-high risk features can be considered for adjuvant RT. Role of RT as definitive treatment, even in unresectable cases, is limited.

Chemotherapy

Few case reports have shown promising results with sorafenib in recurrent and metastatic disease.[103,104] Role of cytotoxic regime such as dacarbazine, dacarbazine with 5-fluorouracil, cyclophosphamide, methotrexate, doxorubicin, cyclophosphamide and lomustine have been reported with limited response.[88]

Recurrent Disease

Recurrent PC is challenging to manage. Surgery forms the main treatment modality even in a recurrent setting. Two preoperative localization techniques must be used before planned surgery.[88] Most patients with PC have an indolent course, and hence the primary aim of recurrent disease management must be complete resection and maximum achievable biochemical cure.

Palliation

Patients with PC have an indolent course, and most succumb to effects of intractable hypercalcemia rather than to the disease itself. When the disease is unresectable, primary aim must be to control calcium levels. Tumor debulking has achieved good control of hypercalcemia and makes patients more responsive to medical management of hypercalcemia.[9,105] Hypercalcemia can be managed with hydration, calcitonin, and cinacalcet. Bone resorption can be inhibited with bisphosphonates (pamidronate and zoledronic acid). Denosumab is a monoclonal antibody, which binds to RANK expressed by osteoclasts and prevents bone resorption.[106]

Prognosis

Inadequate surgery, presence of lymph nodal metastases, and high-risk disease as per Schulte classification are associated with poor prognosis in most studies.[107,108] Rate of recurrence is high (23–51%).[88] However, the overall survival at 5 and 10 years is 78–91% and 60–72% respectively.[88]

Follow-up

Patients must be followed up, throughout their lifetime. Interval of follow-up visits must be once in 6 months for the first 5 years and then annually. At each follow-up visit, serum calcium and PTH level must be monitored.

CONCLUSION

Management of primary hyperparathyroidism has undergone extensive changes with improved cure rates due to the advent of better imaging, localization techniques, operative techniques and even laboratory testing. Intimate knowledge of anatomy, ectopic locations and anomalies is paramount to achieve the best cure rates after surgery. PC is rare and adequate resection during initial surgery is the only curative modality available. Other modalities of treatment are associated with a limited response.

REFERENCES

1. Bushinsky DA, Monk RD. Calcium. Lancet. 1998;352(9124):306-11.
2. Goldstein DA. Serum calcium. In: Clinical Methods: The History, Physical, and Laboratory Examinations, 3rd edition. London: Butterworths; 1990.
3. Payne RB, Little AJ, Williams RB, Milner JR. Interpretation of serum calcium in patients with abnormal serum proteins. Br Med J. 1973;4(5893):643-6.
4. Kumar R, Thompson JR. The regulation of parathyroid hormone secretion and synthesis. J Am Soc Nephrol. 2011;22(2):216-24.
5. Holt EH, Inzucchi SE. Physiology and pathophysiology of the parathyroid glands and preoperative evaluation. In: Surgery of the Thyroid and Parathyroid Glands. Springer, Berlin, Heidelberg; 2007. pp. 235-43.
6. Heaney RP. Ethnicity, bone status, and the calcium requirement. Nutr Res. 2002;22(1-2):153-78.
7. Wilhelm SM, Wang TS, Ruan DT, Lee JA, Asa SL, Duh QY, et al. The American Association of Endocrine Surgeons guidelines for definitive management of primary hyperparathyroidism. JAMA Surg. 2016;151(10):959-68.

8. Wermers RA, Khosla S, Atkinson EJ, Hodgson SF, O'Fallon WM, Melton LJ. The rise and fall of primary hyperparathyroidism: a population-based study in Rochester, Minnesota, 1965-1992. Ann Intern Med. 1997;126(6):433-40.
9. Talat N, Schulte KM. Clinical presentation, staging and long-term evolution of parathyroid cancer. Ann Surg Oncol. 2010;17(8):2156-74.
10. Cetani F, Pardi E, Marcocci C. Update on parathyroid carcinoma. J Endocrinol Invest. 2016;39(6):595-606.
11. Salcuni AS, Cetani F, Guarnieri V, Nicastro V, Romagnoli E, de Martino D, et al. Parathyroid carcinoma. Best Practi Res Clin Endocrinol Metab. 2018;32(6):877-89.
12. Yeh MW, Ituarte PH, Zhou HC, Nishimoto S, Amy Liu IL, Harari A, et al. Incidence and prevalence of primary hyperparathyroidism in a racially mixed population. J Clin Endocrinol Metab. 2013;98(3):1122-9.
13. Nishi SP, Barbagelata NA, Atar S, Birnbaum Y, Tuero E. Hypercalcemia-induced ST-segment elevation mimicking acute myocardial infarction. J Electrocardiol. 2006;39(3): 298-300.
14. Shane E, Dinaz I. Hypercalcemia: pathogenesis, clinical manifestations, differential diagnosis, and management. Primer on the metabolic bone diseases and disorders of mineral metabolism. 2006;26:176.
15. Bringhurst FR, Stern AM, Yotts MA, Mizrahi NE, Segre GV, Potts Jr JT. Peripheral metabolism of PTH: fate of biologically active amino terminus in vivo. Am J Physiol. 1988;255(6): E886-93.
16. Silverman R, Yalow RS. Heterogeneity of parathyroid hormone. Clinical and physiologic implications. J Clin Invest. 1973;52(8):1958-71.
17. Silverberg SJ. Vitamin D deficiency and primary hyperparathyroidism. J Bone Miner Res. 2007;22(S2):V100-4.
18. Shinall M, Dahir K, Broome J. Differentiating familial hypocalciuric hypercalcemia from primary hyperparathyroidism. Endocr Pract. 2013;19(4):697-702.
19. Lappas D, Noussios G, Anagnostis P, Adamidou F, Chatzigeorgiou A, Skandalakis P. Location, number and morphology of parathyroid glands: results from a large anatomical series. Anat Sci Inter. 2012;87(3):160-4.
20. Zanocco K, Angelos P, Sturgeon C. Cost-effectiveness analysis of parathyroidectomy for asymptomatic primary hyperparathyroidism. Surgery. 2006;140(6):874-82.
21. Udelsman R, Pasieka JL, Sturgeon C, Young JE, Clark OH. Surgery for asymptomatic primary hyperparathyroidism: proceedings of the third international workshop. J Clin Endocrinol Metab. 2009;94(2):366-72.
22. Silverberg SJ, Shane E, Jacobs TP, Siris E, Bilezikian JP. A 10-year prospective study of primary hyperparathyroidism with or without parathyroid surgery. New Engl J Med. 1999;341(17):1249-55.
23. Pasieka JL, Parsons LL. Prospective surgical outcome study of relief of symptoms following surgery in patients with primary hyperparathyroidism. World J Surg. 1998;22(6): 513-9.
24. Øgard CG, Engholm G, Almdal TP, Vestergaard H. Increased mortality in patients hospitalized with primary hyperparathyroidism during the period 1977-1993 in Denmark. World J Surg. 2004;28(1):108-11.
25. Vestergaard P, Mollerup CL, Frøkjær VG, Christiansen P, Blichert-Toft M, Mosekilde L. Cardiovascular events before and after surgery for primary hyperparathyroidism. World J Surg. 2003;27(2):216-22.
26. Piovesan A, Molineri N, Casasso F, Emmolo I, Ugliengo G, Cesario F, et al. Left ventricular hypertrophy in primary hyperparathyroidism. Effects of successful parathyroidectomy. Clin Endocrinol. 1999;50(3):321-8.
27. Walker MD, Rundek T, Homma S, DiTullio M, Iwata S, Lee JA, et al. Effect of parathyroidectomy on subclinical cardiovascular disease in mild primary hyperparathyroidism. Eur J Endocrinol. 2012;167(2):277.
28. Wojtczak B, Syrycka J, Kaliszewski K, Rudnicki J, Bolanowski M, Barczyński M. Surgical implications of recent modalities for parathyroid imaging. Gland Surg. 2020;9(Suppl 2):S86.
29. Cheung K, Wang TS, Farrokhyar F, Roman SA, Sosa JA. A meta-analysis of preoperative localization techniques for patients with primary hyperparathyroidism. Ann Surg Oncol. 2012;19(2):577-83.
30. Morita SY, Somervell H, Umbricht CB, Dackiw AP, Zeiger MA. Evaluation for concomitant thyroid nodules and primary hyperparathyroidism in patients undergoing parathyroidectomy or thyroidectomy. Surgery. 2008;144(6): 862-7.
31. Adler JT, Chen H, Schaefer S, Sippel RS. Does routine use of ultrasound result in additional thyroid procedures in patients with primary hyperparathyroidism? J Am Coll Surg. 2010;211(4):536-9.
32. Ruda JM, Hollenbeak CS, Stack Jr BC. A systematic review of the diagnosis and treatment of primary hyperparathyroidism from 1995 to 2003. Otolaryngol Head Neck Surg. 2005;132(3): 359-72.
33. Kösem M, Algün E, Kotan C, Harman M, Öztürk M. Coexistent thyroid pathologies and high rate of papillary cancer in patients with primary hyperparathyroidism: controversies about minimal invasive parathyroid surgery. Acta Chirurgica Belgica. 2004;104(5):568-71.
34. Bentrem DJ, Angelos P, Talamonti MS, Nayar R. Is preoperative investigation of the thyroid justified in patients undergoing parathyroidectomy for hyperparathyroidism?. Thyroid. 2002; 12(12):1109-12.
35. Ryan S, Courtney D, Timon C. Co-existent thyroid disease in patients treated for primary hyperparathyroidism: implications for clinical management. Eur Arch Otorhinolaryngol. 2015;272(2):419-23.
36. Lubitz CC, Hunter GJ, Hamberg LM, Parangi S, Ruan D, Gawande A, et al. Accuracy of 4-dimensional computed tomography in poorly localized patients with primary hyperparathyroidism. Surgery. 2010;148(6):1129-38.
37. Starker LF, Mahajan A, Björklund P, Sze G, Udelsman R, Carling T. 4D parathyroid CT as the initial localization study for patients with de novo primary hyperparathyroidism. Ann Surg Oncol. 2011;18(6):1723-8.
38. Argirò R, Diacinti D, Sacconi B, Iannarelli A, Diacinti D, Cipriani C, et al. Diagnostic accuracy of 3T magnetic resonance imaging in the preoperative localisation of parathyroid adenomas: comparison with ultrasound and 99mTc-sestamibi scans. Eur Radiol. 2018;28(11):4900-8.
39. Jones JM, Russell CF, Ferguson WR, Laird JD. Pre-operative sestamibi-technetium subtraction scintigraphy in primary hyperparathyroidism: experience with 156 consecutive patients. Clin Radiol. 2001;56(7):556-9.
40. Mitchell J, Milas M, Barbosa G, Sutton J, Berber E, Siperstein A. Avoidable reoperations for thyroid and parathyroid surgery: effect of hospital volume. Surgery. 2008;144(6):899-907.
41. Beheshti M, Hehenwarter L, Paymani Z, Rendl G, Imamovic L, Rettenbacher R, et al. 18 F-Fluorocholine PET/CT in the

assessment of primary hyperparathyroidism compared with 99m Tc-MIBI or 99m Tc-tetrofosmin SPECT/CT: a prospective dual-centre study in 100 patients. Eur J Nucl Med Mol Imaging. 2018;45(10):1762-71.
42. Kluijfhout WP, Pasternak JD, Gosnell JE, Shen WT, Duh QY, Vriens MR, et al. 18F fluorocholine PET/MR imaging in patients with primary hyperparathyroidism and inconclusive conventional imaging: a prospective pilot study. Radiology. 2017;284(2):460-7.
43. Kendrick ML, Charboneau JW, Curlee KJ, Van Heerden JA. Risk of parathyromatosis after fine-needle aspiration/Discussion. Am Surg. 2001;67(3):290-3; discussion 293-4.
44. MacFarlane MP, Fraker DL, Shawker TH, Norton JA, Doppman JL, Chang RA, et al. Use of preoperative fine-needle aspiration in patients undergoing reoperation for primary hyperparathyroidism. Surgery. 1994;116(6):959-65.
45. Alwaheeb S, Rambaldini G, Boerner S, Coiré C, Fiser J, Asa SL. Worrisome histologic alterations following fine-needle aspiration of the parathyroid. J Clin Pathol. 2006;59(10):1094-6.
46. Ibraheem K, Toraih EA, Haddad AB, Farag M, Randolph GW, Kandil E. Selective parathyroid venous sampling in primary hyperparathyroidism: a systematic review and meta-analysis. Laryngoscope. 2018;128(11):2662-7.
47. Chaffanjon PC, Voirin D, Vasdev A, Chabre O, Kenyon NM, Brichon PY. Selective venous sampling in recurrent and persistent hyperparathyroidism: indication, technique, and results. World J Surg. 2004;28(10):958-61.
48. Reidel MA, Schilling T, Graf S, Hinz U, Nawroth P, Büchler MW, et al. Localization of hyperfunctioning parathyroid glands by selective venous sampling in reoperation for primary or secondary hyperparathyroidism. Surgery. 2006;140(6):907-13.
49. Arrangoiz R, Cordera F, Caba D, Juárez MM, Moreno E, Luque E. Parathyroid embryology, anatomy, and pathophysiology of primary hyperparathyroidism. Inter J Otolaryngol Head Neck Surg. 2017;6(4):39-58.
50. Randolph GW. Surgery of the thyroid and parathyroid glands: expert consult premium edition-enhanced online features and print. Philadelphia: Elsevier Health Sciences; 2012.
51. Taterra D, Wong LM, Vikse J, Sanna B, Pękala P, Walocha J, et al. The prevalence and anatomy of parathyroid glands: a meta-analysis with implications for parathyroid surgery. Langenbecks Arch Surg. 2019;404(1):63-70.
52. Locker FG, Silverberg SJ, Bilezikian JP. Optimal dietary calcium intake in primary hyperparathyroidism. Am J Med. 1997;102(6):543-50.
53. Shah VN, Shah CS, Bhadada SK, Rao DS. Effect of 25 (OH) D replacements in patients with primary hyperparathyroidism (PHPT) and coexistent vitamin D deficiency on serum 25 (OH) D, calcium and PTH levels: a meta-analysis and review of literature. Clin Endocrinol. 2014;80(6):797-803.
54. Rolighed L, Rejnmark L, Sikjaer T, Heickendorff L, Vestergaard P, Mosekilde L, et al. Vitamin D treatment in primary hyperparathyroidism: a randomized placebo controlled trial. J Clin Endocrinol Metab. 2014;99(3):1072-80.
55. Ahmad S, Kuraganti G, Steenkamp D. Hypercalcemic crisis: a clinical review. Am J Med. 2015;128(3):239-45.
56. Rubin MR, Bilezikian JP, McMahon DJ, Jacobs T, Shane E, Siris E, et al. The natural history of primary hyperparathyroidism with or without parathyroid surgery after 15 years. J Clin Endocrinol Metabol. 2008;93(9):3462-70.
57. Gordon DL, Airan MC, Thomas W, Seidman LH. Parathyroid identification by methylene blue infusion. Br J Surg. 1975;62(9):747-9.
58. Ito F, Sippel R, Lederman J, Chen H. The utility of intraoperative bilateral internal jugular venous sampling with rapid parathyroid hormone testing. Ann Surg. 2007;245(6):959.
59. Rubello D, Pelizzo MR, Boni G, Schiavo R, Vaggelli L, Villa G, et al. Radioguided surgery of primary hyperparathyroidism using the low-dose 99mTc-sestamibi protocol: multi-institutional experience from the Italian Study Group on Radioguided Surgery and Immunoscintigraphy (GISCRIS). J Nucl Med. 2005;46(2):220-6.
60. Norman J, Lopez J, Politz D. Abandoning unilateral parathyroidectomy: why we reversed our position after 15,000 parathyroid operations. J Am Coll Surg. 2012;214(3):260-9.
61. Udelsman R, Lin Z, Donovan P. The superiority of minimally invasive parathyroidectomy based on 1650 consecutive patients with primary hyperparathyroidism. Ann Surg. 2011;253(3):585-91.
62. Rajaei MH, Oltmann SC, Adkisson CD, Elfenbein DM, Chen H, Carty SE, et al. Is intraoperative parathyroid hormone monitoring necessary with ipsilateral parathyroid gland visualization during anticipated unilateral exploration for primary hyperparathyroidism: a two-institution analysis of more than 2,000 patients. Surgery. 2014;156(4):760-8.
63. Lee S, Ryu H, Morris LF, Grubbs EG, Lee JE, Harun N, Feng L, et al. Operative failure in minimally invasive parathyroidectomy utilizing an intraoperative parathyroid hormone assay. Ann Surg Oncol. 2014;21(6):1878-83.
64. Irvin III GL, Dembrow VD, Prudhomme DL. Operative monitoring of parathyroid gland hyperfunction. Am J Surg. 1991;162(4):299-302.
65. Irvin GL, Dembrow VD, Prudhomme DL. Clinical usefulness of an intraoperative "quick parathyroid hormone" assay. Surgery. 1993;114(6):1019-23.
66. Irvin GL, Solorzano CC, Carneiro DM. Quick intraoperative parathyroid hormone assay: surgical adjunct to allow limited parathyroidectomy, improve success rate, and predict outcome. World J Surg. 2004;28(12):1287-92.
67. Richards ML, Thompson GB, Farley DR, Grant CS. An optimal algorithm for intraoperative parathyroid hormone monitoring. Arch Surg. 2011;146(3):280-5.
68. Wharry LI, Yip L, Armstrong MJ, Virji MA, Stang MT, Carty SE, et al. The final intraoperative parathyroid hormone level: how low should it go? World J Surg. 2014;38(3):558-63.
69. Moalem J, Ruan DT, Farkas RL, Shen WT, Miller S, Duh QY, Clark OH, Kebebew E. Prospective evaluation of the rate and impact of hemolysis on intraoperative parathyroid hormone (IOPTH) assay results. Ann Surg Oncol. 2010;17(11):2963-9.
70. Carneiro-Pla D. Contemporary and Practical Uses of Intraoperative Parathyroid Hormone Monitoring. Endocr Pract. 2011;17(Suppl 1):44-53.
71. Moffett J, Suliburk J. Parathyroid autotransplantation. Endocr Pract. 2011;17(Suppl 1):83-9.
72. Feldman AL, Sharaf RN, Skarulis MC, Bartlett DL, Libutti SK, Weinstein LS, et al. Results of heterotopic parathyroid autotransplantation: a 13-year experience. Surgery. 1999;126(6):1042-8.
73. Guerrero MA. Cryopreservation of parathyroid glands. Int J Endocrinol. 2010;2010.
74. Allendorf J, DiGorgi M, Spanknebel K, Inabnet W, Chabot J, LoGerfo P. 1112 consecutive bilateral neck explorations for primary hyperparathyroidism. World J Surg. 2007;31(11):2075-80.

75. Del Valle HB, Yaktine AL, Taylor CL, Ross AC (Eds). Dietary reference intakes for calcium and vitamin D. Washington (DC):National Academies Press; 2011.
76. Brennan MF, Norton JA. Reoperation for persistent and recurrent hyperparathyroidism. Ann Surg. 1985;201(1):40.
77. Udelsman R, Donovan PI. Remedial parathyroid surgery: changing trends in 130 consecutive cases. Ann Surg. 2006; 244(3):471.
78. Thakker RV. Multiple endocrine neoplasia type 1 (MEN1) and type 4 (MEN4). Mol Cell Endocrinol. 2014;386(1-2): 2-15.
79. Thakker RV, Newey PJ, Walls GV, Bilezikian J, Dralle H, Ebeling PR, et al. Clinical practice guidelines for multiple endocrine neoplasia type 1 (MEN1). J Clin Endocrinol Metabol. 2012;97(9):2990-3011.
80. Mizusawa N, Uchino S, Iwata T, Tsuyuguchi M, Suzuki Y, Mizukoshi T, et al. Genetic analyses in patients with familial isolated hyperparathyroidism and hyperparathyroidism-jaw tumour syndrome. Clin Endocrinol. 2006;65(1):9-16.
81. Chen JD, Morrison C, Zhang C, Kahnoski K, Carpten JD, Teh BT. Hyperparathyroidism-jaw tumour syndrome. J Intern Med. 2003;253(6):634-42.
82. Ji YB, Song CM, Sung ES, Jeong JH, Lee CB, Tae K. Postoperative hypoparathyroidism and the viability of the parathyroid glands during thyroidectomy. Clinical Exp Otorhinolaryngol. 2017;10(3):265.
83. Dedivitis RA, Aires FT, Cernea CR. Hypoparathyroidism after thyroidectomy: prevention, assessment and management. Curr Opin Otolaryngol Head Neck Surg. 2017;25(2):142-6.
84. Kakava K, Tournis S, Papadakis G, Karelas I, Stampouloglou P, Kassi E, et al. Postsurgical hypoparathyroidism: a systematic review. In Vivo. 2016;30(3):171-9.
85. Orloff LA, Wiseman SM, Bernet VJ, Fahey III TJ, Shaha AR, Shindo ML, et al; American Thyroid Association Surgical Affairs Committee Writing Task Force. American thyroid association statement on postoperative hypoparathyroidism: diagnosis, prevention, and management in adults. Thyroid. 2018;28(7):830-41.
86. Mannstadt M, Clarke BL, Vokes T, Brandi ML, Ranganath L, Fraser WD, et al. Efficacy and safety of recombinant human parathyroid hormone (1-84) in hypoparathyroidism (REPLACE): a double-blind, placebo-controlled, randomised, phase 3 study. Lancet Diab Endocrinol. 2013;1(4):275-83.
87. Obara T, Fujimoto Y. Diagnosis and treatment of patients with parathyroid carcinoma: an update and review. World J Surg. 1991;15(6):738-44.
88. Rodrigo JP, Hernandez-Prera JC, Randolph GW, Zafereo ME, Hartl DM, Silver CE, et al. Parathyroid cancer: an update. Cancer Treatment Reviews. 2020:102012.
89. Pandya C, Uzilov AV, Bellizzi J, Lau CY, Moe AS, Strahl M, et al. Genomic profiling reveals mutational landscape in parathyroid carcinomas. JCI Insight. 2017;2(6).
90. Yu W, McPherson JR, Stevenson M, van Eijk R, Heng HL, Newey P, et al. Whole-exome sequencing studies of parathyroid carcinomas reveal novel PRUNE2 mutations, distinctive mutational spectra related to APOBEC-catalyzed DNA mutagenesis and mutational enrichment in kinases associated with cell migration and invasion. J Clin Endocrinol Metab. 2015;100(2):E360-4.
91. Schantz A, Castleman B. Parathyroid carcinoma. A study of 70 cases. Cancer. 1973;31(3):600-5.
92. Bondeson L, Sandelin K, Grimelius L. Histopathological variables and DNA cytometry in parathyroid carcinoma. Am J Surg Path. 1993;17(8):820-9.
93. Erickson LA, Mete O. Immunohistochemistry in diagnostic parathyroid pathology. Endocr Pathol. 2018;29(2):113-29.
94. Nam M, Jeong HS, Shin JH. Differentiation of parathyroid carcinoma and adenoma by preoperative ultrasonography. Acta Radiol. 2017;58(6):670-5.
95. Hara H, Igarishi A, Yano Y, Yashiro T, Ueno E, Aiyoshi Y, Ito K, Obara T. Ultrasonographic features of parathyroid carcinoma. Endocr J. 2001;48(2):213-7.
96. Zhang M, Sun L, Rui W, Guo R, He H, Miao Y, et al. Semi-quantitative analysis of 99mTc-sestamibi retention level for preoperative differential diagnosis of parathyroid carcinoma. Quant Imaging Med Surg. 2019;9(8):1394-401.
97. Agarwal G, Dhingra S, Mishra SK, Krishnani N. Implantation of parathyroid carcinoma along fine needle aspiration track. Langenbecks ArchSurg. 2006;391(6):623-6.
98. Shaha AR, Shah JP. Parathyroid carcinoma. A diagnostic and therapeutic challenge. Cancer. 1999;86:378-80.
99. Xue S, Chen H, Lv C, Shen X, Ding J, Liu J, Chen X. Preoperative diagnosis and prognosis in 40 parathyroid carcinoma patients. Clin Endocrinol. 2016;85(1):29-36.
100. Asare EA, Sturgeon C, Winchester DJ, Liu L, Palis B, Perrier ND, et al. Parathyroid carcinoma: an update on treatment outcomes and prognostic factors from the National Cancer Data Base (NCDB). Ann Surg Oncol. 2015;22(12):3990-5.
101. Hsu KT, Sippel RS, Chen H, Schneider DF. Is central lymph node dissection necessary for parathyroid carcinoma? Surgery. 2014;156(6):1336-41.
102. Silva-Figueroa AM, Hess KR, Williams MD, Clarke CN, Christakis I, Graham PH, et al. Prognostic scoring system to risk stratify parathyroid carcinoma. J Am Coll Surg. 2017; 224(5):980-7.
103. Rozhinskaya L, Pigarova E, Sabanova E, Mamedova E, Voronkova I, Krupinova J, et al. Diagnosis and treatment challenges of parathyroid carcinoma in a 27-year-old woman with multiple lung metastases. Endocrinol Diabetes Metab Case Rep. 2017;2017:16-0113.
104. Akirov A, Asa SL, Larouche V, Mete O, Sawka AM, Jang R, et al. The Clinicopathological Spectrum of Parathyroid Carcinoma. Front Endocrinol. 2019;10:731.
105. Harari A, Waring A, Fernandez-Ranvier G, Hwang J, Suh I, Mitmaker E, et al. Parathyroid carcinoma: a 43-year outcome and survival analysis. J Clin Endocrinol Metabol. 2011;96(12):3679-86.
106. Berenson JR. Treatment of hypercalcemia of malignancy with bisphosphonates. Semin Oncol. 2002;29(6):12-8.
107. Sadler C, Gow KW, Beierle EA, Doski JJ, Langer M, Nuchtern JG, et al. Parathyroid carcinoma in more than 1,000 patients: a population-level analysis. Surgery. 2014;156(6): 1622-30.
108. Villar-del-Moral J, Jiménez-García A, Salvador-Egea P, Martos-Martínez JM, Nuño-Vázquez-Garza JM, Serradilla-Martín M, et al. Prognostic factors and staging systems in parathyroid cancer: a multicenter cohort study. Surgery. 2014; 156(5):1132-44.

CHAPTER 25

Sarcomas of the Head and Neck

Vidita Powle, Narayana Subramaniam, Samskruthi P Murthy, Sivakumar Vidhyadharan

INTRODUCTION

Head and neck sarcomas are uncommon neoplasms that arise from mesenchymal elements that account for <1% of all adult tumors. They are a diverse group of malignancies that usually arise from soft tissue bone and cartilage. With over forty subtypes, they can have variable biological behavior, ranging from slow growing indolent tumors with low potential for recurrence to aggressive malignancies with high metastatic potential and poor survival even with multimodal treatment. In this chapter, we describe the management of head and neck sarcomas and the evidence on which it is based.

EPIDEMIOLOGY

Head and neck sarcomas account for 2% of all head and neck malignancies, <10% of sarcomas in the adult and around a third of all pediatric sarcomas.[1,2] Data from the Indian subcontinent is sparse, but shows similar epidemiology.[3] They can present at almost any age; patients with angiosarcomas most often present in the sixth decade of life, while those with rhabdomyosarcomas (RMS) present in the first decade of life.[4] Most series show a slight male preponderance.[5] As these tumors arise from connective tissue elements they are ubiquitous and can arise from virtually any site in the head and neck; clinical features, natural history, and treatment are determined by histology.

ETIOLOGY (TABLE 1)

In a majority of cases, the etiology is poorly understood. Genetic alterations and germline mutations can be associated with sarcomas, and may be associated with

Table 1: Etiologic factors in head and neck sarcomas.[15,16]

Genetic predisposition	*Gene/genes*	*Sarcoma/sarcomas*
Li-Fraumeni syndrome	*TP53*	Bony and soft tissue sarcomas
Hereditary retinoblastoma	*Rb*	Osteosarcoma
DMS-MFH	*LOH at 9p21-22*	Malignant fibrous histiocytoma (MFH)
Werner syndrome	*WMN*	Bony and soft tissue sarcomas
Gardner syndrome	*APC*	Desmoid tumors
Neurofibromatosis type 1	*NF1*	MPNST
Costello syndrome	*HRAS*	Rhabdomyosarcoma
Beckwith-Wiedemann syndrome	*CDKN1, IGF2, H19, KCNQ1OT1*	Rhabdomyosarcoma
Rothmund-Thomson syndrome	*RECQL4*	Osteosarcoma
Paget's disease	Unknown	Osteosarcoma
Ollier and Maffucci syndrome	*IDH1, IDH2*	Chondrosarcoma
Environmental exposure	*Sarcoma/sarcomas*	
Ionizing radiation	Bony and soft tissue sarcomas	
HIV, HHV-8	Kaposi sarcoma	
Industrial waste	Bony and soft tissue sarcomas	
Herbicides and chlorophenols	Bony and soft tissue sarcomas	

Table 2: Sarcomas with their corresponding chromosomal aberrations and fusion genes.[8]

Type of sarcoma	*Chromosomal aberration*	*Fusion gene*
Alveolar rhabdomyosarcoma	t(1;13)(p36;q14) t(2;13)(q36;q14)	*PAX7-FOXO1* *PAX3-FOXO1*
Alveolar soft part sarcoma	t(X;17)(p11;q25)	*ASPSCR1-TFE3*
Angiomatoid fibrous histiocytoma	t(2;22)(q33;q12)	*EWSR1-CREB1*
Clear cell sarcoma	t(12;22)(q13;q12)	*EWSR1-ATF1*
Dermatofibrosarcoma protuberans	t(17;22)(q22;q13)	*COL1A1-PDGFB*
Desmoplastic small round cell tumor	t(11;22)(p13;q12)	*EWSR1-WT1*
Ewing sarcoma family	t(11;22)(q24;q12) ins(21;22)(q22;q12) t(16;21)(p11;q22)	*EWSR1-FLI1* *EWSR1-ERG* *FUS-ERG*
Fibromyxoid sarcoma	t(7;16)(q34;p11)	*FUS-CREB3L2*
Myxoid liposarcoma	t(12;16)(q13;p11) t(12;22)(q13;p12)	*FUS-DDIT3* *EWSR1-DDIT3*
Synovial sarcoma	t(X;18)(p11;q11)	*SS18-SSX*

syndromes such as Li-Fraumeni and neurofibromatosis type I.[6] Li-Fraumeni syndrome is an autosomal dominant disorder resulting from a germline mutation in the p53 tumor suppressor gene, which can also result in breast and central nervous system malignancies, and leukemias. Neurofibromatosis type I is associated with a 10% cumulative lifetime risk of developing malignant peripheral nerve sheath tumors (MPSNT), which usually occur later in adulthood.[7] Gardner's syndrome, nevoid basal cell carcinoma syndrome, Carney's triad, and Werner syndrome have also been associated with soft tissue sarcomas (STS). Up to 20% of patients with sarcomas have identifiable chromosomal translocations, which represent an insult occurring as early as at the stem cell level.[8] These fusion genes can act as diagnosis and serve as potential therapeutic targets.[9] A list of sarcomas, their chromosomal aberrations, and fusion genes is shown in **Table 2**. Environmental exposure has also been associated with sarcoma, including ionizing radiation and chemical exposure. Previous radiotherapy (RT) to the head and neck has been demonstrated to be a risk for developing sarcomas,[9-11] which is a distinct subtype discussed subsequently. Chemical exposure to phenoxyacetic acids and chlorophenols as insecticides has shown to be associated with sarcomas.[12] Occupational chemical exposure with thorotrast, vinyl chloride, and arsenic have also been linked to the risk of developing sarcomas.[13] Chemotherapy with alkylating agents for pediatric cancers also increases the risk of sarcomas. Human herpes virus 8 on a background of human immunodeficiency virus and acquired immune deficiency syndrome (HIV-AIDS) is associated with Kaposi's sarcoma,[14] which is pathognomonic of this infection. In spite of multiple identified causes, only a fraction is associated with these risk factors, with the remaining cases believed to occur due to a complex interaction between genetic susceptibility and environmental exposure.

CLASSIFICATION

The classification of sarcomas is based on the tissue of origin—approximately 80% arise in the soft tissue and 20% in the bone. The classification is as shown in **Table 3**.

CLINICAL FEATURES

Early detection of lesions leads to improved survival, which forms the basis of screening in at-risk individuals, as described later in the chapter. However, diagnosis is often delayed due to presentation with nonspecific symptoms such as jaw swelling or neck lumps in young adults or older patients with no traditional risk factors for malignancy, such as smoking or alcohol intake. Patients can present at virtually any age. Presentation depends on the site of origin of these tumors and the histological subtype. Soft tissue sarcomas often present as painless neck masses, producing symptoms only due to intrinsic compression or local invasion, such as hoarseness, dysphagia or dyspnea. They can also present as scalp lesions, lesions in the subcutaneous tissues of the face, orbital lesions resulting in proptosis, poor vision and swelling, or lesions of the nasal cavity, paranasal sinuses, and skull-base resulting in epistaxis, nasal obstruction or headache. Bony tumors often arise in the maxilla or mandible, resulting in bony expansion, pain, and loosening of teeth. Around 10% of patients have metastases at diagnosis, most often to the lungs, liver, and bone.[18] A 34-year review of MD Anderson data

Table 3: WHO classification of common head and neck sarcomas based on origin.[17]

Tissue type	*Tumor*
Soft tissue sarcomas	
Adipocyte	Liposarcoma (well-differentiated or atypical lipomatous tumor, myxoid, dedifferentiated or pleomorphic)
Fibroblasts and myofibroblasts	Fibrosarcoma (adult and infantile subtypes), myxofibrosarcoma, dermatofibrosarcoma protuberans, extrapleural solitary fibrous tumor
Skeletal muscle	Rhabdomyosarcoma (embryonal, alveolar, pleomorphic, spindle cell, and sclerosing subtypes)
Smooth muscle	Leiomyosarcoma
Vascular elements	Angiosarcoma, Kaposi sarcoma
Nerve sheath elements	Malignant peripheral nerve sheath tumor
Uncertain origin	Synovial sarcoma, alveolar soft part sarcoma
Undifferentiated and unclassified elements	Undifferentiated sarcoma (spindle cell, pleomorphic, round cell, epithelioid, not otherwise specified subtypes)
Bone sarcomas	
Osteogenic elements	Osteosarcoma (conventional, low grade central, telangiectatic, small cell, parosteal, periosteal, high grade surface, extraskeletal subtypes)
Chondrogenic elements	Chondrosarcoma (conventional, dedifferentiated, mesenchymal, clear cell subtypes)
Primitive neuro-ectodermal elements	Ewing sarcoma

comprising over a thousand one hundred patients of head and neck sarcomas show the most common sites of origin were scalp or face (30%), sinonasal tract or anterior skull base (30%), parotid gland and neck (19%), and oral cavity and pharynx (18%).[19] The general principles of management are discussed in general, followed by individual subtypes **(Fig. 1A and B)**.

PATHOLOGY

Head and neck sarcomas are an extremely heterogeneous and diverse group of malignancies with an often indistinct presentation, resulting in the onus of diagnosis falling on the pathologist. Although well-established and studied subtypes exist, there are some very rare variants, necessitating the involvement of experienced specialists in these patients' care. Soft tissue sarcomas are classified based on their lineage, as shown in **Table 3**. In general, soft tissue sarcomas of the head and neck have a lower metastatic potential than elsewhere in

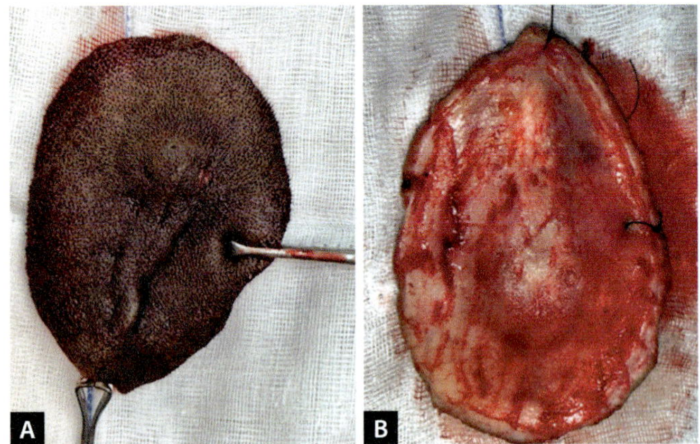

Figs. 1A and B: Dermatofibrosarcoma of the scalp viewed from above (A) and below (B).

the body, and hence have a reasonable chance of cure, if treated appropriately. Bone tumors are most often osteosarcoma and chondrosarcoma, however Ewing's sarcoma and other rare tumors can also occur. Fine-needle aspiration (FNA) of the lesion may be sufficient for establishing a diagnosis by an experienced pathologist, but more often a core needle biopsy under local anesthesia is required. This has the advantage of allowing immunohistochemistry and cytogenetic testing. In 10% of cases, where even repeat core needle biopsy is insufficient to establish a diagnosis, open biopsy is required.[20] In doing so, it is vital to observe oncological principles and avoid tumor seeding; the path to the tumor should be excised in subsequent resection or identifiable for RT planning. Second opinions from pathologists experienced in sarcoma evaluation may prove invaluable.

STAGING

The two important staging systems established for sarcomas are the American Joint Cancer Committee (AJCC)/Union for International Cancer Control (UICC) 8th edition staging system **(Table 4)** and the Memorial Sloan-Kettering Staging System (**Table 5**). In the AJCC system for STS, unlike with other tumors, grade (G), mitotic count and tumor necrosis are of paramount importance, which is a reflection that tumor biology in this group of tumors can be highly variable and is arguably the single most important prognostic determinant. In bone tumors the AJCC system depends on size criteria and grade.

The AJCC 8th edition was shown to better prognosticate patients than the previous edition by an analysis of over thousand seven hundred patients of STS in the SEER (Surveillance Epidemiology End Results) database.[21]

Table 4: AJCC 8th edition staging of head and neck soft tissue sarcomas.

Tx	Primary tumor cannot be assessed
T1	Tumor ≤2 cm
T2	Tumor >2 to ≤4 cm
T3	Tumor >4 cm
T4a	Tumor with orbital invasion, skull base or dura invasion, invasion of central compartment viscera, involvement of facial skeleton or invasion of pterygoid muscles
T4b	Tumor with brain parenchymal invasion, carotid artery encasement, prevertebral muscle invasion or central nervous system involvement via perineural spread
Nx	Regional lymph nodes cannot be assessed
N0	No nodal metastasis
N1	Regional lymph node metastasis
M0	No metastases
M1	Metastatic disease
GX	Grade cannot be assessed
G1	Total differentiation, mitotic count and necrosis score of 2–3
G2	Total differentiation, mitotic count, and necrosis score of 4–5
G3	Total differentiation, mitotic count, and necrosis score of 6–8
Tumor differentiation	
1	Sarcomas resemble normal adult mesenchymal tissue (e.g., low-grade leiomyosarcoma)
2	Sarcomas for which histologic typing is certain (e.g., myxoid/round cell liposarcoma)
3	Embryonal and undifferentiated sarcomas, sarcomas of doubtful type, synovial sarcomas soft tissue osteosarcomas, Ewing's/primitive neuroectodermal tumors
Mitotic count	
1	0–9 mitoses per 10 high power fields
2	10–19 mitoses per 10 high power fields
3	≥20 mitoses per 10 high power fields
Tumor necrosis	
0	No necrosis
1	<50% tumor necrosis
2	≥50% tumor necrosis

Table 5: Memorial Sloan-Kettering staging for soft tissue sarcomas.[22]

Characteristic	*Favorable*	*Unfavorable*
Size (cm)	<5 cm	>5 cm
Depth of invasion	Superficial	Deep
Grade	Low	High
Stage grouping	*Characteristic signs*	
Stage 0	3 favorable signs	
Stage I	2 favorable signs	
Stage II	1 unfavorable sign/1 favorable sign + 2 unfavorable signs	
Stage III	3 unfavorable signs	
Stage IV	Distant metastases	

Table 6: AJCC 8th edition staging for head and neck bone sarcomas.

Tx	Primary tumor cannot be assessed
T0	No evidence of primary tumor
T1	Tumor ≤8 cm in greatest dimension
T2	Tumor >8 cm in greatest dimension
T3	Discontinuous tumors in the primary bone site
Nx	Regional lymph nodes cannot be assessed
N0	No nodal metastasis
N1	Regional lymph node metastasis
M0	No metastases
M1a	Lung metastasis
M1b	Bone or other distant metastasis
GX	Grade cannot be assessed
G1	Well differentiated—low grade
G2	Moderately differentiated—high grade
G3	Poorly differentiated—high grade

This has been shown to be a reliable alternative to the AJCC/UICC staging system **(Table 6)** and has been validated in head and neck STS.[23] Understanding that STS are a diverse group of disorders, the current philosophy is that nomograms are a better way to prognosticate patients, since unlike in other tumors, the need for adjuvant therapy is not dictated by staging.[24]

A size cutoff of 8 cm has been derived from data pertaining to bony sarcomas occurring all over the body;[25] 8 cm bony tumors in the head and neck are very rare. Hence, validations of this staging system in the head and neck are lacking.

IMAGING

Cross-sectional imaging forms a vital part of establishing the diagnosis and staging. Contrast-enhanced computed tomography (CECT) is often the first-line investigation in evaluation of most head and neck tumors. In bony sarcomas, it can identify the origin of the lesion, whether it is the sinus, maxilla, mandible or skull bones. Local invasion to surrounding tissues, intracranial and orbital invasion can be identified. In soft tissue tumors, the origin and extent of lesions can be identified. Large, solitary superficial masses without lymphadenopathy in those with risk factors (genetic susceptibility or previous irradiation) were the most reliable imaging findings in STS of the head and neck.[26] Calcifications are also an important sign associated

Table 7: National Comprehensive Cancer Network (NCCN) approach to evaluation of head and neck sarcomas.[27]

Feature	*Sarcoma*
Imaging features	
Calcified or calcified matrix	Liposarcoma, leiomyosarcoma, synovial sarcoma, undifferentiated sarcoma, osteosarcoma, chondrosarcoma, Ewing's sarcoma
Secondary osseous destruction	Myxofibrosarcoma, rhabdomyosarcoma, synovial sarcoma, undifferentiated sarcoma, osteosarcoma, chondrosarcoma, Ewing's sarcoma
Predominantly cyst-like (high water content)	Myxoid liposarcoma, myxofibrosarcoma
Intense enhancement or flow voids	Solitary fibrous tumor, angiosarcoma, Kaposi's sarcoma, alveolar soft part sarcoma
Intrinsic T1 hyper-intensity to skeletal muscle	Well-differentiated liposarcoma and atypical lipomatous tumor, alveolar soft part sarcoma
Patient age	
Infant	Infantile fibrosarcoma
Child, adolescent, young adult	Rhabdomyosarcoma, synovial sarcoma, alveolar soft part sarcoma, Ewing's sarcoma
Associated clinical findings	
Superficial and subcutaneous lesions	Infantile fibrosarcoma, dermatofibrosarcoma protuberans, leiomyosarcoma, angiosarcoma, Kaposi's sarcoma
Paranasal sinus involvement	Adult fibrosarcoma, rhabdomyosarcoma, leiomyosarcoma, undifferentiated sarcoma, solitary fibrous tumor
History of radiotherapy	Leiomyosarcoma, angiosarcoma, undifferentiated sarcoma, osteosarcoma, fibrosarcoma
Trauma (e.g., tattoo sites)	Dermatofibrosarcoma protuberans
Neurofibromatosis type I	Rhabdomyosarcoma, angiosarcoma, malignant peripheral nerve sheath tumor
Systemic symptoms or paraneoplastic syndrome	Solitary fibrous tumor, Ewing's sarcoma
AIDS	Kaposi's sarcoma, leiomyosarcoma

with STS. Magnetic resonance imaging (MRI) with intravenous gadolinium-based contrast can complement CT findings. The standard MRI sequences are T1- and T2-weighted sequences with fat suppressed T2 or short tau inversion recovery (STIR) sequences. Diffusion-weighted imaging can also provide insight into cellularity and presence of calcification or hemorrhage in the tumor. Screening for distant metastases is important in advanced stage or high-grade tumors; this can be performed with CT of the thorax or the abdomen, to identify deposits in the lungs or liver. Positron emission tomography with CECT (PET CT) is a reasonable alternative for evaluation of the whole body. Technetium scintigraphy is a good tool for evaluation of the skeleton for multiple bony metastases in histologies such as Ewing's sarcoma. An approach to imaging as described by the National Comprehensive Cancer Network (NCCN) is shown in **Table 7**.

OUTCOMES

The prognostic determinants in head and neck sarcomas can be classified in to tumor-related factors, biological factors, molecular factors, and patient-related factors.[28] The tumor-related factors are size, subsite, depth, and margin status after resection. Biological factors include grade and hypoxia, while molecular factors include p53 status, Ki-67 expression, Rb products, and presence of fusion genes. Patient factors include age, comorbidities, and previous irradiation.[28-30] Grade and tumor margins have consistently been shown as the most significant prognostic factors.[19,20,31,32] The pooled results of a meta-analysis of 1,120 patients showed that head and neck STS had a 5-year overall survival of 75% and disease-free survival of around 50%.[33] Results for the Head and Neck Sarcoma Registry reported the long-term results of over 200 patients, noting that histologies such as dermatofibrosarcoma protuberans and chondrosarcoma had nearly 100% survival, while malignant fibrous histiocytoma or fibrosarcoma had a survival of 60–70%, and survival <50% was seen in osteosarcoma, angiosarcoma, RMS, and malignant peripheral nerve sheath tumors.[34] Distant metastasis occurs in 10–30% of patients, lower than those with sarcomas in the extremities, which may be because of biological differences in these tumors or because of the earlier presentation from disruption of head and neck cosmesis or function.[35]

PRINCIPLES OF MANAGEMENT

The major challenge to head and neck sarcomas is the inability to deliver aggressive local therapy (surgery and RT) due to the proximity to critical anatomical structures. For lesions without evidence of distant metastasis, complete surgical excision is the primary modality of choice in most histologies. The role of adjuvant RT and chemotherapy is based on randomized clinical trials that often had limited representation from patients with head and neck tumors. In view of this relative paucity of evidence, multidisciplinary care is important to ensure optimal outcomes. Additionally, when use of one modality has limitations (surgical resection at the skull base), complementary use of other modalities

Flowchart 1: Approach to head and neck sarcoma.

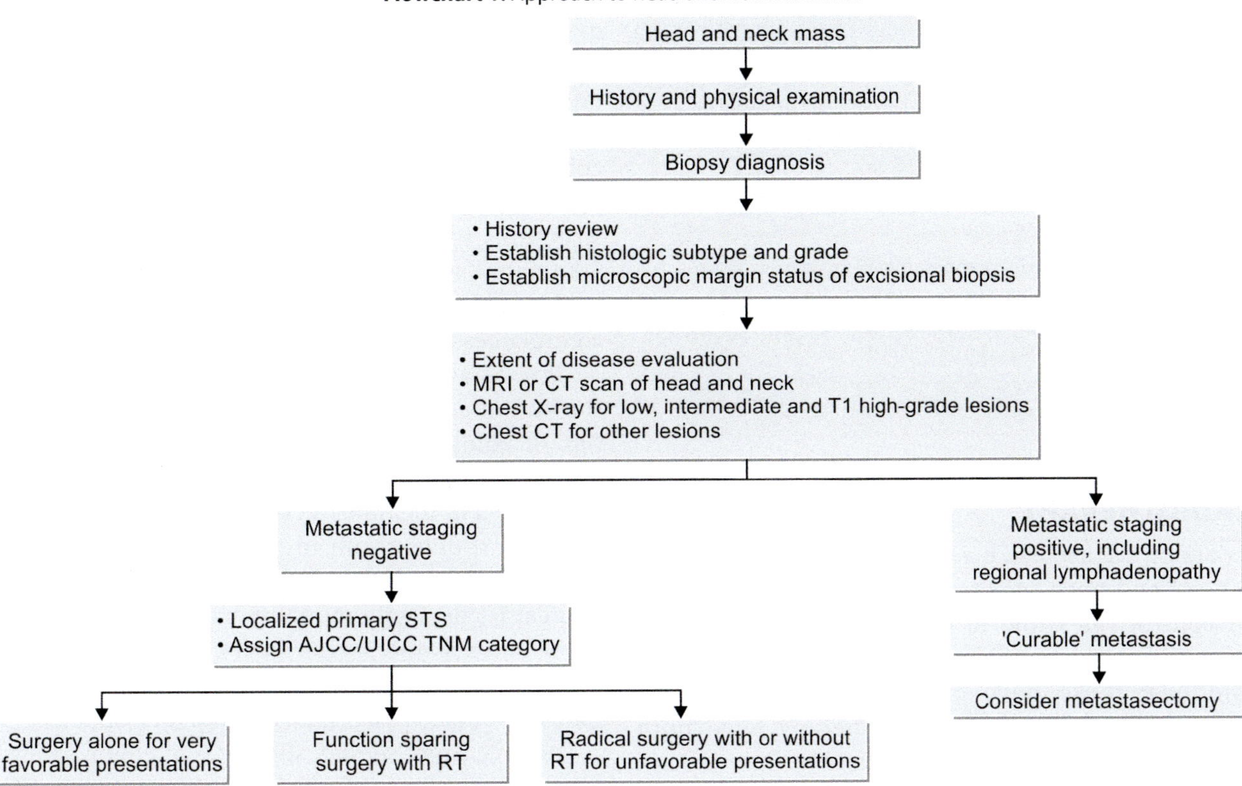

(adjuvant RT) can ensure favorable outcomes; hence early and coordinated involvement of oncologists is vital. An algorithm for management is shown in **Flowchart 1**.

SURGERY

Surgery remains the most common frequent treatment in head and neck sarcomas.[35] The goal of surgery is to achieve an en bloc resection with circumferential margins. The zones of excision in a sarcoma, as shown in **Figure 2**, are the tumor, the reactive zone or pseudocapsule, which contains compressed tumor cells and a fibrovascular zone of reactive inflammatory cells, and the normal zone. Excisions though the pseudocapsule result in a high probability of local recurrence. With time, the recommended margins have reduced; the current recommendation is to aim for margins of 2 cm wherever feasible, but in many subsites of the head and neck, such as the skull base this is not feasible.[36] Hence adequate clearance refers to resection as wide as permitted by surrounding vital structures, commonly accepted as a 1 cm margin, or an anatomical clearance of the next uninvolved anatomical barrier.[27] The standard terms used to describe resections are R0 (microscopically negative margins), R1 (microscopically positive margins), and R2 (grossly positive margins).

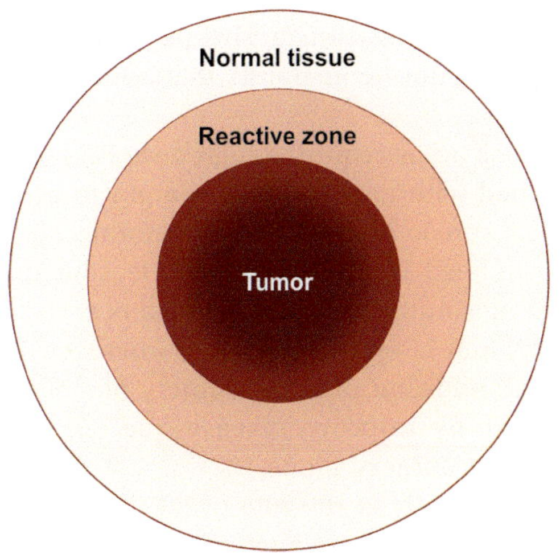

Fig. 2: Zones of excision in a soft tissue sarcoma.

Neck dissection is indicated only when there is evidence of nodal metastasis, which has been demonstrated in RMS, angiosarcoma, clear cell sarcoma, epithelioid sarcoma, malignant fibrous histiocytoma, and synovial sarcoma. Elective neck dissection is not indicated in the absence of nodal spread.

Locally recurrent disease should be resected whenever feasible. An approach to adjuvant therapy in locally recurrent disease is shown in **Table 8**.

Table 8: Approach to locally recurrent sarcomas of the head and neck.[18]

Context	*Approach*
No prior chemotherapy or radiotherapy	Consider combined approach with external beam radiotherapy. In osteosarcoma, consider induction chemotherapy
Prior radiotherapy	Consider combined approach with brachytherapy
Critical structure involvement	Consider preoperative RT or ablative approach
In presence of metastases	If multiple, palliative treatment with aggressive local therapy If few resectable metastatic lesion consider metastatectomy or stereotactic RT

RADIOTHERAPY

The data on RT use has been extrapolated largely from non-head and neck subsites. Historical data had poor local control rates due to dosage constraints in the head and neck; however with improved RT delivery techniques, these have improved. External beam radiotherapy (EBRT) and brachytherapy have both been used in the treatment of head and neck sarcomas. Brachytherapy is more invasive; however treatment times are shorter, typically 4–6 days. EBRT in an adjuvant setting typically uses 60 and 66 Gy in the low and high-risk groups respectively, using a 'shrinking field' technique and the usual dose constraints that apply to head and neck RT.

High-risk areas requiring high dose RT includes the surgical bed with an additional margin to account for subclinical spread of disease; in extremities this is 5 cm, however in head and neck this is not feasible due to the potential morbidity of irradiating organs at risk in close proximity, and is reduced to 2 cm wherever feasible.[37] In general, addition of RT to surgery has been shown to significantly improve disease-free survival when compared to surgery alone (87 vs. 45%).[38] Two trials looked specifically at the role of RT with conservative surgical excision. The National Cancer Institute trial randomized extremity STS to receive either conservative limb-sparing surgery alone or conservative limb-sparing surgery with adjuvant RT, with chemotherapy used depending on the grade. They found local control rates were significantly better with RT (99 vs. 70%).[39] A trial by Memorial Sloan-Kettering Cancer Center evaluated adjuvant brachytherapy used after resection of STS in the extremities and superficial trunk, showing that adjuvant brachytherapy only significantly improved local control in high-grade lesions (89 vs. 66%); disease-specific survival and distant metastasis rates were comparable.[37]

In cases where resections are associated with positive margins (R1/2) or high-grade lesions, adjuvant RT has been shown to significantly improve local control rates in retrospective data.[38,40,41] Local control rates in this setting improved from 25 to 54%[42] or 75%[38] in two cohorts. It has also been shown in limb STS that a planned R1/R2 resection due to proximity to critical structures when administered with adjuvant RT was associated with better results, while an unplanned R1/R2 resection resulting in positive margins had poor control rates even after adjuvant RT.[43]

Preoperative RT is another approach that has been shown to be effective with STS with a potentially lower risk of complications and good local control rates.[44] This is attributed to lower doses (50 Gy), better tissue oxygenated in the undissected bed and smaller field size; however, it does result in higher wound complication rates.[44] This is being offered only in some centers. Radical RT as a sole modality has been shown to have a low efficacy; the 5-year local control rate in patients with tumors <5 cm was around 50%[45] and should not be routinely offered as a primary therapeutic option.

In a recurrent setting, surgery is offered whenever an adequate resection is feasible. In oligometastatic disease involving the lung with a good disease-free interval (>2 years), pulmonary metastatectomy may be considered if complete excision is likely. All other sites of distant metastasis are deemed incurable barring soft tissue metastasis in liposarcoma.

CHEMOTHERAPY

Given the distant metastasis risk, chemotherapy has been studied extensively; however due to the heterogeneity in data available and a lack of consistency in results, its role is still not well established. The Sarcoma Meta-Analysis Collaboration analyzed individual patient data from 14 clinical trials comprising over one and a half thousand patients with resectable STS and concluded that doxorubicin-based chemotherapy improved times to local recurrence and distant metastasis with a trend toward improved overall survival.[46] Other trials have shown similar results, with pooled results showing a modest, nonsignificant improvement in overall survival (54 vs. 50%).[47-49] In contrast, a literature-based meta-analysis by Pervaiz et al. comprising nearly 2,000 patients showed an absolute overall survival benefit of 6% in favor of chemotherapy with doxorubicin and ifosfamide (46 vs. 40%), which was significant.[50] It is to be noted here, however, that short-term and long-term toxicity associated with these two agents necessitates a significant survival benefit to justify their use, except in nonpleomorphic RMS and Ewing's sarcoma, where the role of multiagent chemotherapy is well established.

Induction chemotherapy has also been of significant interest, with the intention of shrinking tumor size allowing less intensive local therapies. Although some series have demonstrated their success, survival impact is doubtful and the risk benefit ratio is unclear, making their role in resectable disease unclear. Induction chemotherapy should be considered in inoperable locally advanced tumors where shrinking the tumor would make an R0/R1 resection more likely or prevent mutilation; a high percentage of tumor necrosis may indicate a favorable prognosis.[51]

In metastatic disease, systemic treatment is most commonly preferred. A meta-analysis showed that single agent doxorubicin is the optimal therapy for metastatic disease.[52] Pazopanib, a novel tyrosine kinase inhibitor, has also showed improvement in overall and disease-free survival in a metastatic setting.[53]

Individual subtypes:

- *Angiosarcoma:* These are rare sarcomas that arise from endothelial cells. They can present at any age in any location, however they are commonly seen in elderly white males (seventh or eight decades of life) as violaceous macules or papules on the scalp. They commonly mimic benign lesions such as bruises or benign vascular lesions. They can often have diffuse involvement beyond the visible extent. Satellite nodules can occur in half of patients and are associated with poor prognosis. Nodal involvement can occur but is still rare (6–10%). Distant metastasis occurs in 36–77%. Angiosarcomas occurring in the head and neck have a worse prognosis than those occurring elsewhere (5-year overall survival of 34 vs. 64%). Multimodal treatment with surgery and RT offer the best chance of local control and survival. R0 resection can be different because of early and diffuse involvement of surrounding tissues. There is an argument against complex reconstruction that may postpone RT, as they may adversely impact survival. Limited evidence is available to support chemotherapy use; however induction taxane-based chemotherapy followed by RT or limited excision has shown promising results.[54-57]
- *Kaposi's sarcoma:* This is locally aggressive endothelial sarcoma associated with human herpesvirus-8 (HHV-8). Several different types are recognized, including classic, endemic, iatrogenic, and AIDS-associated, of which the latter is the most common in the head and neck. They present as multiple purple to brown violaceous patches that may form plaques or nodules on the skin, hard palate or oropharynx. They may ulcerate. Histologically, they show proliferation of small blood vessels with inflammatory cells and spindle cell proliferation. Treatment ranges from observation in those with limited asymptomatic lesions to chemotherapy for extensive lesions. Although it is radiosensitive, local therapies such as RT and surgery are used only in palliation as they do not prevent appearance of new lesions.[58-62]
- *Rhabdomyosarcoma:* RMS arises from myocytes, can present at almost any age; almost half present in the first decade of life and only about 8% present in the sixth decade. It is one of the most common malignancies occurring in children, with about 40% arising in the head and neck in this age group. In the head and neck, a quarter involves the orbit, half are parameningeal, and the remainder occurs in other sites. Orbital RMS presents early and dramatically; however they have excellent outcome since propensity for regional and distant metastasis is low. Parameningeal RMS can have intracranial and leptomeningeal involvement by virtue of their location, and have a higher risk of distant metastasis. Bone metastasis is common and a bone scan may be indicated in patients with a high risk of distant metastasis. Adults can present with RMS of the tongue, mimicking squamous cell carcinoma. In young patients with a good prognosis, the morbidity of treatment needs to be considered; the treatment regimen with the least long-term toxicity needs to be recommended. Surgery can result in major functional and cosmetic morbidity while RT can result in insidious issues that present later on (craniofacial growth abnormalities, cataract, second malignancy risk, and hypopituitarism). Only one local treatment should ideally be offered. Surgery is not usually the treatment of choice as these lesions are generally radiosensitive; it is reserved for residual or recurrent disease. RT offers good control rates, as high as 90% in some series, with 45–60 Gy in conventional fractionation of 2 Gy/day. Coverage of lymph nodal basins is recommended in parameningeal tumors. Several extensive trials have been performed, on the basis of which current treatment strategies are based. The common agents used are vincristine, adriamycin actinomycin-D, and cyclophosphamide. 5-year survival rates are around 70%. Poor prognostic determinants are parameningeal site, intracranial involvement, bone erosion, age <10 years, and FOXO1 translocation.[63-67]

- *Leiomyosarcoma:* These are relatively uncommon in the head and neck. They can arise from arrector pili or other smooth muscles in the head and neck. They have also been described to arise in the oral cavity, parotid, thyroid, and larynx. Review of histology by a pathologist experienced in sarcoma reporting can help confirm the diagnosis. The treatment of choice is complete surgical excision with adjuvant RT (except in small or early lesions where surgery alone may suffice). Nodal spread. Survival depends on the grade of tumor.[68-71]
- *Hemangiopericytoma and solitary fibrous tumor:* These are another rare subtype that arise from pericytes of the blood vessels; however up to 20% of them occur in the head and neck region. Sinonasal lesions are the most common presentation, and these are believed to be biologically less aggressive. Histologically, they are characterized by the presence of small, thin-walled blood vessels arranged in a "staghorn" pattern with perivascular hyalinization. Based on overlapping histology and molecular alterations, these have now been grouped with solitary fibrous tumors; they both often have fibroblastic spindle cells that stain positive for CD34. They are generally slow growing, initially painless, and locally invasive. Surgical therapy is the mainstay, with RT offered in unresectable cases or for palliation of bleeding. Local recurrence is common, occurring in around 20%, with distant metastasis occurring in 15%. The role of chemotherapy is not well defined.[72,73]
- *Desmoid tumor:* These are not sarcomas; they represent the monoclonal proliferations of benign-appearing fibroblasts that often occur deep within soft tissue. They have a locally infiltrative growth pattern with a propensity for local recurrence. They commonly occur in the third to fourth decades of life. History of preceding trauma may be elicited but often this draws the patient's attention to the lesion rather than causing it. In the head and neck, the supraclavicular fossa is the most common site. Differentiation from low-grade sarcomas can be through detection of point mutations in CTNNB1 (beta catenin encoding gene). Observation is a reasonable approach. They can be excised but R0 resection can be challenging. RT can shrink/reduce rate of growth but risk/benefit ratio needs to be considered. Treatment with cytotoxic therapies, anti-inflammatories such as sulindac, tamoxifen, and imatinib has been tried with variable success rates.[74-77]
- *Malignant fibrous histiocytoma:* This is often a diagnosis of exclusion and is a sarcoma with fibroblastic and histiocytic origin. It is synonymous with undifferentiated high-grade pleomorphic sarcoma. It occurs in adults, commonly 40–60 years of age, as a mass in the parotid, neck, scalp, face, skull base or orbit. They may be radiation-induced as well. Distant spread to the lungs has been demonstrated in up to 16%. These tumors require multidisciplinary management; surgical excision is most commonly advised but the high rates of margin positivity necessitate adjuvant RT. The high risk of distant metastasis forms a rationale for induction or adjuvant chemotherapy. 5-year overall survival rates have been shown to be around 50%, with poor prognostic factors positive margins, size >5 cm, high grade, location other than parotid or neck and previous irradiation of the field. Recent evidence suggests that outcomes in the head and neck may be superior to those arising elsewhere.[78-81]
- *Fibrosarcoma:* These are of fibroblastic or myofibroblastic origin and were one of the most common head and neck sarcomas identified until IHC and genetic typing resulting in many of these being reclassified. They have a high risk of local recurrence and nodal involvement is rare. Distant metastasis can occur in around 15% of patients, most commonly to the lungs. They may be a late complication of RT or burn injury. Patients are usually 30–60 years of age and usually present with lesions in the sinonasal tract, neck or jaw. Infantile fibrosarcomas have been identified and have an excellent response to chemotherapy. Identifying gene fusions can help establish the diagnosis. Low-grade lesions can be treated with adequate surgery while high-grade lesions require adjuvant RT even when margins are adequate.[81-84]
- *Liposarcoma*: It is a common STS and presentations in the head and neck are similar to the rest of the body. They are most commonly seen in males, presenting in the subcutaneous tissue of the neck, salivary glands, skin or aerodigestive tract. Their behavior depends on the grade of the tumor. Myxoid liposarcomas have an unusual natural history of metastasis to extrapulmonary soft tissues. Pleomorphic liposarcomas are poorly differentiated with a higher metastatic potential (up to a third of patients). Completely excision is preferred, although they are considered moderately radiosensitive. They are considered chemoresistant, though myxoid tumors are sensitive to trabectedin. Survival is good, with most series reporting a 5-year overall survival of 66–80%.[85-88]
- *Synovial sarcoma:* These are a misnomer; they are a spindle cell mesenchymal malignancy with varying

degrees of epithelial differentiation and do not arise from intra-articular or synovial tissue. They occur commonly in the skull base, prevertebral, parapharyngeal or retropharyngeal spaces as a swelling with or without pain. Laryngeal involvement has also been demonstrated. Calcification is seen on imaging. Local and distant recurrences are common. These tumors are sensitive to chemotherapy, often showing complete responses with ifosfamide and doxorubicin. Surgery with adjuvant RT is the most common treatment protocol followed, with some centers employed induction chemotherapy initially. The largest series shows a 5-year survival of 72%.[89,90]

- *Osteosarcoma:* This is the most common primary bone malignancy, of which about 10% occur in the head and neck. The majority are sporadic, however it may be associated with multiple inherited syndromes as mentioned above. The most common sites are the maxilla, mandible, and calvaria. They commonly present as painless bony swellings that can create symptoms due to expansion. Neuropathic symptoms have been shown to be associated with a poor prognosis. On imaging, plain X-ray, although rarely done now, can demonstrate a lytic or sclerotic lesion within the bone. Cross-sectional imaging can demonstrate "unburst" or "hair-on-end" appearance results from rapid tumor growth, resulting in stretching and perpendicular ossification of Sharpey's fibers perpendicular to the periosteum. "Codman's triangle" refers to a triangular area of subperiosteal new bone formation. Based on the location, osteosarcoma is classified in to medullary (within the bone), from the bone surface (parosteal or periosteal) or extraosseous. Imaging findings are best discussed with mandible as the prototype. CT better demonstrates tumor matrix (destruction or ossification), cortical destruction, and periosteal reaction. MRI better demonstrates soft-tissue involvement and marrow invasion. Ossified tumors show low signal intensity on T1 and T2-weighted sequence, while nonmineralized tumors show intermediate signal intensity on T1, high intensity on T2 and STIR and enhancement with contrast. Low central T1W1 and high T2 signals after injection suggest medullary involvement and can guide resection margins. Parosteal osteosarcomas appear radiodense and homogeneous lobulated tumor attached to the cortical bone but not the medulla, while periosteal osteosarcoma have 1–3 mm wide periosteal radiolucency ("string sign") in a third of cases. On histology, the characteristic appearance is malignant osteoid with sarcomatous spindle to round-shaped anaplastic cells. Based on the stromal component, they are subtyped as osteoblastic, chondroblastic, fibroblastic, giant cell-rich, small cell, epithelioid, and telangiectatic, with variable grades. Tumor resection with surgery is the primary modality of choice, but the definition of an adequate margin is unclear; this ranges from 1 to 3 cm in literature. Adjuvant RT is considered only when margins are close or positive; RT is not considered a primary modality in this tumor. Another approach in high-grade osteosarcoma is to use induction chemotherapy, as shown in the **Flowchart 2**, and plan adjuvant chemotherapy based on the necrosis in the resection specimen. Chemotherapy in the induction or adjuvant setting has been shown to increase disease-free survival from around 20 to >60%. Kassir published a meta-analysis of osteosarcoma in the head and neck suggesting that since the survival was poor (37%), and hence chemotherapy may be beneficial. Smeele responded with another meta-analysis that showed that chemotherapy benefit was most pronounced in those with negative margins, and hence margin status was a potentially major confounding factor. However, another systematic review by Smeele showed that both

Flowchart 2: Induction chemotherapy-based approach to osteosarcoma of the head and neck.

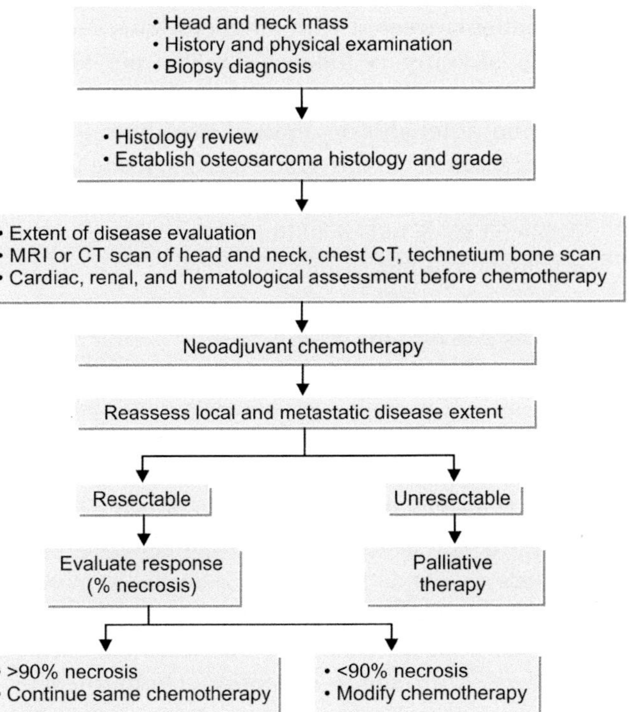

overall and disease-free survival were improved with chemotherapy. The more recent meta-analysis of chemotherapy in craniofacial osteosarcomas by Liang et al. showed that chemotherapy resulted in improved survival in patients with positive margins, high-grade or maxillary tumors. Chemotherapy was most often doxorubicin and cisplatin based.[91-98]

- *Chondrosarcoma:* After osteosarcoma, these are the most common sarcomas arising in bone accounting for around 10%. There are two commonly involved patterns; the first involved the sinonasal tract and are more common in younger patients and women, while the second is the laryngotracheal type that is more common in older men. Regional and distant metastasis is rare. Laryngeal chondrosarcomas have a typical appearance on CT; they appear as calcified masses with a stippled appearance and distorted or enlarged cartilage, most often the posterior cricoid. Histologically, they appear as a collection of malignant chondrocytes in a myxoid matrix with no osteoid formation. They may range for well to poorly differentiated. The recommended treatment is complete surgical resection. In the skull base this may be difficult and the tumor is removed like other skull-base tumors, often piece-meal with final margins negative under frozen section cover. In unresectable lesions, either radical RT or partial resection followed by adjuvant RT may be employed but this is an area of controversy. A large systematic review of skull-base chondrosarcomas showed recurrence rates for patients treated with surgery alone, radical RT alone and surgery followed by RT were 44%, 19%, and 9% respectively. Laryngeal chondrosarcomas may be amenable to limited excisions or partial laryngectomies in low-grade tumors, while laryngectomy may be the only approach in high-grade tumors. Adjuvant RT is indicated in positive margins or when adequate margins cannot be achieved, like in certain areas of the skull base. 5-year survival rates are as high as 87% in some series.[99-103]
- *Ewing's sarcoma:* This is a very rare tumor in the head and neck. It is often seen between 5 and 30 years of age, with a quarter of patients having distant metastasis at presentation. It can involve the mandible, skull or maxilla. Diagnosis is by biopsy and by identifying characteristic gene fusions. Radiologically, these tumors appear as permeative bone destruction with an accompanying soft tissue mass. Treatment mirrors RMS as these are radiosensitive and chemosensitive tumors. Multiagent induction chemotherapy is standard, followed by surgery or RT, often depending on which is less morbid. Adjuvant RT is indicated following surgery, if inadequate. The common chemotherapeutic agents used are vincristine, actinomycin-D, cyclophosphamide, vincristine, and etoposide.[104-106]
- *Radiation-induced sarcomas:* In order to establish causation, the criteria described are the sarcoma should lie within the irradiated field within the area encompassed by the 5% isodense line, it should be histologically distinct from the first malignancy, and several years should have elapsed since irradiation. The exact time gap has been contested, with most authors agreeing a period of 3–4 years. The strongest association seemed to be development of sinonasal tract tumors following nasopharyngeal irradiation. Histology is diverse and virtually any subtype can be associated with this clinical scenario. There are no specific pathological findings that are associated with radiation-induced sarcomas. Surgical excision offers the best chance of cure. Outcomes are poor, with a 5-year disease-free survival of 10–30%. This may be due to difficulty in establishing a diagnosis. Inadequate resection margins in the irradiate wound bed and limitations with radical excision. The benefit of adjuvant chemotherapy is unclear.[107-111]

FOLLOW-UP AND SCREENING

NCCN guidelines suggest clinical and radiological surveillance every 3–6 months for 2–3 years, then every 6 months for 2 years and then annually. For patients who underwent major resection, baseline imaging after surgery (usually 4–6 weeks) results in standard images against which the future images cannot be compared. For those with a high metastatic potential, surveillance with PET CT may be advisable.

REFERENCES

1. Brockstein B. Management of sarcomas of the head and neck. Curr Oncol Rep. 2004;6(4):321-7.
2. Kraus DH, Dubner S, Harrison LB, Strong EW, Hajdu SI, Kher U, et al. Prognostic factors for recurrence and survival in head and neck soft tissue sarcomas. Cancer. 1994;74:697-702.
3. Ramaswamy A, Rekhi B, Bakhshi S, Hingmire S, Agarwal M. Indian data on bone and soft tissue sarcomas: a summary of published study results. South Asian J Cancer. 2016;5(3):138-45.
4. Bajpai J, Khanna N, Vora T, Gulia A, Laskar S, Puri A, et al. An analysis of bone and soft-tissue sarcomas registered during the year 2012 at Tata Memorial Hospital, Mumbai, with clinical outcomes. Indian J Cancer. 2018;55(1):37.
5. Peng KA, Grogan T, Wang MB. Head and neck sarcomas: analysis of the SEER database. Otolaryngol Head Neck Surg. 2014;151:627-33.

6. Malkin D, Li FP, Strong LC, Fraumeni JF Jr., Nelson CE, Kim DH, et al. Germ line p53 mutations in a familial syndrome of breast cancer, sarcomas, and other neoplasms. Science. 1990;250(4985):233-8.
7. Zahm SH, Fraumeni JF Jr. The epidemiology of soft tissue sarcoma. Semin Oncol. 1997;24:504-14.
8. Mitelman F, Johansson B, Mertens F. (2009). Mitelman Database of Chromosome Aberrations in Cancer. [online] Available from http://cgap.nci.nih.gov/Chromosomes/Mitelman. [Last accessed July, 2020].
9. Pierce SM, Recht A, Lingos TI, Abner A, Vicini F, Silver B, et al. Long-term radiation complications following conservative surgery (CS) and radiation therapy (RT) in patients with early stage breast cancer. Int J Radiat Oncol Biol Phys. 1992;23:915-23.
10. Taghian A, de Vathaire F, Terrier P, Le M, Auquier A, Mouriesse H, et al. Long-term risk of sarcoma following radiation treatment for breast cancer. Int J Radiat Oncol Biol Phys. 1991;21:361-7.
11. Murray EM, Werner D, Greeff EA, Taylor DA. Postradiation sarcomas: 20 cases and a literature review. Int J Radiat Oncol Biol Phys. 1999;45(4):951-61.
12. Balarajan R, Acheson ED. Soft tissue sarcomas in agriculture and forestry workers. J Epidemiol Community Health. 1984;38(2):113-6.
13. Eriksson M, Hardell L, Adami HO. Exposure to dioxins as a risk factor for soft tissue sarcoma: a population-based case-control study. J Natl Cancer Inst. 1990;82(6):486-90.
14. Deyrup AT, Lee VK, Hill CE, Cheuk W, Toh HC, Kesavan S, et al. Epstein-Barr virus-associated smooth muscle tumors are distinctive mesenchymal tumors reflecting multiple infection events: a clinicopathologic and molecular analysis of 29 tumors from 19 patients. Am J Surg Pathol. 2006;30(1):75-82.
15. Farid M, Ngeow J. Sarcomas associated with genetic cancer predisposition syndromes: a review. Oncologist. 2016;21(8):1002-13.
16. Parsa N. Environmental factors inducing human cancers. Iran J Public Health. 2012;41(11):1-9.
17. Romañach MJ, León JE, de Almeida OP, Carlos R. Soft tissue sarcomas of the head and neck. SADJ. 2012;67(10):582-4.
18. Harrison LB, Sessions RB, Kies MS. Head and Neck Cancer: A Multidisciplinary Approach, 4th edition. Philadelphia: Lippincott Williams & Wilkins; 2014. p. 844.
19. Shellenberger TD, Sturgis EM. Sarcomas of the head and neck region. Curr Oncol Rep. 2009;11:135-42.
20. Tejani MA, Galloway TJ, Lango M, Ridge JA, Von Mehren M. Head and neck sarcomas: a comprehensive cancer center experience. Cancers (Basel). 2013;5:890-900.
21. Cates JM. Staging soft tissue sarcoma of the head and neck: Evaluation of the AJCC 8th edition revised T classifications. Head Neck; 2019. pp. 1-8.
22. Bentz BG, Singh B, Woodruff J, Brennan M, Shah JP, Kraus D. Head and neck soft tissue sarcomas: a multivariate analysis of outcomes. Ann Surg Oncol. 2004;11:619-28.
23. Shuman AG, Brennan MF, Palmer FL, Kuk D, Moraco N, Singer S, et al. Soft tissue sarcoma of the head & neck: nomogram validation and analysis of staging systems. J Surg Oncol. 2015;111(6):690-5.
24. Callegaro D, Miceli R, Mariani L, Raut CP, Gronchi A. Soft tissue sarcoma nomograms and their incorporation into practice. Cancer. 2017;123(15):2802-20.
25. Bielack S, Carrle D, Casali PG. Osteosarcoma: ESMO clinical recommendations for diagnosis, treatment and follow-up. Ann Oncol. 2009;20(4):137-9.
26. Jaly AA, Thway K, Touska P, Wale A, Miah A, Kerawala C, et al. Imaging Soft-tissue Sarcomas of the Head and Neck: A Tertiary Soft-tissue Sarcoma Unit Experience. Anticancer Res. 2019;39(11):6223-30.
27. National Comprehensive Cancer Network. (2019) NCCN clinical practice guidelines in oncology (NCCN Guidelines) soft tissue sarcoma. Version 4.2019. [online] Available from https://www.nccn.org/professionals/physician_gls/default.aspx. [Last accessed July, 2020]
28. O'Sullivan B, Pisters PWT. Staging and Prognostic factor evaluation in soft tissue sarcoma. Surg Oncol Clin N Am. 2003;12:333-53.
29. Drobnjak M, Latres E, Pollack D, Karpeh M, Dudas M, Woodruff JM, et al. Prognostic implications of p53 nuclear overexpression and high proliferation index of Ki-67 in adult soft-tissue sarcomas. J Natl Cancer Inst. 1994;86:549-54.
30. Heslin MJ, Cordon-Cardo C, Lewis JJ, Woodruff JM, Brennan MF. Ki-67 detected by MIB-1 predicts distant metastasis and tumor mortality in primary, high grade extremity soft tissue sarcoma. Cancer. 1998;83:490–7.
31. Huber GF, Matthews TW, Dort JC. Soft-tissue sarcomas of the head and neck: a retrospective analysis of the Alberta experience 1974 to 1999. Laryngoscope. 2006;116(5):780-85.
32. Lajer CB, Daugaard S, Hansen HS, Kirkegaard J, Holmgaard S, Christensen ME. Soft tissue sarcomas of the head and neck: a single-centre experience. Clin Otolaryngol. 2005;30(2):176-82.
33. Anderson S, Mann H, Krarup-Hansen A, Lajer CB, Gronhoj C. Patient and Tumor Characteristics of Adult Head and Neck Soft Tissue Sarcomas: A Systematic Review and Meta-Analysis. Hindawi Sarcoma; 2019. pp. 1-8.
34. Wanebo HJ, Koness RJ, MacFarlane JK, Eilber FR, Byers RM, Elias EG, et al. Head and neck sarcoma: report of the Head and Neck Sarcoma Registry. Society of Head and Neck Surgeons Committee on Research. Head Neck. 1992;14(1):1–7.
35. Sturgis EM, Potter BO. Sarcomas of the head and neck region. Curr Oncol. 2003;15:239-52.
36. Makary RF, Gopinath A, Markiewicz MR, Fernandes R. Margin Analysis: Sarcoma of the Head and Neck. Oral Maxillofacial Surg Clin N Am. 2017;29:355-66.
37. Pisters PW, Harrison LB, Leung DH, Woodruff JM, Casper ES, Brennan MF. Long-term results of a prospective randomized trial of adjuvant brachytherapy in soft tissue sarcoma. J Clin Oncol. 1996;14:859-68.
38. Tran LM, Mark R, Meier R, Calcaterra TC, Parker RG. Sarcomas of the head and neck. Cancer. 1992;70(1):169-77.
39. Yang JC, Chang AE, Baker AR, Sindelar WF, Danforth DN, Topalian SL, et al. Randomized prospective study of the benefit of adjuvant radiation therapy in the treatment of soft tissue sarcomas of the extremity. J Clin Oncol. 1998;16:197-203.
40. Eeles RA, Fisher C, A' Hern RP, Robinson M, Rhys-Evans P, Henk JM, et al. Head and neck sarcomas: prognostic factors and implications for treatment. Br J Cancer. 1993;68(1):201-7.
41. de Bree R, van der Waal I, de Bree E, Leemans CR. Management of adult soft tissue sarcomas of the head and neck. Oral Oncol. 2010;46(11):786-90.
42. Barker Jr JL, Paulino AC, Feeney S, McCulloch T, Hoffman H. Locoregional treatment for adult soft tissue sarcomas

of the head and neck: an institutional review. Cancer J. 2003;9(1):49-57.

43. Gerrand CH, Wunder JS, Kandel RA, O'Sullivan B, Catton CN, Bell RS, et al. Classification of positive margins after resection of soft-tissue sarcoma of the limb predicts the risk of local recurrence. J Bone Joint Surg (Br). 2001; 83-B:1149-55.
44. O'Sullivan B, Gullane P, Irish J, Neligan P, Gentili F, Mahoney J, et al. Preoperative radiotherapy for adult head and neck soft tissue sarcoma: assessment of wound complication rates and cancer outcome in a prospective series. World J Surg. 2003;27(7):875-83.
45. Kepka L, Delaney TF, Suit HD, Rosenberg AE, Gebhardt MC, Hornicek FJ, et al. Results of radiation therapy for unresected soft-tissue sarcomas. Int J Radiat Oncol Biol Phys. 2005;63: 852-9.
46. Sarcoma Meta-analysis Collaboration (SMAC). Adjuvant chemotherapy for localised resectable soft tissue sarcoma in adults. Cochrane Database Syst Rev. 2000;(4):CD001419.
47. Sarcoma Meta-analysis Collaboration. Adjuvant chemotherapy for localized resectable soft-tissue sarcoma of adults: meta-analysis of individual data. Lancet. 1997;350:1647-54.
48. Verweij J, Seyance C. The reason for confining the use of adjuvant chemotherapy in soft tissue sarcoma to the investigational setting. Semin Radiat Oncol. 1999;9:352-9.
49. Benjamin RS. Evidence for using adjuvant chemotherapy as standard treatment of soft tissue sarcoma. Semin Radiat Oncol. 1999;9:349-51.
50. Pervaiz N, Colterjohn N, Farrokhyar F, Tozer R, Figueredo A, Ghert M. A systematic meta-analysis of randomized controlled trials of adjuvant chemotherapy for localized resectable soft-tissue sarcoma. Cancer. 2008;113:573-81.
51. Blay J-Y, Bonvalot S, Fayette J, Stockle E, Ray-Coquard I, Coindre J-M, et al. Neoadjuvant chemotherapy in sarcoma. Bull Cancer. 2006;93(11):1093-8.
52. Bramwell VH, Anderson D, Charette ML. Doxorubicin-based chemotherapy for the palliative treatment of adult patients with locally advanced or metastatic soft tissue sarcoma. Cochrane Database Syst Rev. 2003;(3):CD003293.
53. van der Graaf WT, Blay JY, Chawla SP, Dong-Wan K, Bui-Nguyen B, Casali PG, et al. Pazopanib for metastatic soft tissue sarcoma (PALETTE): a randomised, double-blind, placebo-controlled phase 3 trial. Lancet. 2012;379:1879-86.
54. Lee KC, Chuang SK, Philipone EM, Peters SM. Characteristics and prognosis of primary head and neck angiosarcomas: a surveillance, epidemiology, and end results program (SEER) analysis of 1250 cases. Head Neck Pathol. 2019;13(3): 378-85.
55. Shin JY, Roh SG, Lee NH, Yang KM. Predisposing factors for poor prognosis of angiosarcoma of the scalp and face: Systematic review and meta-analysis. Head Neck. 2017; 39(2):380-6.
56. Mark RJ, Tran LM, Sercarz J, Fu YS, Calcaterra TC, Juillard GF. Angiosarcoma of the head and neck: the UCLA experience 1955 through 1990. Arch Otolaryngol-Head Neck Surg. 1993;119(9):973-8.
57. Lees KA, Prummer CM, Janus JR. Angiosarcoma. In Evidence-Based Management of Head and Neck Vascular Anomalies. Cham: Springer; 2018. pp. 95-102.
58. Stavrakas M, Nixon I, Andi K, Oakley R, Jeannon JP, Lyons A, et al. Head and neck sarcomas: clinical and histopathological presentation, treatment modalities, and outcomes. J Laryngol Otol. 2016;130(9):850-9.
59. Ramírez-Amador V, Anaya-Saavedra G, Martínez-Mata G. Kaposi's sarcoma of the head and neck: a review. Oral Oncol. 2010;46(3):135-45.
60. Patrikidou A, Vahtsevanos K, Charalambidou M, Valeri RM, Xirou P, Antoniades K. Non-AIDS Kaposi's sarcoma in the head and neck area. Head Neck. 2009;31(2):260-8.
61. Han S, Yin X, Xu W, Wang Y, Han W. The Management of Head and Neck Sarcoma. J Craniofac Surg. 2020;31(2):e189-92.
62. Sanchez IM, DiTommaso LE, Tsoukas MM. Oral Kaposi Sarcoma. JAMA Dermatol. 2019;155(3):370.
63. Orbach D, Mosseri V, Gallego S, Kelsey A, Devalck C, Brenann B, et al. Nonparameningeal head and neck rhabdomyosarcoma in children and adolescents: Lessons from the consecutive International Society of Pediatric Oncology Malignant Mesenchymal Tumor studies. Head Neck. 2017;39(1):24-31.
64. Häußler SM, Stromberger C, Olze H, Seifert G, Knopke S, Böttcher A. Head and neck rhabdomyosarcoma in children: a 20-year retrospective study at a tertiary referral center. J Cancer Res Clinical Oncol. 2018;144(2):371-9.
65. Ladra M, Marcus KJ, Yock T. Rhabdomyosarcoma. In: Target Volume Delineation for Pediatric Cancers. Cham: Springer.; 2019. pp. 125-44.
66. Casey DL, Wolden SL. Rhabdomyosarcoma of the head and neck: a multimodal approach. J Neurol Surg B Skull Base. 2018;79(1):58-64.
67. Radzikowska J, Kukwa W, Kukwa A, Czarnecka AM, Kawecki M, Lian F, Szczylik C, Krzeski A. Management of pediatric head and neck rhabdomyosarcoma: a case-series of 36 patients. Oncology Letters. 2016;12(5):3555-62.
68. Workman AD, Farquhar DR, Brody RM, Parasher AK, Carey RM, Purkey MT, et al. Leiomyosarcoma of the head and neck: a 17-year single institution experience and review of the National Cancer Data Base. Head Neck. 2018;40(4): 756-62.
69. Saluja TS, Iyer J, Singh SK. Leiomyosarcoma: Prognostic outline of a rare head and neck malignancy. Oral Oncol. 2019; 95:100-5.
70. Gootee J, Sioda N, Aurit S, Curtin C, Silberstein P. Important prognostic factors in leiomyosarcoma survival: a National Cancer Database (NCDB) analysis. Clin Trans Oncol; 2019. pp. 1-0.
71. Ko E. Primary oral leiomyosarcoma: a systematic review and update. J Oral Pathol Med. 2019;48(9):780-7.
72. Shaigany K, Fang CH, Patel TD, Park RC, Baredes S, Eloy JA. A population-based analysis of Head and Neck hemangiopericytoma. Laryngoscope. 2016;126(3):643-50.
73. Stanisce L, Ahmad N, Levin K, Deckard N, Enriquez M, Brody J, et al. Solitary fibrous tumors in the head and neck: comprehensive review and analysis. Head Neck Pathol; 2019. pp. 1-9.
74. Collins BJ, Fischer AC, Tufaro AP. Desmoid tumors of the head and neck: a review. Ann Plast Surg. 2005;54(1):103-8.
75. Wang CP, Chang YL, Ko JY, Cheng CH, Yeh CF, Lou PJ. Desmoid tumor of the head and neck. Head Neck. 2006; 28(11):1008-13.
76. De Bree E, Zoras O, Hunt JL, Takes RP, Suárez C, Mendenhall WM, et al A. Desmoid tumors of the head and neck: a therapeutic challenge. Head Neck. 2014;36(10): 1517-26.
77. Santti K, Beule A, Tuomikoski L, Rönty M, Jääskeläinen AS, Saarilahti K, et al. Radiotherapy in desmoid tumors. Strahlenther Onkol. 2017;193(4):269-75.

78. Borucki RB, Neskey DM, Lentsch EJ. Malignant fibrous histiocytoma: Database review suggests a favorable prognosis in the head and neck. Laryngoscope. 2018;128(4): 885-8.
79. Scelsi CL, Wang A, Garvin CM, Bajaj M, Forseen SE, Gilbert BC. Head and neck sarcomas: A review of clinical and imaging findings based on the 2013 World Health Organization Classification. Am J Roentgenol. 2019;212(3): 644-54.
80. Udager AM, Singh R, Billings SD, Patel RM. Malignant Fibrous, Fibrohistiocytic, and Myofibroblastic Tumors. In: Soft Tissue Tumors of the Skin. New York, NY: Springer; 2019. pp. 205-33.
81. Tran N-A, Guenette JP, Jagannathan J. Soft Tissue Special Issue: Imaging of Bone and Soft Tissue Sarcomas in the Head and Neck. Head Neck Pathol. 2020;14(1):132-43.
82. Janz TA, Nagasubramanian R, Wei JL. Pediatric head and neck fibrosarcomas: a demographical, treatment, and survival analysis and review of a rare case. Int J Ped Otorhinolaryngol. 2019;116:92-6.
83. Vijay P, Bajpai M, Pardhe N, Saleem M. Fibrosarcoma of Maxilla. Oral Maxillofac Pathology J. 2018;9(2).
84. Mark RJ, Sercarz JA, Tran L, Selch M, Calcaterra TC. Fibrosarcoma of the head and neck: the UCLA experience. Arch Otolaryngol Head Neck Surg. 1991;117(4):396-401.
85. Golledge J, Fisher C, Rhys-Evans PH. Head and neck liposarcoma. Cancer. 1995;76(6):1051-8.
86. Davis EC, Ballo MT, Luna MA, Patel SR, Roberts DB, Nong X, Sturgis EM. Liposarcoma of the head and neck: The University of Texas MD Anderson Cancer Center experience. Head Neck. 2009;31(1):28-36.
87. Gritli S, Khamassi K, Lachkhem A, Touati S, Chorfa A, Makhlouf TB, et al. Head and neck liposarcomas: a 32 years experience. Auris Nasus Larynx. 2010;37(3):347-51.
88. Barisella M, Giannini L, Piazza C. From head and neck lipoma to liposarcoma: a wide spectrum of differential diagnoses and their therapeutic implications. Curr Opin Otolaryngol Head Neck Surg. 2020;28(2):136-43.
89. Bukachevsky RP, Pincus RL, Shechtman FG, Sarti E, Chodosh P. Synovial sarcoma of the head and neck. Head Neck. 1992;14(1):44-8.
90. Madabhavi I, Bhardawa V, Modi M, Patel A, Sarkar M. Primary synovial sarcoma (SS) of larynx: an unusual site. Oral Oncol. 2018;79:80-2.
91. Smeele LE, Snow GB, van der Waal I. Osteosarcoma of the head and neck: meta-analysis of the nonrandomized studies. Laryngoscope. 1998;108(6):946.
92. Kassir RR, Rassekh CH, Kinsella JB, Segas J, Carrau RL, Hokanson JA. Osteosarcoma of the head and neck: meta-analysis of nonrandomized studies. Laryngoscope. 1997; 107(1):56-61.
93. Smeele LE, Kostense PJ, van der Waal I, Snow GB. Effect of chemotherapy on survival of craniofacial osteosarcoma: a systematic review of 201 patients. J Clin Oncol. 1997;15(1): 363-7.
94. Chen Y, Gokavarapu S, Shen Q, Liu F, Cao W, Ling Y, et al. Chemotherapy in head and neck osteosarcoma: adjuvant chemotherapy improves overall survival. Oral Oncol. 2017; 73:124-31.
95. Vassiliou LV, Lalabekyan B, Jay A, Liew C, Whelan J, Newman L, et al. Head and neck sarcomas: a single institute series. Oral Oncol. 2017;65:16-22.
96. Boon E, van der Graaf WT, Gelderblom H, Tesselaar ME, van Es RJ, Oosting SF, et al. Impact of chemotherapy on the outcome of osteosarcoma of the head and neck in adults. Head Neck. 2017;39(1):140-6.
97. Liang L, Zhang T, You Y, He Q, Fan Y, Liao G. An individual patient data meta-analysis on the effect of chemotherapy on survival in patients with craniofacial osteosarcoma. Head Neck. 2019;41(6):2016-23.
98. Luo Z, Chen W, Shen X, Qin G, Yuan J, Hu B, et al. Head and neck osteosarcoma: CT and MR imaging features. Dentomaxillofac Radiol. 2020;49(2):20190202.
99. Bloch OG, Jian BJ, Yang I, Han SJ, Aranda D, Ahn BJ, et al. Cranial chondrosarcoma and recurrence. Skull Base. 2010; 20(3):149-56.
100. Koch BB, Karnell LH, Hoffman HT, Apostolakis LW, Robinson RA, Zhen W, et al. National cancer database report on chondrosarcoma of the head and neck. Head Neck. 2000;22(4):408-25.
101. Chin OY, Dubal PM, Sheikh AB, Unsal AA, Park RC, Baredes S, et al. Laryngeal chondrosarcoma: a systematic review of 592 cases. Laryngoscope. 2017;127(2):430-9.
102. Ellis MA, Gerry DR, Byrd JK. Head and neck chondrosarcomas: analysis of the Surveillance, Epidemiology, and End Results database. Head Neck. 2016;38(9):1359-66.
103. Piazza C, Paderno A, Nicolai P. Conservative surgery for laryngeal chondrosarcoma: a review of the most recently proposed approaches. Curr Opin Otolaryngol Head Neck Surg. 2017;25(2):93-100.
104. Bouaoud J, Temam S, Cozic N, Galmiche-Rolland L, Belhous K, Kolb F, et al. Ewing's Sarcoma of the Head and Neck: Margins are not just for surgeons. Cancer Med. 2018;7(12):5879-88.
105. Lombardi D, Mattavelli D, Redaelli De Zinis LO, Accorona R, Morassi ML, et al. Primary Ewing's sarcoma of the sinonasal tract in adults: A challenging disease. Head Neck. 2017;39(3):E45-50.
106. Margaix-Muñoz M, Bagán J, Poveda-Roda R. Ewing sarcoma of the oral cavity. A review. J Clin Exp Dent. 2017;9(2): e294-e301.
107. Xi M, Liu MZ, Wang HX, Cai L, Zhang L, Xie CF, et al. Radiation-induced sarcoma in patients with nasopharyngeal carcinoma: a single-institution study. Cancer. 2010;116(23): 5479-86.
108. Thijssens KM, van Ginkel RJ, Suurmeijer AJ, Pras E, van der Graaf WT, Hollander M, et al. Radiation-induced sarcoma: a challenge for the surgeon. Ann Surgs Oncol. 2005;12(3): 237-45.
109. Thiagarajan A, Iyer NG. Radiation-induced sarcomas of the head and neck. World J Clin Oncol. 2014;5(5):973.
110. Tay GC, Iyer NG, Ong WS, Tai D, Ang MK, Ha TC, et al. Outcomes and prognostic factors of radiation-induced and de novo head and neck squamous cell carcinomas. Otolaryngol Head Neck Surg. 2016;154(5):880-7.
111. Giannini L, Incandela F, Fiore M, Gronchi A, Stacchiotti S, Sangalli C, et al. Radiation-induced sarcoma of the head and neck: a review of the literature. Front Oncol. 2018;8:449.

CHAPTER 26

Radiotherapy in Head and Neck Cancer

Vinay Kumar, Suman Bhasker

INTRODUCTION

Radiotherapy is one of the key treatment modalities in head and neck cancer management, in primary, adjuvant, and palliative settings. The most common histology in this region is head and neck squamous cell carcinoma (HNSCC), which is a radiosensitive entity. This chapter is meant to provide a brief overview of radiotherapy in head and neck cancer, namely the principles, different modalities available, and treatment considerations; more details on fields and dosages are covered under individual chapters on respective subsites **(Table 1)**. A thorough understanding of these principles is important for clinicians who treat cancer and allied health professionals who help care for and rehabilitate these patients.

Delineation of radiotherapy targets:[1]

- Gross tumor volume (GTV) is all the palpable/visible tumor on clinical and radiological examination.
- Clinical target volume (CTV) is the area of microscopic spread of tumor.
- Planning target volume (PTV) is extra-area around tumor and microscopic disease to account for daily set-up errors over the course of multifractionated radiotherapy.

IMAGING AND DIAGNOSTIC WORKUP FOR RADIOTHERAPY[2]

The role of clinical physical examination by inspection via indirect laryngoscopy, visualization via fiberoptic laryngoscopy and palpation to assess the extent of lesion and clinical evaluation of neck nodes cannot be overemphasized.

Computed tomography (CT), magnetic resonance imaging (MRI) and hybrid positron emission tomography-CT (PET-CT), ultrasound (USG) with color Doppler are the various imaging modalities with variable utility and advantage with respect to radiotherapy planning.

Use of CT:

- Patients having respiratory compromise due to large aerodigestive tract or neck mass.
- 45-seconds delay axial CT with coronal and sagittal reconstruction help in better mucosal and tumor enhancement and assessing the extent of tumor.
- Avoidance of dental artifacts and respiratory and swallowing artifacts in cases of oral cavity tumor and oropharynx, laryngeal and hypopharyngeal tumors.
- Assessment of malignant nodal involvement. CT is superior to clinical physical examination and MRI.

Use of MRI:

- Assessment of skull base region, nasopharyngeal, sinonasal tumors, and involvement of dura.
- To identify perineural invasion—in such cases target has to be extended along nerve root up to skull base, e.g., parotid tumors.
- For pediatric patients with the intent of reducing radiation dose.
- Patients with contraindication for IV contrast.

Uses of USG:

- Assessment of benign and malignant nodes.
- Biopsy guidance of suspicious nodes and thyroid nodules.

Uses of PET-CT:

- Detects primary in around 10–25% of cases of carcinoma of unknown primary (CUP) after CT, MRI, and endoscopy.
- To detect distant metastasis in locally advanced disease or N3 lesions.
- Decision-making with regards to deferring surgery in view of extensive disease.

Table 1: Subsites in the head and neck and role of radiotherapy.

Site	*Divisions*	*Subsite*	*Radiotherapy consideration*
Oral cavity		• Lip • Commissure of lip, oral commissure • Anterior two-thirds of tongue • Gum (upper and lower) • Floor of mouth • Hard palate • Cheek mucosa (buccal mucosa) • Vestibule of mouth • Retromolar trigone	Radiotherapy is curative in postoperative setting only except in T1 lesions
Pharynx	Nasopharynx		Radiotherapy is radical and best delivered by intensity-modulated radiotherapy (IMRT) considering the volume of irradiation, critical structures surrounding nasopharynx. Stage I treated with radiation alone, stage II and above treated with concurrent chemoradiotherapy (CCRT)
	Oropharynx	• Base of tongue • Lingual tonsil • Soft palate • Tonsillar fossa and pillars • Vallecula • Lateral pharyngeal wall • Uvula • Glossotonsillar sulci	Radiochemotherapy is organ preserving strategy in this cancer. Anti-EGFR targeted therapy along with radiotherapy has also shown good results in this site
	Hypopharynx	• Pyriform sinus • Posterior pharyngeal wall • Postcricoid region	CCRT is an organ preserving strategy in this cancer. However, prognosis is poor as compared to laryngeal cancer due to rich lymphatics
Larynx	Supraglottic larynx	• Epiglottis • Aryepiglottic folds • Ventricular bands (false cords)	CCRT is an organ preserving strategy in this cancer. Surgical salvage followed by fixing artificial voice box in recurrent/residual disease
	Glottis	True vocal cords including anterior and posterior commissures	Local radiotherapy to primary in case of T1 and T2 lesion
	Subglottic larynx	Subglottis	CCRT is an organ preserving strategy in this cancer
Nasal cavity and para-nasal sinus	Maxillary sinus		IMRT with chemotherapy therapy is utilized in both radical (inoperable cases) and postoperative setting. However, particle therapy may have utility in view of Bragg's peak
	Nasal cavity	• Septum • Floor • Lateral wall • Vestibule	Same as above
	Ethmoid sinus		Same as above
Major salivary glands*	• Parotid glands • Submandibular glands • Sublingual glands		Radiotherapy can be administered for pleomorphic adenoma in certain scenarios. Radiotherapy is almost always delivered postoperatively
Thyroid gland*			Radiotherapy for recurrent or metastatic lesions and lesion nonresponding to radioiodine ablation therapy except anaplastic carcinoma that can be treated with chemoradiotherapy
Ear		• Pinna • External auditory canal	Radiotherapy can be radical or postoperative

Key: *usually nonsquamous histology.

- Reassessment after 3–6 months of therapy, evaluation of recurrence, and utility in adaptive radiotherapy (radiotherapy simulation and planning occurs more than once during the course of therapy to account for tumor shrinkage, edema, and loss of weight due to radiation reaction).

RADIATION FRACTIONATION AND RADIOBIOLOGY[3]

Radiotherapy acts on cancer cells and normal tissue through the principal of 5Rs of radiobiology (reoxygenation, repair of sublethal damage, redistribution, repopulation, and radiosensitivity). Cells are most sensitive for effects of radiation in G2/M phase and least sensitive in S phase of cell cycle. There is always certain fraction of cells in proliferation in tumor and radiation kill these actively proliferating cells, results in recruitment of resting cells into cell cycle; this forms the basis of fractionation in radiotherapy. Inter-fraction interval allows for repair of sublethal damage in normal tissue cells and thus recovery. Accelerated repopulation is the triggering of rapid proliferation of cells as tumor shrinks and starts at 4 weeks after start of radiotherapy; it is countered by a dosage of 0.6 Gy per day.

Conventional fractionation: Delivery of daily radiation at 2 Gy/fraction. Prolonging overall treatment time has little effect on late-responding tissue and has sparing effect on acutely reacting tissue.

Hypofractionation: Delivery of daily radiation >2 Gy/ fraction. Late responding tissue ($\alpha/\beta = 3$) is sensitive to larger dose per fraction.

Hyperfractionation: Delivery of more than one fraction per day without increasing biological equivalent dose and overall treatment time. Hyperfractionation has shown to improve in both locoregional control and overall survival, increase acute reaction without increase of late effect.

Accelerated fractionation: Delivery of radiotherapy for more than 5 days in a week and thereby reducing overall treatment time. Local control is increased without additional survival benefit.

Continuous hyperfractionated accelerated radiation therapy (CHART): It is delivery of more than one fraction per day over shorter overall treatment time with inter-fractionation interval of 6 hours. CHART-WEL is delivery of higher dose at inter-fraction interval to 4 hours and omitted weekend. CHART has shown to improve overall survival and local control.

Altered fractionation with chemotherapy: It is still in the phases of clinical trial due to severe acute reaction with altered fractionation alone.

Continuous hyperfractionated accelerated radiation therapy while breathing carbogen and addition of nicotinamide: Acceleration avoided tumor proliferation, hyperfractionation minimized late effects, carbogen breathing to overcome chronic hypoxia, and addition of nicotinamide to overcome acute hypoxia. This strategy has shown improved outcome in advanced laryngeal cancer, but results of randomized control trial are still awaited.

Clinical outcomes with altered fractionation: A meta-analysis published by Bourhis in 2006 considered 6,515 patients of HNSCC in randomized trials with a median follow-up of 6 years. The majority were oropharynx and larynx tumors (74%) with advanced stage. They concluded that altered fractionated radiotherapy conferred a survival benefit of 3.4% at 5 years; Of these, hyperfractionated therapy had the benefit (8% at 5 years). There was also a locoregional control benefit (6.4% at 5 years), most pronounced in patients <50 years.[4] A follow-up meta-analysis by the same group in 2011 of over 24,000 patients in 102 trials also concluded that altered fractionation CCRT and CCRT were the two best treatments, with the former having a slight benefit.[5] However in the context of the RTOG 0129 long-term results showing no benefits of accelerated fractionation CCRT over standard fractionation CCRT,[6] there is insufficient evidence to support the use of altered fractionation in CCRT.

Radiotherapy contouring and definition of target volume and dose:[7]

- Gross disease should receive 70 Gy.
- Positive margins and areas of extranodal extension should receive 60 Gy.
- Levels of lymph nodes harboring microscopic disease (one level above and below the involved positive nodes and tumor bed) should receive 60 Gy.
- Levels of lymph nodes suspected to harbor microscopic disease should receive 50 Gy at 2 Gy per fraction.
- Unilateral neck irradiation is generally sufficient for parotid tumors, well-lateralized early tonsillar and buccal cancers.

Parallel opposed radiotherapy portals for head and neck cancer management:

- To accommodate for penumbra, margins of 0.7–1 cm are planned.
- Portals for head and neck cancer other than oral cavity tumors cover the following structures:
    - Gross tumor, Level IB, Level II, Level III, Level IV, Level V, Level IV up to 44 Gy/22#
    - Gross tumor, Level IB, Level II, Level III, Level IV, Level VI up to 56 Gy/28#
    - Gross tumor and clinically palpable lymph nodes up to 70 Gy/35#
    - In case of postoperative, tumor bed and level of positive lymph node on histopathology are treated up to 60 Gy/30# except T1 and early T2 without adverse radiotherapy prognostic factors such as absence of lymph nodes, <2 mm depth of tumor invasion, no lymphovascular space invasion

- In case of postoperative tumor with positive margin or extranodal extension, tumor bed and lymph node level are treated up to 64 Gy/32#.
- Portals for oral cavity tumor are as follows:
  - Gross tumor, Level IA, Level II, Level III, Level IV, Level V up to 44 Gy/22#
  - Gross tumor, Level IA, Level IB, Level II, Level III, Level IV, Level VI up to 56 Gy/28#
  - Gross tumor and clinically palpable lymph nodes up to 70 Gy/35#
  - Usually unresected oral cavity are treated with palliative intent except for younger patients with good performance status who can be given curative intent doses (most commonly when tumor is not resectable or patient unwilling for surgery).
- Tumors of maxillary sinus, ear (without clinical or imaging lymph nodes) and T1 vocal cord are treated by local radiotherapy alone without elective lymph node irradiation. Perineural invasion or margin positivity, partial maxillectomy becomes indication for radiotherapy up to 64 Gy. In case of lymph node positivity, go for bilateral elective neck irradiation. In case of T3, T4 tumors with N0, M0, and HNSCC, go for unilateral elective neck irradiation up to 50 Gy/25#. All other parameters such as perinodal spread, positive margins becomes indication for 66 Gy/33#.
- Laryngeal and hypopharyngeal cancer:
  - Early T1 glottic cancer—narrow field comprising glottis, popular fractionation is 60 Gy/30# (hypofractionation)
  - Other T1N0 and T2 N0—upper border of thyroid or hyoid to lower border of cricoids with 1–1.5 cm margin all around. T1 N0 is treated up to 66 Gy. T2N0 (and beyond) up to 70 Gy.

TECHNIQUES OF RADIOTHERAPY

Brachytherapy:[7] It is used as primary single modality of treatment in T1/early T2 and N0 lesions of oral cavity, oropharynx, nasal vestibule, and in recurrent settings. As an adjunct single postoperative radiotherapy modality for T1 and early T2 and N0 lesions with high-risk histopathologic features. It is also used as a boost to radiation therapy in node positive oral cavity and node-negative nasopharyngeal cancer.

Brachytherapy can be achieved by inserting nylon catheters in obturator/surface mold (for maxillary sinus cancer and skin cancer respectively), interstitial implantation of plastic catheters in and around the tumor, by use of hairpin technique with gutter guide (soft palate/tonsil), by utilizing balloon brachytherapy technique or implantation of palladium (103Pd) seeds (nasopharyngeal carcinoma). Forward planning or inverse planning is utilized for treatment dosimetry and radiotherapy is usually delivered by high-dose-rate technique.

Dose of 40–48 Gy in 10–12 fractions are delivered at 0.5–1 cm from outer plane of catheter in monotherapy. 20–24 Gy in 7–8 fractions is delivered as boost after EBRT.

Conventional radiotherapy: The general principle of radiotherapy is that 1.5–2 cm of margin around the tumor should be included within the radiation portals. Total radiation dose delivered in head and neck cancers is 70 Gy/35# and 60 Gy/30# for radical and postoperative treatment respectively. Radiotherapy is delivered by shrinking field technique (spinal cord is excluded from radiation field after 44 Gy). A boost of 14 Gy (4–8 Gy for postoperative clear margin (≥1 cm) and positive margin and extranodal extension) is delivered to gross tumor and the postoperative bed. Bilateral neck is irradiated except for T1/early T2 N0 lesions, localized external auditory canal, vocal cord, and maxillary sinus tumors. Conventional technique is utilized for all the sites except parotid, thyroid, and nasal cavity tumors. Due to large volume of irradiation, nasopharyngeal tumors are irradiated by intensity-modulated radiotherapy technique. Radiotherapy portals for head and neck cancer are as follows:

- Upper border is at line joining tragus of ear to maxillary/zygomatic prominence for all nonparotid, nonnasopharyngeal cancer, and unknown primary with secondary neck suspected to be of nasopharyngeal origin.
- Lower border is immediately below the clavicle except for thyroid and postcricoid cancers with esophageal extension.
- Anterior border is in air for oral cavity cancer and those tumors with submandibular lymph nodes. For other sites without submandibular lymph nodes, anterior cortex of mandible with aim to exclude lip after making sure that the portal covers whole of neck.
- Posterior border is at the tip of C2 vertebrae or 1–1.5 cm posterior to the maximum extent of neck lymph node. Electron that has limited range of 5 cm depth and stopped by bone can be used to supplement the dose of radiotherapy for enlarged neck nodes after first phase of radiotherapy to exclude spinal cord.

3D Conformal Radiotherapy (3D CRT):[8] 3D Conformal Radiotherapy (3D CRT) and intensity-modulated radiotherapy (IMRT) are relatively newer radiotherapy techniques. 3D CRT is good for tumors of parotid and thyroid. If we are contemplating limited areas of irradation like in early carcinomas, extensive area of irradiation or proximal critical structures like in nasopharyngeal tumors, complex location like in thyroid cancer, then IMRT is the technique of choice. Conformity of radiation to target and avoidance of critical normal tissue (spinal cord) is the major advantage of IMRT.

Set-up before the delivery of actual radiation can be effected by various means. Conventionally, megavoltage X-ray of treatment position is superimposed on digitally reconstructed radiograph (DRR) of planning CT for regular set-up. However, image-guided radiotherapy (IGRT) utilizing cone-beam CT and hexa-pod couch readjustment, external and internal fiducials placement before simulation and matching the same in treatment position are the various ways of performing IGRT.

If intensity modulated radiotherapy is delivery by path of arc of radiotherapy machine then it is called Volumetric Modulated Arc Therapy (VMAT) or Rapid Arc therapy.

Mucositis, weight loss due to mucositis, and tumor edema during treatment results in change of tumor position relative to critical normal structure. To account for this geographic miss, resimulation, replanning and reset-up is done at interval during the course of radiotherapy. This is called adaptive radiotherapy.

Stereotactic radiotherapy by linear accelerator or linac placed over robotic arms (Cyber-Knife) has very little role in radical treatment of head and neck cancer.

Charged particle radiotherapy:[9] Charged particles interact with electrons of atom to deposit energy and have superior dose distribution as compared to that of photons. Depth-dose curve demonstrates initial plateau region followed by steep dose deposition over very small area known as Bragg peak. Charged particles have characteristics of low- or high-LET (linear energy transfer-rate of energy lost by particle in tissue). X-ray, gamma rays, protons have low-LET whereas heavier charged particles, i.e., carbon ions have high-LET and corresponding value of radiobiological effectiveness (RBE) is 1 and 3 respectively. High-LET radiations are not influenced by oxygenation status, stage of cell cycle, and DNA repair. Particle therapy is particularly helpful for tumors of paranasal sinus in view of their proximity to eyeball, optic nerve.

Neutron radiotherapy:[10] Fast neutrons are generated by accelerating protons with particle accelerators and then impacting them onto beryllium, typically generating 50–70 MeV. Fast neutrons interact with nuclei of atom producing nuclear fragments which in turn produce series of ionization events. RBE for normal tissue, central nervous tissue, and salivary gland tumor is 3, 4, and 8 respectively. Thus fast neutron therapy is beneficial in salivary gland malignancies with therapeutic gain factor between 2.3 and 2.6.

Boron Neutron Capture Therapy:[11] Tumor cells are tagged with ^{10}B (Boron) and cross section of ^{10}B captures the passing low energy of neutrons, results in nuclear transmutation reaction. The disadvantage is capture of neutrons by other atoms in normal tissue.

RADIOSENSITIZERS, RADIOPROTECTORS, BIOREDUCTIVE DRUGS, AND HYPERTHERMIA[12]

Radiation acts on cells by direct (DNA breaks) and indirect [generation of free radicals like hydroxyl (OH^-) and super-oxide (O_3^-) that in turn attack DNA molecules] effect. Unlike in tumor cells, damaged DNA of normal cells with intact DNA repair mechanism are repaired by base excision repair, nucleotide excision repair, single-stranded break repair, double-stranded break repair, and mismatch repair.

Cell cycle has G1, S, G2, and M phase; resistant cells at the beginning of G1 phase become progressively sensitive over the successive phases of cell cycle to become maximally sensitive at M phase. As cells in different phases of cell cycle are killed by fractionated radiotherapy, more and more resting cells enter cell cycle and this phenomenon is called redistribution or reassortment. However, a proportion of the tumor has surviving hypoxia areas. Cells in these hypoxic areas are usually present in the radioresistant resting phase (G0) and tumor control is impossible unless this is overcome.

Overcoming tumor hypoxia:

- Breathing high-oxygen-content gas under normobaric and hyperbaric conditions (around 3 atmospheres) has shown significant local tumor control and subsequent survival under hyperbaric conditions especially in head and neck cancer. Oxygen and carbogen have been used.
- *Hypoxic cell radiosensitizers:* These are agents that mimic oxygen and preferentially sensitize the resistant population. They are not metabolized by tumor cells through which they diffuse, so they can penetrate deeper than oxygen. They are electron-affinity nitroaromatic compounds and were associated with improve locoregional control and disease-free survival. There was a significant improvement in locoregional control over radiotherapy alone.[13,14] Nimorazole has become part of standard radiotherapy practice in Denmark.
- Optimal outcome with radiotherapy is achieved with baseline hemoglobin level of 10–11 g%. However,

patient with low hemoglobin levels have poorer oncologic outcome. Erythropoietin administered to increase hemoglobin levels have been shown to result in poor oncologic control and stimulation of tumor growth.
- Nicotinamide, an analog of vitamin B_3, can prevent disruption in blood flow to tumors that result in hypoxia.
- *Bioreductive agents:* These are agents undergoing intracellular reduction to form active cytotoxic species. Mitomycin C (cross-link DNA) improved local tumor control without increase of toxicity. 2-nitroimidazoles derivatives were found to have dose-limiting gastrointestinal side-effects and other serious side-effects. Organic nitroxides (benzotriazine di-N-oxide-tirapazamine) enhance antitumor effect of cisplatin and have been used in a trial of CCRT in head and neck cancer.

Radioprotectors

Radioprotectors are the agents that selectively protect normal tissue from damage induced by irradiation and by chemotherapy:
- *Amifostine:*[15] This is a sulfhydryl-containing compound with an acceptable toxicity profile. Free radical scavenging by competition with oxygen is the main mechanism of action. However, it has various radioprotective effects on normal tissue. Amifostine has been shown reduce the incidence of acute and chronic xerostomia in postoperative setting. Effect of amifostine on fibrosis and tumor protection is yet to be proven.
- *Pentoxifylline:*[16] Alters red blood cell deformability, inhibit platelet aggregation, and reduce fibrinolytic activity, thereby increase oxygen delivery. This drug appears to increase radiation damage of tumor and decrease the rate and intensity of late radiation effect on normal tissue.
- *Other protectors:* IL-1, TNF-α, and TGF-β may have role in prevention of post-RT fibrosis and may have radioprotector role. Angiotensin converting enzyme inhibitor (captopril), corticosteroids, prostaglandin, and essential fatty acids are the other radio protectors.

Hyperthermia as an Adjunct Therapy[17]

Hyperthermia combined with radiotherapy therapy or chemoradiotherapy in head and neck cancer has resulted in improvement of clinical response rates. Complete response rate, actuarial local control rate, and 5-year survival more than doubled without any increase in toxicity in patients receiving combined therapy with hyperthemia and radiotherapy in locally advanced head and neck cancer.

Clinical Effects of Radiation on Normal Tissues

The effect of radiation on normal tissue is divided into acute (during radiotherapy), subacute (those developing within 6 months of completion of radiotherapy) and late (effects developing after 2 years of radiotherapy). The effect of radiotherapy is seen in all the tissue within and outside the radiation portals; the bystander/abscopal effect[18] is due to release of cytokines of tumors and normal tissue damage. Various metric systems are available to quantify the effects of radiation on normal tissue. Radiation Therapy Oncology Group (RTOG) scale for acute and late toxicities is being gradually replaced by National Cancer Institute (NCI)'s Common Terminology Criteria for Adverse Events (CTCAE) reporting system.

Unique features of CTCAE is replacement of toxicity with new terminology (adverse events), utility of this system both for acute and late normal tissue effect quantification and quantification of effect of all modalities (surgery, radiotherapy, chemotherapy) and all combinations of anticancer treatment.

General grading of clinical features as per CTCAE is as follows:
- Clinical or radiological appearance with apparently no symptoms.
- Mild symptoms requiring pharmacological measures.
- Symptoms needing opioids, antibiotics, hospital admission, and/or elective surgical procedure.
- Symptoms needing emergency surgical procedure impending complication/death.
- Death.

Signs and symptoms of radiation reactions are as follows:
- Mucositis (burning/pain in oral cavity)
- Salivation/drooling of saliva
- Difficulty in swallowing
- Halitosis due to poor oral hygiene
- Skin discoloration
- Pain.

Management of Adverse Events during and after Radiation Therapy for Head and Neck Cancer[19-21]

- Patients can receive prophylactic gargle solution (an example of a popular formulation is ½ tsp of salt, ½ tsp of baking soda added to 1 L of water), benzylamine gargle, and steam inhalation from the first day of radiotherapy to till subsistence of symptoms. This can help with thick salivary secretions and pharyngeal irritation.

- Oral morphine solution can help treat drooling.
- Surface-coating agents such as sucralfate or viscous lignocaine can relieve pain from oral mucositis.
- Fluconazole treats oral candidiasis which may occur during radiotherapy.
- Patients with purulent oral secretions or throat pain without clinical evidence of candidiasis should be administered antibiotics based on throat swab culture and sensitivity report.
- Altered taste sensation and xerostomia can be addressed by modifying food ingredients, drinking lemon juice before food.
- Multivitamins can be added with a view to help mucositis. However, antioxidant property of multivitamin may risk interference with tumor kill.
- Intravenous fluid administration may be required in dehydrated patients.
- Patients who are unlikely to be able to continue eating during radiotherapy should undergo prophylactic nasogastric tube placement (percutaneous endoscopic gastrostomy preferred if use for over a month is anticipated).
- Most symptoms subside with time and lifestyle adjustment, reassurance is important.

REIRRADIATION

Locoregional failure is the predominant pattern of failure in treated patients with advanced tumors. Additionally, a third of patients have second primary tumors. This makes reirradiation an attractive proposition. However it is not without serious risk of morbidity and even mortality. A decision to reirradiate needs multidisciplinary input and multiple considerations, a summary of which are provided below, with treatment strategies as shown in **Flowchart 1**.

Radiobiology of Reirradiation

As a concept, reirradiation may seem counterintuitive in recurrent tumors as it represents a failure or radiotherapy to control the first tumor. It is likely that radioresistance arises in certain clones of cells, through exposure to high-dose radiotherapy.[22] Therefore if irradiation is contemplated, biologically effective and high-dose radiotherapy is required to control disease, often through altered fractionation or with molecular agents to improve efficacy.

The most important rate-limiting factor is tissue tolerance; carotid blowout and spinal cord myelopathy are the disastrous effects of reirradiation. The previous radiotherapy plan, including dose delivery to critical structures is important to review before

Flowchart 1: Reirradiation strategies.

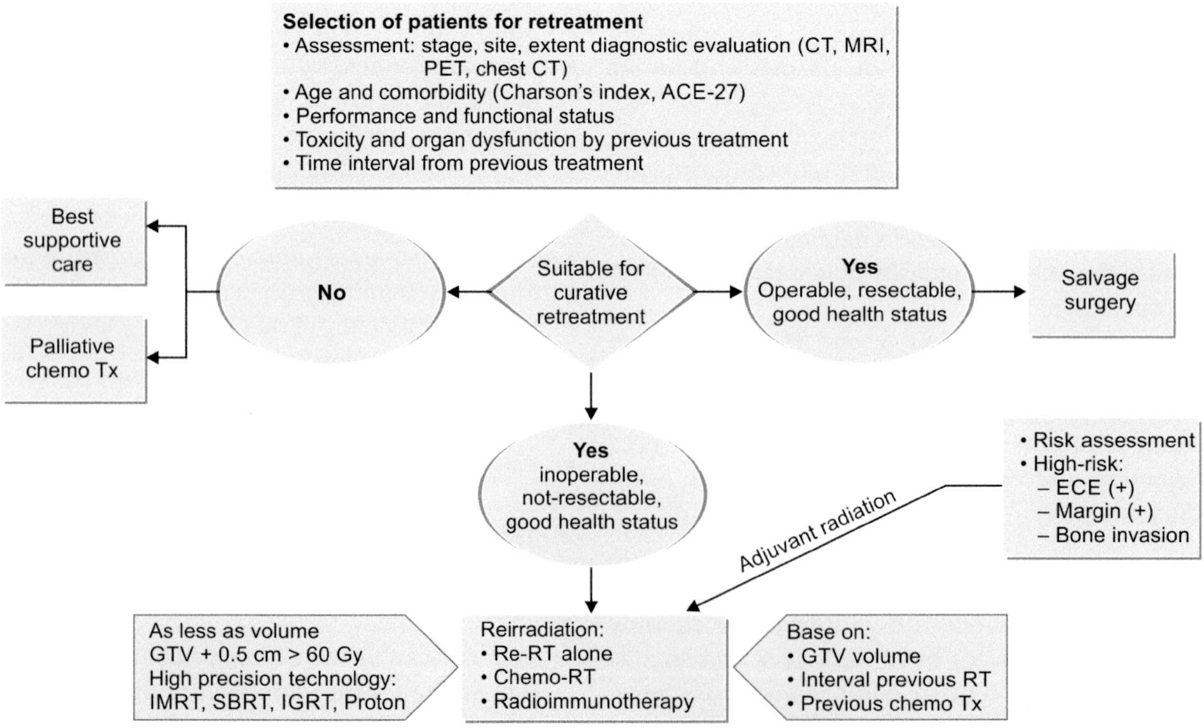

(GTV: gross tumor volume; IGRT: image-guided radiotherapy; IMRT: intensity-modulated radiotherapy; SBRT: stereotactic body radiation therapy; RT: radiotherapy; ECE: extracapsular extension)

contemplating reirradiation. Experimental evidence from rhesus monkeys has shown that spinal cord repair is complete at the 3-year mark after initial radiotherapy.[23] There are no definite guidelines in this situation, each decision has to be taken individually.

Indications for reirradiation:

The treatment strategies for reirradiation are:

- *Adjuvant radiotherapy following salvage resection:* Salvage surgery still offers the best survival benefit in locoregionally recurrent HNSCC. However, a subset of this population is unlikely to have reasonable locoregional control rates unless adjuvant radiotherapy is administered (most commonly those with positive margins or extranodal extension). In the GORTEC trial,[24] previously irradiated patients were randomized to either CCRT or observation after R0 or R1 resection of recurrence HNSCC. Adjuvant chemoradiotherapy significantly improved locoregional control (LRC) and disease-free survival (DFS) but not overall survival (OS), with a 2-year OS of 45%. However, a third of the patients receiving CCRT had grade 3-4 chronic toxicities and 8% had treatment-related death.
- *Reirradiation of unresectable cancers:* The RTOG conducted two prospective phase II trials. In RTOG 9610, 86 patients received hyperfractionated radiotherapy (1.5 Gy/fraction twice a day) concurrently with hydroxyurea and 5-fluorouracil followed by 1 week of rest for four cycles. OS was 15.2% at 2 years with 7.6% treatment-related death and 19.4% grade 3/4 toxicity.[25] In the RTOG 9911 study, 105 patients were reirradiated with IMRT; however, the two arms received either cisplatin or paclitaxel. Grade 3/4 late toxicities were reported in 33.8% and treatment related in 8%. However at 2 years, progression free survival (PFS) and OS were 15.8% and 25.9% respectively, significantly better than RTOG 9610.[26] A more recent phase II trial by Tao et al.[27] included 53 previously irradiated patients of HNSCC who were randomized to monofractionated radiotherapy (60 Gy in 6 cycles of 2 Gy/fraction 5 days/week over 11 weeks with concomitant hydroxyurea and 5-fluorouracil, or hyperfractionated radiotherapy (60 Gy in 1.2 Gy/fraction twice a day for 5 days/week in 5 weeks) with cetuximab. Both arms had reasonable median OS with no significant difference (37.4 and 21.9 months respectively), with no difference in toxicity (40% had grade 3/4 toxicity) or treatment breaks.

Treatment strategies in irradiation:

- *Reducing the treatment field and introducing vascular tissue:* Surgical salvage is still the gold-standard in locoregionally recurrent HNSCC wherever feasible. This allows a smaller field to be irradiated. A review on IMRT in reirradiation showed that radiation treatment volumes >50 cm^3 was associated with a significantly higher risk of grade 3 toxicity; no patients with treatment volumes <25 cm^3 had grade 3 toxicity.[28] Introduction of vascularized tissue in the form of flaps, especially to protect the carotid, may prevent life-threatening hemorrhage.[29]
- *Timing of radiotherapy:* RTOG 9610 showed that the 1-year survival rate for those irradiated within 1 year and 3 years after initial radiotherapy were 35% and 48%. This may be a reflection of disease free interval and tumor biology, or related to radiobiology in the irradiated bed.
- *Choice of radiotherapy technique:* IMRT, stereotactic ablative radiotherapy (SABR), and proton therapy have been shown to have lower toxicity rates in reirradiation.[30-32] This is because they can deliver higher doses to the tumor while sparing surrounding organs-at-risk, preserving quality of life (QoL). Cetuximab and reirradiation with stereotactic ablative radiotherapy (SABR) were studied in two other studies,[33,34] showing that addition of cetuximab improved OS with limited grade 3 toxicity (6%) and no grade 4 toxicity. Addition of cetuximab did reduce QoL scores.

Complications of reirradiation:

- *Acute toxicity:* As discussed earlier, acute grade 3/4 toxicities occur in a third of patients with treatment related death in 5–10%. A reduced functional reserve may also contribute to this toxicity.
- *Late toxicity:* Data is limited as most patients do not survive long enough to experience late toxicity, but the most serious toxicities are:
  - *Spinal cord myelopathy:* Part of the spinal cord is expected to have received 45–50 Gy from previous treatment. With adequate precautions and planning the risk of spinal cord myelopathy is <1%.
  - *Carotid blowout:* Occurs in 3% of patients at a median of 8 months, fatal in three-quarters of patients.[35] Continuous conventional fractionation or hyperfractionation has a lower association with carotid blowout than accelerated fractionation regimens,[36] however patients compared and treatment parameters were heterogenous.
  - *Osteradionecrosis:* Conventional opposed two bilateral port delivery was associated with a risk of 10–15%,[37] however this has reduced with modern techniques like IMRT and SABR (<7%).

Prognosis

Previously discussed prognostic factors include disease free interval and treatment volumes. Anatomical site is also an important determinant; those with nasopharynx, larynx or lateral neck recurrence had better survival than those recurring in the oral cavity or hypopharynx.[28] Second primary tumors also have a better survival than recurrent tumors.[38] Recent publications have aimed to use recursive-partitioning analysis (RPA) to determine which patients are suitable for irradiation. Ward et al. performed a multi-institutional cohort study of IMRT in reirradiation of 412 patients of HNSCC. The three prognostic subgroups they identified were class I (patients reirradiated >2 years after initial treatment who underwent surgical resection, 2-year OS 61.9%), class II (patients reirradiated >2 years after initial treatment who did not undergo resection or those undergoing reirradiation <2 years after initial treatment without tracheostomy or feeding tube dependence, 2-year OS 40%) and class III (remaining patients, 2-year OS 16.8%).[39] They also validated this RPA on another cohort of patients treated with stereotactic body radiotherapy.[40] Another group was unable to validate the RPA model on their cohort of 159 patients.[41] A review of 919 patients from 16 publications concluded that in postoperative irradiation of recurrent and second primary HNSCC should be offered only in the presence of high-risk features (positive margins and ENE) using highly conformal techniques when >50 Gy can be delivered, and in these circumstances local control was 21–100% with a 2-year OS of 48% (range 24–81%).[42]

CONCLUSION

Radiotherapy continues to be an integral part of head and neck cancer management. With technological advances in radiotherapy delivery, the scope of treatment had increased while limiting treatment-related morbidity. A thorough knowledge of the published literature is imperative to ensure to optimize treatment and improve outcomes.

REFERENCES

1. Viswanathan AN, Dizon DS, Gien LT, Koh WJ, Gunderson LL, Tepper JE. Clinical Radiation Oncology, 4th edition. Philidelphia: Elsevier; 2016. pp. 1173-202.
2. Cacicedo J, Fernandez I, Del Hoyo O, Dolado A, Gómez-Suarez J, Hortelano E, et al. Should PET/CT be implemented in the routine imaging work-up of locally advanced head and neck squamous cell carcinoma? A prospective analysis. Eur J Nucl Med Mol Imaging. 2015;42(9):1378-89.
3. Joiner MC, Van der Kogel A. Basic Clinical Radiobiology, 4th edition. Cleveland: CRC press; 2009.
4. Bourhis J, Overgaard J, Audry H, Ang KK, Saunders M, Bernier J, et al. Hyperfractionated or accelerated radiotherapy in head and neck cancer: a meta-analysis. Lancet. 2006;368(9538):843-54.
5. Blanchard P, Hill C, Guihenneuc-Jouyaux C, Baey C, Bourhis J, Pignon JP. Mixed treatment comparison meta-analysis of altered fractionated radiotherapy and chemotherapy in head and neck cancer. J Clin Epidemiol. 2011;64(9):985-92.
6. Brady LW, Perez CA, Wazer DE. Perez & Brady's Principles and Practice of Radiation Oncology. Philadelphia: Lippincott Williams & Wilkins; 2013.
7. Nag S, Cano ER, Demanes DJ, Puthawala AA, Vikram B. The American Brachytherapy Society recommendations for high-dose-rate brachytherapy for head-and-neck carcinoma. Int J Radiat Oncol Biol Phy. 2001;50(5):1190-8.
8. Portaluri M, Fucilli FI, Castagna R, Bambace S, Pili G, Tramacere F, et al. Three-dimensional conformal radiotherapy for locally advanced (stage II and worse) head-and-neck cancer: dosimetric and clinical evaluation. Int J Radiat Oncol Biol Phy. 2006;66(4):1036-43.
9. Castro JR, Reimers MM. Charged particle radiotherapy of selected tumors in the head and neck. Int J Radiat Oncol Biol Phy. 1988;14(4):711-20.
10. Battermann JJ, Breur K. Results of fast neutron teletherapy for locally advanced head and neck tumors. Int J Radiat Oncol Biol Phy. 1981;7(8):1045-50.
11. Barth RF, Vicente MH, Harling OK, Kiger WS, Riley KJ, Binns PJ, et al. Current status of boron neutron capture therapy of high grade gliomas and recurrent head and neck cancer. Radiat Oncol. 2012;7(1):146.
12. Isa AY, Ward TH, West CM, Slevin NJ, Homer JJ. Hypoxia in head and neck cancer. Br J Radiol. 2006;79(946):791-8.
13. Overgaard J, Hansen HS, Overgaard M, Bastholt L, Berthelsen A, Specht L, et al. A randomized double-blind phase III study of nimorazole as a hypoxic radiosensitizer of primary radiotherapy in supraglottic larynx and pharynx carcinoma. Results of the Danish Head and Neck Cancer Study (DAHANCA) Protocol 5-85. Radiother Oncol. 1998; 46(2):135-46.
14. Overgaard J. Hypoxic modification of radiotherapy in squamous cell carcinoma of the head and neck–a systematic review and meta-analysis. Radiother Oncol. 2011;100(1):22-32.
15. Gu J, Zhu S, Li X, Wu H, Li Y, Hua F. Effect of amifostine in head and neck cancer patients treated with radiotherapy: a systematic review and meta-analysis based on randomized controlled trials. PloS One. 2014;9(5):e95968.
16. Futran ND, Trotti A, Gwede C. Pentoxifylline in the treatment of radiation-related soft tissue injury: preliminary observations. Laryngoscope. 1997;107(3):391-5.
17. Datta NR, Rogers S, Ordóñez SG, Puric E, Bodis S. Hyperthermia and radiotherapy in the management of head and neck cancers: a systematic review and meta-analysis. Int J Hyperthermia. 2016;32(1):31-40.
18. Siva S, MacManus MP, Martin RF, Martin OA. Abscopal effects of radiation therapy: a clinical review for the radiobiologist. Cancer Lett. 2015;356(1):82-90.
19. Kahn ST, MAC PA. Management of xerostomia related to radiotherapy for head and neck cancer. Oncology. 2005;19(14).
20. Mealey BL, Semba SE, Hallmon WW. The head and neck radiotherapy patient: Part 2—Management of oral complications. Compendium. 1994;15(4):442-4.
21. Rose-Ped AM, Bellm LA, Epstein JB, Trotti A, Gwede C, Fuchs HJ. Complications of radiation therapy for head and

neck cancers: the patient's perspective. Cancer Nursing. 2002;25(6):461-7.

22. Weichselbaum RR, Beckett MA, Schwartz JL, Dritschilo A. Radioresistant tumor cells are present in head and neck carcinomas that recur after radiotherapy. Int J Radiat Oncol Biol Phys. 1988;15:575-9
23. Ang KK, Jiang GL, Feng Y, Stephens LC, Tucker SL, Price RE. Extent and kinetics of recovery of occult spinal cord injury. Int J Radiat Oncol Biol Phys. 2001;50:1013-20.
24. Janot F, de Raucourt D, Benhamou E, Ferron C, Dolivet G, Hamoir RJB, et al. Randomized trial of postoperative reirradiation combined with chemotherapy after salvage surgery compared with salvage surgery alone in head and neck carcinoma. J Clin Oncol. 2008;26:5518-23.
25. Spencer SA, Harris J, Wheeler RH, Machtay M, Schultz C, Spanos W, et al. Final report of RTOG 9610, a multi-institutional trial of reirradiation and chemotherapy for unresectable recurrent squamous cell carcinoma of the head and neck. Head Neck. 2008;30:281-8.
26. Langer CJ, Harris J, Horwitz EM, Nicolaou N, Kies M, Curran W, et al. Phase II study of lowdose paclitaxel and cisplatin in combination with splitcourse concomitant twice-daily reirradiation in recurrent squamous cell carcinoma of the head and neck: results of Radiation Therapy Oncology Group Protocol 9911. J Clin Oncol. 2007;25: 4800-5.
27. Tao Y, Faivre L, Laprie A, Boisselier P, Ferron C, Jung GM, et al. Randomized trial comparing two methods of re-irradiation after salvage surgery in head and neck squamous cell carcinoma: once daily split-course radiotherapy with concomitant chemotherapy or twice daily radiotherapy with cetuximab. Radiother Oncol. 2018;128(3): 467-71.
28. Takiar V, Garden AS, Ma D, Morrison WH, Edson M, Zafereo ME, et al. Reirradiation of head and neck cancers with intensity modulated radiation therapy: outcomes and analyses. Int J Radiat Oncol Biol Phys. 2016;95:1117-31.
29. Suárez C, Fernández-Alvarez V, Hamoir M, et al. Carotid blowout syndrome: modern trends in management. Cancer Manag Res. 2018;10:5617-28.
30. Kharofa J, Choong N, Wang D, Firat S, Schultz C, Sadasiwan C, et al. Continuous-course reirradiation with concurrent carboplatin and paclitaxel for locally recurrent, non-metastatic squamous cell carcinoma of the head-and-neck. Int J Radiat Oncol Biol Phys. 2012;83:690-5.
31. Siddiqui F, Patel M, Khan M, McLean S, Dragovic J, Jin JY, et al. Stereotactic body radiation therapy for primary, recurrent, and metastatic tumors in the head-and-neck region. Int J Radiat Oncol Biol Phys. 2009;74:1047-53.
32. Cengiz M, Ozyigit G, Yazici G, Doğan A, Yildiz F, Zorlu F, et al. Salvage reirradiaton with stereotactic body radiotherapy for locally recurrent head-and neck tumors. Int J Radiat Oncol Biol Phys. 2011;81:104-9.
33. Heron DE, Rwigema JC, Gibson MK, Burton SA, Quinn AE, Ferris RL. Concurrent cetuximab with stereotactic body radiotherapy for recurrent squamous cell carcinoma of the head and neck: a single institution matched case-control study. Am J Clin Oncol. 2011;34:165-72.
34. Vargo JA, Heron DE, Ferris RL, Rwigema J-C M, Wegner RE, Kalash R, et al. Prospective evaluation of patient-reported quality-of-life outcomes following SBRT ± cetuximab for locally-recurrent, previously-irradiated head and neck cancer. Radiother Oncol. 2012;104:91-5.
35. McDonald MW, Lawson J, Garg MK, Quon H, Ridge JA, Saba N, et al. ACR appropriateness criteria retreatment of recurrent head and neck cancer after prior definitive radiation expert panel on radiation oncology-head and neck cancer. Int J Radiat Oncol Biol Phys. 2011;80:1292-8.
36. Suárez C, Fernández-Alvarez V, Hamoir M, Mendenhall WM, Strojan P, Quer M, et al. Carotid blowout syndrome: modern trends in management. Cancer Manag Res. 2018;10:5617-28.
37. De Crevoisier R, Bourhis J, Domenge C, Wibault P, Koscielny S, Lusinchi A, et al. Full-dose reirradiation for unresectable head and neck carcinoma: experience at the Gustave-Roussy Institute in a series of 169 patients. J Clin Oncol. 1998;16:3556-62.
38. Mendenhall WM, Mendenhall CM, Malyapa RS, Palta JR, Mendenhall NP. Re-irradiation of head and neck carcinoma. Am J Clin Oncol. 2008;31:393-8.
39. Ward MC, Riaz N, Caudell JJ, Dunlap NE, Isrow D, Zakem SJ, et al. Refining patient selection for reirradiation of head and neck squamous carcinoma in the IMRT era: a multi-institution cohort study by the MIRI collaborative. Int J Radiat Oncol Biol Phys. 2018;100(3):586-94.
40. Vargo JA, Ward MC, Caudell JJ, Riaz N, Dunlap NE, Isrow D, et al. A multi-institutional comparison of SBRT and IMRT for definitive reirradiation of recurrent or second primary head and neck cancer. Int J Radiat Oncol Biol Phys. 2018;100(3): 595-605.
41. Orlandi E, Bonomo P, Ferella L, D'Angelo E, Maddalo M, Alterio D, et al. Long-term outcome of re-irradiation for recurrent or second primary head and neck cancer: a multi-institutional study of AIRO—Head and Neck working group. Head Neck. 2019;41(10):3684-92.
42. Merlotti A, Mazzola R, Alterio D, Alongi F, Bacigalupo A, Bonomo P, et al. What is the role of postoperative re-irradiation in recurrent and second primary squamous cell cancer of head and neck? A literature review according to PICO criteria. Crit Rev Oncol Hematol. 2017;111:20-30.

CHAPTER

27 Tracheal Malignancies

Dinesh MG, Samskruthi P Murthy, Narayana Subramaniam, Sivakumar Vidhyadharan

INTRODUCTION

Primary tumors of the trachea are rare, comprising 2% of tumors of the upper aero digestive tract.[1] The low incidence can be attributed to high immune surveillance of trachea. Early detection of these tumors is difficult due to overlapping symptomatology with common airway disorders such as asthma, chronic obstructive pulmonary disease (COPD) and bronchitis,[2] hence most often there is a mean delay of 8 months before diagnosis of malignant tracheal tumor.[3] A varied array of tumors involve trachea, with almost 90% of tumors being malignant. Squamous cell carcinoma (SCC) and adenoid cystic carcinoma (ACC) are the most frequent malignant tumors of the trachea. These tumors are often difficult to treat due to late presentation and scarcity of literature regarding management and outcomes. The following chapter deals with presentation, management, and palliation of primary malignant tracheal tumors.

EPIDEMIOLOGY

Incidence of primary tracheal malignancy is 0.1 in 100,000 population per year, which corresponds to 0.2% of respiratory tract tumors and 0.02–0.04% of all malignant tumors.[4,5] The laminar flow in the tracheal lumen prevents the deposition of carcinogens on to the mucosa; hence the incidence of smoking-induced SCC is significantly lower than those in the lung or larynx.[6] Malignancy of larynx and bronchus occur about 40 and 400 times more often than malignancy of trachea.[7,8]

SURGICAL ANATOMY

The success of the tracheal surgery rests heavily on the surgeon's knowledge of anatomy. The trachea is a cartilaginous tubular structure extending from the lower edge of the cricoid cartilage to the upper end of bronchus. The carina is situated at the level of T4 vertebra, and forms the lower end of the trachea. The length of trachea ranges from 10 to 13 cm. The scaffold of trachea consists of 18–22 D-shaped cartilaginous rings that form the anterior and lateral wall of the trachea with the trachealis muscle running longitudinally forming the posterior wall. It also abuts the anterior wall of the esophagus. The position of the trachea also varies with age; an elderly patient has decreased ascent of trachea on cervical extension than younger patients.[9] There are approximately two rings for every centimeter of the trachea with a wall thickness of 2–3 mm. The external diameter measures 1.8–2.3 cm and the mucosa of the trachea is lined by pseudostratified ciliated columnar epithelium.

Arterial Supply

Understanding the arterial supply of trachea is essential for safe and successful surgery. The fundamental principle of tracheal mobilization and dissection around the trachea is based on the fact that trachea has a segmental blood supply and the feeding artery enters tracheal wall laterally.[10] The segmental arteries further branch into superior and inferior arteries in a longitudinal direction, forming anastomoses with branches from above and below. They pierce the tracheal wall at intercartilaginous ligaments and further branch into anterior and posterior arteries that run circumferentially within the tracheal wall in the submucosal plane. The segmental arrangement of blood supply limits tracheal dissection to no more than 1–2 cm on either side on anastomotic site. The cervical trachea is supplied by tracheoesophageal branches of the inferior thyroid artery. The configuration of the branches differs between individuals, but commonly the first branch supplies lower cervical trachea, the second branch supplies middle, and the third branch supplies upper cervical trachea. The thoracic trachea is supplied by superior, middle and inferior bronchial arteries which are branches of descending arch of aorta; the pattern of bronchial artery branching is highly variable.

Lymphatic Drainage

The path of lymphatic drainage consists of paratracheal nodes, inferior deep cervical nodes, superior tracheobronchial nodes, and carinal nodes. They further drain into bronchopulmonary and hilar nodes, and finally into pulmonary and intrapulmonary nodes.

Relations

The trachea is in close proximity with major blood vessels in the mediastinum. The cervical trachea at the upper end is in close relation to the right and left lobes of the thyroid, which are situated on the anterolateral aspect of the trachea. The thyroid isthmus occupies second or third tracheal ring. The esophagus begins from the level of the cricoid cartilage and runs inferiorly along the left posterior border of the trachea. The right posterior border of the trachea runs over the anterior aspect of the vertebral body. The right and left vagus nerves run inferiorly posterolateral to common carotid artery. The right and left recurrent laryngeal nerves (RLNs) branch off the vagus nerve at the subclavian artery and arch of aorta respectively and loop around them to ascend into the neck along the tracheoesophageal groove.

The brachiocephalic or innominate artery originates from the arch of aorta over the right anterior aspect of the thoracic trachea and then runs superiorly. The left common carotid artery branches off the arch of the aorta just left of the midline of the trachea and runs superiorly over the left anterolateral aspect of trachea. The superior vena cava runs along the right anterior aspect of the trachea. The azygos vein joins superior vena cava at right tracheobronchial angle and can be mistaken for a lymph node. The main pulmonary artery lies anterior and to the left of the carina. Its corresponding branches run laterally on the anterior surface of respective main bronchi.[11]

PATHOLOGY

The pathology of tracheal malignancies tumors is as shown in **Table 1**. SCC comprises one-third of all primary tracheal malignancies. Variants of SCC such as basaloid, verrucous, spindle cell, acantholytic, and adenosquamous have also been described. They commonly grow as polypoidal or ulcerative masses that grow toward the lumen. When associated with smoking, second primary tumors in the lung, larynx or oropharynx are common.

Table 1: Pathology of malignant tracheal tumors.

Epithelial tumors	*Salivary gland tumors*
• Squamous cell carcinoma • Adenocarcinoma • Large-cell undifferentiated carcinoma • Neuroendocrine	• Mucoepidermoid carcinoma • Adenoid cystic carcinoma • Carcinoma ex pleomorphic adenoma
Neuroendocrine tumors	*Mesenchymal tumors*
• Typical and atypical carcinoids • Large-cell neuroendocrine tumor • Small cell carcinoma	• Soft-tissue type sarcomas • Chondrosarcoma • Malignant lymphomas

Tracheal SCC has shown to be well, moderately, and poorly differentiated in 24%, 49%, and 27% of cases respectively.[12]

Adenoid cystic carcinoma accounts for another one-third of tracheal malignancies. As per the WHO classification, ACCs are defined as basaloid tumors comprised of both epithelial and myoepithelial cell with variable morphologic patterns such as tubular, cribriform, and solid. ACC is commonly not associated with smoking. Local perineural spread is a hallmark of ACC, and as with other sites, they have a high propensity for local recurrence. The tumor has a propensity to grow submucosally in longitudinal and circumferential directions far beyond what is clinically and radiologically visible.[13]

PRESENTATION

The symptoms of tracheal malignancy often overlap with symptoms of asthma, developing over months. Dyspnea (58%), cough (54%), hemoptysis (45%), wheeze (36%), and stridor (24%) are commonly seen at presentation.[2] Tumors located closer to subglottic and carina cause respiratory distress earlier than tumors along the length of trachea. SCC tends to grow into the lumen of trachea and hence present earlier than ACC. The delay in presentation also affects management and prognosis, as the symptom duration difference between resectable and unresectable tracheal malignancy is 3.4 months.[2] Tracheal cancer affects men 2–4 times more than women. Nearly 40% of tracheal tumors are associated with tumors of oropharynx, lung, and larynx.[14,15]

EVALUATION

- *Spirometry:* Spirometry values are based on degree, extent, and site of obstruction. The values that aid in diagnosis are peak expiratory flow, maximum inspiratory flow at 50% of the forced vital capacity (MIF_{50}), and maximum expiratory flow at 50% of the forced vital capacity (MEF_{50}). In cases with respiratory distress, pulmonary function test is of no value.

Table 2 represents the spirometry values that can be associated with tracheal malignancies.

- *Bronchoscopy:* Bronchoscopy is the most valuable test in evaluating trachea. With flexible tracheobronchoscopy, the extent of lesion, extent of airway lumen obstruction, relations and distance from carina and cricoid cartilage can be assessed. Biopsies from the lesion can be taken. Bronchoscopy must be performed with caution in patients with acute respiratory distress, as bronchoscopy may worsen symptoms by causing edema and bleeding from the tumor. During bronchoscopy, the larynx must be evaluated to rule out synchronous primary tumors and assess the status of the vocal cord mobility.
- *Computed tomography:* Computed tomography (CT) evaluation is must in all cases, as most cases present late. Serial axial, coronal, and sagittal imaging sections are required to study the extent of the tumor, lymph nodal metastases, and presence of synchronous primaries in the lung or larynx. CT frequently identifies extramural spread while vertical extension of growth is often underestimated. Even with multiplanar reformatting and 3D rendering, CT scan is inferior to bronchoscopy in assessing vertical length of tumor extension.[16]
- *Esophagoscopy:* Esophagoscopy may be required if patient complaints of dysphagia and/or CT shows esophageal involvement.

STAGING

There is no American Joint Committee on Cancer (AJCC) recommended TNM staging for tracheal cancer. The following two staging systems have been proposed[17,18] **(Table 3)**, but their utility and prognostication capacity need to be validated.

TREATMENT

Before deciding on the treatment modality and intent of treatment, preoperative evaluation, and general condition

Table 2: Spirometry values associated with tracheal malignancy.

Tumor or obstruction site	*Type of obstruction*	*MIF_{50}*	*MEF_{50}*	*MIF_{50}/MEF_{50} ratio*
Extrathoracic (cervical trachea)	Fixed (sessile growth)	Decreased	Decreased	1
	Variable (polypoidal growth)	Decreased	Normal or decreased	<1
Intrathoracic (thoracic trachea)	Fixed	Normal or decreased	Decreased	>1

Table 3: Proposed TNM classification systems for tracheal malignancy.

Staging system proposed by Bhattacharyya et al.[17]	
T stage	*N stage*
T1: Primary tumor confined to trachea; size <2 cm *T2:* Primary tumor confined to trachea; size >2 cm *T3:* Primary tumor spread outside the trachea but not to adjacent organs or structures *T4:* Spread to adjacent organs or structures	*N0:* No evidence of regional nodal disease *N1:* Positive regional nodal disease
Staging system proposed by Macchiarini et al.[18]	
T stage	*N stage*
Tis: Any tumor without invasion *T1a:* <3 cm limited to mucosa *T1b:* >3 cm limited to mucosa *T2:* Any tumor that invades cartilage or adventitia *T3:* Any tumor that invades trachea or larynx *T4a:* Any tumor that invades carina or main bronchus *T4b:* Any tumor that invades neighboring structures	*N0:* No evidence of node metastasis *N1:* Local nodes positive *Upper third:* Highest mediastinal nodes; upper paratracheal nodes, prevascular and retrotracheal *Middle third:* Upper paratracheal nodes; prevascular and retrotracheal, lower paratracheal nodes; para-aortic nodes (ascending aorta or phrenic) *Lower third:* Upper paratracheal nodes; prevascular and retrotracheal; subaortic nodes (aortopulmonalis *window)* *N1a:* 1–3 positive nodes in upper third *N1b:* >3 positive nodes in upper third *N2:* Regional nodes positive
M0: No distant metastasis *M1:* Metastasis to nodes other than N1 and N2 *M2:* Distant metastasis (e.g., lung)	*Upper third:* Lower paratracheal nodes; subaortic nodes (aortopulmonary window) *Middle third:* Highest mediastinal nodes; subaortic nodes (aortopulmonalis window) *Lower third:* Upper paratracheal nodes; pulmonary ligament

of the patient must be assessed thoroughly. Surgical excision of the tumor is associated with the best outcomes and has the highest likelihood of cure. Management of tracheal tumors is multidisciplinary with treating team consisting of head and neck surgeon, thoracic surgeon, pulmonologist, medical oncologist, radiation oncologist, and anesthetist familiar with thoracic procedures.

Acute airway obstruction, if present, must be relieved by rigid bronchoscopy and intra-tracheal tumor debulking to enlarge the airway lumen.[19] Potential bleeding that can occur can be detrimental, and hence care must be taken to achieve hemostasis from tumor surface. Further treatment must be planned at the earliest. In the presence of unresectable or metastatic disease, a stent can be placed after tumor debulking, but if surgical excision is contemplated, then stenting, tracheostomy, and preoperative radiotherapy must not be advocated.[20]

SURGERY

Although the history of tracheal surgery dates back to the second and third century, while it was only after 1990 that Grillo established principles of tracheal surgery with success.[14,21] Assessing resectability is paramount, as incomplete resection has a negative effect on survival. A thorough knowledge of anatomy is essential for successful tracheal resection. The principles of tracheal surgery can be divided into:

- *Anesthetic considerations:* Anesthesia during tracheal resection is as crucial as the surgery. A patient with no airway compromise should undergo slow induction with no paralytic agents. On spontaneous ventilation, laryngeal mask airway (LMA) can be inserted, and through the LMA, flexible bronchoscopy is performed to confirm the tumor extent and location. An extra-long endotracheal tube is inserted over the bronchoscope, beyond the tumor. Patients with airway compromise also undergo slow induction without paralytic agent. The airway is established by passing a rigid bronchoscope, and spontaneous ventilation is maintained with rigid bronchoscopy. A core of tumor is de-bulked, and once lumen is established, extra-long endotracheal tube is inserted under fiberoptic bronchoscopic guidance.[22] After resection of the tumor, the orotracheal tube is retracted just above the proximal resected end, and another flexible endotracheal tube is inserted into the distal end of the trachea through the sterile operative field. After anastomosis, the distal flexible tube is removed, and the retracted orotracheal tube is pushed back in place. Postsurgery, a small endotracheal tube is inserted without inflated cuff for postoperative ventilation if required. Air humidification, chest physiotherapy, and upright position during the postoperative period are necessary to manage secretions.[23]
- *Access:* The cervical trachea is the easiest to access. A collar incision is placed in the neck to expose from the level of hyoid superiorly up to sternal notch inferiorly. The sternohyoid and sternothyroid muscles are separated in the midline as in thyroid surgery or divided inferiorly to get better exposure. The thyroid isthmus is resected, and thyroid lobes are retracted laterally. Thyroidectomy is performed when there is involvement of thyroid gland.
  Thoracic trachea and carina can be accessed through right posterolateral thoracotomy (via fourth intercostal space) or median sternotomy with or without left trans-sternal incision (clamshell incision) through third or fourth intercostal space for additional access. Right posterolateral thoracotomy is the most frequent approach for distal trachea and carina. Intrathoracic exposure of trachea is gained by retraction of innominate vein superiorly, lateral retraction of the aorta and superior vena cava. The main pulmonary artery is reflected inferiorly.[22]
- *Principles of resection:* The primary concern during resection is to maintain vascularity of the trachea and prevent injury to the RLN. The cervical course of the RLN is traced adjacent to planned resection segment of trachea. If one of the nerves needs resection, the decision to do so is reserved until the end of surgery as the tumor may be unresectable and resecting an RLN may add significant morbidity. The extent of tumor is marked during bronchoscopy. A plane of dissection is created between trachea and esophagus. The separation of trachea and esophagus is limited only to the segment of resection as microvascular collaterals from esophagus supply posterior membranous part of the trachea. The trachea is looped, and lateral sutures are placed below the level of resection to prevent retraction of distal trachea inferiorly. By blunt dissection, an avascular plane is created between the trachea and pretracheal fascia along the whole visible length of trachea without disrupting the lateral attachments of the trachea; this maneuver helps to mobilize trachea effortlessly. The endotracheal tube positions are then changed. No more than 2 cm of tracheal release is done on either side of the resection margin. Tracheal segment is resected and oriented. The inferior border of the posterior cricoid cartilage is the limit of mobilization,

as RLN is in close approximation superior to lower border of cricoid. If required anterior third of the cricoid ring can be resected, but resection of over a third of the cricoid is not compatible with tracheal resection. The margin of resection has not been defined; either 1 cm margin or one extra tracheal ring is resected as margin. The principle of resection is the same in all segments of the trachea.

- *Anastomosis:* Tracheal resection of up to 5 cm length allows anastomosis without tension. Stay sutures with 2-0 absorbable sutures are placed at 3 o'clock and 9 o'clock positions just above the proximal end and below the distal end of the resected trachea. The neck is flexed, and by approximating the stay sutures, tension on the anastomotic site is assessed. If there is tension, then lengthening maneuvers are employed. The anastomosis is performed with 4-0 absorbable sutures that are placed at corresponding edges of the resection. The alignment of the membranous and cartilaginous portion of trachea must be maintained. Full-thickness bites are placed at 2–3 mm interval to attain an airtight closure **(Fig. 1)**. Two types of suturing technique are described. Circumferential open sutures are placement followed by tying knot externally. The sutures are tied in the reverse order that they are placed. Approximation of the tracheal edges and rotation of the trachea to place sutures under visualization is maintained by stay sutures placed earlier. Another technique involves placing posterior membranous wall sutures first in such a way that the knots lay intraluminal. The anterior wall sutures are placed later on by tying knots exteriorly.[22]
  Carina anastomosis has been described in three ways:
  1. An end-to-end anastomosis between the trachea and left main bronchus and an end-to-side anastomosis between the right main bronchus and trachea
  2. End-to-end anastomosis between the trachea and right main bronchus followed by an end to side anastomosis of left main bronchus and trachea
  3. Approximating the two main bronchus to end of trachea as a unified structure

  The third option is associated with more tension than the other anastomoses options. After anastomosis is complete, an air leak test is performed and if possible a check bronchoscopy. A chin-to-manubrium stitch (Grillo's) stitch is placed to maintain neck in flexion up to 7–10 days postoperatively.
- *Tracheal lengthening maneuvers*: Resections of >5 cm will need tracheal-lengthening maneuvers and only about 6% require trachea-lengthening maneuvers.[24] Suprahyoid release is achieved by releasing the muscular attachments of the mylohyoid, geniohyoid, genioglossus, and medial hyoglossus from the hyoid bone. The fascial sling of the posterior belly of digastric is maintained. The body of the hyoid is freed from the cornu of the hyoid. Attachments of sternohyoid, omohyoid, and thyrohyoid muscles should not be detached from hyoid. The gain of length is 2–3 cm.[25] Alternatively, the pulmonary ligament can be incised at the level of inferior pulmonary vein and pericardium. The pulmonary vasculature is circumscribed to allow upward movement of the right hilum. Releasing left hilum does not aid in gaining additional length.[26] Approximately 2 cm can be gained with a right hilar release. Neck flexion and anterior pretracheal dissection also aids in gaining additional tracheal length.
- *Tracheal reconstruction:* Most resections can be managed with primary anastomosis. Reconstruction or replacement is required in long segment loss of trachea. Autologous grafts are most preferred. Autologous flaps are ideal as they also provide vascular bed and aid in healing. Cutaneous chondromucosal forearm tubular flaps, compound tracheal segments vascularized by sternocleidomastoid muscle, deltopectoral flap with costal cartilage and palatal mucosal grafts and pectoralis major myocutaneous flap with costal cartilage have been described.[27] Use of aortic allografts, foreign material and tissue-engineered tracheal reconstruction have also been described, but their role in tracheal malignancy and the effect of postoperative radiation on the graft is not well defined.

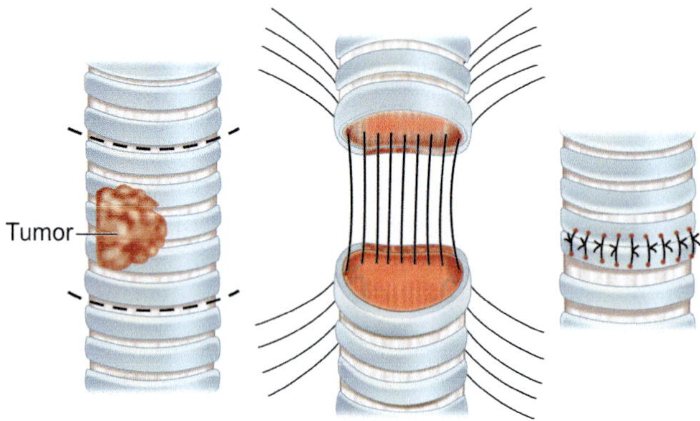

Fig. 1: Tracheal resection.

Cervical exenteration: Cervical exenteration, described initially by Hermes Grillo, is a radical procedure that involves resection of larynx, pharynx, trachea, and esophagus with or without mediastinal tracheostomy.[28] This procedure is described to resect extensive cervical esophageal cancer, invasive thyroid cancer, and stomal recurrence after laryngectomy and primary tracheal malignancy. The cervical access is gained by lower cervical transverse incision just above the heads of the clavicle. This incision allows access to the neck and upper mediastinum. The sternum is divided along midline up to second intercostal space and the resection is completed. If a mediastinal stoma needs to be fashioned, then the upper sternum and medial ends of clavicle (up to 4 cm) and corresponding first two costal cartilage are resected. A tracheostoma is created between the innominate artery and left common carotid artery above their branching off the aorta. Innominate artery, if involved by tumor or under tension by tracheal stump, can be resected under electroencephalographic monitoring. Pharyngeal reconstruction can be performed with gastric pull-up or colonic transposition. The omentum is draped around the innominate artery stump and the tracheal stump. Mobilizing the lower skin flap over the pectoral regions creates a permanent end tracheostoma. Grillo et al. reported a favorable outcome with this procedure.[28]

Contraindications for tracheal resection are patient-related factors such as respiratory failure and poor general condition, tumor-related factors such as extensive mediastinal lymph nodal metastasis, an extension of disease to major vessels and prior radiotherapy to trachea (>55 Gy).[29]

Postoperative complications with tracheal resections can occur at a rate of 9–45%.[30] One of the most dreaded complications is anastomotic dehiscence, which results in mediastinitis, pneumonia, and respiratory insufficiency. Arrhythmias are common in thoracic and carinal resections (15%). Mortality associated with tracheal resections has significantly reduced over the recent years from 21 to 2–3%.[31]

Radiotherapy

Indications for radiotherapy are either as an adjuvant to surgery or in unresectable tumors. Radiotherapy is inferior to surgery in achieving tumor control and survival.

SEER database match pair analysis to determine the efficacy of radiotherapy in malignant tracheal tumor has reported improved survival with radiation therapy, especially in SCC, regional disease, and unresectable disease.[32] However, only 5% in either arm had undergone R0 resection. Hence, the real benefit of postoperative radiotherapy may be higher. The overall survival was significantly better after surgery and postoperative radiotherapy when compared to surgery alone (58 vs. 7%). The benefit was sustained in median survival (91 vs. 12 months). Various studies have reported benefit of radiotherapy, but most include patients from a wide range of time and control rates may be superior with currently used conformal techniques. A total of 55–60 Gy is administered in postoperative radiotherapy.[33] Role of concurrent chemoradiotherapy (CTRT) in adjuvant therapy is sparsely studied, and its benefit may be extrapolated from evidence in head and neck SCC.

In unresectable tumors, radiation alone or concurrent with chemotherapy can be employed. A total radiotherapy dose of 60 Gy is recommended. Concurrent cisplatin is the most common chemotherapy administered. Other regimes containing cisplatin, 5-fluorouracil and etoposide for four cycles concurrent with 60 Gy[34] and cisplatin (80 mg/m^2 on day 1 and 28) and vinorelbine (12 mg/m^2 on day 1,8,15) concurrent with 60 Gy followed by vinorelbine 25 mg/m^2 has also been reported.[33]

Palliative Chemotherapy

Palliative chemotherapy can be administered based on the histology of the tumor. Cisplatin, paclitaxel, cisplatin, and vinorelbine for SCC, and pemetrexed or gemcitabine for adenocarcinoma can be administered. Somatic mutations of EGFR, EML-4-ALK can be tested to consider tyrosine kinase inhibitors.[33]

Palliative Procedures

Endoscopic approaches with laser debulking and stenting are options in unresectable tumors with airway obstructions. Self-expanding metal stents can be used to maintain the airway patent after tumors debulking in patients with expected survival of at least 6 months. Prolonged in situ stents can cause late complications such as dislodgement and esophageal or vascular fistulas; hence stenting must be avoided in cases with expected prolonged survival like in ACC.[29] An Italian series included 2,008 patients with malignant airway obstruction treated with laser excision, stenting, and endoluminal brachytherapy. They reported an improved quality of life in 93%, but the palliation was temporary.[35]

PROGNOSIS

Outcome of tracheal malignancy is dismal with population-based studies reporting 5 and 10-year overall survival of 5–15% and 6–7%.[33] The reason for this may

Table 4: Outcomes in tracheal malignancy.

Study	*Number of patients*	*Period*	*Outcome (5-year overall survival)*	
			Squamous cell carcinoma	*Adenoid cystic carcinoma*
Grillo et al.[14]	198	1962–1989	45%	65%
Gaissert et al.[2]	270	1962–2002	Resectable 39% Unresectable 7%	Resectable 52% Unresectable 33%
Honings et al.[7]	308 (Netherlands Cancer registry)	1989–2002	12%	61%
Urdaneta et al.[36]	573 (SEER Database)	1973–2004	13%	74%

be that most patients present with unresectable disease. Patients who undergo surgical resection have the best survival. Prognostic factors that negatively affect survival are incomplete resection, involvement of adjacent structures (thyroid, extramural disease), lymphatic metastasis, and perineural spread.[29] Studies that have reported outcomes after resection of tracheal malignancy are presented in **Table 4**.

SURVEILLANCE

Primary SCC of the trachea is associated with second primaries in the bronchus or lung and hence must undergo screening CT of the chest and check bronchoscopy during follow-up period. ACC of the trachea is more prone for late local recurrences and metastases, and hence serial evaluation must be directed at ruling out recurrences and lung metastases.

CONCLUSION

Primary tracheal malignancies are rare tumors. Most patients present in an advanced stage, due to delay in diagnosis. A detailed knowledge of tracheal anatomy is essential to perform surgical resection. Surgery achieves best oncologic outcomes. Other treatment modalities have a limited role in the management of tracheal tumors.

REFERENCES

1. Licht PB, Friis S, Pettersson G. Tracheal cancer in Denmark: a nationwide study. Eur J Cardiothor Surg. 2001;19:339-45.
2. Gaissert HA, Grillo HC, Shadmehr MB, Wright CD, Gokhale M, Wain JC, et al. Long-term survival after resection of primary adenoid cystic and squamous cell carcinoma of the trachea and carina. Ann Thorac Surg. 2004;78(6): 1889-97.
3. Perelman MI, Koroleva NS. Primary tumors of the Trachea. In: Grillo HC, Eschapasse H (Eds). Major Challenges, International Trends in General Thoracic Surgery. Philadelphia: Saunders; 1987. pp. 91±106.
4. Manninen MP, Antila PJ, Pukander JS, Karma PH. Occurrence of tracheal carcinoma in Finland. Acta Otolaryngol. 1991; 111(6):1162-9.
5. Young JL, Percy CL, Asire AJ. Incidence and Mortality, Data, 1973-1977. In: U.S. Department of Health and Human Services (Ed). Surveillance, Epidemiology and End Results. Bethesda, Maryland: National Cancer Institute; 1981. pp. 87-91.
6. Bennetts FE. Tracheal tumours. Postgrad Med J. 1969;45(525): 446-54.
7. Honings J, van Dijck JA, Verhagen AF, van der Heijden HFM, Marres HAM. Incidence and treatment of tracheal cancer: a nationwide study in the Netherlands. Ann Surg Oncol. 2007;14:968-76.
8. Honings J, Gaissert HA, van der Heijden HF, Verhagen AFTM, Kaanders JHAM, Henri AMM. Clinical aspects and treatment of primary tracheal malignancies. Acta Otolaryngol. 2010;130:763-72.
9. Furlow PW, Mathisen DJ. Surgical anatomy of the trachea. Ann Cardiothorac Surg. 2018;7(2):255-60.
10. Grillo HC. Surgery of the trachea and bronchi. Hamilton (ON, Canada): BC Decker; 2004. pp. 39-61.
11. Minnich DJ, Mathisen DJ. Anatomy of the trachea, carina, and bronchi. Thorac Surg Clin. 2007;17:571-85.
12. Heffner DK. Diseases of the trachea. In: Barnes L (Ed). Surgical Pathology of the Head and Neck, 2nd edition. New York: Marcel Dekker; 2001. pp. 602-31.
13. Ellis GL, Auclair PL. AFIP atlas of tumor pathology, tumors of the salivary glands. Silver Spring (MD): ARP Press; 2008.
14. Grillo HC, Mathisen DJ. Primary tracheal tumors: treatment and results. Ann Thorac Surg. 1990;49(1):69-77.
15. Pellegrino R, Viegi G, Brusasco V, Crapo RO, Burgos F, Casaburi R, et al. Interpretative strategies for lung function tests. Eur Respir J. 2005;26(5):948-68.
16. Finkelstein SE, Schrump DS, Nguyen DM, Hewitt SM, Kunst TF, Summers RM. Comparative evaluation of super high-resolution CT scan and virtual bronchoscopy for the detection of tracheobronchial malignancies. Chest. 2003; 124(5):1834-40.
17. Bhattacharyya N. Contemporary staging and prognosis for primary tracheal malignancies: a population-based analysis. Otolaryngol Head Neck Surg. 2004;131(5):639-42.
18. Macchiarini P. Primary tracheal tumours. Lancet Oncol. 2006;7(1):83-91.
19. Wood DE. Management of malignant tracheobronchial obstruction. Surg Clin North Am. 2002;82(3):621-42.
20. Gaissert HA. Primary tracheal tumors. Chest Surg Clin N Am. 2003;13(2):247-56.
21. Grillo HC, Suen HC, Mathisen DJ, Wain JC. Resectional management of thyroid carcinoma invading the airway. Ann Thorac Surg. 1992;54(1):3-10.

22. Tracheal Resection and sleeve pneumonectomy. In: Nesbitt JC, Wind GG (Eds). Thoracic Surgical Oncology: Exposures and Techniques. Philadelphia, Lippincott: Williams & Wilkins; 2003.
23. Pinsonneault C, Fortier J, Donati F. Tracheal resection and reconstruction. Can J Anaesth. 1999;46(5 Pt 1):439-55.
24. Donahue DM, Grillo HC, Wain JC, Wright CD, Mathisen DJ. Reoperative tracheal resection and reconstruction for unsuccessful repair of postintubation stenosis. J Thorac Cardiovasc Surg. 1997;114:934-8; discussion 938-9.
25. Montgomery WW. Suprahyoid release for tracheal anastomosis. Arch Otolaryngol. 1974;99:255-60.
26. Grillo HC, Dignan EF, Miura T. Extensive Resection and Reconstruction of Mediastinal Trachea without Prosthesis or Graft: An Anatomical Study in Man. J Thorac Cardiovasc Surg. 1964;48:741-9.
27. Abouarab AA, Elsayed HH, Elkhayat H, Mostafa A, Cleveland DC, Nori AE. Current Solutions for Long-Segment Tracheal Reconstruction. Ann Thorac Cardiovasc Surg. 2017; 23(2):66-75.
28. Grillo HC, Mathisen DJ. Cervical exenteration. Ann Thorac Surg. 1990;49(3):401-9.
29. Madariaga MLL, Gaissert HA. Overview of malignant tracheal tumors. Ann Cardiothorac Surg. 2018;7(2):244-54.
30. Tapias LF, Mathisen DJ. Prevention and management of complications following tracheal resections-lessons learned at the Massachusetts General Hospital. Ann Cardiothorac Surg. 2018;7(2):237-43.
31. Mitchell JD, Mathisen DJ, Wright CD, Wain JC, Donahue DM, Moncure AC, et al. Clinical experience with carinal resection. J Thorac Cardiovasc Surg. 1999;117:39-52; discussion 52-3.
32. Xie L, Fan M, Sheets NC, Chen RC, Jiang GL, Marks LB. The use of radiation therapy appears to improve outcome in patients with malignant primary tracheal tumors: a SEER-based analysis. Int J Radiat Oncol Biol Phys. 2012;84: 464-70.
33. Behringer D, Könemann S, Hecker E. Treatment approaches to primary tracheal cancer. Thorac Surg Clin. 2014;24(1): 73-6.
34. Videtic GM, Campbell C, Vincent MD. Primary chemoradiation as definitive treatment for unresectable cancer of the trachea. Can Respir J. 2003;10(3):143-4.
35. Cavaliere S, Venuta F, Foccoli P, Toninelli C, Face BL. Endoscopic treatment of malignant airway obstructions in 2,008 patients. Chest. 1996;110:1536-42.
36. Urdaneta AI, Yu JB, Wilson LD. Population based cancer registry analysis of primary tracheal carcinoma. Am J Clin Oncol. 2011;34:32-7.

Multidisciplinary Management of Unresectable Head and Neck Cancer

Manish Mair, Hitesh Singhavi, Narayana Subramaniam

INTRODUCTION

A National Cancer Data Base study showed that in the US, 55% of patients with oral cancer presented with advanced stage disease; in tertiary care centers, this was as high as 85%.[1] In developing countries as well, the majority of head and neck cancers have an advanced stage at presentation.[2] Many of these patients are considered inoperable and hence unfit for curative intent therapies. With time, the concept of unresectability has become more indistinct; improved surgical techniques, equipment, and perioperative care has allowed surgeons to safely perform procedures that were unthinkable a decade or so previously.

Unresectability in itself has different components; technical unresectability refers to the inability to achieve negative margins even with the sacrifice of important structures, while the term unresectable/inoperable can refer to the unacceptable morbidity, poor outcomes and poor surgical fitness and physiological reserve that make surgery an unviable option even when negative margins can be achieved. In these cases, the major considerations are symptom control and preservation of quality of life. Multidisciplinary care is essential to achieve optimal outcomes in this cohort. The purpose of this chapter is to describe the evidence that goes into decision making in these patients. For clarity we are restricting the discussion to head and neck squamous cell carcinoma (HNSCC) of the surgically treated subsites. Although HPV-related HNSCC has significantly better outcomes even in the setting of advanced disease,[3-8] the same principles apply.

NOMENCLATURE

Management of locally advanced head and neck cancer begins with accurate staging. It is possible to determine resectability of advanced stage disease with contemporary imaging techniques.

Advanced disease can be classified into:

- Postoperative "high-risk" HNSCC (high risk of morbidity and potential mortality following surgery)
- Potentially resectable advanced disease
- Unresectable disease without distant metastases (disease that cannot be resected without unacceptably high morbidity due to removal of key structures like cervical vertebrae, brachial plexus, deep muscle of the neck, skull base or common carotid artery)
- Disease with distant metastases

Anatomical criteria based on which disease is classified as inoperable/unresectable in each subsite are as follows:

- *Oral cavity:* Involvement of masticator space, pterygoid plates (where achieving margins at skull base not possible), internal carotid artery encasement >270° or extensive skin defect where adequate margins not achievable or where resection causes significant morbidity
- *Oropharynx:* Involvement of lateral pterygoid muscle, pterygoid plates, lateral nasopharynx, skull base or common carotid artery encasement
- *Larynx/hypopharynx:* Involvement of prevertebral space, mediastinal structures or common carotid artery encasement
- *Nasal cavity and paranasal sinus:* Involvement of orbital apex, dura, middle cranial fossa, cranial nerves other than V2, nasopharynx or clivus
- *Salivary glands:* Involvement of skull base, pterygoid plates or encasement of common carotid artery
- *Thyroid:* Gross extrathyroidal extension in anaplastic carcinoma

MASTICATOR SPACE

The masticator space (MS) is a complex anatomic site located below temporal bone. It is a fascia-lined space that is enclosed by the superficial layers of the deep cervical fascia. The superficial layer of the deep cervical fascia splits at the lower border of the mandible, with the inner lip attaching to the skull base, deep to the medial pterygoid muscle, and the superficial layer enclosing the masseter and inserting on to the zygomatic arch. These two layers meet in front of and behind the ramus of the mandible to enclose the MS. The infratemporal fossa (ITF) is bounded anteriorly by the posterior wall of the maxillary sinus, laterally by the ramus of the mandible, medially by the medial pterygoid muscles, and posteriorly by the styloid process and the tympanic part of the temporal bone. A transaxial plane passing between through the notch (sigmoid notch) classifies the space into two parts—space superior to this plane is termed as "high" ITF and below it is known as "low" ITF. Often MS and ITF are used interchangeably, however a clear understanding of the two is important; the ITF is not lined by fascia and encompasses the medial part of the MS and a part of the prestyloid paraparyngeal space.[9]

T4a versus T4b oral cancer: Studies by Liao et al.[10-13] defied the dictum that T4b tumors are inoperable. He classified T4b disease into supra and infra notch, with the former having a higher incidence of locoregional recurrence. Studies by Trivedi et al.[14-16] further classified ITF involvement into class I (low masticator space involving medial pterygoid and masseter muscles, ascending ramus of mandible), class II (intermediate masticator space involving lateral pterygoid and temporalis muscle and lower half of pterygoid plates), and class III (high masticator space with involvement of pterygo-maxillary fissure and intracranial extension). Another large study of 210 advanced buccal cancers by Mair et al.[17] found that T4a and T4b group had similar local recurrence rate when adequate margins were achieved; overall T4b patients had poorer overall survival as compared to T4a thus postulating the need for treatment intensification in T4b group. A study by Pillai et al.[18] on 277 patients on advanced buccal cancers showed there was pathological downstaging of 47% when staging was performed with contrast enhanced CT even when interpreted by experienced radiologists, and that in adequately treated pT4a and pT4b patients the 2-year OS were 57% and 58% respectively.

Surgical challenges: Surgical removal of such extensive disease is a challenging task due to difficulty in visualization and presence of the pterygoid venous plexus. Moreover, achieving clear margin is difficult due to its proximity to the skull base and probable involvement of neural structures.

Compartment resection: The concept of compartment resection was proposed by Trivedi et al.[15] They suggested that the entire anatomic unit of masticator space which includes posterior segment of mandible upper alveolus, masseter muscle, whole of both medial and lateral pterygoid muscles with pterygoid plates and part of temporalis muscle should be removed in an en-bloc fashion. They proposed that this results in minimal bleeding, better reproducibility, and greater chances of achieving negative margins. They also found good survival rates when both pterygoid muscle (lateral pterygoid and medial pterygoid) are involved and pterygoid plates and pterygomaxillary fissure were free, challenging the dogma of lateral pterygoid involvement as a sign of inoperability.

CAROTID ARTERY

Involvement of the internal carotid artery may be a contraindication to surgery. Yousem et al.[19,20] concluded that MRI could effectively evaluate carotid artery involvement. Yoo et al.[21] found carotid artery invasion to be an independent risk factor for poor outcome; they recommended peeling of tumor off rather than resection of carotid when carotid encasement was <180°. The OS for patients with tumor attachment greater and less than 180° were 8.3% and 33% respectively. The MRI imaging criteria that require consideration prior to surgery are involvement >270° that has a higher risk of carotid injury intraoperatively, obliteration of fat between the node and the artery is likely to point to vessel wall invasion, deformation and length of the artery involved can also differentiate abutment and invasion, and in tumors like those of the hypopharynx what appears to be encasement could be involvement anteriorly by the tumor and posteriorly by the nodal disease, which may not preclude complete resection.

PREVERTEBRAL FASCIA

The prevertebral fascia covers the longus muscle complex and constitutes the posterior border of the prevertebral space.[22] Hematogenous dissemination is quite frequent when tumors extends into the prevertebral space. They are also associated with a high rate of retropharyngeal nodal involvement and poor prognosis. Very advanced cancers of the nasopharynx, oropharynx, hypopharynx, larynx, and extensive nodal disease with extracapsular spread lead to prevertebral space involvement. According to Feng et al.,[23] prevertebral muscle invasion was found to be an independent risk factor for recurrence in nasopharyngeal tumor. Similarly, Lee et al.[24] concluded that nasopharyngeal carcinoma with involvement of prevertebral fascia leads to poor overall survival. These patients also had a propensity for distant metastases. From a surgeon's perspective, clinical involvement of prevertebral space is difficult to examine because it requires assessment of tumor mobility independently from movement of the musculature and vertebral column.

EXTENDED SURGICAL RESECTION

- *Carotid resection:* It is difficult to predict surgical resectibility of the tumor or nodal deposit when carotid encasement is 180–270°. It is also important to note that these patients have a poor survival; one study predicted a 2-year OS of 8% in this cohort.[17] Using MRI assessment, for nodal disease >270° carotid involvement, it is virtually improbable that the surgeon would be able to completely dissect the deposit off the carotid artery even with subadventitial dissection (0%).[19] The carotid artery is the last structure to be sacrificed in the extended radical neck dissection. Following are the situations in which carotid should not be sacrificed:
  - When reconstruction of the vessel is not possible
  - In the case of insufficient cerebral collateral circulation
  - Complete removal of tumor is not possible
  - When radiotherapy has been accepted as an alternative therapy.

  In case the internal carotid artery needs to be sacrificed, preoperative neurological testing to access the collateral blood flow should be done. This involves balloon test occlusion with the help of single photon emission computed tomography (SPECT). During surgery, revascularization using bypass or allograft should be performed; this not only reestablishes the cerebral flow but also reduces the chances of subsequent thromoboembolic stroke. When revascularization of the carotid is attempted after resection, the incidence of stroke varies from 0–20%,[25,26] as opposed to up to 58% when no revascularization is attempted. The mortality rate was also reduced (3 vs. 29%).[27,28] Further details of carotid resection are available in the chapter on sinonasal and anterior skull base tumors.
- *Cranial nerve resection:* Resection of multiple cranial nerves such as vagus results in high morbidity with persistent issues such as dysphagia and aspiration. Bilateral resection results in lifelong tracheostomy dependence. Sympathetic chain resection results in Horner's syndrome (miosis, anhidrosis, partial ptosis, and enophthalmos). Extended resections of vital structures are associated with poor quality of life and often negligible improvements in prognosis; with improved reconstruction techniques although most advanced stage tumors are now resectable, it is critical for a multidisciplinary assessment of these patients to determine the best course of treatment. If planned for surgery, ruling out distant metastases and discussing the potential morbidity and mortality associated with extensive resection need to be discussed.

DEFINITIVE RADIOTHERAPY

Radiotherapy alone has a minimal role in the curative management of unresectable head and neck cancer. Literature has shown inferior survival outcomes with radiotherapy alone when compared to combined therapy.[26-28] However, there is a substantial contribution of radiotherapy when it comes to palliative treatment. The most effective palliation is one that relieves symptoms with as little morbidity achievable. The quad shot regimen is said to be effective in palliation setting;[29] it consists of 370 cGy delivered twice daily for 2 consecutive days (total of 1,480 cGy/cycle), repeated every 3–4 weeks for a total of 4,400 cGy in three cycles. For patients who tolerate this regimen well and who continue to respond, additional cycles can be delivered. As one cycle can be delivered in 2 days, it reduces the travel burden on the patients and allows normal cell repopulation. In addition, the dose is calibrated to avoid the threshold dose for mucositis. Literature suggests 72% of the patients experienced better quality of life after the treatment. Toxicity in terms of mucositis, skin reaction and salivary gland toxicities were minimal; symptomatically there was improvement in dysphagia in 85% and reduced or unchanged in 89%. Another review by Grewal et al. recommended palliative radiotherapy in a more personalized manner;[30] in their review they divided the regimen of palliative radiation according to the estimated time of survival. For those having an estimate survival <4 months, quad shot regimen is recommended due to its reduced toxicity, reduced duration of treatment and symptom palliation. For an estimated survival of 4–12 months, longer regimens are recommended, such as 2000 cGy in 5# or 5000 cGy in 20#. A similar regimen (2,000 cGy in 5#) is used for hemostasis in tumor related bleeding. For those with an estimated survival >12 months, 6,000 cGy in 30 days may be more suitable. Another retrospective study by Agrawal et al. suggested that hypofractionated radiotherapy (4,000 cGy in 16 fractions) regimen is an effective treatment modality for sustained symptoms; symptomatic relief was seen in over half of patients with acceptable toxicity.[31]

CHEMORADIOTHERAPY

Previously, radiotherapy was the mainstay of treatment for unresectable cancer. However, survival outcomes after radiation alone when combined with therapy were inferior by about 25%.[32-34] Merlano M et al. published a trial comprising 157 patients of HNSCC randomized to alternating radiotherapy and chemotherapy or radiotherapy alone. They found significantly higher complete response rates (43 vs. 22%) and 5-year OS (25 vs. 10%).[35] Similar results were also shown in a retrospective study by Eursritanakorn et al.[36]

In another trial by the Head and Neck Intergroup, 295 patients were randomized into three groups: group A (single daily fractionated radiotherapy with 70 Gy at 2 Gy/day), group B (concurrent chemoradiation), and group C (split course of radiotherapy and three cycles of concurrent 5-fluorouracil and cisplatin with 30 Gy given with the first cycle and 30–40 Gy given with the third cycle; surgical resection was considered if possible after the second cycle of chemotherapy). Grade 3 or worse toxicity was higher in chemotherapy groups (52% in A vs. 89% in B vs. 77% in C). The percentage of patients who completed treatment were 73% in group A, 85% in group B and 73% in group C. Median OS was superior in group B (19.1 months vs. 12.6 in group A). Group C had intermediate median OS of 13.8 months. 21% of patients in group C underwent surgery with neck dissection in 56%. They concluded that whenever feasible, addition of chemotherapy to radiation alone provides survival advantage with acceptable toxicity.[37]

Induction Chemotherapy Followed by Radiotherapy

It is widely believed that induction chemotherapy (IC) reduces the risk of distant metastases while concurrent chemoradiotherapy (CCRT) improves locoregional control.[37,38] The phase III trials TAX 323[38] and TAX 324[39] studied the feasibility of IC in LAHNSCC. While TAX 323 included only unresectable cases, TAX 324 had patients with technically unresectable tumors and also those with resectable tumors but suitable for organ preservation. Both these trials showed that three drug IC (docetaxel, platinum, and 5-fluorouracil, or TPF) yielded better OS than two drug IC (platinum and 5-fluorouracil, or PF) for locally advanced HNSCC. Patients in TAX 323 trial received radiotherapy after IC while those in TAX 324 receive carboplatin based CCRT after IC. The incidence of grade 3/4 neutropenia (76.9% vs. 52.5% in TAX 323 and 83% vs. 56% in TAX 324) and febrile neutropenia (5.2% vs. 2.8% in TAX 323 and 12% vs. 7% in TAX 324) were higher with TPF IC. A similar benefit in OS, progression free survival (PFS), disease free survival and locoregional control rate of TPF over PF was showed by Blanchard et al. in the meta-analysis published in 2013.[40] A meta-analysis by Pignon et al.[41] on the addition of chemotherapy to showed the most pronounced absolute survival benefit for CCRT (6.5% at 5 years). IC showed an absolute survival benefit of 2.4% at 5 years, which was not significant. However, when trials with PF IC were considered in isolation, the benefit of IC was found to be marginally significant. The only advantage of IC over CCRT was reduced distant failure rate.

To address the issue of whether IC was of value in locally advanced HNSCC, there were two randomized trials were subsequently conducted, DeCIDE[42] and PARADIGM.[43] DeCIDE included patients with advanced nodal disease at presentation (N2/N3, M0), who were randomized to either CCRT with docetaxel, fluorouracil, and hydroxyurea (DFHX) or to IC with 2 cycles of TPF followed by DFHX CCRT. They found no difference in OS (or distant-failure free survival. PARADIGM study compared upfront CCRT and TPF IC followed by CCRT in previously untreated stage III-IVB patients. They found better 3-year PFS (69% vs. 67%) and OS (78% vs. 73%) for the control arm of CCRT, however the difference was not significant. Both these studies showed higher toxicity in the IC arm. It is important to understand that both the studies had poor accrual rates and very ambitious targets with respect to improvement in 3-year OS by 15% (50 vs. 65% in DeCIDE and 55 vs. 70% in PARADIGM).

Another study in 2014 by the Spanish Head and Neck Cancer Cooperative Group[44] comparing TPF IC versus PF IC versus definitive CCRT failed to show any advantage of IC-CCRT over CCRT alone in patients with unresectable locally advanced HNSCC. They randomly assigned 439 unresectable HNSCC patients to three cycles of IC (TPF/PF) followed by CCRT with cisplatin or 7 weeks of CCRT alone. They found no difference in median time to treatment failure, which was 7.9, 7.9, and 8.2 for TPF-CCRT, PF-CCRT, and CCRT respectively. Moreover, there was no difference in OS suggestive of no added benefit of adding IC with CCRT. Another trial consisting of 407 unresectable head and neck cancer patients comparing cetuximab-radiotherapy to IC followed by CCRT showed no difference in recurrence rates, toxicity or locoregional control rates between the two arms.[45]

In an Indian scenario where gingivobuccal cancers predominate, Patil et al. defined technical unresectability as:[45]

- Buccal primary with diffuse margins and peritumoral edema going up to or above the level of the zygomatic arch without any satellite nodules
- Buccal primary with supranotch involvement of the ITF

- Buccal primary with extensive skin infiltration precluding excision with achievement of negative margins
- Oral tongue primary extending up to or below the level of the hyoid bone
- Oral tongue primary extending to the vallecula

They analyzed the effect of IC in 721 patients with unresectable oral cancer who underwent ICT with two or three drugs (taxane + platinum ± 5-fluorouracil) followed by resection if feasible. Resection was possible in 66% and 40% who received the three drug and two drug regimens respectively. Complete resection was achieved in all these patients. The median OS was 19.6 months in patients undergoing surgery and 8.16 months in patients who received nonsurgical treatment, which was significant.[46] Joshi et al. showed the efficacy and impact of IC in 110 T4b oral cavity cancers. Resectability was achieved in 31%. The median OS for patients receiving definitive surgical and non-surgical therapy were 18 and 6.5 months respectively.[47] Another retrospective analysis by Rudresha et al. showed similar results.[48] Joshi et al. analyzed 35 patients with advanced laryngohypopharyngeal cancer who received IC to achieve resectibility. These patients had extensive soft tissue/skin involvement, oropharyngeal involvement or cartilage erosion with extensive skin/soft tissue involvement. Resectability could be achieved in a third of these patients.[49]

TARGETED THERAPY

This literature review has been covered in the chapter on management of recurrent and metastatic head and neck cancers.

RECOMMENDATION AND SUMMARY

The multidisciplinary approach is imperative to manage patients with unresectable head and neck cancers. Patients with good performance status (ECOG 0 or 1) recommendations include CCRT or IC followed by CCRT. One may also consider RT alone or RT with targeted therapy based on the patient's tolerance to chemotherapy. The benefit of adding IC to CCRT is still unclear. Definitive RT with or without concurrent systemic therapy should be considered in patients with an ECOG performance status of 2. Adding chemotherapy in these cases should be done taking into consideration the comorbidities and expected life expectancy of the patients. As the performance status of the patients gets poorer, its treatment goal shifts toward palliative treatment either with RT, single agent systemic therapy, or supportive care. This helps manage symptoms with acceptable toxicity and improvement or maintenance of quality of life.

REFERENCES

1. Patel UA, Lynn-Macrae A, Rosen F, Holloway N, Kern R. Advanced stage of head and neck cancer at a tertiary-care county hospital. Laryngoscope. 2006;116(8):1473-7.
2. Nair D, Singhvi H, Mair M, Qayyumi B, Deshmukh A, Pantvaidya G, et al. Outcomes of surgically treated oral cancer patients at a tertiary cancer center in India. Indian J Cancer. 2017;54(4):616-20.
3. Marur S, D'Souza G, Westra WH, Forastiere AA. HPV-associated head and neck cancer: a virus-related cancer epidemic. Lancet Oncol. 2010;11(8):781-9.
4. Posner MR, Lorch JH, Goloubeva O, Tan M, Schumaker LM, Sarlis NJ, et al. Survival and human papillomavirus in oropharynx cancer in TAX 324: a subset analysis from an international phase III trial. Ann Oncol. 2011;22(5):1071-7.
5. Rischin D, Young RJ, Fisher R, Fox SB, Le QT, Peters LJ, et al. Prognostic significance of p16INK4A and human papillomavirus in patients with oropharyngeal cancer treated on TROG 02.02 phase III trial. J Clin Oncol. 2010;28(27):4142-8.
6. O'Sullivan B, Huang SH, Su J, Garden AS, Sturgis EM, Dahlstrom K, et al. Development and validation of a staging system for HPV-related oropharyngeal cancer by the International Collaboration on Oropharyngeal cancer Network for Staging (ICON-S): a multicentre cohort study. Lancet Oncol. 2016;17(4):440-51.
7. Lydiatt WM, Patel SG, O'Sullivan B, Brandwein MS, Ridge JA, Migliacci JC, et al. Head and neck cancers—major changes in the American Joint Committee on cancer eighth edition cancer staging manual. CA Cancer J Clin. 2017;67(2):122-37.
8. Nguyen-Tan PF, Zhang Q, Ang KK, Weber RS, Rosenthal DI, Soulieres D, et al. Randomized phase III trial to test accelerated versus standard fractionation in combination with concurrent cisplatin for head and neck carcinomas in the Radiation Therapy Oncology Group 0129 trial: long-term report of efficacy and toxicity. J Clin Oncol. 2014;32(34):3858.
9. Standring S. Infratemporal and pterygopalatine fossae and temporomandibular joint. In: Strandring S (Ed). Gray's Anatomy: The Anatomical Basis of Clinical Practice, 14th edition. London: Churchill Livingstone Elsevier; 2011. p. 527.
10. Liao CT, Chang JT, Wang HM, Ng SH, Hsueh C, Lee LY, et al. Surgical outcome of T4a and resected T4b oral cavity cancer. Cancer. 2006;107(2):337-44.
11. Liao CT, Wen YW, Lee SR, Liu TW, Tsai ST, Tsai MH, et al. Clinical Outcomes of Taiwanese Patients with cT4 Oral Cavity Squamous Cell Carcinoma: Toward the Identification of the Optimal Initial Treatment Approach for cT4b Patients. Ann Surg Oncol. 2017;24(3):785-93.
12. Liao CT, Ng SH, Chang JT, Wang HM, Hsueh C, Lee LY, et al. T4b oral cavity cancer below the mandibular notch is resectable with a favorable outcome. Oral Oncol. 2007;43(6):570-9.
13. Liao CT, Wen YW, Yang LY, Lee SR, Ng SH, Liu TW, et al. Comparative clinical outcomes of Taiwanese patients with resected buccal and tongue squamous cell carcinomas. Oral Oncol. 2017;67:95-102.
14. Trivedi NP, Kekatpure VD, Shetkar G, Gangoli A, Kuriakose MA. Pathology of advanced buccal mucosa cancer involving masticator space (T4b). Indian J Cancer. 2015;52(4):611.
15. Trivedi NP, Kekatpure V, Kuriakose MA. Radical (compartment) resection for advanced buccal cancer involving masticator space (T4b): Our experience in thirty patients. Clinical Otolaryngology. 2012;37(6):477-83.
16. Trivedi NP. Oral cancer involving masticator space (T4b): Review of literature and future directions. Head Neck. 2018;40(10):2288-94.
17. Mair MD, Sawarkar N, Nikam S, Sarin R, Nair D, Gupta T, et al. Impact of radical treatments on survival in locally

advanced T4a and T4b buccal mucosa cancers: Selected surgically treated T4b cancers have similar control rates as T4a. Oral Oncol. 2018;82:17-22.
18. Pillai V, Yadav V, Kekatpure V, Trivedi N, Chandrashekhar NH, Shetty V, et al. Prognostic determinants of locally advanced buccal mucosa cancer: Do we need to relook the current staging criteria? Oral Oncol. 2019;95:43-51.
19. Yousem DM, Hatabu H, Hurst RW, Seigerman HM, Montone KT, Weinstein GS, et al. Carotid artery invasion by head and neck masses: prediction with MR imaging. Radiology. 1995;195(3):715-20.
20. Yousem DM, Gad K, Tufano RP. Resectability issues with head and neck cancer. Am J Neuroradiol. 2006;27(10): 2024-36.
21. Yoo GH, Hocwald E, Korkmaz H, Du W, Logani S, Kelly JK, et al. Assessment of carotid artery invasion in patients with head and neck cancer. Laryngoscope. 2000;110(3):386-90.
22. Guo CB, Feng Z, Zhang JG, Peng X, Cai ZG, Mao C, et al. Supraomohyoid neck dissection and modified radical neck dissection for clinically node-negative oral squamous cell carcinoma: a prospective study of prognosis, complications and quality of life. J Craniomaxillofac Surg. 2014;42(8):1885-90.
23. Feng AC, Wu MC, Tsai SY, Chan KY, Cheng SH, Wang A, et al. Prevertebral muscle involvement in nasopharyngeal carcinoma. International J Radiation Oncology Biology Physics. 2006;65(4):1026-35.
24. Lee CC, Chu ST, Chou P, Lee CC, Chen LF. The prognostic influence of prevertebral space involvement in nasopharyngeal carcinoma. Clinical Otolaryngology. 2008;33(5):442-9.
25. Katsuno S, Ishiyama T, Sakaguchi M, Takemae H. Carotid resection and reconstruction for advanced cervical cancer. Laryngoscope. 1997;107(5):661-4.
26. Freeman SB. Advanced cervical metastasis involving the carotid artery. Current opinion in otolaryngology & head and neck surgery. 2005;13(2):107-11.
27. Wright JG, Nicholson R, Schuller DE, Smead WL. Resection of the internal carotid artery and replacement with greater saphenous vein: a safe procedure for en bloc cancer resections with carotid involvement. J Vasc Surg. 1996;23(5): 775-82.
28. Feiz-Erfan I, Han PP, Spetzler RF, Lanzino G, Ferreira MA, Gonzalez LF, Porter RW. Salvage of advanced squamous cell carcinomas of the head and neck: internal carotid artery sacrifice and extracranial-intracranial revascularization. Neurosurg Focus. 2003;14(3):1-5.
29. Corry J, Peters LJ, D'Costa I, Milner AD, Fawns H, Rischin D, et al. The 'QUAD SHOT'—a phase II study of palliative radiotherapy for incurable head and neck cancer. Radiother Oncol. 2005;77(2):137-42.
30. Grewal AS, Jones J, Lin A. Palliative radiation therapy for head and neck cancers. Int J Radiat Oncol Biol Phys. 2019;105(2):254-66.
31. Agarwal JP, Nemade B, Murthy V, Ghosh-Laskar S, Budrukkar A, Gupta T, et al. Hypofractionated, palliative radiotherapy for advanced head and neck cancer. Radiother Oncol. 2008;89(1):51-6.
32. Vokes EE, Weichselbaum RR, Lippman SM, Hong WK. Head and neck cancer. New Engl J Med. 1993;328(3):184-94.
33. Adelstein DJ. Concurrent Chemoradiotherapy. In: Squamous Cell Head and Neck Cancer. New Jersey: Humana Press; 2005. pp. 187-95.
34. Cooper JS, Farnan NC, Asbell SO, Rotman M, Marcial V, Fu KK, et al. Recursive partitioning analysis of 2105 patients treated in Radiation Therapy Oncology Group studies of head and neck cancer. Cancer. 1996;77(9):1905-11.
35. Merlano M, Benasso M, Corvò R, Rosso R, Vitale V, Blengio F, et al. Five-year update of a randomized trial of alternating radiotherapy and chemotherapy compared with radiotherapy alone in treatment of unresectable squamous cell carcinoma of the head and neck. J Natl Cancer Inst. 1996;88(9):583-9.
36. Eursritanakorn S. Survival Rates of Concurrent Chemo-Radiation versus Radiation Alone in Locally Advanced, Unresectable Head and Neck Cancers: A Retrospective Cohort Study. J Med Assoc Thai. 2016;99:S91-8.
37. Adelstein DJ, Li Y, Adams GL, Wagner Jr H, Kish JA, Ensley JF, et al. An intergroup phase III comparison of standard radiation therapy and two schedules of concurrent chemoradiotherapy in patients with unresectable squamous cell head and neck cancer. J Clin Oncol. 2003;21(1):92-8.
38. Vermorken JB, Remenar E, Van Herpen C, Gorlia T, Mesia R, Degardin M, et al. Cisplatin, fluorouracil, and docetaxel in unresectable head and neck cancer. New Engl J Med. 2007;357(17):1695-704.
39. Posner MR, Hershock DM, Blajman CR, Mickiewicz E, Winquist E, Gorbounova V, et al. Cisplatin and fluorouracil alone or with docetaxel in head and neck cancer. New Engl J Med. 2007;357(17):1705-15.
40. Blanchard P, Bourhis J, Lacas B, Posner MR, Vermorken JB, Hernandez JJ, et al. Taxane-cisplatin-fluorouracil as induction chemotherapy in locally advanced head and neck cancers: an individual patient data meta-analysis of the meta-analysis of chemotherapy in head and neck cancer group. J Clin Oncol. 2013;31(23):2854-60.
41. Pignon JP, Le Maitre A, Maillard E, Bourhis J, Mach-Nc Collaborative Group. Meta-analysis of chemotherapy in head and neck cancer (MACH-NC): an update on 93 randomised trials and 17,346 patients. Radiother Oncol. 2009;92(1):4-14.
42. Cohen EE, Karrison T, Kocherginsky M, Huang CH, Agulnik M, Mittal BB, et al. DeCIDE: A phase III randomized trial of docetaxel (D), cisplatin (P), 5-fluorouracil (F)(TPF) induction chemotherapy (IC) in patients with N2/N3 locally advanced squamous cell carcinoma of the head and neck (SCCHN). 2012;30(15).
43. Haddad R, O'Neill A, Rabinowits G, Tishler R, Khuri F, Adkins D, et al. Induction chemotherapy followed by concurrent chemoradiotherapy (sequential chemoradiotherapy) versus concurrent chemoradiotherapy alone in locally advanced head and neck cancer (PARADIGM): a randomised phase 3 trial. Lancet Oncol. 2013;14(3):257-64.
44. Hitt R, Grau JJ, Lopez-Pousa A, Berrocal A, García-Girón C, Irigoyen A, et al. A randomized phase III trial comparing induction chemotherapy followed by chemoradiotherapy versus chemoradiotherapy alone as treatment of unresectable head and neck cancer. Annals Oncol. 2014;25(1):216-25.
45. Patil VM, Prabhash K, Noronha V, Joshi A, Muddu V, Dhumal S, et al. Neoadjuvant chemotherapy followed by surgery in very locally advanced technically unresectable oral cavity cancers. Oral Oncol. 2014;50(10):1000-4.
46. Prabhash K, Patil VM, Noronha V, Joshi A, Dhumal S, Muddu VK, et al. Neoadjuvant chemotherapy in very locally advanced technically unresectable oral cavity cancers. Journal of Clinical Oncol; 2014. pp. e17033-e17033.
47. Joshi A, Patil VM, Noronha V, Juvekar S, Deshmukh A, Chatturvedi P, et al. Is there a role of induction chemotherapy followed by resection in T4b oral cavity cancers?. Indian J Cancer. 2013;50(4):349.
48. Rudresha AH, Chaudhuri T, Lakshmaiah KC, Babu KG, Dasappa L, Jacob LA, et al. Induction chemotherapy in locally advanced T4b oral cavity squamous cell cancers: A regional cancer center experience. Indian J Cancer. 2017;54(1):35.
49. Joshi P, Patil V, Joshi A, Norohna V, Chaturvedi P, Chaukar D, et al. Neo-adjuvant chemotherapy in advanced hypopharyngeal carcinoma. Indian J Cancer. 2013;50(1):25.

Management of Recurrent and Metastatic Head and Neck Cancer

Vijay Kumar Srinivasalu, Narayana Subramaniam, Sivakumar Vidhyadharan, Samskruthi P Murthy

INTRODUCTION

Most patients with head and neck cancer in developing countries such as India present with advanced disease due to a lack of awareness and healthcare access. They often have modest to poor outcomes with a median survival of 6–15 months. In this chapter, we summarize the standard systemic treatment regimens available in this setting and the evidence to support them.

HURDLES TO SYSTEMIC THERAPY

- *Tumor-related factors:* The primary tumor may cause issues with eating, dysphagia, and significant weight loss even prior to diagnosis. Loss of weight leads to poor prognosis when it is >5%.[1] Locally advanced hypopharynx and larynx patients can present with airway obstruction, or develop airway obstruction while on treatment needing an emergency tracheostomy.
- *Patient-related factors:* Tobacco and alcohol addiction, associated comorbidities, and lack of a social network are common patient-related factors that can complicate systemic treatment. As a standard of care in a curative setting with head and neck squamous cell cancer (HNSCC), high-dose platinum is given concurrently with radiotherapy, either as definitive therapy or adjuvant treatment after surgery. Chemotherapy, when added, led to an increase in acute and late or long-term side effects.
- *Treatment-related factors:* In treatment-naive patients, delivering systemic therapy is influenced by multiple factors such as performance status, associated comorbidities, previous initial treatment for the locoregional disease, tumor or tissue programmed death-ligand 1 (PD-L1) combined positive score (CPS), and related prognostic factors. Various active therapeutic drugs are available in our armamentaria, such as checkpoint inhibitor immunotherapy, targeted therapy, and multiple chemotherapeutic agents alone or in combination.

PROGNOSTIC FACTORS

While choosing systemic therapy, various patient-specific factors influencing prognosis needs to be considered. The various factors associated with improved survival are as follows:[2-6]

- Eastern Cooperative Oncology Group (ECOG) performance status
- Human papillomavirus (HPV)-associated oropharyngeal cancers
- Prior response to chemotherapy
- Time since completion of definitive therapy
- Tumor PD L1 expression status [a predictive marker for response to anti-programmed cell death protein 1 (PD 1) therapy].

In contrast, factors associated with a poor prognosis include the following:

- Weight loss
- Poor performance status
- Prior radiation therapy
- Active smoking
- Significant comorbidities.

With the numerical increase in age, there is often an increase in the associated comorbidities. However, survival outcomes have not differed between young and older patients with metastatic and recurrent head and neck cancer, except for increased toxicity in older patients.[7,8]

CHOICE OF THERAPY FOR METASTATIC OR PREVIOUSLY UNTREATED HNSCC

Factors that affect the choice of treatment for patients with advanced head and neck cancer with no prior systemic therapy are the ECOG performance status, symptoms related to locoregional disease burden, PD-L1 CPS from biopsy specimens and associated comorbidities **(Flowchart 1)**.

A metastatic or previously untreated head and neck cancer combines two different groups of patients, the first group, who presents initially with advanced disease and are not suitable or ideal candidates for definitive treatment and the second group consists of those patients who develop metastasis or incurable locally recurrent disease following local treatment (surgery and/or radiotherapy) without receiving any prior chemotherapy.

In metastatic and recurrent head and neck cancers, monotherapy with either immunotherapy or with combination, i.e., pembrolizumab, with or without chemotherapy was assessed in the KEYNOTE-048 study.[9] On adding pembrolizumab to a platinum analog and fluorouracil (5FU) combination, there was an improvement in overall survival. For metastatic tumors with high PD-L1 expression (CPS ≥ 1), pembrolizumab monotherapy improved overall survival compared to cetuximab plus chemotherapy. Still, its benefits are unclear if this is only seen in those with a CPS ≥ 20.

The following is preferred for patients with no prior systemic treatment (either chemotherapy or immunotherapy) based on performance status and associated comorbidities:

- Patients with rapidly progressive disease may benefit from a more rapid treatment response. In such patients, pembrolizumab with platinum plus 5FU (chemoimmunotherapy) is preferred, regardless of CPS. Some oncologists prefer a taxane instead of 5FU based on better tolerability when combined with platinum, but this combination has not been tested in a clinical trial.[10] Considering local therapy before administration of systemic therapy should be encouraged for better control of symptoms.

For a patient without the rapidly progressive disease, the preferred approach is mainly based on CPS on the biopsy:

- *CPS ≥ 20:* Suggestion is for monotherapy with single-agent pembrolizumab
- *CPS ≥ 1 and < 20:* Monotherapy with pembrolizumab, the addition of platinum plus 5FU chemotherapy depends mostly on the performance status. For patients with good performance status, pembrolizumab with chemotherapy can be considered, whereas, for those with a lesser performance status who would prefer to avoid the side effects of chemotherapy, single-agent pembrolizumab can be considered.
- *CPS = 0 or unavailable:* Chemotherapy is considered usually platinum and 5FU based regimen ± pembrolizumab. A doublet cytotoxic chemotherapy regimen, with or without concurrent or sequential cetuximab, can be considered for patients who are eligible for combination therapy but have contraindications to immunotherapy. Two drug regimens, usually platinum with either a taxane or 5FU, contribute to improvement in objective response rate (ORR) alone without any survival benefit when compared to single-agent chemotherapy. Adding cetuximab to cisplatin plus 5FU increased overall survival. Patients who are not eligible for combination chemotherapy plus immunotherapy can be considered for single-agent chemotherapy such as platinum-based compounds (typically carboplatin), taxanes (e.g., paclitaxel, docetaxel or nanoparticle-based paclitaxel), 5FU, methotrexate or monoclonal antibody-like cetuximab.
- *Pembrolizumab with or without chemotherapy:* This combination of pembrolizumab plus chemotherapy improved overall survival compared to cetuximab plus chemotherapy in metastatic or recurrent patients without prior exposure to any systemic treatment. For tumors with high PD-L1 expression, single-agent immunotherapy pembrolizumab improved overall survival with lesser toxicity. Pembrolizumab achieved durable responses either alone or in combination compared to cetuximab plus chemotherapy. The approval for pembrolizumab use by the US FDA for head and neck cancers are along with cisplatin and 5FU and as monotherapy for tumors with PD-L1 CPS ≥ 1. Pembrolizumab immunotherapy is administered for a maximum of 2 years when given as monotherapy or with combination chemotherapy.

The KEYNOTE-048, an open-label phase 3 trial that compared immunotherapy (pembrolizumab) to systemic chemotherapy in which 882 patients with recurrent or metastatic head and neck tumors were randomly assigned to 3 arms on a 1:1:1 basis. Arm A received single-agent immunotherapy with pembrolizumab. Arm B received pembrolizumab plus a platinum and 5FU chemotherapy combination, and arm C received cetuximab plus a platinum and 5FU combination.[9,11] Tumor PD-L1 status was assessed using CPS, which is calculated by combining lymphocytes and other cells that stain in addition to tumor cells. Results were analyzed separately for tumors with CPS ≥ 20, CPS ≥ 1, and the entire study population regardless of CPS.

At a median follow-up of approximately 13 months, pembrolizumab-containing combination therapy,

Flowchart 1: Approach to initial systemic therapy in patients with metastatic or recurrent head and neck squamous cell carcinoma.

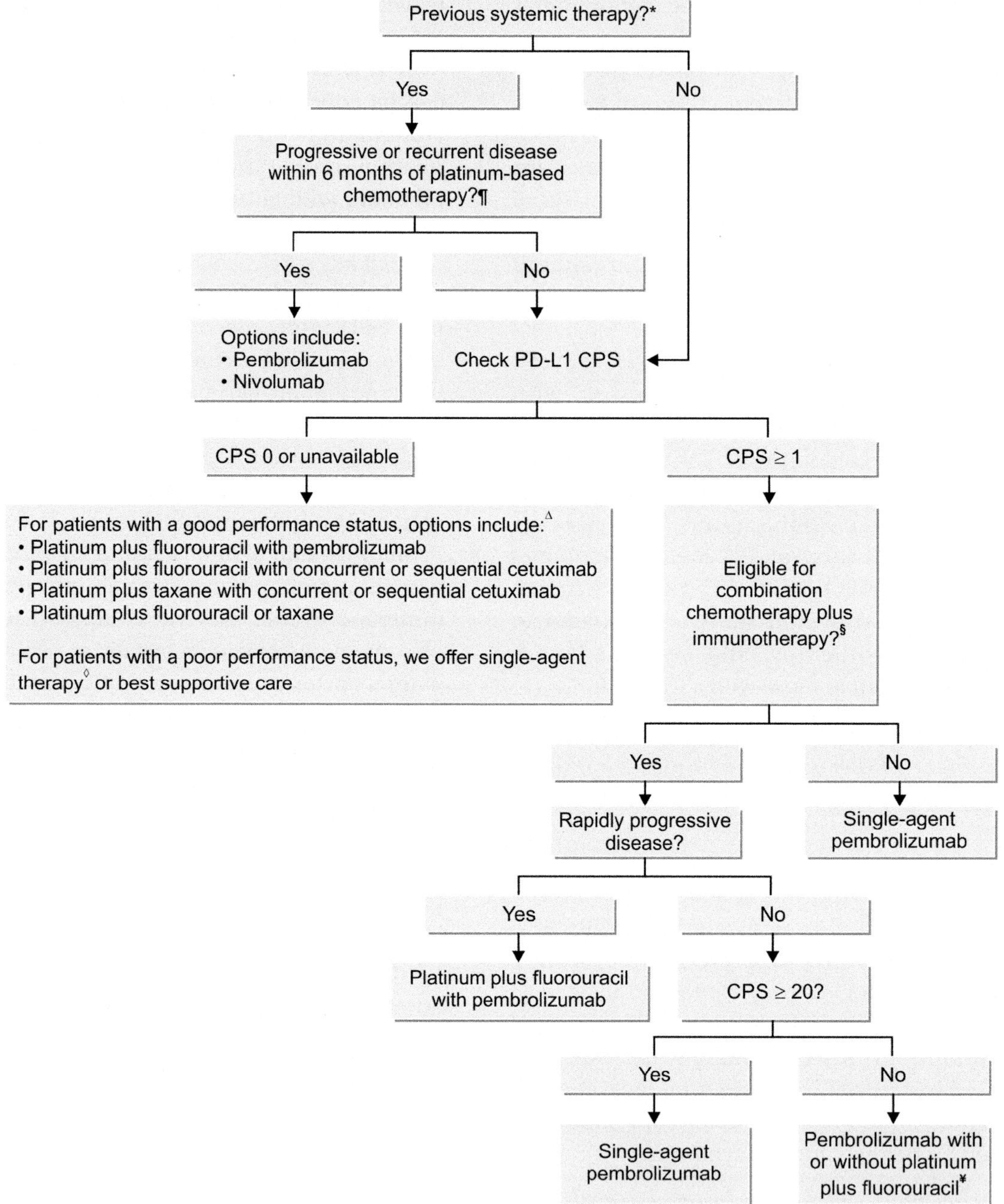

Patients with advanced disease who are ineligible for salvage surgery and/or radiation therapy may be eligible for systemic therapy. The goals of treatment are palliative. The listed treatments are the preferred options, although alternative agents that are not listed may also be effective. Clinical trials are encouraged if available.

* Systemic therapy may have been given with or without radiation therapy for initial management of locoregional disease.

¶ Progressive or recurrent disease within 6 months of receiving platinum-based chemotherapy with or without cetuximab.

Δ The benefit of pembrolizumab in patients with a CPS of 0 is less certain. Patients who are not candidates for pembrolizumab may benefit from the addition of cetuximab to platinum-based chemotherapy. Platinum-based doublet chemotherapy alone may be preferred in patients with an impaired performance status.

◊ Options for single-agent therapy include: Platinum-based chemotherapy (carboplatin preferred); taxanes; cetuximab; fluorouracil; methotrexate; gemcitabine.

§ Eligibility for combination chemotherapy and/or immunotherapy is influenced by patient performance status, comorbidities, and prognostic factors. Combination chemotherapy is defined as doublet platinum-based chemotherapy.

¥ We prefer pembrolizumab with chemotherapy for patients with a good performance status (e.g., ECOG performance status ≤2). For others, we prefer single-agent pembrolizumab.

(PD-Ll: programmed cell death ligand 1; CPS: combined positive score; ECOG: Eastern Cooperative Oncology Group) in comparison with cetuximab-containing combination therapy, demonstrated the following:

- Improvement in overall survival (OS) was seen in patients with CPS ≥ 20 [median 14.7 vs. 11.0 months, 2 year OS 35 vs. 19%, hazard ratio (HR) 0.60, 95% CI 0.45–0.82] and in patients with CPS ≥ 1 (median 13.6 vs. 10.4 month, 2 year OS 31 vs. 17%, HR 0.65, 95% CI 0.53–0.80).
- OS was significantly improved (median 13.0 vs. 10.7 month, 2 year OS 29 vs. 19%, HR 0.77, 95% CI 0.63–0.93).
- Progression-free survival (PFS) was similar in patients with CPS ≥ 20 (median 5.8 vs. 5.2 months, HR 0.73, 95% CI 0.55–0.97) or CPS ≥ 1 (median 5.0 months each, HR 0.82, 95% CI 0.67–1.00).
- Objective response rates (ORR) were similar (43 vs. 38% for CPS ≥ 20, 36% each for CPS ≥ 1).
- Longer duration of response in patients with any positive CPS (7.1 vs. 4.2 months for CPS ≥ 20, 6.7 vs. 4.3 months for CPS ≥ 1).
- Grade ≥ 3 side effects between the two treatment arms were similar (85 vs. 83%).

- *Single-agent pembrolizumab, in comparison with cetuximab-containing combination therapy, the following were observed:*
  - Improvement with OS in patients with CPS ≥ 20 (median 14.9 vs. 10.7 months, 2 year OS 38 vs. 22%, HR 0.61, 95% CI 0.45–0.83) and in patients with CPS ≥ 1 (median 12.3 vs. 10.3 month, 2 year OS 30 vs. 19%, HR 0.78, 95% CI 0.64–0.96).
  - Patients in both the study arms had very similar OS (median 11.5 vs. 10.7 months, 2 year OS 27 vs. 19%, HR 0.83, 95% CI 0.70–0.99).
  - Low PFS in the total population (median 2.3 vs. 5.2 months, HR 1.34), early progressors were more in the pembrolizumab arm.
  - The duration of response was 23 months with pembrolizumab versus 5 months in the combination arm, whereas overall response rates were low (17 vs. 36%).
  - Fewer all grade toxicities (5 vs. 83% grade 3–5 adverse events).
- *Cetuximab with platinum-based chemotherapy:* In patients not eligible for immunotherapy such as lupus nephritis or with various autoimmune conditions, cetuximab with platinum and 5FU or platinum plus a taxane can be considered. The use of epidermal growth factor receptor (EGFR) inhibitor cetuximab is preferred with platinum plus a taxane rather than platinum plus 5FU due to fewer side effects. However, both the regimens had similar efficacy. Cetuximab is a chimeric (mouse/human) monoclonal antibody that acts by targeting the EGFR on the cell surface. Cetuximab, when combined with a platinum-based doublet, leads to an increase in overall survival. The approval of cetuximab in the first-line setting is with platinum-based combination chemotherapy. With cetuximab, the docetaxel-based combination had fewer side effects compared to a fluorouracil-based combination with similar efficacy.[10]
- *Cetuximab with platinum and fluorouracil:* The EXTREME trial assessed the benefits of cetuximab with combination chemotherapy. About 442 recurrent or metastatic HNSCC patients were randomized to platinum-based chemotherapy [cisplatin 100 mg/m^2 on day 1 or carboplatin area under the concentration (AUC) 5 day 1] plus 5FU (1,000 mg/m^2 per day for 4 days) cycled every 3 weeks, with or without cetuximab (400 mg/m^2 for the initial dose, followed by subsequent weekly 250 mg/m^2).[12] In this study, 39% of patients had received chemotherapy as part of their initial definitive treatment at least 6 months prior to randomization. Six cycles of chemotherapy were the maximum allowed, but cetuximab maintenance was permitted until disease progression or toxicity. But, in the chemotherapy arm, crossover to include cetuximab was not allowed.
  - In comparison with chemotherapy alone, the addition of targeted agent cetuximab to chemotherapy significantly improved overall survival (median 10.1 vs. 7.4 months, HR for death 0.80, 95% CI 0.64–0.99) and a significant improvement was noted in the PFS and ORR (median 5.6 vs. 3.3 months and 36 vs. 20%) respectively. Irrespective of the HPV status of the tumor, the responses obtained with cetuximab were similar.[13]
  - There was no increase in grade 3 or 4 adverse events while comparing cetuximab with chemotherapy alone (82 vs. 76%). Severe hypomagnesemia (5 vs. 1%), severe skin reactions (9 vs. <1 %), and sepsis (4 vs. <1%) were noted with cetuximab. Acute infusion-related toxicity was 3% in the study with the administration of cetuximab.
- *Cetuximab with platinum and taxane:* About 539 patients with recurrent or metastatic HNSCC were stratified randoly to receive six cycles of cisplatin and 5FU plus cetuximab versus four cycles of cisplatin and docetaxel plus cetuximab in an open-label phase III trial.[10] Both these regimens, i.e., CF + cetuximab and CD + cetuximab, were then followed by maintenance cetuximab.

- After a median follow-up of two and a half years, the overall survival was similar in both the groups (median 14.5 vs. 13.4 months; 2 years OS 29 vs. 21%; HR 0.87, 95% CI 0.71–1.05). The 5FU containing regimen had fewer toxicity, less delays in administration (10 vs. 27%), less substitution of carboplatin for cisplatin (9 vs. 34%), and more patients receiving maintenance cetuximab (73 vs. 53%) in the 5FU containing regimen.

- *Limited role for other targeted agents:* Cetuximab should not be replaced with either anti-EGFR monoclonal antibody-like panitumumab or anti-vascular endothelial growth factor (VEGF) monoclonal antibody-like bevacizumab in head and neck cancers.
  - *Panitumumab*—In SPECTRUM, a randomized phase 3 trial for previously untreated recurrent or metastatic HNSCC, the addition of panitumumab to cisplatin and 5FU led to an improvement in PFS but no improvement in OS with increased grade ≥3 toxicity.[14]
  - *Bevacizumab*—In a randomized phase III trial (E1305) of previously untreated recurrent or metastatic HNSCC, bevacizumab, when added to the platinum-based doublet, improved both PFS and ORR without any improvement in OS and higher grade ≥3 bleeding.[15]
- *Combination cytotoxic chemotherapy:* Most of the chemotherapy combinations in head and neck cancers include a platinum compound that acts as a backbone for systemic therapy. Improved ORR was seen with combination treatment regimens compared to a single agent without any demonstrable improvement in OS.
  - *Platinum and 5FU:* This combination is a standard regimen used in the palliative setting, i.e., cisplatin (100 mg/m^2 intravenous, day 1) and 5FU (1,000 mg/m^2 per day, continuous infusion, for 4 days). 5FU and cisplatin together had ORR of 30% in phase III studies, which was significant while comparing with single-agent cisplatin or methotrexate.[2,3,16,17] In the South West Oncology Group (SWOG) trial, 261 patients with advanced HNSCC were randomly assigned to one of three regimens: cisplatin with 5FU, carboplatin with 5FU, or single-agent methotrexate.[2] The ORR with doublet was better (32% and 21% vs. 10% with single-agent methotrexate). The median survival was comparable (6.6, 5.0, and 5.6 months, respectively). Cisplatin had more all grade 3 or 4 toxicity followed by carboplatin regimen and single-agent methotrexate (33 vs. 26% and 16% respectively). Due to the toxicity of fluoroquinolones and prolonged duration of administration, platinum plus taxane, or a single agent is preferred as initial therapy in the palliative setting.
  - *Platinum and taxane:* Both platinum analogs have been combined with taxanes (paclitaxel or docetaxel), but no superiority was evident in comparison with cisplatin plus 5FU. The only trial that assessed the role of a platinum-taxane regimen in head and neck cancer was a phase III Eastern Cooperative Oncology Group trial that compared cisplatin plus 5FU to cisplatin plus paclitaxel.[16] At 8 months of median follow-up, there was no difference in OS (8.7 vs. 8.1 months, 1 year OS 41 vs. 32%) or ORR (27 vs. 26%). Patients receiving cisplatin plus 5FU noticed an increase in gastrointestinal and hematologic toxicities. Docetaxel plus cisplatin was cycled every 3 weeks in a phase II study with excellent responses ranging between 32 and 55%. The median response duration was 5 months.[18-21] Incremental response rates were associated with increased toxicities in 70% of patients in the study. Docetaxel, when administered weekly, had lesser side effects with similar efficacy.[22] Replacing cisplatin with carboplatin had multiple advantages such as ease of administration, lesser renal toxicity, neurotoxicity, hearing loss, and emesis. Either paclitaxel or docetaxel has been combined with carboplatin in phase II trials with no phase III randomized trial[23-25] and found to have a response rate of 25–43%.
  - *Cisplatin plus pemetrexed*: In some subsets of patients, there has been some activity with this combination, but is not considered for initial treatment in recurrent or metastatic HNSCC. 795 patients with HNSCC were randomly assigned to either doublet combination of cisplatin plus pemetrexed or cisplatin alone in a phase III trial.[26] No improvement in the overall survival with the two-drug regimen (median 7.3 vs. 6.3 months, HR 0.87, 95% CI 0.75–1.02. In a pre-specified exploratory analysis, OS improved only in patients with good PS (0 or 1) and in tumors of the oropharynx, but a comparison with the current standard of care (a platinum compound combination) was not made.
  - *Triple or quadruple drug regimens:* When we add a third drug to a doublet, there can be an increase in responses, but at the cost of increased side effects, especially neutropenic fever.

Regimens studied in phase II studies include paclitaxel, cisplatin and 5FU,[27-29] cisplatin with docetaxel and 5FU,[30,31] vinblastine, doxorubicin, methotrexate and cisplatin[32] and ifosfamide, paclitaxel, and cisplatin or carboplatin.[33,34] However, there is a lack of evidence to demonstrate the superiority of single or two-drug regimens over the triplet EXTREME regimen.

- *Nonplatinum-based regimens:* These may be useful in patients with renal failure or hearing impairment and are not candidates for platinum-based chemotherapy. A SWOG study with 57 patients with metastatic or recurrent HNSCC, the combination of gemcitabine (3,000 mg/m^2) plus paclitaxel (150 mg/m^2) on day 1 and 15 cycled every showed a 28% ORR[35] with a median PFS of 4 months and OS of 8 months, but not better than single-agent taxane. The combination of paclitaxel and cetuximab administered weekly showed a response rate of 54% with an OS of about 8 months and a PFS of 4 months, as shown in an open-label phase II clinical trial.[36] The efficacy of paclitaxel and cetuximab regimen was consistent with other doublet regimens.

CHOICE OF THERAPY: A RECURRENT SETTING

The selection of subsequent sequential therapy is never constant, and there is no agreed-upon standard of care with clinicians differing in their approach. With immunotherapy being the new standard in the first-line setting, appropriate second-line regimens are less clear. As such, considering enrolments into clinical trials is encouraged, but in our setting, the recruitment of patients into a clinical trial is a major challenge.

Factors to be considered while choosing a drug of choice or the treatment regimens are prior treatment history, performance status, potential toxicities of a proposed regimen, and associated comorbidities. Considering local therapy before administration of systemic therapy should be encouraged for better control of symptoms. The time interval at which the disease progresses or recurs after primary treatment (i.e., chemoradiation with platinum analog with or without cetuximab) and performance status of the patient prior to initiation of systemic therapy are vital determinants of initial therapy.

Key factors that need to be considered prior to initiation of systemic therapy include the following:

- Prior chemotherapy received (either concurrent or induction)
- Response to the initial chemotherapy or chemoradiation regimen
- Immunotherapy exposure
- The time interval between initial treatment and disease progression
- Patient performance status and comorbidities.

1. *For patients with progression on platinum-based chemotherapy (with or without cetuximab) and eligible for immunotherapy (pembrolizumab or nivolumab), should be considered as the drug of choice*

   PD-1 inhibitor immunotherapy: Both pembrolizumab and nivolumab target the PD-1 and noticed to have activity in patients with HNSCC and the US FDA approved checkpoint inhibitors such as pembrolizumab and nivolumab for patients who progressed on platinum-based chemotherapy for metastatic or recurrent HNSCC.

   Pembrolizumab: Novel PD-1 inhibitor that has shown activity in previously treated head and neck cancers. In prospective trials, the reported ORR ranged between 15 and 18%. In patients who responded, the duration of response was beyond 6 months. A modest survival benefit was observed with less toxicity when compared with docetaxel, methotrexate, or cetuximab.

   KEYNOTE-040: Pembrolizumab was compared to standard of care (investigator's choice of docetaxel, methotrexate, or cetuximab) in an open-label, phase 3 clinical trial where patients who failed prior platinum-based regimens were included.[37]

   After a follow-up period of over 7 months, the following observations were as follows:

   - Pembrolizumab arm had fewer adverse events (63 vs. 84%) but more immune-related toxicity (e.g., hypothyroidism, pneumonitis).
   - Patients assigned to pembrolizumab had more tumor responses (15 vs. 10%) but this was not statistically significant; however, the obtained responses were more durable (median duration of response 18 vs. 5 months)
   - Pembrolizumab improved OS for the whole group (1-year survival 37 vs. 27%, the median survival of 8.4 months with immunotherapy vs. 6.9 months with the standard of care, HR 0.80, 95% CI 0.65–0.98).
   - Survival benefit in the 26% of patients with PD-L1 expression ≥50% (HR 0.53, 95% CI 0.35–0.81), and no statistical significance with PD-L1 expression <50% (HR 0.93, 95% CI 0.73–1.17) in a prespecified exploratory analysis.

This study showed the activity of immunotherapeutic drug pembrolizumab in head and neck cancers, with probably added advantage with high PD-L1 expressing tumors.

Evidence on the activity of pembrolizumab was noticed in two large nonrandomized studies in previously treated HNSCC patients:

- KEYNOTE-012 study included 192 patients who were pembrolizumab administered on one of two schedules: 10 mg/kg cycled every 2 weeks, or a fixed dose of 200 mg cycled every 3 weeks.[38-41] Inclusion criteria had a heavily pretreated patient with nearly half the patients having received at least three prior therapies; in this study, the ORR was 18%. Responses lasted for more than 6 months in 85% (range >2 to >30 months), and OS at 1 year was 38%.
- KEYNOTE-055 study had 171 patients who were pembrolizumab administered at a dose of 200 mg cycled every 3 weeks.[42] Inclusion criteria were patients with cetuximab and platinum-refractory HNSCC. The median duration of response was 8 months with a 16% response rate; similar response rates were noted irrespective of HPV status and PD L1 subgroups.

Nivolumab: Novel PD-1 inhibitor with activity in previously treated head and neck patients including those with cetuximab resistance. 13% of ORR was obtained with a modest survival benefit and less toxicity.

Checkmate-141–It is a practice-changing phase III trial where 361 platinum-refractory, recurrent or metastatic head and neck patients were randomly assigned to two arms; arm one received nivolumab (3 mg/kg cycled every 2 weeks), and arm 2 received single-agent investigator's choice of therapy (docetaxel, methotrexate or cetuximab).[43-47]

- At 11.4 months median follow-up, OS was statistically significant with nivolumab (median 7.7 vs. 5.1 months, one-year OS 34.0 vs. 19.7%, HR 0.71, 95% CI 0.55–0.90). Nivolumab increased ORR (13.3 vs. 5.8%)
- Overall survival increased with PD-L1 expression ≥1% (8.7 vs. 4.6 months, HR 0.55, 95% CI 0.36–0.83) with no statistically significant increase in OS for PD-L1 expression <1% (HR 0.89, 95% CI 0.54–1.45).
- OS increased in HPV positive tumors (median 9.1 vs. 4.4 months, HR 0.56, 95% CI 0.32–0.99) with no statistical difference with HPV negative subsets (median 7.5 vs. 5.8 months, HR 0.73, 95% CI 0.42–1.25).
- Nivolumab led to an improvement in overall survival among those without prior cetuximab exposure (median 8.2 vs. 4.9 months, HR 0.52, 95% CI 0.35–0.77)[46] and for those with previous exposure to cetuximab, OS was similar to that seen with chemotherapy (median OS 7.1 vs. 5.1 months, HR 0.84, 95% CI 0.62–1.15) in a subsequent posthoc exploratory analysis.
- Outcomes on quality of life (QOL) questionnaire found no changes with nivolumab and a decrease in 8 out of 15 domains with chemotherapy.[43]

Checkmate 141 led the FDA to approve nivolumab at a dose of 240 mg cycled every 2 weeks.[48] Later on, nivolumab 480 mg administered every 4 weeks got approval based on the pharmacokinetics and safety analysis.[49]

Durvalumab: The newer PD-L1 inhibitor has also been evaluated in phase II trials and found to have some clinical activity in head and neck cancers.[50] Durvalumab either alone or with tremelimumab (a CTLA-4 inhibitor) is compared with chemotherapy, the study results are awaited.

2. *For patients who progress on initial platinum-based compounds (with or without cetuximab) and are ineligible for immunotherapy, single agent or combination chemotherapy can be considered.*

   Options include taxane, platinum agent (preferably carboplatin if previously exposed to cisplatin), methotrexate, docetaxel, 5FU or cetuximab if not exposed prior

   Cytotoxic chemotherapy: For patients who progress on the first-line of chemotherapy, responses obtained to subsequent lines of single-agent cytotoxic chemotherapy are very meager with no survival benefit with second-line treatment. For HNSCC patients with documented evidence of progression on the first line, the choice of drug regimen is based on prior treatment history, performance status, and the associated comorbidities. No data were available to document survival benefit to chemotherapy after first-line immunotherapy or chemoimmunotherapy.[51]

   Single-agent chemotherapy: In a phase III trial on comparison of weekly intravenous methotrexate with gefitinib (an epidermal growth factor receptor tyrosine kinase inhibitor), in a heavily pretreated population, there was a limited activity with single-agent methotrexate.[52] 152 patients were treated with methotrexate with an ORR of 4% and an OS of 7 months.[51] Other single agents chemotherapy drugs mostly platinum analogs such as cisplatin or taxanes such as docetaxel or paclitaxel demonstrated higher response rates when compared to methotrexate in randomized trials but was associated with increased toxicity and no effect on survival.[17,53-55] Gemcitabine may represent a single agent option for some previously treated HNSCC patients and is shown to have some activity in several observational studies.[56,57] Different chemotherapeutic drugs have varying toxicity profiles, and this information is critical when choosing a regimen. For example, mucositis is more common with single-agent methotrexate than cisplatin, but nausea or vomiting are less.[53] When docetaxel administered weekly was compared with methotrexate, there was higher grade 3 or 4 neutropenia in the docetaxel arm (13%) and increased grade 3 or 4 anemia (15%) and mucositis (5%) in the methotrexate arm.[55]

Metronomic chemotherapy with methotrexate: Reports initially suggested that oral metronomic chemotherapy with this drug had good clinical activity, excellent tolerability in platinum-resistant setting, but this has not been tested in patients with prior immunotherapy. Randomized studies have to be designed in the future to incorporate metronomic chemotherapy into routine clinical practice. Metronomic therapy targets the tumor angiogenesis predominantly; it uses frequent and low doses of chemotherapy given over prolonged periods of time with minimal toxicities. Seventy-six patients with platinum-resistant oral cavity tumors were treated with metronomic dosing of methotrexate (9 mg/m^2 cycled weekly) along with celecoxib and erlotinib in phase II clinical trial.[58] In this approach, OS was 61%, and PFS was 35% at 6 months with good tolerability and improvements QOL parameters.

Immunotherapy with cetuximab: After earlier preliminary data,[59,60] Vermoken in a phase II study[61] included 103 patients with progressive disease following two to six cycles of platinum-based therapy to cetuximab at a dose of 400 mg/m^2 given on week 1 (dose 1) followed by 250 mg/m^2 cycled weekly which later became the standard schedule and dose of cetuximab. The ORR was 13% (17 patients) (13%) which included 8 of 79 (10%) patients who had progressed on platinum analog cisplatin and 9 out of 51 (18%) recorded stable disease with a median survival of 7.5 months from the start of cetuximab therapy. The standard approved schedule for cetuximab is 250 mg/m^2 cycled weekly; further dose escalation failed to show any benefit. Cetuximab at a dose of 500 mg/m^2 cycled every 2 weeks was well tolerated with ORR of 11%.[62] On increasing doses to 750 mg/m^2 cycled, there was no improvement with ORR of 8%.

Investigational agents:

- *Palbociclib:* It is an oral CDK4-6 inhibitor that has shown significant survival benefits in metastatic hormone-positive breast cancer, which was evaluated in recurrent or metastatic HNSCC. The biologic basis for assessing CDK4-6 inhibitors in head and neck cancer with suppression of the EGFR pathway had upregulation of cyclin-dependent kinase pathway, and this could be partially reversed when combined with CDK inhibitor.[63] In a phase II study by Atkins et al., HPV negative tumors with resistance to platinum and/or cetuximab were treated with palbociclib in combination with cetuximab.[63-65] PALATINUS, a phase II study, showed that palbociclib plus cetuximab combination could potentially reverse previous cetuximab resistance; however, it did not improve PFS or OS relative to cetuximab plus placebo.[65]
- *Small molecule tyrosine kinase inhibitors (TKI):* Gefitinib, sunitinib, erlotinib, afatinib, and lapatinib are the large array of small molecules tested in head and neck cancers with no clear established role in clinical practice.[52, 66-71] In trials comparing EGFR inhibitors such as gefitinib and afatinib, both alone and in combination with chemotherapy, none of the above-mentioned TKIs demonstrated OS benefit.[52,70-72]

3. *Immunotherapy, when used in the first line and later develops progressive disease with no prior exposure to cetuximab, the combination of platinum plus taxane or platinum plus 5FU ± cetuximab can be considered. Although the addition of cetuximab increased OS when added to platinum plus 5FU in first-line, there is no evidence that this is more effective than using cetuximab sequentially as second-line therapy.*
4. *If progression on combining immunotherapy and platinum plus 5FU-based chemotherapy regimen is documented, then monotherapy with cetuximab or cetuximab with taxane combination can be considered as an optimal regimen. If tumors progress on chemotherapy, then they are more likely to be resistant, and the use of cetuximab can be encouraged.*
5. *Consider the best supportive care for extremely advanced or metastatic head and neck cancers with multiple comorbidities and poor ECOG performance status.*

In patients with rapid progression (progression within 6 months of platinum-based chemotherapy, irrespective of the usage of cetuximab), monotherapy with immunotherapy (pembrolizumab or nivolumab) can be considered as the drug of choice rather than a single agent or combination therapy with a platinum analog, taxane, cetuximab or methotrexate. Further chemotherapy is most likely to fail in this population due to a high likelihood of chemotherapy resistance. If the tumor progresses at or after 6 months of platinum-based chemotherapy following initial definitive treatment that included platinum-based chemotherapy, it is better to consider immunotherapy with or without platinum plus 5FU-based regimens, if the tumor is progressed on cisplatin, carboplatin is the preferred agent.

REFERENCES

1. Fakhry C, Zhang Q, Nguyen-Tân PF, Rosenthal DI, Weber RS, Lambert L, et al. Development and validation of nomograms predictive of overall and progression-free survival in patients with oropharyngeal cancer. J Clin Oncol. 2017;35:4057-65.
2. Forastiere AA, Metch B, Schuller DE, Ensley JF, Hutchins LF, Triozzi P, et al. Randomized comparison of cisplatin plus fluorouracil and carboplatin plus fluorouracil versus methotrexate in advanced squamous-cell carcinoma of the head and neck: a Southwest Oncology Group study. J Clin Oncol. 1992;10:1245-51.
3. Jacobs C, Lyman G, Velez-García E, Sridhar KS, Knight W, Hochster H, et al. A phase III randomized study comparing cisplatin and fluorouracil as single agents and in combination for advanced squamous cell carcinoma of the head and neck. J Clin Oncol. 1992;10:257-63.
4. Morton RP, Rugman F, Dorman EB, Stoney PJ, Wilson JA, McCormick M, et al. Cisplatinum and bleomycin for advanced or recurrent squamous cell carcinoma of the head and neck: a randomized factorial phase III controlled trial. Cancer Chemother Pharmacol. 1985;15:283-9.
5. Recondo G, Armand JP, Tellez-Bernal E, Domenge C, Belehradek M, De Vathaire F, et al. Recurrent and/or metastatic head and neck squamous cell carcinoma: a clinical, univariate, and multivariate analysis of response and survival with cisplatin-based chemotherapy. Laryngoscope. 1991;101:494-501.
6. Argiris A, Li Y, Forastiere A. Prognostic factors and long-term survivorship in patients with recurrent or metastatic carcinoma of the head and neck. Cancer. 2004;101:2222-9.
7. Argiris A, Li Y, Murphy BA, Langer CJ, Forastiere AA. Outcome of elderly patients with recurrent or metastatic head and neck cancer treated with cisplatin-based chemotherapy. J Clin Oncol. 2004;22:262.
8. Forastiere AA, Leong T, Rowinsky E, Murphy BA, Vlock DR, DeConti RC, et al. Phase III comparison of high-dose paclitaxel + cisplatin + granulocyte colony-stimulating factor versus low-dose paclitaxel + cisplatin in advanced head and neck cancer: Eastern Cooperative Oncology Group Study E1393. J Clin Oncol. 2001;19:1088.
9. Burtness B, Harrington KJ, Greil R, Soulières D, Tahara M, de Castro Jr G, et al. Pembrolizumab alone or with chemotherapy versus cetuximab with chemotherapy for recurrent or metastatic squamous cell carcinoma of the head and neck (KEYNOTE-048): a randomised, open-label, phase 3 study. Lancet. 2019;394:1915-28.
10. Guigay J, Fayette J, Mesia R, Lafond C, Saada-Bouzid E, Geoffrois L, et al. TPExtreme randomized trial: TPEx versus Extreme regimen in 1st line recurrent/metastatic head and neck squamous cell carcinoma (R/M HNSCC). J Clin Oncol. 2019;37S.
11. Rischin D, Harrington KJ, Greil R, Soulieres D, Tahara M, de Castro G, et al. Protocol-specified final analysis of the phase 3 KEYNOTE-048 trial of pembrolizumab (pembro) as first-line therapy for recurrent/metastatic head and neck squamous cell carcinoma (R/M HNSCC). J Clin Oncol. 2019; 37S:6000.
12. Vermorken JB, Mesia R, Rivera F, Remenar E, Kawecki A, Rottey S, et al. Platinum-based chemotherapy plus cetuximab in head and neck cancer. N Engl J Med. 2008;359:1116-27.
13. Vermorken JB, Psyrri A, Mesía R, Peyrade F, Beier F, de Blas B, et al. Impact of tumor HPV status on outcome in patients with recurrent and/or metastatic squamous cell carcinoma of the head and neck receiving chemotherapy with or without cetuximab: retrospective analysis of the phase III EXTREME trial. Ann Oncol. 2014;25:801-7.
14. Vermorken JB, Stöhlmacher-Williams J, Davidenko I, Licitra L, Winquist E, Villanueva C, et al. Cisplatin and fluorouracil with or without panitumumab in patients with recurrent or metastatic squamous-cell carcinoma of the head and neck (SPECTRUM): an open-label phase 3 randomised trial. Lancet Oncol. 2013;14:697-710.
15. Argiris A, Li S, Savvides P, P Ohr J, Gilbert J, Levine MA, et al. Phase III randomized trial of chemotherapy with or without bevacizumab in patients with recurrent or metastatic head and neck cancer. J Clin Oncol. 2019;37:3266-74.
16. Gibson MK, Li Y, Murphy B, Hussain MHA, DeConti RC, Ensley J, et al. Randomized phase III evaluation of cisplatin plus fluorouracil versus cisplatin plus paclitaxel in advanced head and neck cancer (E1395): an intergroup trial of the Eastern Cooperative Oncology Group. J Clin Oncol. 2005;23:3562-7.
17. Clavel M, Vermorken JB, Cognetti F, Cappelaere P, de Mulder PH, Schornagel JH, et al. Randomized comparison of cisplatin, methotrexate, bleomycin and vincristine (CABO) versus cisplatin and 5-fluorouracil (CF) versus cisplatin (C) in recurrent or metastatic squamous cell carcinoma of the head and neck. A phase III study of the EORTC Head and Neck Cancer Cooperative Group. Ann Oncol. 1994;5:521-6.
18. Schöffski P, Catimel G, Planting AS, Droz JP, Verweij J, Schrijvers D, et al. Docetaxel and cisplatin: an active regimen in patients with locally advanced, recurrent or metastatic squamous cell carcinoma of the head and neck. Results of a phase II study of the EORTC Early Clinical Studies Group. Ann Oncol. 1999;10:119-22.
19. Glisson BS, Murphy BA, Frenette G, Khuri FR, Forastiere AA. Phase II trial of docetaxel and cisplatin combination chemotherapy in patients with squamous cell carcinoma of the head and neck. J Clin Oncol. 2002;20:1593-9.
20. Specht L, Larsen SK, Hansen HS. Phase II study of docetaxel and cisplatin in patients with recurrent or disseminated squamous-cell carcinoma of the head and neck. Ann Oncol. 2000;11:845.
21. Baur M, Kienzer HR, Schweiger J, DeSantis M, Gerber E, Pont J, et al. Docetaxel/cisplatin as first-line chemotherapy in patients with head and neck carcinoma: a phase II trial. Cancer. 2002;94:2953-8.

22. Guntinas-Lichius O, Appenrodt S, Veelken F, Krug B. Phase II study of weekly docetaxel and cisplatin in patients with advanced recurrent and metastatic head and neck cancer. Laryngoscope. 2006;116:613.
23. Stathopoulos GP, Rigatos S, Papakostas P, Fountzilas G. Effectiveness of paclitaxel and carboplatin combination in heavily pretreated patients with head and neck cancers. Eur J Cancer. 1997;33:1780.
24. Clark JI, Hofmeister C, Choudhury A, Matz G, Collins S, Bastian R, et al. Phase II evaluation of paclitaxel in combination with carboplatin in advanced head and neck carcinoma. Cancer. 2001;92:2334-40.
25. Samlowski WE, Moon J, Kuebler JP, Craig R. Nichols, Gandara DR, et al. Evaluation of the combination of docetaxel/carboplatin in patients with metastatic or recurrent squamous cell carcinoma of the head and neck (SCCHN): a Southwest Oncology Group Phase II study. Cancer Invest. 2007;25:182-8.
26. Urba S, van Herpen CM, Sahoo TP, Shin DM, Licitra L, Mezei K, et al. Pemetrexed in combination with cisplatin versus cisplatin monotherapy in patients with recurrent or metastatic head and neck cancer: final results of a randomized, double-blind, placebo-controlled, phase 3 study. Cancer. 2012;118:4694-705.
27. Worden FP, Moon J, Samlowski W, Clark JI, Dakhil SR, Williamson S, et al. A phase II evaluation of a 3-hour infusion of paclitaxel, cisplatin, and 5-fluorouracil in patients with advanced or recurrent squamous cell carcinoma of the head and neck: Southwest Oncology Group study 0007. Cancer. 2006;107:319.
28. Hussain M, Gadgeel S, Kucuk O, Du W, Salwen W, Ensley J. Paclitaxel, cisplatin, and 5-fluorouracil for patients with advanced or recurrent squamous cell carcinoma of the head and neck. Cancer. 1999;86:2364-9.
29. Benasso M, Ponzanelli A, Merlano M, Numico G. Paclitaxel, cisplatin and 5-fluorouracil in recurrent squamous cell carcinoma of the head and neck: a phase II trial from an Italian cooperative group. Acta Oncol. 2006;45:168-74.
30. Janinis J, Papadakou M, Xidakis E, Boukis H, Poulis A, Panagos G, et al. Combination chemotherapy with docetaxel, cisplatin, and 5-fluorouracil in previously treated patients with advanced/recurrent head and neck cancer: a phase II feasibility study. Am J Clin Oncol. 2000;23:128-31.
31. Baghi M, Hambek M, Wagenblast J, May A, Gstoettner W, Knecht R. A phase II trial of docetaxel, cisplatin and 5-fluorouracil in patients with recurrent squamous cell carcinoma of the head and neck (SCCHN). Anticancer Res. 2006;26:585-90.
32. Okuno SH, Mailliard JA, Suman VJ, Edmonson JH, Creagan ET, Nair S, et al. Phase II study of methotrexate, vinblastine, doxorubicin, and cisplatin in patients with squamous cell carcinoma of the upper respiratory or alimentary passages of the head and neck. Cancer. 2002;94:2224-31.
33. Shin DM, Glisson BS, Khuri FR, Ginsberg L, Papadimitrakopoulou V, Lee JJ, et al. Phase II trial of paclitaxel, ifosfamide, and cisplatin in patients with recurrent head and neck squamous cell carcinoma. J Clin Oncol. 1998;16:1325-30.
34. Shin DM, Khuri FR, Glisson BS, Ginsberg L, Papadimitrakopoulou VM, Clayman G, et al. Phase II study of paclitaxel, ifosfamide, and carboplatin in patients with recurrent or metastatic head and neck squamous cell carcinoma. Cancer. 2001;91:1316-23.
35. Malhotra B, Moon J, Kucuk O, Clark JI, Urba SG, Wolf GT, et al. Phase II trial of biweekly gemcitabine and paclitaxel with recurrent or metastatic squamous cell carcinoma of the head and neck: Southwest Oncology Group study S0329. Head Neck. 2014;36:1712-7.
36. Hitt R, Irigoyen A, Cortes-Funes H, Grau JJ, García-Sáenz JA, Cruz-Hernandez JJ, et al. Phase II study of the combination of cetuximab and weekly paclitaxel in the first-line treatment of patients with recurrent and/or metastatic squamous cell carcinoma of head and neck. Ann Oncol. 2012;23:1016-22.
37. Cohen EEW, Soulières D, Le Tourneau C, Dinis J, Licitra L, Ahn M-J, et al. Pembrolizumab versus methotrexate, docetaxel, or cetuximab for recurrent or metastatic head-and-neck squamous cell carcinoma (KEYNOTE-040): a randomised, open-label, phase 3 study. Lancet. 2019;393:156-67.
38. Mehra R, Seiwert TY, Gupta S, Weiss J, Gluck I, Eder JP, et al. Efficacy and safety of pembrolizumab in recurrent/metastatic head and neck squamous cell carcinoma: pooled analyses after long-term follow-up in KEYNOTE-012. Br J Cancer. 2018;119:153-9.
39. KEYTRUDA® (pembrolizumab) for injection, for intravenous use KEYTRUDA® (pembrolizumab) injection, for intravenous use Initial U.S. Approval: 2014. [online] Available from: http://www.accessdata.fda.gov/drugsatfda_docs/label/2016/125514s009lbl.pdf. [Last accessed July, 2020]
40. Seiwert TY, Burtness B, Mehra R, Weiss J, Berger R, Eder JP, et al. Safety and clinical activity of pembrolizumab for treatment of recurrent or metastatic squamous cell carcinoma of the head and neck (KEYNOTE-012): an open-label, multicentre, phase 1b trial. Lancet Oncol. 2016;17:956-65.
41. Chow LQ, Haddad R, Gupta S, Mahipal A, Mehra R, Tahara M, et al. Antitumor activity of pembrolizumab in biomarker-unselected patients with recurrent and/or metastatic head and neck squamous cell carcinoma: results from the phase Ib KEYNOTE-012 Expansion Cohort. J Clin Oncol. 2016; 34(32):3838-45.
42. Bauml J, Seiwert TY, Pfister DG, Worden F, Liu SV,, Gilbert J et al. Pembrolizumab for platinum- and cetuximab-refractory head and neck cancer: results from a single-arm, phase II study. J Clin Oncol. 2017;35:1542.
43. Harrington KJ, Ferris RL, Blumenschein G Jr, Colevas AD, Fayette J, Licitra L, et al. Nivolumab versus standard, single-agent therapy of investigator's choice in recurrent or metastatic squamous cell carcinoma of the head and neck (CheckMate 141): health-related quality-of-life results from a randomised, phase 3 trial. Lancet Oncol. 2017;18:1104.
44. Gillison ML, Blumenschein G Jr, Fayette J, Guigay J, Colevas AD, Licitra L, et al. CheckMate 141: 1-year update and subgroup analysis of nivolumab as first-line therapy in patients with recurrent/metastatic head and neck cancer. Oncologist 2018;23:1079.
45. Haddad R, Concha-Benavente F, Blumenschein G Jr, Fayette J, Guigay J, Colevas AD, et al. Nivolumab treatment beyond RECIST-defined progression in recurrent or metastatic squamous cell carcinoma of the head and neck in CheckMate 141: A subgroup analysis of a randomized phase 3 clinical trial. Cancer. 2019;125:3208-18.
46. Ferris RL, Licitra L, Fayette J, Even C, Blumenschein G Jr, Harrington KJ, et al. Nivolumab in patients with recurrent or metastatic squamous cell carcinoma of the head and neck: efficacy and safety in CheckMate 141 by prior cetuximab use. Clin Cancer Res. 2019;25:5221-30.
47. Ferris RL, Blumenschein G Jr, Fayette J, Guigay J, Colevas AD, Licitra L, et al. Nivolumab for recurrent squamous-cell

carcinoma of the head and neck. N Engl J Med. 2016; 375:1856-67.
48. OPDIVO (nivolumab) injection, for intravenous use Initial U.S. Approval: 2014. [online] Available from: http://www.accessdata.fda.gov/drugsatfda_docs/label/2016/125554s022lbl.pdf. [Last accessed July, 2020].
49. OPDIVO (nivolumab) injection, for intravenous use Initial U.S. Approval: 2014. [online] Available from: https://www.accessdata.fda.gov/drugsatfda_docs/label/2018/125554s048s049s050s051s052s061s062s064s065s066lbl.pdf (Accessed on March 26, 2018). [Last accessed July, 2020].
50. Zandberg DP, Algazi AP, Jimeno A, Good JS, Fayette J, Bouganim N, et al. Durvalumab for recurrent or metastatic head and neck squamous cell carcinoma: results from a single-arm, phase II study in patients with ≥25% tumour cell PD-L1 expression who have progressed on platinum-based chemotherapy. Eur J Cancer. 2019;107:142.
51. Saleh K, Daste A, Martin N, Pons-Tostivint E, Auperin A, Herrera-Gomez RG, et al. Response to salvage chemotherapy after progression on immune checkpoint inhibitors in patients with recurrent and/or metastatic squamous cell carcinoma of the head and neck. Eur J Cancer. 2019;121:123-9.
52. Stewart JS, Cohen EE, Licitra L, Van Herpen CML, Khorprasert C, Soulieres D, et al. Phase III study of gefitinib compared with intravenous methotrexate for recurrent squamous cell carcinoma of the head and neck [corrected]. J Clin Oncol. 2009;27:1864-71.
53. Hong WK, Schaefer S, Issell B, Cummings C, Luedke D, Bromer R, et al. A prospective randomized trial of methotrexate versus cisplatin in the treatment of recurrent squamous cell carcinoma of the head and neck. Cancer. 1983; 52:206-10.
54. A phase III randomised trial of cistplatinum, methotrextate, cisplatinum + methotrexate and cisplatinum + 5-FU in end stage squamous carcinoma of the head and neck. Liverpool Head and Neck Oncology Group. Br J Cancer. 1990;61:311-5.
55. Guardiola E, Peyrade F, Chaigneau L, Cupissol D, Tchiknavorian X, Bompas E, et al. Results of a randomised phase II study comparing docetaxel with methotrexate in patients with recurrent head and neck cancer. Eur J Cancer. 2004;40:2071-6.
56. Raguse JD, Gath HJ, Bier J, Riess H, Oettle H. Gemcitabine in the treatment of advanced head and neck cancer. Clin Oncol (R Coll Radiol). 2005;17:425-9.
57. Catimel G, Vermorken JB, Clavel M, de Mulder P, Judson I, Sessa C, et al. A phase II study of gemcitabine (LY 188011) in patients with advanced squamous cell carcinoma of the head and neck. EORTC Early Clinical Trials Group. Ann Oncol. 1994;5:543-7.
58. Patil VM, Noronha V, Joshi A, Dhumal S, Mahimkar M, Bhattacharjee A, et al. Phase I/II study of palliative triple metronomic chemotherapy in platinum-refractory/early-failure oral cancer. J Clin Oncol. 2019;37:3032.
59. Herbst RS, Arquette M, Shin DM, Dicke K, Vokes EE, Azarnia N, et al. Phase II multicenter study of the epidermal growth factor receptor antibody cetuximab and cisplatin for recurrent and refractory squamous cell carcinoma of the head and neck. J Clin Oncol. 2005;23:5578-87.
60. Baselga J, Trigo JM, Bourhis J, Tortochaux J, Cortés-Funes H, Hitt R, et al. Phase II multicenter study of the antiepidermal growth factor receptor monoclonal antibody cetuximab in combination with platinum-based chemotherapy in patients with platinum-refractory metastatic and/or recurrent squamous cell carcinoma of the head and neck. J Clin Oncol. 2005;23:5568-77.
61. Vermorken JB, Trigo J, Hitt R, Koralewski P, Diaz-Rubio E, Rolland F, et al. Open-label, uncontrolled, multicenter phase II study to evaluate the efficacy and toxicity of cetuximab as a single agent in patients with recurrent and/or metastatic squamous cell carcinoma of the head and neck who failed to respond to platinum-based therapy. J Clin Oncol. 2007;25:2171-7.
62. Fury MG, Sherman E, Lisa D, Agarwal N, Algazy K, Brockstein B, et al. A randomized phase II study of cetuximab every 2 weeks at either 500 or 750 mg/m2 for patients with recurrent or metastatic head and neck squamous cell cancer. J Natl Compr Canc Netw. 2012;10:1391-8.
63. Michel L, Ley J, Wildes TM, Schaffer A, Robinson A, Chun S-E, et al. Phase I trial of palbociclib, a selective cyclin dependent kinase 4/6 inhibitor, in combination with cetuximab in patients with recurrent/metastatic head and neck squamous cell carcinoma. Oral Oncol. 2016;58:41-8.
64. Adkins D, Ley J, Neupane P, Worden F, Sacco AG, Palka K, et al. Palbociclib and cetuximab in platinum-resistant and in cetuximab-resistant human papillomavirus-unrelated head and neck cancer: a multicentre, multigroup, phase 2 trial. Lancet Oncol. 2019;20:1295-305.
65. Adkins D, Lin JC, Sacco AG, Le JC. Palbociclib plus cetuximab versus placebo plus cetuximab in platinum-resistant, cetuximab-naive, HPV-unrelated head and neck cancer: a double-blind randomized phase II trial (PALATINUS). J Clin Oncol. 2019;37:15S.
66. Cohen EE, Rosen F, Stadler WM, Recant W, Stenson K, Huo D, et al. Phase II trial of ZD1839 in recurrent or metastatic squamous cell carcinoma of the head and neck. J Clin Oncol. 2003;21:1980-7.
67. Cohen EE, Kane MA, List MA, Brockstein BE, Mehrotra B, Huo D, et al. Phase II trial of gefitinib 250 mg daily in patients with recurrent and/or metastatic squamous cell carcinoma of the head and neck. Clin Cancer Res. 2005;11:8418-24.
68. Kirby AM, A'Hern RP, D'Ambrosio C, Tanay M, Syrigos KN, Rogers SJ, et al. Gefitinib (ZD1839, Iressa) as palliative treatment in recurrent or metastatic head and neck cancer. Br J Cancer. 2006;94:631-6.
69. Soulieres D, Senzer NN, Vokes EE, Hidalgo M, Agarwala SS, Siu LL. Multicenter phase II study of erlotinib, an oral epidermal growth factor receptor tyrosine kinase inhibitor, in patients with recurrent or metastatic squamous cell cancer of the head and neck. J Clin Oncol. 2004;22:77-85.
70. Machiels JP, Haddad RI, Fayette J, Licitra LF, Tahara M, Vermorken JB, et al. Afatinib versus methotrexate as second-line treatment in patients with recurrent or metastatic squamous-cell carcinoma of the head and neck progressing on or after platinum-based therapy (LUX-Head & Neck 1): an open-label, randomised phase 3 trial. Lancet Oncol. 2015;16:583-94.
71. Argiris A, Ghebremichael M, Gilbert J, Lee JW, Sachidanandam K, Kolesar JM, et al. Phase III randomized, placebo-controlled trial of docetaxel with or without gefitinib in recurrent or metastatic head and neck cancer: an eastern cooperative oncology group trial. J Clin Oncol. 2013;31:1405-14.
72. Guo Y, Ahn MJ, Chan A, Wang C-H, Kang J-H, Kim S-B, et al. Afatinib versus methotrexate as second-line treatment in Asian patients with recurrent or metastatic squamous cell carcinoma of the head and neck progressing on or after platinum-based therapy (LUX-Head & Neck 3): an open-label, randomised phase III trial. Ann Oncol. 2019;30:1831-9.

CHAPTER 30

Head and Neck Cancer Management in the Geriatric Patient

Manish Mair, Hitesh Singhavi, Narayana Subramaniam

INTRODUCTION

Aging has been defined as "progressive, generalized impairment of function resulting in a loss of adaptive response to stress and in a growing risk of age-associated disease."[1] However, "elderly" or "old age" has no standard definition. The United Nations has defined an older population as one aged is >60–65 years, however, this varies significantly in different parts of the world. Most developed countries accept a chronological age of over 65 years as an elderly or old population, which may not apply to developing countries. By 2050, all developing countries will face a major demographic shift, with 80% of all the elderly population living in low- and middle-income countries. With this demographic shift in the population and an increased life expectancy, we are likely to face a tremendous rise in the incidence of head and neck cancer in elderly patients.

According to the 2018 GLOBOCAN report,[2] 30% of all head and neck cancers were registered in patients over 65 years, estimated to increase by 100% by 2040. In spite of a heavy huge disease burden in the elderly population, treatment paradigms for such patients are not well-defined. This is mainly due to the lack of dedicated randomized control trials (RCTs) or under-representation of this population in them **(Tables 1 and 2)**. In a meta-analysis by Pignon et al. consisting of 93 clinical trials, only 692 of 17,346 patients (4%) were >70 years of age.[3] As a result, most management protocols have been developed from subset analysis.

Additional considerations in the elderly are physiological capacity, frailty, age-related reduction in renal function, and susceptibility to drug toxicity aging of the renal system to dehydration or drug-related toxicity. A comprehensive geriatric assessment is of prime

Table 1: Trials in head and neck cancer (HNC) comparing radiotherapy and chemoradiotherapy and their age limits for recruitment.

Trial	*Year of publication*	*Median age of patients*	*Age limit (years)*	*Patient population*
RTOG 9501[4]	2004	56	None; 6% of patients >70	High-risk HNC
EORTC 22931[5]	2004	54	18–70	Stage III/IV HNC
Racadot et al.[6]	2008	56	18–75	Node positive HNC
Tobias et al.[7]	2010	58	32–81	Advanced HNC

Table 2: Definitive concurrent chemoradiotherapy trials in head and neck cancer (HNC).

Trial	*Year of publication*	*Median age*	*Age limit (years)*	*Subsite*
Veterans' Affairs Trial[8]	1991	62	24–79	Advanced laryngeal cancer
RTOG-91-11[9]	2003	59	26–79, 50% were >60	Stage III/IV laryngeal cancer
EORTC 24954[10]	2009	55	35–76	Stage III/IV laryngeal cancer
GORTEC[11]	1999	55	32–74	Oropharynx
RTOG 97-03[12]	2004	56	21–83	Advanced HNC
Bonner et al.[13]	2006	57	34–83	Advanced HNC

importance, as some elderly patients may be vulnerable and cancer or its therapy may decompensate an underlying frailty. On the other hand, a fit elderly patient may not be offered optimal treatment purely due to age compromising on their best chance of cure. This chapter highlights the key considerations in management of head and neck cancer in the elderly and the evidence that can aid decision-making.

GERIATRIC ASSESSMENT SCALES AND EVALUATION OF THE ELDERLY

Comprehensive geriatric assessment is defined as a systematic method to identify medical, psychosocial, and functional limitations of a frail older person in order to develop a coordinated plan to maximize overall health and to further optimize treatment procedures. Health care of elderly individuals' goes beyond conventional medical management; the majority of geriatric assessment scales examine functional status, activities of daily living (ADL), comorbidities, cognition, mental health, social support, nutrition, geriatric syndromes, and polypharmacy. There are many validated tools available for geriatric assessment, however, it is difficult to define which among them is the most accurate as this differs with region, local resource availability, and healthcare structures.

It is a standard recommendation that all patients over 70 years undergo a formal geriatric assessment[14,15] as it is an important tool that may help identify concerns missed during routine oncological evaluation. Systematic reviews that included several geriatric assessment domains such as performance status, geriatric depression scale, and nutritional status, showed that these assessments independently predicted mortality.[16-19] Additionally, it has been shown that geriatric assessment could identify abnormalities missed in routine consultations in over half of patients; these issues included poor physical functioning, poor nutritional status, falls, depression, and cognitive impairment. These impairments have all been independently associated with worse outcomes in patients with cancer.[20-22] Routine implementation of these formal assessments in oncology has been difficult due to them being a lengthy process, posing logistical issues. To circumvent this, different screening tools assess that frailty have been introduced, such as the geriatric 8 (G8), Groningen frailty index (GFI), Senior Adult Oncology Program 2 (SAOP2), Triage Risk Screening Tool (TRST), and Vulnerable Elders Survey-13 (VES-13) (details in **Table 3**). These assessments typically take under 10 minutes to administer and some have been shown to accurately predict functional decline and poorer survival.[23-25] These have been proved to be a useful compromise when complete geriatric assessment is not possible. They also highlight the patient's perception of their underlying health status with responses on individual components of the screening tools serving to unmask underlying impairment. This may also allow clinicians to focus on particular problem areas during a more comprehensive assessment. A summary of comprehensive geriatric assessment is shown in **Table 4**.

Functional Status

Eastern Cooperative Oncology Group (ECOG) or Karnofsky Performance Status Scales often assess functional status. However, in older people, evaluating the ADL and instrumental activities of daily living (IADL) are of importance. ADL explores six basic functions of everyday life: (1) bathing, (2) dressing, (3) using the toilet, (4) continence, (5) transferring, and (6) feeding. The score ranges from 6 (patient independent) to 0 (patient very dependent). IADL scale is a measure of more elaborate functional activities in elderly patient.[26] It includes eight items: (1) ability to use the phone,

Table 3: Screening tools in geriatric assessment.

Tool	*Domains*	*Time taken to perform (min)*	*Score range*	*Abnormal score*
Geriatric 8	Nutritional status, weight loss, body mass index, motor skills, psychological status, number of medications, and self-perception of health and one item relative to age of patient (<80 years, 80–85 years and >85 years)	4.4	0–17	≤14
Triage Risk Screening Tool	Cognitive impairment, walking ability, number of medications, emergency department attendance in the last 30 days or hospitalization during the previous 90 days, and whether subject lives alone	2	0–6	≥1
Vulnerable Elders-13 Survey	Perception of health status, examples of everyday activity, difficulty performing activities related to his health or physical condition	4	0–10	≥3
Groningen Frailty Index	Mobility, nutrition, vision, comorbidity, hearing, cognition, psychosocial and physical fitness	2	0–15	≥4

Table 4: Comprehensive geriatric assessment.

Functional status
• *Activities of daily living:* Walking, bathing, dressing, grooming, feeding, and continence • *Instrumental activities of daily living:* Shopping, transportation, using the telephone, managing finances, managing medication, cooking, and cleaning • Karnofsky Performance Status Scale of 0–100 • Self-reported number of falls in different time frames • Timed up and go assessment of gait speed; threshold of 0.8 m/s • *Short physical performance battery:* Gait speed, lower extremity strength, and balance
Comorbidity
• Physical health section • Charlson Comorbidity Index • Cumulative Illness Rating Scale—geriatrics include geriatric syndromes
Nutritional status
• Body mass index • Weight loss in past 6 months • *Mini Nutritional Assessment:* Appetite loss, weight loss, mobility, psychological stress, neurophysiological problems, and body mass index
Psychological state
• Mental health inventory-17 • Geriatric Depression Scale Depression screening • Distress thermometer visual analog scale of 0–10
Cognition
• *Blessed orientation memory concentration test:* Orientation, registration, and attention • *Mini-Mental State Examination:* Orientation, attention, memory, language, constructional ability, and calculation • Mini-Cog Brief screening test
Polypharmacy
Total number of medications
Social support and function
Emotional support, financial support, and positive social interaction

(2) shopping, (3) food preparation, (4) housekeeping, (5) laundry, (6) mode of transportation, (7) responsibility for own medications, and (8) ability to handle finances. The score ranges from 8 (high function, independent) to 0 (low function, dependent). In addition to this, gait speed, grip strength, balance, and leg strength, are associated with overall survival in older people.[27]

Comorbidity

Comorbidity has been shown to be a reliable predictor of mortality and treatment tolerance in head and neck cancer.[28] It has also been shown that this is independent of performance status, suggesting that patients may be high functioning but can decompensate significantly after treatment.[29] The common tools to assess comorbidity are the Charlson Comorbidity Index (CCI), Adult Comorbidity Evaluation (ACE), and Cumulative Illness Rating Scale (CIRS) for geriatrics. CCI accounts for the comorbid condition, severity and risk of death, and has been applied suitably to head and neck cancer in a prospective and retrospective setting.[30] The ACE-27 comprises 27 different comorbidities and has been validated in head and neck cancer, accurately predicting survival,[31] however, it is unsuitable for retrospective use.

Cognition

There is a risk of mild cognitive impairment, dementia, and delirium with increasing age. These are best evaluated using formal cognitive assessments, patient observations, and accounts from caregivers.[32] If cognition is impaired, it may hamper the patient's ability to fully understand a complex decision-making process. Impaired cognition is also a risk factor for delirium. In addition, it is also important to understand that decision-making can be preserved in individuals with cognitive decline.[33] Addressing cognitive impairments is important to enhance response to treatment and improve quality of life.

Mental Health

Psychological distress, depression, and anxiety are common among elderly patients with cancer. Distress, depression and anxiety were seen in 41%, 30%, and 20% of elderly cancer patients.[34-36] These symptoms can significantly impair quality of life and functional status of the patient. Poor psychological state can interrupt or halt definitive cancer treatment impacting survival.[11]

Social Support

Lack of social support is a significant factor impacting survival outcomes in elderly patients. In a study of nearly 3,000 breast cancer patients, socially isolated women had a higher rate of mortality.[37] The availability of caregivers and financial support during cancer treatment should also be taken into consideration. Realistic patient treatment goals should be discussed and appropriate management plan should be formulated based on these considerations.

Nutrition

Malnutrition and weight loss correlate with increased complication rates and poor survival outcomes in older people.[38] Cancer patients are often malnourished and this is one of the most common reasons for alteration of cancer specific therapies.[39] Malnutrition can be assessed by Mini Nutritional Assessment (MNA) tool that can predict the nonhematological complications of chemotherapy.[36] Nutritional evaluation is a crucial component of the initial geriatric assessment.

Polypharmacy

Polypharmacy can be defined as the use of an increased number of medications, inappropriate medication use, or medication duplication. In a study of elderly population, 48% of the patients used five or more medications at the time of starting treatment.[40] Clinicians should assess polypharmacy and counsel regarding stoppage of inappropriate medications to avoid interference with therapy and limit treatment-related morbidity.

PRETREATMENT PREPARATION

As per the National Comprehensive Cancer Network guidelines,[41] the first approach to management of a senior patient is to consider their life expectancy. Older patients can be classified into three groups: (1) young-old (65–74 years), (2) middle-old (75–84 years), and (3) oldest-old (≥85 years). Life expectancy estimated using life table data given by Walter and Schonberg estimates that the 25th percentile of healthiest 70-year-old males will live >19 years, 50% will live at least 13 years and 25% <8 years.

If the life expectancy is low in the context of completion of cancer treatment, supportive or palliative care is the best treatment option. If the patient has a good life expectancy, then one has to consider whether the patient has the mental capacity to consent for cancer treatment. It is important to note in addition to chronological age, functional reserve, and complications of the treatment should be considered to formulate an appropriate treatment plan. Based on demographic data and self-reported functional reserves, Lee et al. developed a tool to estimate 4-year mortality risk,[32] which is an example of a tool that can help in treatment planning.

Additionally, it is important to assess patient's goals and values with respect to cancer management. If the patient's goal is to consider cancer treatment then they need a geriatric assessment as discussed earlier. Appropriate referral based on detection of impairment should be made as shown in **Table 5**. Clinicians should also understand that communications with elderly population need optimization; written material should be simple with large font size and enhanced with pictures for better understanding and oral communication should involve feedback and also use of the teach-back method. In this method, the patient describes back what they have understood in their own words.

Table 5: Intervention requirements based on impairments identified on geriatric assessment.

Impairment	*Intervention*
Functional status	• Physiotherapy • Occupational therapy • Frequency of fall • Encourage exercise and physical activity
Cognition	• Involve family members • Prevent delirium • Avoid inappropriate medications
Social support	• Transportation • Home safety assessment • Social care reference
Depression	• Appropriate medications • Psychology reference
Nutrition	• Dietician reference • Speech and swallowing reference • Oral care • Physiotherapy

The surgical and anesthetic team should be equally involved before performing oncologic surgery on elder patients. Comorbidities need to be optimally controlled before surgery for better outcomes. Anesthetic concerns are covered in a different chapter. There is no conclusive evidence suggesting differences in outcome between regional and general anesthesia in the elderly,[42] but rarely in head and neck cancer, surgery can be performed under regional anesthesia. It also important to understand fluid management in elderly patients, as they are sensitive to volume shifts, especially with underlying cardiac conditions.[43]

Elderly patients are also at increased risk of a stroke during neck dissection due to pre-existing condition of carotid stenosis and/or atherosclerosis.[44,45] Carotid Doppler may be recommended as a screening tool, but literature has not showed any benefit and it is not a routine practice.[44] However, surgeon should be aware of this and cautious when positioning the neck and handling carotid sheath during neck dissection.

Treating an elderly patient needs to be a multidisciplinary decision. Curative treatment in elderly patient requires due consideration but only when the patient has the ability to tolerate the treatment, experience a good chance of cure and continue to enjoy a reasonable quality of life. Clinicians should also offer alternative treatment options to the patient, especially if they do not desire radical treatment and its accompanying morbidity.

CONSIDERATIONS IN SURGICAL MANAGEMENT

Surgery is the primary modality of treatment for most head and neck cancers. In spite of the survival benefit, surgery is not without morbidity, which can be significant. Multiple studies have demonstrated similar survival outcomes among the elderly and young patients.[46-49] However, survival outcomes have been shown to be poorer in patients over 80 years.[47] Another Surveillance, Epidemiology, and End Results (SEER) database compared survival outcomes of 2,548 surgically managed patients over 70 years of age with glottic, tongue, or tonsillar squamous cell carcinomas to younger controls. There was a significant decrease in overall survival and disease-specific survival in the glottis and anterior tongue subgroups but not the tonsillar subgroup.[50,51] A summary of results has been shown in **Table 6**.

POSTOPERATIVE COMPLICATIONS

Most of the studies show no increase in the postoperative complications with increasing age. Morgan demonstrated a higher 30-day mortality rate for older patients but the two cohorts were not matched for stage or comorbidity.[51] Bridger showed a higher complication rate in elderly patients when they had more than two pre-existing comorbidities.[55]

Free Flaps in the Elderly

Free flap surgery has been shown to be reliable in the elderly, however, they come at the cost of prolonged surgery and a higher propensity for postoperative complications. Two retrospective studies showed that there is no increase in the incidence of surgical complications in elderly patients. Nonetheless, medical complications were seen which were related to the

Table 6: Studies showing impact of age on outcomes in head and neck cancer surgery.

Author	*Patient population*	*Results*
Kowalski et al.[46]	115 patients ≥70 years matched with 115 younger patients	5-year survival rates were 43% in older, 55.6% in younger (NS)
Clayman et al.[47]	43 patients ≥80 years vs. 79 years similar patients ≤65 years	5-year survival rates were 33% in older, 63% in younger ($p = 0.001$)
McGuirt et al.[48]	215 patients >65 years	5-year survival rates were 53.4% in 65–71 years, 58.9% in 72–74 years, 55.1% in 75–80 years, and 46.3% in >81 years
Shaari et al.[49]	52 patients >70 years and 35 patients ≤70 years	• Overall complications in older patients 48% vs. 52% in younger patients (NS) • Mortality rate 6% in older vs. 0% in younger
Laccourreye et al.[50]	69 patients >65 years	5-year survival and local control were 68% and 93.9%, respectively
Morgan et al.[51]	810 patients ≥65 years and 963 patients <65 years	• 30-day mortality was 3.5% in older and 0.8% in younger (NS) • Complication rate 32% in older and 21% in younger
Sesterhenn et al.[52]	56 patients ≥75 years and 112 patients <60 years	• Postoperative mortality was 3.6% in older and 0% in young • Complication rate was 12.5% in older and 9.8% in younger (NS)
Milet et al.[53]	29 patients age ≥70 years and 232 patients <70 years	Postoperative mortality 13% in older and 2.5% in younger
Zabrodsky et al.[54]	24 patients ≥70 years	Overall complication rate 63%
Sanabria et al.[30]	242 patients ≥70 years	Complication rate 56.6%, male sex, bilateral neck dissection, more than two comorbidities, reconstruction and stage IV were predictors of complications
Bridger et al.[55]	26 patients ≥70 years and 91 patients <70 years	Surgical complications—42% in older and 37% in younger; medical complications—54% in older and 29% in younger (NS)
Bhattacharyya et al.[56]	1,882 glottic, 426 oral tongue, 200 tonsillar cancer patients >70 years matched with 5069 controls	Elderly patients had worse survival in oral tongue and glottis cancers but comparable survival in tonsillar cancer
Blackwell et al.[57]	13 patients ≥80 years and 99 younger patients	Medical complication 64% in elderly and 15% in young, cost of treatment higher in elderly
Subramaniam et al.[58]	115 patients >70 years matched with 115 patients 50–60 years	Elderly patients had reduced performance status and more comorbid illnesses but similar postoperative course. Longer median hospital stay, tracheostomy and feeding tube dependence, ICU stay and more nonfatal cardiac events

patient's comorbidities.[55,56] Blackwell showed higher risk of postoperative complications in 13 patients over 80 years undergoing free flap surgery even after controlling for comorbidities.[57] Based on this retrospective literature, one can infer that free flap surgery is safe in the elderly but the choice of patient is important; here preoperative screening tools and geriatric assessments play a role in an objective standardized evaluation of fitness for surgery.

Quality of Life

Quality of life is an important consideration after definitive surgical therapy. Khafif et al. used the University of Washington Quality of Life Questionnaire for patients 65–75 years and those over 75 years. Surgical intervention improved pain and discomfort while physical functioning was a product of age. Additionally, older patients tended to score less on several other quality of life domains. This can likely be attributed to an inability to resume normal life due to emotional and physical limitations, and the sense of burden on their caregivers.[59] However, Dhiwakar et al. found no difference in the change of quality of life between young and older patients.[60]

CONSIDERATIONS IN NONSURGICAL MANAGEMENT

The distinct advantages of radiotherapy in head and neck cancer are its potential for organ preservation in the curative setting and for managing micrometastasis in an adjuvant setting.[49] The most commonly used radiotherapy regimen for curative treatment is 1.8–2.0 Gy per fraction, 5 days a week over 7 weeks, to a total dose of 70 Gy, while in an adjuvant setting the dose is up to 60 Gy in 1.8–2 Gy per fraction, 5 days a week for 6 weeks.

Radiotherapy and chemotherapy are suitable treatment options for elderly patients with advanced head and neck cancers. The combination of chemotherapy and radiotherapy has also been shown to influence disease free survival in the elderly patient with acceptable toxicities.[61] Literature shows that in addition to age, smoking status, glomerular filtration rate, and Karnofsky status played a significant role in influencing overall survival.

Hyperfractionated radiation: It is used to increase the radiation dose with fractionation of 1.5 Gy more than once daily, reducing the number of days for completion of treatment and potentially improving locoregional control. Hyperfractionated radiation therapy was shown to be effective in the meta-analysis conducted by Bourhis et al. but with increasing age there was deceased compliance and tolerance, with higher incidence of noncancer-related deaths in patients >70 years.[62]

Toxicity in elderly individuals: It is generally believed that treatment toxicities are higher in elderly individual. Pignon et al. registered a significant increase in radiation-induced mucositis in older individuals.[63] Similarly, Allal et al. found that older patients had more unplanned treatment breaks than the young.[64] An Indian retrospective study concluded that patients over age of 70 years had difficulty in completion or receiving appropriate adjuvant radiotherapy.[65] Another Indian study done in unresectable locally advanced oral cavity cancers and oropharyngeal cancers suggested higher treatment-related toxicity including acute mucositis, xerostomia, acute skin and pharyngeal toxicities in elderly individuals. However, it did not achieve statistical significance and age cut-off was controversial.[66] Huang et al. compared 238 patients over 75 years of age to 1,249 younger patients and showed no difference in treatment interruptions or late toxicities.[67] Other western studies also suggest acceptable toxicity rates.[68,69] It has been shown that radiotherapy can be delivered without dose reduction in elderly individuals with completion rates of up to 80%.[70] Elderly patients should be watched closely for acute toxicities but should be considered for curative intent radiotherapy wherever appropriate.

CONSIDERATIONS IN CHEMOTHERAPY ADMINISTRATION

The role of chemotherapy in head and neck cancer is expanding. Currently, it has three main roles: (1) neoadjuvant chemotherapy in borderline resectable cancer, (2) definitive treatment in combination with radiotherapy, and (3) palliative chemotherapy. Standard chemotherapy for head and neck is combination of platinum-based agents (cisplatin/carboplatin), paclitaxel and 5-fluorouracil. It achieves a response rate of 40–50% in metastatic settings while in definitive settings its response rates of up to 85% have been reported.[71]

Neoadjuvant Chemotherapy in Elderly Individuals

The evidence on benefits and tolerance of neoadjuvant chemotherapy in the elderly for head and neck cancers is limited; however, an Indian study has shown that individualized treatment selection (chemotherapy drug chosen based on patients comorbidities) is associated with high compliance rate of 73% when used for organ preservation and 82% when used for technically unresectable disease, with a response rate of 41%.[72] Thus, in a select group of elderly head and neck cancer, individualized neoadjuvant chemotherapy can be delivered with satisfactory compliance creating a window of opportunity for clinicians and patients.

Concurrent Chemoradiotherapy

Literature on survival benefits of combining chemotherapy with radiotherapy in elderly individuals is evolving. In a large meta-analysis by Pignon et al.[3] showed that adding chemotherapy to locoregional treatment was most beneficial between 18 and 50 years. For patients over 70 years there was no benefit in survival. This could be attributed to an increased number of noncancer-related deaths in this group thus overshadowing the effect of concomitant systemic therapy.

Chemotherapy in an Adjuvant Setting

The addition of chemotherapy to radiotherapy in an adjuvant setting has shown maximum benefit in the presence of extranodal extension and positive margins. An analysis of 1,199 patients of head and neck squamous cell carcinoma aged ≥70 years from the National Cancer Data Base was performed by Yoshida et al.[73] All these patients underwent surgery and received adjuvant therapy for positive margins or extranodal extension. They showed that 3-year overall survival for chemoradiotherapy and radiotherapy was 52.4% and 43.4%, respectively (p = 0.012) in propensity-score matched cohorts. The survival benefit of chemotherapy was primarily in those with N2-3 nodal disease. From this study one can infer that is reasonable to consider elderly individuals with good performance for concomitant chemoradiotherapy, especially when they have a high nodal burden.

RECURRENT AND METASTATIC HEAD AND NECK CANCER

Argiris et al. evaluated 53 patients >70 years of age with recurrent or metastatic head and neck cancers. The data was collected from two mature phase III randomized trials conducted by the ECOG trials (E1393 and E1395).[74] They concluded that elderly patients had a significantly higher incidence of severe nephrotoxicity, diarrhea, and thrombocytopenia. However, survival outcomes were similar to that of younger patients.

TARGETED THERAPY

Platinum-based chemotherapy may not be suitable for elderly individuals with underlying renal, cardiac, and other comorbidities. In such a scenario, epidermal growth factor receptor (EGFR) inhibitors can be offered concurrently with radiotherapy. Two recent trials, namely De-ESCALaTE and RTOG 1016 trials comparing concomitant cetuximab with cisplatin during radiotherapy in human papillomavirus (HPV)-positive oropharyngeal carcinoma demonstrated that EGFR inhibitors were inferior in terms of overall and progression-free survival, which would suggest that although addition of cetuximab to radiotherapy is more effective than radiotherapy alone, it is still not as effective as concurrent chemoradiotherapy with cisplatin.[75,76] Interestingly, a randomized trial undertaken by the Magrini et al.[77] comparing radiotherapy with either concurrent cisplatin or cetuximab; those on cetuximab experienced as much morbidity as those treated with cisplatin and needed more nutritional support. This is a clear indication that cetuximab is not without toxicity. One should also note that there is evolving literature on the benefits of nimotuzumab, currently only as an adjuvant agent with concurrent chemoradiotherapy.

CONCLUSION

Elderly patients should always undergo geriatric assessment using screening tools followed by comprehensive assessment if required. This may help evaluate the functional status of the patients to better stratify patients, predict treatment toxicity, and guide treatment decisions. G8 and VES-13 are the most widely used screening tools for geriatric assessment. Special consideration needs to be given to the patient's wishes, goal, social support, comorbidities, and nutrition in older patients. Conventional surgical and radiotherapy have been safely applied in the geriatric population with good results. Addition of chemotherapy has also shown benefit but it comes with a risk of increased toxicity and treatment breaks, leading to poor survival outcomes. Alternative treatment options should always be considered in these patients.

REFERENCES

1. Franceschi C, Garagnani P, Morsiani C, Conte M, Santoro A, Grignolio A, et al. The continuum of aging and age-related diseases: common mechanisms but different rates. Front Med (Lausanne). 2018;5:61.
2. Bray F, Ferlay J, Soerjomataram I, Siegel RL, Torre LA, Jemal A. Global cancer statistics 2018: GLOBOCAN estimates of incidence and mortality worldwide for 36 cancers in 185 countries. CA Cancer J Clin. 2018;68(6):394-424.

3. Pignon JP, le Maître A, Maillard E, Bourhis J, MACH-NC Collaborative Group. Meta-analysis of chemotherapy in head and neck cancer (MACH-NC): an update on 93 randomised trials and 17,346 patients. Radiother Oncol. 2009;92(1):4-14.
4. Bernier J, Cooper JS, Pajak TF, van Glabbeke M, Bourhis J, Forastiere A, et al. Defining risk levels 1 in locally advanced head and neck cancers: a comparative analysis of concurrent postoperative radiation plus chemotherapy trials of the EORTC (# 22931) and RTOG (# 9501). Head Neck. 2005; 27(10):843-50.
5. Bernier J, van Glabbeke M, Domenge C, Wibault P, Ozsahin M, Matuszewska K, et al. Results of EORTC phase III trial 22931 comparing, postoperatively, radiotherapy (RT) to concurrent chemo-radiotherapy (RT-CT) with high dose cisplatin in locally advanced head and neck (H&N) carcinomas (SCC). Eur J Cancer. 2001;37:S267.
6. Racadot S, Mercier M, Dussart S, Dessard-Diana B, Bensadoun RJ, Martin M, et al. Randomized clinical trial of post-operative radiotherapy versus concomitant carboplatin and radiotherapy for head and neck cancers with lymph node involvement. Radiother Oncol. 2008;87(2):164-72.
7. Tobias JS, Monson K, Gupta N, MacDougall H, Glaholm J, Hutchison I, et al. Chemoradiotherapy for locally advanced head and neck cancer: 10-year follow-up of the UK Head and Neck (UKHAN1) trial. Lancet Oncol. 2010;11(1):66-74.
8. Department of Veterans Affairs Laryngeal Cancer Study Group, Wolf GT, Fisher SG, Hong WK, Hillman R, Spaulding M, et al. Induction chemotherapy plus radiation compared with surgery plus radiation in patients with advanced laryngeal cancer. N Engl J Med. 1991;324(24):1685-90.
9. Forastiere AA, Goepfert H, Maor M, Pajak TF, Weber R, Morrison W, et al. Concurrent chemotherapy and radiotherapy for organ preservation in advanced laryngeal cancer. N Engl J Med. 2003;349(22):2091-8.
10. Lefebvre J, Horiot J, Rolland F, Tesselaar M, Leemans CR, Geoffrois L, et al. Phase III study on larynx preservation comparing induction chemotherapy and radiotherapy versus alternating chemoradiotherapy in resectable hypopharynx and larynx cancers. EORTC protocol 24954-22950. J Clin Oncol. 2007;25(18 Suppl):LBA6016.
11. Denis F, Garaud P, Bardet E, Alfonsi M, Sire C, Germain T, et al. Late toxicity results of the GORTEC 94-01 randomized trial comparing radiotherapy with concomitant radiochemotherapy for advanced-stage oropharynx carcinoma: comparison of LENT/SOMA, RTOG/EORTC, and NCI-CTC scoring systems. Int J Radiat Oncol Biol Phys. 2003;55(1): 93-8.
12. Garden AS, Harris J, Vokes EE, Forastiere AA, Ridge JA, Jones C, et al. Preliminary results of Radiation Therapy Oncology Group 97-03: a randomized phase II trial of concurrent radiation and chemotherapy for advanced squamous cell carcinomas of the head and neck. J Clin Oncol. 2004; 22(14):2856-64.
13. Bonner JA, Harari PM, Giralt J, Azarnia N, Shin DM, Cohen RB, et al. Radiotherapy plus cetuximab for squamous-cell carcinoma of the head and neck. N Engl J Med. 2006;354(6): 567-78.
14. VanderWalde N, Jagsi R, Dotan E, Baumgartner J, Browner IS, Burhenn P, et al. NCCN guidelines insights: older adult oncology, version 2.2016. J Natl Compr Canc Netw. 2016; 14(11):1357-70.
15. Extermann M, Aapro M, Bernabei R, Cohen HJ, Droz JP, Lichtman S, et al. Use of comprehensive geriatric assessment in older cancer patients: recommendations from the task force on CGA of the International Society of Geriatric Oncology (SIOG). Crit Rev Oncol Hematol. 2005;55(3):241-52.
16. Hamaker ME, Vos AG, Smorenburg CH, De Rooij SE, van Munster BC. The value of geriatric assessments in predicting treatment tolerance and all-cause mortality in older patients with cancer. Oncologist. 2012;17(11):1439-49.
17. Giantin V, Valentini E, Iasevoli M, Falci C, Siviero P, De Luca E, et al. Does the Multidimensional Prognostic Index (MPI), based on a Comprehensive Geriatric Assessment (CGA), predict mortality in cancer patients? Results of a prospective observational trial. J Geriatr Oncol. 2013;4(3): 208-17.
18. Kenis C, Bron D, Libert Y, Decoster L, Van Puyvelde K, Scalliet P, et al. Relevance of a systematic geriatric screening and assessment in older patients with cancer: results of a prospective multicentric study. Ann Oncol. 2013;24(5):1306-12.
19. Soubeyran P, Fonck M, Blanc-Bisson C, Blanc JF, Ceccaldi J, Mertens C, et al. Predictors of early death risk in older patients treated with first-line chemotherapy for cancer. J Clin Oncol. 2012;30(15):1829-34.
20. Hurria A, Rosen C, Hudis C, Zuckerman E, Panageas KS, Lachs MS, et al. Cognitive function of older patients receiving adjuvant chemotherapy for breast cancer: a pilot prospective longitudinal study. J Am Geriatr Soc. 2006; 54(6):925-31.
21. Robb C, Boulware D, Overcash J, Extermann M. Patterns of care and survival in cancer patients with cognitive impairment. Crit Rev Oncol Hematol. 2010;74(3):218-24.
22. Goodwin JS, Zhang DD, Ostir GV. Effect of depression on diagnosis, treatment, and survival of older women with breast cancer. J Am Geriatr Soc. 2004;52(1):106-11.
23. Klepin HD, Geiger AM, Tooze JA, Kritchevsky SB, Williamson JD, Pardee TS, et al. Geriatric assessment predicts survival for older adults receiving induction chemotherapy for acute myelogenous leukemia. Blood. 2013; 121(21):4287-94.
24. Owusu C, Margevicius S, Schluchter M, Koroukian SM, Schmitz KH, Berger NA. Vulnerable elders survey and socioeconomic status predict functional decline and death among older women with newly diagnosed nonmetastatic breast cancer. Cancer. 2016;122(16):2579-86.
25. Kenis C, Decoster L, Van Puyvelde K, De Greve J, Conings G, Milisen K, et al. Performance of two geriatric screening tools in older patients with cancer. J Clin Oncol. 2014;32(1):19-26.
26. Soubeyran P, Bellera C, Goyard J, Heitz D, Curé H, Rousselot H, et al. Screening for vulnerability in older cancer patients: the ONCODAGE Prospective Multicenter Cohort Study. PloS One. 2014;9(12):e115060.
27. Lawton MP, Brody EM. Assessment of older people: self-maintaining and instrumental activities of daily living. Gerontologist. 1969;9(3):179-86.
28. Cesari M, Kritchevsky SB, Newman AB, Simonsick EM, Harris TB, Penninx BW, et al. Added value of physical performance measures in predicting adverse health-related events: results from the Health, Aging and Body Composition Study. J Am Geriatr Soc. 2009;57(2):251-9.
29. Vitzthum LK, Feng CH, Noticewala S, Hines PJ, Nguyen C, Zakeri K, et al. Comparison of comorbidity and frailty indices in patients with head and neck cancer using an online tool. JCO Clin Cancer Inform. 2018;2:1-9.
30. Sanabria A, Carvalho AL, Vartanian JG, Magrin J, Ikeda MK, Kowalski LP. Comorbidity is a prognostic factor in elderly

patients with head and neck cancer. Annals of surgical oncology. 2007;14(4):1449-57.
31. Reid BC, Alberg AJ, Klassen AC, Samet JM, Rozier RG, Garcia I, et al. Comorbidity and survival of elderly head and neck carcinoma patients. Cancer. 2001;92(8):2109-16.
32. Piccirillo JF. Importance of comorbidity in head and neck cancer. Laryngoscope. 2000;110(4):593-602.
33. Slater H, Young J. A review of brief cognitive assessment tests. Rev Clin Gerontol. 2013;23(2):164-76.
34. Braun M, Gurrera R, Karel M, Armesto J, Moye J. Are clinician's ever biased in their judgments of the capacity of older adult's to make medical decisions? Generations. 2009;33(1): 78-91.
35. Hurria A, Li D, Hansen K, Patil S, Gupta R, Nelson C, et al. Distress in older patients with cancer. J Clin Oncol. 2009; 27(26):4346-51.
36. Caillet P, Canoui-Poitrine F, Vouriot J, Berle M, Reinald N, Krypciak S, et al. Comprehensive geriatric assessment in the decision-making process in elderly patients with cancer: ELCAPA study. J Clin Oncol. 2011;29(27):3636-42.
37. Decoster L, Van Puyvelde K, Mohile S, Wedding U, Basso U, Colloca G, et al. Screening tools for multidimensional health problems warranting a geriatric assessment in older cancer patients: an update on SIOG recommendations. Ann Oncol. 2015;26(2):288-300.
38. Tomaka J, Thompson S, Palacios R. The relation of social isolation, loneliness, and social support to disease outcomes among the elderly. J Aging Health. 2006;18(3):359-84.
39. Magnuson A, Allore H, Cohen HJ, Mohile SG, Williams GR, Chapman A, et al. Geriatric assessment with management in cancer care: current evidence and potential mechanisms for future research. J Geriatr Oncol. 2016;7(4):242-8.
40. Extermann M, Boler I, Reich RR, Lyman GH, Brown RH, DeFelice J, et al. Predicting the risk of chemotherapy toxicity in older patients: the Chemotherapy Risk Assessment Scale for High-Age Patients (CRASH) score. Cancer. 2012; 118(13):3377-86.
41. Colevas AD, Yom SS, Pfister DG, Spencer S, Adelstein D, Adkins D, et al. NCCN guidelines insights: head and neck cancers, version 1.2018. J Natl Compr Canc Netw. 2018; 16(5):479-90.
42. Maggiore RJ, Dale W, Gross CP, Feng T, Tew WP, Mohile SG, et al. Polypharmacy and potentially inappropriate medication use in older adults with cancer undergoing chemotherapy: effect on chemotherapy-related toxicity and hospitalization during treatment. J Am Geriatr Soc. 2014;62(8):1505-12.
43. Lee SJ, Lindquist K, Segal MR, Covinsky KE. Development and validation of a prognostic index for 4-year mortality in older adults. JAMA. 2006;295(7):801-8.
44. Nosan DK, Gomez CR, Maves MD. Perioperative stroke in patients undergoing head and neck surgery. Ann Otol Rhinol Laryngol. 1993;102(9):717-23.
45. Thompson SK, Southern DA, McKinnon JG, Dort JC, Ghali WA. Incidence of perioperative stroke after neck dissection for head and neck cancer: a regional outcome analysis. Ann Surg. 2004;239(3):428-31.
46. Kowalski LP, Alcantara PS, Magrin J, Parise Júnior O. A case-control study on complications and survival in elderly patients undergoing major head and neck surgery. Am J Surg. 1994;168(5):485-90.
47. Clayman GL, Eicher SA, Sicard MW, Razmpa E, Goepfert H. Surgical outcomes in head and neck cancer patients 80 years of age and older. Head Neck. 1998;20(3):216-23.
48. McGuirt WF, Davis SP 3rd. Demographic portrayal and outcome analysis of head and neck cancer surgery in the elderly. Arch Otolaryngol Head Neck Surg. 1995;121(2): 150-4.
49. Shaari CM, Buchbinder D, Costantino PD, Lawson W, Biller HF, Urken ML. Complications of microvascular head and neck surgery in the elderly. Arch Otolaryngol Head Neck Surg. 1998;124(4):407-11.
50. Laccourreye O, Malinvaud D, Holsinger FC, Consoli S, Ménard M, Bonfils P. Trade-off between survival and laryngeal preservation in advanced laryngeal cancer: the otorhinolaryngology patient's perspective. Ann Otol Rhinol Laryngol. 2012;121(9):570-5.
51. Morgan RF, Hirata RM, Jaques DA, Hoopes JE. Head and neck surgery in the aged. Am J Surg. 1982;144(4): 449-51.
52. Sesterhenn AM, Schotte TL, Bauhofer A, Timmesfeld N, Wiegand S, Werner JA, et al. Head and neck cancer surgery in the elderly: outcome evaluation with the McPeek score. Ann Otol Rhinol Laryngol. 2011;120(2):110-5.
53. Milet PR, Mallet Y, El Bedoui S, Penel N, Servent V, Lefebvre JL. Head and neck cancer surgery in the elderly-does age influence the postoperative course? Oral Oncol. 2010;46(2):92-5.
54. Zabrodsky M, Calabrese L, Tosoni A, Ansarin M, Giugliano G, Bruschini R, et al. Major surgery in elderly head and neck cancer patients: immediate and long-term surgical results and complication rates. Surg Oncol. 2004;13(4):249-55.
55. Bridger AG, O'Brien CJ, Lee KK. Advanced patient age should not preclude the use of free-flap reconstruction for head and neck cancer. Am J Surg. 1994;168(5):425-8.
56. Bhattacharyya N. A matched survival analysis for squamous cell carcinoma of the head and neck in the elderly. Laryngoscope. 2003;113(2):368-72.
57. Blackwell KE, Azizzadeh B, Ayala C, Rawnsley JD. Octogenarian free flap reconstruction: complications and cost of therapy. Otolaryngol Head Neck Surg. 2002;126(3): 301-6.
58. Subramaniam N, Balasubramanian D, Rka P, Rathod P, Murthy S, Vidhyadharan S, et al. Peri-operative outcomes following major surgery for head and neck cancer in the elderly: institutional audit and case-control study. J Laryngol Otol. 2018;132(8):742-7.
59. Khafif A, Posen J, Yagil Y, Beiser M, Gil Z, Ben-Yosef R, et al. Quality of life in patients older than 75 years following major head and neck surgery. Head Neck. 2007;29(10): 932-9.
60. Dhiwakar M, Khan NA, McClymont LG. Surgery for head and neck skin tumors in the elderly. Head Neck. 2007;29(9): 851-6.
61. Haehl E, Rühle A, David H, Kalckreuth T, Sprave T, Stoian R, et al. Radiotherapy for geriatric head-and-neck cancer patients: what is the value of standard treatment in the elderly? Radiat Oncol. 2020;15(1):31.
62. Bourhis J, Overgaard J, Audry H, Ang KK, Saunders M, Bernier J, et al. Hyperfractionated or accelerated radiotherapy in head and neck cancer: a meta-analysis. Lancet. 2006; 368(9538):843-54.
63. Pignon T, Scalliet P. Radiotherapy in the elderly. Eur J Surg Oncol. 1998;24(5):407-11.
64. Allal AS, Maire D, Becker M, Dulguerov P. Feasibility and early results of accelerated radiotherapy for head and neck carcinoma in the elderly. Cancer. 2000;88(3):648-52.

65. Malik A, Mishra A, Chopda P, Singhvi H, Nair S, Nair D, et al. Impact of age on elderly patients with oral cancer. Eur Arch Otorhinolaryngol. 2019;276(1):223-31.
66. Biswas R, Halder A, Ghosh A, Ghosh SK. A comparative study of treatment outcome in younger and older patients with locally advanced oral cavity and oropharyngeal cancers treated by chemoradiation. South Asian J Cancer. 2019;8(1): 47-51.
67. Huang SH, O'Sullivan B, Waldron J, Lockwood G, Bayley A, Kim J, et al. Patterns of care in elderly head-and-neck cancer radiation oncology patients: a single-center cohort study. Int J Radiat Oncol Biol Phys. 2011;79(1):46-51.
68. Schofield CP, Sykes AJ, Slevin NJ, Rashid NZ. Radiotherapy for head and neck cancer in elderly patients. Radiother Oncol. 2003;69(1):37-42.
69. Zachariah B, Balducci L, Venkattaramanabalaji GV, Casey L, Greenberg HM, DelRegato JA. Radiotherapy for cancer patients aged 80 and older: a study of effectiveness and side effects. Int J Radiat Oncol Biol Phys. 1997;39(5):1125-9.
70. Wasil T, Lichtman SM, Gupta V, Rush S. Radiation therapy in cancer patients 80 years of age and older. Am J Clin Oncol. 2000;23(5):526-30.
71. Bhide SA, Ahmed M, Barbachano Y, Newbold K, Harrington KJ, Nutting CM. Sequential induction chemotherapy followed by radical chemo-radiation in the treatment of locoregionally advanced head-and-neck cancer. Br J Cancer. 2008;99(1):57-62.
72. Patil VM, Noronha V, Joshi A, Ramaswamy A, Dhumal S, Juvekar S, et al. Neoadjuvant chemotherapy in geriatric head and neck cancers. Head Neck. 2017;39(5):886-92.
73. Yoshida EJ, Luu M, David JM, Kim S, Mita A, Scher K, et al. Postoperative chemoradiotherapy in patients with head and neck cancer aged 70 or older with positive margins or extranodal extension and the influence of nodal classification. Head Neck. 2018;40(6):1228-36.
74. Argiris A, Li Y, Murphy BA, Langer CJ, Forastiere AA. Outcome of elderly patients with recurrent or metastatic head and neck cancer treated with cisplatin-based chemotherapy. J Clin Oncol. 2004;22(2):262-8.
75. Gillison ML, Trotti AM, Harris J, Eisbruch A, Harari PM, Adelstein DJ, et al. Radiotherapy plus cetuximab or cisplatin in human papillomavirus-positive oropharyngeal cancer (NRG Oncology RTOG 1016): a randomised, multicentre, non-inferiority trial. Lancet. 2019;393(10166):40-50.
76. Mehanna H, Robinson M, Hartley A, Kong A, Foran B, Fulton-Lieuw T, et al. Radiotherapy plus cisplatin or cetuximab in low-risk human papillomavirus-positive oropharyngeal cancer (De-ESCALaTE HPV): an open-label randomised controlled phase 3 trial. Lancet. 2019; 393(10166):51-60.
77. Magrini SM, Buglione M, Corvò R, Pirtoli L, Paiar F, Ponticelli P, et al. Cetuximab and radiotherapy versus cisplatin and radiotherapy for locally advanced head and neck cancer: a randomized phase II trial. J Clin Oncol. 2016;34(5):427-35.

Molecular Biology of Head and Neck Cancer

Vijay Kumar Srinivasalu, Narayana Subramaniam, Sivakumar Vidhyadharan, Samskruthi P Murthy

INTRODUCTION

Molecular mechanism of any cancer includes complex alterations of genetic, epigenetic, transcriptomic and proteomic make-up, and evolutionary process of potentially any cell type. The process can extend from understanding the driver and passenger genetic alterations to actionable alterations in coherent cell signaling pathways. One of the major factors for the complexity is molecular heterogeneity in cancer.

Molecular heterogeneity can be within different clones of cell types representing different molecular changes in the same tumor tissue (intratumoral or clonal) or between different tumor types giving different molecular pattern in the same tissue or organ (intertumoral). Intertumoral has been further understood as different molecular profiles of two metastatic lesions of the same primary (intermetastatic) or different clones of one metastatic lesion of a primary tumor (intrametastatic) and at a organismal level, heterogeneity can be due to different molecular profiles of the same tumor in different subjects (interpatient).[1]

With the availability of high-resolution cellular imaging, next generation sequencing, and rapid multiomic experimental methods, currently there has been a rapid expansion of knowledge on molecular changes happening in cancer cells, during the transformative initiation of normal cells to cancer cells, the evolution during natural history as well as treatment and finally the uncontrollable expansion and metastasis. In this chapter, we summarize the molecular mechanisms of cancer development in head and neck cancers.

CENTRAL MOLECULAR PATHOPHYSIOLOGY OF CANCERS

The molecular pathophysiology of three stages of cancer, such as initiation, progression and metastasis dealt with altered molecular signaling pathways that regulate key physiological functions of normal cell such as growth and proliferation, differentiation, stress response, deoxyribonucleic acid (DNA) repair, metabolism and cell survival. Alterations in molecular signaling pathways can also alter the reaction of tumor cells to the adjacent stromal microenvironment, immune cells, tissue macrophages, and vascular endothelial cells. Because of all these changes, carcinogenesis is a dynamic process happening within a set of distinctive signaling streams/traits that are complementary to each other in cell(s). There are about 10 of these traits that have been characterized so far.[2]

HALLMARKS OF CANCER

Hallmark 1: Enabling Replicative Immortality

The key feature acquired by cancer cells to evade senescence and to allow endless replication following disruption of the cell cycle:[3-7]

- *Human papillomavirus (HPV)-negative head and neck squamous cell carcinoma (HNSCC)*: *TP53*, *CCND1*, and *CDKN2A* are established cancer genes in HPV-negative
- *Human papillomavirus-positive HNSCC: TP53* and the genes encoding the Rb family [comprising *RB1*, *RBL1* (which encodes *p107*), and *RBL2* (which encodes *p130*)] are established cancer genes in HPV-positive HNSCC

Human papillomavirus-driven carcinogenesis: High-risk HPV types encode virulent alleles of two viral proteins, E6 and E7, which endow viral oncogenic potential by targeting molecular pathways that underlie neoplastic transformation.

Downstream consequences of high-risk HPV E6 and E7 action include the promotion of cell cycle progression, disruption of keratinocyte differentiation, keratinocyte immortalization, genomic instability, and neoplastic transformation.[7]

A central advance in the understanding of HPV-related carcinogenesis arose with the elucidation of mechanisms for the oncogenic potential of E6. High-risk HPV E6 proteins bind to p53 and induce ubiquitin-dependent proteolysis of the p53 tumor suppressor protein.[8] p53 is the protein product of the *TP53* gene, a regulator of the DNA-damage response,[9] G2/M cell cycle transition,[10] and the most commonly mutated tumor suppressor gene in cancer **(Fig. 1)**.[11]

Only E6 alleles from high-risk HPV types bind p53 and the strength of the binding affinity of E6 alleles for p53 correlates with that HPV type's oncogenic potential. For example, HPV16, which is responsible for more HPV-related HNSCC than HPV18,[12] encodes for an E6 allele that binds p53 with twice the affinity of the HPV18 E6 allele.[13]

The Cancer Genome Atlas (TCGA) consortium which presented the most comprehensive HNSCC genome-wide analysis to date[14] showed analysis of 279 HNSCC, of which 36 were HPV-positive, identified recurring activating mutations in *PIK3CA* in HPV-positive HNSCC.[15] *PIK3CA* encodes the catalytic subunit of phosphoinositol-3-kinase (PI3K) of the AKT/PI3K/AKT/mTOR pathway, which is essential for protein synthesis, cell growth, proliferation, and survival.[16] Overexpression and constitutive activation of *PIK3CA* leads to inhibition of apoptosis and, thus further tipping the balance toward carcinogenesis. TCGA found 56% of HPV-positive HNSCC showed activating mutations in this gene.

Amplification of the *E2F1* was another important HPV-specific finding. *E2F1* encodes a mitogenic transcription factor. *E2F1* target genes encode for proteins that are critical for progression of the cell cycle through the G1/S transition.[17,18] Interestingly, *E2F1* is regulated by the Rb tumor suppressor,[18] a target of HPV E7.[19] Overexpression of *E2F1* leads to dysregulation of this cell cycle checkpoint, pushing the cell toward carcinogenesis. TCGA found activating mutations in *E2F1* in 19% of HPV-positive HNSCC, compared to 2% in HPV-negative HNSCC.

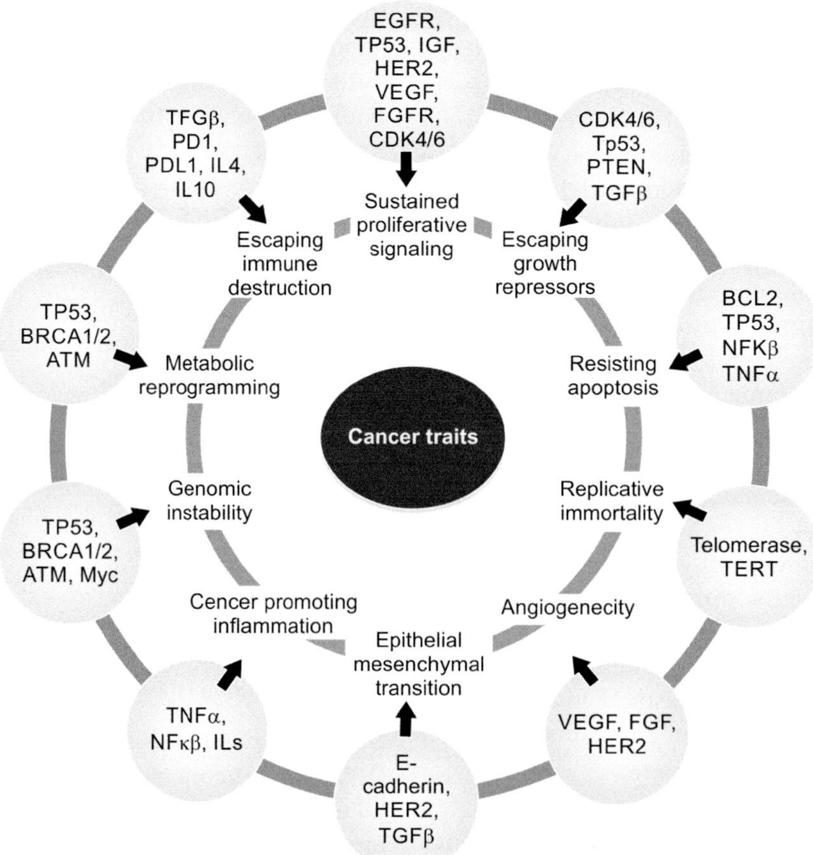

Fig. 1: Cancer traits. (ATM: ataxia telangiectasia-mutated; EGFR: epidermal growth factor receptor; FGF: fibroblast growth factor; FGFR: fibroblast growth factor receptor; IGF: insulin-like growth factor; IL: interleukins; NFκβ: nuclear factor kappa B; TNFα: tumor necrosis factor alpha; VEGF: vascular endothelial growth factor)

In a study pioneered by Seiwert et al., they found that HPV-positive tumors showed a distinct genetic profile with unique mutations in *DDX3X*, *CYLD*, and fibroblast growth factor receptor (FGFR), as well as enrichment for PI3K pathway alterations and rarer KRAS mutations common for HPV-negative HNSCC tissues.

In HPV-negative HNSCC, there were several mutations noted in *TP53*, *CDKN2A*, *MLL2*, *CUL3*, *NSD1*, and *PIK3CA* genes, with copy number increases in epidermal growth factor receptor (EGFR), *CCND1* and *FGFR1*. There were also identifiable somatic aberrations in DNA-repair genes (*BRCA1/2*, *Fanconi anemia* genes, and ataxia telangiectasia-mutated (ATM) that may play a role in the susceptibility of these tumours to treatment. These DNA-repair genes mutations were more common in HPV associated tumors with no significant history of smoking.[20] Considering a recent report that *RAD51B*, a *BRCA2* cofactor,[21] was a potential integration target for HPV16 leading to loss of its DNA-repair function, may indicate that the role of DNA-repair gene disruption in HPV-positive HNSCC carcinogenesis warrants further investigation.

The emerging role of ErbB family proteins in HPV-positive HNSCC: ErbB family proteins are encoded by four genes that play a central role in carcinogenesis: *ERBB1* (also known as *HER1* or *EGFR*), *ERBB2* (also known as *HER2* or *CD340*), *ERBB3* (also known as *HER3*), and *ERBB4* (also known as *HER4*).[22,23] Pollock showed that *HER2* and *HER3* expression were increased in HPV-positive HNSCC.[24] They also reported that afatinib, an anti-ErbB family small molecule inhibitor, significantly inhibited cell growth compared to cetuximab in HPV-positive cetuximab-resistant HNSCC cell lines. These findings suggested that targeting ErbB family receptor tyrosine kinases might be a potentially effective treatment for HPV-positive HNSCC.

However, these results were not supported by the LUX Head and Neck phase 1 trial,[25,26] which showed that both patients with p16-positive tumors and patients whose tumors progressed after cetuximab therapy derived less benefit from afatinib. One possible explanation for this apparent discrepancy was a difference in definitions, e.g., the LUX study considered previous exposure to cetuximab equivalent to cetuximab-resistance.

The discrepancy was addressed with a recent study investigating the relationship between HPV oncoproteins and HER3-mediated signaling, and the role of HER3 as a potential molecular target in HPV-positive HNSCC.[27] This study proposed a novel mechanism by which HPV can promote tumor growth through the mTOR/AKT/PI3K pathway. HER3 expression was found to be significantly increased in HPV-positive cell lines compared to HPV-negative cell lines.

Brand et al. then investigated the role of E6 and E7 oncoproteins in HER3 expression. They found that *E6/E7* gene silencing led to diminished HER3 production, while increased E6/E7 oncoprotein production led to increased HER3 production. The results indicate a relationship between HPV infection and HER3 expression that is mediated by the E6 and E7 oncoproteins.[27]

HER3 expression might also affect cellular proliferation and tumor growth in HPV-positive HNSCC cell lines. Genetic ablation of HER3 resulted in significantly reduced cellular proliferation (21–55%) and HER3 knockdown led to reduction in phosphorylation of AKT and RPS6.[27] The reduction of these proteins, which are components of the same mTOR/AKT/PI3K pathway, suggests that HER3 exerts its proliferative effect by signaling through the mTOR/AKT/PI3K signaling pathway.

- Ectopic expression of telomerase reverse transcriptase
- *Cancer stem cells (CSCs)*: These are a highly tumorigenic subpopulation of cells within the tumor (constituting <10% of the whole tumor[9] with the capability to self-renew, undergo differentiation and proliferate. They are an important factor in treatment resistance and metastasis; it is believed that they are a common cause of recurrence after treatment

NANOG (inhibitor of self-differentiation and chemotherapy resistance), OCT-4 (for self-renewal and pluripotency), BMI1 (in self-renewal), and Snail and Twist and Wnt signaling (in epithelial to mesenchymal transition, which is important in metastasis) and ABC (in drug efflux and chemotherapy resistance) are believed to be the important genetic and transcription factors associated with CSCs.[10,11]

Hallmark 2: Changes in Growth Factor Signaling

Epidermal growth factor receptor pathway: Dysregulation of the EGFR pathway is responsible for initiation, proliferation, and resistance to treatment of the tumors. EGFR is overexpressed in >80% of HNSCC.[13,28] However, all subsites do not have the same expression levels, with laryngeal having the lower levels of expression than oral or oropharyngeal tumors.[28]

Epidermal growth factor receptor binding results in autophosphorylation, and downstream activation of many oncogenic signal transduction pathways such as Ras, Raf, mitogen-activated protein (MAP)-kinase-pathway, JAK-STAT, and PI3K/AKT pathways. This is turn lead to cellular proliferation, angiogenesis, and an inhibition of apoptosis.[29-31] Patients with high-EGFR expression are associated with advanced stage, poorer differentiation and treatment resistance; however, some studies have shown that it may be associated with more radiation sensitivity.[32,33]

In view of this pivotal role that EGFR plays in HNSCC several targeted agents have been studied, with only cetuximab and nimotuzumab showing some therapeutic benefit.[34] However, unlike in lung cancer, EGFR expression was not associated with prognostic significance and is not a biomarker for treatment response with targeted agents.

Hallmark 3: Insensitivity to Growth Inhibitory Signals

Transforming growth factor beta (TGF-β) pathway: It acts through the TGF-β receptors[35-37] and then through the intracellular signal transduction mediators *SMAD2, SMAD3* and *SMAD4*[38,39] that regulate target gene transcription and downregulates proliferation while increasing apoptosis.

Hallmark 4: Evading Apoptosis—PI3K/PTEN/AKT

This is a signal transduction pathway involved in 10–20% of HNSCC through activation of *PIK3CA* mutations, inactivating mutations or deletions of PTEN.[40]

Hallmark 5: Invasion and Metastasis

Lymph node metastasis is arguably the single most important prognostic determinant in HNSCC. Dissemination occurs through the disruption of the extracellular matrix, which depend on activation of a cascade of matrix metalloproteinases (MMPs).

Epithelial-to-mesenchymal Transition

This is a pathological process through which epithelial cells undergo alteration, leading to tissue invasion and metastasis. EMT is a result of transcriptional and translational events leading to reprogramming of cells. Cells lose their cell–cell adherence, acquiring increased cell mobility and with a higher incidence of tissue invasion and metastasis.[41-43] Its exact clinical relevance is still unknown.[44]

Hallmark 6: Angiogenesis

Nutrient and oxygen supply and elimination of waste are rate-limiting steps in tumor proliferation. In order to grow beyond a certain size, all tumors require the development of blood vessels that can do this.[45,46] This is contingent on the presence of growth factors such as vascular endothelial growth factor (VEGF). VEGF immunohistochemistry (IHC) expression in HNSCC has been shown to be linked to prognosis.[46] However, the impact of HPV status on this relation is unknown.[47] Anti-VEGF-targeted therapies although initially promising, showed very little value in HNSCC. Drugs such as sunitinib and sorafenib have a definite role in thyroid cancers.

Hallmark 7: Replicative Immortality

Replicative immortality is achieved by upregulating telomerase enzyme. This would add nucleotide repeats and/or maintains the telomere length to provide replicative immortality. Also, this upregulation was found to be associated with poor prognosis with chemotherapy in certain cancers.

Hallmark 8: Cancer Promoting Inflammation

It is due to immune cell infiltration and expression and secretion of growth and survival factors to the tumor microenvironment causing propagation and invasion of tumors.

Hallmark 9: Genomic Instability

It can occur in different ways. Mutations in gatekeeper genes such as *TP53* and *RB1* are significantly higher in cancer cells and this can cause overall genomic instability which causes clonal evolution and selective growth advantage.[48] Mutations in caretaker genes, which are involved in DNA repair is called *mutator phenotype*, can give rise to more mutations in other part causing genomic instability in sporadic cancers when collapse of DNA replication occurs due to oncogene activations.[49]

Accordingly, somatic mutations in tumor cells are divided into driver and passenger mutations. Variations in *TP53, CDKN2A, SMAD4, PIK3CA, EGFR, PTEN,* and *MET* are the prominent driver mutations in head and neck cancers.[50] Passenger mutations are generally synonymous (without any amino acid change) variation and without any direct role in proliferation.

Hallmark 10: Metabolic Reprogramming

To adapt to cell proliferation and survival is an important change in biochemical physiology. According to Warburg phenomenon, cancer cells tap cellular energy via anaerobic glycolysis.[51] This is to adapt to hypoxic microenvironment and mitochondrial dysfunction and ATP depletion.[52]

PIK3CA mutations, which are seen in HNSCC, causes abnormal PI3K/Akt signaling pathway stimulating hexokinase and phosphor-fructokinase to drive glycolysis by activation or induction (via mTOR pathway).[53]

EPIGENETIC MODIFICATION

Direct damage to the genome may not always be the cause for development of tumors. Alternatively, in the absence of alteration of gene sequence, altered gene expression may be associated with tumorigenesis. Hypermethylation of tumor suppressor genes has been demonstrated to be associated with the development of HNSCC in this way.[50]

The evidence for epigenetic modification was seen in the TCGA analysis which showed in both HPV-positive and negative tumors contained recurrent focal amplifications for 3q26/28, a region that involves, among others, the squamous lineage transcription factor SOX2.[14]

This factor controls gene expression in pluripotent stem cells, contributing to the continuation of their pluripotency. Additionally, it plays a role in the reprogramming of somatic cells, reversing their epigenetic configuration back to the pluripotent embryonic state.[54]

Evidence of amplification of this gene provides a mechanism for conversion of squamous cells to CSCs, a concept that has been supported by other studies.[55]

In HPV-driven HNSCC, additional amplification of the host genome at the site of HPV integration,[14] and dysregulation of *p53* and Rb tumor-suppressor genes by HPV oncoproteins E6 and E7 do not fully account for the genome-wide spectrum of gene expression changes in HPV-positive HNSCC. Chromatin structure and epigenetic modifications, such as DNA methylation and histone-modifications, regulate gene expression, and their changes may explain genome-wide dysregulation found in HPV-positive HNSCC.

Sartor et al. showed HPV-positive HNSCC overall were found to have greater DNA methylation, both in terms of targeted genic methylation and global methylation, compared to HPV-negative HNSCC. The group found higher promoter methylation of polycomb repressive complex 2 target genes and increased expression of *DNMT3A*, in HPV-positive cells, implicating this DNA methyltransferase in the methylation patterns observed in HPV-positive HNSCC.

RUNX2, *IRS-1*, and *CCNA1* had higher methylation and lower expression in HPV-positive cells, whereas p16 (the surrogate marker of HPV infection) and *KRT8* had higher methylation and lower expression in HPV-negative cells.[56,57]

CONCLUSION

Although progress has been made in the areas of diagnostics and therapeutics of HNSCC, second tumors and metastases still remain a cause for low 5-year survival and high rates of morbidity and mortality. Combined approaches have seen improvement in the overall survival of patients, but advanced cancers require a trade-off between good cure rates and treatment-related morbidity. Thus, there is a desperate need for new and improved approaches in cancer treatment.

In HPV-driven carcinogenesis the current literature suggests that viral oncoproteins lead to significant epigenetic cascades and that aberrant chromatin structure plays an important role in the integration of HPV into the host genome. A "chicken and the egg" question remains unanswered for the potentially interdependent phenomena of HPV integration and HNSCC aberrations in chromatin structure, and requires further mechanistic investigation.

Head and neck squamous cell carcinoma is a highly heterogeneous malignancy, and the successful personalized therapy would allow for better prognostication of patients to allow less intensive morbid treatment regimens for the biologically favorable tumors and more intensive regimens, preferably with targeted therapy, for the more biologically aggressive tumors. The integration of molecular diagnostics and the molecular risk-based approach to cancer treatment that has become standard of care in other malignancies needs to be further developed and explored in head and neck cancer.

REFERENCES

1. Vogelstein B, Papadopoulos N, Velculescu VE, Zhou S, Diaz LA Jr, Kinzler KW. Cancer genome landscapes. Science. 2013;339:1546-58.
2. Hanahan D, Weinberg RA. Hallmarks of cancer: the next generation. Cell. 2011;144:646-74.
3. Kastan MB, Bartek J. Cell-cycle checkpoints and cancer. Nature. 2004;432:316-23.
4. Balz V, Scheckenbach K, Götte K, Bockmühl U, Petersen I, Bier H. Is the p53 inactivation frequency in squamous cell carcinomas of the head and neck underestimated? Analysis of p53 exons 2-11 and human papillomavirus 16/18 E6 transcripts in 123 unselected tumor specimens. Cancer Res. 2003;63:1188-91.
5. Opitz OG, Suliman Y, Hahn WC, Harada H, Blum HE, Rustgi AK. Cyclin D1 overexpression and p53 inactivation immortalize primary oral keratinocytes by a telomerase-independent mechanism. J Clin Invest. 2001;108:725-32.
6. Rheinwald JG, Hahn WC, Ramsey MR, Wu JY, Guo Z, Tsao H, et al. A two-stage, p16(INK4A)- and p53-dependent keratinocyte senescence mechanism that limits replicative potential independent of telomere status. Mol Cell Biol. 2002;22:5157-72.

7. Smeets SJ, van der Plas M, Schaaij-Visser TB, van Veen EA, van Meerloo J, Braakhuis BJ, et al. Immortalization of oral keratinocytes by functional inactivation of the p53 and pRb pathways. Int J Cancer. 2011;128:1596-605.
8. Chen C, Wei Y, Hummel M, Hoffmann TK, Gross M, Kaufmann AM, et al. Evidence for epithelial-mesenchymal transition in cancer stem cells of head and neck squamous cell carcinoma. PLoS One. 2011;6:e16466.
9. Jacobs JJ, Kieboom K, Marino S, DePinho RA, van Lohuizen M. The oncogene and polycomb-group gene bmi-1 regulates cell proliferation and senescence through the ink4a locus. Nature. 1999;397:164-8.
10. Yu CC, Lo WL, Chen YW, Huang PI, Hsu HS, Tseng LM, et al. Bmi-1 regulates snail expression and promotes metastasis ability in head and neck squamous cancer-derived ALDH1 positive cells. J Oncol. 2011;2011:609259.
11. Clay MR, Tabor M, Owen JH, Carey TE, Bradford CR, Wolf GT, et al. Single-marker identification of head and neck squamous cell carcinoma cancer stem cells with aldehyde dehydrogenase. Head Neck. 2010;32:1195-201.
12. Thariat J, Milas L, Ang KK. Integrating radiotherapy with epidermal growth factor receptor antagonists and other molecular therapeutics for the treatment of head and neck cancer. Int J Radiat Oncol Biol Phys. 2007;69:974-84.
13. Citri A, Yarden Y. EGF-ERBB signalling: towards the systems level. Nat Rev Mol Cell Biol. 2006;7:505-16
14. Global Burden of Disease Cancer Collaboration, Fitzmaurice C, Allen C, Barber RM, Barregard L, Bhutta ZA, et al. Global, regional, and national cancer incidence, mortality, years of life lost, years lived with disability, and disability-adjusted life-years for 32 cancer groups, 1990 to 2015: a systematic analysis for the Global Burden of Disease Study. JAMA Oncol. 2017;3:524-48.
15. Cancer Genome Atlas Network. Comprehensive genomic characterization of head and neck squamous cell carcinomas. Nature. 2015;517:576-82.
16. Laplante M, Sabatini DM. mTOR signaling in growth control and disease. Cell. 2012;149:274-93.
17. Johnson DG, Schwarz JK, Cress WD, Nevins JR. Expression of transcription factor E2F1 induces quiescent cells to enter S phase. Nature. 1993;365:349-52.
18. Sellers WR, Rodgers JW, Kaelin WG Jr. A potent transrepression domain in the retinoblastoma protein induces a cell cycle arrest when bound to E2F sites. Proc Natl Acad Sci USA. 1995;92:11544-8
19. Boyer SN, Wazer DE, Band V. E7 protein of human papilloma virus-16 induces degradation of retinoblastoma protein through the ubiquitin-proteasome pathway. Cancer Res. 1996;56:4620-4.
20. Seiwert TY, Zuo Z, Keck MK, Khattri A, Pedamallu CS, Stricker T, et al. Integrative and comparative genomic analysis of HPV-positive and HPV-negative head and neck squamous cell carcinomas. Clin Cancer Res. 2015;21:632-41.
21. Cousineau I, Abaji C, Belmaaza A. *BRCA1* regulates *RAD51* function in response to DNA damage and suppresses spontaneous sister chromatid replication slippage: implications for sister chromatid cohesion, genome stability, and carcinogenesis. Cancer Res. 2005;65:11384-91.
22. Subramaniam D, He AR, Hwang J, Deeken J, Pishvaian M, Hartley ML, et al. Irreversible multitargeted ErbB family inhibitors for therapy of lung and breast cancer. Curr Cancer Drug Targets. 2015;14:775-93.
23. Androutsopoulos G, Adonakis G, Liava A, Ravazoula P, Decavalas G. Expression and potential role of ErbB receptors in type II endometrial cancer. Eur J Obstet Gynecol Reprod Biol. 2013;168:204-8.
24. Pollock NI, Wang L, Wallweber G, Gooding WE, Huang W, Chenna A, et al. Increased Expression of HER2, HER3, and HER2:HER3 heterodimers in HPV-positive HNSCC using a novel proximity-based assay: Implications for targeted therapies. Clin Cancer Res. 2015;21:4597-606.
25. Machiels JP, Galot R, Schmitz S. HER2 and HER3 in HPV+ and HPV–HNSCC—Letter. Clin Cancer Res. 2016;22:1825.
26. Machiels JP, Haddad RI, Fayette J, Licitra LF, Tahara M, Vermorken JB, et al. Afatinib versus methotrexate as second-line treatment in patients with recurrent or metastatic squamous-cell carcinoma of the head and neck progressing on or after platinum-based therapy (LUX-Head & Neck 1): an open-label, randomised phase 3 trial. Lancet Oncol. 2015;16:583-94.
27. Brand TM, Hartmann S, Bhola NE, Peyser ND, Li H, Zeng Y, et al. Human papillomavirus regulates HER3 expression in head and neck cancer: implications for targeted HER3 therapy in HPV+ patients. Clin Cancer Res. 2017;23:3072-83.
28. Kalyankrishna S, Grandis JR. Epidermal growth factor receptor biology in head and neck cancer. J Clin Oncol. 2006; 24:2666-72.
29. Ciardiello F, Tortora G. EGFR antagonists in cancer treatment. N Engl J Med. 2008;358:1160-74.
30. Herbst RS, Giaccone G, Schiller JH, Natale RB, Miller V, Manegold C, et al. Gefitinib in combination with paclitaxel and carboplatin in advanced non-small-cell lung cancer: A phase III trial—INTACT 2. J Clin Oncol. 2004;22:785-94.
31. Grandis JR, Tweardy DJ. TGF-alpha and EGFR in head and neck cancer. J Cell Biochem Suppl. 1993;17F:188-91.
32. Takes RP, Baatenburg de Jong RJ, Schuuring E, Litvinov SV, Hermans J, Van Krieken JH. Differences in expression of oncogenes and tumor suppressor genes in different sites of head and neck squamous cell. Anticancer Res. 1998;18: 4793-800.
33. Ang KK, Berkey BA, Tu X, Zhang HZ, Katz R, Hammond EH, et al. Impact of epidermal growth factor receptor expression on survival and pattern of relapse in patients with advanced head and neck carcinoma. Cancer Res. 2002;62:7350-6.
34. Kim S, Grandis JR, Rinaldo A, Takes RP, Ferlito A. Emerging perspectives in epidermal growth factor receptor targeting in head and neck cancer. Head Neck. 2008;30:667-74.
35. Ouban A, Muraca P, Yeatman T, Coppola D. Expression and distribution of insulin-like growth factor-1 receptor in human carcinomas. Hum Pathol. 2003;34:803-8.
36. Jones HE, Goddard L, Gee JM, Hiscox S, Rubini M, Barrow D, et al. Insulin-like growth factor-I receptor signalling and acquired resistance to gefitinib (ZD1839; Iressa) in human breast and prostate cancer cells. Endocr Relat Cancer. 2004; 11:793-814.
37. Wang D, Song H, Evans JA, Lang JC, Schuller DE, Weghorst CM. Mutation and downregulation of the transforming growth factor beta type II receptor gene in primary squamous cell carcinomas of the head and neck. Carcinogenesis. 1997;18:2285-90.
38. Huntley SP, Davies M, Matthews JB, Thomas G, Marshall J, Robinson CM, et al. Attenuated type II TGF-beta receptor signalling in human malignant oral keratinocytes induces a less differentiated and more aggressive phenotype that

is associated with metastatic dissemination. Int J Cancer. 2004;110:170-6.

39. Qiu W, Schönleben F, Li X, Su GH. Disruption of transforming growth factor beta-Smad signaling pathway in head and neck squamous cell carcinoma as evidenced by mutations of *SMAD2* and *SMAD4*. Cancer Lett. 2007;245:163-70.
40. Kozaki K, Imoto I, Pimkhaokham A, Hasegawa S, Tsuda H, Omura K, et al. *PIK3CA* mutation is an oncogenic aberration at advanced stages of oral squamous cell carcinoma. Cancer Sci. 2006;97:1351-8.
41. Hugo H, Ackland ML, Blick T, Lawrence MG, Clements JA, Williams ED, et al. Epithelial—mesenchymal and mesenchymal—epithelial transitions in carcinoma progression. J Cell Physiol. 2007;213:374-83.
42. Moustakas A, Heldin CH. Signaling networks guiding epithelial-mesenchymal transitions during embryogenesis and cancer progression. Cancer Sci. 2007;98:1512-20.
43. Mani SA, Guo W, Liao MJ, Eaton EN, Ayyanan A, Zhou AY, et al. The epithelial-mesenchymal transition generates cells with properties of stem cells. Cell. 2008;133:704-15.
44. Chung CH, Parker JS, Ely K, Carter J, Yi Y, Murphy BA, et al. Gene expression profiles identify epithelial-to-mesenchymal transition and activation of nuclear factor-kappaB signaling as characteristics of a high-risk head and neck squamous cell carcinoma. Cancer Res. 2006;66:8210-8.
45. Kerbel RS. Tumor angiogenesis. N Engl J Med. 2008;358: 2039-49.
46. Kyzas PA, Cunha IW, Ioannidis JP. Prognostic significance of vascular endothelial growth factor immunohistochemical expression in head and neck squamous cell carcinoma: a meta-analysis. Clin Cancer Res. 2005;11:1434-40.
47. Fei J, Hong A, Dobbins TA, Jones D, Lee CS, Loo C, et al. Prognostic significance of vascular endothelial growth factor in squamous cell carcinomas of the tonsil in relation to human papillomavirus status and epidermal growth factor receptor. Ann Surg Oncol. 2009;16:2908-17.
48. Greaves M, Maley CC. Clonal evolution in cancer. Nature. 2012;481:306-13.
49. Negrini S, Gorgoulis VG, Halazonetis TD. Genomic instability—an evolving hallmark of cancer. Nat Rev Mol Cell Biol. 2010;11:220-8.
50. Worsham MJ, Chen KM, Meduri V, Nygren AO, Errami A, Schouten JP, et al. Epigenetic events of disease progression in head and neck squamous cell carcinoma. Arch Otolaryngol Head Neck Surg. 2006;132:668-77.
51. Warburg O, Wind F, Negelein E. The Metabolism of Tumors in the Body. J Gen Physiol. 1927;8:519-30.
52. Pelicano H, Martin DS, Xu RH, Huang P. Glycolysis inhibition for anticancer treatment. Oncogene. 2006;25:4633-46.
53. Jones RG, Thompson CB. Tumor suppressors and cell metabolism: a recipe for cancer growth. Genes Dev. 2009;23: 537-48.
54. Takahashi K, Yamanaka S. Induction of pluripotent stem cells from mouse embryonic and adult fibroblast cultures by defined factors. Cell. 2006;126:663-76.
55. Keysar SB, Le PN, Miller B, Jackson BC, Eagles JR, Nieto C, et al. Regulation of head and neck squamous cancer stem cells by PI3K and SOX2. J Natl Cancer Inst. 2017;109:1-12.
56. Riethdorf S, Neffen EF, Cviko A, Loning T, Crum CP, Riethdorf L. *p16INK4A* expression as biomarker for HPV 16-related vulvar neoplasias. Hum Pathol. 2004;35:1477-83.
57. Sartor MA, Dolinoy DC, Jones TR, Colacino JA, Prince ME, Carey TE, et al. Genome-wide methylation and expression differences in HPV(+) and HPV(–) squamous cell carcinoma cell lines are consistent with divergent mechanisms of carcinogenesis. Epigenetics. 2011;6:777-87.

CHAPTER 32

Personalized Medicine in Head and Neck Cancer Therapy

Vineeth Sukrithan

INTRODUCTION

Exposure to alcohol and smoking are the classical risk factors linked to the occurrence of head and neck squamous cell cancers (HNSCC). Infections with oncogenic strains of human papillomavirus (HPV), mainly HPV-16, are seen in an increasing proportion of mainly oropharyngeal SCC (OPSCC), with tonsillar crypt SCC having the highest attributable fraction of HPV positivity (47%).[1] The prevalence of HPV-attributable OPSCC has increased from 7.2% in 1990–1994 to 32.7% in 2010–2012.[2]

The eight edition of the AJCC/IUCC TNM staging for oropharyngeal cancers includes p16^{INK4A} immunostaining as a surrogate for HPV status. HPV-positive OPSCC are now staged differently as they may be candidates for de-escalation therapy due to their overall good prognosis. E7 viral protein expression results in de-repression of the cyclin-dependent kinase inhibitor 2A (*CDKN2A*) gene encoding p16^{INK4A} making it a surrogate marker for HPV-driven OPSCC. However, false positives are high in non-OPSCC cases due to a lower prevalence of oncogenic HPV in non-OPSCC subsites. A study of HPV involvement in non-OPSCC assessed by HPV DNA polymerase chain reaction (PCR) plus E6 and E7 mRNA expression found that only 3.9 and 3.1% for oral and laryngeal cancers, respectively, had oncogenic HPV infections.[1] Therefore, routine testing of p16, HPV DNA, or mRNA is not routinely undertaken in non-OPSCC cancers.

The stark differences in the mutational landscape between HPV-positive and -negative tumors have fueled interest in gaining a better understanding of the genomic attributes of HNSCC with the aim of developing personalized therapies with better efficacy and lesser toxicity.

MOLECULAR SUBTYPES OF HEAD AND NECK SQUAMOUS CELL CANCERS

In a landmark study from 2015, The Cancer Genome Atlas (TCGA) released data from the molecular profiling of 279 HNSCC cases. Four major molecular subtypes of HNSCC which had previously been described based on gene expression patterns, namely basal, mesenchymal, atypical, and classical,[3,4] were subsequently validated from the TCGA cohort:[5]

1. The basal subtype is characterized by activating *HRAS* mutations, inactivation of *NOTCH1* and *CASP8* with intact oxidative stress signaling.
2. The mesenchymal subtype has an epithelial to mesenchymal transition (EMT) signature and high expression of CD56 and human leukocyte antigen (HLA) class I mutations.
3. The atypical subtype consisted of HPV-positive tumors with high expression of *CDKN2A*, *LIG1*, and *RPA2* with activating mutations in the *PIK3CA* helical domain and a low level of EGFR amplification.
4. The classical subtype showed a tobacco-induced gene expression signature characterized by a high number of mutations clustered in the oxidative stress pathway, such as the nuclear factor erythroid 2-related factor 2 gene (*NFE2L2*, also known as *NRF1*), *KEAP1*, and *CUL3*.[5] Loss-of-function mutations in *TP53*, *CDKN2A* loss, and chromosome 3q (containing *PIK3CA*) amplification are also seen in this subtype.

A distinct subset of HPV-negative tumors with a reduced number of Copy Number Alteration (CNA-silent) was noted in the TCGA cohort that bore a wild-type *TP53* with fewer copy CNAs. Another group had previously shown that these tumors were DNA mismatch repair proficient and seemed to occur more frequently in non-smoking females without antecedent alcohol consumption and was associated with a better prognosis.[5,6]

HPV-positive tumors on the other hand can be further subclassified based on RNA sequencing into two groups, namely mesenchymal with immunological response genes (named HPV-IMU) and keratinocyte differentiation with oxidative stress genes (named HPV-KRT). The second group had more frequently integrated HPV and was enriched for 3q CNAs and *PIK3CA* mutations, while HPV-IMU tumors were enriched for chromosome 16q losses.[7] However, unlike the HPV-negative CNA-silent tumors, prognostic differences are yet to be shown for these two subgroups.

Gene expression patterns also differ based on the anatomic location of HNSCC. Next-gen sequencing (NGS) of exomes of 50 Indian tobacco-exposed patients exclusively with gingivo-buccal squamous cell carcinoma from the India Cohort of the TCGA revealed novel mutations (*USP9X, MLL4, ARID2, UNC13C,* and *TRPM3*) not routinely found in other anatomic locations. The prevalence of *TP53* mutations was nearly equal in both HPV-positive and HPV-negative cases (65%) which was a novel finding. *FAT1* mutations that promote aberrant Wnt activation occurred in up to 28% (compared to earlier reports of <12%). Three major molecular subgroups of gingiva-buccal SCC patients were identified. One subgroup harbored mutations in *CASP8* and *NOTCH1* with or without mutations in *FAT1* and *ARID2*. Another subgroup comprised patients with mutated *TP53*, while patients belonging to the third subgroup had *MLL4* and *USP9X* mutations. Patients in the first and third groups had significantly better disease-free survival (by 8 months) compared with the mean for the entire population.[8]

Cytogenetic Alterations

Cytogenetic alterations in the chromosomal patterns in HNSCC largely follow the patterns of gene deletion and amplification. Amplifications of 1q, 3q, 5p, and 8q and deletions of 3p, 5q, and 11q are seen regardless of the HPV status.

HPV-positive tumors have amplifications of 3q26/28 region containing transcription factors of squamous origin, *TP63, SOX2,* and *PIK3CA*. HPV-specific losses of chromosomal loci 14q32 and 9q, which contain the tumor necrosis factor receptor-associated factor 3 (*TRAF3*) and ataxia telangiectasia mutated (*ATM*) genes, have been reported.[9] The 7p region that includes EGFR is less amplified in HPV-positive tumors indicating less reliance on EGFR signaling.

In contrast, HPV-negative tumors have deletions in 9p21.3 while 11q13 containing *CCND1, FADD,* and *CTTN* and 11q22 containing *BIRC2* and *YAP1* are amplified.[5]

Mutational Landscape and Targeted Agents in HNSCC

Cell Cycle Regulation: CDKN2A, TP53, and CCND1

Loss of function of *TP53* and *CDKN2A* with *CCND1* amplifications is the major mechanism for cell cycle dysregulation in HPV-negative tumors. *TP53* is mutated in up to 87% and *CDKN2A* gene alterations are seen in up to 57%.[10,11] Epigenetic changes such as hypermethylation of promoters at CpG islands can also reduce the overall *CDKN2A* protein expression which is lost in almost all HPV-negative tumors.[12] MYC amplifications are seen in 5–15% of HPV-negative tumors. Overall HPV-negative tumors are not associated with the good prognosis typical of HPV-positive tumors. However, a small subset of HPV-negative oral cavity SCC harboring activating *HRAS* mutations and inactivating *CASP8* mutations do show a favorable prognosis.

The co-occurrence of *CDKN2A* mutations with *TP53* mutations allows HPV-negative tumors to bypass the two major cell-cycle checkpoints, namely G1-S and G2-M. *CDKN2A*, a tumor suppressor gene, encodes the p16INK4A protein, which binds and disrupts the cyclin D–CDK4 and cyclin D–CDK6 complexes. Loss of *CDKN2A* combined with the amplification of cyclin D1 (*CCND1*) located on 11q13 drives cells through the G1–S checkpoint. p53 protein is a key tumor suppressor that induces p21, another cyclin-dependent kinase (CDK) inhibitor that arrests the cell cycle at the G2-M checkpoint, and loss of p53 activity is associated with the accumulation of defective DNA.

In HPV-positive tumors, E6 and E7 viral oncogenic proteins lead to ubiquitination of *TP53* and *RB1* with focal amplification of *E2F1*, obviating the need for loss-of-function mutations in *TP53* or *CDKN2A*. *RB1* mutations, although rare at <10%, are seen predominantly in HPV-positive tumors.

Targeted Strategies Aimed at Disrupting Cell Cycle Regulation

Cyclin-dependent kinase inhibitors are being studied in patients with *CCND1* amplifications with extensive pre-clinical and clinical evidence of benefit in breast cancers. CDK4/6 inhibitors (Ribociclib and Palbociclib) act at the G2 to M phase checkpoint and enhance apoptosis induced by DNA damaging agents in *TP53* mutant HNSCC.[12]

Inhibition of *CDK1* phosphorylation by a WEE-1 kinase inhibitor, AZD1775, also disrupts the G2 checkpoint and is currently being tested in HNSCC in the neo-adjuvant setting in combination with chemotherapy

(NCT02508246) and in the locoregionally advanced setting combined with chemoradiotherapy (NCT02585973). Inhibition of checkpoint kinase 1/2 (CHK1/2) can induce cell death in *TP53* mutant HNSCC in vitro.[13]

PI3K-PTEN-AKT-mTOR Pathway

PI3K signaling pathway affects translation and transcription of multiple targets that are involved in various cellular properties such as proliferation, survival, and motility. PI3K alterations are already manifest in dysplastic lesions of the head and neck region in patients without evidence of invasive cancer and may mark cancer precursor lesions with a high risk of malignant transformation, irrespective of the HPV status.[14]

Activating mutations and amplifications, *PIK3CA* which encodes the catalytic p110α subunit is the most commonly altered oncogene in HNSCC. 41% of patients in the TCGA cohort had a *PIK3CA* mutation or amplification. The presence of mutations in the *PIK3CA* helical domain is a unique feature of HPV-positive tumors, whereas in HPV-negative tumors, mutations occur throughout the gene.

PTEN mutations or deletions are seen in 11% of HPV-positive HNSCC and 5% of HPV-negative HNSCC.[15,16] PI3K-PTEN-AKT-mTOR pathway is dysregulated in ~30% of HNSCC.[17]

Targeted Strategies Aimed at PI3K-PTEN-Akt-mTOR Pathway

Activating gain-of-function mutations in *PI3KCA* are considered more targetable as compared to inactivating loss-of-function mutations such as those seen in tumor suppressors. However, no significant improvement in clinical outcomes was seen with PX-866, an irreversible PI3K inhibitor, in unselected population of HNSCC when combined with docetaxel or cetuximab.[18]

BYL719, a PI3K class Iα isoform inhibitor, showed signals of activity when combined with cetuximab in a phase Ib study.[19] Another phase I study studying Buparlisib in combination with cisplatin-based chemoradiotherapy in a locoregionally advanced setting is currently underway. Mammalian target of rapamycin (mTOR) inhibitors such as temsirolimus and everolimus have limited antitumor activity in platinum-refractory recurrent or metastatic HNSCC, and more research is required to study the mechanisms behind primary and secondary refractoriness in these novel targeted agents.[20,21]

Receptor Tyrosine Kinase and MAP Kinase Pathway—EGFR, ERBB, FGFR, MET

EGFR, FGFR1, IGF1R, MET, and *HRAS* mutations are predominantly seen in HPV-negative tumors while *FGFR2* and *FGFR3* alterations and *KRAS* mutations are more frequent in HPV-positive tumors. *ERBB2* alterations are seen in 3–4% of both subtypes. Overexpression of *EGFR* was seen in >90% of HNSCC and associated with a poor prognosis.[22,23] MET amplification is found in 2–13% of HNSCC and mutated in ~6% patients.[24] Acquired MET amplification is also a primary mechanism of resistance to EGFR inhibition.[25] EGFR has pleiotropic functions and links to MAPK signaling, PI3K signaling,[26] and direct nuclear signaling.[27] Interestingly, one of the targets of MAPK signaling is cyclin D1. Mutually exclusive mutational status is seen in growth factor receptors with cyclin D1 indicating functional synergy and hence a potential for synthetic lethality.

Targeted Strategies Aimed at Receptor Tyrosine Kinase and MAP Kinase Pathway

Cetuximab, an anti-EGFR monoclonal antibody, improves survival in both locoregionally advanced and recurrent or metastatic settings when combined with radiotherapy and chemotherapy.[28,29] Various molecularly targeted therapies are currently being studied in combination with cetuximab in many phase 1 and 2 clinical trials. Afatinib, an irreversible pan-ERBB inhibitor, was shown to improve progression-free survival in a non-selected population of recurrent or metastatic HNSCC when compared to methotrexate in the second-line setting.[30] Dacomitinib, another irreversible pan-ERBB inhibitor, also demonstrated a single agent response rate of ~13% in a phase 2 study.[31] FGFR inhibitors are currently in the early stages of clinical development. A phase II study of foretinib, an oral multikinase inhibitor of *MET* and *VEGFR2*, was conducted in an unselected HNSCC population and no signals of clinical activity were noted.[32]

DNA Damage Response Pathway: BRCA, ATM, ATR

Mutations in *BRCA1, BRCA2,* and *ATR* are seen in 6, 7, and 10% of HNSCC, respectively. *ATM* mutations are also seen in up to 16% of HPV-positive HNSCC. These proteins are important for DNA damage repair through homologous recombination. An HPV-specific genetic change is loss of chromosome 9q, which contains *ATM* genes.[9]

Targeted Strategies Aimed at DNA Damage Response Pathway

PARP inhibitors and ATR inhibitors, in combination with radiotherapy or cisplatin, are being studied in patients with a homologous repair deficient genotype. ATR inhibitors, AZD6738 and VX-970, are in the early phase of development in HNSCC (NCT02264678; NCT02567422).

WNT Signaling

NOTCH1 is mutated in 11–19% of HNSCC.[33,34] NOTCH signaling is important for cell differentiation, proliferation, angiogenesis, and survival.[35,36] Significant geographic variations have been reported with a predominance of inactivating mutations in the TCGA cohort compared to activating gain-of-function mutations with over-expression of downstream effectors in a Chinese series.[37,38]

There are four receptors of the Notch family named *NOTCH1–NOTCH4*. The Notch receptors bind to membrane-bound ligands on other cells and are cleaved, and the Notch intracellular domain translocates to the nucleus and acts as a transcription factor.[39,40] *NOTCH1* was identified as a tumor-suppressor gene in HNSCC. Notch and β-catenin have a direct interaction: Membrane-bound Notch can bind to active β-catenin[41] and regulate its expression level by degradation. Subsequently, increased β-catenin activity leads to downstream activation of a variety of transcription factors that are linked to tumor progression by controlling cellular proliferation or cell death.

FAT1 gene is mutated in 23% of HNSCC cases. It encodes a large membrane protein belonging to the cadherin family of calcium-dependent transmembrane adhesion proteins which are linked to cell–cell contact, actin activity and WNT signaling. *FAT1* also binds β-catenin and sequesters it at the membrane, inhibiting its function in nuclear transcription. Knockdown of *FAT1* expression caused β-catenin release and β-catenin-mediated signaling.[42]

Co-occurrence of inactivating *FAT1* and *NOTCH1* alterations in HNSCC suggests that the carcinogenic route through inactivation of *FAT1* is associated with inactivation of *NOTCH1* to further increase β-catenin levels.

Targeted Strategies Aimed at WNT Signaling

A phase I study reported a response rate of 13% in 15 HNSCC patients treated with the combination of a NOTCH inhibitor MK-0752 with mTOR inhibitor ridaforolimus.[43] LGK974, a drug that targets Porcupine, a Wnt-specific acyltransferase, is currently being studied in a phase I study focused on patients with Wnt-dependent cancers including HNSCC.

Pathways Related to Immune-evasion

The discovery of the efficacy of checkpoint inhibitors as a modality of cancer treatment is a paradigm shift that holds the potential for durable responses in tumors that are amenable to immune targeting. No satisfactory biomarkers of response to immune strategies exist and surrogates in current use such as PD-L1 staining, tumor mutation burden, and levels of tumor infiltrating lymphocytes are of suboptimal predictive value. HNSCCs also tend to exhibit a low frequency of mutations in immune-responsive genes involved in antigen presentation such as *HLA-A*, *HLA-B*, and *B2M* in both HPV-positive and HPV-negative tumors.

Targeted Strategies Aimed at Immune-evasion

A randomized phase III study ("Checkmate 141") comparing nivolumab, an anti-PD-1 antibody, in 361 patients with platinum-resistant recurrent or metastatic HNSCC with the investigator's choice of therapy showed a survival benefit (7.5 vs. 5.1 months) with a 30% reduced risk of death.[44]

Much work is currently underway in identifying subsets of patients who may benefit from immune checkpoint inhibitor (ICI) therapy. 75% of HPV-positive HNSCC and 23% of HPV-negative HNSCC in the combined University of Chicago and TCGA cohort ($N = 558$) were described as having an "inflamed" phenotype defined as an enrichment of immune response genes related to CD8+ T lymphocyte infiltration, PD-L1, CTLA-4, LAG3, PD-L2, and IDO expression.[45] No prospective randomized data is available to suggest if this phenotype is predictive of response. Preliminary evidence also indicates that there may be a correlation between inflamed tumor phenotype and mesenchymal subtype, thereby providing a rationale for their targeting by immune strategies.[46]

Pathways Related to Epigenetic Programming

Gene expression is controlled epigenetically by the modulation of chromatin accessibility to transcription factors by methylation or acetylation of histones and at the DNA level by a pattern of methylation of cytosine residues at CpG islands. In HPV-negative HNSCC, decreased expression of micro-RNAs, miR-let-7c-5p, and miR-100-5p was shown to be inversely correlated with the expression of genes encoding proteins involved in cell cycle control indicating an important role for micro-RNAs in the evolution of HNSCC.[47]

Targeting Epigenetic Programming

An ongoing phase Ib/II study is studying the combination of azacytidine, a hypomethylating agent, with Anti-PD-L1 and CTLA-4 antibody in patients with relapsed/refractory metastatic HNSCC (NCT03019003).

In conclusion, personalized treatment based on genomics and epigenomics holds promise in the management of HNSCC. Much work remains to be done in discovering and refining biomarkers that predict for response with these targeted strategies. Lastly, the explosion of research interest in immunotherapies will need to be channeled toward rational combinations of various agents to improve rates of durable survival with acceptable tolerability profiles.

REFERENCES

1. Castellsagué X, Alemany L, Quer M, Halec G, Quirós B, Tous S, et al. HPV involvement in head and neck cancers: Comprehensive assessment of biomarkers in 3680 patients. J Natl Cancer Inst. 2016;108(6):djv403.
2. D'Souza G, Kreimer AR, Viscidi R, Pawlita M, Fakhry C, Koch WM, et al. Case-control study of human papillomavirus and oropharyngeal cancer. N Engl J Med. 2007;356(19): 1944-56.
3. Chung CH, Parker JS, Karaca G, Wu J, Funkhouser WK, Moore D, et al. Molecular classification of head and neck squamous cell carcinomas using patterns of gene expression. Cancer Cell. 2004;5(5):489-500.
4. Walter V, Yin X, Wilkerson MD, Cabanski CR, Zhao N, Du Y, et al. Molecular subtypes in head and neck cancer exhibit distinct patterns of chromosomal gain and loss of canonical cancer genes. PLoS One. 2013;8(2):e56823.
5. Lawrence MS, Sougnez C, Lichtenstein L, Cibulskis K, Lander E, Gabriel SB, et al. Comprehensive genomic characterization of head and neck squamous cell carcinomas. Nature. 2015;517(7536):576-82.
6. Smeets SJ, Braakhuis BJM, Ylstra B, Leemans CR, Brakenhoff RH. TP53 mutations are associated with a particular pattern of genomic imbalances in head and neck squamous cell carcinoma. Cell Oncol. 2007;29:160.
7. Zhang Y, Koneva LA, Virani S, Arthur AE, Virani A, Hall PB, et al. Subtypes of HPV-positive head and neck cancers are associated with HPV characteristics, copy number alterations, PIK3CA mutation, and pathway signatures. Clin Cancer Res. 2016;22(18):4735-45.
8. Maitra A, Biswas NK, Amin K, Kowtal P, Kumar S, Das S, et al. Mutational landscape of gingivo-buccal oral squamous cell carcinoma reveals new recurrently-mutated genes and molecular subgroups. Nat Commun. 2013;4:2873.
9. Hayes DN, Van Waes C, Seiwert TY. Genetic landscape of human papillomavirus-associated head and neck cancer and comparison to tobacco-related tumors. J Clin Oncol. 2015;33(29):3227-34.
10. Seiwert TY, Zuo Z, Keck MK, Khattri A, Pedamallu CS, Stricker T, et al. Integrative and comparative genomic analysis of HPV-positive and HPV-negative head and neck squamous cell carcinomas. Clin Cancer Res. 2015;21(3):632-41.
11. Chung CH, Guthrie VB, Masica DL, Tokheim C, Kang H, Richmon J, et al. Genomic alterations in head and neck squamous cell carcinoma determined by cancer gene-targeted sequencing. Ann Oncol. 2015;26(6):1216-23.
12. Lim AM, Do H, Young RJ, Wong SQ, Angel C, Collins M, et al. Differential mechanisms of CDKN2A (p16) alteration in oral tongue squamous cell carcinomas and correlation with patient outcome. Int J Cancer. 2014;135(4):887-95.
13. Gadhikar MA, Sciuto MR, Alves MVO, Pickering CR, Osman AA, Neskey DM, et al. Chk1/2 inhibition overcomes the cisplatin resistance of head and neck cancer cells secondary to the loss of functional p53. Mol Cancer Ther. 2013;12(9): 1860-73.
14. Verlaat W, Snijders PJ, van Moorsel MI, Bleeker M, Rozendaal L, Sie D, et al. Somatic mutation in PIK3CA is a late event in cervical carcinogenesis. J Pathol Clin Res. 2015; 1(4):207-11.
15. Pedrero JMG, Carracedo DG, Pinto CM, Zapatero AH, Rodrigo JP, Nieto CS, et al. Frequent genetic and biochemical alterations of the PI 3-K/AKT/PTEN pathway in head and neck squamous cell carcinoma. Int J Cancer. 2005;114(2): 242-8.
16. Shao X, Tandon R, Samara G, Kanki H, Yano H, Close LG, et al. Mutational analysis of the PTEN gene in head and neck squamous cell carcinoma. Int J Cancer. 1998;77(5):684-8.
17. Lui VWY, Hedberg ML, Li H, Vangara BS, Pendleton K, Zeng Y, et al. Frequent mutation of the PI3K pathway in head and neck cancer defines predictive biomarkers. Cancer Discov. 2013;3(7):761-9.
18. Jimeno A, Bauman JE, Weissman C, Adkins D, Schnadig I, Beauregard P, et al. A randomized, phase 2 trial of docetaxel with or without PX-866, an irreversible oral phosphatidylinositol 3-kinase inhibitor, in patients with relapsed or metastatic head and neck squamous cell cancer. Oral Oncol. 2015;51(4):383-8.
19. Gonzalez-Angulo AM, Juric D, Argilés G, Schellens JHM, Burris HA, Berlin J, et al. Safety, pharmacokinetics, and preliminary activity of the α-specific PI3K inhibitor BYL719: Results from the first-in-human study. J Clin Oncol. 2013; 31(15 Suppl):2531.
20. Grünwald V, Keilholz U, Boehm A, Guntinas-Lichius O, Hennemann B, Schmoll HJ, et al. TEMHEAD: a single-arm multicentre phase II study of temsirolimus in platin- and cetuximab refractory recurrent and/or metastatic squamous cell carcinoma of the head and neck (SCCHN) of the German SCCHN Group (AIO). Ann Oncol. 2015;26(3):561-7.
21. Massarelli E, Lin H, Ginsberg LE, Tran HT, Lee JJ, Canales JR, et al. Phase II trial of everolimus and erlotinib in patients with platinum-resistant recurrent and/or metastatic head and neck squamous cell carcinoma. Ann Oncol. 2015;26(7): 1476-80.
22. Hama T, Yuza Y, Saito Y, Ouchi J, Kondo S, Okabe M, et al. Prognostic significance of epidermal growth factor receptor phosphorylation and mutation in head and neck squamous cell carcinoma. Oncologist. 2009;14(9):900-8.
23. Keren S, Shoude Z, Lu Z, Beibei Y. Role of EGFR as a prognostic factor for survival in head and neck cancer: a meta-analysis. Tumour Biol. 2014;35(3):2285-95.
24. Seiwert TY, Jagadeeswaran R, Faoro L, Janamanchi V, Nallasura V, El Dinali M, et al. The MET receptor tyrosine kinase is a potential novel therapeutic target for head and neck squamous cell carcinoma. Cancer Res. 2009;69(7): 3021-31.
25. Engelman JA, Zejnullahu K, Mitsudomi T, Song Y, Hyland C, Park JO, et al. MET amplification leads to gefitinib resistance

in lung cancer by activating ERBB3 signaling. Science. 2007;316(5827):1039-43.
26. Normanno N, De Luca A, Bianco C, Strizzi L, Mancino M, Maiello MR, et al. Epidermal growth factor receptor (EGFR) signaling in cancer. Gene. 2006;366(1):2-16.
27. Lin S-Y, Makino K, Xia W, Matin A, Wen Y, Kwong KY, et al. Nuclear localization of EGF receptor and its potential new role as a transcription factor. Nat Cell Biol. 2001;3(9):802-8.
28. Vermorken JB, Mesia R, Rivera F, Remenar E, Kawecki A, Rottey S, et al. Platinum-based chemotherapy plus cetuximab in head and neck cancer. N Engl J Med. 2008;359(11):1116-27.
29. Bonner JA, Harari PM, Giralt J, Azarnia N, Shin DM, Cohen RB, et al. Radiotherapy plus cetuximab for squamous-cell carcinoma of the head and neck. N Engl J Med. 2006;354(6):567-78.
30. Machiels J-PH, Haddad RI, Fayette J, Licitra LF, Tahara M, Vermorken JB, et al. Afatinib versus methotrexate as second-line treatment in patients with recurrent or metastatic squamous-cell carcinoma of the head and neck progressing on or after platinum-based therapy: an open-label, randomised phase 3 trial. Lancet Oncol. 2015;16(5):583-94.
31. Abdul Razak AR, Soulières D, Laurie SA, Hotte SJ, Singh S, Winquist E, et al. A phase II trial of dacomitinib, an oral pan-human EGF receptor (HER) inhibitor, as first-line treatment in recurrent and/or metastatic squamous-cell carcinoma of the head and neck. Ann Oncol. 2013;24(3):761-9.
32. Seiwert T, Sarantopoulos J, Kallender H, McCallum S, Keer HN, Blumenschein G. Phase II trial of single-agent foretinib (GSK1363089) in patients with recurrent or metastatic squamous cell carcinoma of the head and neck. Invest New Drugs. 2013;31(2):417-24.
33. Stransky N, Egloff AM, Tward AD, Kostic AD, Cibulskis K, Sivachenko A, et al. The mutational landscape of head and neck squamous cell carcinoma. Science. 2011;333(6046):1157-60.
34. Agrawal N, Frederick MJ, Pickering CR, Bettegowda C, Chang K, Li RJ, et al. Exome sequencing of head and neck squamous cell carcinoma reveals inactivating mutations in NOTCH1. Science. 2011;333(6046):1154-7.
35. Hori K, Sen A, Artavanis-Tsakonas S. Notch signaling at a glance. J Cell Sci. 2013;126(Pt 10):2135-40.
36. Kerbel RS. Tumor angiogenesis. N Engl J Med. 2008;358(19):2039-49.
37. Song X, Xia R, Li J, Long Z, Ren H, Chen W, et al. Common and complex Notch1 mutations in Chinese oral squamous cell carcinoma. Clin Cancer Res. 2014;20(3):701-10.
38. Sun W, Gaykalova DA, Ochs MF, Mambo E, Arnaoutakis D, Liu Y, et al. Activation of the NOTCH pathway in head and neck cancer. Cancer Res. 2014;74(4):1091-104.
39. Ntziachristos P, Lim JS, Sage J, Aifantis I. From fly wings to targeted cancer therapies: A centennial for notch signaling. Cancer Cell. 2014;25(3):318-34.
40. Kopan R, Ilagan MXG. The canonical Notch signaling pathway: Unfolding the activation mechanism. Cell. 2009;137(2):216-33.
41. Kwon C, Cheng P, King IN, Andersen P, Shenje L, Nigam V, et al. Notch post-translationally regulates β-catenin protein in stem and progenitor cells. Nat Cell Biol. 2011;13(10):1244-51.
42. Morris LGT, Kaufman AM, Gong Y, Ramaswami D, Walsh LA, Turcan Ş, et al. Recurrent somatic mutation of FAT1 in multiple human cancers leads to aberrant Wnt activation. Nat Genet. 2013;45(3):253-61.
43. Piha-Paul SA, Munster PN, Hollebecque A, Argilés G, Dajani O, Cheng JD, et al. Results of a phase 1 trial combining ridaforolimus and MK-0752 in patients with advanced solid tumours. Eur J Cancer. 2015;51(14):1865-73.
44. Ferris RL, Blumenschein G, Fayette J, Guigay J, Colevas AD, Licitra L, et al. Nivolumab for Recurrent Squamous-Cell Carcinoma of the Head and Neck. N Engl J Med. 2016;375(19):1856-67.
45. Rabinowits G, Haddad RI. Overcoming resistance to EGFR inhibitor in head and neck cancer: a review of the literature. Oral Oncol. 2012;48(11):1085-9.
46. Saloura V, Zuo Z, Koeppen H, Keck MK, Khattri A, Boe M, et al. Correlation of T-cell inflamed phenotype with mesenchymal subtype, expression of PD-L1, and other immune checkpoints in head and neck cancer. J Clin Oncol. 2014;32(15 Suppl):6009.
47. Lubov J, Maschietto M, Ibrahim I, Mlynarek A, Hier M, Kowalski LP, et al. Meta-analysis of microRNAs expression in head and neck cancer: uncovering association with outcome and mechanisms. Oncotarget. 2017;8(33):55511-24.

CHAPTER 33

Nuclear Medicine in Head and Neck Cancer

Smitha Chinmay Kulkarni, Samskruthi P Murthy

INTRODUCTION

Nuclear medicine (NM) forms an essential component in present-day oncology. NM utilizes radiopharmaceutical agents and instrumentation to study physiological process of tumors that help to diagnose, localize, stage, prognosticate tumors and aid in optimizing cancer therapy. With the advent of newer molecular radiotracers in nuclear imaging that will enable accurate noninvasive in vivo tumor characterization based on which treatment decisions can be individualized in the future.

PART A: FUNDAMENTALS OF NUCLEAR MEDICINE

Imaging Methods

Imaging modality in NM consists of three types, namely (1) planar scintigraphy, (2) single-photon emission computed tomography (SPECT), and (3) positron emission tomography (PET):

- *Planar scintigraphy:* It is the most basic form of imaging which provides a single two-dimensional (2D) image. It utilizes a single gamma camera that identifies gamma rays emitted by radiotracer decay in the body. Planar scintigraphy has a very low spatial resolution but has extremely high sensitivity with the ability to detect nanograms of injected radioactive material.[1]
- *Single-photon emission computed tomography:* SPECT provides a three-dimensional image, utilizing 2–3 gamma cameras that identify gamma rays emitted by radiotracer decay from the body. The cameras reconstruct the signal acquired to provide cross-sectional images of the distribution of injected molecules. The main advantage of SPECT is that multiple probes can be used to study separate isotopes. SPECT has lower sensitivity than PET.[2]
- *Positron emission tomography:* PET utilizes the photon capture by a ring of detectors around the patient. PET uses positron-emitting isotope as radiotracers. Emitted positron annihilates with electron to emit two photons in opposite direction that gets picked up by the detector. The ring of detectors collects all events and reconstructs image to provide a cross-sectional imaging and reliable information about the concentration of radioisotope.[3]

Radionuclides

Radionuclides are radioactive elements that are used in both diagnostic and therapeutic applications in NM. The choice of radionuclide is based on the indication of whether it is used for diagnostic or therapeutic use. For diagnostic purposes, a radionuclide that emits gamma rays which penetrate deep are chosen while for therapeutic purposes radionuclide that emits radiation which travels a short distance to deposit their energy to minimize nontarget tissue radiation is chosen.[3]

Types of Radionuclide

- *Photon emitters:* They emit gamma rays (30–300 KeV). They are commonly used in SPECT imaging. They have longer half-life of several hours to days. Examples are technetium-99m, gallium-67, indium-111, and iodine-123.
- *Positron emitters:* They are positron-emitting radionuclides used in PET. They have a very short half-life that allows high-dose administration and allows repeated administration in a day.[3] Examples are carbon-11 (t½ 20.4 min), nitrogen-13 (t½ 9.96 min), oxygen-15 (t1½ 2.05 min), fluorine 18 (t½ 109.7 min), and gallium-68 (t½ 68 min).
- *Beta emitters:* They are used in therapeutics as they have a long path of transit (0.8–5 mm) and low

linear energy transfer (0.2 KeV/μm).[4] Examples are lutetium-177, holmium-166, rhenium-186, copper-67, promethium-149, gold-199, and rhodium-105.
- *Alpha emitters:* They are radionuclides that emit higher energy (4–9 MeV) with short travel (40–100 μm).[5] Alpha emitters lose 100–1,000 times more energy than external beam radiation while traversing DNA.[6] Examples are bismuth-213, astatine-211, radium-223, and actinium-255.

Radiotracers

These are compounds in which one atom or more have been replaced with radionuclides in order to study function based on the pattern of radiodecay. The types of radiotracers are:
- *Small molecules:* Radiolabeled glucose analog ^{18}F (fluorine-18)-2-fluoro-2-deoxy-D-glucose (2FDG) is one of the most common radiotracer used (>90%).[7] It not specific to any tissue but is specific to tissues with high glucose metabolism. Further details of ^{8}F (fluorine-18)-2-fluoro-2-deoxy-D-glucose (2FDG) is described in detail in the following section.
- *Targeting agents:* Antibodies are targeted agents that bind to known receptors. Commonly studied antibody radiotracers are antivascular endothelial growth factor (anti-VEGF), antiepidermal growth factor receptor (anti-EGFR) antibody.[3] Protein scaffolds that bind to a wide range of proteins such as insulin, tumor necrosis factor-alpha, and HER-2 are being studied. They possess high tumor penetration because of their relatively small size. Aptamers are molecules that have the ability to fold into a complex structure. Oligonucleotides are commonly used as aptamers but have a high rate of degradation in cells and blood.[8]

Chelators

Chelators are molecules that covalently bind to biologically active targeting molecule. They are used to bind to a radionuclide to prevent hydrolysis and aid in effectively supplying site-specific radioactive substance. Examples are diethylenetriamine pentaacetic acid (DTPA), 1,4,7,10-tetraazacyclododecane-1,4,7,10-tetraacetic acid (DOTA).[9]

The role of nuclear imaging is vital in present-day oncology practice. They aid in determining the extent of disease, assess disease progression, and also aid in treatment decision-making. The role of radiopharmaceuticals in therapeutics of cancer has emerged in various fields. Their therapeutic use, when appropriate, has been discussed in respective chapter. The following chapter focuses primarily on diagnostic approaches that are commonly used in head and neck tumors.

PART B: POSITRON EMISSION TOMOGRAPHY

Positron emission tomography-computed tomography (PET-CT) in combination with anatomical imaging modalities as computed tomography (PET-CT) and magnetic resonance imaging (PET-MRI) using ^{18}F-fluorodeoxyglucose (^{18}F-FDG) is a primary diagnostic tool for evaluation and management of head and neck malignancies, primarily squamous cell carcinomas (HNSCC) and thyroid malignancies. It is used in multiple clinical scenarios, such as pretreatment staging, radiotherapy planning, therapy-response assessment, and post-therapy follow-up. In the following section, we have attempted to highlight the practical aspects of performing a routine fluorodeoxyglucose positron emission tomography-computed tomography (FDG PET-CT) and PET-MRI, utility, strengths and limitations of each modality.

Radiopharmaceuticals

^{18}F-fluorodeoxyglucose is the most commonly used radiopharmaceutical in oncological practice. It has a relatively longer half-life of positron emitter fluorine-18 (110 min) that allows time for this radiopharmaceutical to be transported from the site of production (medical cyclotron) to the imaging facilities.

The use of FDG in oncology is based on the principle that many tumor cells demonstrate increased glucose metabolism compared to normal cells due to overexpression of glucose membrane transporters, especially glucose transporter 1 (GLUT1), and have enhanced hexokinase activity. Thus, ^{18}F-FDG, an analog of glucose, is transported and phosphorylated to ^{18}FDG-6-phosphate, which unlike glucose, does not undergo further enzymatic reactions and remains trapped in the cell. Most tumors and normal tissues have relatively low glucose-6-phosphatase activity, and so with minimal dephosphorylation of ^{18}FDG, the accumulation of this compound is proportional to the glycolytic rate. The relatively high tumor to background ratio and the superior resolution of PET systems are the main advantages of FDG imaging. Its combination with contrast-enhanced computed tomography (CECT) significantly improves the diagnostic efficiency in head and neck malignancies.

Patient Preparation

- *Hydration:* Good hydration should be ensured to promote good clearance of FDG from the pelvicalyceal system. If patient is receiving intravenous (IV) fluids, the fluid should not contain dextrose or lactose.
- *Diet:* Patients should be fasting except for water for 4–6 hours. This encourages low insulin levels, thus reducing FDG uptake in normal muscles and adipose tissue and maximizes FDG uptake in the tumor cells, thereby increasing the tumor to background ratio.
- *Glycemic control:* High serum glucose levels can substantially degrade image quality and diagnostic accuracy by competing with FDG uptake. For optimal image quality, the blood glucose level should be ≤150 mg/dL if possible. PET usually is rescheduled if glucose is above 200 mg/dL. Euglycemic status should be achieved in diabetic patients before the study:
  - *Insulin:* Intermediate and long-acting insulin should not be given on the day of the scan. It is to be remembered that insulin administration will increase FDG uptake in the heart, skeletal muscles, and liver. This might degrade image quality and can reduce the sensitivity. If required, rapidly acting insulin (2–5 units) can be given if glucose is elevated with a minimum time interval of 1 hour which is necessary between insulin administration and FDG injection. Glucose should be rechecked before FDG injection.
  - *Oral hypoglycemic agents:* Metformin reduces hepatic gluconeogenesis and has no direct action on insulin secretion hence should not interfere with FDG uptake. Other oral antidiabetic drugs, such as sulfonylureas (tolbutamide, glyburide, and glipizide) lower plasma glucose primarily by stimulating insulin secretion and should be stopped before FDG PET study.
- *Strenuous exercise:* It should be avoided on the day of the study to minimize muscle uptake and exposure to cold temperature and drugs that stimulate the sympathetic nervous system (such as nicotine and ephedrine) should be avoided for 48 hours to minimize brown fat uptake.

Ideal Time Interval to Positron Emission Tomography Imaging

- *Biopsy:* Around 1 week
- *Surgical procedure:* Around 6 weeks. Depends on the invasiveness of the procedure
- *Chemotherapy:* 2–4 weeks (PET-CT usually ordered a day or two before the next cycle)
- *Radiation:* 2–6 months
- *Granulocyte colony-stimulating factor:* 1–4 weeks.

Chemoradiotherapy can cause both false-positive results from inflammation as well as false-negative results possible "stunning" of the viable tumor. FDG uptake can be reduced within 1 day of starting chemotherapy, hence baseline studies should be performed.

Physiological Uptake of Fluorodeoxyglucose

- *Brain:* The normal brain has high FDG uptake in the gray matter and basal ganglia. Mild focal areas of increased activity can be seen normally in the frontal eye fields.
- *Head and neck:* Lymphatic tissue including Waldeyer's ring in head and neck region may show moderate FDG uptake, which is a normal phenomenon. Normal uptake can be seen in mylohyoid muscles and sublingual glands, soft palate and palatine, and lingual tonsils (especially prominent in children in cold weather). Nasopharyngeal uptake may be normal. In children, adenoid tissues may be visualized at the base of the tongue. Occasionally tongue uptake can be seen, especially if the patient speaks after injection of FDG. Laryngeal muscle and vocal cord uptake is a common normal variant, especially if the patient speaks soon after FDG administration. Normal activity is most pronounced posteriorly. Cervical paraspinal muscles, longus colli and longus capitis, extraocular muscles, temporalis muscle, and muscles of mastication may show diffuse minimally increased FDG uptake sometimes.
- *Myocardium:* It may show variable intense to no FDG uptake depending upon the patient's diet, glycemic and insulin status. Liver may show moderate homogeneous FDG uptake. There may be physiological FDG distribution in the intestinal loops (especially in patients on metformin).

Fluorodeoxyglucose Uptake in Benign Conditions

- *Thermogenic adipose tissue:* Moderate to intense FDG uptake in brown fat which may mimic muscle activity, lymph nodes or malignancy is a significant problem encountered during PET-CT study. Focal uptake in brown fat may be seen in posterior cervical, paraspinal, supraclavicular, axillary, mediastinal, and suprarenal regions.
- Asymmetric uptake in the lateral pharyngeal recesses may be inflammatory.
- Asymmetric laryngeal uptake may be secondary to postoperative changes or vocal cord paralysis.

- Benign tumors such as Warthin's tumor may show moderate FDG uptake.
- Diffuse thyroid gland uptake may be seen in Graves' disease and chronic thyroiditis (especially Hashimoto's thyroiditis). Focal FDG uptake may be seen in benign or malignant nodule.
- Postsurgical and postradiation inflammatory changes may cause minimal to moderate FDG uptake. Postradiation therapy complications such as osteonecrosis and chondronecrosis. Osteomyelitis may have variable FDG uptake. Correlating with the corresponding CT findings, careful study of the pattern and intensity of FDG uptake will guide in correct diagnosis.

Indications of FDG PET-CT in Head and Neck Malignancies

The major indications of FDG PET-CT in head and neck oncology are as follows:

- *Carcinoma of unknown primary:* Isolated cervical nodal metastases are predominantly squamous cell carcinomas. According to literature, even after an extensive diagnostic workup which includes physical examination, CT/MRI of the neck, fine-needle biopsy of lymph nodes, panendoscopy and blind and directed biopsies, the detection rate of primary tumor is <50%.[10] The reported sensitivity of FDG PET is 8–74% in literature.[11,12] False-positive results may be due to inflammatory processes and false-negative results are generally superficial lesions with depth <4 mm.[13]
- *Staging:* Recent studies have shown that ^{18}F-FDG PET-CT is essential in the staging workup in head and neck malignancies, as its performance resulted in a change of the management in approximately 33% of patients:[14,15]
  - *Locoregional staging:* The sensitivity of ^{18}F-FDG PET-CT for the detection of primary HNSCC is >95%. However, the extent of the primary tumor assessment is generally performed with clinical examination, endoscopy, and MRI. CECT is essential to assess the extent of the tumor and its relationship with the adjacent structures. With the advancements in the CT quality of PET-CT machines and the introduction of PET-MRI hybrid imaging, better tumor delineation can be obtained, and the metabolic parameters can also be correlated.[16]

    Positron emission tomography-computed tomography is useful in clinically N0 neck in oral or oropharyngeal cancers, with T1-T3 disease, where it can reduce the probability of occult neck metastases to <15%. PET-CT can also guide in surgical planning, as the specificity of PET-CT is high. The patient can undergo sentinel lymph node biopsy if FDG PET is negative and a neck dissection may be planned if FDG PET shows positive lymph nodes, thereby it may help in reducing the number of unnecessary neck dissections. False-negative results may be due to small lymph nodal lesions with micrometastases, due to lower spatial resolution (4–6 mm), and false-positive results from inflamed lymph nodes.
  - *Distant staging:* Most frequent sites of distant metastases in HNSCC are lungs, liver, and bones. Oral cavity tumors are known to have distant metastases even with clinical N0 neck. FDG PET-CT shows a high accuracy in detecting distant metastases. Characterization of very small-sized lung nodules may be a limitation.
  - *Prognostication:* The semiquantitative parameters such as standardized uptake value (SUV), metabolic tumor volume (MTV), and total lesion glycolysis (TLG) may be independent indicators of recurrence-free survival and overall survival.[17]
- *Recurrence:* FDG PET-CT has a very high negative predictive value in the recurrence setting. Role of CT or MRI may be limited in postoperative neck due to anatomical distortion. The specificity and sensitivity of FDG PET-CT are very high (<90%) for identifying regional and distant recurrences. The sensitivity of FDG PET-CT is high for local recurrence detection (97%), but the specificity is lower (79%) due to false-positive results because of infection and inflammation.[18] Biopsy may not be required if FDG PET-CT is negative. Dual point imaging (delayed imaging) may help to differentiate between recurrence and inflammation. PET-CT may be delayed for about 4 months after radiation therapy to avoid false-negative results from "stunning."
- *Therapy response evaluation:* Useful in assessing the residual disease postradiotherapy or chemotherapy for predicting the need for post-treatment neck dissection in order to reduce regional recurrence. High SUV of the residual lesion may indicate poor survival. Pitfalls are false-positive results from post-chemo-/radiotherapy inflammation, osteonecrosis of the jaw, infections and false-negative results from tumor stunning and microscopic diseases.
- *Radiotherapy planning:* PET-CT is helpful in the assessment of gross tumor volume and intensity-modulated radiation therapy planning.

Limitations:
- Cystic carcinomas of head and neck and their metastatic deposits may be FDG less or nonavid.
- Warthin's tumor and pleomorphic adenomas of the parotid gland may show increased FDG uptake. Thus, FDG PET alone will not be able to differentiate between benign and malignant lesions of salivary glands.
- Misregistration between PET and CT images, movement artifacts and artifacts due to metallic implants may cause difficulty in interpreting the images.

Positron Emission Tomography-Magnetic Resonance Imaging[19]

Advantages: (a) Excellent soft-tissue contrast with detailed anatomical information, (b) increased diagnostic accuracy, (c) reduced radiation dose when compared to PET-CT, and (d) advanced MR imaging techniques such as diffusion-weighted imaging, dynamic contrast-enhanced imaging, functional MRI (fMRI), and MR spectroscopy help in lesion characterization.

Disadvantages: (a) Challenge in claustrophobic patients and (b) increased motion artifacts due to longer acquisition timings.

Nonfluorodeoxyglucose Tracers in Head and Neck Cancer Imaging[20]

Radiolabeled amino acids may be labeled with positron emitters carbon-11 in forms such as L-[methyl-11C]-methionine (MET), L-1-[11C]-tyrosine (TYR), or fluorine-18, in forms such as L-3-[^{18}F]-fluoro-alpha-methyltyrosine (FMT) or O-[2-(^{18}F)-fluoroethyl]-L-tyrosine (FET) for utility in head and neck cancers. These may be better suited to differentiate between residual lesion and postradiation inflammatory changes. Hypoxia agents such as 18-fluorine misonidazole may be useful in radiation therapy planning. Radiolabeled monoclonal antibodies targeted against specific molecular processes such as cell proliferation, angiogenesis, tumor invasion, differentiation, cell death and apoptosis, and metastasis may have potential application in the future.

PART C: IMAGING IN NEUROENDOCRINE TUMORS

Medullary Thyroid Cancer

Medullary thyroid cancer (MTC) is a rare neuroendocrine tumor arising from the parafollicular C cells of the thyroid. Surgery remains the primary mode of treatment with total thyroidectomy and neck dissection being the standard operative procedure. Elevated postoperative serum calcitonin and carcinoembryonic antigen (CEA) levels suggest persisting tumor or metastases. Morphologic imaging methods are often insufficient either because of the small size of the tumor or difficulty of interpretation in a surgically distorted neck anatomy.[21] Somatostatin is a regulatory peptide hormone with an inhibitory role in hormone release and neurotransmitter modulation.[22] MTC secretes and stores somatostatin and expresses its receptors, which are also thought to play a role in the growth of neuroendocrine tumors.[23]

Somatostatin receptor (SSTR) scintigraphy is useful in diagnosing these tumors as they generally exhibit increased expression of SSTRs. This technique helps in localization of primary neuroendocrine tumors and unsuspected metastases in approximately 90% of patients. Subsequently, SSTR expressing patients may be considered for peptide receptor radioligand therapy (PRRT) using an alpha- or a beta-emitting radionuclide.

Imaging

Single-photon emitting computed tomography using indium-111-diethylenetriaminepentaacetic acid (DTPA)-octreotide (OctreoScan) was traditionally used for imaging of NETs. However, it has been found less sensitive than the conventional imaging modalities due to poor imaging characteristics of the tracer indium 111.[23] Also, it gives a higher radiation dose to the patient. Recently, the octreotide analogs have been labeled with positron-emitting radionuclide gallium-68 (half-life—68 hours) with the help of chelator (DOTA) to produce excellent quality of images with high lesion to background ratio. The SSTR analogs commonly used are TOC [D-Phe-cyclo(Cys-Tyr-D-Trp-Lys-Thr-Cys) Thr(ol)], TATE [D-Phe-cyclo(Cys-Tyr-D-Trp-Lys-Thr-Cys)Thr], and NOC [D-Phe-cyclo(Cys-1-Nal-D-Trp-Lys-Thr-Cys) Thr(ol)]. Gallium-68 (68Ga) is synthesized from its parent radiopharmaceutical, germanium-68 by elution of an in-house 68Ge-68Ga generator and labeled with peptide using a synthesis module; hence the logistical issues do not come into the picture. 68Ga can be labeled with different somatostatin analogs with the help of a chelator DOTA to form radiolabeled peptides 68Ga-DOTA-TOC, 68Ga-DOTA-NOC, 68Ga-DOTA-TATE that have different affinity profile with various subtypes of SSTR receptors. 68Ga-DOTA-NOC has wider affinity profile (SSTR subtype 2, 3, and 5).

Patient Preparation and Procedure[24]

Fasting before injection is not essential. However, in case a CECT has to be combined, the patient requires fasting for 4 hours. Discontinuation of "cold" octreotide (if any, when possible and not contraindicated) to avoid possible SSTR receptor blockade (1 day is suggested for short-lived and 3–4 weeks for long-acting octreotide analogs). The activity is intravenously administered with a dose ranging from 100 to 200 MBq [2.5–5.5 mCi (millicurie)]. Voiding before scanning will reduce the background noise and radiation dose to the kidneys and bladder. Physiological uptake of Ga-DOTA peptides seen in pituitary gland, spleen, bilateral adrenal gland, the uncinate process of the pancreas, proximal intestinal loops, kidneys and urinary bladder.

Performance of 68Ga-DOTA Peptide Study in Medullary Thyroid Carcinoma

In a prospective study, 68Ga-DOTA-NOC PET-CT showed a sensitivity of 80.7% and a positive predictive value of 100% for detecting recurrent MTC. When 68Ga-DOTA-NOC was compared to ^{18}F-FDG PET-CT, it showed superior results with a higher sensitivity (75.61 and 63.4% respectively).[25] It is also superior to ^{111}In-DTPA-octreotide scan, demonstrating a significantly higher number of lesions.

Other tracers for medullary thyroid cancer:

- *Technetium-99m (^{99m}Tc)-labeled pentavalent dimercaptosuccinic acid [^{99m}Tc(V)-DMSA]:* It is a nonspecific tumor imaging radiopharmaceutical. Uptake mechanism of ^{99m}Tc(V)-DMSA depends on blood flow and phosphate groups on tumor and the pH of the medium. The advantages being cost-effectiveness, in-house preparation, and lower radiation exposure dose to the patient and personnel, and better image quality. However, this radiopharmaceutical is not commercially available in many countries.
- *^{18}F-DOPA:* Fluorine-18-L-dihydroxyphenylalanine (^{18}F-DOPA) is analog of natural L-dopa (dopamine precursor) a neutral amino acid. Uptake is via large amino acid transporter, overexpressed in neuroendocrine tumors, and is further decarboxylated with aromatic amino acid decarboxylase, which is upregulated in neuroendocrine tumors has been found to be a sensor for detection of locoregional and distant MTC metastases.[26]
- *^{18}F-FDG PET-CT:* Fluorine-18-fluorodeoxyglucose (FDG) uptake in neoplastic cells correlates with poor differentiation and high proliferative activity. Neuroendocrine tumors usually show an indolent course and consequently low FDG uptake. However, when these tumors undergo dedifferentiation and become more aggressive, they may show increased FDG uptake.

Choice of Nuclear Imaging in Suspected Medullary Thyroid Cancer Recurrence

If calcitonin is rising with a faster rate than CEA, it is advisable to request for a Ga-68-DOTA-NOC PET-CT or F-DOPA PET-CT, whereas it is better to go for FDG PET-CT first if CEA is rising faster than calcitonin, which indicates possible dedifferentiation.

Head and Neck Paragangliomas

Performance of 68Ga-DOTA peptide study in head and neck paragangliomas: In a study conducted in 20 consecutive patients of head and neck paragangliomas, 68Ga-DOTA-NOC PET-CT detected total 38 lesions, while [^{18}F]-FDOPA PET/CT identified 37/38 and CT/MRI identified 22/38 lesions.[27] Other tracers for head and neck paragangliomas include [^{18}F]-fluorodihydroxyphenylalanine (FDOPA), iodine-131 meta-iodobenzylguanidine (I-131 MIBG) that is taken up by the paraganglioma such as noradrenaline and accumulates in sympathomedullary cells. Further details are covered in the chapter on paragangliomas.

PART D: PARATHYROID SCINTIGRAPHY

Hyperparathyroidism may present as recurrent renal stones, weakness, fatigue, and bone pain or may present as elevated serum calcium levels with patients being asymptomatic. The challenge in imaging of parathyroid glands is their smaller size and location in close proximity with the thyroid gland. About 80–85% of parathyroid adenomas are found adjacent to the thyroid while others are ectopically placed in the superior mediastinum, intrathymic or adjacent to the thymus, along the esophagus, carotid sheath, or rarely at the carotid bifurcation. This variation results in false-negative results on conventional anatomical imaging. Presence of single or multiple hyperfunctioning adenomas accounts for 80–85% of cases of primary hyperparathyroidism, hyperplasia occurs in 12–15% of cases and parathyroid carcinomas for about 1–3% of cases. Technetium-99m sestamibi is the radiopharmaceutical of choice for imaging parathyroid adenomas. The ^{99m}Tc in this radiopharmaceutical has an advantage of having good energy characteristics for imaging and sestamibi gets localized in the mitochondria of parathyroid tissue.

^{99m}Tc-sestamibi has yielded sensitivity rates of about 90% in primary hyperparathyroidism.

Procedure[28]

- *Preparation:* No special patient preparation is necessary before this scan. Local examination is necessary to palpate for thyroid nodules and other neck lesions
- *Radiopharmaceutical:* ^{99m}Tc-sestamibi (hexakis-2-methoxyisobutylisonitrile)
- *Dose:* 15–20 mCi
- *Route of administration:* Intravenous
- *Mechanism of uptake:* It is a lipophilic cationic isonitrile derivative that accumulates in the mitochondria-rich oxyphil cells. The main driving factor for sestamibi retention is negative transmembrane potential of the mitochondria.

Protocols

- *Dual-phase imaging:* ^{99m}Tc-sestamibi initially concentrates in normal thyroid tissue, thyroid adenomas, parathyroid adenomas, and hyperplastic parathyroid glands. The tracer activity significantly decreases with time in the normal thyroid tissue. Also, the intensity of uptake fades off from thyroid nodules and hyperplastic parathyroid glands. There is preferential increased tracer uptake in most of the parathyroid adenomas in the initial images when compared to normal thyroid tissue with insignificant retention of the tracer on the delayed images. Majority of parathyroid adenomas (>500 mg) can be detected by this method. Additional SPECT-CT images improve contrast resolution and help in the localization of uptake focus, thereby improving sensitivity and specificity.
- *Dual tracer imaging (subtraction method):* Additionally a second tracer, which is taken up by the thyroid gland only, such as ^{99m}Tc-pertechnetate ($^{99m}TcO_4^-$) or ^{123}I may be injected following a sestamibi scintigraphy. The distributions of the two tracers can be visually compared and also the thyroid scan can be digitally subtracted from the parathyroid scan to remove the thyroid activity and enhance the visualization of parathyroid tissue. Alternatively ^{99m}TC-tetrofosmin can also be used instead of ^{99m}Tc-sestamibi. Scintigraphically, it is not able to differentiate between parathyroid adenoma and parathyroid carcinoma:
    - *False-positive results:* Solid thyroid nodules, sarcoidosis, thyroid carcinoma, lymphoma other neck tumors, and brown tumors.
    - *False-negative results:* Size <500 mg, multidrug resistance-related protein (MRP) or P-glycoprotein expression which is responsible for efflux of sestamibi from the adenoma,[29] secondary parathyroidism, cells in G0 phase (show less uptake than those in G2 and S phase), and oncocytic variety of parathyroid adenoma.

Positron Emission Tomography Tracers for Parathyroid Gland Imaging

11C-methionine: (t½ 20 min). Its uptake is related to amino acid reflux into stimulated parathyroid tissue. Uptake in inflammatory conditions may cause problem while interpreting images.

^{18}F-FDG: (t½ 110 min). ^{18}F-FDG reflects the glucose metabolism. There is a differential concentration of FDG in abnormal parathyroid tissue. Its major limitation is accumulation in other malignant and benign lesions and inflamed or infected tissue.

^{18}F-fluorocholine: (t½ 110 min)—*Mechanism of uptake*: Choline on phosphorylation by choline kinase gets trapped to form a major membrane phospholipid called phosphatidylcholine. There is upregulation in the choline kinase activity in neoplastic cells such as parathyroid adenoma. Hence, increased cell proliferation in the adenoma or hyperplasia possibly leads to increased choline uptake. Studies have shown that fluorocholine is superior to sestamibi for detection of parathyroid adenomas.[30]

Minimally Invasive Parathyroidectomy[31]

Recurrent hyperparathyroidism is seen in 10% of patients due to inadequate localization preoperatively. Nowadays limited neck exploration has become the surgical strategy. Accurate preoperative localization of adenoma is necessary for success of minimally invasive parathyroidectomy. Its advantages include a small incision with minimal dissection, minimal postoperative complications, shorter hospital stay, less costly, can be performed as a daycare procedure under local anesthesia. This can be done as a single-day protocol where imaging and surgery are done on the same day or on two separate days (this involves performing ^{99m}Tc-MIBI scintigraphy up to a few days before surgery to localize the adenoma). On the day of surgery, a small dose of ^{99m}Tc-MIBI (2–3 mCi) is injected in the theater before the start of the operation, followed by a search in the relevant area using the gamma probe. The major advantages of the separate day protocol are a small amount of radioactivity is required and, therefore, the surgical team is exposed to less radiation. Also, the maximum tracer distribution time in the adenoma is already known by means of imaging, thereby facilitating the surgeon to know the time interval between the injection and incision.

Procedure: After IV injection of the radiopharmaceutical, external scanning over the neck should be done with the gamma probe to locate the highest radioactive spot on the skin surface. Then a small incision is made and the probe is inserted over the presumed location of the adenoma. The location of the highest radioactivity corresponds to the site of high-pitch sound signals produced by the gamma. Presence of adenoma is suggested by a parathyroid-to-thyroid radioactivity ratio higher than 1.5. After the excision of the lesion, the surgical bed has to be scanned again to ensure complete removal of establishing a new level of background radioactivity.

Indications: Solitary parathyroid adenoma with significant ^{99m}Tc-sestamibi uptake, no coexisting ^{99m}Tc-MIBI-avid thyroid nodules, no history of familial hyperparathyroidism or multiple endocrine neoplasia, and no history of previous neck surgery or irradiation.

PART E: SENTINEL LYMPH NODE BIOPSY IN ORAL CANCER

Two important applications of the sentinel lymph node biopsy (SLNB) in the head and neck region are (1) melanoma and (2) squamous cell carcinomas of the oral cavity. A positive sentinel node is an unfavorable prognostic factor in oral cancers. Practical problem in head and neck sentinel lymph nodal mapping is the complex anatomy and unpredictable lymphatic drainage.[32] The radiological technique of using ultrasound-guided fine-needle aspiration cytology (FNAC) has the disadvantage of having reduced sensitivity.[33]

Indications

Patients with transoral resectable T1-T2 tumors and clinical and radiological negative lymph node assessment (including FNAC) are generally candidates for SLNB.

Preparation

No specific preparation is needed for the injection or imaging procedure.

Procedure

Frequently used radiocolloids for lymphoscintigraphy are technetium-99 (^{99m}Tc)-nanocolloid (dose: 1.5–2 mCi in a total volume of 0.4 mL) or filtered ^{99m}Tc-sulfur colloid (dose: 0.5–0.8 mCi in 0.4 mL volume).

Injection Technique

A local anesthetic application of (10% xylocaine spray) a few minutes before radiocolloid injection may be considered for tumors of the oral cavity. Radiocolloid is injected into the intact mucosa around the primary lesion in three or four sites. Patient must be asked to spit out the excess saliva in the mouth in order to minimize tracer entry into the oropharynx and esophagus by swallowing, causing confusion in scan interpretation.

Imaging

Planar dynamic imaging (depicting sequential images of lymphatic drainage) has to be performed immediately due to the short distance between the injection site and the sentinel lymph nodes in the head and neck region. Static planar images (anterior and lateral views) acquired after 5–15 minutes usually identify the first draining lymph node. Delayed images (2–3 hours after injection) may help in differentiating sentinel and second-tier nodes. Planar image is a 2D overview, and the sentinel lymph node can be localized and marked on the patient's skin with the use of an external radioactive marker (cobalt-57-source pen). The skin marking is preferably done based on the oblique lateral images in order to reproduce the patient's position during surgery. If available, it is recommended to perform SPECT-CT, as it provides a 3D representation of a planar image and helps in anatomical localization of sentinel lymph node and second-tier nodes. It also differentiates nonnodal radioactivity accumulation (leakage or contamination) from radioactive nodes.

Intraoperative Probing

Intraoperatively, a gamma-ray detection hand-held probe, is used for detection of sentinel lymph nodes. The probe provides an acoustic signal when pointed toward the radioactive lymph node. The position of the sentinel lymph node has to be checked before the skin incision. Few practical difficulties are detection of deeply located sentinel lymph nodes due to tissue attenuation and overriding of counts by a relatively large amount of radioactivity at the site of the primary lesion that may be close to the sentinel lymph node (especially in the submandibular region). Blue dye may be used as an additional indicator of lymphatic flow. However, its rapid transit through lymphatic channels limit its use in head and neck cancers.

Intraoperative Imaging

Recently portable and hand-held mini gamma cameras have been developed for intraoperative imaging.

The images provide an overview of all the hot spots in the surgical field. Sentinel lymph nodes located close to the primary site, which may be easily missed by counting probe, can be visualized with a gamma camera. It ensures the completeness of the procedure, and in 20% of the cases, an immediate postoperative imaging reveals additional sentinel lymph nodes.[34]

Technical Limitations

- Differences in patient neck positions and markings between the imaging and surgery; these can be addressed by using an intraoperative gamma probe or the portable gamma camera.
- Misregistration between SPECT and CT images resulting in spurious anatomical localization, which can be taken care of by proper immobilization of head.
- Contaminations and leaked radioactivity, which can be differentiated by acquiring SPECT-CT images.

Accuracy

In a prospective cohort study to validate SLNB against elective lymph node dissection (ELND), the sensitivity of the lymphoscintigraphy by imaging and probing was found to be 93 and 100% respectively with a negative predictive value of 100%.[35] In a multicentric trial including 140 patients of T1-T2 oral squamous cell carcinomas (95 tongue, 26 floor of the mouth, and 19 other cancers), the negative predictive value of SLNB was 96%.[36]

CONCLUSION

Nuclear medicine is a vital component of present-day oncology practice. Nuclear imaging plays an important role in determining the extent of disease, assess disease progression and also aid in prognostication of disease. With the advent of newer molecular radiotracers in nuclear imaging that enable accurate noninvasive in vivo tumor characterization, better more individualized therapies are expected in the future.

REFERENCES

1. Brenner AI, Koshy J, Morey J, Lin C, DiPoce J. The bone scan. Semin Nucl Med. 2012;42(1):11-26.
2. Rahmim A, Zaidi H. PET versus SPECT: strengths, limitations and challenges. Nucl Med Commun. 2008;29(3):193-207.
3. Kramer-Marek G, Capala J. The role of nuclear medicine in modern therapy of cancer. Tumour Biol. 2012;33(3):629-40.
4. Bethge WA, Sandmaier BM. Targeted cancer therapy using radiolabeled monoclonal antibodies. Technol Cancer Res Treat. 2005;4(4):393-405.
5. Milenic DE, Brechbiel MW. Targeting of radio-isotopes for cancer therapy. Cancer Biol Ther. 2004;3(4):361-70.
6. Hall EJ, Giaccia AJ. Radiobiology for the Radiologist, 6th edition. Philadelphia: Lippincott Williams & Wilkins; 2006.
7. van Dongen GA, Visser GW, Lub-de Hooge MN, de Vries EG, Perk LR. Immuno-PET: a navigator in monoclonal antibody development and applications. Oncologist. 2007;12(12): 1379-89.
8. Levy-Nissenbaum E, Radovic-Moreno AF, Wang AZ, Langer R, Farokhzad OC. Nanotechnology and aptamers: applications in drug delivery. Trends Biotechnol. 2008;26(8):442-9.
9. Price EW, Orvig C. Matching chelators to radiometals for radiopharmaceuticals. Chem Soc Rev. 2014;43(1):260-90.
10. Mendenhall WM, Mancuso AA, Parsons JT, Stringer SP, Cassisi NJ. Diagnostic evaluation of squamous cell carcinoma metastatic to cervical lymph nodes from an unknown head and neck primary site. Head Neck. 1998;20(8):739-44.
11. Greven KM, Keyes JW Jr, Williams DW III, et al. Occult primary tumors of the head and neck: lack of benefit from positron emission tomography imaging with 2-[F-18] fluoro-2-deoxy-D-glucose. Cancer. 1999;86(1):114-8.
12. Kresnik E, Mikosch P, Gallowitsch H, Kogler D, Wieser S, Heinisch M, et al. Evaluation of head and neck cancer with (18)F-FDG PET: a comparison with conventional methods. Eur J Nucl Med. 2001;28(7):816-21.
13. Hannah A, Scott AM, Tochon-Danguy H, et al. Evaluation of 18F-fluorodeoxyglucose positron emission tomography and computed tomography with histopathologic correlation in the initial staging of head and neck cancer. Ann Surg. 2002;236(2):208-17.
14. Czernin J, Allen-Auerbach M, Schelbert HR. Improvements in cancer staging with PET/CT: literature-based evidence as of September 2006. J Nucl Med. 2007;48(Suppl 1):78S-88S.
15. Mak D, Corry J, Lau E, Rischin D, Hicks RJ. Role of FDG-PET/CT in staging and follow-up of head and neck squamous cell carcinoma. Q J Nucl Med Mol Imaging. 2011;55(5):487-99.
16. Buchbender C, Heusner TA, Lauenstein TC, Bockisch A, Antoch G. Oncologic PET/MRI, part 1: tumors of the brain, head and neck, chest, abdomen, and pelvis. J Nucl Med. 2012;53(6):928-38.
17. Pak K, Cheon GJ, Nam HY, Kim SJ, Kang KW, Chung JK, et al. Prognostic value of metabolic tumor volume and total lesion glycolysis in head and neck cancers: a systematic review and meta-analysis. J Nucl Med. 2014;55(6):884-90.
18. Wong RJ, Lin DT, Schöder H, Patel SG, Gonen M, Wolden S, et al. Diagnostic and prognostic value of [(18)F] fluorodeoxyglucose positron emission tomography for recurrent head and neck squamous cell carcinoma. J Clin Oncol. 2002;20(20): 4199-208.
19. Jadvar H, Colletti PM. Competitive advantage of PET/MRI. Eur J Radiol. 2014;83(1):84-94.
20. Wedman J, Pruim J, Roodenburg JL, Halmos GB, Langedijk JA, Dierckx RA, et al. Alternative PET tracers in head and neck cancer. a review. Eur Arch Otorhinolaryngol. 2013; 270(10):2595-601.
21. Scollo C, Baudin E, Travagli JP, Caillou B, Bellon N, Leboulleux S, et al. Rationale for central and bilateral lymph node dissection in sporadic and hereditary medullary thyroid cancer. J Clin Endocrinol Metab. 2003;88(5):2070-5.
22. Mato E, Matías-Guiu X, Chico A, Webb SM, Cabezas R, Berná L, et al. Somatostatin and somatostatin receptor subtype gene expression in medullary thyroid carcinoma. J Clin Endocrinol Metab. 1998;83(7):2417-20.
23. Lodish M, Dagalakis U, Chen CC, Sinaii N, Whitcomb P, Aikin A, et al. (111)In-octreotide scintigraphy for identification of metastatic medullary thyroid carcinoma in

children and adolescents. J Clin Endocrinol Metab. 2011; 97(2):E207-E212.
24. Virgolini I, Ambrosini V, Bomanji JB, Baum RP, Fanti S, Gabriel M, et al. Procedure guidelines for PET/CT tumor imaging with 68Ga-DOTA-conjugated peptides: 68Ga-DOTA-TOC, 68Ga-DOTA-NOC, 68Ga-DOTA-TATE. Eur J Nucl Med Mol Imaging. 2010;37(10):2004-10.
25. Naswa N, Sharma P, Suman Kc S, Lata S, Kumar R, Malhotra A, et al. Prospective evaluation of 68Ga-DOTA-NOC PET-CT in patients with recurrent medullary thyroid carcinoma: comparison with 18F-FDG PET-CT. Nucl Med Commun. 2012;33(7):766-74.
26. Golubic AT, Pasini Nemir E, Zuvic M, Mutvar A, Kusacic Kuna S, Despot M, et al. The value of 18F-DOPA PET/CT in patients with medullary thyroid carcinoma and increased calcitonin values. Nucl Med Commun. 2017;38(7):636-41.
27. Janssen I, Chen CC, Taieb D, Patronas NJ, Millo CM, Adams KT, et al. 68Ga-DOTATATE PET/CT in the localization of head and neck paragangliomas compared with other functional imaging modalities and CT/MRI. J Nucl Med. 2016;57(2): 186-91.
28. Hindié E, Ugur O, Fuster D, O' Doherty M, Grassetto G, Ureña P, et al. 2009 EANM parathyroid guidelines. Eur J Nucl Med Mol Imaging. 2009;36(7):1201-16.
29. Kao A, Shiau YC, Tsai SC, Wang JJ, Ho ST. Technetium-99m methoxyisobutylisonitrile imaging for parathyroid adenoma: relationship to P-glycoprotein or multidrug resistance-related protein expression. Eur J Nucl Med Mol Imaging. 2002;29(8):1012-5.
30. Prabhu M, Damle NA. Fluorocholine PET imaging of parathyroid disease. Indian J Endocrinol Metab. 2018;22(4): 535-41.
31. Starker LF, Fonseca AL, Carling T, Udelsman R. Minimally invasive parathyroidectomy. Int J Endocrinol. 2011;2011: 206502.
32. Shoaib T, Soutar DS, MacDonald DG, Gray HW, Ross GL. The nodal neck level of sentinel lymph nodes in mucosal head and neck cancer. Br J Plast Surg. 2005;58(6):790-4.
33. Hart RD, Nasser JG, Trites JR, Taylor SM, Bullock M, Barnes D. Sentinel lymph node biopsy in N0 squamous cell carcinoma of the oral cavity and oropharynx. Arch Otolaryngol Head Neck Surg. 2005;131(1):34-8.
34. Vermeeren L, Olmos RA, Klop WM, Balm AJ, van den Brekel MW. A portable γ-camera for intraoperative detection of sentinel nodes in the head and neck region. J Nucl Med. 2010;51(5): 700-3.
35. Stoeckli SJ. Sentinel node biopsy for oral and oropharyngeal squamous cell carcinoma of the head and neck. Laryngoscope. 2007;117(9):1539-51.
36. Civantos FJ, Zitsch RP, Schuller DE, Agrawal A, Smith RB, Nason R, et al. Sentinel lymph node biopsy accurately stages the regional lymph nodes for T1-T2 oral squamous cell carcinomas: results of a prospective multi-institutional trial. J Clin Oncol. 2010;28(8):1395.

Robotic Surgery in Head and Neck Cancer

Sivakumar Vidhyadharan, Narayana Subramaniam, Samskruthi P Murthy

INTRODUCTION

In 1495, Leonardo da Vinci designed the first robot which was a mechanical, armored knight used for the purposes of entertaining royalty.[1] Many centuries later, robots appeared first in popular science fiction.[2] The term "robot" originates from the Czech word "robota" which means laborer, which introduced the concept of robots in lay people's minds. It was coined in a play called Rossum's Universal Robots in 1921, written by Karel Capek.[3]

In 2003, a California-based surgical robotics company Intuitive Surgical, Inc. (Sunnyvale, CA, USA) acquired Computer Motion, Inc. and monopolized the robotic surgery market worldwide with the da Vinci surgical robot platform. Although da Vinci robot was originally designed for endoscopic cardiac surgery, it is primarily utilized for robotic prostatectomy. Since its introduction in 1997 and the Food and Drug Administration (FDA) approval in 2001, it has been used in a variety of surgical procedures. The surgical robot has been a commercial success due the various benefits it tenders over the conventional endoscopic or laparoscopic surgery. The da Vinci Surgical System is presently the leading robotic surgery platform and is considered the yardstick against which other systems are measured.[3-5] **Figure 1** shows milestones in robotic head and neck surgery.

The da Vinci's latest model, the Xi, released by Intuitive Surgical in 2014, is composed of an operational cart with four arms, a mobile platform, and a master console. Manipulation of the surgical instruments is facilitated by cable-driven joints located on the distal ends of each robotic arm. The EndoWrist system mimics the movements of the human wrist and has seven degrees of freedom.[6,7] An 8-mm camera allows clear visualization and magnification.[6-9] Inhibitory drawbacks are the system costs and large amount of space required for its use.[10,11] The da Vinci platform also lacks haptic feedback but surgeons compensate for the lack of haptic feedback with excellent visual feedback, which gives the user a sense of touch.[6]

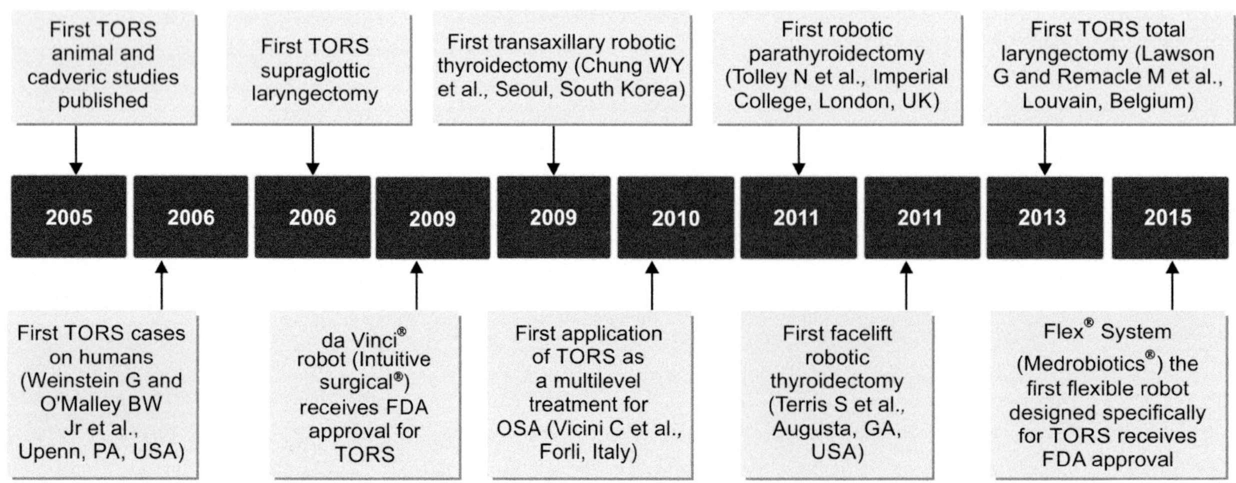

Fig. 1: Milestones in robotic surgery.

In resource constricted areas, large size, and high cost of the da Vinci system pose significant barriers to the utilization of robotic surgery.[10,11] In spite of Intuitive's market dominance with the current robotic platform, technologies such as hepatic feedback or biometric integration such as eye tracking cameras or head-tracking robotic arms that may enhance surgical skills they have not incorporated and hopefully they would do so in future.[5,8,12-14] For better understanding, this chapter is divided into two main parts.

PART A: TRANSORAL ROBOTIC SURGERY

The first use of robotic surgery in head and neck tumors to resect a vallecular cyst.[15] Preclinical feasibility for laryngopharyngeal surgery was then established.[16] Rather than inserting the instruments through a laryngoscope, as it was routinely done with transoral laser microsurgery (TLM) and by McLeod and Melder in their vallecular cyst excision, Hockstein and colleagues established that oral and oropharyngeal retractors more reliably facilitated surgery without external collisions.[16,17]

After the success of completion of preclinical studies, robotic surgery was introduced in the clinical specialty setting in otorhinolaryngology and head and neck surgery by Professors Gregory Weinstein and Bert O'Malley at the University of Pennsylvania in 2006. They demonstrated the safety and feasibility of transoral robotic resection for tongue base using the da Vinci surgical robot, thereby coining the term "TORS" (as an acronym for transoral robotic surgery). By providing a less safe access to the pharynx, parapharyngeal space, and larynx without the morbidity of lip-splitting neck incisions and accompanying disruption of the pharyngeal musculature or the limitations associated with TLM, TORS benefitted on the presence of the oral cavity as an access point for natural orifice transluminal endoscopic surgery (NOTES).

By 2009, indications for TORS rapidly grew to include a number of benign and malignant neoplasms involving the different anatomical subsites within the head and neck. At present, TORS represents an important treatment approach for tumors of the oropharynx, hypopharynx, parapharyngeal space, supraglottic larynx, and nasopharynx. It has also been implemented in the management of unknown primary tumors and also total laryngectomy (TL). Besides head and neck cancers, it plays the role of a valuable tool, as part of multilevel surgical treatment for obstructive sleep apnea (OSA) in patients who cannot tolerate continuous positive airway pressure. This is due to the excellent access to oropharynx it offers, which was first described by Professor Claudio Vicini at the University of Pavia in 2010.[3,4]

Suitability of Patients for TORS

In the absence of adequate exposure, TORS is a poor choice. The factors required to ensure proper endoscopic access in patients undergoing either TORS or TLM are (eight "Ts"): Teeth, Trismus, Transverse dimensions (mandibular), Tori, Tongue, Tilt (atlanto-occipital extension), Treatment (prior radiation), and Tumor.[18,19] To allow standardized, uniform and adequate resection, Weinstein et al. proposed specific contraindications which were derived from their experience with over 1,400 patients who had undergone TORS resections at the University of Pennsylvania[20] (described in chapter on Oropharynx).

Surgical Procedure

During a TORS procedure, after prior intubation by the anesthetist, the surgeon positions, or "docks," the robot at the surgical site, inserting two dissecting arms and the camera arm through the oral cavity with a retractor in place. Nasotracheal intubation provides some additional space in the oral cavity in most cases. The endotracheal tube must be secured intraorally with a suture to the mandible to prevent accidental extubation if orotracheal intubation is performed. The angles of the two dissecting robotic arms form an acute angle of 30–45°, with the endoscope positioned between them; it becomes more acute during resection of larynx or hypopharyngeal subsites. The axis of rotation of each arm is placed near the oral commissure.[21] Generally, a 5-mm grasping instrument is used in one arm and monopolar electrocautery on the other. Otherwise, a second grasper may be used to hold a laser fiber.[22]

The 0° or 30° endoscope is attached depending on the location of the tumor and anatomical exposure. The surgeon then sits at a remote console with binocular, high-definition eyepieces to control the actions of the robot. An assistant sits at the bedside to provide countertraction, provide suction, and to assist with hemostasis as needed. Dissection proceeds in a similar fashion to traditional transoral or open techniques, focusing on resection margins and hemostasis. Either prior to or after TORS, unilateral or bilateral neck dissection may be performed concomitantly under the same anesthesia, depending on surgeon preference.[23] Ligation of distal branches of the external carotid artery may be performed to decrease the risk of significant postoperative bleeding.[24]

- ***Tonsil cancer:*** The aim of resecting tonsil tumors with TORS is to ensure compartmental resection of the tonsil, the constrictor bed it sits on along with a cuff of soft palate and the tongue base to ensure histologically negative margins. An incision is made through the pterygomandibular raphe to identify the parapharyngeal space with the help of the medial pterygoid tendon, separating the constrictor muscles from the parapharyngeal fat, mobilizing the superior pole of the tonsil with an adequate cuff of tissue from the soft palate, progressive dissection in the parapharyngeal space to free the stylopharyngeus and pharyngeal constrictors, mobilizing tongue base mucosa, and deep tissue between the anterior and posterior tonsillar pillars, resecting at least a centimeter segment of styloglossus to ensure a histologically negative margin, making index cuts on the posterior pharyngeal wall to avoid resection of excessive amounts of mucosa and progressive transection of the constrictor muscle along with the stylopharyngeal musculature to achieve an en bloc resection. Postoperatively the tonsil defect is left to heal on its own and complete mucosalization normally takes place within 6 weeks. Patients commence oral much before 6 weeks and are decannulated off their nasogastric (NG) tube.[25-28] **Figures 2 and 3** show a TORS lateral oropharyngectomy procedure. **Figure 4** shows a tonsil tumor extending to the base tongue.
- ***Tongue base cancer:*** Exposure of the tongue base tumor performed using relevant retractors which is based on the patient's anatomy and ease of access. Assessment of the preoperative scans is imperative to assess the precise location, lateralization, and depth of the tumor. Patients with tumors crossing the midline are not good candidates for TORS. Incision is made along the posterior one-third of the tongue and is deepened followed by a midline cut toward the vallecula. The vallecula identifies the depth of the resection needed, and the lateral margin is established which may involve part of the lower third of the tonsil. The lingual artery is encountered as the dissection into the tongue base progresses. The bedside assistant ligates vessel with Ligaclips, applied transorally. Once resected out, the tumor is orientated for the pathologist, and a NG tube is routinely inserted which is decannulated a few weeks later.[27]
- ***Supraglottic laryngectomy:*** The following three steps are the main components of the standard complete

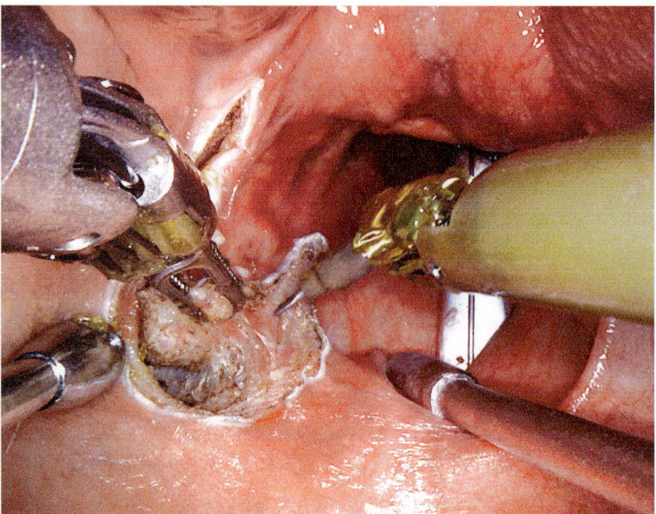

Fig. 2: Incision for left lateral oropharyngectomy.

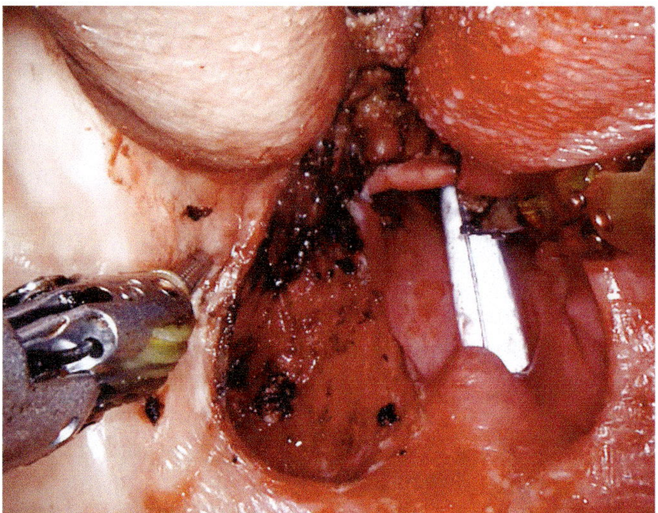

Fig. 3: Left lateral oropharyngectomy defect.

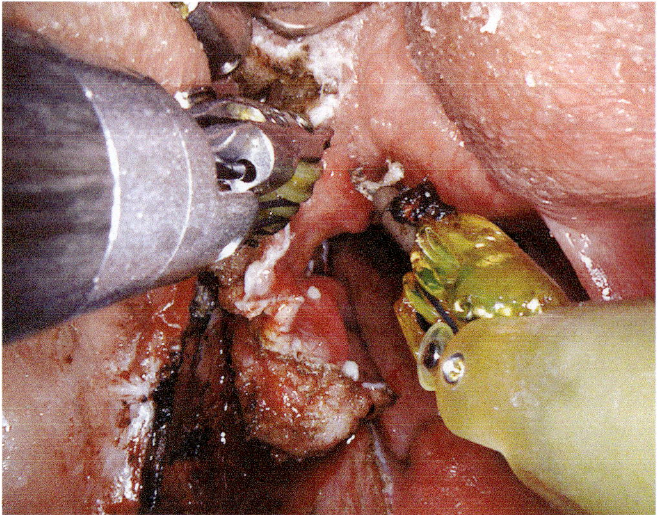

Fig. 4: Left tonsil carcinoma extending to base of tongue (T2).

TORS-SGL (transoral robotic surgery-supraglottic laryngectomy) for a supraglottic laryngeal cancer which can be performed in any order, on condition that exposure is adequate and allows for a complete visualization of the tumor for oncological en bloc resection.[22,29,30] Weinstein recommended resecting each half of the supraglottis separately.[29,31] The transvallecular approach to the pre-epiglottic space is through the vallecular mucosa, identification of the hyoid bone, dissection of the thyrohyoid membrane, and identification of the thyroid cartilage. Laterally, superior laryngeal vascular bundles need to be delineated in the lateral pharyngoepiglottic folds and divided. The pre-epiglottic space is then dissected. Aryepiglottic folds are divided above and laterally to the arytenoid. The dissection is followed between the arytenoid cartilages and ventricular bands to the level of the ventricles, allowing for resection of the false vocal cords and the upper paraglottic spaces above the ventricles within the specimen. Horizontal sectioning is performed through the ventricles, exposing the ventricular floors, and the vocal cords. Anteriorly, the petiole is transected just above the anterior commissure, and the transection is connected to the dissection of the lower pre-epiglottic space. After completion of these three steps, the specimen can readily be removed and the margins are determined from frozen sections if required. A tracheostomy is only needed in the presence of gross edema. In most patients, a tracheostomy is not required and extubation can be within 24 hours.[32-34] **Figure 5** shows a supraglottic tumor while **Figure 6** shows the resultant defect after excision.

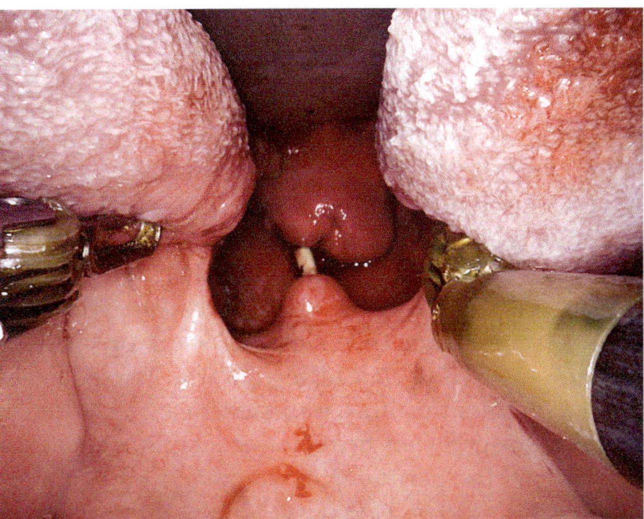

Fig. 5: T2 supraglottic tumor visualized through the robotic endoscope.

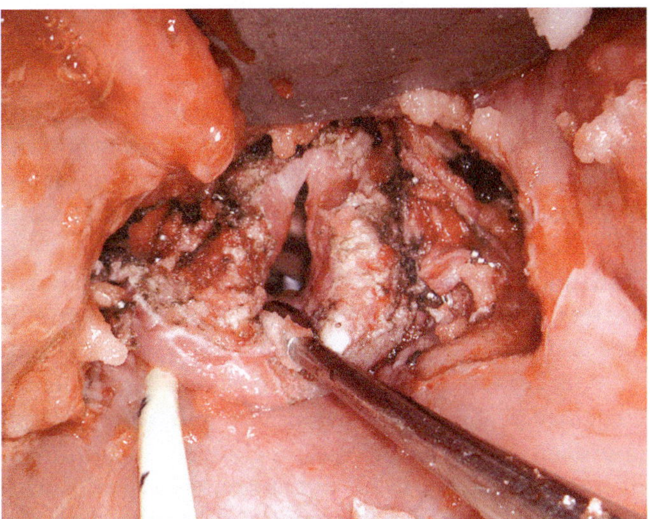

Fig. 6: TORS supraglottic carcinoma resection defect.

- ***Nasopharyngectomy:*** Wei and Ho described a transoral robotic nasopharyngectomy for recurrent nasopharyngeal carcinoma, similar to the first TORS nasopharyngectomy approach described by Ozer and Waltonen.[35,36] A midline soft palate split allows good exposure. The entire nasopharynx mucosa and both eustachian tube openings were resected to delineate the clivus and prevertebral fascia. The robotic approach avoided incisions on the face and mandibulotomy.[36,37] Hanna et al. described in four human cadavers a novel robotic surgical approach that allows adequate endoscopic access for resection of tumors involving the anterior and central skull base. By making, bilateral sublabial incisions and wide anterior maxillary antrostomies (Caldwell-Luc) and bilateral wide middle meatal antrostomies with posterior septectomy. They were able to gain adequate access to the anterior and central skull base, including the cribriform plate, fovea ethmoidalis, medial orbits, planum sphenoidale, sella turcica, suprasellar and parasellar regions, nasopharynx, pterygopalatine fossa, and clivus and all their cadaveric dissections. The three-dimensional (3D) visualization obtained by the dual-channel endoscope at the surgeon's console provided excellent depth perception. The most significant advantage was the ability of the surgeon to perform two-handed tremor-free endoscopic closure of dural defects. Their novel approach also allowed for 3D, two-handed, tremor-free endoscopic dissection, and precise closure of dural defects. They were of the opinion that these advantages may expand the indications of minimally invasive endoscopic approaches to the skull base.[38]

Margins in TORS

Similar to any oncologic surgery, margin status is of great importance in robotic head and neck surgery. Hanna et al. studied the positive margin rate and predictors in TORS, they reported that rate of positive margins dramatically increased with consecutively higher T classifications. Patients with T1 and T2 cancer had positive margin rate of under 20% (13.0% and 17.1%, respectively), while patients with T3 cancer had a rate of 28.2%, and margins of almost half of patients with T4 cancer were positive after surgery (47.9%). The difference among T classifications was statistically significant and was a significant predictor of margin status after accounting for pertinent demographic and clinicopathologic features. Following TORS, T3 tumors were three times more likely than T1 tumors to have positive margins, and T4 tumors were seven times more likely to result in positive margins. From these results, the authors were of the opinion that, it may be extremely difficult to achieve positive margins with high T classifications in TORS. Further research is needed regarding the functional and oncologic outcomes of TORS patients with T3 and T4 cancer to understand the utility of TORS in these patients. They also found that TORS procedures yielded a positive margin rate of 15.3% at academic centers as compared to 24.5% at nonacademic centers, but it was not significant on multivariable analysis.[39]

With regards to intraoperative margin assessment, a combination of the "specimen-driven" and "defect-driven" approach is practiced. Intraoperatively, a minimum of a 5-mm margin in all dimensions is aimed during resection. This can be estimated using the diameter of the 5-mm EndoWrist instrument (Intuitive Surgical Inc. Sunnyvale, CA). When energy devices are used to cut tissue and tissue necrosis between 250 and 500 µm occurs, with shrinkage occurring to the magnitude of 25% after the incision[13,40] and formalin fixation causes further shrinkage of 10%. Hence, for tongue base resections, a 2-mm margin on the formalin-fixed paraffin-embedded specimen should be the aim during the resection. This is not possible in tonsillar tumors, especially after formalin fixation because the thickness of the irradiated constrictor bed will not measure 2 mm. Hence, it is important to examine all aspects of the specimen once it is completely resected.[41-43]

Feasibility and Outcomes with TORS

- *Oropharyngeal cancer:* Traditionally, the treatment for oropharyngeal cancer was open surgical resection with or without flap reconstruction, or radiotherapy with or without neck dissection. Parsons et al. analyzed data from 51 studies with 6,400 patients that compared surgery with radiotherapy[44] showing that survival and local control of oropharyngeal cancer was similar between the two treatment types, but the rate of fatal or severe complications was significantly greater for patients who underwent surgery. Furthermore, a large, phase III randomized controlled trial, which randomized 226 patients with advanced oropharyngeal cancer to receive radiotherapy alone or radiotherapy with concomitant carboplatin and fluorouracil, showed that concomitant chemotherapy provided a survival benefit, with significantly increased overall survival (22% vs. 16%) and locoregional control (48% vs. 25%).[45] Hence, nonsurgical management became the standard of care in the management of oropharyngeal cancer.

  However, over time, the number of patients suffering toxicity from the radical doses of radiotherapy to the head and neck increased and worsened when combined with chemotherapy.[46,47] The long-term side-effects of radiation therapy include pharyngeal stenosis leading to dysphagia, and laryngeal scarring causing dysphonia. Very severe stenosis may lead to the requirement for tracheostomy. Severe late radiation toxicity effects include dry mouth, scarring of soft tissues, and osteoradionecrosis of the mandible.[48] Difficulties with teeth and oral hygiene, mouth opening, and dry mouth or sticky saliva may be severe and debilitating.[46] Dysphagia is now identified as one of the major side effects of nonsurgical management, with several patients requiring supplementary enteral feeding or nutritional assistance, with a permanent gastrostomy or NG tube.[49-51] Symptoms of dry mouth are significantly reduced by employing parotid sparing plans in intensity-modulated radiotherapy. These toxicity risks, along with the development of minimally invasive surgical techniques, have led to a resurgence of interest in the primary surgical management of oropharyngeal squamous cell carcinoma (OPSCC).[52]

  Moore et al. reported outcomes of OPSCC treated with TORS.[53] Their study involved 45 patients with stage T1-T4a OPSCC. The authors found no major complications, concluding that TORS was safe with acceptable oncological outcomes.[15,54]

  Weinstein et al. conducted a multicenter study to determine the safety, feasibility, and the adequacy of surgical margins for TORS.[55] They reviewed the results from independent institutional review board-approved clinical trials in three separate institutions and found that TORS appeared to be safe, feasible, and plays an important role in the multidisciplinary management of head and neck cancer, among the 177 patients studied with majority of their tumors arising in the oropharynx and larynx. Their positive margin rate was 4.3%. Tracheostomy was performed in 12.4% of all patients with only 2.3% retaining the tracheostomy tube at last follow-up. Their percutaneous endoscopic gastrostomy dependency rate was 5.0% for patient who had undergone primary TORS and the average hospital stay was 4.2 days.

Since the introduction of TORS as a treatment paradigm for early T-stage oropharyngeal carcinoma, concerns have surrounded this technology and its comparative effectiveness to existing treatment. Human papillomavirus (HPV)-associated OPSCC has been recognized as a pathological entity distinct from other tumors of the head and neck, including smoking induced OPSCC.

Park et al. published a systematic review to determine safety and efficacy of TORS versus open surgery for oropharyngeal cancer. They found that primary TORS has an advantage for disease-free survival and lowering the free flap reconstruction rate and has the reduction of time to decannulation and the length of hospital stay. They also reported that TORS patient had lower risks of pharyngocutaneous fistulas as compared to open surgery.[56]

Swallowing function in TORS was shown to better than with open surgery in OPSCC. Outcome data at 1-year follow-up, comparing transoral primary surgical and nonsurgical approaches to OPSCC, shows significantly improved swallowing function in patients treated with primary surgery with the majority of patients reporting normal swallowing.[57] In another study, oncological outcomes for TORS for OPSCC were comparable to both open surgery and concurrent chemoradiotherapy (CCRT).[58]

Moore et al. reported a locoregional recurrence-free survival rate was 92% with an overall survival rate of 86% at 5 years in a large series of OPSCC undergoing TORS.[22]

TORS is currently used and approved by the FDA for T1 and T2 cancers in the USA with a small proportion of T3 and T4 tumors also included. TORS radical tonsillectomy was first reported in 2007 by Weinstein et al. that included a cohort of 27 patients with tonsil carcinomas staged T1–T3. They had a negative margin of 93%, 0% mortality and an acceptable complication rate with 4% gastrostomy dependence at 6 months.[43] de Almeida JR et al. conducted a multi-institutional study[18] that gathered outcomes for 410 patients from 11 centers showed 2-year locoregional control rates of 92% and disease-free survival of 91%.[59]

In 2014, de Almeida's meta-analysis[24] compared TORS, neck dissection and adjuvant therapy as appropriate, with IMRT (intensity-modulated radiotherapy, with or without chemotherapy) and salvage surgery as appropriate. 772 patients who underwent TORS were compared with 1,287 patients who had received primary IMRT treatment. Their oncological outcomes were comparable (2-year overall survival estimates ranged from 84 to 96% for IMRT and from 82 to 94% for TORS). But, the main difference lay in the reports of adverse effect. Patients who had undergone IMRT treatment had esophageal stenosis (4.8%), osteoradionecrosis (2.6%), and gastrostomy tubes insertion (43%), whereas those who received primary surgery experienced hemorrhage (2.4%), fistula (2.5%), and gastrostomy tubes insertion at the time of surgery (1.4%) or during adjuvant treatment (30%). About 12% of patients required tracheostomy tubes at the time of surgery, but most were decannulated prior to discharge.[15]

Even with the mounting popularity of TORS in the treatment of OPSCC, there are some potential drawbacks, such as the use of TORS which does not obviate the need for postoperative radiotherapy in many cases and common and serious complications of postoperative hemorrhage with an incidence rate ranging from 3 to 8%.[15,24,60,61] However, postoperative bleeding can be reduced ligating the ipsilateral external carotid artery during the surgery.[15,26]

Patients with HPV-negative OPSCC are more likely to present with large-volume primary disease that is less amenable to minimal access surgery. Patient selection for TORS is based on both tumor and patient characteristics and follow similar contraindications as mentioned before. There is little data investigating the role of TORS specifically for HPV-negative OPSCC, and it remains unclear whether surgery should play a role in intensifying treatment for this patient population. TORS potentially offers a surgical option to intensify treatment for HPV-negative OPSCC patients with low-volume primary disease.[62]

A randomized phase II, two-arm trial (RTOG 1221), was designed to compare survival outcomes in patients with T1-2, N1-2b HPV-negative OPSCC. The experimental arm was to receive transoral surgery (TORS or TLM) for the primary tumor with neck dissection. Adjuvant IMRT (54–60 Gy) with or without concurrent chemotherapy was planned depending on margin status, extracapsular extension, lymphovascular or perineural invasion. The control arm treatment consisted of IMRT (70 Gy) with concurrent chemotherapy.[46] This trial was discontinued in view of poor recruitment. The failure of RTOG 1221 to accrue suggests that physicians and patients may be unwilling to be randomized between surgical and nonsurgical approaches.[62,63]

In one retrospective study, Cohen et al. reported on 13 patients with HPV-negative OPSCC who underwent primary TORS and staged neck dissection. Adjuvant IMRT with or without concurrent cisplatin-based chemotherapy was given based on pathologic characteristics including margin status, extracapsular spread, and nodal burden. Eleven of the 13 patients had T1 or 2 tumors. Four patients had N0, seven patients had N1, and two patients had N2b nodal disease. Six patients received adjuvant concurrent chemoradiation, two received radiation alone, and five received no adjuvant therapy. After a mean follow-up of 23 months, no patients had local recurrence, and one patient had both local and distant recurrence. HPV status did not impact disease-free or overall survival in this study.[64]

de Almeida et al. reported results of a collaborative cohort of OPSCC that was primarily HPV-positive. This study found no significant survival difference based on HPV status. This study representing the largest reported series of HPV-negative OPSCC treated with TORS found favorable survival in HPV-negative patients with 2-year locoregional control and overall survival of 92 and 94%, respectively.[65]

Moore et al. reported on a small HPV-negative OPSCC cohort which had good survival, comparable to those with HPV-associated OPSCC.[66]

Dabas et al. in their cohort of HPV-negative OPSCC with a single modality, deintensified treatment using TORS showed a disease-free survival of 89.6% and overall survival of 93.8%.[67]

In addition, Dabas et al. also studied the long-term oncological outcome of multimodal treatment with TORS for stage IV HPV-negative OPSCC. Of 86 patients with stage IVa disease, patients received TORS followed by adjuvant RT/CCRT and had a disease-free survival of 76.7% and an overall survival of 88.4% on a mean follow-up of 34 months.[67,68]

TORS as a single modality treatment also allows cure in early resectable tumors that may be poor responders to radiotherapy. TORS can be used to deintensify the treatment of early-stage OPSCC and avoid morbidity associated with adjuvant treatment.[68] Hence, TORS may be a good option to improve functional outcomes even in selected HPV-negative patients with OPSCC.

- *Unknown primary tumors:* Robotically-assisted surgical removal of the tongue base, tongue base mucosectomy (TBM), has been shown to improve diagnostic yield in the detection of carcinoma of unknown primaries (CUP). TORS-assisted TBM has emerged as a novel diagnostic strategy to further decrease the number of patients classified as CUP. The improved vision and maneuverability of the robotic instruments allows comprehensive sampling of the tongue base mucosa in a way that has not been previously possible. Winter SC, et al. reported their diagnostic hit rate for tongue base primaries using this technique as 53%.[69] **Figure 7** shows the tongue base mucosectomy specimen while **Figure 8** shows a typical superficial tongue base mucosectomy defect.

Although positron emission tomography-computed tomography (PET-CT) offers the highest sensitivity and specificity compared to CT or MRI alone, it has the lowest sensitivity in the tongue base, manifesting the small volume of disease in occult cases and the surrounding uptake of radiolabeled isotope in the surrounding lingual tonsils.[70]

Excision of the lingual tonsil is reported using the laser with diagnostic identification of the primary site ranging between 75 and 89%. However, with TORS, the improved visualization in the robotic-assisted technique combined with the absence of limitations of access and line of sight operating (as with the laser) make this attractive option in a larger subset of patients.[71] Mehta et al. reported that a retrospective

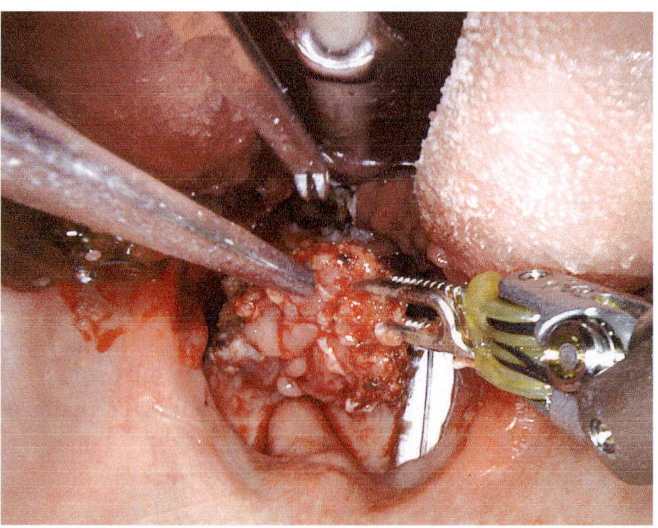

Fig. 7: Orientation of left tongue base mucosectomy specimen.

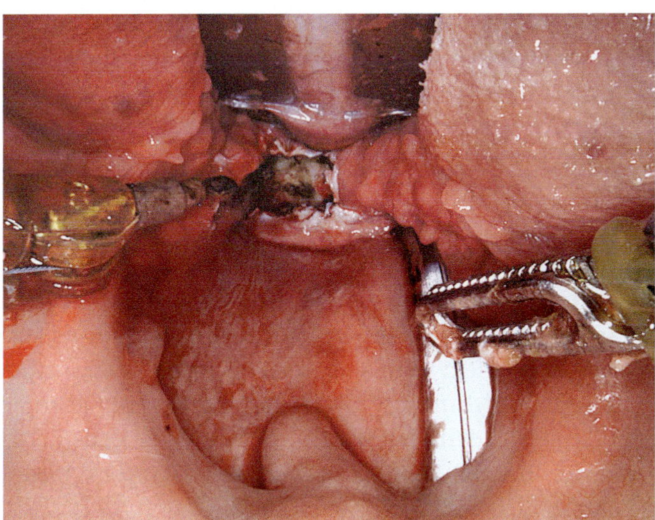

Fig. 8: Left tongue base of mucosectomy defect.

series of 10 cases identified 90% of primary tumor in the base of tongue.[71] Patel et al., in their retrospective series of 47 patients had a detection rate of 72% in their series; although the majority were in the base of tongue, 13 tumors were identified in the tonsil.[72] Krishnan et al. performed TORS TBM in 7 cases of CUP, identifying the base of tongue as the primary site in 5 (71.4%). They reported the average time before return to normal swallowing function was 2.7 days with no major surgical complications.[73]

- *Laryngeal and hypopharyngeal cancer:* With reference to the technical limitations of TORS, de Virgilio et al. defined their approaches based on TORS for 22 hypopharyngeal cancers, 19 glottic cancers, and seven supraglottic cancers to optimize exposure of larynx and hypopharynx during TORS. They recommended the following: (1) during the initial diagnostic laryngoscopy, a trial of the Feyh-Kastenbauer (FK) retractor system and 30° telescope should be performed for exposure, (2) muscle relaxants are to be used intraoperatively, (3) tracheostomy to be routinely performed prior to the TORS, (4) 30° robotic endoscope should be positioned as far from the operative site as possible, (5) the 30° endoscope should be positioned at an acute angle at the posterior pharyngeal wall, (6) retraction of the tongue anteriorly, and (7) an ipsilateral epiglottectomy should be performed for pyriform sinus lesions. Exposure outcomes for larynx were mixed, with four patients deemed "good" exposure, 21 "fair" and one "poor." while exposure for hypopharynx was frequently either poor or fair.[31,74]

Most common application of TORS is being SGL with growing number of studies reporting success with TORS for laryngeal cancer. TORS-SGL should allow for complete oncological resection of the supraglottic tumor, while preserving laryngeal functionality, hence TORS-SGL are reserved for selected T1 and T2, and rarely T3 cancers.[31,74-76] Early T-stage tumors (T1 and T2) are usually situated in suprahyoid epiglottis and laryngeal aspects of the aryepiglottic folds. However, resection of these tumors is associated with a high aspiration risk.

In tumors of the anterior laryngeal vestibule or infrahyoid epiglottis, the pre-epiglottic space (PES) needs to be cleared for oncological reasons. Also, tumors of the infrahyoid epiglottis may extend to the ventricular bands, which then require resection along with the paraglottic space. Early T-stage tumors of the vallecula may have occult extension into the tongue base or epiglottic folds, which can be challenging and require surgical expertise to obtain clear margins. Frozen sections should be performed routinely to confirm clearance.[77,78] About a third of the published undergoing TORS-SGL had cT1 disease while a little over half had cT2 disease.[31,76,77]

Absolute contraindications to TORS-SGL encompass: inadequate transoral exposure (e.g., inter-incisor distance <3 cm, trismus, and difficult exposure), invasion of the thyroid and/or cricoid cartilage, impaired vocal cord mobility or arytenoid mobility, paraglottic space invasion, invasion of posterior commissure with extension to the glottic larynx, involvement of >2 cm of the base of the tongue mucosa or invasion of muscles of tongue base. Relative contraindications to TORS-GL are unfit patients and those unlikely to tolerate aspiration in the early postoperative period.[31]

Weinstein first described TORS-SGL.[78] Mendelsohn et al. reported 2-year outcomes in their 18 patients with a mean follow-up of 28 months. Their locoregional control, disease-specific survival, and overall survival were 83, 100, and 89%, respectively. Three patients had recurrence in the neck, and four failed distantly. About 50% of patients received adjuvant therapy for advanced neck disease.[79] Park et al. reported TORS-SGL with a 2-year disease-free survival rate of 91%. However, only two patients enrolled had a follow-up of >20 months. And 50% of their patients underwent adjuvant therapy; 19% with radiation only (for pT3 disease) and 31% with chemoradiotherapy.[32] Mendelsohn et al. and Olsen et al. reported 2-year overall survival ranging from 66.7 to 88.9%.[79,80]

In 2016, Razafindranaly et al. reported outcomes of TORS-SGL in 84 patients. Although oncological outcomes were good, 9.5% of patients needed feeding tubes and a quarter needed a temporary tracheostomy with 1% requiring a permanent one. Also, aspiration pneumonia was diagnosed in nearly a quarter of patients and postoperative bleeding occurred in 18% of patients. From the results, the authors concluded that although TORS was safe and achieved good functional outcomes, serious complications are common. They stressed the importance of identifying appropriate candidates to reduce treatment-related toxicity.[81]

The feasibility of TORS-SGL was evaluated by Alon et al. by utilizing this approach in seven patients with T1-T3 lesions using the FK retractor with the laryngeal blade. Four of their patients underwent tracheostomy, which remained in place for a range of 4 days to being permanent, and five patients had prolonged tube feeding, two had gastrostomies and three had prolonged NG tube placements for 38–56 days. Also, follow-up duration was too brief to assess survival.[82]

Resection of early-stage glottic carcinomas has been performed with TORS, however, the literature is limited.[31] Vural et al. reported a TORS glottic resection by completely removing the paraglottic spaces up to the upper border of cricoid cartilage in a recurrent cancer following radiotherapy.[76] Lallemant et al. published a series of 13 patients who had undergone TORS for glottic carcinoma, staged T1a-T2 in 13 patients.[83] At the same time, de Virgilio et al. published a review of approaches used at their center to improve TORS exposure in this setting.[46,83] Wang et al. reported on a series of eight patients operated on with TORS for glottic carcinoma with anterior commissure involvement, that was either stage T1 (n = 3) or stage T2 (n = 5, of whom two had a recurrent disease after previous TLM). With a mean follow-up of 40 months, all patients survived with their larynx preserved and no local recurrence, tracheostomy, or tube feeding dependence. The purpose of Wang's study was to report the treatment results of TORS in type V to type VI endoscopic cordectomy (as classified by the European Laryngological Society) for early glottic cancer with anterior commissure involvement and, therefore, to evaluate the clinical feasibility of this surgical organ-preservation strategy.[84]

As an endoscopic approach, TLM has several limitations, such as a narrow working field, the need for long and cumbersome instruments, and the line of sight issue of the laser beam. However, with TORS for being applied for laryngeal operations, the endowristed instrument could conquer the limitations inherent in the direct line-of-site approach used in TLM.[78]

TORS-total laryngectomy (TORS-TL) is a procedure in evolution, and limited case series have been published. To date, this procedure has been primarily in cases of salvage laryngectomy not requiring concurrent neck dissection. Careful patient selection is required, as the exposure considerations are more pertinent to this procedure given the dissection deeper within the pharynx. This procedure is technically demanding, and should not be considered if the surgeon is not experienced in transoral tumor surgery.[85]

Although only a very small number of patients have been operated transoral robotic total laryngectomy has been shown to be feasible. The reported goal is to reduce postoperative morbidity by decreasing the risk of postoperative fistula as a result of better preservation of the pharyngeal mucosa and by limiting the lateral dissection between the pharyngeal and vascular spaces, thus decreasing the risk of a carotid blow-out. A minimally invasive approach to the laryngeal site in patients requiring bilateral neck dissection seems counterintuitive and indications require refinement.[86,87]

Krishnan et al. reported good survival and outcomes in three patients who underwent TORS-TL.[85-87]

Hypopharyngeal cancers can also be approached with TORS. Park et al. found no significant differences in overall and disease-specific survival at 3 years on comparing oncologic and functional outcomes in patients who underwent TORS-assisted hypopharyngectomy (n = 30) versus open surgery (n = 26).[88]

Park et al. reported an 89% overall survival and 84% disease-free survival at 3 years in 23 patients of hypopharyngeal cancer resected with TORS. They showed that 96% of the patients had favorable swallowing abilities.[89]

- *Nasopharyngeal cancer:* Tsang et al. published a series of 12 patients who underwent robotic nasopharyngectomy. The 2-year overall survival, disease-free survival, and local control were 83, 61, and 86%, respectively. This early result of robotic nasopharyngectomy showed a high local control rate with the operating time was comparable to open surgery and morbidities were low. The median operating time was 225 minutes, slightly <4 hours that compared favorably with open resection.[37]

- *Parapharyngeal tumors:* Chan et al. concluded in a systematic review of TORS in parapharyngeal tumors that the advantages over open surgery were absence of an external scar and avoiding first-bite syndrome. However, this approach does carry the risk of capsule rupture. The position of the carotid artery is also key, it is ideal for lesions medial to the carotid where vessel retraction is feasible.[90,91] Ansarin et al. reported a series of parapharyngeal space tumors in the poststyloid compartment resected with TORS approach and Vidhyadharan et al. reported the use of TORS for resection of a second branchial arch cyst medial to the carotid vessels.[92,93]
- *Salvage resections:* Early evidence suggests that TORS may be associated with reduced postoperative morbidity in a salvage setting when compared to traditional open techniques.[15,25,65] Significant expertise with TORS is needed before embarking on these procedures for recurrent oropharyngeal cancers. It must be understood that cross-sectional imaging, especially for the tongue base, is done with the tongue in the resting position in the mouth. During TORS, the tongue is brought out for access and the blades of the mouth retractor will distort tongue anatomy. Hence, the depth of the tumor as seen on MRI may not be accurately defined, and in cases where the tumor is ill-defined, additional techniques will be needed to define the cancer extent on table. Adjuncts such as intraoral ultrasound may help define the tumor thickness and boundaries in these patients, as the interface between tumor tissue and normal tissue is not clearly defined. When adequately performed, significant specimen sizes can be resected with adequate resection margins. Given that the oropharynx is already compromised by the scarring and diminished function from previous CCRT, patients will need prolonged rehabilitation. Free flap reconstruction is not required in majority of cases, as the defect will heal by secondary intention. Published literature noted that free flap reconstruction, independent of T-stage, has an adverse effect on functional outcomes. In situations where the resection is through into the neck or where the tissue is felt to be unhealthy, a TORS-assisted free flap inset is needs to be performed. The neck should be dealt with as appropriate, and in cases where no neck disease is present, the relevant feeding vessels to the operated region should be ligated.[27]

  Surgical salvage using TORS is a reasonable alternative to open surgical procedures for recurrent/residual head and neck cancer cases. It is associated with acceptable limited morbidity, reduced rates of PEG and tracheostomy dependence, quicker operative time, minimal blood loss, and shorter hospital stay. White et al. showed a significant difference in 2-year overall survival between the TORS (74%) and open surgical approach (43%), which was due to higher positive margins reported in the open surgical arm. They reported higher incidence of tracheostomy tube insertion in open surgery arm (79%) at the time of surgery as compared to TORS (23%). Most of the patients in the TORS arm were decannulated of the tracheostomy tube in 1–2 weeks.[93] Dabas et al. reported a median survival with TORS of 19 months and the median time to recurrence in was 3 months. They reported that a total of 56.7% patients were successfully salvaged with TORS.[94]

  Paleri et al. studied the role of TORS in the management of residual and recurrent oropharyngeal cancer and showed an overall survival of 48.2%, local control of 76.6%, and disease-specific survival of 77.1% at 42.6 months. They concluded that TORS is an appropriate treatment option in selected patients with good oncological outcomes and added advantages such as intraoperative ultrasound imaging and avoiding mandibulotomy. Issues specific to recurrent cancers that are encountered during TORS resection and the innovative technical refinement for TORS of residual and recurrent oropharyngeal cancer of the tongue base are described in this study.[41]
- *Retropharyngeal node:* Metastatic infiltration of pharyngeal squamous cell cancers to the retropharyngeal nodes was initially explained by Ballantyne. It is the first echelon nodal station for nasopharyngeal cancers and it been involved may worsen prognosis. Moore EJ, et al. reported that retropharyngeal node involvement will be identified during imaging (PET-CT/MRI) in about 10% of patients with oropharyngeal cancers and hence advised retropharyngeal node dissection during TORS for the primary tumor. The nodes not identified by imaging, in the presence of other adverse features for oropharyngeal carcinoma, will be covered by postoperative radiation fields.[95] Byeon HK et al., Givi B et al., and Petruzzi G et al.[96-98] demonstrated the feasibility of transoral robotic retropharyngeal lymph node (RPLN) dissection technique in their case series, respectively. Givi B et al. also mentioned that patients with OPSCC had higher short-term complication risk as compared to those with papillary thyroid carcinoma.[97] However, Byeon HK, et al. reported favorable outcomes in their series of patients with OPSCC.[96]

Complications in TORS

Hemorrhage is one of the most common postoperative complications following TORS causing 30% of readmissions to the hospital.[60,99,100] The intensity of postoperative TORS hemorrhage can range from minor bleeding managed with just observation to catastrophic hemorrhage necessitating an emergency tracheostomy for airway management and leading to even death. Chia et al. performed a survey of self-reported complications following TORS on a total of 2,015 patients that revealed a catastrophic bleed rate of 3.5% and mortality rate of 0.3%.[8] Several studies have identified factors associated with postoperative TORS hemorrhage, including larger primary tumors, greater extent of surgery, prior radiation, and perioperative anticoagulation.[61,101-103] Stokes et al. in their recent systematic review concluded that overall incidence of postoperative TORS hemorrhage in high-volume centers is low (5.78%) and that the combined incidence of major hemorrhage requiring emergent embolization, transcervical arterial ligation or tracheostomy to control hemorrhage is much lower (2.90%). They also reported that transcervical arterial ligation of either the external carotid artery or its branches to reduce the arterial blood flow to the surgical bed does not reduce the overall incidence of postoperative TORS hemorrhage but may lead to fewer major postoperative hemorrhages.[26,104,105] Other TORS-related complications were local pain, dysphagia, and aspiration pneumonia.[28,104,105]

PART B: ROBOTIC NECK SURGERY

Another important area is robotic neck surgery, which relates to scarless-in-the-neck thyroid and parathyroid surgery. There has been a tremendous evolution in the surgical approaches for thyroidectomy over the past two decades. The first endoscopic thyroidectomy was performed over two decades ago, following which robotic surgery begun to be used for a transaxillary approach. Robotic parathyroidectomy soon followed, with newer approaches such as the facelift and transoral approach representing further evolution in technique.[15,106,107]

Some of the limitations of the endoscopic procedures such as reduced range of motion and impaired eye-hand coordination due to unstable 2D view is overcome by using the robotic platform. Several studies have described the safety of the remote-access robotic thyroidectomy procedures and have showed comparable oncologic outcomes between the robotic and traditional open thyroidectomy.[106]

Classification of Robotic and Endoscopic Thyroidectomy

Since the initial transaxillary approach, many new approaches have been developed. Approaches are now defined based on the use of CO_2 insufflation and the anatomical approach. Techniques associated with insufflation are the cervical approach, axillary approach, breast approach, anterior chest approach, transoral approach, and various axillo-breast approaches such as the axillo-bilateral breast approach (ABBA), bilateral axillo-breast approach (BABA), and unilateral or BABA. The techniques that do not use gas insufflation are minimally invasive video-assisted thyroidectomy (MIVAT), the anterior chest approach, axillary approach, postauricular facelift approach, and transoral approach. Several modifications and combinations of these approaches have also been published in the literature.[108]

The selection of approach is mainly dependent on the training and comfort of surgeon and patient characteristics. Both the transaxillary and retroauricular approaches are performed in a gasless fashion, while the transoral technique requires CO_2 gas insufflation for the procedure. It is advisable to use intraoperative nerve monitoring (IONM) in robotic thyroidectomy. Displacing the IONM tube with patient position and manipulation is common and should be anticipated **(Table 1)**.[106,109]

Indications and Contraindications

According to the experience of the surgeon, the disease status, and the approach, the indications for robotic and

Table 1: Classification of robotic and endoscopic thyroidectomy.[108]

CO_2 insufflation method	*Gasless method*
Cervical approach	Minimally invasive video-assisted thyroidectomy
Anterior chest approach	Anterior chest approach
Axillary approach	Video-assisted neck surgery
Breast approach with parasternal approach	*Axillary approach*: • Axillary approach with anterior chest port • Single incision axillary approach • Gasless unilateral axillo-breast or axillary approach
Axillo-breast approach: • Axillo-bilateral-breast approach • Bilateral axillo-breast approach • Unilateral/bilateral axillo-breast approach	Facelift (retroauricular) approach
Transoral approach	Transoral approach

endoscopic thyroidectomy can be changed and expanded. Accepted indications include benign lesions <5 cm in size and differentiated thyroid cancer <4 cm in size. As the surgeon progresses, they may be more comfortable extending the indications to more challenging clinical situations such as larger benign lesions and malignancy with limited extrathyroidal extension. With approaches such as the transoral approach, specimen delivery is a major consideration with larger lesions.[109-111]

Contraindications for these approaches are advanced malignancies with local invasion, large lesions, and previously operated or irradiated fields.[13,14] Thyroiditis is a relative contraindication as the tissue is inflamed and prone for bleeding which can obscure vision.[109-110]

Operative Techniques in Remote Access Thyroidectomy

The gasless transaxillary approach, BABA, postauricular facelift approach, and transoral vestibular approach are most commonly used. Using the da Vinci Robot, regardless of the selected approach, there are three consistent steps to robotic thyroidectomy are forming the working space, docking, and console stages.[106]

Gasless Unilateral Axillary Approach

The patients is placed in supine position with a slight neck extension and arm at the side and raised to allow axillary exposure. A 5–6 cm incision is placed in the fossa and under vision the flap is raised superficial to the pectoral fascia and then subplatysmally until the two heads of the sternocleidomastoid muscle, and subsequently below the sternothyroid muscle, which is the point of access into the thyroid bed. An external retractor is placed which maintains this working space till the surgery is completed. A second smaller axillary skin incision is placed inferiorly to insert another trocar; this allows limiting the size of the initial incision. Three robotic arms are then docked within the main incision. A 30° face-down robotic endoscope is placed in the center, with a ProGrasp forceps above the camera port, a harmonic scalpel in the dominant hand, and a Maryland dissector in the nondominant hand through the second incision. Dissection is performed from the superior pole below, adequately sealing the vessels and keeping the field bloodless to identify the parathyroids and the laryngeal nerves. The gland is retracted medially to finally divide the isthmus and free the specimen. Subsequently, the central compartment can be accessed. The arms are then removed and the incision is closed over a suction drain.[106,109,110]

Bilateral Axillo-breast Approach

The patient is positioned supine with neck, slightly extended using a shoulder roll. For inserting the trocars, both arms are abducted slightly. Instillation of adrenaline solution subcutaneously can limit bleeding during dissection. Two incisions are placed in the upper circumareolar regions to begin dissecting the plane using a vascular tunneler. This plane is dissected up to the thyroid cartilage superiorly and both sternocleidomastoids laterally. After creating a suitable working space, an endoscope is inserted through the 12 mm right breast port and the left 12 mm breast port is used for the operating instruments. Both axillae are used to inserted smaller cannulas. CO_2 insufflation at a pressure of 5–6 mm Hg is used to maintain the working space. The gland is removed through the larger breast port and the robot arms and ports are removed. Valsalva maneuver performed and midline of the strap muscles is reapproximated and the incisions are closed in layers over a suction drain.[106,109-111]

Postauricular or Retroauricular Facelift Approach

The patient is in supine position with head turned toward the opposite side of the thyroid lesion. An incision is made in the skin over the postauricular sulcus, curving posteriorly at the upper third of the auricle and continued toward the occipital hairline.[23,26] Under vision, the flaps are raised subcutaneously and then subplatysmally to the lower border of the mandible above, the sternal notch below and the sternocleidomastoid medially. An external retractor (Koh's retractor) is placed to maintain the working space only after the omohyoid, sternohyoid, and sternothyroid muscles are dissected and retracted upward to expose the thyroid gland under direct vision. The instrumentation is similar to other approaches. In this approach, lateral retraction of the sternocleidomastoid, commonly with a self-retaining retractor, allows adequate working space. The remainder of the dissection is as described previously.[106-109,112]

Transoral Vestibular Approach

The patient is placed in a supine position with neck extension and a 1.5–2 cm in placed in the gingivolabial sulcus. Lateral incisions are made on either side carefully to avoid injury to the mental nerves. Dilute adrenaline can be infiltrated to prevent bleeding during dissection with a blunt tunneler. A 30° rigid endoscope is placed centrally with the smaller trocars on either side for the instrumentation. A pressure of 5–6 mm is maintained for CO_2 insufflation. The working plane is dissected subplatysmally under vision, laterally till the sternocleidomastoid muscles and inferiorly to the suprasternal notch. The 30° robotic endoscope and two instruments such as a bipolar Maryland forceps or monopolar scissors are placed. If a third instrument is required, an axillary port is placed. To allow exposure, external stitches may be placed to retract the strap muscles outward and laterally. Dissection is as described before, and the gland is removed in a specimen bag through the oral incision. Drains are not usually used in this technique.[106,108,113]

Advantages and Disadvantages of Remote Access Thyroidectomy

Among the four most common remote access thyroidectomy procedures, it is difficult to conclude which approach is best as each one has its own advantages and disadvantages. CO_2 insufflation techniques have the advantage of smaller skin incisions and less dissection, and may have better cosmesis in the immediate postoperative period. However, these techniques can result in CO_2 embolism, hypercapnia, respiratory acidosis, subcutaneous emphysema, and cerebral edema. Gasless methods have the advantages of maintaining a clear surgical field without gas fumes, and the absence of complications related to CO_2 insufflation, additionally enabling the surgeons to use the conventional instruments employed in conventional thyroidectomy to dissect skin flaps and control hemostasis.[114]

Remote access thyroid surgery is not minimally invasive surgery (MIS) in terms of skin flap elevation for creating the working space; it only avoids an external incision on the neck. Exposure in different techniques is similar, however, the transaxillary and retroauricular facelift approaches permit performing lateral selective neck dissection without altering patient position. Central neck dissection can be done in all four approaches, although it is relatively difficult in the BABA due to an inadequate angle of approach. Cosmetic outcome is excellent irrespective of the technique employed.

The techniques also have their own unique morbidity profiles. Patients have described contractures of fibrous bands in the operative field after surgery.[115,116] Cost is often prohibitively expensive.[117-120] Remote access thyroidectomy is technically challenging, and the prolonged learning curve can result in serious patient morbidity.

Complications, Feasibility and Safety in Robotic Thyroidectomy

Complications

Large series that demonstrate the safety of remote access thyroidectomy do not reflect the relatively high complication rates that most surgeons account early in the learning curve. Serious complications, such as tracheal and esophageal injury and CO_2 embolisms have been documented. The safety of patients must be the first priority. Strict patient selection criteria are needed for successful surgical outcomes, especially during the steep learning curve also necessitating an appropriate training program for surgeons. Patients need to be aware of the possibility of converting to open surgery for safety reasons.

In meta-analyses by Lang et al. and Kandil et al., recurrent laryngeal nerve paralysis and hypoparathyroidism were comparable in robotic and open thyroidectomy.[120-123] However, in subgroup analyses by Kandil et al., transient recurrent laryngeal nerve paralysis was higher in the robotic procedure than the conventional procedure[54] and injury was more frequent early in the learning curve and with low-volume surgeons.[121] Remote access surgery was more commonly associated with seroma, which occasionally needed multiple outpatient aspirations.[106,108]

Unusual complications, such as, transient brachial plexus injury, have been reported in the transaxillary approach, which can be minimized through appropriate positioning. Marginal mandibular nerve can be damaged in the postauricular approach and the mental nerve in the transoral approach.[113,114]

Operative Time

Sung et al. showed that the transaxillary and the facelift approach required similar operative times on average.[111] Kandil et al. reporting that robotic approaches added 43.5 minutes to operative time. Robotic and endoscopic procedures roughly required the same operative times.[121] As the surgical experience for robotic thyroidectomy increases the total operative time may decrease. Both Lee et al. and Song et al. estimated the learning curve for robotic thyroidectomy via the transaxillary approach to be between 35 and 50 cases and Liu et al. reported the learning curve of the BABA to be about 40 cases.[124-126] The reason for needing to operate on the proposed number of cases to overcome the learning curve is due to the intricacies of flap dissection and manipulation of the robotic instruments.

Surgical Adequacy

Surgical completeness of total thyroidectomy can be an issue with limited vision and poor access. Thyroglobulin (Tg) levels are often considered surrogate markers for the surgical and have been shown to be significantly higher in robotic approaches than in open surgery in a meta-analysis.[108] Lee et al. stated that surgical clearance with BABA was comparable to open approaches;[127] however, Lang et al. in their meta-analysis showed that lymph node yield in the robotic approach was significantly lower.[123]

Oncologic Outcomes

This should be the paramount consideration in the treatment of malignancy. Studies by Tae, Lee, and Song et al., showed that oncological outcomes were comparable between robotic transaxillary thyroidectomy and conventional thyroidectomy,[128-130] but follow-up period was limited. Given the recent history of these approaches and the long follow-up required in thyroid cancer, further studies are required to address this issue Definitively.

Cosmetic and Functional Outcomes and Quality of Life

The most important reason for patients and surgeons to choose robotic thyroidectomy is for its superior cosmetic results as compared to conventional thyroidectomy. In the transaxillary approach, long-term cosmetic satisfaction is higher than in open thyroidectomy.[131] In terms of voice outcomes, although one study reported similar postoperative voice outcomes in both transaxillary and conventional thyroidectomy, there was better subjective voice recovery and results for acoustic parameters of voice pitch in robotic thyroidectomy via the gasless transaxillary approach than conventional surgery.[132,133] However, well-designed prospective studies are required to evaluate this. Some studies also assessed postoperative swallowing function after robotic thyroidectomy, but there is no definitive evidence available. Patients who have undergone gasless transaxillary thyroidectomy have longer pain and sensory disturbance in the anterior chest area than patients who have undergone conventional thyroidectomy.[134] Minimizing anterior chest dissection may help address this issue. QoL after transaxillary robotic thyroidectomy has been shown to be comparable to QoL after open thyroidectomy.[135]

Robotic Lateral Neck Dissection

Robotic thyroid surgery has been expanded to lateral neck dissection for thyroid cancers with lateral compartment lymph node metastasis by performing a gasless transaxillary approach or postauricular facelift approach. Song et al. recommended from their study that ultrasound-guided charcoal tattooing prior to surgery is useful for identifying metastatic lymph nodes during robotic lateral neck dissection. However, its oncologic safety needs further evaluation as there has been no long-term follow-up study after robotic lateral neck dissection.[108,136]

Kang et al. used robot-assisted thyroidectomies and concomitant robotic radical neck dissections in 33 patients with thyroid cancer and lymph node metastases.[136,137] They had transient hypocalcemia in 17 patients which resolved within 2 months. Two patients reported transient hoarseness which also subsided within 3 months, with reports of no nerve damage intraoperatively. Four patients had seromas and three more patients had minor chyle leaks. Likewise, Koh et al. reported a case of robot-assisted neck dissection through a modified facelift approach after nonrobotic squamous cell carcinoma resection without complications.[138]

Tae K et al. published a study comparing robot-assisted selective neck dissection via a posterior facelift approach for squamous cell carcinoma in 11 patients to the conventional open technique in 19 patients. They showed that the average operative time was significantly longer in the robotic group; however, patient in the robot-assisted neck dissection group had improved cosmetic satisfaction.[139]

Similarly, Lee et al. published their study comparing the conventional supraomohyoid neck dissection through an external cervical incision in 16 patients with robotic-assisted neck dissection in 10 patients for oral squamous cell carcinoma. They did not observe any significant difference in clinical outcome between the groups. The conventional group had significantly shorter average operative time. There was an observed statistically significant improvement in cosmetic satisfaction in the robot-assisted group. Lee et al. were of the opinion that the prolonged operative times was due to inadequate dissection achieved by pulling the tissue and cutting with harmonic curved shears or a monopolar coagulator.[140]

Park et al. and Song et al. investigated the use of the robot in neck dissection, primary tumor resection, and subsequent reconstruction. In the study by Park et al., robot-assisted neck dissections by a modified facelift or retroauricular approach was performed in seven patients with head and neck cancer. TORS primary tumor resection followed by neck dissection and then either robot-assisted or conventional reconstruction using a radial forearm free flap or anterior lateral thigh free flap was done. They noted decreased cervical scarring but greater dissection and a larger skin flap elevation leading to increase invasive nature of surgery with robotic-assisted neck dissection via the modified facelift and retroauricular approaches as compared to conventional transcervical techniques.[141]

NEWER ROBOTIC SURGERY SYSTEMS

- *Flex robotic system:* The Flex robotic system (Medrobotics Corp., Raynham, MA, USA) is a newer robotic platform that has been designed to improve access in relatively inaccessible areas of the human body. Unlike in the da Vinci, the endoscope is flexible, and allows for cauterization and irrigation. It has a cart to carry the scope and console, which controls the scope, which has access ports for insertion of semiflexible instruments. The visual output is 2D.[5,142-144]

  The Flex robotic system performs a diverse range of transoral surgery in the oropharynx, hypopharynx and larynx, while occupying less physical space than most other systems. It has recently been approved for NOTES.[5] Mattheis S et al. published a report where the Flex robotic system was used successfully to resect lesions of the oropharynx, hypopharynx, or supraglottic larynx in 40 patients with no adverse events.[145]

  Lang and colleagues conducted a prospective single armed, clinical follow-up multicenter study of the Medrobotics Flex Robotic System for access and visualization of the oropharynx, hypopharynx, and larynx as well as for resection of benign and malignant lesions. They found it a good tool for exposure and resection with difficulty only in exposing the false and true cords.[146]

- *da Vinci single port:* The original design of the da Vinci robotic system had some constraints including the inability to use all four instruments at once, the rigid, straight orientation and size of instruments, and the challenge in docking the patient side cart. Hence, to tackle these problems, a new, flexible, single-arm robotic surgical system (da Vinci SP Surgical system, Model SP999; Intuitive Surgical Inc.) was created and first assessed clinically on 19 patients undergoing genitourinary surgery in a prospective clinical trial in 2010.[147]

  The da Vinci SP Surgical system houses a stereoscopic binocular camera and three 6 mm instruments within a 2.5 cm circular cannula and individually articulate within the surgical field. These instruments embody a snake-like appearance similar to the 5-mm multiport EndoWrist instruments merged with an additional elbow joint giving these instruments their flexibility. This allows exposure to with a transoral approach and use of existing retractor.[148-150]

  Chan YK et al. determined it was safe and effective in surgery of the oropharynx, larynx, hypopharynx, and nasopharynx. The limitation they noted is the limited space for an assistant to suction and a lack of bone instrumentation for the nasopharynx and skull base. They concluded that the da Vinci SP robotic system appeared to be safe and feasible for use in transoral endoscopic head and neck surgery and may offer great potential to advance the range of MIS.[151]

SUMMARY

The traditional morbid approaches for accessing and resecting tumors of the upper aerodigestive tract are often replaced with MIS with focus on functional outcomes in the form of TORS. Nonetheless, it is important to keep in mind that the present indications for TORS are limited and long-term data on the safety and oncological outcomes are required to better appreciate the true role of TORS in treatment of head and neck cancer. The development of new flexible, miniaturized robots is likely to further expand the indications for TORS to tumors involving the nasopharynx and skull base as well as those located in the glottic and subglottic larynx. At the same time, with the advent of numerous companies developing multiple robotic platforms the costs might also be driven down due to market competition. The situation in robotic thyroid and parathyroid surgery is less clear. However, they do signify a viable option when a neck scar is undesirable for cultural or biological reasons. Until costs are sufficiently reduced or indications expanded for robotic neck surgeries, the role of these procedures is likely to remain for niche group of patients.

Acknowledgments: The primary author would like to thank Dr Suren Krishnan, Department of Otolaryngology, Royal Adelaide Hospital, Australia, for providing the operative photographs for this chapter which were taken during his fellowship.

REFERENCES

1. Kim KH, Choi HG JY. Head and neck robotic surgery: pros and cons. Head Neck Oncol. 2013;5:26.
2. Hockstein NG, Gourin CG, Faust RA, Terris DJ. A history of robots: from science fiction to surgical robotics. J Robot Surg. 2007;1:113-8.
3. Garas G, Arora A. Robotic head and neck surgery: history, technical evolution and the future. ORL J Otorhinolaryngol Relat Spec. 2018;80:117-24.
4. Garas G, Tolley N. Robotics in otorhinolaryngology—head and neck surgery. Ann R Coll Surg Engl. 2018;100:34-41.
5. Khandalavala K, Shimon T, Flores L, Armijo PR, Oleynikov D. Emerging surgical robotic technology: a progression toward microbots. Ann Laparosc Endosc Surg. 2020;5:3.
6. Peters BS, Armijo PR, Krause C, Choudhury SA, Oleynikov D. Review of emerging surgical robotic technology. Surg Endosc. 2018;32:1636-55.
7. van den Bedem LJM. Realization of a demonstrator slave for robotic minimally invasive surgery. Eindhoven: Technische Universiteit Eindhoven; 2010. doi: 10.6100/IR684835.

8. Freschi C, Ferrari V, Melfi F, Ferrari M, Mosca F, Cuschieri A. Technical review of the da Vinci surgical telemanipulator. Int J Med Robot. 2013;9:396-406.
9. Rao PP. Robotic surgery: new robots and finally some real competition! World J Urol. 2018;36:537-41.
10. Rassweiler JJ, Autorino R, Klein J, Mottrie A, Goezen AS, Stolzenburg JU, et al. Future of robotic surgery in urology. BJU Int. 2017;120:822-41.
11. Leung T, Vyas D. Robotic surgery: applications. Am J Robot Surg. 2014;1:1-64.
12. Cadeddu JA. Re: Early experience with the Senhance®—laparoscopic/robotic platform in the US. J Urol. 2019;202: 642-3.
13. Rassweiler JJ, Teber D. Advances in laparoscopic surgery in urology. Nat Rev Urol. 2016;13:387-99.
14. Escobar PF, Bedaiwy MA, Fader AN, Falcone T. Laparoendoscopic single-site (LESS) surgery in patients with benign adnexal disease. Fertil Steril. 2010;93:2074.e7-10.
15. Golunsiński W. Functional organ preservation surgery in head and neck cancer: transoral robotic surgery and beyond. Front Oncol. 2019;9:293.
16. Adelstein DJ, Ridge JA, Brizel DM, Holsinger FC, Haughey BH, O'Sullivan B, et al. Transoral resection of pharyngeal cancer: summary of a National Cancer Institute Head and Neck Cancer Steering Committee Clinical Trials Planning Meeting, November 6–7, 2011, Arlington, Virginia. Head Neck. 2012;34:1681-703.
17. Vasan N, Sharum M, Rodney JP. Potential of robotic systems in phonosurgery. Robot Surg. 2019;6:3-8.
18. Dowthwaite SA, Franklin JH, Palma DA, Fung K, Yoo J, Nichols AC. The role of transoral robotic surgery in the management of oropharyngeal cancer: a review of the literature. ISRN Oncol. 2012;2012:945162.
19. Rich JT, Milov S, Lewis JS Jr, Thorstad WL, Adkins DR, Haughey BH. Transoral laser microsurgery (TLM) +/– adjuvant therapy for advanced stage oropharyngeal cancer: outcomes and prognostic factors. Laryngoscope. 2009;119:1709-19.
20. Weinstein G, O'Malley BW Jr, Rinaldo A, Silver CE, Werner JA, Ferlito A. Understanding contraindications for transoral robotic surgery (TORS) for oropharyngeal cancer. Eur Arch Otorhinolaryngol. 2015;272:1551-2.
21. Byrd JK, Ferris RL. Is there a role for robotic surgery in the treatment of head and neck cancer? Curr Treat Options Oncol. 2016;17:29.
22. Solares CA, Strome M. Transoral robot-assisted CO_2 laser supraglottic laryngectomy: experimental and clinical data. Laryngoscope. 2007;117:817-20.
23. Kucur C, Durmus K, Gun R, Old MO, Agrawal A, Teknos TN, et al. Safety and efficacy of concurrent neck dissection and transoral robotic surgery. Head Neck. 2016;38(Suppl 1): E519-23.
24. Mandal R, Duvvuri U, Ferris RL, Kaffenberger TM, Choby GW, Kim S. Analysis of post-transoral robotic-assisted surgery hemorrhage: frequency, outcomes, and prevention. Head Neck. 2016;38(Suppl 1):E776-82.
25. Weinstein GS, O'Malley BW Jr, Snyder W, Sherman E, Quon H. Transoral robotic surgery: radical tonsillectomy. Arch Otolaryngol Head Neck Surg. 2007;133:1220-6.
26. Gleysteen J, Troob S, Light T, Brickman D, Clayburgh D, Andersen P, et al. The impact of prophylactic external carotid artery ligation on postoperative bleeding after transoral robotic surgery (TORS) for oropharyngeal squamous cell carcinoma. Oral Oncol. 2017;70:1-6.
27. Paleri V, Fox H, Winter S. Transoral robotic surgery for oropharyngeal cancer. ORL J Otorhinolaryngol Relat Spec. 2018;80:156-70.
28. Nichols AC, Theurer J, Prisman E, Read N, Berthelet E, Tran E, et al. Radiotherapy versus transoral robotic surgery and neck dissection for oropharyngeal squamous cell carcinoma (ORATOR): an open-label, phase 2, randomised trial. Lancet Oncol. 2019;20:1349-59.
29. Dziegielewski PT, Ozer E. Transoral robotic surgery: supraglottic laryngectomy. Oper Tech Otolaryngol Head Neck Surg. 2013;24:86-91.
30. Ozer E, Alvarez B, Kakarala K, Durmus K, Teknos TN, Carrau RL. Clinical outcomes of transoral robotic supraglottic laryngectomy. Head Neck. 2013;35:1158-61.
31. Smith RV. Transoral robotic surgery for larynx cancer. Otolaryngol Clin North Am. 2014;47:379-95.
32. Park YM, Kim WS, Byeon HK, Lee SY, Kim SH. Surgical techniques and treatment outcomes of transoral robotic supraglottic partial laryngectomy. Laryngoscope. 2013;123: 670-7.
33. Kayhan FT, Kaya KH, Sayin I. Transoral robotic cordectomy for early glottic carcinoma. Ann Otol Rhinol Laryngol. 2012;121:497-502.
34. Remacle M, Matar N, Lawson G, Bachy V, Delos M, Nollevaux MC. Combining a new CO_2 laser wave guide with transoral robotic surgery: a feasibility on four patients with malignant tumors. Eur Arch Otorhinolaryngol. 2010;269: 1833-7.
35. Ozer E, Waltonen J. Transoral robotic nasopharyngectomy: a novel approach for nasopharyngeal lesions. Laryngoscope. 2008;118:1613-6.
36. Wei WI, Ho WK. Transoral robotic resection of recurrent nasopharyngeal carcinoma. Laryngoscope. 2010;120:2011-4.
37. Yin Tsang RK, Ho WK, Wei WI. Combined transnasal endoscopic and transoral robotic resection of recurrent nasopharyngeal carcinoma. Head Neck. 2012;34:1190-3.
38. Hanna EY, Holsinger FC, DeMonte F, Kupferman M. Robotic endoscopic surgery of the skull base: a novel surgical approach. Arch Otolaryngol Head Neck Surg. 2007;133: 1209-14.
39. Hanna J, Morse E, Brauer P, Judson B, Mehra, S. Positive margin rates and predictors in transoral robotic surgery after federal approval: a national quality study. Head Neck. 2019;41:3064-72.
40. Oleynikov D. Robotic surgery. Surg Clin North Am. 2008;88: 1121-30.
41. Paleri V, Fox H, Coward S, Ragbir M, McQueen A, Ahmed A, et al. Transoral robotic surgery for residual and recurrent oropharyngeal cancers: exploratory study of surgical innovation using the IDEAL framework for early-phase surgical studies. Head Neck. 2018;40:512-25.
42. Johnson RE, Sigman JD, Funk GF, Robinson RA, Hoffman HT. Quantification of surgical margin shrinkage in the oral cavity. Head Neck. 1997;19:281-6.
43. Mistry RC, Qureshi SS, Kumaran C. Post-resection mucosal margin shrinkage in oral cancer: quantification and significance. J Surg Oncol. 2005;91:131-3.
44. Parsons JT, Mendenhall WM, Stringer SP, Amdur RJ, Hinerman RW, Villaret DB, et al. Squamous cell carcinoma of the oropharynx: surgery, radiation therapy, or both. Cancer. 2002;94:2967-80.
45. Denis F, Garaud P, Bardet E, Alfonsi M, Sire C, Germain T, et al. Final results of the 94–01 French Head and Neck Oncology and Radiotherapy Group randomized trial comparing radiotherapy alone with concomitant radiochemotherapy in advanced-stage oropharynx carcinoma. J Clin Oncol. 2004; 22:69-76.
46. Abendstein H, Nordgren M, Boysen M, Jannert M, Silander E, Ahlner-Elmqvist M, et al. Quality of life and head and

neck cancer: a 5-year prospective study. Laryngoscope. 2005; 115:2183-92.
47. Rogers SN, Ahad SA, Murphy AP. A structured review and theme analysis of papers published on 'quality of life' in head and neck cancer: 2000–2005. Oral Oncol. 2007;43:843-68.
48. Denis F, Garaud P, Bardet E, Alfonsi M, Sire C, Germain T, et al. Late toxicity results of the GORTEC 94–01 randomized trial comparing radiotherapy with concomitant radiochemotherapy for advanced-stage oropharynx carcinoma: comparison of LENT/SOMA, RTOG/EORTC, and NCI-CTC scoring systems. Int J Radiat Oncol Biol Phys. 2003;55:93-8.
49. Wilson JA, Carding PN, Patterson JM. Dysphagia after non-surgical head and neck cancer treatment: patients' perspectives. Otolaryngol Head Neck Surg. 2011;145:767-71.
50. Paleri V, Patterson J. Use of gastrostomy in head and neck cancer: a systematic review to identify areas for future research. Clin Otolaryngol. 2010;35:177-89.
51. Moor JW, Patterson J, Kelly C, Paleri V. Prophylactic gastrostomy before chemoradiation in advanced head and neck cancer: a multiprofessional web-based survey to identify current practice and to analyse decision making. Clin Oncol (R Coll Radiol). 2010;22:192-8.
52. Hamilton D, Khan MK, O'Hara J, Paleri V. The changing landscape of oropharyngeal cancer management. J Laryngol Otol. 2017;131:3-7.
53. Ramos AC, de Souza Bastos EL, Kim KC. Perspectives of robotic bariatric surgery. In: Joel F, Salomao F (Eds.) Obesity and Diabetes: New Surgical and Nonsurgical Approaches. Switzerland, Cham: Springer International Publishing; 2015. pp. 69-87.
54. Moore EJ, Olsen KD, Kasperbauer JL. Transoral robotic surgery for oropharyngeal squamous cell carcinoma: a prospective study of feasibility and functional outcomes. Laryngoscope. 2009;119:2156-64.
55. Dowthwaite S, Panizza B, O'Neill J, Porceddu S, Jackson JE, Benjamin C. Outcomes of primary trans-oral surgical management of early tonsillar squamous cell carcinoma with risk-adapted adjuvant radiotherapy. Aust J Otolaryngol. 2019;2:7.
56. Park DA, Lee MJ, Kim SH, Lee SH. Comparative safety and effectiveness of transoral robotic surgery versus open surgery for oropharyngeal cancer: a systematic review and meta-analysis. Eur J Surg Oncol. 2020;46:644-9.
57. Chen AM, Daly ME, Luu Q, Donald PJ, Farwell DG. Comparison of functional outcomes and quality of life between transoral surgery and definitive chemoradiotherapy for oropharyngeal cancer. Head Neck. 2015;37:381-5.
58. Ward MC, Koyfman SA. Transoral robotic surgery: the radiation oncologist's perspective. Oral Oncol. 2016;60: 96-102.
59. De Almeida JR, Byrd JK, Wu R, Stucken CL, Duvvuri U, Goldstein DP, et al. A systematic review of transoral robotic surgery and radiotherapy for early oropharynx cancer: a systematic review. Laryngoscope. 2014;124:2096-102.
60. Chia SH, Gross ND, Richmon JD. Surgeon experience and complications with transoral robotic surgery (TORS). Otolaryngol Neck Surg. 2013;149:885-92.
61. Zenga J, Suko J, Kallogjeri D, Pipkorn P, Nussenbaum B, Jackson RS. Postoperative hemorrhage and hospital revisit after transoral robotic surgery. Laryngoscope. 2017;127: 2287-92.
62. Sload R, Silver N, Jawad BA, Gross ND. The role of transoral robotic surgery in the management of HPV negative oropharyngeal squamous cell carcinoma. Curr Oncol Rep. 2016;18:53.
63. Holsinger F, Thorstad W, Fontenla S, et al. Randomized phase II trial of transoral endoscopic head and neck surgery followed by risk-based IMRT and weekly cisplatin versus IMRT and weekly cisplatin for HPV negative oropharynx cancer RTOG 1221; 2014.
64. Cohen MA, Weinstein GS, O'Malley BW Jr, Feldman M, Quon H. Transoral robotic surgery and human papillomavirus status: oncologic results. Head Neck. 2011;33:573-80.
65. De Almeida J, Li R, Magnuson JS, Smith RV, Moore E, Lawson G, et al. Oncologic outcomes after transoral robotic surgery: a multi-institutional study. JAMA Otolaryngol Head Neck Surg. 2015;141:1043-51.
66. Moore EJ, Olsen SM, Laborde RR, García JJ, Walsh FJ, Price DL, et al. Long-term functional and oncologic results of transoral robotic surgery for oropharyngeal squamous cell carcinoma. Mayo Clin Proc. 2012;87:219-25.
67. Dabas S, Gupta K, Ranjan R, Sharma AK, Shukla H, Dinesh A. Oncological outcome following de-intensification of treatment for stage I and II HPV negative oropharyngeal cancers with transoral robotic surgery (TORS): a prospective trial. Oral Oncol. 2017;69:80-3.
68. Gupta K, Dabas S. Oncological outcome following intensification of treatment by transoral robotic surgery (TORS) for HPV negative stage IV oropharyngeal cancer: a Prospective trial. (3380). Ann Oncol. 2017;28(Suppl 10):x100-x110.
69. Winter SC, Ofo E, Meikle D, Silva P, Fraser L, O'Hara J, et al. Trans-oral robotic assisted tongue base mucosectomy for investigation of cancer of unknown primary in the head and neck region. The UK experience. Clin Otolaryngol. 2017;42:1247-51.
70. Rusthoven KE, Koshy M, Paulino AC. The role of fluorodeoxyglucose positron emission tomography in cervical lymph node metastases from an unknown primary tumor. Cancer. 2004;101:2641-9.
71. Mehta V, Johnson P, Tassler A, Kim S, Ferris RL, Nance M, et al. A new paradigm for the diagnosis and management of unknown primary tumors of the head and neck: a role for transoral robotic surgery. Laryngoscope. 2013;123:146-51.
72. Patel SA, Magnuson JS, Holsinger FC, Karni RJ, Richmon JD, Gross ND, et al. Robotic surgery for primary head and neck squamous cell carcinoma of unknown site. JAMA Otolaryngol Head Neck Surg. 2013;139:1203-11.
73. Krishnan S, Connell J, Ofo E. Transoral robotic surgery base of tongue mucosectomy for head and neck cancer of unknown primary. ANZ J Surg. 2017;87:E281-E284.
74. De Virgilio A, Park YM, Kim WS, Baek SJ, Kim SH. How to optimize laryngeal and hypopharyngeal exposure in transoral robotic surgery. Auris Nasus Larynx. 2013;40:312-9.
75. Iro H, Waldfahrer F, Altendorf-Hofmann A, Weidenbecher M, Sauer R, Steiner W. Transoral laser surgery of supraglottic cancer: follow-up of 141 patients. Arch Otolaryngol Head Neck Surg. 1998;124:1245-50.
76. Vural E, Tulunay-Ugur OE, Suen JY. Transoral robotic supracricoid partial laryngectomy with cartilaginous framework preservation. J Robot Surg. 2012;6:363-6.
77. Vilaseca-Gonzalez I, Bernal-Sprekelsen M, Blanch-Alejandro JL, Moragas-Lluis M. Complications in transoral CO_2 laser surgery for carcinoma of the larynx and hypopharynx. Head Neck. 2003;25:382-8.
78. Gorphe P. A contemporary review of evidence for transoral robotic surgery in laryngeal cancer. Front Oncol. 2018;8: 121.
79. Mendelsohn AH, Remacle M, Van Der Vorst S, Bachy V, Lawson G. Outcomes following transoral robotic surgery: supraglottic laryngectomy. Laryngoscope. 2013;123:208-14.

80. Olsen SM, Moore EJ, Koch CA, Price DL, Kasperbauer JL, Olsen KD. Transoral robotic surgery for supraglottic squamous cell carcinoma. Am J Otolaryngol. 2012;33:379-84.
81. Razafindranaly V, Lallemant B, Aubry K, Moriniere S, Vergez S, Mones ED, et al. Clinical outcomes with transoral robotic surgery for supraglottic squamous cell carcinoma: experience of a French evaluation cooperative subgroup of GETTEC. Head Neck. 2016;38:E1097-101.
82. Alon EE, Kasperbauer JL, Olsen KD, Moore EJ. Feasibility of transoral robotic-assisted supraglottic laryngectomy. Head Neck. 2012;34:225-9.
83. Lallemant B, Chambon G, Garrel R, Kacha S, Rupp D, Galy-Bernadoy C, et al. Transoral robotic surgery for the treatment of T1-T2 carcinoma of the larynx: preliminary study. Laryngoscope. 2013;123:2485-90.
84. Wang CC, Liu SA, Wu SH, Lin WJ, Jiang RS, Wang L. Transoral robotic surgery for early glottic carcinoma involving anterior commissure: preliminary reports. Head Neck. 2016;38:913-8.
85. Smith RV, Schiff BA, Sarta C, Hans S, Brasnu D. Transoral robotic total laryngectomy. Laryngoscope, 2013;123:678-82.
86. Lawson G, Mendelsohn AH, van der Vorst S, Bachy V, Remacle M. Transoral robotic surgery total laryngectomy. Laryngoscope. 2013;123:193-6.
87. Krishnan G, Krishnan S. Transoral robotic surgery total laryngectomy: evaluation of functional and survival outcomes in a retrospective case series at a single institution. ORL J Otorhinolaryngol Relat Spec. 2017;79:191-201.
88. Park YM, Byeon HK, Chung HP, Choi EC, Kim SH. Comparison study of transoral robotic surgery and radical open surgery for hypopharyngeal cancer. Acta Otolaryngol. 2013;133:641-8.
89. Park YM, Kim WS, De Virgilio A, Lee SY, Seol JH, Kim SH. Transoral robotic surgery for hypopharyngeal squamous cell carcinoma: 3-year oncologic and functional analysis. Oral Oncol. 2012;48:560-6.
90. Tsang RK, To VS, Ho AC, Ho WK, Chan JY, Wei WI. Early results of robotic assisted nasopharyngectomy for recurrent nasopharyngeal carcinoma. Head Neck. 2015;37:788-93.
91. Chan JYK, Tsang RK, Eisele DW, Richmon JD. Transoral robotic surgery of the parapharyngeal space: a case series and systematic review. Head Neck. 2015;37:293-8.
92. Ansarin M, Tagliabue M, Chu F, Zorzi S, Proh M, Preda L. Transoral robotic surgery in retrostyloid parapharyngeal space schwannomas. Case Rep Otolaryngol. 2014;2014: 296025.
93. Vidhyadharan S, Krishnan S, King G, Morley A. Transoral robotic surgery for removal of a second branchial arch cyst: a case report. J Robot Surg. 2012;6:349-53.
94. Dabas S, Dewan A, Ranjan R, Dewan AK, Shukla H, Sinha R. Salvage transoral robotic surgery for recurrent or residual head and neck squamous cell carcinoma: a single institution experience. Asian Pac J Cancer Prev. 2015;16:7627-32.
95. Moore EJ, Ebrahimi A, Price DL, Olsen KD. Retropharyngeal lymph node dissection in oropharyngeal cancer treated with transoral robotic surgery. Laryngoscope. 2013;123:1676-81.
96. Byeon HK, Duvvuri U, Kim WS, Park YM, Hong HJ, Koh YW, et al. Transoral robotic retropharyngeal lymph node dissection with or without lateral oropharyngectomy. J Craniofac Surg. 2013;24:1156-61.
97. Givi B, Troob SH, Stott W, Cordeiro T, Andersen PE, Gross ND. Transoral robotic retropharyngeal node dissection. Head Neck. 2016;38:E981-6.
98. Petruzzi G, Zocchi J, Moretto S, Pichi B, Cristalli G, Mercante G, et al. Transoral robotic retropharyngeal lymph node dissection in a recurrent head and neck carcinoma. Head Neck. 2019; 41:4051-3.
99. Hay A, Migliacci J, Karassawa D, O'Boyle J, Singh Bhuvanesh, Wong RJ, et al. Complications following transoral robotic surgery (TORS): a detailed institutional review of complications. Oral Oncol. 2017;67:160-6.
100. Parhar HS, Gausden E, Patel J, Prisman E, Anderson DW, Durham JS, et al. Analysis of readmissions after transoral robotic surgery for oropharyngeal squamous cell carcinoma. Head Neck. 2018;40:2416-23.
101. Hay A, Migliacci J, Karassawa Zanoni D, Boyle JO, Singh B, Wong RJ, et al. Haemorrhage following transoral robotic surgery. Clin Otolaryngol. 2018;43:638-44.
102. Pollei TR, Hinni ML, Moore EJ, Hayden RE, Olsen KD, Casler JD, et al. Analysis of postoperative bleeding and risk factors in transoral surgery of the oropharynx. JAMA Otolaryngol Head Neck Surg. 2013;139:1212-8.
103. Kubik M, Mandal R, Albergotti W, Duvvuri U, Ferris RL, Kim S. Effect of transcervical arterial ligation on the severity of postoperative hemorrhage after transoral robotic surgery. Head Neck. 2017;39:1510-5.
104. Stokes W, Ramadan J, Lawson G, Ferris RL, Holsinger FC, Turner MT. Bleeding complications after transoral robotic surgery: a meta-analysis and systematic review. Laryngoscope. 2020;doi: 10.1002/lary.28580. Online ahead of print.
105. Asher SA, White HN, Kejner AE, Rosenthal EL, Carroll WR, Magnuson JS. Hemorrhage after transoral robotic-assisted surgery. Otolaryngol Head Neck Surg. 2013;149:112-7.
106. Chang EHE, Kim HY, Koh YW, Chung WY. Overview of robotic thyroidectomy. Gland Surg. 2017;6:218-28.
107. Terris DJ, Singer MC, Seybt MW. Robotic facelift thyroidectomy: II. Clinical feasibility and safety. Laryngoscope. 2011; 121:1636-41.
108. Thankappan K. Robotic retro-auricular thyroidectomy: indications and technique. J Head Neck Phys Surg. 2019;7: 6-10.
109. Tae K, Ji YB, Song CM, Ryu J. Robotic and endoscopic thyroid surgery: evolution and advances. Clin Exp Otorhinolaryngol. 2019;12:1-11.
110. Tae K, Ji YB, Jeong JH, Lee SH, Jeong MA, Park CW. Robotic thyroidectomy by a gasless unilateral axillo-breast or axillary approach: our early experiences. Surg Endosc. 2011;25:221-8.
111. Tae K, Ji YB, Cho SH, Lee SH, Kim DS, Kim TW. Early surgical outcomes of robotic thyroidectomy by a gasless unilateral axillo-breast or axillary approach for papillary thyroid carcinoma: 2 years' experience. Head Neck. 2012;34:617-25.
112. Sung ES, Ji YB, Song CM, Yun BR, Chung WS, Tae K. Robotic thyroidectomy: comparison of a postauricular facelift approach with a gasless unilateral axillary approach. Otolaryngol Head Neck Surg. 2016;154:997-1004.
113. Kim HY, Chai YJ, Dionigi G, Anuwong A, Richmond JD. Transoral robotic thyroidectomy: lessons learned from an initial consecutive series of 24 patients. Surg Endosc. 2018;32:688-94.
114. Kim KN, Lee DW, Kim JY, Han KH, Tae K. Carbon dioxide embolism during transoral robotic thyroidectomy: a case report. Head Neck. 2018;40:E25-8.
115. Kwak DH, Kim WS, Kim HK, Bae TH. A band-like neck scar contracture after bilateral axillo-breast approach robotic thyroidectomy. Arch Plast Surg. 2016;43:614-5.
116. Kim JH, Park JW, Gong HS. Axillary web syndrome after transaxillary robotic thyroidectomy. J Robot Surg. 2014;8: 281-3.
117. Berber E, Bernet V, Fahey TJ 3rd, Kebebew E, Shaha A, Stack BC Jr, et al. American thyroid association statement on remote-access thyroid surgery. Thyroid. 2016;26:331-7.
118. Broome JT, Pomeroy S, Solorzano CC. Expense of robotic thyroidectomy: a cost analysis at a single institution. Arch Surg. 2012;147:1102-6.

119. Cabot JC, Lee CR, Brunaud L, Kleiman DA, Chung WY, Fahey TJ 3rd, et al. Robotic and endoscopic transaxillary thyroidectomies may be cost prohibitive when compared to standard cervical thyroidectomy. Surgery. 2012;152:1016-24.
120. Lang BH, Wong CK, Tsang JS, Wong KP, Wan KY. A systematic review and meta-analysis comparing surgically-related complications between robotic-assisted thyroidectomy and conventional open thyroidectomy. Ann Surg Oncol. 2014;21:850-61.
121. Kandil E, Hammad AY, Walvekar RR, Hu T, Masoodi H, Mohamed SE, et al. Robotic thyroidectomy versus nonrobotic approaches: a meta-analysis examining surgical outcomes. Surg Innov. 2016;23:317-25.
122. Sun GH, Peress L, Pynnonen MA. Systematic review and meta-analysis of robotic vs conventional thyroidectomy approaches for thyroid disease. Otolaryngol Head Neck Surg. 2014;150:520-32.
123. Lang BH, Wong CK, Tsang JS, Wong KP, Wan KY. A systematic review and meta-analysis evaluating completeness and outcomes of robotic thyroidectomy. Laryngoscope. 2015;125: 509-18.
124. Lee J, Yun JH, Nam KH, Soh EY, Chung WY. The learning curve for robotic thyroidectomy: a multicenter study. Ann Surg Oncol. 2011;18:226-32.
125. Song CM, Jang YI, Ji YB, Park JS, Kim DS, Tae K. Factors affecting operative time in robotic thyroidectomy. Head Neck. 2018;40:893-903.
126. Liu SY, Kim JS. Bilateral axillo-breast approach robotic thyroidectomy: review of evidences. Gland Surg. 2017;6: 250-7.
127. Lee KE, Koo DH, Im HJ, Park SK, Choi JY, Paeng JC, et al. Surgical completeness of bilateral axillo-breast approach robotic thyroidectomy: comparison with conventional open thyroidectomy after propensity score matching. Surgery. 2011;150:1266-74.
128. Tae K, Song CM, Ji YB, Sung ES, Jeong JH, Kim DS. Oncologic outcomes of robotic thyroidectomy: 5-year experience with propensity score matching. Surg Endosc. 2016;30:4785-92.
129. Lee SG, Lee J, Kim MJ, Choi JB, Kim TH, Ban EJ, et al. Long-term oncologic outcome of robotic versus open total thyroidectomy in PTC: a case-matched retrospective study. Surg Endosc. 2016;30:3474-9.
130. Sung TY, Yoon JH, Han M, Lee YH, Lee YM, Song DE, et al. Oncologic safety of robot thyroid surgery for papillary thyroid carcinoma: a comparative study of robot versus open thyroid surgery using inverse probability of treatment weighting. PLoS One. 2016;11:e0157345.
131. Ji YB, Song CM, Bang HS, Lee SH, Park YS, Tae K. Long-term cosmetic outcomes after robotic/endoscopic thyroidectomy by a gasless unilateral axillo-breast or axillary approach. J Laparoendosc Adv Surg Tech A. 2014;24:248-53.
132. Song CM, Yun BR, Ji YB, Sung ES, Kim KR, Tae K. Long-term voice outcomes after robotic thyroidectomy. World J Surg. 2016;40:110-6.
133. Tae K, Kim KY, Yun BR, Ji YB, Park CW, Kim DS, et al. Functional voice and swallowing outcomes after robotic thyroidectomy by a gasless unilateral axillo-breast approach: comparison with open thyroidectomy. Surg Endosc. 2012;26: 1871-7.
134. Song CM, Ji YB, Bang HS, Park CW, Kim H, Tae K. Long-term sensory disturbance and discomfort after robotic thyroidectomy. World J Surg. 2014;38:1743-8.
135. Song CM, Ji YB, Bang HS, Park CW, Kim DS, Tae K. Quality of life after robotic thyroidectomy by a gasless unilateral axillary approach. Ann Surg Oncol. 2014;21:4188-94.
136. Song CM, Park JS, Park W, Ji YB, Cho SH, Tae K. Feasibility of charcoal tattooing for localization of metastatic lymph nodes in robotic selective neck dissection for papillary thyroid carcinoma. Ann Surg Oncol. 2015;22:S669-75.
137. Kang SW, Lee SH, Ryu HR, Lee KY, Jeong JJ, Nam KH, et al. Initial experience with robot-assisted modified radical neck dissection for the management of thyroid carcinoma with lateral neck node metastasis. Surgery. 2010;148: 1214-21.
138. Koh YW, Chung WY, Hong HJ, Lee SY, Kim WS, Lee HS, et al. Robot-assisted selective neck dissection via modified face-lift approach for early oral tongue cancer: a video demonstration. Ann Surg Oncol. 2012;19:1334-5.
139. Tae K, Ji YB, Song CM, Jeong JH, Cho SH, Lee SH. Robotic selective neck dissection by a postauricular facelift approach: comparison with conventional neck dissection. Otolaryngol Head Neck Surg. 2014;150:394-400.
140. Lee HS, Kim WS, Hong HJ, Ban MJ, Lee D, Koh YW, et al. Robot-assisted supraomohyoid neck dissection via a modified face-lift or retroauricular approach in early-stage cN0 squamous cell carcinoma of the oral cavity: a comparative study with conventional technique. Ann Surg Oncol. 2012;19: 3871-8.
141. Park YM, Lee WJ, Yun IS, Lee DW, Lew DH, Lee JM, et al. Free flap reconstruction after robot-assisted neck dissection via a modified face-lift or retroauricular approach. Ann Surg Oncol. 2013;20:891-8.
142. Friedrich DT, Dürselen L, Mayer B, Hacker S, Schall F, Hahn J, et al. Features of haptic and tactile feedback in TORS—a comparison of available surgical systems. J Robot Surg. 2018;1:103-8.
143. Funk E, Goldenberg D, Goyal N. Demonstration of transoral robotic supraglottic laryngectomy and total laryngectomy in cadaveric specimens using the Medrobotics Flex System. Head Neck. 2017;39:1218-25.
144. Persky MJ, Issa M, Bonfili JR, Goyal N, Goldenberg D, Duvvuri U. Transoral surgery using the Flex Robotic System: initial experience in the United States. Head Neck. 2018;40:2482-86.
145. Mattheis S, Hasskamp P, Holtmann L, Schäfer C, Geisthoff U, Dominas N, et al. Flex Robotic System in transoral robotic surgery: the first 40 patients. Head Neck. 2017;39:471-5.
146. Lang S, Mattheis S, Hasskamp P, Lawson G, Guldner C, Mandapathil M, et al. A European multicenter study evaluating the flex robotic system in transoral robotic surgery. Laryngoscope. 2017;127:391-5.
147. Kaouk JH, Haber GP, Autorino R, Crouzet S, Ouzzane A, Flamand V, et al. A novel robotic system for single-port urologic surgery: first clinical investigation. Eur Urol. 2014;66: 1033-43.
148. Holsinger FC. A flexible, single-arm robotic surgical system for transoral resection of the tonsil and lateral pharyngeal wall: next-generation robotic head and neck surgery. Laryngoscope. 2016;126:864-9.
149. Tsang RK, Holsinger FC. Transoral endoscopic naso-pharyngectomy with a flexible next-generation robotic surgical system. Laryngoscope. 2016;126:2257-62.
150. Chen MM, Orosco RK, Lim GC, Holsinger FC. Improved transoral dissection of the tongue base with a next-generation robotic surgical system. Laryngoscope. 2018;128:78-83.
151. Chan JY, Tsang RK, Holsinger FC, Tong MC, Ng CW, Chiu PW, et al. Prospective clinical trial to evaluate safety and feasibility of using a single port flexible robotic system for transoral head and neck surgery. Oral Oncol. 2019;94:101-5.

Management of Tumor-like Lesions of the Head and Neck

CHAPTER 35

Odontogenic Lesions and Tumors

Sushma Mehta, Narayana Subramaniam, Samskruthi P Murthy, Sivakumar Vidhyadharan

INTRODUCTION

Lesions arising from the embryonic elements of the tooth-forming apparatus are relatively rare but a common feature in head and neck surgery practice. They are a diverse group of disorders with overlapping features but often very varied management principles. Odontogenic lesions are broadly classified as cysts, which are pathological epithelial-lined cavities and tumors, which are solid but not necessarily neoplastic. They can arise in either the maxilla or the mandible. The purpose of this chapter is to enumerate the various lesions, clinical features, and the evidence related to their management.

ODONTOGENIC CYSTS

These are pathological epithelial-line cavities formed from embryonic elements of the tooth-forming apparatus, including the enamel epithelium, rests of Malassez and the dental lamina. These account for 90% of cysts arising in the jaw and are most commonly radicular cysts (55%), dentigerous cysts (21%), and odontogenic keratocysts (OKCs) (12%).[1,2] The classification based on tissue of origin is as follows:

- *Derived from rests of Malassez:*
  - Periapical cyst
  - Residual cyst
- *Derived from enamel epithelium:*
  - Dentigerous cyst
  - Eruption cyst
- *Derived from dental lamina:*
  - Odontogenic keratocyst
  - Lateral periodontal cyst
  - Glandular odontogenic cyst
  - Gingival cyst of newborn
  - Gingival cyst of adult
- *Unclassified:*
  - Paradental cyst
  - Calcifying odontogenic cyst

Dentigerous Cyst[3-5]

Also known as follicular cyst, they arise from the epithelium of the enamel. They enclose the crown of an unerupted tooth through follicular expansion. They commonly occur early in life, even in the first decade; this is because they involve the third molars of the mandible and the permanent maxillary canines, which develop early. They have a slight predilection for male gender. Clinically, they may grow to a large size before becoming apparent. They are often detected on radiographs if a tooth is missing or is unerupted. They may also have a history of jaw swelling or pain if the cyst gets infected.

Radiographically they are unilocular radiolucent lesions at the crown of unerupted teeth. Unless infected, the border is well defined. A large cyst may appear multiloculated due to bony trabeculae persisting at the cementoenamel junction. As shown in **Figures 1A to C**, they can be central (where the crown covers the crown symmetrically), lateral (where there is follicular expansion eccentrically) or circumferential (where the entire tooth is enveloped by the cyst).

Histologically, the cyst has a thin fibrous wall, comprising young fibroblasts with stroma and ground substance rich in acid mucopolysaccharide. The epithelial lining is derived from enamel epithelium, which is nonkeratinized and a 2–4 cell thick layer of flat or cuboidal cells. There are islands of odontogenic epithelium and there may be foci of inflammatory infiltrate if infected.

They are treated based on patient age, site, and size of the cyst and likelihood of normal eruption of the involved tooth. The cyst is usually enucleated, with an extraction of the involved tooth if it is unlikely to be useful or if space required is insufficient. The tooth is preserved wherever possible, and if it is unlikely to be aligned after eruption, orthodontic treatments can be used. Decompression is

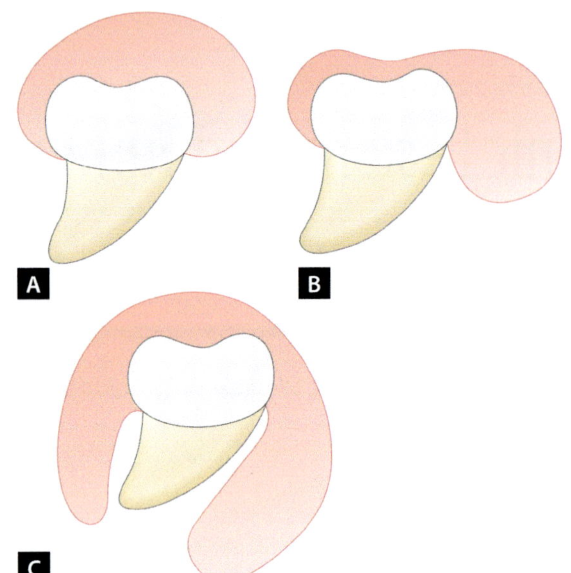

Figs. 1A to C: Radiologic types of dentigerous cyst: (A) Central; (B) Lateral; and (C) Circumferential.

used when there is a large cyst impinging on the inferior alveolar nerve.

Recurrence potential is low when managed appropriately.

Odontogenic Keratocyst

Formerly known as "primordial cyst," OKC arises from the primordial odontogenic epithelium. It is a clinically important entity as it has potential for recurrence after surgical treatment. Derived from dental lamina remnants or reduced enamel epithelium in the dental follicle, it commonly occurs in the angle of ascending ramus of the mandible. They commonly occur in the second and third decades of life. Often they are asymptomatic, growing to a large size before becoming apparently, or picked up on routine radiographs for other indications. Some patients can complain of jaw pain, swelling or discharge, especially in the background of fracture of infection. They may also report paresthesia of the lower lip or teeth or displaced eruption of teeth.[6-14] Rarely they may prevent with aggressive bony expansion and erosion, mimicking malignancy.[15-17] Gorlin–Goltz syndrome, an autosomal dominant disorder presents with multiple nevoid basal-cell carcinomas, OKC (65–75% of patients), congenital skeletal defects, palmar and plantar pits, central nervous system, and ocular defects. A thorough evaluation in addition to radiographs of the jaws, chest and skull, MRI brain and pelvic ultrasound in women is indicated.

Radiologically, lesions are round or ovoid with radiolucency and sclerotic margins. They can be unilocular or multilocular with scalloped margins occurring when there is uneven growth. Cortical plate expansion is unusual, with resorption and perforation commonly leading to fractures. Main postulated there are four radiological variants, envelopmental (embraces adjacent unerupted tooth), replacement (formed in place of a normal tooth), extraneous (arises in the ramus away from teeth), and collateral (adjacent to tooth roots).[18]

Histologically, the wall of the cyst is thin in the absence of inflammation. It is characteristic, with a parakeratinized corrugated or rippled appearance, a uniform thickened epithelium 6–10 cells thick. The basal layer is palisaded with a "tombstone" appearance.

Thorough evaluation and assessment is required before planning treatment. Factors affecting treatment decisions are age, size, location, symptomatology, soft tissue involvement, and if the lesion is recurrent. Enucleation and cryotherapy with liquid nitrogen showed good control rates over 2–10 years in modest cohorts.[19] Subsequent papers suggested that enucleation was sufficient with liquid nitrogen being required in high-risk lesion for recurrence or where complete enucleation was not feasible due to location or adjacent critical structures.[20] Stoelinga proposed a strategy based on the behavior patterns of OKC.[21] According to their publication, unilocular cysts in the mandible and maxilla require enucleation except for those in the ascending ramus (due to fracture risk). They proposed that all large posterior maxillary cysts should be considered OKC until proven otherwise. In addition to enucleation, Carnoy's solution can be used in the alveolar region but not within the maxillary sinus due to fear of necrosis of the maxillary sinus walls. They recommended incision biopsies for all multilocular lesions, with enucleation and excision of the overlying mucosa, followed by application of Carnoy's solution or electrocoagulation at the point of attachment of the cyst to the soft tissues. Marsupialization is not considered as a safe surgical procedure in these patients due to the high risk of recurrence. Although it is suspected that recurrence is more a result of incomplete removal than intrinsic growth in biology, recurrent lesions were found to have Ki-67 values in the epithelial lining twice as high as those with primary lesions, suggesting that genetic or biological factors may play a role in recurrence.[22] Although there are cases of malignancy arising within OKC, this is still considered as a rare occurrence.

Eruption Cyst

This is a dentigerous cyst occurring in the soft tissue, as opposed to around the crown of an unerupted tooth within the bone. In an eruption cyst, the tooth is impeded in the process of eruption into the soft tissue overlying the bone. These are more common in children than in adults,[23,24] commonly aged between 1–12 (mean 4.4) years. They are most commonly found in relation to the maxillary permanent dentition, and often present as a smooth swelling over an erupting tooth, which may have a bluish tinge. It is painful, soft, and fluctuant when infected.

Radiologically, it is seen as a soft tissue shadow with no bone involvement except for a dilated and open crypt.

Histologically, the cyst lining is 2–3 layers thick often with a few foci of irregular thickening when there is a history of inflammation. The gingival connective tissue is acellular with an eosinophilic hue, while the follicular connective tissue is more densely cellular with a basophilic hue.

These are commonly treated with marsupialization[25] with extraction of teeth only when required. When the cyst roof is excised exposing the crown, the tooth may proceed to erupt normally.

Lateral Periodontal Cyst

These arise in between teeth due to their origin from dental lamina rests within the inter-radicular crestal or midroot-level bone. They commonly occur in the mandible or maxilla around the premolars and canine areas. They occur in adults with a slight male preponderance. The adjacent teeth are often vital, nonmobile, and may have divergence of the roots without resorption. Soft tissue swelling does not occur commonly.[26]

Radiographically, these lesions present as round or tear-drop-shaped unilocular radiolucencies between teeth.

Histologically, they are lined by thin squamous epithelium of 2–3 layers thick resembling enamel epithelium with interspersed plaques. Clear cells may be seen within plaques. Cyst wall attachment to fibrous wall is tenuous.

The cyst is enucleated after raising a labial mucoperiosteal flap. A large defect after enucleation can be addressed with bone grafts or membranes that will allow bone healing and prevent soft tissue ingrowth [such as expanded polytetrafluoroethylene (ePTFE)].[27,28]

Botryoidal odontogenic cysts are a variety of these that are commonly polycystic, expansive, and have a high propensity for recurrence if not treated appropriately. They require careful and thorough excision and follow-up.

Calcifying Odontogenic Cyst[29-32]

First described by Gorlin,[33,34] it can occur both centrally and laterally in both the mandible and the maxilla. The canine-premolar region of the maxilla is commonly involved. They often present as swelling with little to no pain, or on routine radiographs. There may be bony expansion from intraosseous lesions. There may also be perforation of the cortical plate to involve soft tissues. Extraosseous lesions are pink-red, circumscribed and <4 cm in diameter.

Radiographically, lesions are radiolucent and unilocular with well-delineated borders with areas of opacity due to calcified material.

Histologically, the lining epithelium shows a basal layer of columnar cells, a thick overlying cellular layer and deposits of "ghost" epithelial cells that may be calcified.

They are managed with enucleation; conservative removal is often adequate. Recurrences are rare.

Radicular Cyst[35-37]

These are inflammatory cysts that arise from inflammatory foci within the epithelial residues of the periodontal ligament from periodontitis. They arise most commonly in the apices of involved teeth and can be left behind within the bone after removal of the offending tooth, when it is referred to as a residual cyst. They occur both in the maxilla and mandible within the tooth-bearing areas. They are often asymptomatic, enlarging in size slowly. Initially, the bony enlargement is hard but subsequently the covering bone thins out with characteristic "eggshell crackling."

Radiographically, they are round/oval lucencies with narrow opaque margins extending to the lamina dura of the underlying tooth.

Histologically, they are lined by stratified squamous epithelium. The lining can vary significantly in thickness. Characteristic of hyaline/Rushton's hyaline bodies is found in 10% of patients. Foci of inflammation are common, along with deposits of cholesterol crystals.

Treatment is often through an apicectomy, where the apex of the tooth and soft tissue are removed and replaced with a filling material. Small lesions may undergo resolution spontaneously after root canal treatments.

Glandular Odontogenic Cyst[38-40]

These are jaw cysts with mucinous glandular elements within them or complete glandular elements. Recent literature has described them as more aggressive lesions which often to grow to a larger size. There is also a lack on clarity as to the overlap between these lesions and low-grade mucoepidermoid carcinoma. They may represent a true cyst of glandular origin from trapped nests of salivary glands, a metaplastic differentiation to glandular epithelium, or a low-grade mucoepidermoid carcinoma arising within the cyst epithelium.

Radiologically, they have no pathognomonic features.

Histologically, these are often multilocular with epithelium of varying thickness with a bland interface between the epithelium and the connective tissue. The glandular epithelium is cuboidal to columnar with eosinophilic cytoplasm. Like periodontal cysts, they may have plaque-like thickening. Inflammatory components are unusual.

Treatment is by enucleation and curettage, however serial sectioning of the tumor is required to rule out a mucoepidermoid carcinoma. If malignancy is confirmed a wide excision with at least a 1-cm circumferential gross margin is recommended.

NONODONTOGENIC CYSTS[41-44]

Although involving continuous anatomical areas, these are not derived from embryonic dental elements.

- *Nasolabial cysts:* These arise in the soft tissue of the nasolabial fold, possibly arising from the embryonic remnants of the nasolacrimal duct. They cause swelling and can get infected and rupture. Radiologically, these are well delineated and arise lateral to the pyriform fossa, and on histology, these are lined by pseudostratified columnar epithelium. They need complete enucleation that can often be performed by a sublabial approach.
- *Nasopalatine duct cysts:* These arise from nasopalatine duct remnants in the lines of fusion of the embryonic facial processes. These present during adulthood and present as swellings in the premaxilla that can displace teeth. It is important to distinguish periapical lesions by testing the viability of the incisor teeth. Radiologically, they can appear as large lesions that extend intranasally and cause destruction of adjacent bone. They are treated with surgical enucleation.
- *Aneurysmal bone cysts:* Their presentation in the head and neck are similar to that elsewhere in the body (long bones and spine). They can involve both the maxilla and the mandible, and present as swelling and malocclusion. Swellings can be associated with sudden increase in size and painful in half of patients. A recent history of replacement of teeth may be noted. When the lesion perforated the cortex and is covered only by periosteum it may exhibit eggshell crackling. Temporomandibular joint capsule impingement may interfere with mouth opening. Radiographically, there is a characteristic "ballooning" growth pattern seen with a radiolucent area and "blown-out" cortical expansion. Histologically, there are capillaries and blood-filled spaces lined by spindle cells separated by fibrous tissue. Excision is by curettage but a quarter can recur.

ODONTOGENIC TUMORS (FIG. 2)

These are a group of cellular proliferations with highly variable biology and clinical behaviors. Regezi[45] proposed a biological classification of these tumors (**Table 1**).

Epithelial Odontogenic Tumors

Ameloblastoma[46-52]

First described by Malassez, this term was used to describe unicystic ameloblastomas that develops within the lining, lumen or wall of a cyst, and invasive ameloblastomas. They arise from odontogenic epithelial remnants such as dental lamina rests of Serres and Malassez. As they are neoplastic lesions, they are able to invade and resorb bone, overcome the confines of bone, and invade surrounding soft tissue. This is unlike OKC, which invade bone but do not involve soft tissue. Rather than an individual tumor, these are a group of tumors that are described under the following headings:

- *Ameloblastoma in situ and microinvasive ameloblastoma:* These arise within the lining or within the lumen of a dentigerous cyst. Initially the lesion may involve a focal area of the cyst wall (mural). If it grows to involve only the cyst wall, it is referred to as intraluminal, while if it grows down into connective tissue, it is referred to as transmural. When it involves the connective tissue in the form islands or strands, it is referred to as microinvasive. When it involves the underlying bone, it is overtly invasive.
- *Invasive ameloblastoma:* This is considered to be the prototype of a benign odontogenic neoplasm and will result in progressive bone destruction if untreated. It is common in all ages, more common in the second and third decades of life. The mandible is involved in three quarters of patients with the third molar region of the mandible, which is the most common site of occurrence. Common symptoms are bony swelling and resultant facial asymmetry. Pain is an occasional feature.

  Radiologically, these are expansile radiolucencies that are uni- or multilocular with well-demarcated borders. There can be displacement of the inferior alveolar canal inferiorly and the sinus membrane

Tumor ameloblastoma

Intraosseous

Epithelial origin

Mural ameloblastoma in situ

Transmural

Intraluminal

Invasive

Normal odontogenesis

Epithelial cap

Stellate reticulum

Ameloblasts

Adenomatoid odontogenic tumor or cyst

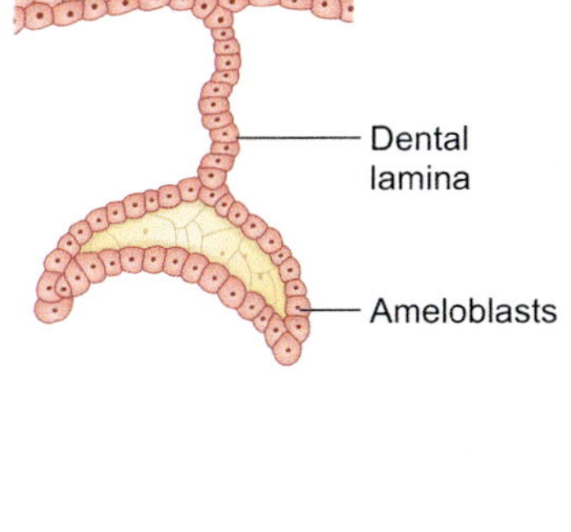

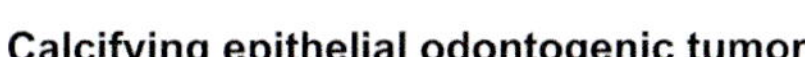

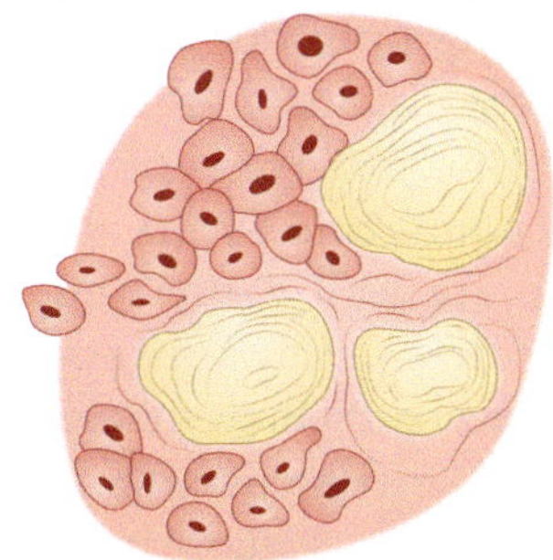

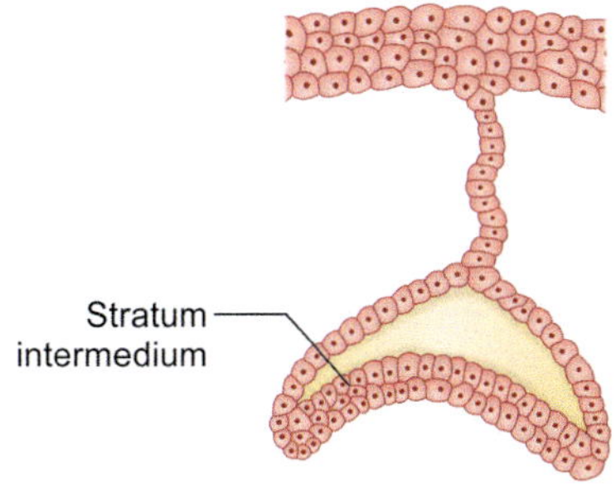

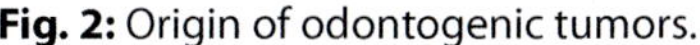

Fig. 2: Origin of odontogenic tumors.

Table 1: Biological classification of tumors.

Benign with no recurrence potential	*Benign with some recurrence potential*	*Benign with high recurrence potential*	*Malignant*
Squamous odontogenic tumor	Unicystic ameloblastoma	Ameloblastoma	Malignant ameloblastoma
Adenomatoid odontogenic tumor	Calcifying epithelial odontogenic tumor	Clear cell odontogenic tumor	Ameloblastic carcinoma
Cementoblastoma	Central odontogenic fibroma	Odontogenic ghost cell tumor	Primary intraosseous carcinoma
Odontoma	Ameloblastic fibroma and fibro-odontoma	Odontogenic myxoma	Odontogenic ghost cell carcinoma
Periapical cemento-osseous dysplasia		Odontoameloblastoma	Ameloblastic fibrosarcoma

superiorly toward the orbit. Mixed lucency is seen in a quarter of desmoplastic ameloblastomas.

Histologically, there are six subtypes of ameloblastoma: acanthomatous, basal cell, desmoplastic, follicular, granular cell, and plexiform. Follicular is the most common pattern. There are epithelial islands that are interspersed with collagenous fibrous stroma. Squamous metaplasia is not uncommon. Cystic degeneration is not uncommon. Plexiform ameloblastoma have epithelial proliferation in a network of anastomosing strands. Basal cell pattern refers to the presence of basaloid cells in a fibrous stroma. Pathological variants have an impact on recurrence rates; follicular type, plexiform and acanthomatous have recurrence rates of 29.5%, 16.7%, and 4.5%, respectively.

Curative intent resection requires bony resection with 1–1.5 cm bony margins and an uninvolved anatomical barrier. Enucleation and curettage is suitable only to palliate symptoms.

Prognosis is good in adequately resected (control rates 98% and higher). Curettage can result in recurrence in 15–30%.

- *Peripheral ameloblastomas:* These are a variant of invasive ameloblastoma that have the histological appearance of intraosseous ameloblastoma but occur within the soft tissues overlying the tooth-bearing regions of the jaws. It is considered more of a hamartoma than a true neoplasm. They present in the fifth and sixth decades of life as swelling associated with but not invading the bone. It may be associated with HPV infection, however, this is not firmly established. They are treated with complete excision with at least 2–3 mm margins. There is believed to be a higher risk of malignant transformation to ameloblastic carcinoma.
- *Desmoplastic ameloblastoma:* This is another variety of invasive ameloblastoma with distinct histopathological and radiographic features. Radiographically, it has mixed radiolucent-radiopaque lesions. Histologically, they have thickened bony trabeculae and dense scar-like fibroblastic stroma, occasionally with well-developed islands like in follicular pattern lesions. They are managed like other invasive ameloblastomas.

Odontoameloblastoma[53-55]

This is a rare tumor that represents an invasive ameloblastoma with elements of an odontoma. It presents as a painless jaw tumor that is multilocular with mixed lucency. The odontoma component is denser than bone. Histology is similar to ameloblastoma with formation of dentin and enamel. Resection is with 1–1.5 cm bony margins and one uninvolved anatomical barrier.

Calcifying Epithelial Odontogenic Tumor[56-58]

Calcifying epithelial odontogenic tumor (CEOT) is an unusual neoplasm with biologic aggression lying on a spectrum between mildly invasive and invasive disease. It is believed to arise from the stratum intermedium of the enamel. It is common in the fourth decade of life and presents as a hard expansile mass that is commonly painless. Mandible involvement is more common. Radiologically, the tumor is completely lucent initially, commonly developing mixed lucency as it progresses. A "soap bubble" appearance is common in multilocular disease. Lesions may also be heavily calcified, appearing denser than adjacent bone. Borders of the lesion may be sclerotic with the bone-tumor interface being ill or well defined. Histologically, they are unencapsulated infiltrating tumors with distinct epithelial components comprising sheets and islands of polygonal cells. Concentric calcification is common, in the form of Liesegang rings. Stromal cells have homogeneous eosinophilic deposits. Treatment is by resection with 1–1.5 cm margins and one uninvolved anatomical barrier.

Squamous Odontogenic Tumor[59-61]

This is considered as a hamartomatous proliferation of epithelial cells arising from the rests of Malassez. It presents as a painless expansion of alveolar process with displacement, loosening of root resorption of teeth. It presents in adults and favors the mandible. Radiologically, these are well-delineated unilocular radiolucencies. Histology shows islands of well-differentiation squamous epithelium that are bland and uniform. Keratinized cells may be present. Stroma shows collagenous fibrous tissue. Enucleation and curettage are sufficient treatment, however, up to 20% develop new lesions in other locations.

Odontogenic Carcinomas[62-64]

These are epithelial malignancies that arise from odontogenic epithelium with varying levels of undifferentiation due to genetic alterations.

- *Primary intraosseous carcinoma ex odontogenic cysts:* These represent a malignant transformation of an underlying odontogenic cyst, which is determined on the final histology. These are common in patients over 50. This entity should be considered when an older patient develops an expanded follicle or radiolucency on the background of a residual impacted tooth. Histologically, it is an odontogenic cyst where there invasive malignancy has developed within the cyst lining. It has a potential for lymphatic spread and distant metastases and needs appropriate staging and management, similar to oral squamous cell carcinoma.

- *Primary intraosseous carcinoma de novo:* These are clinically aggressive lesions that present with radiologically destructive bone lucencies and irregularity of the adjacent bone. There may be varying degrees of tooth root absorption. Paresthesia and anesthesia are common. Histology shows an epithelial malignancy with no underlying component of odontogenic cyst or mucosa. Histology may be similar to ameloblastic carcinoma.
- *Malignant ameloblastomas:* This refers to a benign ameloblastoma with characteristic root resorption but with a concomitant metastatic focus as determined by focused imaging, with or without histology. Although the primary tumor is in itself benign, there is metastasis to lymph nodes or to distant sites such as lungs through vascular invasion, spread and seeding, to form an independent colony with its own histological appearance, growth rate and biology. Treatment is by surgical excision; thoracoscopic resection of lung metastases wherever feasible is preferred.
- *Ameloblastic carcinomas:* These are malignant tumors with marked cytological atypia of the primary site and is associated with local and regional metastasis (they do not need distant metastasis to establish the diagnosis unlike malignant ameloblastoma). These often present like advanced malignant tumors, with large masses of the jaw with loosening of teeth, soft tissue ulceration, and bone resorption. Histology showed marked features of malignancy, on a background of ameloblastoma features. Hypercellularity, cellular atypia, and mitosis are common. Prognosis is often guarded as they are aggressive with distant metastatic potential. Treatment requires wide excision with 2–3 cm margins due to extensive soft tissue involvement; more information on "adequacy" of margins is unavailable. Neck dissection and adjuvant radiotherapy are often indicated. Chemotherapy is administered for metastatic disease; effective agents have been shown to be cyclophosphamide, methotrexate, 5-fluorouracil, vinblastine, cisplatin, bleomycin, adriamycin, and paclitaxel in varying combinations.[65]

Mesenchymal Odontogenic Tumors

- *Odontogenic myxomas:*[66,67] These are benign neoplasms that are similar to ameloblastoma however they arise from the mesenchymal odontogenic elements. They can arise at any age, commonly during adolescence. They often present either as slow growing asymptomatic lesions but can result in pain, displacement and loss of teeth. They are often distributed evenly in both jaws. Radiologically, they present as multilocular "honeycombed" lucencies. Histologically, they are unencapsulated gelatinous tumors with scanty cellularity and indistinct borders. They seem to arise from fibroblasts and stroma is rich in mucopolysaccharides. Inactive rests of odontogenic epithelium may be seen. Curative treatment is by resection with 1–1.5 cm margins. Enucleation and curettage have high recurrence rates and are suitable only as palliative efforts.
- *Cemetoblastomas:*[68-70] These are a hamartomatous proliferation of cementoblasts resulting in disordered growth of cementum around the apical tooth root. They are generally hard expansions of the premolar or molar regions of either jaw with intact overlying soft tissues seen in adolescent and young adults. There may be dull aching pain from bone expansion. Radiologically, these are spherical, radiopaque masses that replace the apices of tooth roots. Histologically, they have a thin fibrous capsule that is in continuation with the periodontal membrane. The tumor has sheets of cementum-like material with vascular supportive stroma. Removal of the lesion with the offending tooth prevents recurrence.
- *Odontogenic fibroma:*[71,72] This is a rare lesion arising from odontogenic mesenchyme. The prototype is the central odontogenic fibroma. It results in a painless expansion that result in displacement or resorption of tooth roots. Radiologically, it presents as unilocular or multilocular radiolucent lesions with well-delineated margins. Histologically, there are two patterns; the first has delicate fibrous tissue with varying amounts of collagen, while the second is well-demarcated and encapsulated with cellular fibrous tissue and myxoid areas. Cementum-like material may be present. Treatment is by enucleation and curettage, bony invasion does not generally occur. Peripheral odontogenic fibromas arise from the periodontal membrane and they do not have bony erosion. They can be excised without bony resection.

Mixed Epithelial and Mesenchymal Odontogenic Tumors (Table 2)

- *Ameloblastic fibromas:*[73-75] These behave as hamartomas or true neoplasms, arising from the epithelium of the enamel and mesenchymal components of the dental pulp. They can present in childhood as

Table 2: Differential diagnosis of odontogenic lesions based on radiological appearance.

Unilocular inter-radicular radiolucency	• Radicular cyst • Lateral periodontal cyst • Adenomatoid odontogenic tumor • Ameloblastoma • CEOT • Squamous odontogenic tumor
Unilocular radiolucency around crown of impacted tooth	• Dentigerous cyst • Ameloblastoma • CEOT • Squamous odontogenic tumor
Unilocular or multilocular radiolucency	• Glandular odontogenic cyst • Keratocystic odontogenic tumor • Central giant cell lesion • Ameloblastoma • Squamous odontogenic tumor
Unilocular radiolucency periapical or lateral root	• Radicular cyst • Central odontogenic fibroma • Squamous odontogenic tumor
Ill-defined angular radiolucency	• Langerhans cell histiocytosis • Squamous odontogenic tumor
Unilocular radiolucency in edentulous area	• Residual cyst • Ameloblastoma • Keratocystic odontogenic tumor
Ill-defined radiolucency involving tooth roots	• Plasmacytoma • Multiple myeloma • Keratocystic odontogenic tumor

(CEOT: calcifying epithelial odontogenic tumor)

a painless jaw expansion. Radiologically, they are radiolucent with well-demarcated borders. They may be associated with impacted teeth. Histologically, there are clear epithelial and mesenchymal components. Treatment is with through enucleation and curettage. Regeneration of the bone within the cavity almost always occurs when removed in children.

- *Adenomatoid odontogenic fibromas:*[76,77] They account for 3–7% of odontogenic tumors and are believed to arise from remnants of the dental lamina. They are common between 10 and 20 years of age. Pericoronal lesions present early as the concerned tooth fails to erupt. Extraosseous lesions can also present as gingival lesions, which have a striking female preponderance (14:1). Most central lesions are identified incidentally on radiographs but they can also present as swelling. Radiographically, these appear as intraosseous well-demarcated radiolucent lesions. Pericoronal lesions may have radiolucency extend beyond the cement-enamel junction. Histologically, there are multinodular proliferations of spindle, cuboidal and columnar cells with duct-like elements and a fibrous capsule. Complete surgical excision through enucleation and curettage is the treatment of choice.

CONCLUSION

Odontogenic lesions although rare can present in a variety of ways. A systematic approach to diagnosis with expertise and specialized knowledge in radiology and pathology is needed for appropriate management. Identifying malignancy is a crucial; benign lesions often require a step-by-step approach to limit treatment-related morbidity.

REFERENCES

1. Chapelle KA, Stoelinga PJ, de Wilde PC, Brouns JJ, Voorsmit RA. Rational approach to diagnosis and treatment of ameloblastomas and odontogenic keratocysts. Br J Oral Maxillofac Surg. 2004;42:381-90.
2. Stoelinga PJ, Bronkhorst FB. The incidence, multiple presentation and recurrence of aggressive cysts of the jaws. J Craniomaxillofac Surg. 1988;16:184-95.
3. Lustmann J, Bodner L. Dentigerous cysts associated with supernumerary teeth. Int J Oral Maxillofac Surg. 1988;17:100-2.
4. Jones AV, Craig GT, Franklin CD. Range and demographics of odontogenic cysts diagnosed in a UK population over a 30-year period. J Oral Pathol Med. 2006;35:500-7.
5. Kaugars GE, Miller ME, Abbey LM. Odontomas. Oral Surg Oral Med Oral Pathol. 1989;67:172-6.
6. Robinson HB. Classification of cysts of the jaws. Am J Orthodont Oral Surg. 1945;31:A370-5.
7. Philipsen HP. Keratocystic odontogenic tumour. In: Barnes L, Eveson JW, Reichart P, Sidransky D (Eds). WHO Classification of Tumours, Pathology and Genetics of Head and Neck Tumours. Lyon: IARC; 2005. pp. 306-7.
8. Reichart PA, Philipsen HP. Aneurysmal bone cavity (cyst). In: Reichart PA, Philipsen HP (Eds). Odontogenic Tumors and Allied Lesions. Germany: Quintessence Publishing; 2004. pp. 335-41.
9. Pogrel MA. The keratocystic odontogenic tumour (KCOT)—an odyssey. Int J Oral Maxillofac Surg. 2015;44:1565-8.
10. Pindborg JJ, Philipsen HP, Henriksen J. Studies on odontogenic cyst epithelium. In: Butcher EO, Sognnaes RF (Eds). Fundamentals of Keratinization. Washington, D.C.: American Association for the Advancement of Science; 1962. pp. 151-60.
11. Pindborg JJ, Hansen J. Studies on odontogenic cyst epithelium: 2. Clinical and roentgenologic aspects of odontogenic keratocysts. Acta Pathologica Microbiologica Scandinavica. 1963;58:283-94.
12. Pindborg JJ, Kramer JR, Torloni H. Histological Typing of Odontogenic Tumours, Jaw Cysts, and Allied Lesions. Geneva: World Health Organization; 1971. pp. 1-44.
13. Shear M, Speight PM. Cysts of the Oral and Maxillofacial Regions, 4th edition. New York: John Wiley and Sons; 2008.
14. Shear M, Altini M. The possible inductive role of ectomesenchyme in the pathogenesis of some odontogenic lesions. J Dent Assoc S Afr. 1976;31:749-54.
15. Partridge M, Towers JF. The primordial cyst (odontogenic keratocyst): its tumour-like characteristics and behaviour. Br J Oral Maxillofac Surg. 1987;25:271-9.
16. Jackson IT, Potparic Z, Fasching M, Schievink WI, Tidstrom K, Hussain K. Penetration of the skull base by dissecting keratocyst. J Craniomaxillofac Surg. 1993;21:319-25.
17. Rippin JW, Woolgar JA. The odontogenic keratocyst in BCNS and non-syndrome patients. In: Browne RM (Ed).

Investigative Pathology of Odontogenic Cysts. Boca Raton, Fl: CRC Press; 1991. pp. 212-32.
18. Main DM. Epithelial jaw cysts: a clinicopathological reappraisal. Br J Oral Maxillofac Surg. 1970;8(2):114-25.
19. Schmidt BL, Pogrel MA. The use of enucleation and liquid nitrogen cryotherapy in the management of odontogenic keratocysts. J Oral Maxillofac Surg. 2001;59(7):720-5.
20. Schmidt BL. The use of liquid nitrogen cryotherapy in the management of the odontogenic keratocyst. Oral Maxillofac Surg Clin. 2003;15(3):393-405.
21. Stoelinga PJ. Excision of the overlying, attached mucosa, in conjunction with cyst enucleation and treatment of the bony defect with carnoy solution. Oral Maxillofac Surg Clin. 2003;15(3):407-14.
22. Li TJ, Browne RM, Matthews JB. Epithelial cell proliferation in odontogenic keratocysts: a comparative immunocytochemical study of Ki67 in simple, recurrent and basal cell naevus syndrome (BCNS)-associated lesions. J Oral Pathol Med. 1995;24(5):221-6.
23. Bodner L. Cystic lesions of the jaws in children. Int J Pediatr Otorhinolaryngol. 2002;62(1):25-9.
24. Aguiló L, Cibrián R, Bagán JV, Gandía JL. Eruption cysts: retrospective clinical study of 36 cases. ASDC J Dent Child. 1998;65(2):102-6.
25. Woldenberg Y, Goldstein J, Bodner L. Eruption cyst in the adult—a case report. Int J Oral Maxillofac Surg. 2004;33(8):804-5.
26. Altini M, Shear M. The lateral periodontal cyst: an update. J Oral Pathol Med. 1992;21(6):245-50.
27. Rasmusson LG, Magnusson BC, Borrman H. The lateral periodontal cyst. A histopathological and radiographic study of 32 cases. Br J Oral Maxillofac Surg. 1991;29(1):54-7.
28. Kerezoudis NP, Donta-Bakoyianni C, Siskos G. The lateral periodontal cyst: aetiology, clinical significance and diagnosis. Endod Dent Traumatol. 2000;16(4):144-50.
29. Prætorius F, Hjørting-Hansen E, Gorlin RJ, Vickers RA. Calcifying odontogenic cyst: range, variations and neoplastic potential. Acta Odontologica Scandinavica. 1981;39(4):227-40.
30. Prætorius F, Ledesma-Montes C. Calcifying cystic odontogenic tumour. In: Barnes L, Eveson JW, Reichart P, Sidransky D (Eds). Pathology and Genetics. Head and Neck Tumours. Lyon: World Health Organization Classification of Tumours, IARC Press; 2005. p. 313.
31. Fejerskov O, Krogh J. The calcifying ghost cell odontogenic tumor-or the calcifying odontogenic cyst. J Oral Pathol. 1972;1(6):273-87.
32. Li TJ, Yu SF. Clinicopathologic spectrum of the so-called calcifying odontogenic cysts: a study of 21 intraosseous cases with reconsideration of the terminology and classification. Am J Surg Pathol. 2003;27(3):372-84.
33. Gorlin RJ, Pindborg JJ, Odont, Clausen FP, Vickers RA. The calcifying odontogenic cyst—a possible analogue of the cutaneous calcifying epithelioma of Malherbe. An analysis of fifteen cases. Oral Surg Oral Med Oral Pathol. 1962;15(10):1235-43.
34. Gorlin RJ, Pindborg JJ, Redman RS, Williamson JJ, Hansen LS. The calcifying odontogenic cyst. A new entity and possible analogue of the cutaneous calcifying epithelioma of Malherbe. Cancer. 1964;17(6):723-9.
35. Brave D, Madhusudan AS, Ramesh G, Brave VR. Radicular cyst of anterior maxilla. Int J Dent Clin. 2011;3(2):16-7.
36. Trope M, Pettigrew J, Petras J, Barnett F, Tronstad L. Differentiation of radicular cyst and granulomas using computerized tomography. Endod Dent Traumatol. 1989;5(2): 69-72.
37. Lustmann J, Shear M. Radicular cysts arising from deciduous teeth: Review of the literature and report of 23 cases. Int J Oral Surg. 1985;14(2):153-61.
38. Gardner DG, Kessler HP, Morency R, Schaffner DL. The glandular odontogenic cyst: an apparent entity. J Oral Pathol. 1988;17(8):359-66.
39. Kaplan I, Gal G, Anavi Y, Manor R, Calderon S. Glandular odontogenic cyst: treatment and recurrence. J Oral Maxillofac Surg. 2005;63(4):435-41.
40. Hussain K, Edmondson HD, Browne RM. Glandular odontogenic cysts: diagnosis and treatment. Oral Surg Oral Med Oral Pathol Oral Radiol Endod. 1995;79(5):593-602.
41. Kransdorf MJ, Sweet DE. Aneurysmal bone cyst: concept, controversy, clinical presentation, and imaging. Am J Roentgenol. 1995;164(3):573-80.
42. Jaffe HL, Lichtenstein L. Solitary unicameral bone cyst: with emphasis on the roentgen picture, the pathologic appearance and the pathogenesis. Arch Surg. 1942;44(6):1004-25.
43. Lysell L, Molin L. Tomography in diagnosis of incisive canal cysts. Sven Tandlak Tidskr. 1972;65(6):321-6.
44. de Redaelli Zinis LO, Mortini P, Farina D, Mossi F. Expansile lesions arising from structures and spaces adjacent to the paranasal sinuses. In: Maroldi R, Nicolai P (Eds). Imaging in Treatment Planning for Sinonasal Diseases. Berlin, Heidelberg: Springer; 2005. pp. 221-54.
45. Regezi JA. Odontogenic cysts, odontogenic tumors, fibro-osseous, and giant cell lesions of the jaws. Mod Pathol. 2002;15(3):331-41.
46. Eversole LR, Leider AS, Hansen LS. Ameloblastomas with pronounced desmoplasia. J Oral Maxillofac Surg. 1984;42(11): 735-40.
47. Reichart PA, Philipsen HP. Odontogenic Tumors and Allied Lesions. London: Quintessence Publishing; 2004.
48. Kahn MA. Ameloblastoma in young persons: a clinicopathologic analysis and etiologic investigation. Oral Surg Oral Med Oral Pathol. 1989;67(6):706-15.
49. Baden E, Doyle JL, Petriella V. Malignant transformation of peripheral ameloblastoma. Oral Surg Oral Med Oral Pathol. 1993;75(2):214-9.
50. Reichart PA, Philipsen HP, Sonner S. Ameloblastoma: biological profile of 3677 cases. Eur J Cancer B Oral Oncol. 1995;31(2):86-99.
51. Sehdev MK, Huvos AG, Strong EW, Gerold FP, Willis GW. Ameloblastoma of maxilla and mandible. Cancer. 1974;33(2): 324-33.
52. Ghandhi D, Ayoub AF, Pogrel MA, MacDonald G, Brocklebank LM, Moos KF. Ameloblastoma: a surgeon's dilemma. J Oral Maxillofac Surg. 2006;64(7):1010-4.
53. Gupta DS, Gupta MK. Odontoameloblastoma. J Oral Maxillofac Surg. 1986;44(2):146-8.
54. Mosqueda-Taylor A, Carlos-Bregni R, Ramírez-Amador V, Palma-Guzmán JM, Esquivel-Bonilla D, Hernández-Rojas LA. Odontoameloblastoma. Clinico-pathologic study of three cases and critical review of the literature. Oral Oncol. 2002;38(8):800-5.
55. Dive A, Khandekar S, Bodhade A, Dhobley A. Odontoameloblastoma. J Oral Maxillofac Pathol. 2011;15(1):60-4.
56. Franklin CD, Pindborg JJ. The calcifying epithelial odontogenic tumor: a review and analysis of 113 cases. Oral Surg Oral Med Oral Pathol. 1976;42(6):753-65.
57. Houston GD, Fowler CB. Extraosseous calcifying epithelial odontogenic tumor: report of two cases and review of the literature. Oral Surg Oral Med Oral Pathol Oral Radiol Endod. 1997;83(5):577-83.

58. Pindborg JJ. A calcifying epithelial odontogenic tumor. Cancer. 1958;11(4):838-43.
59. Pullon PA, Shafer WG, Elzay RP, Kerr DA, Corio RL. Squamous odontogenic tumor: report of six cases of a previously undescribed lesion. Oral Surg Oral Med Oral Pathol. 1975; 40(5):616-30.
60. Leventon GS, Happonen RP, Newland JR. Squamous odontogenic tumor. Am J Surg Pathol. 1981;5(7):671-7.
61. Philipsen HP, Reichart PA. Squamous odontogenic tumor (SOT): a benign neoplasm of the periodontium: a review of 36 reported cases. J Clin Periodontol. 1996;23(10):922-6.
62. Elzay RP. Primary intraosseous carcinoma of the jaws: review and update of odontogenic carcinomas. Oral Surg Oral Med Oral Pathol. 1982;54(3):299-303.
63. Eversole LR. Malignant epithelial odontogenic tumors. Semin Diagn Pathol. 1999;16(4):317-24
64. Scheer M, Koch AM, Drebber U, Kübler AC. Primary intraosseous carcinoma of the jaws arising from an odontogenic cyst—a case report. J Craniomaxillofac Surg. 2004;32(3):166-9.
65. Amzerin M, Fadoukhair Z, Belbaraka R, Iraqui M, Boutayeb S, M'rabti H, et al. Metastatic ameloblastoma responding to combination chemotherapy: case report and review of the literature. J Med Case Rep. 2011;5(1):491.
66. Chi AC, Neville BW. Odontogenic cysts and tumors. Surg Pathol Clin. 2011;4(4):1027-91.
67. Gupta S, Grover N, Kadam A, Gupta S, Sah K, Sunitha JD. Odontogenic myxoma. Natl J Maxillofac Surg. 2013;4(1):81-3.
68. Huber AR, Folk GS. Cementoblastoma. Head Neck Pathol. 2009;3(2):133-5.
69. Slootweg PJ. Cementoblastoma and osteoblastoma: a comparison of histologic features. J Oral Pathol Med. 1992;21(9): 385-9.
70. Sankari LS, Ramakrishnan K. Benign cementoblastoma. J Oral Maxillofac Pathol. 2011;15(3):358-60.
71. Gardner DG. Central odontogenic fibroma current concepts. J Oral Pathol Med. 1996;25(10):556-61.
72. Kaffe I, Buchner A. Radiologic features of central odontogenic fibroma. Oral Surg Oral Med Oral Pathol. 1994;78(6): 811-8.
73. Takeda Y. Ameloblastic fibroma and related lesions: current pathologic concept. Oral Oncol. 1999;35(6):535-40.
74. Kobayashi K, Murakami R, Fujii T, Hirano A. Malignant transformation of ameloblastic fibroma to ameloblastic fibrosarcoma: case report and review of the literature. J Craniomaxillofac Surg. 2005;33(5):352-5.
75. Nelson BL, Folk GS. Ameloblastic fibroma. Head Neck Pathol. 2009;3(1):51-3.
76. Ladeinde AL, Ajayi OF, Ogunlewe MO, Adeyemo WL, Arotiba GT, Bamgbose BO, et al. Odontogenic tumors: a review of 319 cases in a Nigerian teaching hospital. Oral Surg Oral Med Oral Pathol Oral Radiol Endod. 2005;99(2):191-5.
77. Olgac V, Koseoglu BG, Aksakallı N. Odontogenic tumours in Istanbul: 527 cases. Br J Oral Maxillofac Surg. 2006;44(5): 386-8.

CHAPTER 36

Vascular Malformations of the Head and Neck

Radhika Kapahtia, Sivakumar Vidhyadharan, Narayana Subramaniam, Samskruthi P Murthy

INTRODUCTION

Vascular lesions are among the most common congenital and neonatal abnormalities, and can be divided into tumors [vascular tumors (VT)] or malformations [venous malformation (VM)]. VM are defined by proliferating endothelium and have a more indolent course. VM include capillary malformation (CM), VM, lymphatic malformation (LM), arteriovenous malformation (AVM), and their combinations. VMs are more common, accounting for 65% of anomalies. AVMs occur in both genders with an equal incidence. Around half of AVMs are identified at birth, with another third presenting in early childhood.[1] About two-thirds of VMs occur in the head and the neck region and are often difficult to manage due to anatomical complexity. A comprehensive understanding of etiology, classification, and management results is crucial for appropriate management and good outcomes.[2]

CLASSIFICATION

Virchow first described vascular lesions in 1863 based on their microscopic appearance. Since then there have been multiple modifications to the classifications, with the most widely accepted classification, currently the International Society for the Study of Vascular Anomalies (ISSVA) classification (**Table 1**). This made significant progress in removing the confusion in etiology and taxonomy.[3,4]

The terms "congenital" and "acquired" should be used with caution in describing vascular anomalies. Congenital should be restricted to a vascular lesion that is completely expressed at birth. Hemangioma can be nascent or fully grown in a neonate. Vascular malformations, although present at birth at a cellular level, may not manifest until childhood or in adult life. "Acquired" is often a term used for cutaneous lesions that appear after 1 year of life, and is inappropriate for a vascular anomaly that is present but not clinically apparent at birth.[5]

VASCULAR TUMORS

Infantile Hemangioma

This is a benign endothelial tumor which is associated with an early and rapid growth pattern followed by regression and no risk of recurrence. It is believed that infantile hemangioma (IH) arises from vascular progenitor cells rather than through angiogenesis.[6] The precursor cell has been identified as a multipotent hemangioma-derived stem cell (HemSC), which is a mesenchymal cell marker expressing CD90.[7] They have also been shown to express glucose transporter 1 (GLUT1) receptors and are believed to respond to hypoxia.[6] The exact mechanism by which IH regress is not understood and may be apoptosis resulting from falling levels of maternal estrogens after birth.[8]

Clinically, they are common in the Caucasian population, occurring in 4–5% of infants, and are more frequent in premature and female infants.[9,10] Head and neck are the sites of involvement in two-thirds of cases and most of these are solitary.[11] These lesions often present within the first 2 weeks of life, with about 10% causing resultant deformity; they may cause ulceration of the eyelid, lip/nose/scalp, brow involvement can result in alopecia, subglottic involvement can cause stenosis, and periorbital or corneal involvement can disrupt vision.[12]

There are three stages in the life cycle of IH which are as follows:

1. *Proliferating phase:* This is in the first years of life with maximum growth in the first 9 months of life. Involvement of the superficial dermis results in reddish lesions; as they grow larger, they appear bluish.

Table 1: International Society for the Study of Vascular Anomalies (ISSVA) classification of vascular malformations.

	Malformations	
Tumors	*Slow flow*	*High flow*
1. *Infantile hemangioma (IH)* 2. *Congenital hemangioma (CH)* – Rapidly involuting infantile hemangioma (RICH) – Noninvoluting infantile hemangioma (NICH) 3. *Hemangioendotheliomas* – Kaposiform hemangioendothelioma (KHE) – Others 4. *Pyogenic granuloma (PG)*	*Capillary malformation*	*Arterial malformation:* • Aneurysm • Atresia • Ectasia • Stenosis
	Lymphatic malformation: • Microcystic • Macrocystic • Primary lymphedema	*Arteriovenous malformation:* • Capillary malformation arteriovenous malformation • Hereditary hemorrhagic telangiectasia • PTEN-associated vascular anomaly
	Venous malformation: • Cerebral cavernous malformation (CCM) • Cutaneomucosal venous malformation (CMVM) • Glomuvenous malformation (GVM) • Verrucous hemangioma (VH)	*Combined malformation:* • CCM • CMVM • GVM • VH
	Combined malformations: • Capillary venous malformation (CVM) • Capillary lymphatic malformation (CLM) • Capillary lymphatic venous malformation (CLVM) • Lymphatic venous malformation (LVM)	

(PTEN: phosphatase and tensin homolog)

Histologically, plump endothelial cells are identified with vascular channels and connective tissue elements.[13,14]

2. *Involuting phase:* This occurs from 1 to 4 years of life. By the beginning of this phase, the growth has reached a plateau, with the lesions flattening and color fading. Histologically, the endothelial cells flatten out and the blood vessels appear mature, with deposition of pericytes and connective tissue.[15,16]
3. *Involuted phase*: This occurs after 4 years of age, with half of the patients resulting in deformity with scarring, residual telangiectasia, and skin redundancy. Histologically, the vascular tissue is replaced with connective tissue components and adipose.[16]

Around 2% of IH are associated with PHACES (posterior fossa brain malformations. hemangioma, arterial cerebrovascular anomalies, coarctation of the aorta and cardiac defects, eye or endocrine abnormalities or sternal defects). This predisposes to stroke in infancy and MRI (magnetic resonance imaging) should be performed to rule this out.[17]

Diagnosis is commonly established by the history and examination findings. Color Doppler shows fast flow and ultrasound shows a soft tissue mass and increased venous outflow.[18] MRI shows a tumor that is isointense on T1, hyperintense of T2 during the proliferating phase, with replacement of vascular tissue with adipose tissue during involution **(Table 2)**. Biopsy shows a characteristic appearance as described before, with GLUT1 immunohistochemistry specific for these lesions.[19]

Treatment options: Nonoperative management options are observation (appropriate in as many as 90%), conservative wound care, intralesional corticosteroid (3 mg/kg which results in shrinkage in three quarters of patients), and systemic therapy (propranolol, prednisolone, vincristine, and interferon). Pulsed dye laser is used to remove residual pigmented lesions.[20-26]

Surgical intervention is reserved for failure of pharmacotherapy, well-localized tumors in anatomically favorable areas or if surgical excision is likely to be unavoidable.[27,28] Circular lesions in cosmetically important areas are managed with circular excision and purse-string closure, which results in better scarring.[29] Lenticular excision results in a linear scar but is associated with better scarring in the lips and eyelids.

Congenital Hemangiomas

These are hemangiomas that develop in utero and do not progress after delivery. They typically look red and violaceous with areas of coarse telangiectasia, a pallor in the center of the lesion and peripherally. These are relatively rarer in the head and neck when compared to IH. These are two forms commonly identified,

Table 2: Characteristics of vascular malformations.

Vascular malformations	*Presentation*	*MR imaging characteristics*	*Additional helpful imaging characteristics*
Capillary	Cutaneous lesions that often follow a dermal pattern	• Limited utility of imaging • Can be used to exclude complicating components not obvious on physical examination • Additional imaging can be performed if a syndrome is suspected	
Macrocystic lymphatic	• Present at birth or by 2 years of age • Soft large translucent nontender mass	Complex multioculated cystic mass with fluid-fluid levels. Cysts typically larger than >2 cm. Enhancement of the walls and septa on post-contrast imaging	US: large cystic structures without internal vascularity
Microcystic lymphatic	• Present at birth or by 2 years of age • Grow slowly in proportion to growing child • May appear as several small, raised sacs on the skin	Transpatial T1 hypointense T2 hyperintense lesion with multiple small cysts typically less than 2 cm. No enhancement	
Venous	• Most common type of vascular malformation. Slow flow vascular malformation presents as a non-pulsatile compressible soft tissue prominence or discrete mass typically with blueish-purple hue • Often tracking along muscle groups or nerves. These are responsive to changes in flow, i.e., Valsalva	• T2 hyperintense serpiginous tubules that enhance on delayed phase • T2 hypointense focal phleboliths	CT: serpiginous lesions that enhance on postcontrast imaging. More sensitive for phlebolith identification
Venolymphatic	• Present with characteristics of both lymphatic and venous malformation • Classically soft nontender mass can have a blueish-purple hue	Multiloculated cystic mass with fluid-fluid levels. Some enhancement on delayed phase images. Phleboliths can be present	CT: serpiginous lesions, some areas can enhance on post-contrast imaging. More sensitive for phlebolith identification
AVM	• Can present with CHF, embolism, pain, or bleeding depending on location • High flow vascular malformation can present with pulsating lesion or thrill on examination. May feel warm on palpation	Serpiginous tangle of vessels with enhancement on postcontrast imaging and early enhancement of the draining veins	• DSA remains the gold standard • Serpiginous tangle or mass of vessels with enhancement on postcontrast imaging and early enhancement of the enlarged draining veins
AVF	• Symptoms depend on location and what vessels are involved. Can be asymptomatic and incidentally found • Increased collateralization commonly seen	• Abnormal connection between an artery and vein, may present as abnormal dilation and fistulous tract on postcontrast imaging • Best seen on MRA which demonstrates abnormal early venous enhancement	DSA remains the gold standard and demonstrates direct communication of an artery with an abnormal early filling draining vein

(AVM: arteriovenous malformation; AVF: arteriovenous fistula; CHF: congestive heart failure; DSA: digital subtraction angiography; MRA: magnetic resonance angiography; MR: magnetic resonance)

rapidly involuting congenital hemangioma (RICH) and noninvoluting congenital hemangioma (NICH). RICH, as the name suggests, involutes rapidly after birth, usually by the first 7 months. They usually as fully involuted by a year of birth, without an adipose component like in IH. RICH usually do not require management except for corticosteroid or embolization; however, they may be associated with congestive cardiac failure, which needs to be evaluated. NICH does not regress and has persistent fast-flow. These require resection if symptomatic.[30,31]

Kaposiform Hemangioendothelioma

Kaposiform hemangioendothelioma (KHE) is a rare neoplasm that has a propensity for local aggression but no risk of metastases.[32,33] They resemble Kaposi's sarcoma and around half of these presenting at birth, and the remaining developing during the first year of life. Clinically, apparent lesions are large (>5 cm), flat, and reddish-purple. These are symptomatic and they partially regress by 2 years. Half of the patients have associated Kasabach-Merritt phenomenon.[34-36] MRI is used to confirm the extent of the lesion, showing T2-hyperintensity, vascular enhancement, and flow voids.[37,38] Histologically, they are characterized by slit-like vascular spaces with red cell fragments. They are excised if symptomatic; however, waiting for regression is reasonable as the extent of resection required may reduce.

Pyogenic Granuloma

This is solitary reddish papule that is small and pedunculated, arising during the 6th or 7th year of life. They commonly present with bleeding or ulceration. They can involve both the skin and mucous membranes. Within the head and neck they can involve the cheek, oral cavity, face, lips, or scalp.[39] Limited excision methods include curettage, shave, or laser therapy.[40] However, the more limited approaches have a higher recurrence rate; full thickness excision is more effective.

VASCULAR MALFORMATIONS

Capillary Malformations

Formerly known as "port-wine" stain, and the most formidable theory on pathogenesis is the neurovegetative theory. It is believed that they result from embryonic insults in autonomic nervous system development. They commonly affect the branches of the trigeminal nerve.[41]

Clinically, CMs can occur anywhere in the body, and can be solitary or generalized, as in Sturge-Weber syndrome. They involve both genders equally. The discoloration from these lesions may not be visible at birth due to physiological erythema of newborn skin. They may overlie the occipital area or spine, which may herald an underlying vascular malformation of the brain or spine.[42]

These lesions may be treated early in childhood for ideal cosmetic outcomes. Pulse dye laser can help lighten these lesions with minimal scarring. Large lesions may need surgical excision.[42,43]

Lymphatic Malformations

These can be characterized based on the size of the channels involved (microcystic, macrocystic, and combined). They are usually identified within the first 2 years of life, with large lesions presenting at birth but small lesions that grow slowly presenting as late as adulthood. They may even be identified on antenatal ultrasound.[44]

Lesions are soft and compressible on examination, with the overlying skin normal, bluish, or vesicular. Smaller lesions can cause cosmetic disfiguration, while large lesions can cause bleeding, infection, or disruption of tongue function such as speech and swallowing. Most are identified reliably by clinical examination with imaging reserved for large lesions that need their extent delineated. MRI does not show diffuse enhancement and lesions are hyperintense on T2.

Intervention is not mandatory in these lesions; very often these are observed. Intervention is reserved for lesions that result in cosmetic deformity or functional issues. Sclerotherapy is considered the first choice in macrocystic and combined lesions. These lesions are aspirated and injected with sclerotherapy agents (doxycycline, sodium tetradecyl sulfate, bleomycin, and OK432).[45] Ethanol may cause systemic symptoms and should be avoided. Resection is reserved for symptomatic lesions, failed sclerotherapy, or well-localized lesions. Large lesions should be managed with staged resection.

Venous Malformations

These are lesions resulting from aberrant growth in vascular development. These are thin-walled lesions with sponge-like vessels. The endothelium lining of these lesions appears normal but there may be an irregular deposition of smooth muscle fibers.[46] Around half of the patients have mutations in the endothelial receptor TIE2[47] and 10% of these patients have a familial pattern of inheritance.[47]

Clinically, these have a characteristic appearance. They are soft and compressible and may have palpable phleboliths. Larger lesions may involve the surrounding tissue, including muscle or joints. Ulceration and bleeding may occur when the overlying skin is eroded. They may also be associated with deep-seated malformations which can predispose to thrombosis and pulmonary emboli.

Small lesions may not need a diagnostic workup. Ultrasound shows compressible anechoic-hypoechoic channels with intervening areas of variable echogenecity. MRI shows hyperintensity on T2-weighted sequences with intervening flow voids due to phleboliths.[48-50] Histology is not indicated unless there is a suspicion of malignancy.

Patients at risk of thrombosis require heparin or antiplatelet therapies. Sclerotherapy is a good first approach to smaller lesion. For larger, diffuse lesions, specific areas are targeted with sclerotherapy. Often repeated injections are required. Surgical intervention is restricted to symptomatic lesions, although these are difficult to remove completely and have a high chance of recurrence due to hidden channels. Sclerotherapy prior to surgery helps prevent ecurrence.[51-54] An approach to VMs is seen in **Flowchart 1**.[55]

Flowchart 1: Approach to venous malformations.[56]

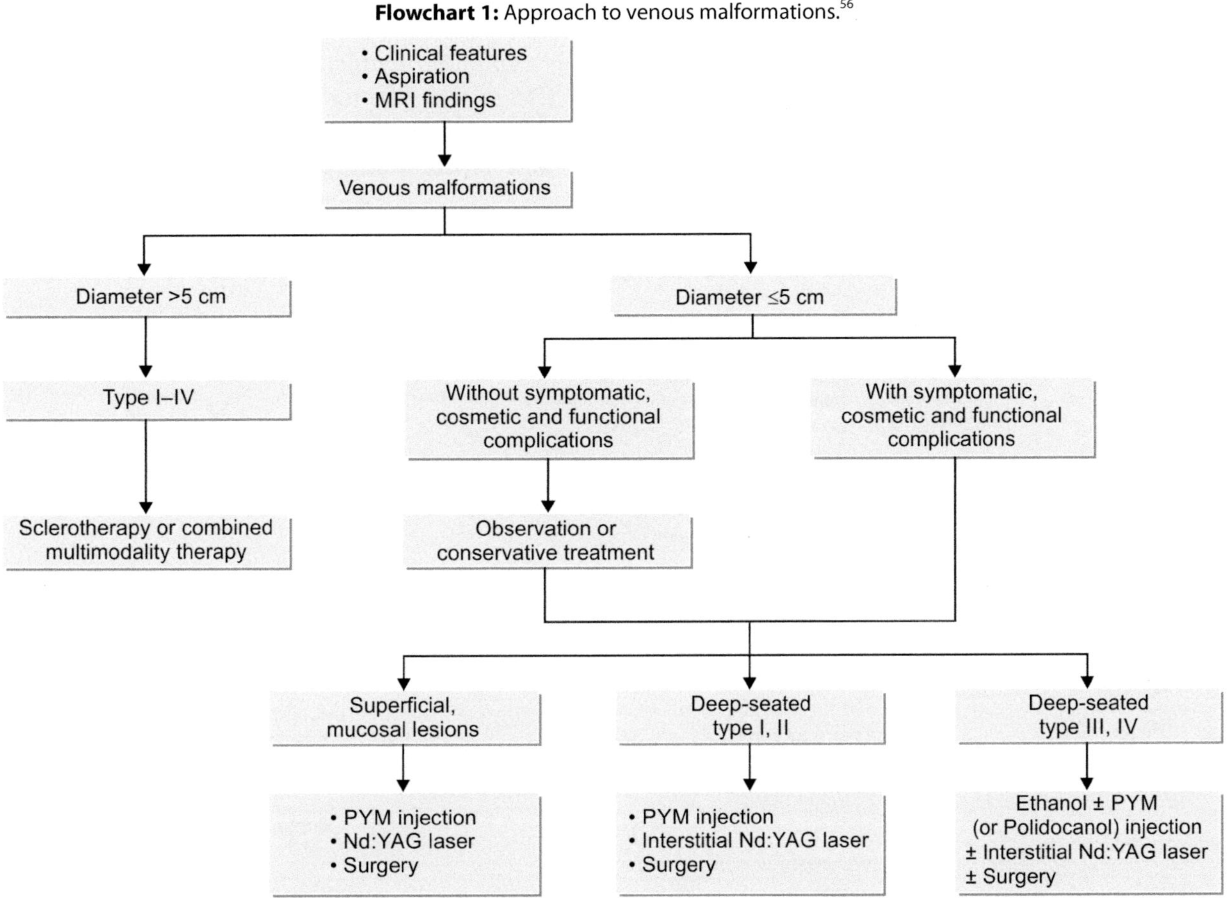

(MRI: magnetic resonance imaging; PYM: pingyangmycin; Nd:YAG: neodymium-doped yttrium aluminum garnet)

Arteriovenous Malformations

These result from disruptions in vascular development occurring in utero; it is believed that primitive channels between arteries and veins that are supposed to regress fail to do so.[56] AVMs can result from a fistula (that directly connect an artery to a vein) or a nidus (abnormal channels that bridge a feeding artery to its feeding veins). As a result of increased blood flow, venous channels become dilated and ectatic with collaterals, followed by opening latent arteriovenous shunts and vasculogenesis. As the pressure continues to increase, aneurysms may form. This progression is common during adolescence.[56-59]

The head and neck are the most common sites of involvement. Unless they are large, they present until childhood or early adolescence. They present initially like IH without thrill or bruit. As they progress, they may cause bleeding and erosion of surrounding structures. According to the Schobinger staging system,[60] the stages are:

- *Stage I or quiescence:* They are warm, pink-blue, and Doppler shows shunting.
- *Stage II or expansion:* There is enlargement, pulsation, thrill, bruit, and tortuous veins.
- *Stage III or destruction:* There are dystrophic skin changes, bleeding, ulceration, and pain.
- *Stage IV or decompensation:* There is cardiac failure.

Diagnosis can be confirmed with ultrasound and Doppler which shows fast flow. MRI shows dilated feeding arteries and draining veins with enhancement and flow voids.[61] Angiography is performed as a precursor to embolization. Biopsy is contraindicated except in suspicion of malignancy.

The goal of therapy is to limit expansion and morbidity from the lesion and/or treatment. Stage I-II lesions are observed unless they can be resected completely. Stage III-IV lesions require intervention as they have a high likelihood of progression. Embolization allows permanent occlusion of the nidus, resulting in shrinkage and resolution. This is often performed before surgical excision, where there is occlusion of the nidus but not the proximal arterial inflow as it will result in collateralization and prevent further endovascular access.[61,62] Resection should be approached with caution because involvement of surrounding areas is often extensive and recurrence rates are high. Additionally, they can result in life-threatening intraoperative hemorrhage. Algorithmic approaches to vascular malformations are shown in **Flowcharts 2 and 3.**[63]

Sturge–Weber Syndrome

This is a sporadic neurocutaneous disorder characterized with CM in the trigeminal nerve distribution, ocular abnormalities (glaucoma and choroidal vascular anomalies) and leptomeningeal vascular malformations.[64]

Flowchart 2: Algorithm for management of congenital vascular anomalies.

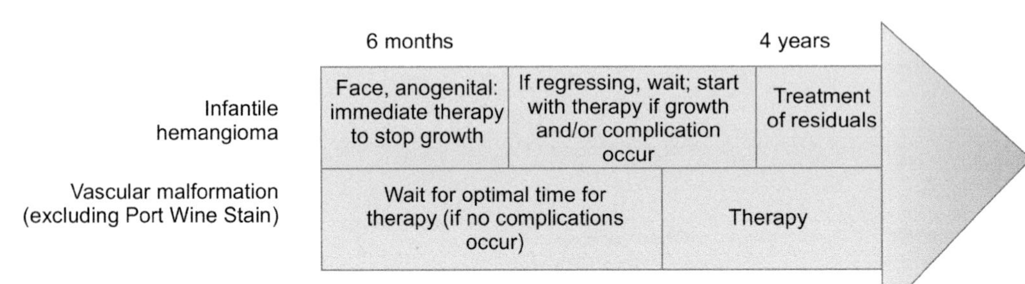

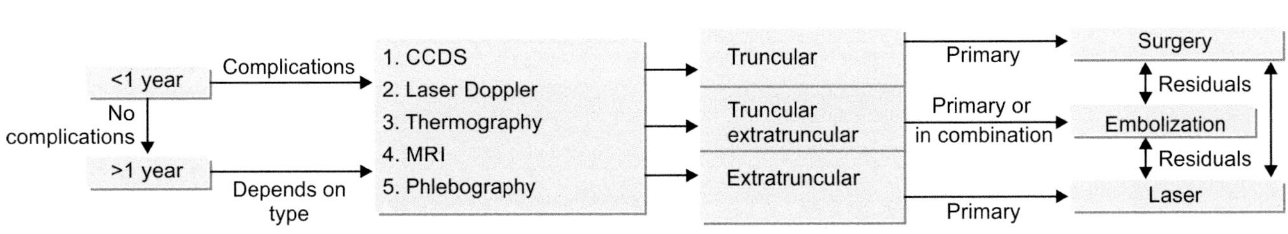

(CCDS: color-coded Doppler sonography; CVA: cerebrovascular accident)

Flowchart 3: Algorithm for management of vascular anomalies.

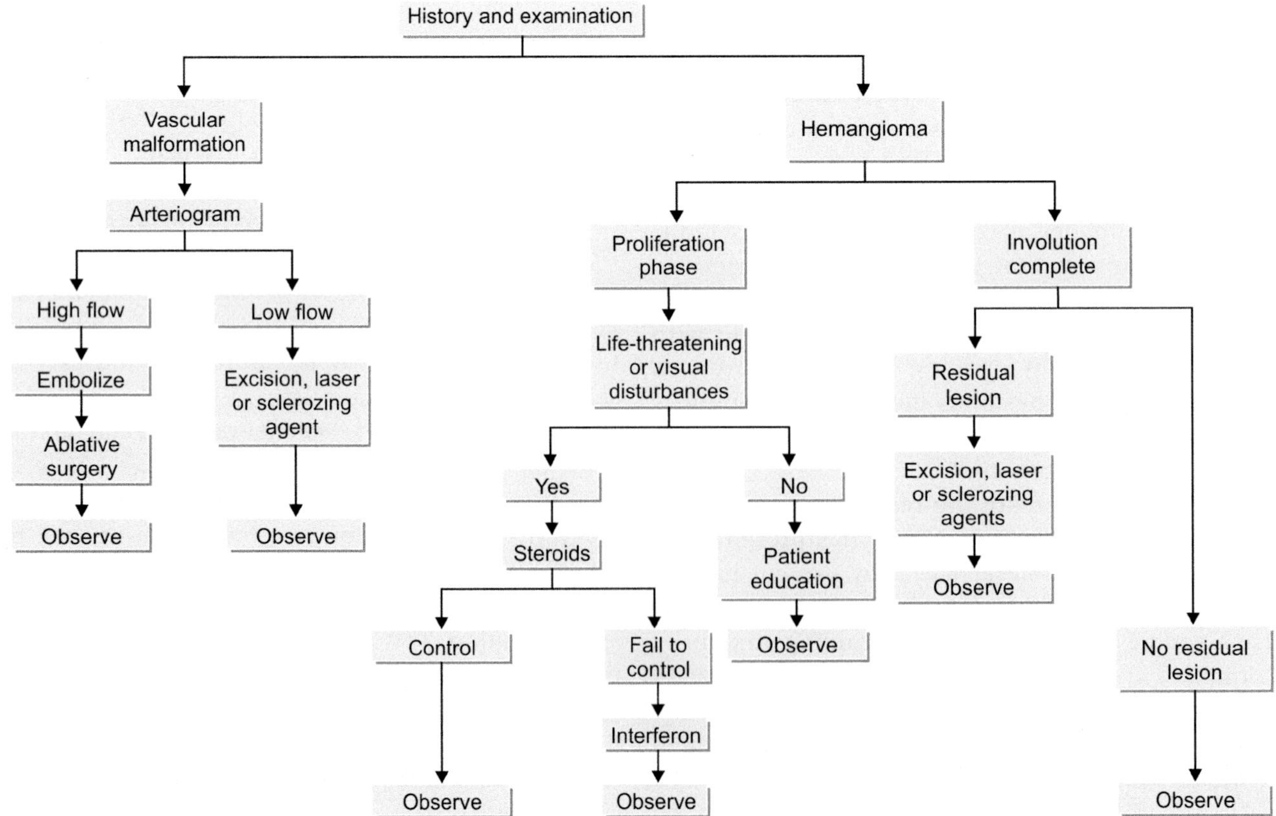

They may also have soft tissue or bony overgrowth and neurological issues.

CONCLUSION

Vascular malformations are characterized by disorders in angiogenesis that can present with a wide array of signs and symptoms. A detailed understanding of these lesions is important to manage them effectively. Recent advances in management limit morbidity while retaining quality of life.

REFERENCES

1. Garzon MC, Huang JT, Enjolras O, Frieden IJ. Vascular malformations: part I. J Am Acad Dermatol. 2007;56(3): 353-70; 371-4.
2. Syed NM. Vascular lesions of head and neck: a literature review. Indian J Dent Sci. 2016;8(3):176-82.
3. Connor SE, Flis C, Langdon JD. Vascular masses of the head and neck. Clin Radiol. 2005;60(8):856-68.
4. Hand JL, Frieden IJ. Vascular birthmarks of infancy: resolving nosologic confusion. Am J Med Genet. 2002;108(4):257-64.
5. Finn MC, Glowacki J, Mulliken JB. Congenital vascular lesions: clinical application of a new classification. J Pediatr Surg. 1983;18(6):894-900.
6. Boscolo E, Bischoff J. Vasculogenesis in infantile hemangioma. Angiogenesis. 2009;12(2):197-207.
7. Khan ZA, Boscolo E, Picard A, Psutka S, Melero-Martin JM, Bartch TC, et al. Multipotential stem cells recapitulate human infantile hemangioma in immunodeficient mice. J Clin Invest. 2008;118(7):2592-9.
8. Razon MJ, Kräling BM, Mulliken JB, Bischoff J. Increased apoptosis coincides with onset of involution in infantile hemangioma. Microcirculation. 1998;5(2-3):189-95.
9. Kilcline C, Frieden IJ. Infantile hemangiomas: how common are they? A systematic review of the medical literature. Pediatr Dermatol. 2008;25(2):168-73.
10. Drolet BA, Swanson EA, Frieden IJ. Infantile hemangiomas: An emerging health issue linked to an increased rate of low birth weight infants. J Pediatr. 2008;153(5):712-5.
11. Amir J, Metzker A, Krikler R, Reisner SH. Strawberry hemangioma in preterm infants. Pediatr Dermatol. 1986; 3(4):331-2.
12. Chang LC, Haggstrom AN, Drolet BA, Baselga E, Chamlin SL, Garzon MC, et al. Growth characteristics of infantile hemangiomas: implications for management. Pediatrics. 2008;122(2):360-7.
13. Smoller BR, Apfelberg DB. Infantile (juvenile) capillary haemangioma: a tumor of heterogeneous cellular elements. J Cutan Pathol. 1993;20(4):330-6.
14. Mancini AJ, Smoller BR. Proliferation and apoptosis within juvenile capillary hemangiomas. Am J Dermatopathol. 1996;18(5):505-14.
15. Höpfel-Kreiner I. Histogenesis of hemangiomas: an ultrastructural study on capillary and cavernous hemangiomas of the skin. Pathol Res Pract. 1980;170(1-3):70-90.
16. Dethlefsen SM, Mulliken JB, Glowacki J. An ultrastructural study of mast cell interactions in hemangiomas. Ultrastruct Pathol. 1986;10(12):175-83.
17. Metry DW, Garzon MC, Drolet BA, Frommelt P, Haggstrom A, Hall J, et al. PHACE syndrome: current knowledge, future directions. Ped Derm. 2009;26(4):381-98.
18. Paltiel H, Burrows PE, Kozakewich HPW, Zurakowski D, Mulliken JB. Soft-tissue vascular anomalies: utility of US for diagnosis. Radiology. 2000;214(3):747-54.
19. Burrows PE, Laor T, Paltiel H, Robertson RL. Diagnostic imaging in the evaluation of vascular birthmarks. Dermatol Clin. 1998;16(3):455-88.
20. Chamlin SL, Haggstrom AN, Drolet BA, Baselga E, Frieden IJ, Garzon MC, et al. Multicenter prospective study of ulcerated hemangiomas. J Pediatr. 2007;151(6):684-9.
21. Sloan GM, Renisch JF, Nichter LS, Saber WL, Lew K, Morwood DT, et al. Intralesional corticosteroid therapy for infantile hemangiomas. Plast Reconstr Surg. 1989;83(3):459-67.
22. Barlow CF, Priebe C, Mulliken JB, Barnes PD, Donald DM, Folkman J, et al. Spastic diplegia as a complication of interferon-alfa-2a treatment of hemangiomas of infancy. J Pediatr. 1998;132(3):527-30.
23. Haisley-Royster C, Enjolras O, Frieden IJ, Garzon M, Lee M, Oranje A, et al. Kasabach-Merritt phenomenon: a retrospective study of treatment with vincristine. J Pediatr Hematol Oncol. 2002;24(6):459-62.
24. Goswamy J, Rothera MP, Bruce IA. Failure of propranolol in the treatment of childhood haemangiomas of the head and neck. J Laryngol Otol. 2011;125(11):1164-72.
25. Lawley LP, Siegfried E, Todd JL. Propranolol treatment for hemangioma of infancy: risks and recommendations. Pediatr Dermatol. 2009;26(5):610-4.
26. Batta K, Goodyear HM, Moss C, Williams HC, Hiller L, Waters R. Randomized controlled study of early pulsed dye laser treatment of uncomplicated childhood haemangiomas: results of a 1-year analysis. Lancet. 2002;360(9332):521-7.
27. Scarcella JV, Dykes ER, Anderson R. Hemangiomas of the parotid gland. Plast Reconstr Surg. 1965;36:38-47.
28. Mulliken, JB, Fishman SJ, Burrows PE. Vascular Anomalies. Curr Prob Surg. 2000;37(8):517-84.
29. Mulliken JB, Rogers GF, Marler JJ. Circular excision of hemangioma and purse-string closure: the smallest possible scar. Plast Reconstr Surg. 2002;109(5):1544-54.
30. Boon LM, Enjolras O, Mulliken JB. Congenital hemangioma: evidence of accelerated involution. J Pediatr. 1996; 128(3):329-35.
31. Enjolras O, Mulliken JB, Boon LM, Wassef M, Kozakewich HP, Burrows PE, et al. Noninvoluting congenital hemangioma: a rare cutaneous vascular anomaly. Plast Reconstr Surg. 2001; 107(7):1647-54.
32. Kasabach HH, Merritt KK. Capillary hemangioma with extensive purpura: report of a case. Am J Dis Child. 1940; 59(5):1063-70.
33. Zukerberg LR, Nikoloff BJ, Weiss SW. Kaposiform hemangioendothelioma of infancy and childhood: an aggressive neoplasm associated with Kasabach–Merritt syndrome and lymphangiomatosis. Am J Surg Pathol. 1993;17(4):321-8.
34. Lyons LL, North PE, Mac-Moune Lai F, et al. Kaposiform hemangio endothelioma: a study of 33 cases emphasizing its pathologic, immunophenotypic, and biologic uniqueness from juvenile hemangioma. Am J Surg Pathol. 2004;28(5): 559-68.
35. Karnes JC, Lee BT, Phung T, Alomari AI, Mulliken JB, Greene AK, et al. Adult-onset kaposiform hemangioendothelioma in a post-traumatic site. Ann Plast Surg. 2009;62(4):456-8.
36. Debelenko LV, Perez-Atayde AR, Mulliken JB, Liang MG, Archibald TH, Kozakewich HPW, et al. D2-40 immunohistochemical analysis of pediatric vascular tumors reveals positivity in kaposiform hemangio-endothelioma. Mod Pathol. 2005;18(11):1454-60.

37. Enjolras O, Mulliken JB, Wassef M, Frieden IJ, Rieu PN, Burrows PE, et al. Residual lesions after Kasabach-Merritt phenomenon in 41 patients. J Am Acad Dermatol. 2000; 42(2 Pt 1):225-35.
38. Mentzel T, Mazzoleni G, Dei Tos AP, Fletcher CD. Kaposiform hemangioendothelioma in adults. Clinicopathologic and immune-histochemical analysis of three cases. Am J Clin Pathol. 1997;108(4):450-5.
39. Patrice SJ, Wiss K, Mulliken JB. Pyogenic granuloma (lobular capillary hemangioma): a clinicopathologic study of 178 cases. Pediatr Dermatol. 1991;8(4):267-76.
40. Kirschner RE, Low DW. Treatment of pyogenic granuloma by shave excision and laser photocoagulation. Plast Reconstr Surg. 1999;104(5):1346-9.
41. Cunha e Sa M, Barroso CP, Caldas MC, Edvinsson L, Gulbenkian S. Innervation pattern of mal-formative cortical vessels in Sturge-Weber disease: a histochemical, immunohistochemical, and ultrastructural study. Neurosurgery. 1997; 41(4):872-6.
42. Jessen RT, Thompson S, Smith EB. Cobb syndrome. Arch Dermatol. 1977;113(11):1587-90.
43. Tan OT, Sherwood K, Gilchrest BA. Treatment of children with port-wine stains using the flashlamp-pulsed tunable dye laser. N Engl J Med. 1989;320(7):416-21.
44. Edwards PD, Rahbar R, Ferraro NF, Burrows PE, Mulliken JB. Lymphatic malformation of the lingual base and oral floor. Plast Reconstr Surg. 2005;115(7):1906-15.
45. Florez-Vargas A, Vargas SO, Debelenko LV, Perez-Atayde AR, Archibald T, Kozakewich HPW, et al. Comparative analysis of D2-40 and LYVE-1 immunostaining in lymphatic malformations. Lymphology. 2008;41(3):103-10.
46. Mulliken JB, Young A. Vascular Birthmarks: Hemangiomas and Malformations. Philadelphia: WB Saunders; 1988.
47. Limaye N, Wouters V, Uebelhoer M, Tuominen M, Wirkkala R, Mulliken JB, et al. Somatic mutations in angiopoietin receptor gene TEK cause solitary and multiple sporadic venous malformations. Nat Gen. 2009;41(1):118-24.
48. Upton J, Coombs CJ, Mulliken JB, Burrows PE, Pap S. Vascular malformations of the upper limb: A review of 270 patients. J Hand Surg (Am). 1999;24(5):1019-35.
49. Hein KD, Mulliken JB, Kozakewich HP, Upton J, Burrows PE. Venous malformations of skeletal muscle. Plast Reconstr Surg. 2002;110(7):1625-35.
50. Choi DJ, Alomari AI, Chaudry G, Orbach DB. Neurointerventional management of low-flow vascular malformations of the head and neck. Neuroimag Clin N Am. 2009;19(2):199-218.
51. Adams DM, Wentzel MS. The role of the hematologist/oncologist in the care of patients with vascular anomalies. Pediatr Clin N Am. 2008;55(2):339-55.
52. Dompmartin A, Acher A, Thibon P, Tourbach S, Hermans C, Deneys V, et al. Association of localized intravascular coagulopathy with venous malformations. Arch Dermatol. 2008;144(7):873-7.
53. Berenguer B, Burrows PE, Zurakowski D, Mulliken JB. Sclerotherapy of craniofacial venous malformations: Complications and results. Plast Reconstr Surg. 1999;104(1): 1-11.
54. Burrows PE, Mason KP. Percutaneous treatment of low flow vascular malformations. J Vasc Interv Radiol. 2004;15(5): 431-45.
55. Zheng JW, Mai HM, Zhang L, Wang YA, Fan XD, Su LX, et al. Guidelines for the treatment of head and neck venous malformations. Int J Clin Exp Med. 2013;6(5):377-89.
56. Halsted W. Congenital arteriovenous and lymphaticovenous fistulae: unique clinical and experimental observations. Proc Natl Acad Sci USA. 1919;5(3):76-9.
57. Masuda H, Zhuang YJ, Singh TM, Kawamura K, Murakami M, Zarins CK, et al. Adaptive remodeling of internal elastic lamina and endothelial lining during flow-induced arterial enlargement. Arterioscler Thromb Vasc Biol. 1999;19(10): 2298-307.
58. Karunanyaka A, Tu J, Watling A, Storer KP, Windsor A, Stoodley MA, et al. Endothelial molecular changes in a rodent model of arteriovenous malformation. J Neurosurg. 2008;109(6):1165-72.
59. Liu AS, Mulliken JB, Zurakowski D, Fishman SJ, Greene AK. Extracranial arteriovenous malformations: natural progression and recurrence after treatment. Plast Reconstr Surg. 2010;125(4):1185-94.
60. Kohout MP, Hansen M, Pribaz JJ, Mulliken JB. Arteriovenous malformations of the head and neck: Natural history and management. Plast Reconstr Surg. 1998;102(3): 643-54.
61. Wu IC, Orbach DB. Neurointerventional management of high-flow vascular malformations of the head and neck. Neuroimag Clin N Am. 2009;19(2):219-40.
62. Sturge WA. A case of partial epilepsy apparently due to a lesion of one of the motor centers of the brain. Trans Clin Soc London. 1879;12:112.
63. Nair SC. Vascular anomalies of the head and neck region. J Maxillofac Oral Surg. 2018;17(1):1-12.
64. Comi AM. Pathophysiology of Sturge-Weber syndrome. J Child Neurol. 2003;18(8):509-16.

Reconstruction in Head and Neck Cancer

CHAPTER 37

Microvascular Reconstruction in Head and Neck Cancer: Principles, Practice and Commonly Used Free Flaps

Narayana Subramaniam, Samskruthi P Murthy, Sivakumar Vidhyadharan

INTRODUCTION

Microvascular free flap reconstruction is a cornerstone of comprehensive head and neck cancer management. In experienced hands, microvascular reconstruction is safe, effective, and successful. With technical advancements in surgery and perioperative care, microvascular reconstruction has allowed successful surgical management of tumors that were previously considered unresectable and untreatable, especially in a salvage setting. But crucial to this success is an in-depth understanding of physiology, appropriate decision-making, and technical expertise. The purpose of this chapter is to provide a brief overview of microvascular reconstruction in head and neck cancer; as site-wise defects and individual flaps have been discussed elsewhere, this chapter will describe literature on intra- and perioperative "best practices," with an organized and practical approach to re-exploration and flap salvage.

PREOPERATIVE CONSIDERATIONS

Patient Selection

Surgical fitness is the primary, most important consideration. Some of the factors associated with increased risk of complications in microvascular flap reconstruction are American Society of Anesthesiologists score ≥2, obesity, and peripheral vascular disease.[1] Age is a controversial issue; although older patients are believed to have poorer wound healing and vessel quality, several authors have shown excellent outcomes in patients older than 70 years of age,[2-4] implying that careful selection of elderly patients ensures success. Smoking has also been shown to be associated with increased risk of complications due to increased thrombogenicity, reduced cutaneous blood flow, and poor wound healing;[5,6] however, large series have shown that flap success rates are not affected by prior tobacco exposure; there were however a higher risk of donor site complications and poor healing at the flap-body interface.[7,8]

Diseases such as diabetes mellitus and chronic kidney disease which are associated with microangiopathy may be associated with a higher risk of flap compromise;[9] however, these are not contraindications to microvascular surgery, this decision needs to be made on an individual patient basis, considering surgical fitness and the functional outcomes associated with alternate reconstructive options such as pedicled flaps. Previous radiotherapy is also a very important factor; prior radiotherapy has been shown to affect the intimal narrowing and dysfunction in the tissue bed, prothrombotic processes, and higher risk of wound complications,[10,11] In these patients, although microvascular flaps may be indicated to introduce healthy vascularized tissue from outside the radiotherapy field, the risk of complications are significant often with the course of treatment prolonged, which the surgeon and patient must be prepared for.

Preoperative Imaging and Vessel Selection

Preoperative imaging is important to determine resectability of the tumor and plan the extent and nature of reconstruction required. It is crucial in previously operated cases, especially when neck dissection has been performed, to determine if the internal jugular vein or carotid artery have been sacrificed; in a vessel depleted neck (the term used when previous neck dissection, flap reconstruction, or irradiation leaves scarce availability of vessels for microvascular free flap reconstruction), an angiogram or venogram may be indicated. In bony reconstruction, preoperative imaging is crucial, especially if dental rehabilitation is planned; this helps determine the extent of bony sacrifice, the osteotomies required in the flap and the plating.[12]

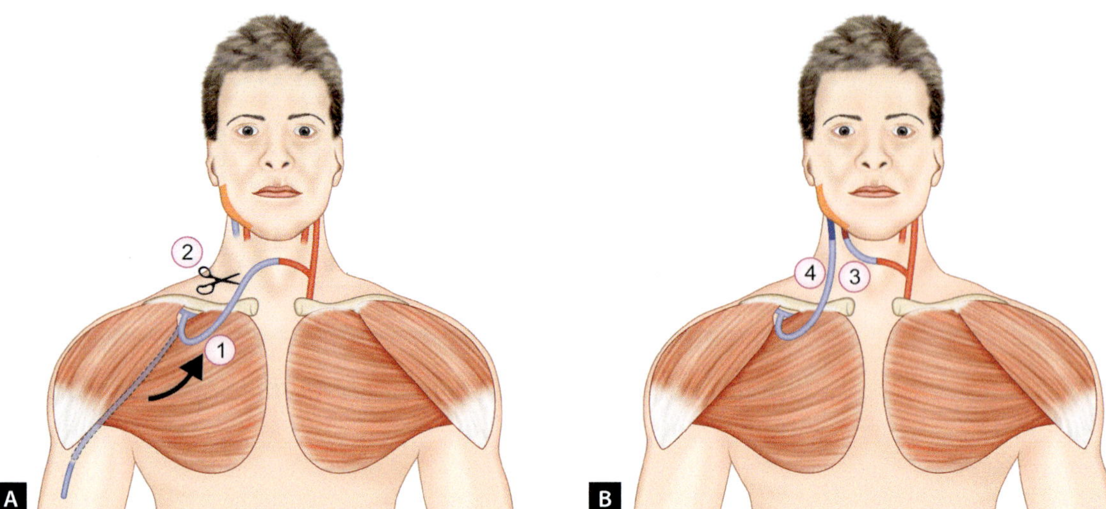

Figs. 1A and B: Corlett loop. 1: Appropriate length of cephalic vein transected and transposed to contralateral external carotid to form arteriovenous fistula (AVF); 2: AVF transected at appropriate length; 3: Short stump used for arterial supply for flap; 4: Long stump used as venous drainage for flap.

In the previously undissected neck, the choices of vessels for microvascular reconstruction are numerous. The primary considerations are the size of caliber in relation to the flap vessels, distance from flap pedicle allowing a tension-free anastomosis, and the lie of a potential anastomosis avoiding any kinks or acute angulation.[13] The common arterial choices are the facial, superior thyroid, lingual, or transverse cervical arteries. In defects of the scalp or upper third of face, the superficial temporal artery is also a popular choice. For venous drainage, internal jugular vein tributaries (often from the thyrolinguofacial trunk) are commonly used. As an alternative, the external jugular vein can be used although it may be more prone to external compression.[14] In a third of cases, the external jugular vein drains into the internal jugular venous system instead of the subclavian vein,[15] which needs to be ruled out in cases where the internal jugular vein have been sacrificed or thrombosed and the anastomosis has been planned to the external jugular vein.

In the vessel depleted neck, the vessels that can be considered are the superficial temporal vessels (occasionally the vein may be absent and not suitable when external carotid has been sacrificed), the transverse cervical artery, internal mammary artery (requires substernal dissection), and thoracoacromial vessels (this means sacrificing the pectoralis major myocutaneous flap as a salvage option).[16] For the vein anastomosis, a vein graft may be required to reach donor vessels (often the great saphenous vein), which increases the number of anastomosis and the chance of failure[17] or a cephalic "flip" where the cephalic vein distal end in the arm is carefully dissected as far as required and flipped up into the neck, keeping the proximal drainage into the axillary vein intact.[18] In a desperate situation, a Corlett loop has been described,[19] where the distal cephalic vein is anastomosed to the external carotid artery initially, and then divided in a single- or two-step procedure, so that the external carotid-cephalic segment acts as the arterial supply and the remaining cephalic stump acts as the venous drainage for the flap **(Figs. 1A and B)**. If the common carotid artery is being sacrificed, the vein graft being used for reconstruction can be harvested with an appropriate tributary for the arterial anastomosis.

Intraoperative Considerations

Technical Aspects

The ideal anastomosis should comprise approximation of the two vessels with watertight closure in a tension-free manner with the anastomosis forming a gentle curve. There are multiple techniques described; however, interrupted suturing techniques are probably the most practiced.[20] Continuous suturing has been shown to have an equal efficacy;[21] however, the concerns as narrowing of the vascular lumen and loosening/breakage of a single stitch leading to compromise of the entire anastomosis.[22,23] The sutures most commonly used are nonabsorbable (nylon or prolene), in a size range of 7-0 to 10-0 depending on the vessel caliber.

End-to-end anastomosis is the most commonly performed technique. With a size discrepancy, up to a 2:1 mismatch may be adjusted for with dilatation of the smaller vessel but not the larger one, while a larger mismatch requires an oblique cut of the smaller vessel wall or end-to-side anastomosis.[24,25] A significant size mismatch is of concern especially in vein anastomosis, where obstruction to flow across the anastomosis results in turbulent and thrombogenic blood flow. End-to-side anastomosis is also favored in venous anastomoses, as there is a concern that manipulation of the carotid artery required for end-to-side arterial anastomosis can result in intimal damage and a higher risk of thrombosis due to the high flow rate.[26]

Ischemia Time and No-reflow Phenomenon

Microvascular tissue transfer requires a certain degree of tolerance to ischemia; however, this time period, known as ischemia time, is multifactorial and can vary between patients and flap composition. Skin and subcutaneous tissue are the most resistant to ischemia, with intracellular pH changes reversible up to 24 hours,[27] while in muscle irreversible damage takes place after 6 hours,[28] while in bowel, this damage sets in after 2 hours.[29] As the ischemia time is prolonged, the tissue begins to suffer ischemia-related damage till a point where even after circulation is re-established, the tissue can no longer be re-perfused, known as "no-reflow phenomenon"; this is believed to be due to cellular swelling within the vascular endothelium, aggregation of platelets within the vascular compartment and extravasation of fluid into the interstitial space.[30] The aim of any reconstructive surgeon should be to restrict ischemia time to as short a period as possible, as the exact threshold of safety is unknown; this can be done by keeping the donor vessels dissected and ready and performing only partial inset before commencing the microvascular anastomosis. Several studies have failed to establish a range of "safe" ischemia time;[31-33] however, as a rule of thumb, it is believed that the ischemia times of enteric, muscle, bone, and skin flaps are 2 hours, 3 hours, 4 hours, and 6 hours, respectively.[34] There are several methods that have been studied to increase this, such as protective hypothermia and ischemic preconditioning but all of these remain experimental techniques.[35,36]

Device-assisted Closure

Several devices have been developed to aid microvascular anastomosis with the intention of increasing the ease of performance, reducing surgical time, and improving patency rates; these include cuffs, splints, couplers, staplers, and automatic stapling devices.[37-40] When compared to conventional suturing technique, they have shown a reduced operating time; however, most studies do not show a significant difference in flap survival rates.[41-43] It is to be noted that these devices cannot be used in certain clinically challenging situations such as small (<1 mm) vessels and atherosclerotic or fragile vessels, necessitating the development of high-quality conventional suturing techniques.

Postoperative Management

Clinical Flap Monitoring

The protocol for postoperative flap monitoring is highly variable between institutions; however, it is unequivocal that regular flap monitoring, especially in the early postoperative period (<72 hours), can detect early vascular compromise and improve chances of salvage. Routine postoperative surveillance includes skin color, temperature, turgor, and capillary refill, wherever possible. Flap prick or scratch to assess bleeding is also followed in some institutions.

Measuring Blood Flow in Microvascular Flaps

Devices that monitor blood flow in microvascular flaps are also used routinely in postoperative surveillance. They have the advantages of often more objective assessment that can be performed by less skilled staff, and the ability to monitor buried flaps without any external component that can be used for monitoring (such as enteric flaps for laryngopharyngeal reconstruction). They can be used to identify flow within the anastomosis itself or downstream, viz., to assess flow in the flap which indirectly reflects anastomotic patency. These are acoustic Doppler sonography, color Doppler ultrasound, implantable Doppler probes, flow couplers (microvascular couplers with an inbuilt mini-Doppler probe), laser Doppler flowmetry, and near-infrared spectroscopy. Other than the acoustic Doppler sonography that is used somewhat universally, the remaining are potential tools that can be used in conjunction with clinical examination, but are not without significant cost. Also, malfunction in them can lead to unnecessary re-exploration. Hence, it is unclear if the routine use of the more sophisticated flap monitoring devices is justified.[44]

Anticoagulation Protocols

Routine postoperative anticoagulation is another contentious topic amongst microsurgeons, with institutional policies varying significantly. The rationale, however, is sound; disrupted endothelial surfaces (at the anastomotic site and areas where the vessels were handled) act as foci for platelet aggregation, followed by intravascular activation of the coagulation pathway, placing the flap at risk of ischemic damage, especially in the early postoperative period.[45,46] Heparin was one of the first agents used prophylactically to prevent postoperative thrombosis, but has a significant risk of postoperative bleeding, hematoma, and paradoxically flap compromise.[45-47] Other agents that have been used are low molecular weight heparins, dextran, and aspirin. There are two important considerations in these patients;

firstly, deep vein thrombosis prophylaxis is important in these patients given the prolonged duration of surgery, risk of thrombosis due to malignancy and immobilization, and needs to be administered. And secondly, the risk of anticoagulation should not outweigh its benefits. Routine anticoagulation may not improve flap outcomes; in a review of 73 centers performing routine microsurgery in 22 countries, the success rates in centers using routine anticoagulation protocols were equivalent to centers that did not.[48] A recent systematic review of anticoagulation in head and neck free flap reconstruction concluded that there was insufficient evidence to describe an "optimal" protocol, with similar outcomes amongst all agents studied.[49]

Flap Re-exploration and Salvage

Etiology as Related to Occurrence of Compromise

- *Intraoperative:* When the compromise occurs intra-operatively, soon after completion of the anastomosis, it is important to rule out compression or kinking of the pedicle throughout its length; often it may be within the "tunnel" under the mandible or within the floor of the mouth. Immediately after release of the clamps following completion of the anastomosis, it should be left undisturbed for 5–10 minutes to allow vasospasm from handling to settle. Topical lignocaine or papaverine have also been applied to help relieve spasm. Hypothermia and hypotension need to be reversed, if present. The "milking test" is then performed; if there is no flow across the anastomosis, the sutures can be loosened or the donor vessel can be opened with a small arteriotomy or venotomy to visualize the anastomosis or insert a microcatheter. If no flow is seen and there are no identifiable systemic causes of poor flow, the anastomosis needs to be taken down and redone.
- *Early postoperative (≤72 hours):* This compromise can initially be due to vasospasm from rough handling of the vessels. Patient positioning leading to compression of the vessels (more commonly the vein) by the flap, drain, or dressings is not uncommon. Post-operative hypotension, increased blood viscosity, and hematoma formation can also produce early compromise.
- *Late postoperative (>72 hours):* This is rarely due to technical issues with the anastomoses and can be a result of hematoma compressing the pedicle or infection. Flap loss after 7 days is uncommon but by no means unheard of.

Management of the Compromised Flap

Surgical Management

- Once the decision is made to re-explore, no time should be wasted; if there is a compressive hematoma compressing the flap pedicle, a few skin sutures can be released before reaching the theater to at least partially decompress the neck.
- *Anesthetic optimization is critical:* Blood products may need to be arranged. Volume replacement can avoid inotropes that can cause vasoconstriction of the microvasculature, aiming for a hemoglobin of 9 g%. Heparinization may be indicated if thrombosis has occurred in the flap pedicle, between 500 and 1,000 IU/h, aiming for an activated partial thromboplastin time (aPTT) of 60–80 seconds. Broad-spectrum antibiotics are indicated if there is suspicion of a salivary leak and potential infection.
- If a vein graft is likely to be required, the patient should be appropriately prepared and draped. Similarly, if a second flap is planned, an extra pair of hands may be invaluable.
- Sutures are first released over the pedicle, for immediate decompression. Warm saline is used for flush out a hematoma, with low power suction to avoid accidentally suctioning the pedicle. Re-exploration is ideally done under the microscope for adequate magnification. The pedicle should be examined in detail and handled gently to avoid further injury or avulsion; blunt instruments are used.
- It is important to determine if the cause for poor flap perfusion is extrinsic (external compression to the pedicle from dressings, head position or drain, internal compression due to a hematoma or physiological disruptions such as hypotension, anemia, hyperviscosity, or hypothermia) or intrinsic (poor anastomotic flow due to spasm, tension, torsion, or thrombosis).
- If the anastomosis is not flowing, the decision is made to take the anastomosis down. If there is torsion, the vessels are cut at the anastomotic site. If there is an identifiable thrombosis, a proximal opening can be made to inspect the anastomosis. Milking a thrombus across the anastomosis is generally ill-advised as it can embolize, causing microthrombi and irreversible damage in the flap microvasculature.
- If the issue is with the donor vessels, new donor vessels need to be identified; in a previously irradiated case or in the presence of florid infection or inflammation, the contralateral neck vessels may have to be used.

- *Less is more:* The aim should be to get the flap working with as little disruption and secondary ischemia as possible.
- Salvage is abandoned when there has been ≥6 hours without any arterial inflow (≥3 hours for functional muscle transfers and ≥2 hours for enteric flaps).

Nonsurgical Management

- Thrombolytic agents have been used to lyse thrombi present in microcirculation and help re-establish blood flow, but timing of intervention and potential averse features is a major concern. Streptokinase/urokinase 100–250 kU or tissue plasminogen activator 15 mg have infused into the artery of free flap after disconnecting the vein (to prevent escape of the agent into systemic circulation). In one of the largest series, the use of thrombolytic agents was unclear and not seen to be more effective than heparin administration.[50]
- Fogarty catheters have been used to perform embolectomy in free flaps; however, their exact role is unknown; a size 2 or 3 catheter has been used with varied success—not all flaps that underwent a successful embolectomy were ultimately salvaged. Additionally, in head-to-head comparisons, embolectomy was shown to be inferior to direct thrombectomy, where the thrombus was removed through an arteriotomy or venotomy.[51-53]
- Leech therapy has been used in cases where there is persistent venous congestion, since the saliva of *Hirudo medicinalis* has hirudin and two other inhibitors of platelet aggregation and vasoconstriction. They decongest venous blood, acting as a temporary shunt to improve microcirculation. 1–10 leeches are applied per day, for up to two sessions each lasting 6 hours, for 2–6 days. The patient's hemoglobin needs to be monitored every 4 hours and transfusion is required if it drops below 8 g%.[54,55]

Outcomes

Large series show flap survival rates in excess of 97%. The common causes of flap failure are infection, hematoma, hypotension, pedicle kinking or compression, problems with flap design or harvest, and in almost a fifth of cases, the cause of failure is unknown.[56,57] It is important to note that each surgeon's learning curve is different, and the success of a microvascular reconstructive surgery program is as dependent on postoperative monitoring and care, and early return to theater when required, as it is on technical expertise and finesse of the operating surgeon.

Performing a Second Flap

The approach to a failed free flap has been described by Hanasono et al.[56] as the "reverse reconstructive ladder," where the choices in descending order of preference are a second free flap, regional flap, skin graft, and primary closure/vacuum-assisted closure. The exceptions may be in septic or hypotensive patient where shorter operative time is imperative, and a simpler reconstructive plan is preferred.

Technical Considerations

- A similar flap is preferred when a second free flap is being performed; like is best replaced with like. This results in lesser long-term functional disturbances and a lower likelihood of needing revision surgery.
- A larger flap dimension may be required if the tissue at the junction of the defect is healthy and needs debridement.
- A longer pedicle length is crucial to facilitate using contralateral neck vessels or vessels outside the zone of trauma; reusing the same vessels is avoided as they may have vasculitic changes and intimal damage.
- The success rate in experienced hands is still as high as 94%.

COMMONLY PERFORMED FREE FLAPS FOR HEAD AND NECK RECONSTRUCTION

Radial Forearm Flap (Fig. 2)

- *Vascular supply:* Radial artery and accompanying venae comitantes or cephalic vein.
- *Salient anatomy:* The flap is centered over the skin of the volar forearm that is generally thin and pliable, especially distally, which has variable hair growth. The main arterial supply comes from the radial artery, which originates from the brachial artery in the medial cubital fossa 1 cm below the elbow crease and medial to the biceps tendon. It then traverses downward in the lateral intermuscular septum between the flexor and extensor compartments, with the radial artery pulse being palpated most reliably just medial to the styloid process of the radius. There are a variable number of septocutaneous perforators (average of 12) throughout its course in the forearm. The radial artery can be safely harvested in a majority of patients as the ulnar artery is the dominant supply of the hand and the deep palmar arch ensures good collateral circulation, determined by Allen test. It also supplies the distal radius bone periosteally via branches to deep flexor pollicis longus and pronator quadratus. The flap is usually

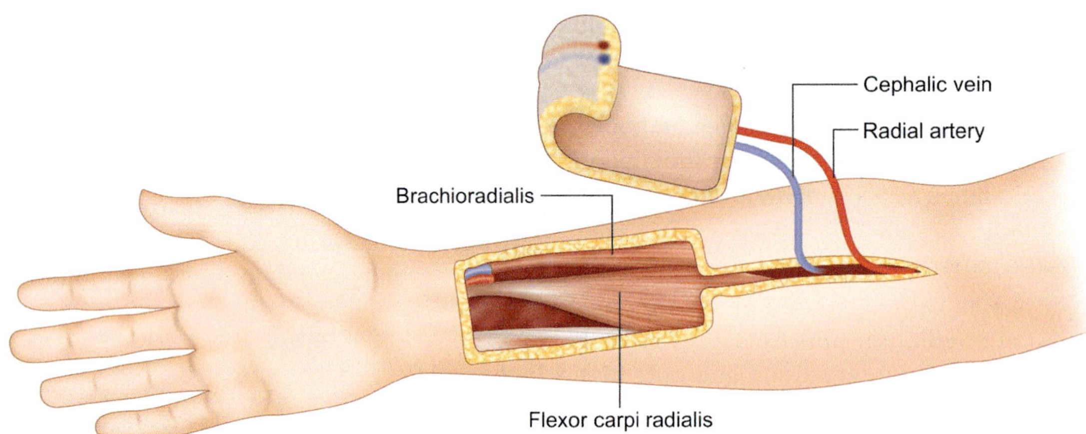

Fig. 2: Radial forearm free flap.

drained with venae comitantes (commonly 2), which accompany the radial artery. The cephalic vein can be incorporated into the flap design but in a minority of cases may not adequately drain the flap necessitating additional anastomosis of the venae comitantes. The lateral antebrachial cutaneous nerve commonly supplies the overlying skin of the flap and can be used for sensory innervation. The palmaris longus tendon (absent in 13%) can be harvested for use as a sling in labial and orbital reconstruction. The distant 10–12 cm of the anterolateral radius can be harvested for bony reconstruction but this needs to be done carefully as harvesting too much bone can result in postoperative fractures.

- *Anatomical variations:* Superficial venous system is highly variable but is not is easily mapped using a tourniquet to engorge the venous system and trace their course. In a series of 750 cadaveric dissections, McCormack[58] found radial and ulnar arteries in all cases. In cases of incomplete deep palmar arches, the thumb and the index finger have the highest risk of developing ischemia, which occurs only when there is also a lack of communication between the superficial and deep palmar arches.[59] Aberrant radial arteries have been described but are exceedingly rare.[60-62]
- *Components and variants:* Most commonly fascio-cutaneous, however, can be modified to include bone (unicortical segment of radius), vascularized tendon, vascularized tendon, or brachioradialis muscle. May also be innervated when harvested with lateral antebrachial cutaneous nerve.
- *Flap design and utilization:* The vascular territory is the volar aspect of the forearm, with the flap most commonly centered over the radial artery with or without the cephalic vein. However, the entire skin of the flexor aspect of the forearm may be harvested safely, from the antecubital fossa to the flexor crease of the wrist. As mentioned above, various chimeric elements can be harvested if the concerned perforators are carefully preserved.
- *Common use:* Replacement of mucosal or soft tissue for defects that are intraoral (tongue, floor of mouth, buccal, and oropharyngeal), intranasal, defects of lip, esophagus, hypopharynx, external skin, and orbit. Bone component can be used for limited alveolar defects or nasal bone defects. Palmaris longus tendon if present can be used as a sling to suspend lower lip to modiolus.
- *Advantages:*
  - Versatile with multiple chimeric components possible
  - Reliable anatomy
  - Pliable, thin skin; good for oropharynx where bulk not desirable
  - Long pedicle length
  - Relatively easy to raise
  - Can be innervated
  - Allows two-team approach
  - Large distal size of vessel allows it to be used as a "flow-through-flap" in double flap reconstruction.
- *Limitations:*
  - Skin quality may be poor; in obese individuals, flap may be very bulky (especially proximally) with variable thickness
  - Donor site morbidity if skin graft is lost leading to tendon exposure and poor cosmetic result, albeit rare
  - Vascular compromise in hand after harvest: rare with a positive Allen test, but has been known to occur.
- *Preoperative assessment and planning:*
  - Modified Allen test is used to determine patency of the palmar arches. In a normal positive test, the hand flushes and color reappears between

5 and 15 seconds. Performing the test with a pulse oximeter and assessing oxygen saturation may improve sensitivity. A negative Allen test is a relative contraindication and this flap should not be harvested due to risk of postoperative hand ischemia.
  - The hand being used should undergo cannulation to avoid vessel trauma or spasm.
  - The nondominant hand is preferred but this is not always possible.
- *Intraoperative considerations:*
  - The marking should generally be performed beyond the flexor crease to allow hiding the scar below a long-sleeved shirt.
  - The more medial aspect of volar forearm is hairless in most individuals and is preferred.
  - If the cephalic vein is being considered for venous drainage, avoid placing the flap too medially.
  - Placing the flap too laterally results in poor cosmesis and more chance of exposure of superficial branch of radial nerve and postoperative pain and discomfort.
  - Most surgeons prefer the suprafascial plane to raise the flap allowing better graft healing and less donor site morbidity; paratenon needs to be preserved to prevent graft loss.
  - Tourniquet is commonly used, elevated to 100 mm Hg above the patient's blood pressure, used for up to 90 minutes.
  - Superficial branch of radial nerve needs to be identified early on and preserved.
  - Proximally, the bifurcation of the brachial artery needs to be identified with the takeoff of the ulnar artery before dividing the radial artery for harvest; the radial recurrent artery is distal to this and is a fairly reliable landmark.
  - Before detaching the flap after releasing the tourniquet, it is imperative to check the pedicle for bleeding; after detaching it and tunneling the pedicle, these may not be easily identified.
  - The donor area is closed circumferentially using a purse-string suture or with subcutaneous quilting sutures to attach the edges of the skin defect to the deep fascia and stabilize the skin graft; partial or full-thickness skin grafts can be used.
  - The graft needs to be anchored down meticulously to the bed, which is often undulating and irregular.
- *Postoperative care:*
  - Monitoring the hand with pulse oximetry over the thumb allows early identification of any ischemia in the hand.
  - Immobilization of the hand with a slab or cast can help prevent graft loss.
  - After the skin graft has taken, the hand can be mobilized with a full range of movement.

Anterolateral Thigh Flap

- *Vascular supply:* Descending branch of the lateral circumflex femoral artery and its vena comitantes.
- *Salient anatomy:* Only the anterior compartment of the thigh is encountered while raising this flap. The descending branch of the lateral circumflex artery supplies the flap through musculocutaneous (85%) or septocutaneous (15%) perforators. The lateral circumflex femoral artery usually arises from the profunda femoris but may rarely arise directly from the femoral artery. The ascending branch of the lateral circumflex femoral artery passes underneath the tensor fascia lata muscle and anastomoses with branches of the deep circumflex iliac artery, while the descending branch runs below the rectus femoris along the anterior aspect of the vastus lateralis. An oblique branch of the lateral circumflex artery occurs in 35% of legs and enters the vastus lateralis in its proximal third. The transverse branch of the lateral circumflex femoral artery passes over the vastus intermedius and pierces the vastus lateralis.
- *Anatomical variations:* After marking a line running between the anterior superior iliac spine and the lateral aspect of the patella, the midpoint is marked. The most common perforators are named "B" (which is reliably present in 90% as is located the midpoint of the line), "A" (which is about 5 cm proximal to "B" and present in 50%), and "C" (which is 5 cm distal to "B" and present in 60%). About 50% of legs have at least two perforators and 25% have one or three perforators; 1% have no perforators.
- *Components and variants:* Commonly fasciocutaneous or adipofascial, however, can include vastus lateralis muscle as one contiguous segment or multiple segments with individual perforators. Osteocutaneous harvest with partial thickness of the femur has been described but is not routine.
- *Flap design and utilization:* With the likely position of perforators being along the line joining the anterior superior iliac spine and lateral patella, the Doppler markings are used to identify potential perforators on which the skin paddle is based. Most commonly, an exploratory incision is used with a gentle curve to allow maximum likelihood of capturing skin perforators; after identifying these, the final skin paddle can be designed having committed to the lateral skin incision. The width of skin paddle that can be harvested

still allowing primary closure can be determined by pinching the skin of edges of the proposed defect together. It is helpful to aim to center the flap around the main perforator wherever possible to avoid marginal necrosis or accidental injury to the perforator during the final steps of harvest and detachment. Large areas (up to 10 × 25 cm) have been safely raised on a single skin perforator but skin bleeding in large flaps needs to be assessed thoroughly before detaching them, especially when raised on a single perforator.

- *Common use:* Replacement of mucosal or soft tissue for defects that are intraoral (tongue, floor of mouth, buccal, and oropharyngeal), reconstruction of defects associated with laryngectomy (circumferential or noncircumferential), neck skin following radical neck dissection, large skull base, and temporal bone defects.
- *Advantages:*
  - Minimal functional and cosmetic donor site morbidity
  - Large size of skin (10 × 25 cm) can be reliably harvested with primary closure.
  - Good length of pedicle.
  - Two-team approach can be used.
  - Innervation can be performed when harvested with lateral cutaneous nerve of thigh.
  - Versatile, with multiple chimeric options.
- *Limitations:*
  - In obese and big-built patients can be prohibitively thick and bulky.
  - Vascular and perforator anatomy can be variable and challenging, especially in novice surgeons.
  - Scar may be long and unsightly.
- *Preoperative assessment:*
  - No specific assessments; identification of previous surgical scars or trauma in the region prevents nasty surprises.
  - Assessment of tissue bulk and muscle tone allows better surgical planning.
- *Intraoperative considerations:*
  - The thigh needs to be exposed from anterior superior iliac spine to patella; this allows adapting to variations and exploration of the whole vascular territory. Good transverse exposure allows undermining the skin edges for primary closure.
  - In spite of picking up good Doppler signals suggestive of perforator location, committing to a skin paddle is best avoided until the perforators are reliably identified.
  - In very muscular patients, the incision can be erroneously placed laterally; the bony landmarks are more reliable than the palpation of the intermuscular septum. The rectus femoris muscle is identified as having a "fish-tail" configuration of muscle fibers with the "arrows" pointing toward the groin.
  - The anteromedial thigh flap perforators will often be exposed during the exploration of the incision and should not be divided until other perforators are identified; they may serve as a lifeboat in the absence of suitable anterolateral thigh flap perforators.
  - Similarly, tensor fascia lata perforators should not be divided until one is certain that they are not required; in most cases, the flap can be raised without disrupting them.
  - In the rare case, that there are no suitable skin perforators and no other perforators are available, the contralateral anterolateral thigh flap may be raised; in these patients there is still a 66% chance of the opposite side having suitable perforators.
  - Perforator dissection requires very gentle dissection and no energy sources near the vessels except for focused low-power bipolar cautery where required; thermal injury can result in a nonviable flap or subsequent flap loss.
  - Some surgeons prefer leaving a small cuff of muscle on either side of the perforator intact as it may avoid kinking or torsion.
  - Harvesting muscle requires carefully identification and preservation of perforators that supply the muscle to prevent patchy loss.
  - The vascular pedicle needs to be dissected meticulously throughout its length to identify aberrant branches and variation; often the artery and vein diverge courses and need to be dissected out separately.
  - Dermal closure is critical to avoid wound breakdown; if tension associated with closure is excessive, skin grafting can be used for closure; drain placement avoids seroma formation and collections in what is often a large dead space.
- *Postoperative care:*
  - Immobilization is not required in most cases; if a graft is used, a crepe bandage may help stabilize the wound bed and prevent graft migration.
  - Although drain volume may be low, early removal of drains, especially when there is a large dead space, may result in seromas or hematomas that are difficult to manage; wait till patients are adequately mobilized to remove drains.

Superficial Circumflex Iliac Artery Perforator Flap (Fig. 3)

- *Vascular supply:* Superficial circumflex iliac artery and a cutaneous vein which usually drains into the saphenous system.
- *Salient anatomy:* The superficial circumflex iliac artery, which is usually a branch of the superficial femoral or external iliac arteries, supplies the flap. The venous drainage is by a cutaneous vein that drains into the saphenous system below the inguinal ligament. The sartorius is a key landmark; the superficial circumflex iliac artery pierces the fascia at the medial aspect of the sartorius muscle, along which the pedicle is traced.
- *Anatomical variations:* The perforator always exists; in a series of over 200 cases, there were none where the perforator was absent.[63] However, the superficial circumflex iliac artery can have a variable point and pattern of origin, between 2.5 and 5 cm below the inguinal ligament, making pinpoint preoperative localization impossible. The draining vein can be variable in diameter and no vein should be divided until the anatomy of the flap is satisfactorily delineated.
- *Components and variants:* Skin and fat can be harvested. Although the classical flap only incorporates these two, a modified flap can encompass up to 15 cm of the proximal sartorius (sartorius-cutaneous groin flap).
- *Flap design and utilization:* The flap is centered on the origin of the superficial circumflex iliac artery. The "two-finger rule" has been described to plan the flap.[64] The anterior superior iliac spine and pubic tubercle are marked first, and then joined by a line to mark the inguinal ligament. The femoral artery is marked as the medial aspect of the flap. The origin of the superficial circumflex iliac artery origin is marked as two fingerbreadths below the junction of the femoral artery and inguinal ligament. Two fingerbreadths medial to the anterior superior iliac spine, the superficial circumflex iliac artery splits into its superficial branch (which gives off the perforator to the skin) and the deep branch that enters the sartorius. The upper extent of the flap is two fingerbreadths above the inguinal ligament, while the lower extent is two fingerbreadths below the origin of the superficial circumflex iliac artery. The lateral extent is the anterior superior iliac spine, with extension beyond this using a 1:1 length-to-width ratio. Up to 12 cm, width can be harvested with primary closure, which is always preferred.

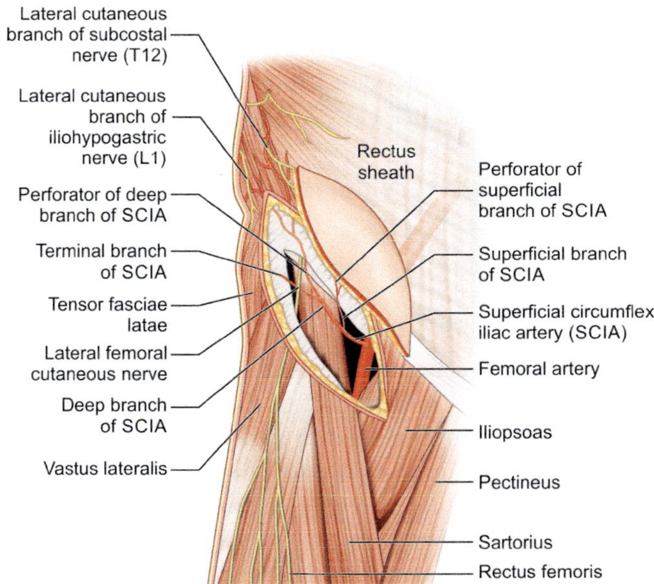

Fig. 3: Superficial circumflex iliac artery perforator flap.

- *Common use:* Thin pliable tissue is quite versatile, can be used for oral and oropharyngeal defects, limited external skin defects, and eyelid and external auditory canal defects.
- *Advantages:*
  - Thin pliable skin in lean built individuals
  - Minimal donor morbidity as scar is hidden and donor area can be closed primarily
- *Limitations:*
  - Pedicle length is short (2–5 cm) and vessel diameter is small with artery usually 1–2 mm in size.
  - Lateral femoral cutaneous nerve may need to be transected depending on relation to pedicle, resulting in anesthesia of anterolateral thigh.
  - In obese patients, bulk often precludes use.
- *Preoperative assessment:* Locating the signal of the superficial circumflex iliac artery with Doppler may be helpful. Identifying the hair-bearing and hairless areas in the groin before shaving the area may help better plan the flap.
- *Intraoperative considerations:*
  - Most surgeons prefer the lateral to medial approach to identify the skin perforator as the lateral course of the artery is constant, while the medial origin is variable.
  - The vessel is best protecting by harvesting the anterior sartorius fascia, even this may put the lateral femoral cutaneous nerve at risk.
  - The sartorius is a key landmark to identify the branching of the superficial circumflex iliac artery into superficial and deep branches.

- Pedicle dissection is crucial to ensure adequate length and vessel caliber; harvesting a cuff of femoral artery or splitting a "Y"-bifurcation longitudinally to form a large "V" may help address caliber issues.
- Donor area can be closed with slight undermining if under tension; if still under tension, the hip can be flexed to facilitate closure with gradual extension over the course of a few days.

- *Postoperative care:* Immobilization is not usually necessary, early ambulation helps with wound healing.

Rectus Abdominis Flap

- *Vascular supply:* Deep inferior epigastric artery and vein.
- *Salient anatomy:* The major component of this flap is rectus abdominis muscle with overlying fat and skin as required. When harvesting this flap, the anterior rectus sheath is incised and the muscle harvested while preserving the posterior rectus sheath (which is deficient below the arcuate line); hence, the anterior rectus sheath should not be excised below the arcuate line, which would make the abdominal wall weak and prone to herniation. The inferior epigastric artery arises from the external iliac artery and courses superiorly in an extraperitoneal plane, crossing the lateral border of the rectus to pierce the transveralis fascia between the rectus muscle and posterior rectus sheath. The vein accompanies the artery. The highest density of skin perforators is periumbilical.
- *Anatomical variations:* Rare, although there have been reports of absent deep inferior epigastric arteries[64] and intramuscular course of the pedicle.[65]
- *Components and variants:* Can be harvested as muscle and fat only, or with a reliable overlying skin paddle; usually, the skin perforators do not require identification and dissection.
- *Common use:* Used where a large volume of soft tissue is required for reconstruction, such as total glossectomy, maxillectomy, and skull base defects.
- *Advantages:*
  - Technically straightforward and quick flap to harvest
  - Anatomy usually consistent
  - Two-team approach is possible
  - Good pedicle length and vessel diameter (2–4 mm)
  - Good volume of soft tissue available for reconstruction
  - Low donor site morbidity
- *Limitations:*
  - Can be very bulky in obese patients
  - In patients who underwent previous abdominal surgery, the anatomy can be distorted and unreliable.
- *Preoperative assessment:* Other than inspecting for previous scar, musculature and presence of hernia, no specific assessment is indicated.
- *Intraoperative considerations:*
  - *Adequate exposure is important*: The abdomen needs to be exposed from above the xiphoid to below the inguinal ligament to facilitate harvesting the whole muscle.
  - Around 8–10 cm of skin can be harvested allowing primary closure, with the periumbilical skin having the highest perforator density.
  - The anterior rectus fascia should be incised first superiorly.
  - A cuff of anterior rectus fascia is left behind to facilitate closure.
  - The muscle volume harvested should be 20–30% larger than the defect to allow for postoperative atrophy and shrinkage.
  - Dissection down to the origin of the pedicle is useful to facilitate adequate length and also to confirm anatomy.
  - Anterior rectus sheath closed with strong nonabsorbable suture such as polypropylene, careful not to snag the underlying peritoneum or its contents; if it cannot be closed, a mesh is used to strengthen the abdominal wall.
- *Postoperative care:*
  - A drain is important to prevent postoperative collection.
  - The patient can be mobilize early but no strenuous activities involving the abdominal wall should be delayed for 6 weeks to allow uninterrupted healing.

Medial Sural Artery Perforator Flap

- *Vascular supply:* Medial sural artery arises from the popliteal artery (a common sural trunk in 30%), accompanied by a vein.
- *Salient anatomy:* First described as a refinement of the medial gastrocnemius flap, the vascular territory is roughly the medial half of the upper third of the posterior calf. The medial sural artery arises most commonly from the popliteal artery and after a few centimeters of its proximal course enters the medial belly of the gastrocnemius to supply the overlying skin via its perforators (2–4 each about 1 mm in diameter). The artery is usually about 2 mm in diameter at

its origin, with the pedicle having a length of 9–16 cm depending on the vascular anatomy.

- *Anatomical variations:* The medial sural artery has three distinct branching patterns within the medial gastrocnemius, with one (31%), two (59%), or three or more (10%) main branches and a variable intramuscular course, none of which preclude the use of this flap; however, the technical difficulty of harvest varies significantly.[66]
- *Components and variants:* This is a skin flap however some gastrocnemius flap can be harvested with its perforating branches.
- *Flap design and utilization:* Exploratory incisions are preferred with some surgeons marking the perforators preoperatively while others choosing not to. Small flaps (5–6 cm) which allow primary closures of the donor site are preferable.
- *Common use:* As an alternative to radial forearm free flap when thin pliable tissue is required for reconstruction.
- *Advantages:*
  - Limited donor morbidity and hidden scar
  - Pedicle length reasonable in most individuals
- *Limitations:*
  - Difficult to raise for inexperienced microvascular surgeons.
  - Perforators can be small and extremely delicate; mishandling them results in nonviability of the flap.
  - Pedicle can have long tortuous intramuscular course and small diameter.
- *Preoperative assessment:* Should not be performed in patients with peripheral vascular disease, clinical assessment to exclude this mandatory.
- *Intraoperative considerations:*
  - Marking of the perforators using Doppler may provide guidance, however, these are not always reliable; exploratory incisions are preferred to committing to the skin paddle around the suspected perforator locations early on in the operation.
  - The perforator is not handled as far as possible; gentle pedicle dissection without traction avoids spasm.
  - The motor nerve to medial belly of gastrocnemius should be identified as spared.
  - The short saphenous vein can be harvested along the skin paddle to aid venous drainage.
  - About 5–6 cm width can be closed primarily, a larger area requires a skin graft; when grafting, immobilization is crucial to avoid graft loss.
- *Postoperative care:* Early ambulation is important but use of a boot that prevents ankle flexion may prevent delayed graft loss after ambulation.

Parascapular System of Flaps (Fig. 4)

- *Vascular supply:* Descending branch of the circumflex scapular artery and its accompanying vein.
- *Salient anatomy:* The circumflex scapular artery is a branch of the subscapular artery that originates from the axillary artery; rarely, it arises directly from the axillary artery. After entering the triangular space, it gives off a transverse scapular branch and a vertical parascapular branch, the latter responsible for the vascular supply to this flap. The descending branch of the circumflex scapular artery, that supplies this flap, has a good caliber (2–4 mm), if traced all the way to its origin. The pedicle length is limited, typically 3–7 cm.
- *Anatomical variations:* As discussed under latissimus dorsi flap.
- *Components and variants:* This flap has skin, subcutaneous fat, and fascia. The lateral border of the scapular and a muscle component can be included with the harvest if required.
- *Flap design and utilization:* A large skin paddle (up to 15 × 25 cm in size has been described) can be harvested.

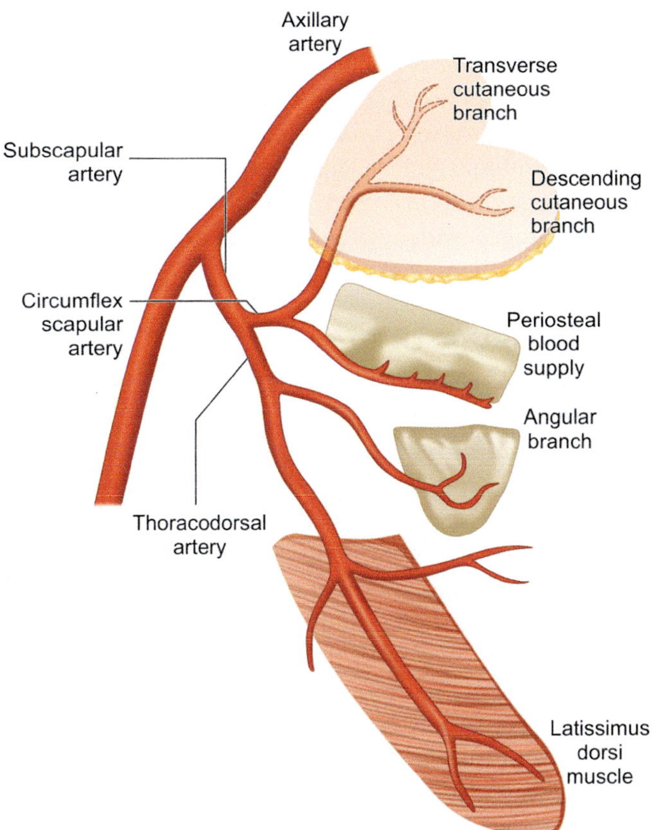

Fig. 4: Parascapular free flap system.

- *Common use:* For soft tissue defects without extensive tissue loss, the thickness of the skin in a moderately built person would be comparable to or slightly thicker than to the anterolateral thigh flap.
- *Advantages:*
  - Low donor morbidity
  - Multiple chimeric components can be raised on a single pedicle
- *Limitations:*
  - Pedicle length may be limited
  - Often requires patient repositioning; two-team harvest may be difficult.
- *Preoperative assessment:* Routine evaluation for altered anatomy and previous surgery or trauma.
- *Intraoperative considerations:*
  - Lateral decubitus position is preferred, with a beanbag below the contralateral shoulder, and the ipsilateral shoulder and arm free.
  - The flap marking is over the triangular space (a point roughly one fingerbreadth below the midpoint of the scapula on the lateral aspect of the scapula), with some surgeons marking the position of the pedicle with a Doppler.
  - The flap is raised from inferior to superior superficial to the deep fascia until the triangular space is encountered, then the deep fascia is incised to trace the pedicle.
  - Numerous branches are isolated and divided to trace the pedicle origin at the circumflex scapular artery, and the subscapular artery, if the additional pedicle length is required.
- *Postoperative care:* Early ambulation of the arm is encouraged, with a suction drain kept in place to avoid seroma or hematoma formation.

Latissimus Dorsi Flap

- *Vascular supply:* Thoracodorsal artery and venae comitantes (usually single).
- *Salient anatomy:* Latissimus dorsi is the largest muscle in the body, up to 20 × 40 cm in size. It originates along the iliac crest and thoracolumbar fascia, inserting into the bicipital groove of the humerus, responsible for extension of the shoulder and medial rotation and adduction of the humerus; hence, this flap is avoided in avid or professional rock climbers because this activity can be hampered. The nerve supply is through the thoracodorsal nerve; in C7 dysfunction, this muscle may be affected. Essentially most of the muscle can be harvested as a flap, with a suitable skin paddle centered over the muscle. The thoracodorsal pedicle is sizeable; the artery is 1.5–4 mm in diameter and vein is 2.5–4 mm in diameter, with the pedicle 5–15 (average 9) cm in length. As soon as the thoracodorsal artery enters the latissimus dorsi muscle, it is divided into horizontal and vertical branches, allowing two discrete paddles to be raised on the same pedicle. Skin perforator density is highest 2 cm behind the anterior edge of the muscle, and like the pectoralis major myocutaneous flap, these perforators are not routinely dissected out. The distal third of the muscle receives blood supply from the thoracic and lumbar intercostal arteries that need to be divided for flap harvest, making the blood supply of the distal third of the muscle unreliable when harvested off the thoracodorsal pedicle alone.
- *Anatomical variations:* The thoracodorsal artery originates from the subscapular artery, which in turn arises from the third part of the axillary artery after it crosses the pectoralis major. There can be variations within the system but the subscapular artery divides into the circumflex scapular artery and the thoracodorsal arteries. The circumflex scapular artery comes up into the triangular space (between teres major, teres minor, and long head of triceps) to supply the lateral aspect of the scapula and the scapular artery, while the thoracodorsal artery continues downward to supply the latissimus dorsi muscle after giving off branches to the tip of the scapula (angular artery) and a branch to the serratus anterior. Variants have been reported such as origin of the thoracodorsal artery arising from the thoracoacromial artery[67] or origin of the latissimus dorsi pedicle from the circumflex scapular artery;[68] however, these variations are exceedingly rare.
- *Components and variants:* The upper two-thirds of the muscle can safely be raised on the dominant pedicle. A relatively large skin paddle can be raised on the muscle without delineation of the skin perforators. Chimeric flaps can be raised on the subscapular system as described earlier, with independent muscle paddles, and bone (scapular tip) as required.
- *Flap design and utilization:* The entire muscle is marked out first with flap design depending on if a skin paddle is required, if required the exploratory incision is placed so as to not disrupt the intended skin paddle. A large incision is usually used to ensure adequate exposure and harvest of this large muscle.
- *Common use:* Used for soft tissue or mucosal defects (depending on the whether a skin paddle is raised or not). It is versatile flap that can be used to cover large surface areas (often scalp or lateral temporal bone defects) that do not need significant bulk, as this is a relatively thin muscle except in climbers.

- *Advantages:*
  - Fairly easy to learn to harvest
  - Very large area of muscle available without much bulk
  - Pedicle length good (5–15 cm) if dissected up to origin from subscapular artery
  - Donor site morbidity is minimal
  - Can be harvested with multiple chimeric components based on the subscapular system
- *Limitations:*
  - Two-team harvest difficult for head and neck defects, patient often needs to be repositioned
  - Risk of hematoma or seroma in donor site due to large dead space created
- *Preoperative assessment:* Routine preoperative assessment to ensure normal anatomy and muscle bulk, and no previous trauma or surgery is crucial.
- *Intraoperative considerations:*
  - Draping to allow the arm to remain mobile is very helpful to maximize pedicle exposure.
  - If harvesting a skin paddle, excessive retraction while raising the flap can shear off the perforators.
  - The superior edge of the muscle is more difficult to delineate as it often fuses with fibers of teres major.
  - Blunt dissection is preferred to delineate the latissimus dorsi muscle from the chest wall.
  - Inferiorly, the muscle fibers fuse with serratus anterior and external oblique; the inferior third of the muscle may not be reliable to harvest off the thoracodorsal pedicle.
  - The pedicle is often dissected from proximal to distal to avoid injury.
  - To increase pedicle length, the superficial circumflex scapular artery and branch to serratus anterior muscle may have to be divided as long as they are not being used for a chimeric component of the flap.
- *Postoperative care:*
  - Drain is left in-situ till output diminished and dead space has been obliterated, this can take as long as 2 weeks.
  - Arm can be mobilized within a day or two as long as there is no tension in the wound closure.

Lateral Arm Flap

- *Vascular supply:* Posterior radial collateral artery and its accompanying vena comitantes.
- *Salient anatomy:* The flap is supplied by the radial collateral artery, which originates from the brachial artery. It wraps around the posterior aspect of the humerus, descending on its lateral aspect, branching into anterior and posterior segments with the latter supplying the lateral arm and forearm flaps. The posterior radial collateral artery provides at least four fascial branches from 1 to 15 cm proximal to the lateral epicondyle. The artery finally divides into an anterior branch that is the nutrient flap to the vessel, and a posterior branch. The flap is based on the long axis of the humerus, with the perforator entering the flap through the septum between the triceps laterally and the biceps, brachioradialis, and brachialis medially. Proximally, the radial nerve crosses the pedicle from lateral to medial and needs to be carefully preserved. The posterior cutaneous nerve of the forearm originates as a branch of the radial nerve and joins the pedicle of the flap, and can be used for innervation.
- *Anatomical variations:* Unusual, however, the most common anomaly is duplication of the posterior radial collateral artery, which can lead to flap failure if unrecognized.
- *Components and variants:* Skin, fat, and fascia are the usual components. A short unicortical segment of the humerus can be harvested along with the soft tissue.
- *Flap design and utilization:* The axis of the flap is marked along the humerus from the deltoid insertion to the lateral epicondyle. Usually, 4–5 cm width is all that can be harvested allowing primary closure. The more distal the skin paddle harvest, the thinner is the skin available.
- *Common use:* Where soft tissue reconstruction is required without too much tissue bulk; commonly intraoral, midface, and skin defects.
- *Advantages:*
  - Hidden scar and low donor site morbidity
  - Two-team harvest is possible.
  - Pliable thin tissue in moderately built patients
- *Limitations:*
  - Pedicle is short (2–6 cm).
  - Pedicle caliber is small (1–2 mm in size).
  - Risk of radial nerve neuropraxia.
- *Preoperative assessment:* Routine preoperative examination indicated; the posterior radial collateral artery can be localized with a Doppler probe preoperatively.
- *Intraoperative considerations:*
  - The posterior flap is elevated first, with the deep fascia lifted off the triceps muscle.
  - The distal pedicle is divided and the inferior aspect of the flap is elevated next; after identifying the supplying vessels and staying deep to them, the septum is divided to free the flap from the deeper layers.
  - Proximal dissection is continued to allow pedicle length and caliber.

- While doing this, the brachialis and triceps are retracted to expose the muscular branches which are divided carefully, without traction on or injury to the radial nerve.
- If bone is being harvested, there is a risk of postoperative supracondylar fracture, leading to prophylactic stabilization of the bone with a locking compression condyle plate.

- *Postoperative care:* No immobilization is usually required when a soft tissue flap is harvested.

Fibula Osteocutaneous Flap (Fig. 5)

- *Vascular supply:* Peroneal artery and its venae comitantes.
- *Salient anatomy:* The fibula osteocutaneous flap is a robust flap supplied by the peroneal artery and its venae comitantes, comprising the vascularized fibula bone, with muscle (flexor hallucis longus and soleus) and a skin paddle as required. The popliteal artery divides into the anterior and posterior tibial arteries with the peroneal artery arising from the latter. The peroneal vessels lie in close proximity to the medial aspect of the fibula, between the tibialis posterior muscle anteriorly and the flexor hallucis longus muscle posteriorly. Except for the proximal and distal 5–6 cm, the entire fibula can be harvested as vascularized bone (≥25 cm in length). In order to harvest the flap, the peroneal muscles need to be detached from the lateral aspect of the fibula, the extensor digitorum longus and extensor hallucis longus from the anterior aspect of the fibula, and the tibialis posterior and flexor hallucis longus muscles from the medial aspect of the fibula. There are several important structures that need to be preserved: the superficial peroneal nerve along the anterior skin incision, the sural nerve along the posterior skin incision, the anterior tibial vessels and nerve deep to the extensor digitorum and extensor hallucis longus muscles, and the common peroneal nerve superiorly near the neck of the fibula during the osteotomy.
- *Anatomical variations:* The peronea arteria magna is a situation where there is a single artery supplying the leg and foot, with hypoplastic anterior and posterior tibial arteries. The incidence is 5%[69] and when it is harvested along with the fibula flap can result in ischemia of the foot. This can be reliably identified in preoperative Doppler ultrasonography or angiography; however, some authors have argued that clinical evaluation of lower limb pulses is adequate to identify this anomaly and routine radiological evaluation is not indicated.[70]
- *Components and variants:* The vascularized bone can be harvested with a skin paddle (supplied by perforators traversing through the peroneal muscles) and components of the flexor hallucis longus and soleus muscles.
- *Flap design and utilization:* The classical incision is marked on the posterior crural intermuscular septum (between the peroneal muscles and the soleus), with skin perforators marked along this line using a Doppler. The skin paddle is centered on the position of these perforators, but usually an exploratory incision is placed to identify perforators before committing to the skin paddle. The skin paddle can be up to 12 cm wide, and donor site closure is performed with split skin grafting if too large to be closed primarily.

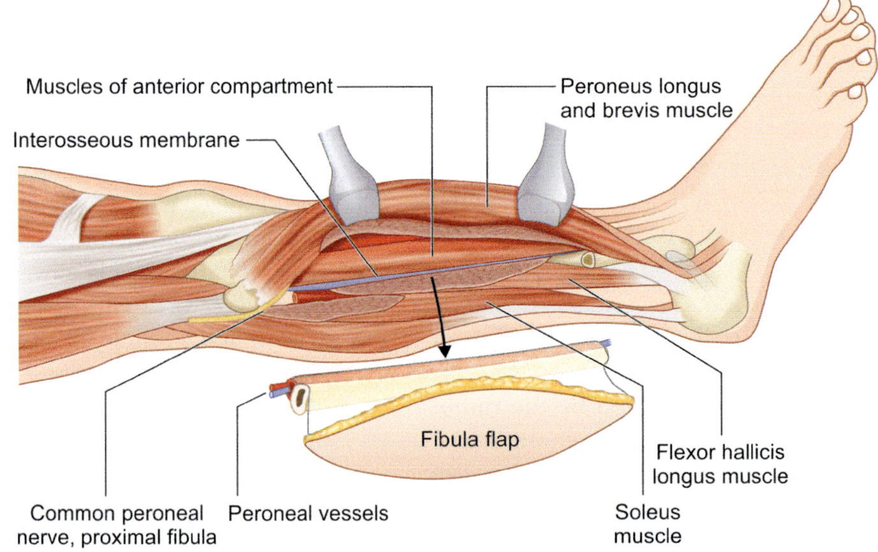

Fig. 5: Fibula osteocutaneous flap.

- *Common use:* For bony reconstruction of the maxilla, mandible, midface, and orbit. The soft tissue components can also be well addressed using this flap.
- *Advantages:*
  - Long length and stock of vascularized bone (suitable for implant placement)
  - Long pedicle length and vessel caliber (1.5–4 mm)
  - Reliable skin and muscle components
  - Two-team harvest is possible
  - Multiple osteotomies can be reliably performed.
- *Limitations:*
  - Poor choice in peripheral vascular disease
  - Donor site morbidity common when grafted
  - Skin paddle has limited thickness and can be poor quality in obesity and peripheral vascular disease.
- *Preoperative assessment:* Many surgeons perform routine angiography or Doppler ultrasonography of the lower limb to rule out vascular anomalies. The choice of leg is not rigid; however, if the surgeon wishes the pedicle to run posteriorly in a mandible reconstruction, the ipsilateral leg is used when the skin paddle is to reconstruct an external skin defect and the contralateral leg is used when the skin paddle is to reconstruct an intraoral defect.
- *Intraoperative considerations:*
  - The leg is draped till above the level of the knee, allowing it to remain mobile. The knee is usually flexed and the ankle is rested on a stirrup or a large saline infusion bag for support.
  - A tourniquet is used at the mid-thigh level, inflated 100 mm Hg above the systolic blood pressure, with most surgeons deflating it after 90 minutes.
  - The anterior incision is placed first, identifying the perforators, dividing the peroneal muscles to leave only a cuff to protect the perforators.
  - The incision is deepened though the deep fascia after identifying the superficial peroneal nerve to prevent injury.
  - The extensor hallucis and extensor digitorum longus muscles are divided close to the fibula free edge, with retraction superiorly, in order to avoid injuring the anterior tibial pedicle.
  - The anterior crural intermuscular septum is divided prior to the osteotomy to provide adequate exposure.
  - The osteotomies can be performed before or after the posterior dissection; different techniques have been described.
  - A stump of 5–6 cm of fibula is preserved superiorly and 5–6 cm inferiorly to prevent injury to the common peroneal nerve above and destabilization of the ankle joint below.
  - After dividing the tibialis posterior muscle to expose the peroneal vessels, care is taken to avoid shearing the pedicle away from the bone, which will compromise its blood supply.
  - The pedicle is dissected superiorly and care is taken to avoid injuring the posterior tibial pedicle.
  - Osteotomies are performed carefully to avoid devascularization of the bone; unnecessary osteotomies and bony segments ≤1.5 cm are avoided.
- *Postoperative care:*
  - A drain is placed to prevent seroma or hematoma formation.
  - Closure is performed primarily or with split skin grafting; mobilization and weight-bearing is initiated early with a boot to stabilize the ankle and allow the graft a stable bed to heal.

Deep Circumflex Iliac Artery Flap

- *Vascular supply:* Deep circumflex iliac artery and the venae comitantes.
- *Salient anatomy:* The deep circumflex iliac artery supplies a large and concave segment of the cancellous iliac crest bone (in contrast to fibula which is exclusively cortical bone). The artery arises from the external iliac artery near the junction with the femoral artery. The vein empties into the saphenous vein or a tributary, terminating in the femoral vein. The internal oblique and iliacus muscle inserted on the concavity of the iliac crest can be harvested as soft tissue cover to the flap.
- *Anatomical variations:* The deep circumflex iliac artery arises laterally or posterolaterally from the external iliac artery behind the inguinal ligament. It is usually adjacent to the inferior epigastric artery origin. The deep circumflex iliac artery runs along the iliac crest to divide into two major branches, the horizontal branch and the ascending branch. The variations are related to the origin of the deep circumflex iliac artery and its terminal branches; however, this does not usually interfere with flap harvest.[71]
- *Components and variants:* Iliac crest bone with adjacent periosteum, iliacus muscle and soft tissue, can be harvested with or without an overlying skin paddle.
- *Flap design and utilization:* Depending on the skin paddle requirement, the incision is either placed in accordance with this or along the inguinal ligament. The contiguous skin paddle is often of poor quality and some surgeons do not routinely harvest it.

- *Common use:* Used for bony reconstruction of the maxilla, mandible, and floor of the orbit
- *Advantages:*
  - The curvature of the iliac crest is a good match for that of the maxilla and mandible, often without the need for an osteotomy
  - Good vessel caliber (1.5–3 mm)
  - Two-team approach is possible.
- *Limitations:*
  - Soft tissue component of this flap is limited
  - May result in postoperative inguinal hernia in up to 9% of patients[72]
  - Delayed mobilization, often takes up to a month for patients to have the full range of pain-free mobility
  - Pedicle length is limited (4–7 cm).
- *Preoperative assessment:* Patients with a high risk of inguinal hernia are not good candidates for harvest of this flap.
- *Intraoperative considerations:*
  - After placing the skin incision, the external oblique aponeurosis is exposed and then the muscle; the avascular plane between the external and internal oblique is delineated.
  - The internal oblique muscle is then incised to isolate it from the transversalis muscle, which is aided by a change in the direction of muscle fibers.
  - This allows identification of the ascending branch of the deep circumflex iliac artery, which is traced proximally to the main pedicle, superficial to the iliacus muscle and transversalis fascia.
  - For the bone harvest, the transversalis muscle and iliacus are divided at the intended sites of osteotomy; the bone harvested can be unicortical or bicortical and the anterior superior iliac spine is usually avoided to preserve all the muscular attachments.
  - In order to better contour the bone, the lateral cortex and crest of the ilium can be "outfractured" while preserving the inner cortex, like a greenstick fracture, to avoid pedicle compromise.
  - The internal oblique and iliacus can be used for soft tissue replacement.
  - Closure needs to be meticulous and in layers, with suction drains. If there is a risk of postoperative hernia, closure is performed with a polypropylene mesh.
- *Postoperative care:*
  - Mobilization is gradual and adequate analgesia is imperative.
  - At least 6 weeks of limited physical activity is crucial to allow healing and prevent a postoperative hernia.

Scapula Bone Flap

- *Vascular supply:* Two alternate bone supplies: the angular scapular branch of the thoracodorsal artery or bone branches from the circumflex scapular system to the mid-portion of the lateral edge of the scapula.
- *Salient anatomy:* The subscapular arterial system supplies the lateral aspect of the scapula, which is harvested as the scapula bone flap. The angular branch of the thoracodorsal system supplies the inferolateral edge and tip of the scapula (up to 2 cm of bone width can be harvested safely). The perforating branches to the bone need to be carefully preserved to ensure that the bone is vascularized. A good length of bone is available (up to 14 cm in males and 10 cm in females) which can be harvested.
- *Anatomical variations:* As discussed under latissimus dorsi flap.
- *Components and variants:* Versatile flap that allows complex chimeric flap design off a single pedicle. Two bone components are possible, the lateral edge of the scapula or the scapula tip. Additional components can be harvested in conjunction with flaps of the parascapular, latissimus, serratus, or thoracodorsal artery perforator flap systems.
- *Flap design and utilization:* The skin paddle can be designed to overlap the lateral border of the scapula and the triangular space.
- *Common use:* Has been used for bony reconstruction of the maxilla, mandible, and orbital floor, with simultaneous reconstruction of soft tissue defects with the chimeric skin and muscle components. The scapular tip flaps are used for short segment maxilla or mandible defects.
- *Advantages:*
  - Versatile system with multiple chimeric components available for harvest
  - Good pedicle length (when harvested up to the subscapular vessel)
  - Low donor morbidity
- *Limitations:*
  - Two-team harvest is difficult and may need repositioning.
  - The bone width may be insufficient for implant placement in dental rehabilitation (controversial).
- *Preoperative assessment:* To rule out anatomical variations, altered anatomy or previous surgery and/or trauma.
- *Intraoperative considerations:*
  - The initial soft tissue dissection is similar to the parascapular flap, till the triangular space is identified.

- The bony perforators are identified and preserved early on; if the scapular tip is desired, the angular artery is preserved, while if the lateral border of the bone is desired, the lateral bone branches of the thoracodorsal arterial system are preserved.
- The teres minor and long head of triceps need to be released from the lateral scapular border to harvest bone; from 1 cm below the glenohumeral joint to the scapular tip can be safely harvested without destabilizing the shoulder joint.
- The site of the osteotomies are exposed in the subperiosteal plane.
- A small oscillating saw is used to create the osteotomies; not >2 cm width of bone is usually harvested.
- The infraspinatus and subscapularis muscles may need to be divided to release the bone.
- The teres muscle and long head of triceps may be resutured to the remaining scapula with drill holes; however, if the teres major does not appear vascular, it should be removed.

- *Postoperative care:*
  - Early mobilization is important to prevent shoulder dysfunction.
  - Premature drain removal may result in seroma or hematoma formation.

REFERENCES

1. Dolan RT, Butler JS, Murphy SM, Cronin KJ. Health-related quality of life, surgical and aesthetic outcomes following microvascular free flap reconstructions: an 8-year institutional review. Ann R Coll Surg Engl. 2012;94(1):43-51.
2. Chick LR, Walton RL, Reus W, Colen L, Sasmor M. Free flaps in the elderly. Plast Reconstr Surg. 1992;90(1):87-94.
3. Shestak KC, Jones NF. Microsurgical free-tissue transfer in the elderly patient. Plast Reconstr Surg. 1991;88(2):259-63.
4. Subramaniam N, Balasubramanian D, Rka P, Rathod P, Murthy S, Vidhyadharan S, et al. Perioperative outcomes following major surgery for head and neck cancer in the elderly: institutional audit and case-control study. J Laryngol Otol. 2018;132(8):742-7.
5. Lawrence WT, Murphy RC, Robson MC, Heggers JP. The detrimental effect of cigarette smoking on flap survival: an experimental study in the rat. Br J Plast Surg. 1984;37(2):216-9.
6. Nolan J, Jenkins RA, Kurihara K, Schultz RC. The acute effects of cigarette smoke exposure on experimental skin flaps. Plast Reconstr Surg. 1985;75(4):544-51.
7. Chang LD, Buncke G, Slezak S, Buncke HJ. Cigarette smoking, plastic surgery, and microsurgery. J Reconstr Microsurgery. 1996;12(7):467-74.
8. Reus WF, Colen LB, Straker DJ. Tobacco smoking and complications in elective microsurgery. Plast Reconstr Surg. 1992;89(3):490-4.
9. Barr LC, Joyce AD. Microvascular anastomoses in diabetes: an experimental study. Br J Plast Surg. 1989;42(1):50-3.
10. Deganello A, Gitti G, Parrinello G, Muratori E, Larotonda G, Gallo O. Cost analysis in oral cavity and oropharyngeal reconstructions with microvascular and pedicled flaps. Acta Otorhinolaryngol Ital. 2013;33(6):380-7.
11. Hanasono MM, Corbitt CA, Yu P, Skoracki RJ. Success of sequential free flaps in head and neck reconstruction. J Plast Reconstr Aesthet Surg. 2014;67(9):1186-93.
12. Rodby KA, Turin S, Jacobs RJ, Cruz JF, Hassid VJ, Kolokythas A, et al. Advances in oncologic head and neck reconstruction: systematic review and future considerations of virtual surgical planning and computer aided design/ computer aided modeling. J Plast Reconstr Aesthet Surg. 2014;67(9):1171-85.
13. Yazar S. Selection of recipient vessels in microsurgical free tissue reconstruction of head and neck defects. Microsurgery. 2007;27(7):588-94.
14. Bianchi B, Ferri A, Ferrari S, Copelli C, Perlangeli G, Leporati M, et al. Reconstruction of mandibular defects using the scapular tip free flap. Microsurgery. 2014;35(2):101-6.
15. Hollinshead WH. Anatomy for Surgeons, 3rd edition. New York: Harper & Row; 1982. pp. 467-9.
16. Wong KK, Higgins KM, Enepekides DJ. Microvascular reconstruction in the vessel-depleted neck. Curr Opin Otolaryngol Head Neck Surg. 2010;18(4):223-6.
17. Vasilakis V, Patel HD, Chen HC. Head and neck reconstruction using cephalic vein transposition in the vessel-depleted neck. Microsurgery. 2009;29(8):598-602.
18. Horng SY, Chen MT. Reversed cephalic vein: a lifeboat in head and neck free flap reconstruction. Plast Reconstr Surg. 1993;92(4):752-3.
19. Ethunandan M, Cole R, Flood TR. Corlett loop for microvascular reconstruction in a neck depleted of vessels. Br J Oral Maxillofac Surg. 2007;45(6):493-5.
20. Griffin JR, Thornton JF. Microsurgery: free tissue transfer and replantation. Selected Readings Plast Surg. 2005;10:1-41.
21. Cordeiro PG; Santamaria E. Experience with the continuous suture microvascular anastomosis in 200 consecutive free flaps. Ann Plast Surg. 1998;40(1):1-6.
22. Schlechter B, Guyuron B. A comparison of different suture techniques for microvascular anastomosis. Ann Plast Surg. 1994;33(1):28-31.
23. Hamilton RB, O'Brien BM. An experimental study of microvascular patency using a continuous suture technique. Br J Plast Surg. 1979;32(3):153-4.
24. Biemer E. Vein grafts in microvascular surgery. Br J Plast Surg. 1977;30(3):197-9.
25. Brener BJ, Raines JK, Darling RC. The end-to-end anastomosis of blood vessels of different diameters. Surg Gynecol Obstet. 1974;138(2):249-50.
26. Shimizu F, Lin MP, Ellabban M, Evans GR, Cheng MH. Superficial temporal vessels as a reserve recipient site for microvascular head and neck reconstruction in vessel-depleted neck. Ann Plast Surg. 2009;62(2):134-8.
27. Eriksson E, Anderson WA, Replogle RL. Effects of prolonged ischemia on muscle microcirculation in the cat. Surg Forum. 1974;25(0):254-5.
28. Thomason PR, Matzke HA. Effects of ischemia on the hind limb of the rat. Am J Phys Med. 1975;54(3):113-31.
29. Chen SH, Tang YB, Chen HC. Survival of transferred ileum after ischemia time longer than 1 hour: a clinical result different from animal studies. J Am Coll Surg. 2013;217(2): 300-5.
30. Ames A III, Wright RL, Kowada M, Thurston JM, Majno G. Cerebral ischemia: II. The no-reflow phenomenon. Am J Pathol. 1968;52(2):437-53.

31. Shaw WW, Ko CY, Ahn CY, Markowitz BL. Safe ischemia time in free-flap surgery: a clinical study of contact-surface cooling. J Reconstr Microsurg. 1996;12(7):421-4.
32. Gürlek A, Kroll SS, Schusterman MA. Ischemic time and free flap success. Ann Plast Surg. 1997;38(5):503-5.
33. Chang EI, Chang EI, Soto-Miranda MA, Zhang H, Nosrati N, Crosby MA, et al. Comprehensive evaluation of risk factors and management of impending flap loss in 2138 breast free flaps. Ann Plast Surg. 2016;77(1):67-71.
34. Wei FC, Mardini S. Flaps and Reconstructive Surgery E-Book. Elsevier Health Sciences; 2016.
35. Addison PD, Neligan PC, Ashrafpour H, Khan A, Zhong A, Moses M, et al. Noninvasive remote ischemic preconditioning for global protection of skeletal muscle against infarction. Am J Physiol Heart Circ Physiol. 2003;285(4):H1435-43.
36. Moses MA, Addison PD, Neligan PC, Ashrafpour H, Huang N, Zair M, et al. Mitochondrial KATP channels in hind limb remote ischemic preconditioning of skeletal muscle against infarction. Am J Physiol Heart Circ Physiol. 2005;288(2):H559-67.
37. Ragnarsson R, Berggren A, Klintenberg C, Ostrup L. Microvascular anastomoses in irradiated vessels: a comparison between the Unilink system and sutures. Plast Reconstr Surg. 1990;85(3):412-8.
38. Berggren A, Ostrup LT, Ragnarsson R. Clinical experience with the Unilink/3M Precise microvascular anastomotic device. Scand J Plast Reconstr Surg. 1993;27(1):35-9.
39. Ahn CY, Shaw WW, Berns S, Markowitz BL. Clinical experience with the 3M microvascular coupling anastomotic device in 100 free-tissue transfers. Plast Reconstr Surg. 1994;93(7):1481-4.
40. Blair WF, Morecraft RJ, Steyers CM, Maynard JA. A microvascular anastomotic device: II. A histologic study in arteries and veins. Microsurgery. 1989;10(1):29-39.
41. Shindo ML, Costantino PD, Nalbone VP, Rice DH, Sinha UK. Use of a mechanical microvascular anastomotic device in head and neck free tissue transfer. Arch Otolaryngol Head Neck Surg. 1996;122(5):529-32.
42. Barker EV, Enepekides DJ. The utility of microvascular anastomotic devices in head and neck reconstruction. Curr Opin Otolaryngol Head Neck Surg. 2008;16(4):331-4.
43. Pratt GF, Rozen WM, Westwood A, Hancock A, Chubb D, Ashton MW, et al. Technology-assisted and sutureless microvascular anastomoses: Evidence for current techniques. Microsurgery. 2012;32(1):68-76.
44. Chao AH, Meyerson J, Povoski SP, Kocak E. A review of devices used in the monitoring of microvascular free tissue transfers. Expert review of medical devices. 2013;10(5):649-60.
45. Spate TH, Gaynor E. Vascular endothelial damage and thrombosis. Adv Cardiol. 1969;4:147-66.
46. Tangelder GJ, Goude Egbrink M, Slaaf DW, Reneman RS, et al. Blood platelets: An overview. J Reconstr Microsurg. 1989; 5(2):167-71.
47. Johnson PC. Platelet-mediated thrombosis in microvascular surgery: new knowledge and strategies. Plast Reconstr Surg. 1990;86(2):359-67.
48. Davies DM. A world survey of anticoagulation practice in clinical microvascular surgery. Br J Plast Surg. 1982;35(1):96-9.
49. Barton BM, Riley CA, Fitzpatrick JC, Hasney CP, Moore BA, McCoul ED. Postoperative anticoagulation after free flap reconstruction for head and neck cancer: a systematic review. Laryngoscope. 2018;128(2):412-21.
50. Yii NW, Evans GR, Miller MJ, Reece GP, Langstein H, Chang D, et al. Thrombolytic therapy: What is its role in free flap salvage? Ann Plast Surg. 2001;46(6):601-4.
51. Egozi D, Fodor L, Ullmann Y. Salvage of compromised free flaps in trauma cases with combined modalities. Microsurgery. 2011;31(2):109-15.
52. Hong KY, Chang LS, Chang H, Minn KW, Jin US. Direct thrombectomy as a salvage technique in free flap breast reconstruction. Microsurgery. 2017;37(5):402-5.
53. Bui DT, Cordeiro PG, Hu QY, Disa JJ, Pusic A, Mehrara BJ. Free flap reexploration: indications, treatment, and outcomes in 1193 free flaps. Plast Reconstr Surg. 2007;119(7):2092-100.
54. Valauri FA. The use of medicinal leeches in microsurgery. Blood Coagul Fibrinolysis. 1991;2(1):185-7
55. Nguyen MQ, Crosby MA, Skoracki RJ, Hanasono MM. Outcomes of flap salvage with medicinal leech therapy. Microsurgery. 2012;32(5):351-7.
56. Chang EI, Zhang H, Liu J, Yu P, Skoracki RJ, Hanasono MM. Analysis of risk factors for flap loss and salvage in free flap head and neck reconstruction. Head Neck. 2016;38(S1):E771-5.
57. Urken ML, Weinberg H, Buchbinder D, Moscoso JF, Lawson W, Catalano PJ, et al. Microvascular free flaps in head and neck reconstruction: report of 200 cases and review of complications. Arch Otolaryngol Head Neck Surg. 1994;120(6):633-40.
58. McCormack L, Cauldwell E, Anson B. Brachial and antebrachial patterns: a study of 750 extremities. Surg Gynecol Obstet. 1953;96(1):43-54.
59. Coleman SS. Arterial patterns in the hand based upon a study of 650 specimens. Surg Gynecol Obstet. 1961;113:409-24.
60. Hedén P, Gylbert L. Anomaly of the radial artery encountered during elevation of the radial forearm flap. J Reconstr Microsurg. 1990;6(02):139-41.
61. Otsuka T, Terauchi M. An anomaly of the radial artery—relevance for the forearm flap. Br J Plast Surg. 1991;44(5):390-1.
62. Small JO, Millar R. The radial artery forearm flap: an anomaly of the radial artery. Br J Plast Surg. 1985;38(4):501-3.
63. Chuang DC, Colony LH, Chen HC, Wei FC. Groin flap design and versatility. Plast Reconstr Surg. 1989;84(1):100-7.
64. Ridha H, Thompson MK, Cameron MG, Durrani AJ. Anatomical variation in deep inferior epigastric pedicles and implications for harvest of lower abdominal flaps. Br J Oral Maxillofac Surg. 2011;49(3):233-4.
65. Wong CH, Song C. The "intramuscular" rectus abdominis pedicle. Plast Reconstr Surg. 2007;119(6):1964-5.
66. Dusseldorp JR, Pham QJ, Ngo Q, Gianoutsos M, Moradi P. Vascular anatomy of the medial sural artery perforator flap: A new classification system of intra-muscular branching patterns. J Plast Reconstr Aesthet Surg. 2014;67(9):1267-75.
67. Marall T, Celik H, Hayran M, Kecik A. An anatomical variation of the thoracodorsal artery with comments on flaps based on the axillary artery. Eur J Plast Surg. 1993;16(4-5):231-3.
68. Satoh K, Ohkubo F, Tojima Y. A variation of the vascular pedicle of the latissimus dorsi muscle. Plast Reconstr Surg. 1991;88(6):1081-4.
69. Rosson GD, Singh NK. Devascularizing complications of free fibula harvest: peronea arteria magna. J Reconstr Microsurg. 2005;21(8):533-8.
70. Lutz BS, Wei FC, Ng SH, Chen IH, Chen SH. Routine donor leg angiography before vascularized free fibula transplantation is not necessary: a prospective study in 120 clinical cases. Plast Reconstr Surg. 1999;103(1):121-7.
71. Ghassemi A, Furkert R, Prescher A, Riediger D, Knobe M, O'dey D, et al. Variants of the supplying vessels of the vascularized iliac bone graft and their relationship to important surgical landmarks. Clin Anat. 2013;26(4):509-21.
72. Kim HS, Kim JY, Hur H, Nam W. Herniation after deep circumflex iliac artery flap: two cases of rare complication. Maxillofac Plast Reconstr Surg. 2016;38(1):10.

CHAPTER 38

Principles of Oral Cavity Reconstruction

Radhika Kapahtia, Narayana Subramaniam, Sivakumar Vidhyadharan, Samskruthi P Murthy

INTRODUCTION

The oral cavity has a complex three-dimensional anatomy and a host of functions that makes reconstruction after ablative surgery challenging. However, surgery forms the mainstay in the management of oral cancer, making understanding these principles vital. An ideal reconstruction aims to reconstruct defects with similar tissue quality and quantity to restore form and function. The major goals of oral cavity reconstruction are restoration of swallowing, mastication, and speech. The frequent use of adjuvant radiotherapy in oral cancer also poses a formidable challenge. In this chapter, we describe the principles of reconstruction following oral cavity ablation for malignancy and evidence that supports them.

GENERAL PRINCIPLES IN ORAL CAVITY RECONSTRUCTION

- *Replacing "like" with "like"*: Whenever possible, it is important to reconstruct defects with similar tissue (e.g., bone with bone). Use of local tissue may help with ideal functional and cosmetic restoration.
- *Oncological outcomes take precedence*: In advanced oral cancer where adjuvant radiotherapy is indicated, it should be commenced within 6–8 weeks after surgery. Reconstruction is meant to enable rather than hamper this. Often simpler reconstruction is planned with secondary procedures and revisions later on.
- *Likelihood of success should impact choice of reconstruction*: Simple straightforward options are preferably in oncological reconstruction. Although technically feasible complex plans should be avoided wherever feasible.[1]

Preoperative Decision-making

- Most defects in advanced oral cancer are composite and require detailed planning with the ablative surgeon, including the need for frozen sections where margins may be more extensive.
- Assessment of the defect, available donor sites, previous radiotherapy details, and other systemic issues that may influence outcomes.[2,3]
- Other issues (such as diabetes, smoking, and vasculitis) that can impact free flap healing need to be managed aggressively perioperatively.[4,5]

Choice of Recipient Vessels

The four paired arteries commonly used as donor vessels are facial, superior thyroid, superficial temporal, and transverse cervical arteries. The external carotid is rarely used in an end-to-side configuration due to the high pressure and risk of blow out. Contralateral vessels are used in the dissected or irradiated neck. The veins used are the common facial, external jugular, and internal jugular veins.

TONGUE RECONSTRUCTION

The tongue is median organ that is symmetrical on either side of the midline raphe. Each half comprises extrinsic (hyoglossus, styloglossus, genioglossus, and palatoglossus) and intrinsic (longitudinal and transverse) muscles and a neurovascular bundle. The functions of the tongue are speech (achieved through palatal contact), swallowing (oral and oropharyngeal phases), mastication (through mixing of the bolus with saliva), and airway maintenance.[6] The aims of tongue reconstruction are to reconstruct the complex anatomy, restoration of swallowing and speech, restoring tissue bulk, allowing sensation and mobility, preventing restriction in mobility of remnant tongue, preventing formation of orocervical fistula when the floor of mouth is resected, and allowing for cosmesis **(Table 1)**.[7] An example of total glossectomy reconstruction is shown in **Figures 1A to C**.

Table 1: Reconstructive options in tongue defects.[12]

Tongue defect		Considerations	Preferred options	Alternatives
Hemi		Thin, pliable skin flap, motility	• Radial forearm flap • Medial sural artery perforator flap • Pectoralis major myocutaneous flap	• Ulnar forearm flap • Anterolateral thigh fasciocutaneous flap • Pectoralis major myocutaneous flap
Subtotal	Anterior two-thirds	Bulky skin flap	Anterolateral thigh fasciocutaneous flap	• Rectus abdominis musculocutaneous flap • Pectoralis major myocutaneous flap
	Anterior three-quarters	Bulky musculocutaneous flap	Anterolateral thigh fasciocutaneous flap	• Rectus abdominis musculocutaneous flap • Pectoralis major myocutaneous flap
Total glossectomy		Large musculocutaneous flap with adequate volume for swallowing	Anterolateral thigh musculocutaneous flap	

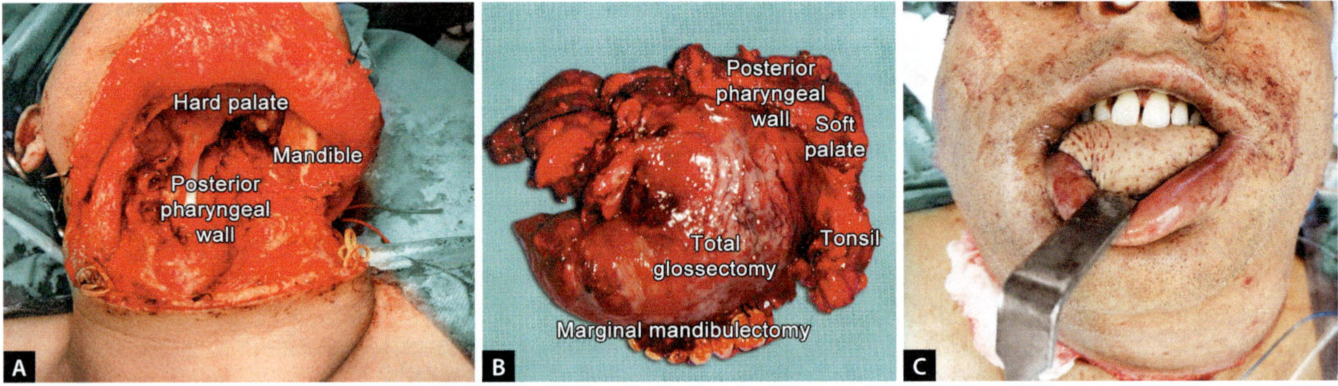

Figs. 1A to C: Total glossectomy. (A) Defect post-resection; (B) Excised specimen; (C) Defect reconstructed with fasciocutaneous anterolateral thigh flap.

SURGICAL CONSIDERATIONS

- Defects involving the floor of the mouth require thin pliable tissue that prevents tethering of the native tongue, while bulky tissue is chosen for large defects of the oral tongue to aid swallowing.
- Flaps can be neurotized either to provide sensation or to aid motor function if muscle flaps are used; in theory, this can aid in mastication, oral hygiene and quality of life, but outcomes have been modest.[8,9]
- The tongue tip should be preserved and not distorted wherever possible to aid speech.
- For posterior defects, bulky flaps that aid glossopalatal contact is important for swallowing.[10]
- Cosmetic outcomes were not significant in these patients.[11]

Buccal Mucosa Reconstruction

The buccal mucosa is continuous with the mucosal lining of the upper and lower lip anteriorly and the retromolar trigone and oropharyngeal mucosa posteriorly **(Fig. 2)**. Laterally, it continues with the gingival mucosa, resulting in advanced lesions being referred to as gingivobuccal sinus cancers as they involve multiple contiguous areas. The mucosa is stratified nonkeratinizing squamous epithelium, with a submucosal lamina propria and minor salivary glands. Deep to this lies the buccinator that is considered the minimum depth to which invasive cancers required to be excised.[12] The infratemporal fossa is often part of the resection in T4 lesions. A defect classification describing thickness, superoinferior plane, and anteroposterior plane is shown in **Table 2**.

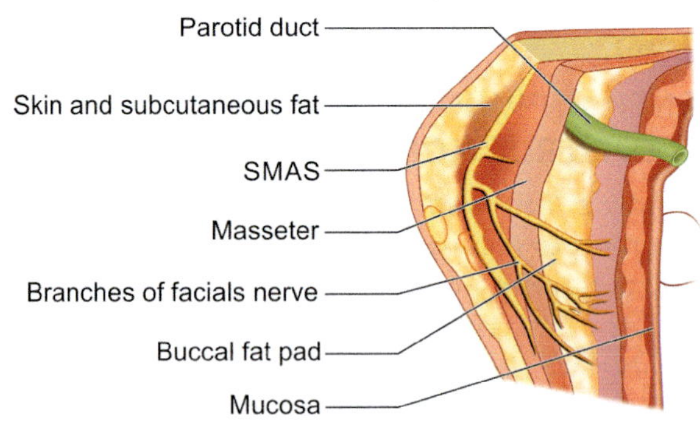

Fig. 2: Cross-section of buccal mucosa. (SMAS: superficial musculo-aponeurotic system)

Table 2: Classification of buccal defects.[12]

Thickness	P: Partial thickness defects—the skin and subcutaneous planes are intact F: Full thickness defects—the overlying skin has been resected
Superoinferior plane	I: Limited buccal defect without bony resection: a: <3 cm in greatest dimension b: >3 cm in greatest dimension II: Minimal bone resection—upper alveolectomy and/or marginal mandibulectomy, no palatal or floor of the mouth defect III: Defect involving segmental mandibulectomy with or without subtotal maxillectomy below the zygomatic arch IV: Extensive bone defect with segmental mandibulectomy and subtotal/total maxillectomy extending above the zygomatic arch
Anteroposterior plane	A: Limited buccal defect without involvement of commissure, infratemporal fossa (ITF), or masticatory space B: Anterior defect with involvement of commissure +/– lip, but not ITF or masticatory space C: Posterior defect with involvement of ITF or masticatory space with or without posterior pharyngeal wall defect without commissure involvement D: Defect extending from lip to ITF or masticatory space with or without posterior pharyngeal wall

Principles of Reconstruction

The aims of reconstruction in these patients are orocutaneous separation, prevention of orocervical fistula, allow adequate mouth opening, facilitate chewing and swallowing, and to restore facial form.[13]

SITE-SPECIFIC RECONSTRUCTIVE OPTIONS

- *Buccal mucosa and cheek defects:*
  - *Small superficial defects:* Split thickness skin graft
  - *Local flaps:* Nasolabial or tongue flap
  - *Regional flaps:* Submental or forehead flap
  - *Free flaps:* Radial forearm or anterolateral thigh flap depending on thickness and surface area required
- *Retromolar trigone:*
  - *Only buccal mucosa:*
    - *Local flaps:* Buccal fat or tongue flap
    - *Regional flaps:* Nasolabial and forehead flap
    - *Free flaps:* Radial forearm and anterolateral thigh flap
  - *Buccal mucosa with marginal mandibulectomy or posterior segmental mandibulectomy:*
    - *Regional flaps:* Pectoralis major, submental, and forehead flap
    - *Free flaps:* Anterolateral, thoracodorsal artery perforator, deep inferior epigastric perforator, and medial sural artery perforator flaps
  - *Buccal mucosa with marginal mandibulectomy or posterior segmental mandibulectomy and skin*:
    - *Regional flaps:* Bipaddle pectoralis major flap
    - *Free flaps:* Radial forearm, anterolateral thigh, thoracodorsal artery perforator, and deep inferior epigastric perforator flaps
- *Buccal mucosa with infratemporal fossa:*
  - *Free flaps:* Latissimus dorsi or rectus abdominis flaps

Surgical Considerations

- The size of the defect should be considered with the mouth maximally open to avoid subsequent trismus.
- A soft and pliable reconstruction is required for mouth opening speech and mastication.
- The reconstructed cheek should not be lax as it is insensate and food tends to collect in it.
- The gingivobuccal sulcus should be reconstructed to allow for dental rehabilitation.
- Lip reconstruction is important to prevent either oral incompetence or microstomia.
- Coverage of mandibulectomy defects is important to prevent bone exposure or osteoradionecrosis.
- Chimeric components can be used for reconstruction of composite internal and external defects.
- Obliteration of the maxillary defect is important to avoid postoperative fluid collection and infection.
- When combined with oropharyngeal defects, nasal regurgitation and hypernasality of speech can be prevented by addressing velopharyngeal incompetence.[14]
- An example of reconstruction of an advanced gingivobuccal cancer resection defect is seen in **Figures 3A to C**.

LIP RECONSTRUCTION

The lip has a trilaminar structure consisting of mucosa, muscle, and skin. At the junction of the mucosa and skin is the mucocutaneous ridge or vermilion border. The V-shaped indentation along the mucocutaneous ridge of the upper lip is called Cupid's bow, with philtral ridges above. There are two aesthetic units in the upper lip and one in the lower lip. Blood supply is from the facial arteries that give off the superior and inferior labial arteries, and are innervated by the maxillary

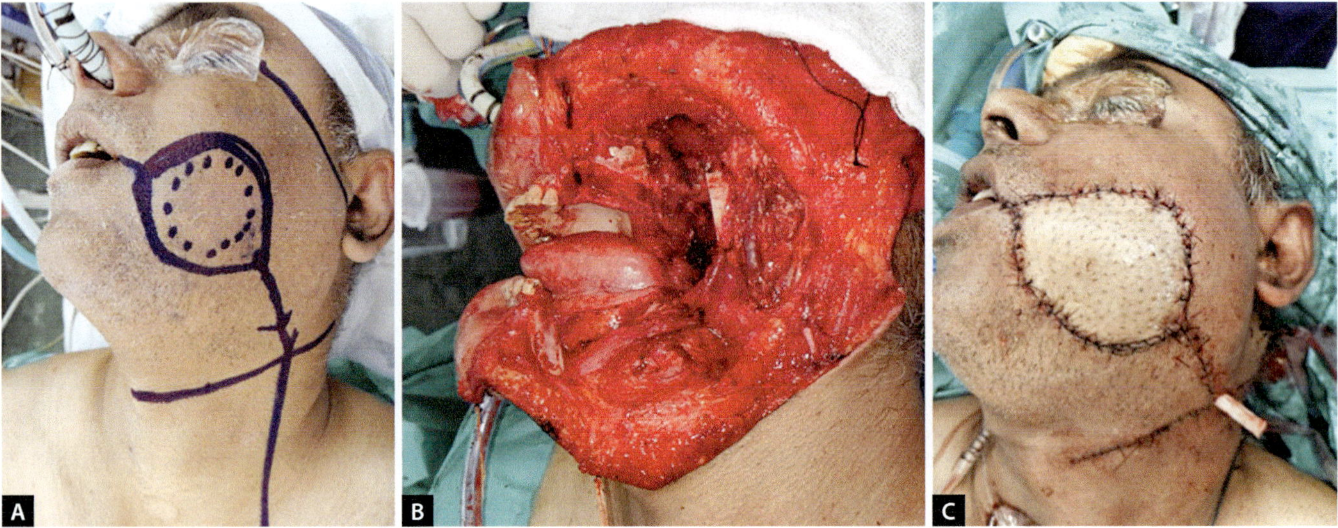

Figs. 3A to C: Compartmental resection and reconstruction of advanced gingivobuccal cancer. (A) Incision marked based on skin involvement, vertical limb of neck incision marked if required; (B) Defect after segmental mandibulectomy, infrastructure maxillectomy, masticator space resection and cheek skin excision; (C) Final appearance after reconstruction with bipaddled anterolateral thigh free flap.

and mandibular branches of the trigeminal nerves.[15] The muscles can be grouped in to upper lip elevators, retractors, and depressors of the lower lip, mentalis (elevation and pouting of the lower lip), and orbicularis oris (sphincteric action). The aims of reconstruction are preservation of function, reconstitution of the orbicularis oris, three-layered closure, vermilion alignment, maintaining the relationship of the upper and lower lips, and optimization of aesthetics.[16]

Surgical Considerations

- *Vermilion reconstruction:*
  - The vermilion border needs to be reconstituted very carefully since discrepancies are easily noticeable; avoiding anesthetic injection as it can disrupt muscle tone.
  - Alternatively methylene blue tattooing of the white roll before administering local anesthetic injections can aid this.
  - Local flaps are ideally harvested from the same lip; however, if unavailable, a unipedicle vermilion flap from the opposite lip can be harvested and inset, with division of the pedicle after 10–14 days.
  - Random local flaps can also be harvested from the buccal mucosa, around 1 cm wide myomucosal flaps can be rotated by 120° for closure of lower lip vermilion defects.
  - Alternatively, a facial artery myomucosal flap can be based superiorly or inferiorly and rotated to reconstruct these defects.
- *Partial thickness defects:*
  - Superficial defects can be managed with primary closure, local flaps, or skin grafting.
  - Partial thickness defects may benefit from conversion into full thickness defects.
  - Local flaps are either advancement or transposition flaps using the cheek or adjacent lip tissue.[17]
- *Small full thickness defects:*
  - Primary closure possible in many cases due to innate elasticity
  - Up to 40% defects can be reapproximated in layers in the lower lip but only 25% in the upper lip because of the landmarks that should not be disrupted.
  - For central upper lip defects involving the philtrum, closure with an Abbe flap is preferable even when primary closure is possible.[18]
  - In men, a linear upper lip scar can be concealed within the moustache; however, in women it may be prominent and disfiguring.
- *Large full thickness defects:*
  - Tissue for large lip defects can be obtained from the opposite lip or the adjacent cheek tissue.
  - Lip switches are composite and give good functional and cosmetic outcomes, as restoration of orbicularis oris has the best likelihood of neurotization and oral competence and allow correction of lip length discrepancy. However, in extensive resections, these are insufficient and can result in microstomia.
  - Cheek flaps have a lower likelihood of microstomia even though aesthetics are worse. However,

adequate cheek laxity is required for these flaps which may not be the case in scarring or previous radiotherapy.

- Large central upper lip defects are best reconstructed with an Abbe flap from the central segment of the lower lip.
- When an Abbe flap is inadequate, it can be combined with cheek advancement.
- Karapandzic, modified Bernard, or nasolabial flaps are better alternatives for larger defects.
- For large lateral and commissure defects medially based rotation-advancement flaps such as the reverse Estlander flap are used, with the flap size of half the defect width to correct proportions and a secondary commissuroplasty.[19-21]

- *Total lip reconstruction:*
  - For defects >80%, the Karapandzic flap results in microstomia **(Figs. 4A to C)**, so bilateral Bernard **(Figs. 5A and B)** or nasolabial flaps are better choices if laxity permits.
  - Functional sequelae with lower lip reconstruction are worse due to incompetence.
  - Radial forearm free flap with a palmaris longus tendon can provide a good surface area with oral competence.[22]
  - Approaches to upper lip reconstruction are shown in **Flowcharts 1 and 2**.[23]

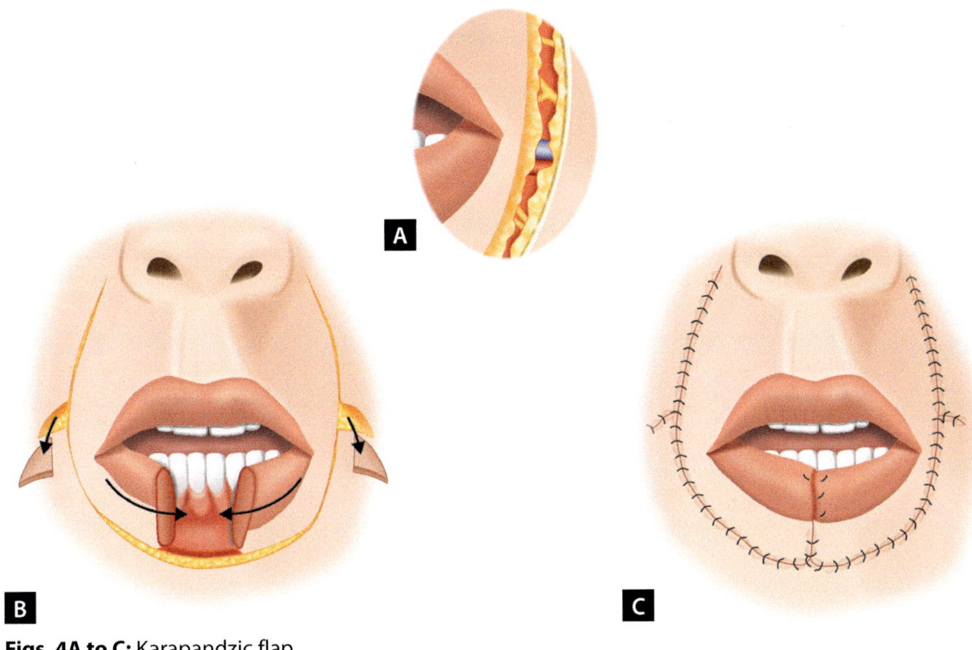

Figs. 4A to C: Karapandzic flap.

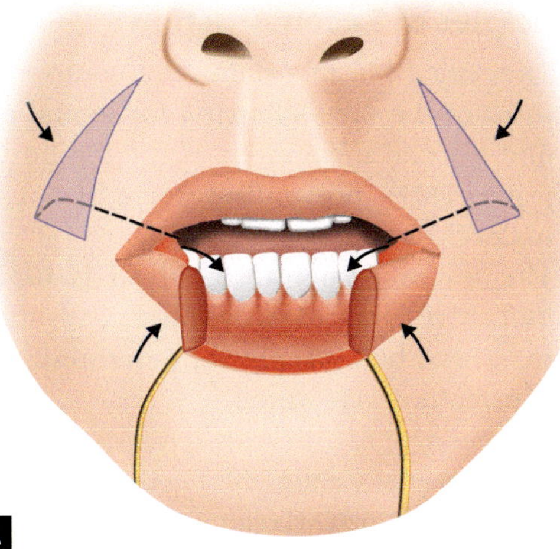

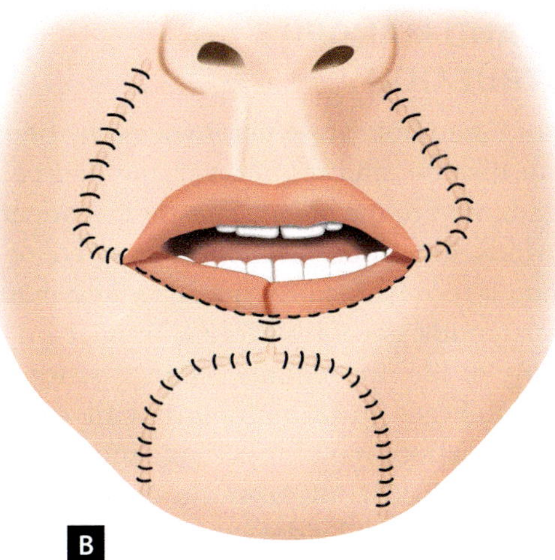

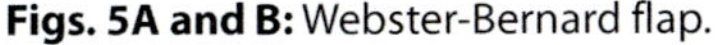

Figs. 5A and B: Webster-Bernard flap.

Flowchart 1: Approach to upper lip reconstruction.

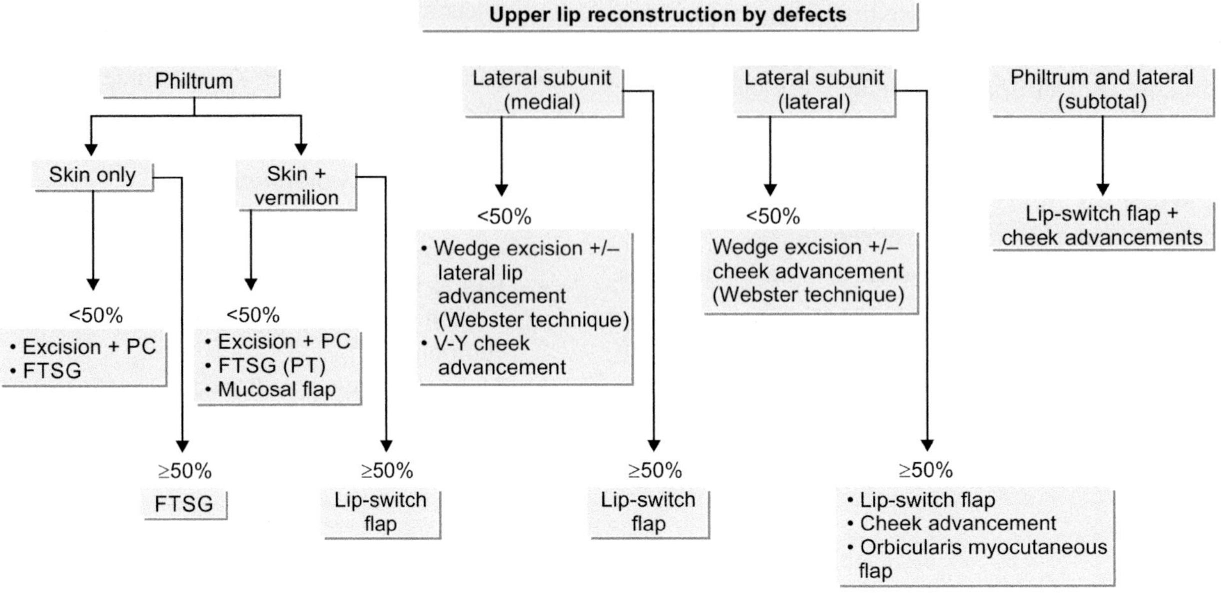

(FTSG: full-thickness skin graft; PC: primary closure; PT: partial-thickness)

Flowchart 2: Approach to lower lip reconstruction.

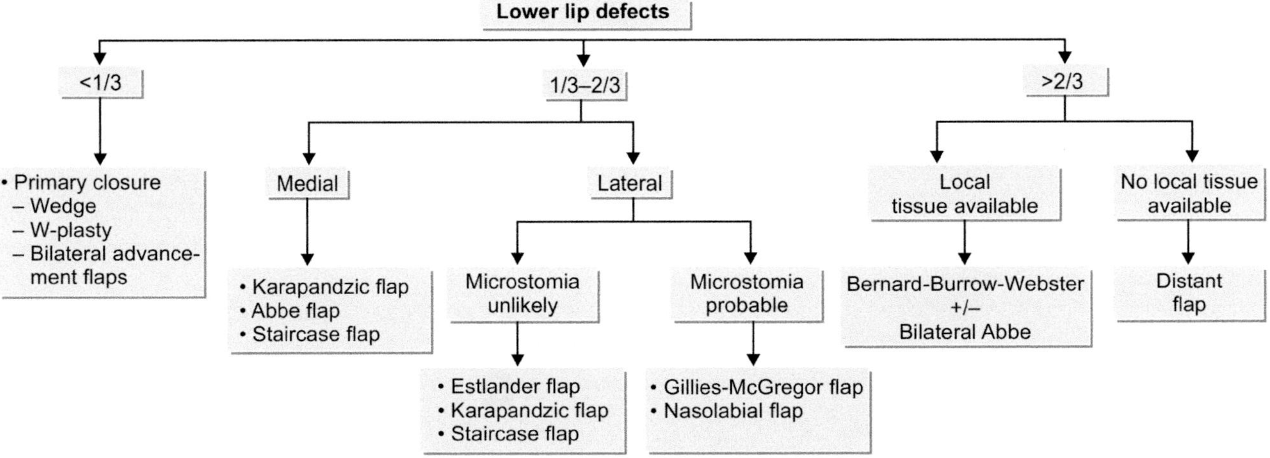

MAXILLA AND MANDIBLE RECONSTRUCTION

The maxilla and mandible are often involved by benign and malignant disease, and require varying degrees of resection. In addition to the obvious aesthetic concerns, there are various functional aspects that need to be addressed in their reconstruction—maxillary and mandibular reconstructions have a profound impact on the patient's quality of life. Inadequate reconstruction can cause varying degrees of impediment with speech, swallowing, mastication, mouth opening, and cosmetic disfigurement **(Table 3)**. An example of a marginal mandibulectomy and lower lip defect following resection of a lower alveolus tumor is seen in **Figures 6A to D**.

Principles of Reconstruction

- The mandible maintains the contour of the lower third of the face, allowing for dental rehabilitation and normal movement of the temporomandibular joint (TMJ), preventing deviation of the jaw and malocclusion.
- The major principle involved is bridging of the defect with vascularized bone, with the segment of mandible being replaced determining the number of osteotomies required.
- Involvement of the condyle is an important consideration, especially if the TMJ needs to be rehabilitated.
- The options for TMJ reconstruction can either be autogenous or prosthetic; autogenous options include

Table 3: Classification of maxillary and mandibular defects.

Maxilla	
Author	*Classification*
Okay et al.[24]	*Class Ia:* Defects involving the hard palate but not the tooth-bearing alveolus *Class Ib:* Defects that involve any portion of the maxillary alveolus and dentition posterior to the canines or that involved the premaxilla *Class II:* Defects that involve any portion of the hard palate and tooth-bearing maxillary alveolus and only one canine, and transverse palatectomy defects that involve <50% of the hard palate *Class III:* involve any portion of the hard palate and tooth-bearing maxillary alveolus including both canines. This includes total and transverse palatectomy defects that involve over 50% of the hard palate
Brown et al.[25]	*Surgical component (vertical)* *Class I:* Minimal loss of alveolar bone without an oroantral fistula, with loss of hard palate only *Class II:* Loss of alveolus and antral walls with no extension to orbital rim or adnexae *Class III:* Class II with orbital floor or medial wall involvement *Class IV:* Maxillectomy with orbital exenteration *Dental component (horizontal)* *A:* Less than or equal to half of the dental alveolus *B:* More than half the dental alveolus or crossing the midline *C:* The entire maxillary alveolus
Mandible	
Jewer et al.[26]	*H:* Unilateral condyle but may cross the midline, *C:* both canines, *HC:* lateral aspect and condyle including both canines, *LC:* lateral and both canines, *LCL:* bilateral defects including canines but not condyles, *HCL:* condyle, lateral, central, and contralateral, and *HCH:* entire mandible
Urken et al.[27]	*C:* condyle, *R:* ramus, *B:* body, *S:* symphysis, S^H: stops at the midline
Brown et al.[28]	*Class I (angle):* Lateral defect not including ipsilateral canine or condyle *Class Ic (angle and condyle):* Lateral defect including condyle *Class II (angle and canine):* Hemimandibulectomy including ipsilateral but not contralateral canine or condyle *Class IIc (angle, canine and condyle):* Hemimandibulectomy including condyle *Class III (both canines):* Anterior mandibulectomy includes both canines but neither angle *Class IV (both canines and at least one angle):* Extensive anterior mandibulectomy including both canines and one or both angles *Class IVc (both canines and at least one condyle):* Extensive anterior mandibulectomy including both canines and one or both condyles

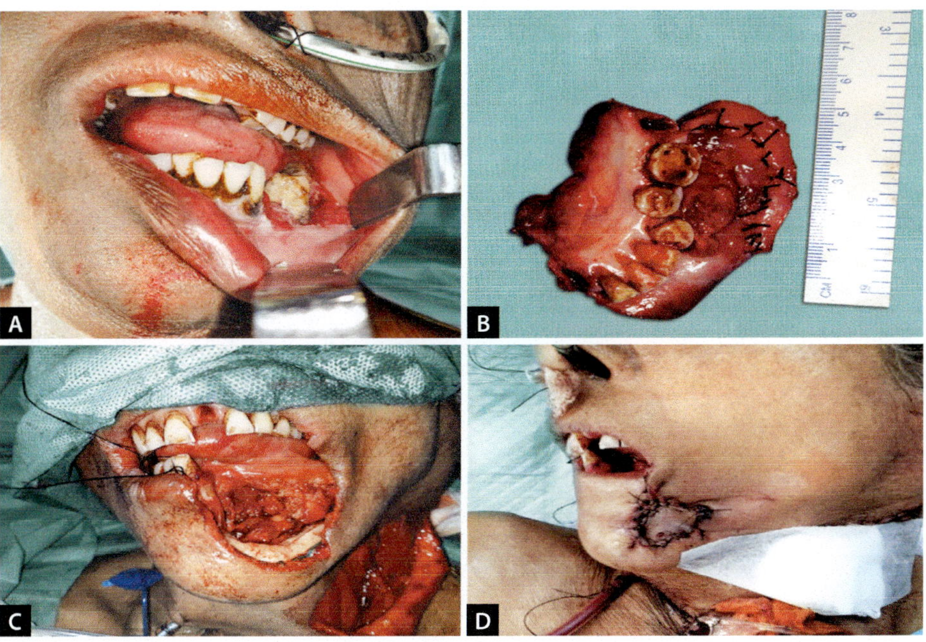

Figs. 6A to D: Carcinoma of lower alveolus extending on to the lip. (A) Lesion; (B) Excised en-bloc specimen; (C) Effect included marginal mandibulectomy, lip resection and excision of external skin; (D) Reconstruction with bipaddled radial forearm free flap.

the deep circumflex iliac artery flap, sternoclavicular free flap, and costochondral free flap.

- In a total maxillectomy, the goals of reconstruction are oronasal separation, orbital support, dental rehabilitation, and restoration of facial contour.
- The classification of maxillary defects by Brown was designed to address these goals where class II defects require oronasal separation and class III defects require orbital support and a separate (horizontal) component exists for dental rehabilitation.
- For vertical class I defects without an oroantral fistula having minimal alveolar bone loss, local flaps such as palatal island flaps, or microvascular soft tissue flaps such as radial forearm flaps can be used. In vertical class II defects, there is loss of alveolus and antral walls without orbital rim disruption. This requires bony reconstruction with a microvascular flap (such as the fibula free flap, scapular free flap, or deep circumflex iliac flap), with the bony component used to reconstruct the alveolar defect and the skin paddle providing oronasal separation. In vertical class III defects, reconstruction is more complex, requiring bony reconstruction of the alveolar and support for the orbit. In class IV defects with orbital exenteration, there is a removal of the globe and periorbita, so the aim of reconstruction is to cover the orbital bone with soft tissue to provide a cavity conducive to place an ocular prosthesis, possibly with osseointegration. **Figures 7A to E** show a posterior hard palate defect reconstructed with a soft tissue flap.
- Okay's classification is more suitable for prosthodontic rehabilitation. In classes I and II, the remnant palate allows stable anchoring of an obturator with a clip, while in class III, obturation is not an option as it cannot be anchored to the remnant palate.
- The ideal choice for maxillary reconstruction is free tissue transfer wherever possible; previous criticisms such as the role of cavity inspection in

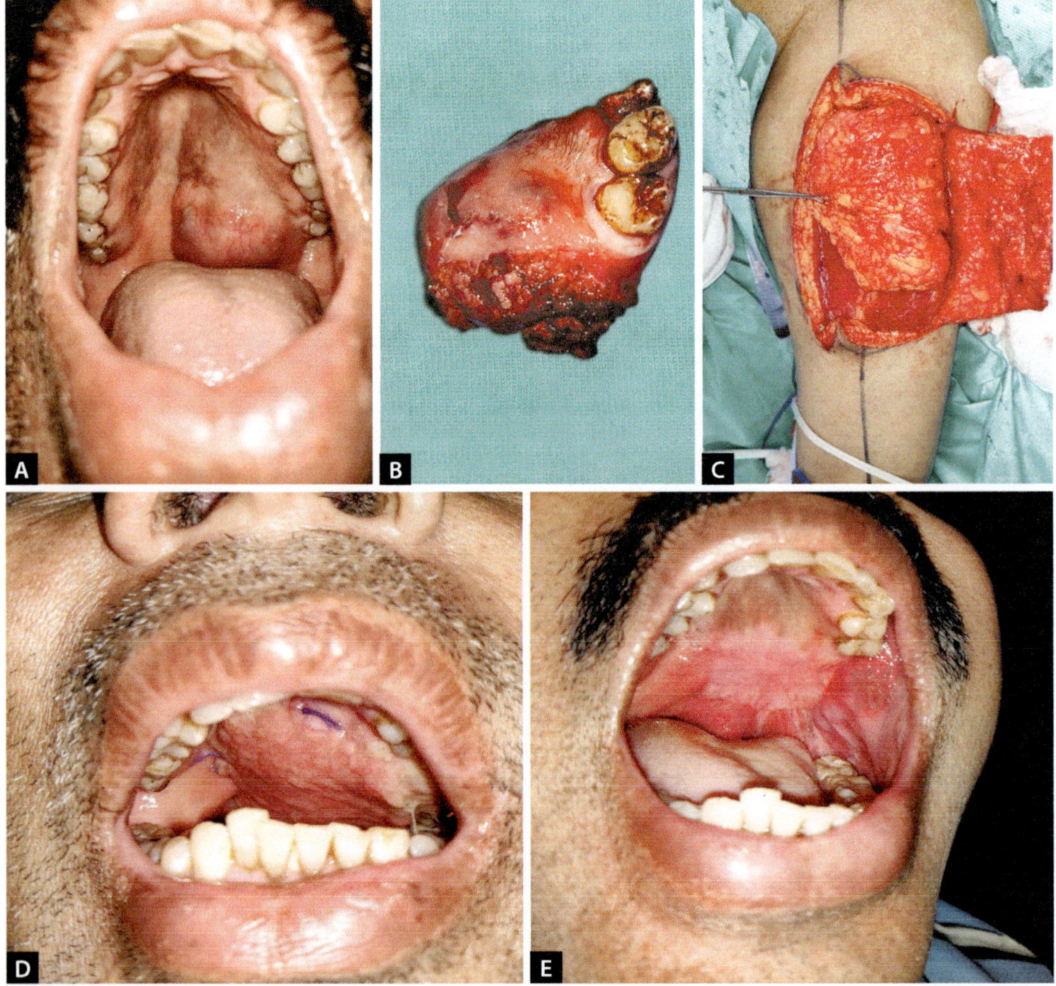

Figs. 7A to E: Adenocarcinoma of left hard palate. (A) Clinical picture; (B) Excised specimen; (C) Adipofascial anterolateral thigh flap used for reconstruction; (D) Clinical image 2 weeks postoperatively; (E) Clinical image 4 months postoperatively.

disease surveillance have not been validated with evidence. Moreover, availability of cross-sectional imaging and routine endoscopy enable effective surveillance.

Surgical Considerations

- *The advantages of the fibula flap in oral cavity reconstruction are well established:*
  - Adequate length and bone volume for extensive reconstruction and osseointegrated dental implant placement
  - A sturdy periosteal and endosteal blood supply allowing one or multiple osteotomies
  - A reliable skin paddle with adequate skin to resurface both intraoral and external skin defects
  - A distant donor site allowing for a two-team approach
  - Low donor site morbidity
- *Despite these benefits, the potential drawbacks are:*
  - Lack of available soft tissue once extensive composite mandibular or maxillary defects present
  - Wide excision of intraoral tumors can result in defects involving the bone, oral lining, external skin, tongue, and masseter muscle.
  - Despite an initial acceptable reconstruction, radiotherapy often leads to thinning of the skin paddle and subsequent contraction, producing a loss.
- The other important aspect is determination which side of the neck is to be used for microvascular anastomosis. In most cases, the anastomosis is performed on the same side of the defect; however, on occasion, this may not be feasible due to a paucity of neck vessels (e.g., if a radical neck dissection is performed or if the neck is irradiated). In these cases, the anastomosis must be performed on the side of the neck opposite to the defect.
- For the anastomosis to be performed on the same side, the pedicle must lie posteriorly to avoid kinking. In this situation, the skin from the fibula free flap will be needed for either external skin defect closure or intraoral mucosal defect closure. If external skin defect closure is required, the *ipsilateral* fibula free flap is harvested, and if intraoral mucosal defect closure is required, *contralateral* fibula free flap is harvested. For the vascular anastomosis to be performed on the opposite side of the neck, the pedicle must lie anteriorly to avoid kinking. In this situation, the converse applies—for an external skin defect requiring closure, the contralateral fibula free flap is harvested, while for an intraoral mucosal defect, the ipsilateral fibula free flap is harvested.
- *Osteotomies:* After division of the proximal peroneal pedicle, further osteotomies are performed with an electric saw according to the tailored paper ruler template. The skin paddle can be separated into two flaps based on each perforator if two septocutaneous perforators are available. The pedicle is skeletonized with removal of unnecessary proximal periosteum and bone. Respect the geometry of the fibula osteoseptocutaneous (OSC) flap to obtain good outcomes in mandibular reconstruction.[29,30] It is important to protect the vascular pedicle and septocutaneous perforators during this process to avoid injury. Gentle handling as the vascularity of the skin paddle can be compromised during flap inset if the septum and its perforators are stretched over the fibula bone and the plate to reach the defect. The minimal recommended bone segment length for osteotomy is 2.5 cm to ensure the adequate inclusion of tiny perforators nourishing the periosteum and subsequently the bone. The more osteotomies are made, the more the decrease of vascularity to the distal segment can be encountered as periosteal sources as well as nutrient arteries supply the proximal bone segments, while the distal segments are nourished only by periosteal sources. In addition, when plating is applied on top of the periosteum to fix the bone segments, there is a concern of possible decrease in periosteal vascular flow to the distal bone segments.
- A piece of flexor hallucis longus or soleus muscle is harvested and placed on top of the fibula and reconstruction plate to improve cosmesis and prevent osteoradionecrosis and plate exposure after postoperative radiation.
- It is recommended to keep the ischemia time for fibular osteocutaneous flaps to <5 hours to reduce partial flap loss and other complication rates.[31]
- *Stereolithographic modeling:* Here, the patient undergoes high-resolution computed tomography (CT) of the facial bones and bilateral fibulae. The images are then reconstructed on to get a three-dimensional understanding of the defect. The reconstructed images are then used to print a rapid prototyping (RPT) model of both the face and the fibula. Mock surgery is then performed on the models to ensure accuracy; after determining the exact positions of the osteotomies, a cutting guide can be fabricated for intraoperative use to save time. The reconstruction plates are also present to ensure accuracy and reduce operative time. For mandibular reconstruction, the RPT modeling technique, mock surgery, and cutting guide fabrication remain

the same. The defect in the mandible is spanned with the osteotomized fibula. Here, 1.7 mm profile thickness mandibular reconstruction plates are used with 2 mm locking screws.

COMMONLY USED LOCAL AND REGIONAL FLAPS FOR ORAL RECONSTRUCTION

Submental Flap

- *Vascular supply:* Submental artery, which is a continuous branch of the facial artery.
- *Salient anatomy:* The submental flap, as indicated by the name, is located in the submental area. Its blood supply derives from the submental artery, which is a continuous branch of the facial artery, located 5–6.5 cm away from the origin of the facial artery. This branch penetrates deep to the submandibular gland through the mylohyoid muscle below the mandible angle, extending medially deep to the anterior belly of the digastric muscle. As the vessel travels along the mandible margin, it sends off cutaneous perforators through the platysma muscle to the skin.
- *Anatomical variations:* The anatomy of the vessel is constant, and the flow it provides to the submental skin is reliable.
- *Components and variants:* The flap comprises skin, subcutaneous fat, platysma muscle, submental fat, and lymph nodes; the anterior belly of digastric and mylohyoid muscles may also be included.
- *Flap design and utilization:* An ellipse of marked centered over the midline in the submental area. A pinch test is used to determine the flap width that can be harvested with primary closure of the donor area. The neck dissection incision is planned around this incision; preservation of the facial artery is critical. Incision can be started from either the inferior or superior margin flap directly through the platysma muscle. Then, the dissection is carried out with division of the anterior belly of the digastric muscle, which is included in the flap to ensure inclusion of the submental pedicle. When the pedicle is identified, its branches to the submandibular gland should be ligated carefully. Finally, when reaching the inferior border of the mandible, care should be taken not to injure the marginal mandibular nerve. The pedicle is then skeletonized and the flap is ready to be transferred. If the flap is going to be transferred as a free flap, dissection of the pedicle can be continued to the facial vessels to obtain a better size and length for anastomosis.[32]
- *Common use:* Replacement of mucosal or soft tissue for defects that are intraoral (tongue, floor of mouth, buccal, and oropharyngeal), defects of face skin, esophagus, and hypopharynx.
- *Advantages:*
    - The arc of the submental flap is used for rotating it to the lower third of the face and the entire oral cavity, making it a suitable pedicle flap for oral cavity reconstruction.
    - Concealed scar in the neck
    - Simple and rapid flap to harvest
    - Provides a relatively thin, well-vascularized piece of tissue in a single stage operation, and obviates the need for a second stage to divide the pedicle, or sophisticated microsurgical techniques.
- *Limitations:*
    - The submental artery is small and dissection of the submental flap is challenging.
    - The venae comitantes are also small and easily injured and therefore temporary venous congestion in the flap is not unusual in the immediate postoperative period.
    - In some cases, the pedicle may be too short to allow the flap to reach the defect, to achieve even greater mobility, the flap can be converted to a reverse flow flap based on retrograde flow through the facial vessels by dividing these vessels proximal to the origin of the submental vessels.
    - Risk of injury to marginal mandibular nerve
- *Preoperative assessment and planning:*
    - Laxity of the skin in the neck should be assessed by “pinch test” to facilitate primary closure of the donor site.
- *Intraoperative considerations:*
    - Including anterior belly of digastric increases the vascularity of the flap
- *Postoperative care:*
    - Flap monitoring

Supraclavicular Flap

- *Vascular supply:* The supraclavicular artery that originates from the transverse cervical artery
- *Salient anatomy:* The supraclavicular flap is a pedicled fasciocutaneous flap with a reliable axial pattern, based on the supraclavicular artery. Its two venae comitantes drain in to the transverse cervical vein. The supraclavicular artery generally originates from the transverse cervical artery. Infrequently, it arises from the suprascapular artery. In 70–90% of cases its origin is in the area of mid-third of the clavicle remaining cases, it branches in the area of the lateral

third of the clavicle. It travels perpendicularly from the transverse cervical artery and pierces the deep fascia of the deltoid muscle 3 cm distally. After its exit from the deep fascia, it runs in a superficial plane and continues its course over the acromioclavicular joint, at the junction of the middle and lateral thirds of the clavicle. At this level, the artery generally divides into numerous branches over the deltoid muscle. These branches develop multiple anastomoses with the vascular network of the thoracoacromial artery, the posterior circumflex humeral artery, and the superficial branch of the transverse cervical artery. These consistent number of perforators interconnected by direct and indirect linking vessels through the subdermal plexus and over the deltoid muscle, the direct linking vessels support the distal supraclavicular artery. After the insertion of the deltoid muscle, their numbers decline and the vascularization of the distal flap relies on the indirect linking vessels and recurrent flow.[2] Hence, beyond this point, it becomes a random pattern flap with higher chances of distal flap necrosis.

- *Components and variants:* The flap comprises skin, subcutaneous fat, and fascia.
- *Flap design and utilization:* The origin of the supraclavicular artery is to be marked in the triangle bounded inferiorly by the clavicle, medially by the posterior border of the sternocleidomastoid muscle and laterally by the external jugular vein. It is found approximately 2.5–4 cm above the clavicle and on average 2 cm posterior to the sternocleidomastoid muscle and 6.5–10 cm from the sternoclavicular joint. The flap can be used as a rotation flap, tunneled flap, supercharged flap, and as a free microvascular transfer flap. If a neck dissection is performed, then vessels to the distal external jugular vein and the transverse cervical artery need to be preserved. A Doppler probe is used to identify the origin of the pedicle in the triangle. Usually, an elliptical skin paddle is designed over the supraclavicular and shoulder region. The insertion of the deltoid muscle is the farthest point from where the flap can be safely elevated without the complication of distal skin paddle necrosis. The flap is elevated the from distal-to-proximal manner in a subfascial plane over the deltoid muscle using sharp dissection or Colorado cautery tip; once the area of the pedicle is approached, bipolar cautery can be used for dissection. The periosteum of the clavicle can be elevated so as to avoid injury to the pedicle, there is no need to skeletonize the pedicle always unless being used for a free tissue transfer. The supraclavicular flap can be supercharged if a larger size is needed. The technique has been described using mostly the posterior circumflex artery. According to Vinh et al.,[33] the anterior humeral artery, lateral thoracic artery perforator, or the thoracoacromial artery perforator can be appropriate for supercharging.
- *Common use:* Replacement of mucosal or soft tissue for defects that are intraoral (tongue, floor of mouth, buccal, and oropharyngeal), defects of face skin, esophagus, hypopharynx, and lateral skull base
- *Advantages:*
  - Excellent color match
  - Skin properties being similar to the surrounding skin
  - Pliable and thin
  - Hairless, excellent for mucosal reconstruction
  - It reaches distant sites, such as oropharynx, because of its long pedicle and broad arc of rotation.
  - It can also be used for large defects, since the flap can reach a considerable size, with maximum dimensions of approximately 10 × 20 cm.
  - Salvage procedure either after radiotherapy or after another flap failure, as transverse cervical artery is not a part of radiation field.
- *Limitations:*
  - Distal flap necrosis can occur
  - Incisional dehiscence
  - Minimal shoulder dysfunction
- *Preoperative assessment and planning:*
  - Laxity of the skin should be assessed by "pinch test" to facilitate primary closure of the donor site.

Nasolabial Flap

- *Vascular supply:* Angular artery terminal branch of facial artery
- *Salient anatomy:* The anatomy of the nasolabial region is complex. The nasolabial crease runs from approximately 1 cm superior to the lateral alar rim to approximately 1 cm lateral to the corner of the mouth. Medial to the crease in the region of the corner of the mouth is the orbicularis oris muscle. Superior and lateral to the crease is the cheek. The buccal and zygomatic branches of the facial nerve primarily innervate the muscles surrounding the nasolabial crease. More recent studies by Pogrel et al. based on cadaveric dissections have described the existence of very superficial muscle fibers below the fold that insert into the underside of the dermis.[34] The artery resides in the dense fibrous tissue at the oral

commissure and continues along the superior border of the upper lip to the nasal ala. It then continues in a medial course along the nasofacial groove toward the medial canthus of the eye. Arterial perforators are especially concentrated in the inferior two-thirds of the nasolabial groove. The subdermal plexus is supplied by feeder vessels from the branches of the facial artery and provides the blood supply to the nasolabial muscle and skin. This allows for high viability and permits bold thinning and shaping. The nasolabial flap is typically classified as an axial pattern flap given that the angular artery runs deep to the flap. The skin of the nasolabial fold has a superior and inferior blood supply allowing for a superiorly or inferiorly based flap. The facial artery is the arterial supply of the inferiorly based flap. The supralabial and alar branches of the facial artery nourish the skin of the nasolabial fold. As the facial artery courses over the dorsum of the nose, it becomes the angular artery. These branches form the distal arterial supply of the inferiorly based flap. The infraorbital artery and the transverse facial artery supply the superolateral skin of the nasolabial region and form the basis of the superiorly based nasolabial flap.[35] A study of the vascularization of the cheek has demonstrated that although the lower three quarters of the nasolabial fold skin has a reliable subcutaneous vascular distribution, the distal third should be considered to have a random distribution.[36]

- *Components and variants:* The flap comprises skin, subcutaneous fat, and fascia.
- *Flap design and utilization:* Before flap harvest, the length requirement and the arc of rotation of the flap must be considered to avoid distal necrosis. Necrosis occurs from excessive length of the flap, from tension on the flap, or from constriction of the arterial supply or venous outflow. Once the dimensions of the defect are established, plans for harvesting the nasolabial flap can be made. A simple technique to determine whether the nasolabial flap will reach the defect with an acceptable amount of tension is to use a piece of gauze to simulate the length, width, and rotation of the nasolabial flap. By holding one end of the gauze at the base of the flap, the gauze can be rotated to simulate rotation of the flap. The flap can then be outlined. If the flap length is short and the base is adequately wide, a random pattern flap can be harvested. Dissection is carried to the depth of the subcutaneous tissue. A generous amount of subcutaneous tissue should be harvested. To limit the thickness of the flap, subcutaneous fat can be removed. The subcutaneous tissue of the donor site usually requires undermining to allow for primary closure; this undermining is best done on the cheek side of the donor site. Harvesting of an axial pattern flap typically requires dissection to the level of the periosteum. Once the flap is harvested, the tension on the flap and the torsion on the arterial supply should be evaluated carefully before suturing the flap in place. Small incisions paralleling the long axis of the flap can be made in the periosteum beyond the base of the flap to reduce tension on the flap; however, care must be taken to not disrupt the arterial supply. After the flap is sutured in place, the distal end should be evaluated for color and turgor.
- *Modifications of the inferiorly based nasolabial flap:*
  - *Floor of mouth reconstruction:* Rose[37] described the one-staged arterialized nasolabial island flap for floor of mouth reconstruction. The skin portion of the flap was centered on the nasolabial fold and extended from the medial canthal area to 2 cm superior to the mandibular margin. The described nasolabial flap contained subcutaneous tissue and facial muscles with the associated vessels. Harvesting of the associated vessels made the flap considerably more reliable than the subcutaneous flap. In addition, harvesting of the underlying muscles added to the mobility of the flap.
  - *Total lip reconstruction:* The flaps are oriented so that the ends abut one another in a straight or staggered line or they are tunneled subcutaneously and sutured one on top of the other.[38] Combinations of flaps can be used for total lip reconstruction; Panje[39] described the use of full-thickness nasolabial flaps with a lower lip switch procedure to reconstruct a total lip defect. Regardless of the technique, closure was achieved; however, the healed lip was tight, and the cosmetic result was often compromised. Prosthesis wear has been suggested during the healing period to reduce the degree of contracture.
  - *Intraoral reconstruction:* Hair growth on the flap can be a problem for intraoral reconstruction in men. The skin flap is designed to include skin under the eyelid and extended laterally to the nasolabial fold. Following incision of the skin along the periphery, the superior incision was carried deep to the periosteum. The dissection is carried inferiorly and was deep to the facial muscles and associated angular vessels. The inferior incision is carried through subcutaneous tissue. A relieving incision is then created along the nasolabial fold. The vascular pedicle

was dissected and released, starting along the caudal margin. With this modification, a circular area of hairless skin 3–5 cm in diameter could be harvested. Passage of the flap into the oral cavity was performed through a tunnel. Insetting of the flap can then be performed easily. Garatea et al.[40] described the use of this flap for the reconstruction of defects of buccal mucosa and the maxillary tuberosity region. A cheek rotation flap, as described by Mustarde was used to close the donor site.[41]

- *Modifications of the superiorly based nasolabial flaps:*
  - Da Silva[42] described reconstruction of the columella using a superiorly based nasolabial flap. The flap was tunneled underneath the alar base to reach the columella. Division of the flap and tunnel closure was performed at a second stage. The advantage of a transnasal approach was the use of a shorter flap.
  - Bilateral nasolabial flaps based on a superior and inferior subcutaneous pedicle have been tunneled translabially for columellar reconstruction in a single stage. Nasolabial flaps with modifications have been used to reconstruct subtotal and total lip defects.
  - Daya and colleagues have described reconstruction of a significant defect of the upper and lower lip in addition to the oral commissure secondary to a severe electrical burn with the use of a submental flap and nasolabial flap. Defects resulting from traumatic tissue avulsion or scarring can also be addressed with the superiorly based nasolabial flap.[43]
- *Common use:* Replacement of mucosal or soft tissue for defects that are intraoral (tongue, floor of mouth, buccal, and oropharyngeal) and defects of face skin
- *Advantages:*
  - Easy to harvest
  - Scar gets concealed in the nasolabial fold
  - Robust blood supply
  - It does not impair speech and causes only minimal donor site morbidity.
  - The flap is not overly time consuming or technically difficult to master; however, knowledge of the relevant anatomy is essential.
- *Disadvantages:*
  - Staged procedure is required in some cases.
  - Partial flap necrosis
  - Nasomaxillary crease and the creation of an edematous and bulky flap

Facial Artery Myomucosal Flap

- *Vascular supply:* Facial artery branch of external carotid artery
- *Salient anatomy:* The facial artery, a collateral branch of the external carotid artery, exits the submandibular region of the neck and ascends over the inferior border of the mandible through the antegonial notch. The facial artery follows an ascending and tortuous route toward the medial angle of the eye. On its path, it passes laterally to the buccinator (deepest layer) and medially to the risorius, zygomaticus major, and superficial lamina of the orbicularis oris. The venous drainage relies on submucosal plexus. Hence, the identification of the facial vein is not mandatory during harvest; however, the base of the flap needs to be wide enough (approximately 2 cm) to ensure a good venous drainage.
- *Components and variants:* The flap comprises mucosa, submucosa, buccinators, underlying facial artery, and submucosal venous plexus.
- *Flap design and utilization:* The flap is designed over the facial artery trajectory with an oblique orientation, from the retromolar trigone to the level of the ipsilateral labial sulcus. The flap can be designed as inferiorly based flap (antegrade flow) or the superiorly based flap (retrograde flow). The length of the flap is tailored proportionally to the size of the defect. The Stensen duct limits the width of the flap posteriorly, which is kept under 3 cm to avoid tension of closure of donor site. Anteriorly, the incision lies 1 cm posterior to the oral commissure. A Doppler ultrasound is used to mark the course of the facial artery. The dissection starts with the localization of the facial artery. It can be done either through an incision in the most distal part of the flap to directly locate the facial artery, or through an incision in the labial commissure area to identify the superior labial artery, and that could be traced back to the facial artery. The initial incision is done through the mucosa, submucosa, and buccinator. The flap is then elevated and should include the facial artery, the overlying buccinator, and a small portion of the orbicularis oris close to the oral commissure. The facial artery is kept attached to the overlying tissues in the entire length of the flap. The donor site is to be closed in two layers, taking care not to suture the Stensen duct in the closure
- *Common use:* Replacement of mucosal defects that are intraoral (tongue, floor of mouth, buccal, and oropharyngeal), lip and intranasal defects

- *Advantages:*
    - Elastic cushion for prosthetic apparatus, remains malleable, and does not shrink postoperatively
    - Reliability
    - Ease of harvest
    - Proximity to the defect
    - Similar mucosal lining
    - Absence of external scar
    - Low rate of significant complications such as weakness of facial musculature.
- *Limitations:*
    - A second-stage procedure is often needed to reduce the bulky mucosal paddle at the base of the flap, to increase the depth of the vestibule and to allow greater mobility of the mobile tongue.

Lateral Forehead Flap

- *Vascular supply:* Superficial temporal artery and accompanying venae comitantes
- *Salient anatomy:* The lateral forehead flap receives axial blood supply through the branches of the superficial temporal artery. The anterior branch of the superficial temporal artery runs forward into the forehead where it supplies the skin, muscles, and pericranium, finally anastomosing with supratrochlear and supraorbital arteries. The posterior branch runs into the parietal scalp and anastomoses with the posterior auricular and occipital arteries.
- *Components and variants:* The flap comprises skin, subcutaneous tissue, loose areolar tissue, and pericranium.
- *Flap design and utilization:* The entire width of the forehead is generally used and the donor defect is covered with a skin graft. The anterior branch of the superficial temporal artery can be traced into the flap before marking out the flap design. The flap is raised to the depth of the pericranium. The base of the flap is kept broad to allow robust supply. If used for external cover, the pedicle can be divided after 2 weeks or so; to ensure that blood supply is adequate before division, the pedicle can be compressed for 2–3 minutes to ensure that the distal flap is still perfused.
- *Common use:* Replacement of mucosal or soft tissue for defects that are intraoral (tongue, floor of mouth, and buccal) and defects of face skin
- *Advantages:*
    - Robust, large block of tissue
    - Early to harvest
    - The underside can be skin grafted for bipaddled reconstruction.
- *Limitations:*
    - Poor cosmetic outcome when forehead is skin grafted
    - Graft take is good but even partial loss leads to even worse cosmesis; this flap is reserved as a last resort.

REFERENCES

1. Blondeel PN, Morris SF, Hallock GG, Neligan PC. Perforator flaps: anatomy, techniques and clinical applications. St Louis: Quality Medical Publishing; 2005.
2. Ninkovic M, Harpf C, Schwabegger AH, Rumer-Moser A. The lateral arm flap. Clin Plast Surg. 2001;28(2):367-74.
3. Song YG, Chen GZ, Song YL. The free thigh flap: a new free flap concept based on the septocutaneous artery. Br J Plast Surg. 1984;37(2):149-59.
4. Koshima I, Saisho H, Kawada S, Hamanaka T, Umeda N, Moriguchi T. Flow-through thin latissimus dorsi perforator flap for repair of soft-tissue defects in the legs. Plast Reconstr Surg. 1999;103(5):1483-90.
5. Kim JT, Koo BS, Kim SK. The thin latissimus dorsi perforator-based free flap for resurfacing. Plast Reconstr Surg. 2001; 107(2):374-82.
6. Engel H, Huang JJ, Lin CY, Lam W, Kao HK, Gazyakan E, et al. A strategic approach for tongue reconstruction to achieve predictable and improved functional and aesthetic outcomes. Plast Reconstr Surg. 2010;126(6):1967-77.
7. Hsiao HT, Leu YS, Liu CJ, Tung KY, Lin CC. Radial forearm versus anterolateral thigh flap reconstruction after hemiglossectomy: functional assessment of swallowing and speech. J Reconstr Microsurg. 2008;24(2):85-8.
8. Kuriakose MA, Loree TR, Spies A, Meyers S, Hicks W. Sensate radial forearm free flaps in tongue reconstruction. Arch Otolaryngol Head Neck Surg. 2001;127(12):1463-6.
9. De Vicente JC, de Villalain L, Torre A, Pena I. Microvascular free tissue transfer for tongue reconstruction after hemiglossectomy: a functional assessment of radial forearm versus anterolateral thigh flap. J Oral Maxillofac Surg. 2008; 66(11):2270-5.
10. Hsiao HT, Leu YS, Chang SH, Lee JT. Swallowing function in patients whounderwent hemiglossectomy: comparison of primary closure and free radial forearm flap reconstruction with videofluoroscopy. Ann Plast Surg. 2003;50(5):450-5.
11. Mannelli G, Arcuri F, Agostini T, Innocenti M, Raffaini M, Spinelli G. Classification of tongue cancer resection and treatment algorithm. J Surg Oncol. 2018;117(5):1092-9.
12. Shetty V, Hedne N, Kekatpure V, Chavre S. Reconstruction of Cheek Defects. In: Contemporary Oral Oncology. Cham: Springer; 2017. pp. 171-95.
13. Wong CH, Wei FC. Microsurgical free flap in head and neck reconstruction. Head Neck. 2010;32(9):1236-45.
14. Balasubramanian D, Thankappan K, Kuriakose MA, Duraisamy S, Sharan R, Mathew J, et al. Reconstructive indications of simultaneous double free flaps in the head and neck: a case series and literature review. Microsurgery. 2012;32(6):423-30.
15. Pinar YA, Bilge O, Govsa F. Anatomic study of the blood supply of perioral region. Clin Anat. 2005;18(5):330-9.
16. Coppit GL, Lin DT, Burkey BB. Current concepts in lip reconstruction. Curr Opin Otolaryngol Head Neck Surg. 2004;12(4):281-7.

17. Webster JP. Crescentic peri-alar cheek excision for upper lip flap advancement with a short history of upper lip repair. Plas Reconstr Surg. 1955;16(6):434-64.
18. Abbe R. A new plastic operation for the relief of deformity due to double harelip. Plastic Reconstr Surg. 1968;42(5):481-3.
19. Karapandzic M. Reconstruction of lip defects by local arterial flaps. Br J Plas Surg. 1974;27(1):93-7.
20. Webster RC, Coffey RJ, Kelleher RE. Total and partial reconstruction of the lower lip with innervated muscle-bearing flaps. Plast Reconstr Surg. 1960;25(4):360-71.
21. Raskob GE, Zitsch III RP, Park CW, Renner GJ, Rea JR JL. Outcome analysis for lip carcinoma. Otolaryngol Head Neck Surg. 1995;113(5):589-96.
22. Harii K, Ohmori K, Ohmori S, Goldwyn RM. Successful clinical transfer of ten free flaps by microvascular anastomoses. Plast Reconstr Surg. 1974;53(4):469.
23. Salibian AA, Zide BM. Elegance in upper lip reconstruction. Plast Reconstr Surg. 2019;143(2):572-82.
24. Okay DJ, Genden E, Buchbinder D, Urken M. Prosthodontic guidelines for surgical reconstruction of the maxilla: a classification system of defects. J Prosthet Dent. 2001;86(4): 352-63.
25. Brown JS, Rogers SN, McNally DN, Boyle M. A modified classification for the maxillectomy defect. Head Neck. 2000;22(1):17-26.
26. Jewer DD, Boyd JB, Manktelow RT, Zuker RM, Rosen IB, Gullane PJ, et al. Orofacial and mandibular reconstruction with the iliac crest free flap: a review of 60 cases and a new method of classification. Plast Reconstr Surg. 1989;84(3): 391-405.
27. Urken ML, Weinberg H, Vickery C, Buchbinder D, Lawson W, Biller HF. Oromandibular reconstruction using micro-vascular composite free flaps. Report of 71 cases and a new classification scheme for bony, soft-tissue, and neurologic defects. Arch Otolaryngol Head Neck Surg. 1991;117(7): 733-44.
28. Brown JS, Barry C, Ho M, Shaw R. A new classification for mandibular defects after oncological resection. Lancet Oncol. 2016;31(1):23-30.
29. Sharma M, Wakure A, Thankappan K, Mathew J, Jairaj D, Dudipala RR, et al. Anatomic basis for an algorithmic approach for free fibula flap donor side selection in composite oromandibular defects. Indian J Plast Surg. 2015;48(1): 43-7.
30. Yagi S, Kamei Y, Torii S. Donor side selection in mandibular reconstruction using a free fibular osteocutaneous flap. Ann Plast Surg. 2006;56(6):622-7.
31. Chang SY, Huang JJ, Tsao CK, Nguyen A, Mittakanti K, Lin CY, et al. Does ischemia time affect the outcome of free fibula flaps for head and neck reconstruction? A review of 116 cases. Plast Reconstr Surg. 2010;126(6):1988-95.
32. Pistre V, Pelissier P, Martin D, Baudet J. The submental flap: its uses as a pedicled or free flap for facial reconstruction. Clin Plast Surg. 2001;28(2):303-9.
33. Vinh VQ, Van Anh T, Ogawa R, Hyakusoku H. Anatomical and clinical studies of the supraclavicular flap: analysis of 103 flaps used to reconstruct neck scar contractures. Plast Reconstr Surg. 2009;123(5):1471-80.
34. Pogrel MA, Shariati S, Schmidt B, Faal ZH, Regezi J. The surgical anatomy of the nasolabial fold. Oral Surg Oral Med Oral Pathol Oral Radiol Endod. 1998;86(4):410-5.
35. Cormack G, Lamberty B. The Arterial Anatomy of Skin Flaps, 2nd edition. Edinburgh: Churchill Livingston; 1994.
36. Herbert DC, DeGeus J. Nasolabial subcutaneous pedicle flaps. Br J Plast Surg. 1975;28(2):90-6.
37. Rose EH. One-stage arterialized nasolabial island flap for floor of mouth reconstruction. Ann Plast Surg. 1981;6(1): 71-5.
38. Meyer R, Abul Failat AS. New concepts in lower lip reconstruction. Head Neck Surg. 1982;4(3):240-5.
39. Panje WR. Lip reconstruction. Otolaryngol Clin North Am. 1982;15(1):169-78.
40. Garatea J, Buenechea R, Bescos C, Gonzalez E, Bassas C. Intraoral reconstruction with the nasolabial island flap: a modified technique. J Craniomaxillofac Surg. 1991;19(3): 119-22.
41. Mustard J. PerdidA de tejidos profundos. Barcelona; 1982.
42. Hagan WE, Walker LB. The nasolabial musculocutaneous flap: clinical and anatomical correlations. Laryngoscope. 1988;98(3):341-6.
43. Daya M, Mahomva O, Madaree A. Multistaged reconstruction of the oral commissures and upper and lower lip with an island submental flap and a nasolabial flap. Plast Reconstr Surg. 2001;108(4):968-71.

CHAPTER 39

Principles of Skull Base Reconstruction

Radhika Kapahtia, Narayana Subramaniam, Sivakumar Vidhyadharan, Samskruthi P Murthy

INTRODUCTION

Cranial base surgery has evolved and outcomes have steadily improved as increasingly reliable reconstructive techniques have been adapted to repair the challenging wounds in this complex anatomic region. Appropriate reconstruction of skull base defects following tumor resection is of paramount importance to avoid serious and life-threatening complications. The introduction and refinement of microvascular free tissue transfer to the skull base along with the advances in alloplast technology (bone substitutes, titanium hardware, and resorbable plate fixation) are the most significant recent developments. In brief, the goal of reconstruction is to seal the intracranial space off from adjacent cavities and to restore complex craniofacial defects resulting from tumor excision.[1]

COMPLICATIONS OF SKULL BASE SURGERY

One must be aware of the complications of skull base surgery so as to understand the importance of reconstruction and the role of the reconstructive surgeon. The overall rate of complications ranges widely from 11.5 to 63% with most studies falling between 25 and 50%.[2]

Early complications following skull base surgery include:

- Dural exposure
- Cerebrospinal fluid (CSF) leak
- Pneumocranium
- Wound infection
- Ascending intracranial infection (e.g., meningitis, epidural abscess, and brain abscess).

Inadequate or failed skull base reconstruction carries a high risk of morbidity and mortality due to the seriousness of early complications.[3]

Late complications:

- Globe malposition
- Diplopia
- Malocclusion
- Nasopharyngeal stenosis
- Trismus
- Chronic sinusitis
- Nasal obstruction
- Facial deformity[4,5]

This decrease in morbidity parallels the implementation of free tissue transfer to the skull base in more challenging defects.[6]

GOALS OF SKULL BASE RECONSTRUCTION

- To create a safe wound by sealing the intracranial compartment from the subjacent spaces
- and To obliterate dead space cover vital structures with vascularized tissue
- To maximize postoperative function (vision, mastication, speech, and sinonasal physiology) and restore optimal cosmesis by providing structural support and adequate soft tissue bulk[7]

BASIC PRINCIPLES OF SKULL BASE RECONSTRUCTION

The basic considerations required before the surgeon embark on reconstruction a skull base defect are as follows:[8]

- *Site of reconstruction:* The skull base can be divided into four regions: anterior, middle, posterior, and midline/central **(Fig. 1)**. Each site has unique features that influence the reconstruction.
- *Defect evaluation:* The defect needs to be considered in terms of the size of the dural defect, the degree of communication between the cranial contents and the aerodigestive tract, and the extent of skin, soft tissue, bone, and mucosal resection.
- *Resection of key structures:* These include orbit, auricle, mandible, maxilla, and palate.

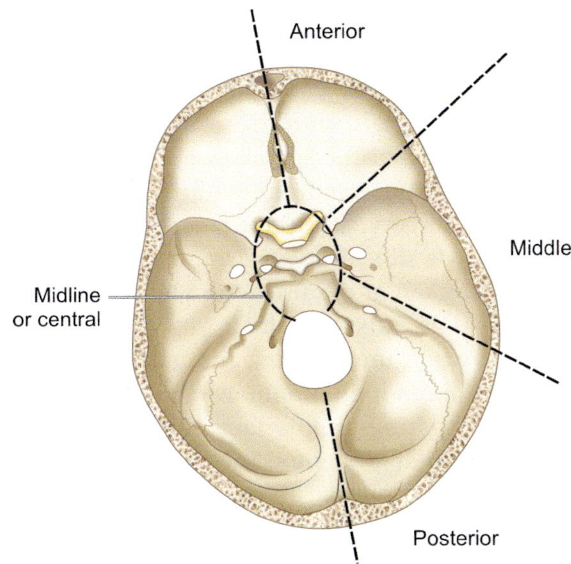

Fig. 1: Divisions of skull base for reconstruction.

- *General factors:* These impact local wound healing and the availability of local tissues for repair, and include prior or intended radiotherapy, previous surgery or scarring, and systemic issues that may interfere with wound healing.

OBJECTIVES OF SKULL BASE RECONSTRUCTION

The objectives that must be met to achieve the goals are as follows:

- *Watertight repair of dural openings and defects:* The risks of direct communication between dura and the upper aerodigestive tract cannot be overemphasized. Persistent CSF leaks pose a threat for meningitis, which can occur in 8.6–41%.[9] Factors thought to contribute to CSF leak include large dural defects, inadequate dural closure, dural openings in areas difficult to access (e.g., planum sphenoidale, cavernous sinus, central and posterior skull base), and dead space adjacent to the cranial cavity leaving dura in contact with air cavities. Every attempt should be made to repair the dural defects with watertight closure either through direct repair (which includes interrupted sutures or a running locking suture using meticulous technique) or patching (which includes autograft, pericranium, or temporalis fascia are readily available and well suited for virtually any defect that may be encountered). Other options for patching are allogenic dura and fascia lata; fibrin glue has proven to be an excellent adjunct, it provides a rapidly setting biologic adhesive to bond onlay grafts or fascial flaps to the underlying dural layer. As a final step in dural repair, it is frequently advisable to suture the dura to drill holes around the periphery of the craniotomy. This simple maneuver is used in pneumatic dissection of the dura in the case of tension pneumocranium.[10]
- *Interposition of vascularized tissue between exposed dura and adjacent spaces:* The placement of vascularized tissue prevents wide dural exposure to adjacent dead spaces or the aerodigestive tract, which if present can result in air desiccation with the risk of necrosis, wound contamination, infection, or CSF leak. Vascular tissue also allows the separation of the intracranial contents from the subcranial spaces, which is essential in cases where nonvital grafts have been used to patch the dura.[11] The specific vascularized flap used depends on the location and size of the defect and the presence of associated defects that must be reconstructed.
- *Replacement of lost skin cover:* Skull base surgery results in associated defects of adjacent structures, requiring composite tissue reconstruction to restore a combination of skin, soft tissue, bone, or mucosa, which local tissue flaps do not provide. The reconstructive surgeon must resort to either pedicled or revascularized free tissue transfer. Many authors have stated that regional pedicled flaps are inferior to free flaps in reconstructing the skull base.[6] Patients undergoing repair with local flaps have a higher rate of acute perioperative problems and late wound breakdown than those undergoing revascularized free tissue repair of the skull base;[12] hence, whenever feasible, free tissue transfer is preferred.[13]
- *Provision of stable skeletal support:* The indications for rigid/osseous reconstruction are as follows:
  - Extremely large bony defects of the skull base that will result in gross brain herniation
  - Near-total or complete orbital roof defects that may result in pulsatile exophthalmos due to pressure from the herniating brain on the globes
  - Orbital wall or orbital floor defects that carry a high risk of enophthalmos
  - Cranio-orbital defects that will result in inadequate soft tissue support and deformity
  - Associated maxillary or mandibular/glenoid fossa defects that will result in facial deformity, malocclusion, and masticatory dysfunction

Sinha et al. describe a three-layer closure of the anterior skull base using titanium mesh, calvarial bone grafts, and pericranial flaps.[14] Badie et al., on the other hand, used titanium alone without bone grafting for a similar repair of the anterior fossa floor.[15] Some authors have reported problems with postoperative infection requiring removal of nonvital grafts or alloplastic implants.[16] To overcome this problem, there are authors who have proposed the use of vascularized bone grafts in conjunction with the temporal/temporoparietal or galeal/pericranial system of flaps.[17] When an isolated bone defect of the cranial base warrants repair, it is generally easier to use alloplastic materials that are completely covered with vascularized soft tissue, such as titanium mesh. Extensive defects of the skull base requiring bony repair are associated with osseous defects of the adjacent craniomaxillofacial skeleton plus defects of skin cover, soft tissue bulk, or mucosa; such defects are treated with osseous composite revascularized free tissue transfer such as the scapular system, fibula osteomyocutaneous, or radial forearm flaps.[18]

- *Filling dead space with adequate soft tissue bulk:* Extensive soft tissue resections mandate reconstruction with flaps capable of returning adequate vascularized tissue bulk to prevent large dead spaces in the cranial base and to maintain adequate surface anatomic contour of the face. Filling of dead spaces is required in temporal fossa, infratemporal fossa, parotid bed, and midfacial region. Local flaps are often insufficient, and microvascular flaps are required. One has to make a choice between muscle (e.g., latissimus or rectus abdominis) and other flaps containing primarily skin or fat (e.g., parascapular or anterolateral thigh). Some authors have described the use of vascularized fat tissue for obliteration of dead spaces.[19] The major disadvantages of using muscle flaps are that the muscle will undergo an unpredictable amount of denervation atrophy over time, rendering it difficult to judge the appropriate degree of bulk to place at the time of reconstruction and the fibrosis that accompanies muscle atrophy can result in stenosis of adjacent spaces such as the nasopharynx or oropharynx.
- *Restoration of resected mucosal lining:* The lining with a lubricated mucosal surface instead of a skin surface is to avoid crusting and accumulation of debris. Flaps such as the gastro-omental flap are ideal to achieve this. If a musculocutaneous or a fasciocutaneous flap is being used, one should consider removing the skin cover on the segment of the flap facing the aerodigestive tract in the hopes that it will mucosalize by ingrowth from the adjacent mucosa.
- *Cranial nerve rehabilitation:* One may encounter temporary or permanent neuropathies involving one or more of cranial nerves V, VII, IX, X, XI, and XII. The resultant impact on facial movement, speech, and swallowing can vary from mild to devastating, and if indicated surgical intervention is required (e.g., eye rehabilitation in VII nerve sacrifice).
- *Esthetic rehabilitation:* Key esthetic anatomic structures such as the ear, nose, eyes, and orbits that are frequently resected during the course of ablative skull base surgery. Definitive reconstruction of these structures is not always warranted and is usually not undertaken at the time of initial reconstruction. However, one must bear their future reconstruction in mind when undertaking the primary skull base repair.[20] Due to the limitations of autogenous tissue in reconstructing unique facial anatomy, currently the best available method for replacement involves a prosthesis anchored to osseointegrated titanium implants.

ANTERIOR SKULL BASE RECONSTRUCTION

Pericranial and galeopericranial flaps are the workhorse for straightforward anterior skull base reconstruction.[21] The blood supply of these flaps is from the deep, and to a lesser extent, the superficial branches of the supraorbital and supratrochlear arteries. The reliability of the blood supply, particularly to a pericranium-only fascial flap, is controversial. It has been shown that incorporating the galea and the frontalis muscle anteriorly in the form of a myofascial flap results in an improved blood supply over the pericranial flap. To maximize the reach of the flap, it should be dissected to the level of the supraorbital rims.[21]

Free grafts are advantageous due to easy harvest and minimal donor site morbidity. Some examples of free grafts are middle turbinate mucosa, temporalis fascia, fascia lata, and palatal mucosa. The free grafts get completely integrated with surrounding tissue after 8 weeks, but the grafts need to be 25% larger than the defect, due its 20% reduction in size during healing process.

For the repair of anterior cranial base defects, instead of free tissue grafts (autograft or allograft), recent developments in endoscopic skull base surgery encompasses the utility of vascularized pedicled flaps. A pedicled flap, is a type of flap which is connected to its donor site and transferred to another area retaining its intact pedicle. The primary workhorse for endoscopic skull base reconstruction remains to be posteriorly-based pedicled nasoseptal flap (NSF) or Hadad-Bassagaisteguy flap for clival defect and high flow cerebrospinal fluid leaks. The other intranasal pedicled flaps are inferior turbinate flap and middle turbinate flap which can be considered as a second option. The limitation of the NSF is its inability to reach certain anterior defects which involve the posterior table or the anterior cribriform plate.

Free flaps can be considered if either the size or location of the skull base defect which is to be repaired exceeds the limits of the pedicled flap or if there is prior sacrifice of the pedicled flap during tumor ablation. The size of the NSF may also be affected by septal spurs and underdeveloped septum especially in patients less than 10 years of age.

Galeopericranial flaps are indicated in most anterior skull base cases where the bony defect is limited to one or more of the following: cribriform plate, ethmoid roof, planum sphenoidale, one or both of the orbital roofs. Its advantages are as follows:

- For patients who have not been previously operated or irradiated, it provides a thin, reliable, and vascularized sheet of fascia that can reach well back into the depths of the anterior skull base.
- It effectively reinforces any dural repair that has been undertaken and separates the anterior fossa from the sinonasal tract below.
- The flap can be sutured to the deep and lateral margins of the bony defect for stabilization.
- It can be passed beneath the supraorbital rims if a one-piece fronto-orbital osteotomy is used to access the skull base; or above the supraorbital rims in the gap between the fronto-orbital bandeau and the frontal bone segment if a two-piece osteotomy or a classic anterior craniofacial approach is used.

The indications for free flap reconstructions are as follows:

- Patients who have had prior surgery and no longer have a reliable galeopericranial flap available
- Those with associated orbital exenteration, maxillectomy, rhinectomy, or facial skin resection
- Patients with failed reconstruction where secondary repair of an open wound with intracranial exposure or CSF leak is necessary

Depending on the situation, many free flaps can be planned keeping in mind the soft tissue bulk and the length, as well as the caliber of the vascular pedicle and the unique feature of the defect. If simple soft tissue obliteration with skin cover is the goal of reconstruction, the rectus abdominis, latissimus dorsi, or parascapular flap can be used. If bony reconstruction of maxillectomy and orbital defects is desired, osseous reconstruction must be performed with either bone grafts placed in combination with free flap coverage or with bone-containing free flaps.[22] Calvarial or iliac bone grafts used to reconstruct key areas of the craniofacial skeleton must be fully wrapped with transferred revascularized free tissue, rectus abdominis and radial forearm free flaps are most commonly used. Of the osseous free flaps, the scapular osteomyocutaneous free flap provides the greatest versatility when reconstructing complex orbitomaxillary-palatal defects that result in association with skull base defects. In selected anterior skull base defects, it may be necessary to provide revascularized free tissue to simply seal the intracranial cavity from the extracranial spaces, the radial forearm fascial/fasciocutaneous or omental free flap can be used to great advantage.[23]

LATERAL SKULL BASE RECONSTRUCTION

The workhorse flaps in this region of skull base defects is the temporal system of flaps. The advantages of the temporal system of flaps are as follows:

- The temporalis system can be raised as a myogenous, fascial, or myofascial flap by incorporating any combination of the temporalis muscle, temporoparietal fascia, or extensions of galea, pericranium, and temporoparietal fascia medial to the temporal line.
- Calvarial bone can be included to yield a composite vascularized pedicled flap.
- The temporalis muscle flap has the greatest utility in reconstructing relatively straightforward defects of the infratemporal fossa.

The indications for free flap reconstruction in lateral skull base defects are as follows:

- For larger and complex defects of the lateral skull base
- Particularly cases in which skin cover, soft tissue bulk, or mucosal lining of the pharynx are to be replaced.

Depending on the nature of the defect, a variety of options can be used. Rectus abdominis, latissimus dorsi, scapular-parascapular, or gastro-omental flaps have been successfully used. Izquierdo et al. described the different uses of the rectus abdominis free flap as the myocutaneous and the de-epithelized types; the myocutaneous design is useful in repairing complex defects needing skin coverage, while the de-epithelized type is useful for defects extending medially across the midline. These authors showed that the subcutaneous vascularized fat of the flap can be shaped to act as a "cork" over the repaired and unrepaired dura.[24] Schramm and Imola described the successful use of the gastro-omental free flaps after infratemporal fossa resections as they provide an abundant supply of well-vascularized, mobile bulk for soft tissue replacement, and a moist mucosal barrier for nasopharyngeal reconstruction.[19]

POSTERIOR SKULL BASE RECONSTRUCTION

Defects of the posterior skull base are typically limited to the bone of the squamous portion of the temporal bone, mastoid prominence, and occipital region. They are not commonly associated with soft tissue defects. Repair of this area therefore is usually accomplished with repair of dural defects whenever possible and the use of free fat grafts to bolster the dural defect. If vascularized soft tissue coverage is warranted to seal the intracranial space, this is easily accomplished using either a temporalis muscle or temporoparietal fascia flap. Bony defects can be successfully closed with hydroxyapatite cement.

ALLOPLASTS IN SKULL BASE RECONSTRUCTION

The alloplasts that are used with greatest success include titanium mesh, hydroxyapatite cement, porous polyethylene, and resorbable plate fixation. Alloplastic materials should be used selectively in skull base reconstruction and caution should be exercised in patients with compromised wound healing, such as those who have undergone prior surgery or radiation, or those planned to undergo postoperative radiation. As a general rule, alloplasts should be well covered by vascularized soft tissue and should not be left exposed to air in the sinonasal or nasopharyngeal cavities.

- *Titanium mesh:* Versatile in craniofacial and skull base reconstruction, it is biocompatible and is easily adapted to the complex contours of the cranial base and orbital cavity. It serves as a relatively rigid reconstruction of bony walls in the skull base region or can be used in conjunction with other implant materials.[25]
- *Hydroxyapatite cement:* It is a bone-substitute material composed of interlinked calcium phosphate chains. It is supplied as a powder and liquid that are mixed intraoperatively to yield a moldable putty that can then be contoured into the required shape. Once the cement has set, it acts as an osteoconductive material and is touted as undergoing incorporation and eventually replacement by bony ingrowth.[26]
- *Porous polyethylene:* Implants are characterized by ingrowth of fibrovascular tissue and have been used successfully in craniofacial trauma reconstruction for several years. They are particularly well suited to reconstruct the orbital walls; however, care should be taken to provide adequate soft tissue coverage or else extrusion of the implant is a distinct possibility.[27] Resorbable plating can be applied to skull base tumor removal in the pediatric patient and it allows for application of the preplating principle when performing the osteotomies. Bioabsorbable implants have also been used to repair defects following transsphenoidal surgery.[28]

ENDOSCOPIC RECONSTRUCTION

It has gained in popularity as both the equipment and experience of surgeons has improved. It is used for small anterior skull base and sphenoid defects (<3 cm). Defects resulting from iatrogenic injury during sinus surgery, trauma, and tumor extirpation have been successfully repaired with endoscopic approaches using a variety of materials including septal bone/cartilage, nasal mucosa, temporalis fascia, cranial bone, and alloderm.[29]

CONCLUSION

Skull base surgery and reconstruction have become commonplace in many academic centers. The evolution of more reliable reconstructive techniques that allow the separation of the intracranial compartment from extracranial structures has moderated complications from extensive skull base procedures. The use of free tissue transfer can provide dependable, vascularized tissue to fill volume defects created by skull base resections as well as reinforce dural closures to prevent CSF leaks and meningitis. Local flaps are a powerful adjunct to free tissue reconstruction and in select cases may be sufficient alone for skull base reconstruction. Regional flaps for skull base reconstruction should probably be reserved for cases where local flaps and free flaps are not a viable alternative.

REFERENCES

1. Imola MJ, Sciarretta V, Schramm VL. Skull base reconstruction. Curr Opin Otolaryngol Head Neck Surg. 2003;11(4): 282-90.
2. Urken ML, Catalano PJ, Sen C, Post K, Futran N, Biller HF. Free tissue transfer for skull base reconstruction analysis of complications and a classification scheme for defining skull base defects. Arch Otolaryngol Head Neck Surg. 1993;119(12):1318-25.
3. Catalano PJ, Hecht CS, Biller HF, Lawson W, Post KD, Sachdev V, et al. Craniofacial resection. An analysis of 73 cases. Arch Otolaryngol Head Neck Surg. 1994;120(11):1203-8.
4. Irish JC, Gullane PJ, Gentili F, Freeman J, Boyd JB, Brown D, et al. Tumors of the skull base: outcome and survival analysis of 77 cases. Head Neck. 1994;16(1):3-10.
5. Janecka IP, Sen C, Sekhar LN, Ramasastry S, Curtin HD, Barnes EL, et al. Cranial base surgery: results in 183 patients. Otolaryngol Head Neck Surg. 1994;110(6):539-46.
6. Neligan PC, Mulholland S, Irish J, Gullane PJ, Boyd JB, Gentili F, et al. Flap selection in cranial base reconstruction. Plast Reconstr Surg. 1996;98(7):1159-66.
7. Solero CL, DiMeco F, Sampath P, Mattavelli F, Pizzi N, Salvatori P, et al. Combined anterior craniofacial resection for tumors involving the cribriform plate: early postoperative complications and technical considerations. Microsurgery. 2000;47(6):1296-304.
8. Fliss DM, Gil Z, Spektor S, Leider-Trejo L, Abergel A, Khafif A, et al. Skull base reconstruction after anterior subcranial tumor resection. Neurosurg Focus. 2002;12(5):e10.

9. Costa H, Cerejo A, Baptista A, Vaz R, Gonçalves M, Guimarães A, et al. The galea frontalis myofascial flap in anterior fossa CSF leaks. Br J Plast Surg. 1993;46(6): 503-7.
10. Fisher J, Jackson IT. Microvascular surgery as an adjunct to craniomaxillofacial reconstruction. Br J Plast Surg. 1989; 42:146-54.
11. Chang DW, Langstein HN, Gupta A, De Monte F, Do KA, Wang X, et al. Reconstructive management of cranial base defects after tumor ablation. Plast Reconstr Surg. 2001;107(6):1346-55.
12. Heth JA, Funk GF, Karnell LH, McCulloch TM, Traynelis VC, Nerad JA, et al. Free tissue transfer and local flap complications in anterior and anterolateral skull base surgery. Head Neck. 2002;24(10):901-11.
13. Kraus DH, Shah JP, Arbit E, Galicich JH, Strong EW. Complications of craniofacial resection for tumors involving the anterior skull base. Head Neck. 1994;16(4):307-12.
14. Sinha UK, Johnson TE, Crockett D, Vadapalli S, Gruen P. Three-layer reconstruction for large defects of the anterior skull base. Laryngoscope. 2002;112(3):424-7.
15. Badie B, Preston JK, Hartig GK. Use of titanium mesh for reconstruction of large anterior cranial base defects. J Neurosurg. 2000;93(4):711-4.
16. Nibu K, Sasaki T, Kawahara N, Sugasawa M, Nakatsuka T, Yamada A, et al. Complications of craniofacial surgery for tumors involving the anterior cranial base. Neurosurgery. 1998;42(3):455-62.
17. Undt G, Hollmann K, Schuster H, Rasse M. Pedicled calvarial bone flap for reconstruction of the anterior skull base following tumor resection. Plast Reconstr Surg. 1996;98(4): 730-4.
18. Goel A. Vascularized osteomyoplastic flaps for skull base reconstruction. Br J Neurosurg 1994;8(1):79-82.
19. Schramm VL Jr, Imola MJ. Management of nasopharyngeal salivary gland malignancy. Laryngoscope. 2001;111(9):1533-44.
20. Day TA, Davis BK. Skull base reconstruction and rehabilitation. Otolaryngol Clin North Am. 2001;34(6):1241-57.
21. Potparic Z, Fukuta K, Colen LB, Jackson IT, Carraway JH. Galeopericranial flaps in the forehead: a study of blood supply and volumes. Br J Plast Surg. 1996;49(8):519-28.
22. Kyutoku S, Tsuji H, Inoue T, Kawakami K, Han F, Ogawa Y. Experience with the rectus abdominis myocutaneous flap with vascularized hard tissue for immediate orbitofacial reconstruction. Plast Reconstr Surg. 1999;103(2):395-402.
23. Schwartz MS, Cohen JI, Meltzer T, Wheatley MJ, McMenomey SO, Horgan MA, et al. Use of the radial forearm microvascular free-flap graft for cranial base reconstruction. J Neurosurg. 1999;90(4):651-5.
24. Izquierdo R, Leonetti JP, Origitano TC, al-Mefty O, Anderson DE, Reichman OH. Refinements using free-tissue transfer for complex cranial base reconstruction. Plast Reconstr Surg. 1993;92(4):567-74.
25. Janecka IP. New reconstructive technologies in skull base surgery: role of titanium mesh and porous polyethylene. Arch Otolaryngol Head Neck Surg. 2000;126(3):396-401.
26. Zide MF, Kent JN, Machado L. Hydroxylapatite cranioplasty directly over dura. J Oral Maxillofac Surg. 1987;45(6): 481-6.
27. Kaptain GJ, Vincent DA, Laws ER Jr. Cranial base reconstruction after transsphenoidal surgery with bioabsorbable implants. Neurosurgery. 2001;48(1):232-3.
28. Mola MJ, Schramm VL. Resorbable fixation in pediatric cranial base surgery: How I do it. Laryngoscope. 2002;112(10): 1897-901.
29. Bolger WE, Mclaughlin K. Cranial bone grafts in cerebrospinal fluid leak and encephalocele repair: A preliminary report. Am J Rhinology. 2003;17(3):153-8.

CHAPTER 40

Principles of Pharyngeal and Tracheal Reconstruction

Dimpy Sharma, Narayana Subramaniam, Sivakumar Vidhyadharan, Samskruthi P Murthy

INTRODUCTION

The upper aerodigestive tract forms a common functional pathway for oral intake, breathing, and speech. Articulation of speech is a result of coordinated movements by the larynx, epiglottis, pharyngeal walls, soft and hard palate, tongue, teeth, and lips. Owing to its rich lymphoid tissue, the pharynx also plays an important role in immunological defense of the upper aerodigestive tract. Pharyngeal reconstruction, following cancer resection, poses a challenge for the reconstructive surgeon. Edgerton introduced the concept of primary reconstruction, following oncological resection in head and neck in 1951.[1] Various local and regional flaps have been used to reconstruct the pharyngeal defect. These are laterally based forehead flap[2] and deltopectoral flap.[3] The pectoralis major myocutaneous flap[4] has its advantage of providing a well-vascularized cover for large defects involving upper aerodigestive tract, skull base as well as face. The other myocutaneous flaps that have been used are the pedicled latissimus dorsi musculocutaneous flap[5-7] and the superior trapezius musculocutaneous flap.[8,9]

Tracheal reconstruction poses other challenges; the trachea has a semi-rigid structure anteriorly to prevent collapse during inspiration and flexible posterior wall to allow esophageal transit. With improvements in tracheal reconstruction techniques and the advent of tracheal transplantation, tumors that were previously not amenable to radical surgery can now be resected, offering patients good oncological outcomes and quality of life. With advancement in the field of microsurgery, the surgical treatment of advanced head and neck cancers has become less debilitating. The free tissue transfer provides flap options that have more reliable vascularity and allow replacement of large volumes of tissue in a single stage. It also allows unparalleled degrees of freedom in flap positioning and orientation without the tethering effect produced by the pedicled flaps. This chapter covers the principles of pharyngeal and tracheal reconstruction following oncological resection and the evidence pertaining to it.

LARYNGEAL AND HYPOPHARYNGEAL RECONSTRUCTION

As with other sites, the reconstructive surgeon needs to consider the following factors before embarking on a plan for reconstruction:

- *Tumor-related:* Size of the tumor, extent of resection, and types of tissue involved (skin, soft tissue, and pharyngeal mucosa)
- *Vessel status:* Availability of donor vessels in the ipsilateral or contralateral neck if free flap reconstruction is planned
- *Previous radiotherapy:* This predisposes to high complication rates and substantial vascularized tissue from outside the field of radiation is often required to circumvent this. If the carotid vessels are at risk of exposure, soft tissue or muscle interposition between the vessels and neck skin is required.
- *Patient-related factors:* Nutritional status, comorbidities affecting wound healing, and ability to tolerate prolonged general anesthesia administration impact decision-making. Smoking impacts wound healing, increases risk of postoperative infection, and affects microvascular blood flow.

GOALS OF RECONSTRUCTION

As partial laryngectomies and their reconstruction have been covered in the chapter on laryngeal cancers, this chapter will be restricted to total laryngectomy with or without pharyngectomy. The goals of laryngopharyngeal reconstruction are as follows:

- Maintaining a patent airway and protection from aspiration
- Re-establishing the integrity of the pharyngeal pathway to allowing swallowing and adequate caloric intake
- Voice and speech rehabilitation

Ideally patients will have all three of these goals addressed but if this is not feasible, this is the order in which they must be addressed; airway patency and aspiration are life-threatening issues, while oral intake is not. In the background of pharyngocutaneous fistulae (PCF) and chronic wound healing issues, patients often cannot have voice rehabilitation addressed for long periods of time and should be made aware of this prior to surgical intervention. Preoperative nutrition status is critical in wound healing; if nutritionally depleted, a period of intensive rehabilitation with tube feeding prior to surgery may be valuable if feasible.

- *Primary closure:* In this case, after total laryngectomy, there is no defect in the hypopharyngeal mucosa. This commonly occurs in glottis and supraglottic endolaryngeal tumors. Several methods of closure have been described, including interrupted or continuous suturing, lock-and-key figure suturing, T-shaped and vertical closure. However, it is unlikely that any particular technique has an advantage over other techniques. The surgical principles that need to be followed are ensuring that the mucosal edge is vascular, gentle handling, and tension free but watertight closure. It is generally accepted that in the nonirradiated patient, 3 cm of stretched mucosa is adequate for pharyngeal closure without any additional tissue.[10] For defects larger than this, additional tissue may be required to avoid dysphagia and poor speech.

  Whether addition of vascularized tissue (such as pectoralis major muscles flap), reduced PCF after total laryngectomy in the irradiated patient has been studied for over two decades. A systematic review showed that incorporation of vascularized tissue in this situation reduced PCF rates by a third (from 31.2 to 22.2%),[11] and it is reasonable to utilize this approach in salvage laryngectomy, especially those who are at a higher risk of PCF.
- *Larger defects:* Disa classified pharyngeal defects into:[12]
  - *Type I:* Partial defects involving ≤50% of the pharyngeal circumference
  - *Type II:* Circumferential defects involving >50% of pharyngeal circumference
  - *Type III:* Extensive noncircumferential defects involving multiple other anatomical sites (such as skin)

The limitation of this system is that it does not distinguish whether partial defects involve the larynx or base tongue.

The approach to reconstruction of laryngopharyngeal defects is shown in **Flowchart 1.**[13] The main factors influencing the choice of reconstruction are: the size of the defect, donor tissue availability, and the general condition of the patient. Prolonged intraoperative period add to increase the morbidity of the patient. Also, it is an additional stress on the patient's cardiovascular and respiratory status if laparotomy is done or chest myocutaneous flap is harvested. Regional and distant flaps have advantage that these can be raised simultaneously as a two-team approach, to reduce the length of surgery. Summaries of flaps that can be used are discussed

Flowchart 1: Approach to reconstruction of laryngopharyngeal defects.

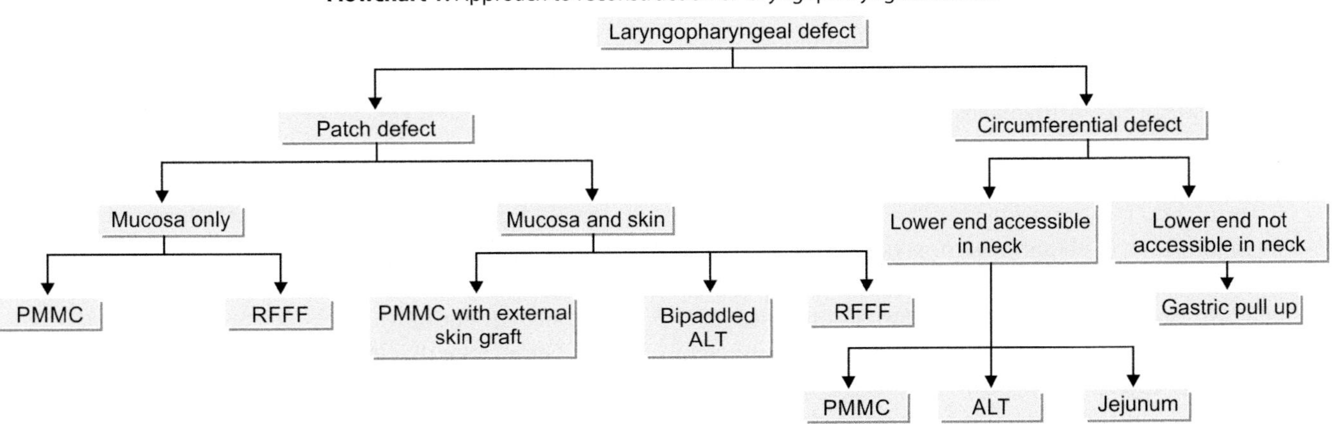

(ALT: anterolateral thigh; PMMC: pectoralis major myocutaneous; RFFF: radial forearm free flap)

below (the remainder are described in the chapter on microvascular reconstruction).

PECTORALIS MAJOR FLAP

- *Vascular supply:* Pectoral branches of the thoracoacromial vessels.
- *Salient anatomy:* The flap comprises the pectoralis major muscle with or without the overlying skin and may include the underlying ribs. This muscle originates from the anterior aspect of the medial half of the clavicle, anterior sternum, true ribs, and external oblique aponeurosis with a twisted spiral insertion in the lateral lip of the bicipital groove of the humerus. This is an axial flap based on the pectoral branch of the thoracoacromial artery and its accompanying veins. There is a clear fascial plane that allows the surgeon to lift the flap and its underlying pedicle off of the pectoralis minor, violation of which can result in disruptions in blood flow. In most patients, there is an additional supply medially through the internal mammary vessels or laterally through the long thoracic vessels, which can be spared or sacrificed depending on the arc of rotation required for inset. The lateral pectoral nerve passes along with the pedicle and the medial pectoral nerve passes through the pectoralis minor to innervate the pectoralis major from below. These are generally divided to prevent contraction in the wound bed, but this results in a loss of tone and bulk over time. The surface marking of the pedicle is through intersection of a line from the acromion process to the xiphisternum and second line drawn from the midpoint of the clavicle to meet the first line.
- *Anatomical variations:* Poland syndrome is associated with absence of the pectoralis major muscle and hypoplasia of the chest wall on one side, and this can be identified easily on clinical examination.
- *Components and variants:* Most commonly myocutaneous, however, can be modified to include bone (rib or sternum). A myofascial flap is also used when skin lining is not required.
- *Flap design and utilization:* The skin paddle, if required, is centered over the pectoralis major muscle, which is palpable in most patients. In women, an inframammary or parasternal skin paddle helps exclude breast tissue from the flap. Up to 2.5 cm of skin beyond the edge of the pectoralis major muscle can be included with good vascularity; beyond this the vascular supply becomes more unpredictable.
- *Common use:* Replacement of mucosal or soft tissue for defects that are intraoral (tongue, floor of mouth, buccal, and oropharyngeal), hypopharynx, and external skin (following radical neck dissection it provides coverage of the vessel with muscle and skin). It can be "tubed" for circumferential defects. A myocutaneous flap placed over the pharyngeal closure following total laryngectomy has been shown to reduce the risk of PCF. Rib component has been used for tracheal defects.
- *Advantages:*
  - Versatile with multiple components possible
  - Reliable anatomy
  - Good thick muscle available when bulk is required
  - Good amount of skin available
  - Relatively easy to raise
- *Limitations:*
  - Flap may be very thick in well-built patients (due to muscle hypertrophy) or the obese (due to subcutaneous fat deposition).
  - Poor donor cosmetic outcome, especially when skin grafting is performed.
  - Some patients report shoulder dysfunction, which is worse when combined with neck dissection.[14]
  - As with all regional flaps, the pedicle orientation and tension dictate flap positioning.

JEJUNAL FREE FLAP

- *Vascular supply:* Branches of the superior mesenteric artery and accompanying vein
- *Salient anatomy:* The flap comprises a loop of jejunum with its blood supply. The jejunum begins at the ligament of Treitz and extends distally for about 6–8 feet. The blood supply is through the superior mesenteric artery and vein, which branch off to form jejunal arterial segmental branches that communicate with the vasa recta. This allows the surgeon to identify a segment of jejunum (10–20 cm) with its vascular supply tracing back to a single pedicle **(Figs. 1A to C)**.
- *Flap design and utilization:* It is used for circumferential reconstruction of pharyngeal and upper esophageal defects, most commonly following total laryngectomy.
- *Advantages:*
  - Reduced risk of stricture when compared to skin-lined flaps
  - Quality of tissue closest to pharynx structurally and functionally
  - Good vascularity; healing issues rare except in failure
- *Limitations:*
  - Sensitive to hypoxia, ischemic time beyond 3 hours likely to result in flap failure

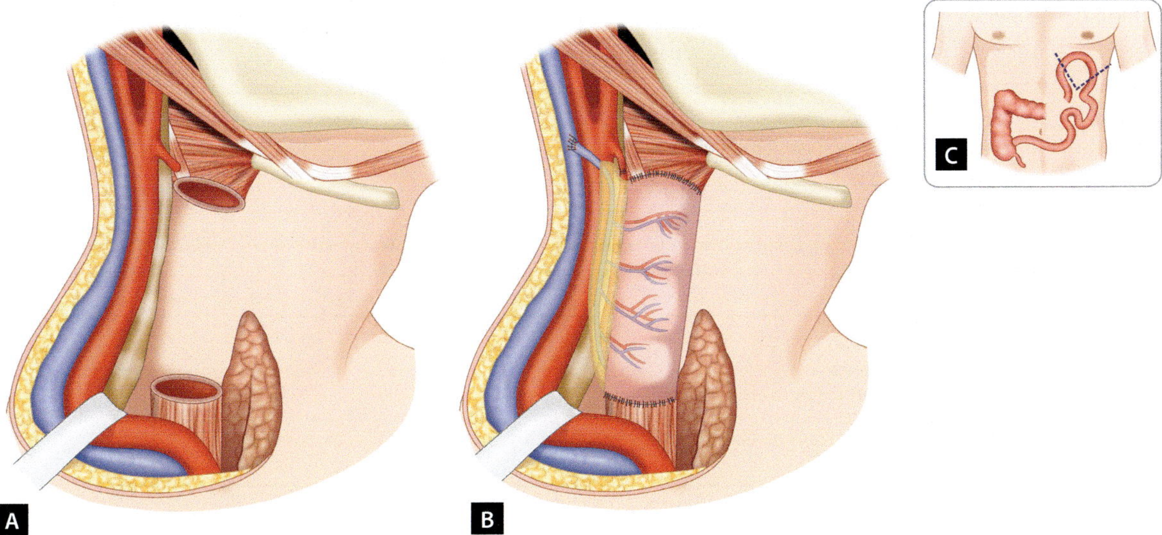

Figs. 1A to C: Free jejunal transfer for pharyngeal reconstruction.

  - History of previous laparotomy
  - Requires an additional laparotomy or laparoscopic procedure for harvest with its own morbidity and physiological stress
  - Pedicle length is short (average 4–6 cm).
  - Vein is thin walled and fragile.
  - Monitoring is difficult requiring a sentinel loop to be brought externally or by allowing a "window" to observe the flap.
  - Poor quality of tracheoesophageal puncture valve speech when compared to skin-lined speech
- *Additional considerations:*
  - *Flap failure:* As the monitoring is difficult, the early recognition of a failing flap can be missed, especially in cases of visceral flap. The most important clinical sign of a jejunal flap failure is per oral bleeding.[15] If diagnosed early, salvage of the flap must be attempted by debridement and revision of anastomosis. When there is microsurgical failure or gross contamination and infection, regional flap or a second free flap reconstruction can be done, after debridement and once the infection has subsided. Management of a failed gastric pull up can be very challenging with a high risk of mortality and an approach is shown in **Flowchart 2.**[16]
  - *Pharyngocutaneous fistula:* PCF are a common complication occurring after pharyngeal reconstruction. The incidences in a primary and salvage setting around 10–15% and 30–35%, respectively.[17] The factors affecting the rate of PCF are previous radiotherapy and chemotherapy, advanced tumors, neck dissection, and hypothyroidism.[18] The incidence of fistula formation has been observed higher in fasciocutaneous flaps. This can be attributed to addition seam suture line for tubing of the flap or the tension on the most vital part of the pedicled flap. A persistent low postoperative albumin in early postoperative period (as early as day 3) and elevated total leukocyte count may be suggestive of an early leak.[19] Fistulas are mostly managed conservatively, mainly by diverting the leak away from the great vessels of neck. Small fistulas usually heal spontaneously within 1–2 weeks. Fistulas with significant leaks require debridement of sloughed necrotic tissue and a well-vascularized cover. In such situation, regional flaps such as pectoralis major, deltopectoral and latissimus dorsi are often the best options.[20-22] Prophylactic antibiotics and proton pump inhibitors help in reducing infection and gastric reflux, therefore reducing the chances of fistula formation. It is unclear if early feeding causes/worsens PCF; a systematic review showed too much heterogeneity to reach an unequivocal conclusion.[23]
  - *Stricture formation:* Distal anastomotic strictures are more common and may occur several months or years after surgery. Previous radiation exposure increases the chances on stricture formation due to extensive fibrosis. Kinking of the bowel segment at the anastomotic site, due to long jejunal segment, can also lead to stricture formation. The patient commonly complains of dysphagia, more for solids than liquids. Strictures can be treated with endoscopic balloon dilatation. Repeated dilatation

Flowchart 2: Management of suspected leak following gastric pull up.

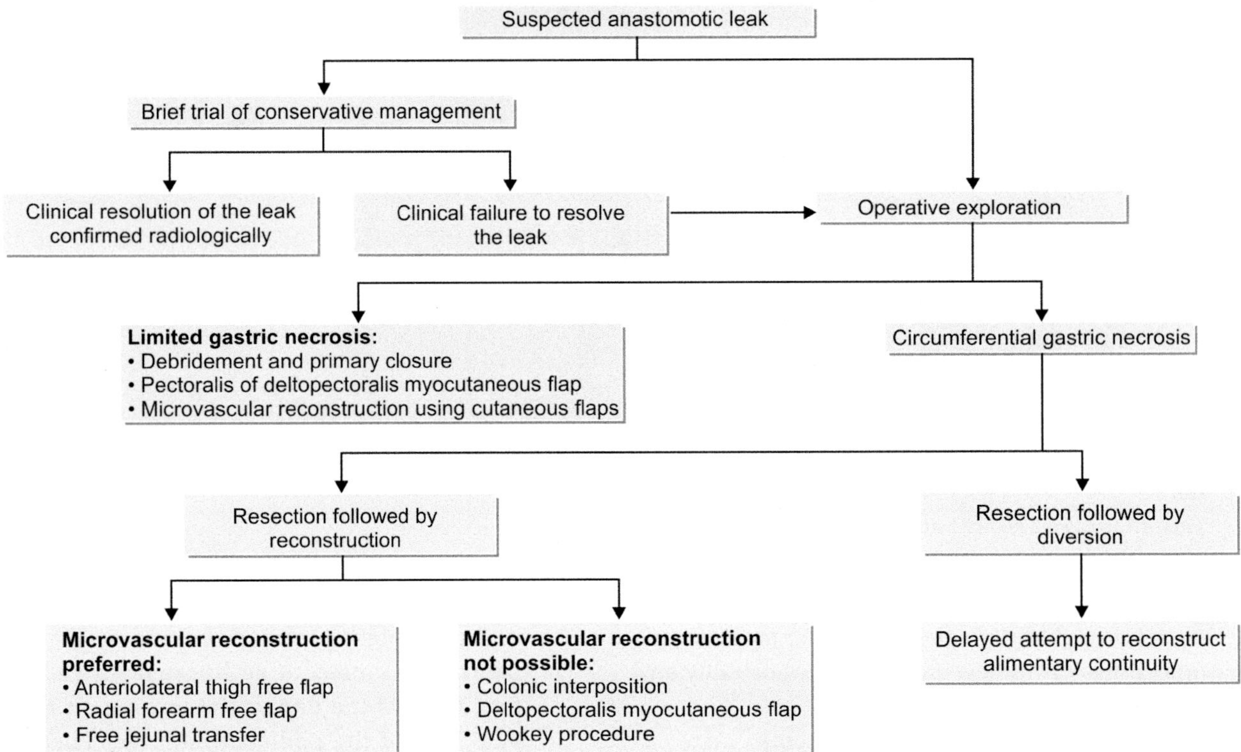

may be required in most of the cases. In refractory cases, surgical repair can be achieved with a free flap reconstruction but this can be very challenging in a reoperative setting.

- *Voice rehabilitation:* There is debate whether primary or secondary tracheoesophageal puncture (TEP) valve placement is superior in the setting of salvage laryngectomy, primarily due to the risk of PCF and the risk that the puncture may accentuate this leading to more wound complications.[24] Good voice quality can be achieved with fasciocutaneous flap reconstruction; however, it is generally accepted that enteric flaps have a poorer quality "gurgling" or "wet voice" due to mucous secretion.
- *Salivary bypass tubes:* A salivary bypass tube is a silicone tube that directs the saliva into the distal esophagus. It helps the tissue to heal by avoiding constant exposure to saliva. It can be used as a stent during the primary reconstruction of pharyngeal defects, using fasciocutaneous free flap, helping in reducing the postoperative complications.[25] Another advantage of this tube is that a nasogastric tube can be inserted through this tube for feeding. It has shown to be very helpful in cases of fistula or stricture formation. Those who support it suggest that it may bridge the tract, allowing for spontaneous closure of PCF, while critics argue it may increase the risk of PCF. No evidence currently supports their use in reducing the risk of complications.[26]

OROPHARYNGEAL RECONSTRUCTION

Oropharyngeal reconstruction may involve primarily closing the wound, flap reconstruction, or allowing healing of wound by secondary intention.[28] The aims of oropharyngeal reconstruction are restoration of the mucosal epithelium, separation of pharynx from the neck with soft tissue, and obliteration of dead space.[27] When there is no communication between pharynx and neck or exposure of bone, small tonsillar, tongue base or palatal defects may either be closed primarily or left to heal by secondary intention. Reconstructive options have been described by Sabri et al. in **Table 1**.[28]

The limitations of the regional flaps for some oropharyngeal reconstructions as compared to the free flaps are their arc of rotation, length of pedicle, and bulkiness, but many modifications have suggested ways to overcome these.[27] Overall, the armamentarium of flaps for oropharyngeal defect reconstruction is the same as those for oral cavity.

Table 1: Reconstructive options in oropharyngeal defects.

Small defects	• Healing by secondary intention • Primary closure • Split thickness skin graft • Buccal mucosa flap • Submental island flap • Palatal island flap
Moderate defects	• Healing by secondary intention • Primary closure • Split thickness skin graft • Pectoralis major myocutaneous flap • Lower trapezius flap • Pedicled latissimus dorsi flap
Large defects	• Large pedicled flaps • Microvascular free flaps (radial forearm, lateral arm, rectus abdominis, jejunum, gastro-omental, and latissimus dorsi)
Large composite bone defects	• Scapula osteocutaneous free flap • Fibula free flap

Reconstruction of the soft palate after resection requires a lot of surgical planning because of its function and difficulty in placing obturators as an alternative (in contrast to hard palate defects). Lv et al. proposed a revision of soft palate defect classification (initially described by Urken) comprising four classes: type I (the defect area of the soft palate is 25% or less), type II (the defect area of the soft palate is more than 25%, but 50% or less), type III (the defect area of the soft palate is more than 50%, but 75% or less), and type IV (the defect area of the soft palate is more than 75%, but 100% or less).[29]

Along with the lateral oropharyngeal walls, the soft palate helps with the functioning of the physiological oropharyngeal valve and also aid in the generation of pressure for resonance of speech and food bolus propulsion during the pharyngeal stage of swallowing. Hence, it is imperative to seek to recreate the mobility of the oropharynx during reconstruction. An immobile reconstructed oropharynx gets further static after adjuvant treatment such as radiation therapy. Several studies report that the pliable radial forearm free flap (RFFF), with or without a palmaris tendon sling, is very useful in the three-dimensional reconstruction of the partial or total defects of soft palate. Most effective reconstruction of the palate was for partial palatal resection defect, where there was some compensation of mobility by the intact lateral oropharyngeal walls and remnant soft palate for the immobile flap within the defect.[30]

To minimize the size of the velopharyngeal opening and reduce the probability of nasal regurgitation of feeds, studies by Yoshida et al. and Brown et al. suggest lining the oropharyngeal surface of the soft palate with an RFFF and then either suturing the lateral oropharyngeal to the nasopharyngeal surface of the soft palate remnant or use a superiorly based posterior oropharyngeal wall mucosal flap to resurface the nasopharyngeal surface of the RFFF suspending the reconstructed soft palate in a suitable level.[31,32]

Seikaly et al. reported that inset of the folded RFFF flap in anatomical soft palate position provides lining to the nasopharyngeal and oropharyngeal lining of the soft palate, with the middle de-epithelialized part of the flap sutured to the posterior oropharyngeal wall to serve as a bridge and reduce the velopharyngeal aperture. This reconstructive method can be used in whole or near total soft palate resections, where the soft palate mobility and position are compromised greatly and when a palmaris tendon sling is not sufficient. Function derangement of soft palate by loss of active elevation and contracture of the reconstructed plate, due to inadequate velopharyngeal closure or large velopharyngeal opening during swallowing and speech, may cause velopharyngeal insufficiency and gives a nasal twang to speech.[33]

Similarly, complex defect reconstruction of the lateral and superior lateral walls of the oropharynx is also very challenging as the resection results in functional reduction of normal speech and swallowing. The extent of postoperative rehabilitation of function is dependent on the extent of the defect and reconstruction technique. Large and wide defects can be managed well by static reconstruction with regional pedicled flaps and mounting of prosthesis. Also, in combination of with the described technique of reconstruction and pharyngeal mucosa, flap can be combined to help narrow the velopharyngeal aperture. With the advantage of simultaneous flap harvest during tumor resection, the various wide oropharyngeal defects may also be reconstructed with RFFF, anterolateral thigh (ALT) flaps, or rectus abdominis myocutaneous flaps.[34]

There is significant swallowing and speech dysfunction when half of base of tongue with oral tongue is excised. The goal of reconstruction for such a defect is to provide satisfactory bulk to the base of tongue for it to come in contact with the soft palate and posterior oropharyngeal wall during swallowing and to sustain the movement of the remnant tongue. The efficiency of swallowing function is inversely proportional to the extent of base of tongue excised. To compensate for the volume of the resulting dead space and prevent "tied down" effect on the remnant functional tongue, flaps such as a radial forearm flap, an ALT flap, a deep epigastric inferior artery perforator flap or a groin flap, and an anteromedial thigh flap may be used.

Total glossectomy is indicated as a primary treatment modality for very advanced cancers involving both oral and oropharyngeal tongue and also may be a curative intent treatment option for patients with recurrent squamous cell carcinoma or salivary gland carcinomas. A reasonable quality of life may be obtained with total glossectomy with preservation of larynx in selected patients. The flap for the tongue defect should be able to provide satisfactory bulk along with suspension of larynx for adequate functional outcome. Flaps that are wide and thick such as the rectus abdominis or a pectoralis major need to be designed with their width about 30% more than that of the defect. In cases where supraglottis is included along with the defect, a total laryngectomy is definitely warranted to prevent the patient from having recurrent aspiration. Free deep inferior epigastric perforator (DIEP) or latissimus dorsi flaps can also be used. Tracheostomy and feeding tube decannulation and some intelligibility of speech are achievable in 70–80% of patients with laryngeal preservation.

The posterior oropharyngeal wall is vital for the swallowing function and reconstruction of the defect at that subsite of oropharynx with a bulky flap can lead to poor quality of life due to frequent aspiration risks. Most of the patients may be dependent on gastrostomy tube feeding and only about a third of patients who have undergone reconstruction might achieve adequate oral intake. As an alternative to free flaps, pedicled thin platysma myocutaneous may be used in these defects.[27] An approach to oropharyngeal defect reconstruction is show in **Flowchart 3**.

In summary, in order to enhance the postoperative swallowing and speech function, several reconstructive techniques are described in the literature with variable results and outcomes. For reconstruction of extensive or complex oropharyngeal defects, microvascular free tissue transfer or regional pedicled flap are safe and reliable. When surgery is the primary treatment modality, about two-thirds of patients may be partially dependent on feeding tube for some time during the postoperative period. However, with early and adequate rehabilitation, most patients achieve decannulation and functional speech. Also, among patients in whom primary closure was performed for small oropharyngeal defects, studies report that partly intelligible conversational speech is attainable.[35]

NASOPHARYNGEAL RECONSTRUCTION

For residual or recurrent nasopharyngeal cancers, salvage surgery is a very tool in prolongation of survival. Song et al. studied the outcomes of four different types of flaps (RFFF, fibula, free flap, pectoralis major myocutaneous flap, and tongue flap) used to reconstruct nasopharyngeal defects after salvage resection. Although a small number of patients had slurring of speech, the rest of their patients had normal or normal or intelligible speech. All of their reconstructed patients were able to tolerate diets of usual consistencies between liquid to solids. They observed that with regards to recipient vessels, the facial artery was usually affected by irradiation for nasopharyngeal cancer and suggested instead use of the superior thyroid artery in the anterior neck as this region usually receives lesser dosage of radiation.[36]

Flowchart 3: Algorithm for oropharyngeal reconstruction after oncological resection.

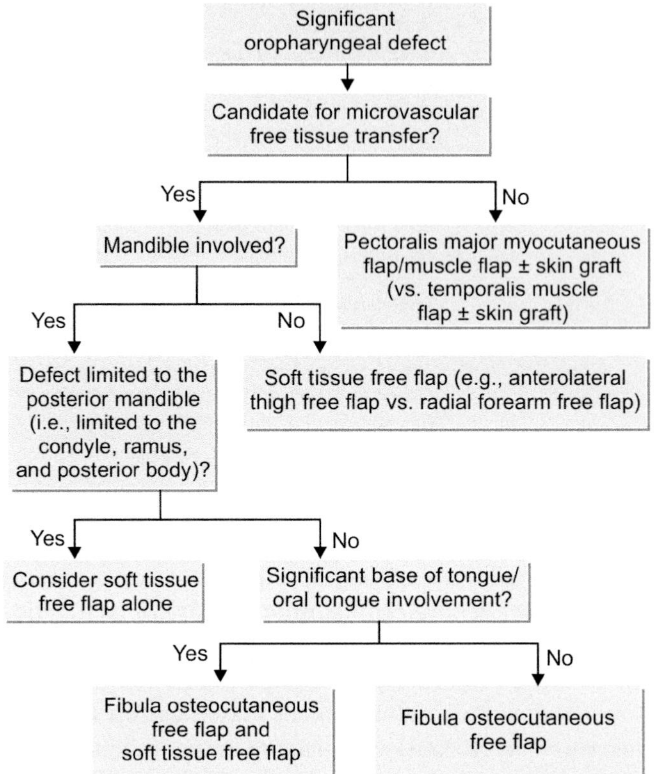

TRACHEAL RECONSTRUCTION

Tracheal reconstruction after oncological resection is challenging as the trachea allows flow of air with the structural integrity to prevent collapse during inspiration while remaining flexible enough to allow neck flexion. The additional functions such as humidification of air and immunity are crucial and impossible to replicate in reconstruction. An approach to tracheal reconstruction is shown in **Flowchart 4.**[37] Tracheal transplantation has only been attempted once in the context of oncological resection; however, the authors did not consider it a success and did not advocate this approach in its current form.

Flowchart 4: Algorithm for tracheal reconstruction after oncological resection.

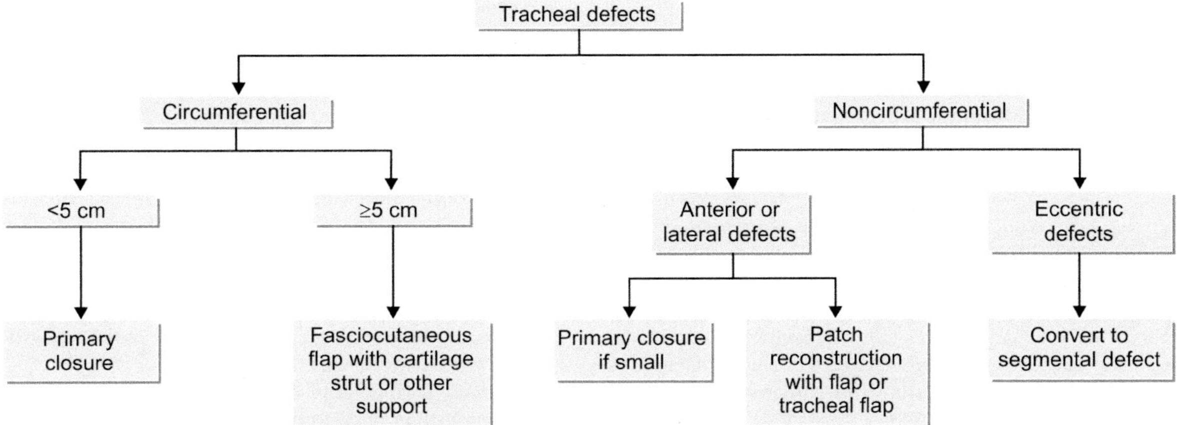

CONCLUSION

Although challenging, with good planning, sound surgical technique and knowledge, the vast majority of these defects can be adequately reconstructed. Managing a patient's expectations is important and a frank and detailed discussion regarding complications and likely functional outcomes is warranted, especially in the setting of secondary reconstruction. Advances in surgical technique and perioperative care allow safe treatment of patients previously considered inoperable. Early and aggressive rehabilitation of swallowing and speech is important for patients to retain good quality of life after major surgery.

REFERENCES

1. Edgerton Jr MT. Replacement of lining to oral cavity following surgery. Cancer. 1951;4(1):110-9.
2. McGregor IA. The temporal flap in intra-oral cancer: its use in repairing the post-excisional defect. Br J Plast Surg. 1963;16:318-35.
3. Bakamjian VY. A two-stage method for pharyngoesophageal reconstruction with a primary pectoral skin flap. Plast Reconstr Surg. 1965;36(2):173-84.
4. Ariyan S. The pectoralis major myocutaneous flap. Plast Reconstr Surg. 1979;63(1):73-81.
5. Quillen CG, Shearin JJ, Georgiade NG. Use of the latissimus dorsi myocutaneous island flap for reconstruction in the head and neck area: case report. Plast Reconstr Surg. 1978; 62(1):113-7.
6. Quillen CG. Latissimus dorsi myocutaneous flaps in head and neck reconstruction. Plast Reconstr Surg. 1979;63(5): 664-70.
7. Barton JF, Spicer TE, Byrd HS. Head and neck reconstruction with the latissimus dorsi myocutaneous flap: anatomic observations and report of 60 cases. Plast Reconstr Surg. 1983;71(2):199-204.
8. McCraw JB, Dibbell DG. Experimental definition of independent myocutaneous vascular territories. Plast Reconstr Surg. 1977;60(2):212-20.
9. Ariyan S. One-stage repair of a cervical esophagostome with two myocutaneous flaps from the neck and shoulder. Plast Reconstr Surg. 1979;63(3):426-9.
10. Hanasono MM, Lin D, Wax MK, Rosenthal EL. Closure of laryngectomy defects in the age of chemoradiation therapy. Head Neck. 2012;34(4):580-8.
11. Paleri V, Drinnan M, Van Den Brekel MW, Hinni ML, Bradley PJ, Wolf GT, et al. Vascularized tissue to reduce fistula following salvage total laryngectomy: a systematic review. Laryngoscope. 2014;124(8):1848-53.
12. Disa JJ, Pusic A, Hidalgo DA, Cordeiro PG. Microvascular reconstruction of the hypopharynx: Defect classification, treatment algorithm, and functional outcome based on 165 consecutive cases. Plastic and Reconstructive Surgery 2003;111(2):652-60.
13. Balasubramanian D, Subramaniam N, Rathod P, Murthy S, Sharma M, Mathew J, et al. Outcomes following pharyngeal reconstruction in total laryngectomy—institutional experience and review of literature. Indian J Plast Surg. 2018;51(2):190-5.
14. Refos JW, Witte BI, de Goede CJ, de Bree R. Shoulder morbidity after pectoralis major flap reconstruction. Head Neck. 2016;38(8):1221-8.
15. Keereweer S, Sewnaik A, Kerrebijin J, Meeuwis CA, Tilanus HW, de Wilt JHW. Salvage or what follows failure of a free jejunal transfer for reconstruction of the hypopharynx. J Plast Reconstr Aesthet Surg. 2010;63(6):976-80.
16. Butskiy O, Anderson DW, Prisman E. Management algorithm for failed gastric pull up reconstruction of laryngopharyngectomy defects: case report and review of the literature. J Otolaryngol Head Neck Surg. 2016;45(1):41.
17. Ganly I, Patel S, Matsuo J, Singh B, Kraus D, Boyle J, et al. Postoperative complications of salvage total laryngectomy. Cancer. 2005;103(10):2073-81.
18. Dedivitis RA, Aires FT, Cernea CR, Brandão LG. Pharyngocutaneous fistula after total laryngectomy: systematic review of risk factors. Head Neck. 2015;37(11):1691-7.
19. Chan JYW, Liu LHL, Wei WI. Early prediction of anastomotic leakage after free jejunal flap reconstruction of circumferential pharyngeal defects. J Plast Reconstr Aesthet Surg. 2013;66(3):376-81.
20. McLean JN, Nicholas C, Duggal P, Chen A, Grist WG, Losken A, et al. Surgical management of pharyngocutaneous fistula after total laryngectomy. Ann Plast Surg. 2012;68(5):442-5.

21. Makitie AA, Irish J, Guallane PJ. Pharyngocutaneous fistula. Curr Opin Otolaryngol Head Neck Surg. 2003;11:78-84.
22. Virtaniemi JA, Kumpulainen EJ, Hirvikoski PP, Johansson RT, Kosma VM. The incidence and etiology of postlaryngectomy pharyngocutaneous fistulae. Head Neck. 2001;23(1):29-33.
23. Hay A, Pitkin L, Gurusamy K. Early versus delayed oral feeding in patients following total laryngectomy. Adv Otolaryngol. 2014;2014:1-10.
24. Emerick KS, Tomycz L, Bradford CR, Lyden TH, Chepeha DB, Wolf GT, et al. Primary versus secondary tracheoesophageal puncture in salvage total laryngectomy following chemoradiation. Otolaryngol Head Neck Surg. 2009;140(3):386-90.
25. Lopez F, Obeso S, Camporro D, Fueyo A, Suarez C, Llorente JL. Outcomes following pharyngolaryngectomy with fasciocutaneous free flap reconstruction and salivary bypass tube. Laryngoscope. 2013;123(3):591-6.
26. Hone RWA, Rahman E, Wong G, Annan Y, Alexander V, Kiran AA, et al. Do salivary bypass tubes lower the incidence of pharyngocutaneous fistula following total laryngectomy? A retrospective analysis of predictive factors using multivariate analysis. Eur Arch Otorhinolaryngol. 2017;274(4): 1983-91.
27. de Bree R, Rinaldo A, Genden EM, Suárez C, Rodrigo JP, Fagan JJ, et al. Modern reconstruction techniques for oral and pharyngeal defects after tumor resection. Eur Arch Otorhinolaryngol. 2008;265(1):1-9.
28. Sabri A. Oropharyngeal reconstruction: current state of the art. Curr Opin Otolaryngol Head Neck Surg. 2003;11(4):251-4.
29. Lv M, Shen Y, Li J, Zhang C, Zhu H, Sun J. Immediate reconstruction of soft palate defects after ablative surgery and evaluation of postoperative function: an analysis of 45 consecutive patients. J Oral Maxillofac Surg. 2014;72(7):1397-406.
30. McCombe D, Lyons B, Winkler R, Morrison W. Speech and swallowing following radial forearm flap reconstruction of major soft palate defects. Br J Plast Surg. 2005;58(3):306-11.
31. Yoshida H, Michi K, Yamashita Y, Ohno K. A comparison of surgical and prosthetic treatment for speech disorders attributable to surgically acquired soft palate defects. J Oral Maxillofac Surg. 1993;51(4):361-5.
32. Brown JS, Zuydam AC, Jones DC, Rogers SN, Vaughan ED. Functional outcome in soft palate reconstruction using a radial forearm free flap in conjunction with a superiorly based pharyngeal flap. Head Neck. 1997;19(6):524-34.
33. Seikaly H, Rieger J, Wolfaardt J, Moysa G, Harris J, Jha N. Functional outcomes after primary oropharyngeal cancer resection and reconstruction with the radial forearm free flap. Laryngoscope. 2003;113(5):897-904.
34. Kimata Y, Uchiyama K, Sakuraba M, Ebihara S, Hayashi R, Haneda T, et al. Velopharyngeal function after microsurgical reconstruction of lateral and superior oropharyngeal defects. Laryngoscope. 2002;112(6):1037-42.
35. Zafereo ME, Weber RS, Lewin JS, Roberts DB, Hanasono MM. Complications and functional outcomes following complex oropharyngeal reconstruction. Head Neck. 2010;32(8): 1003-11.
36. Song M, Chen WK, Zhang Q, Chen SW, Zhuang SM, Yang AK. Irradiation of the recipient site does not adversely affect successful free flap transfer in the repair of head and neck defects after salvage surgery for recurrent nasopharyngeal carcinoma originally treated with radiotherapy. J Plast Surg Hand Surg. 2013;47(1):40-5.
37. Iyer S, Subramaniam N, Vidhyadharan S, Thankappan K, Balasubramanian D, Balasubramoniam KR, et al. Tracheal allotransplantation—lessons learned. Indian J Plast Surg. 2020;53:306-8.

CHAPTER 41

Facial Nerve Disorders and their Management in Head and Neck Cancer

Dimpy Sharma, Federico Bolognesi, Narayana Subramaniam, Federico Biglioli

INTRODUCTION

Facial nerve palsy, either congenital or acquired, leads to facial disfigurement of varying degrees. The facial nerve supplies the facial musculature that is responsible for facial symmetry and expression of emotions. Injury to the facial nerve is a devastating condition for the patient and a complex and challenging problem for the reconstructive surgeon. With improvements in surgical techniques, the goal of facial reanimation surgery has evolved from tarsorrhaphy (for prevention of corneal ulcers) to attempting restoration of facial symmetry and function, and spontaneous blink.

ANATOMY

The facial nerve is the VIIth cranial nerve and the nerve of 2nd brachial arch. The course of the nerve can be described under following headings:

Intracranial Course

Facial nerve arises from four nuclei situated in the lower pons:

- *Parasympathetic:*
  - Motor nucleus
  - Superior salivatory nucleus
  - Lacrimatory nucleus
- *Gustatory:*
  - Nucleus of tractus solitarius

It is a mixed nerve originating as two roots:

1. Motor root
2. Sensory root (nervus intermedius)

The voluntary motor fibers arise from the precentral gyrus, just medial to VIII cranial nerve. Both cranial nerves VII and VIII run together laterally and forward to enter the internal acoustic meatus. In the region of cerebello-pontine angle, the anterior inferior cerebellar artery lies in close proximity to these nerves. It might either loop around or pass in between the two nerves. The anterior inferior cerebellar artery gives a branch, the labyrinthine artery, which passes in to the internal acoustic meatus along with the nerves. Just before entering the internal acoustic meatus, both the roots fuse to form a single nerve trunk. The forehead has bilateral cortical representation as the fibers destined for the upper face ramify to the ipsilateral facial nerve nucleus; therefore, the function of forehead is preserved in upper motor neuron facial palsy.

Intratemporal Course

Intratemporal course has the longest course of any nerve through bone (30 mm). The geniculate ganglion itself is approximately 1.8 mm long.[1] There are two important considerations with respect to the intratemporal course of facial nerve. Firstly, the ratio of nerve to bony canal diameter is 25–50%.[2,3] This ratio is lower in children therefore the need for decompression for entrapment of the nerve in Bell's palsy is much.[4] In Bell's palsy, compression within the bony canal occurs initially and is most severe in the labyrinthine segment, where the mean diameter of the canal is only 1.42 mm (compared to the mean diameter in other tracts).[5,6] Therefore, while decompressing the nerve in Bell's palsy, the labyrinthine segment should be the main target. The second consideration is the lack of consistent intraneural spatial orientation in the facial nerve. Sunderland attempted to study the individual fibers of facial nerve in cadavers and concluded that there was no set arrangement of fibers.[7] These findings were subsequently confirmed by others.[8-10] This lack of scheme of fibers distribution makes it difficult to avoiding synkinesis and mass movement following degeneration and subsequent recovery.

The intratemporal segment of the facial nerve is divided into three parts by two curves:

1. *Labyrinthine (length 5-6 mm):* The nerve is directed laterally above the vestibule and then bends sharply over the anterosuperior part of promontory. This sharp curve is known as genu and this is where it relays into geniculate ganglion. The first branch of the facial nerve, the greater petrosal nerve, leaves the geniculate ganglion to bring parasympathetic secretory fibers to the nose, mouth, and lacrimal gland, and sensory taste fibers from the palate.
2. *Tympanic (length 8-11 mm):* The nerve then runs backward in relation to medial wall above the promontory. It extends from the geniculate ganglion to the bend at the lateral semicircular canal. Here, it gives a branch to stapedius muscle.
3. *Mastoid or vertical (length 9-12 mm):* The nerve is then directed vertically downward and behind the promontory, gives a branch named chorda tympani and reaches the stylomastoid foramen.

Extratemporal Course

As the nerve trunk exits the stylomastoid foramen, it crosses the lateral side of the base of styloid process. Here the main trunk becomes superficial making it susceptible to injury. It then enters the parotid gland through the posteromedial surface and divides into two main trunks that divide into several branches. Each branch subdivides into several branches and gives off five terminal branches including the temporal, orbicularis oculi, zygomatic, buccal, marginal mandibular, and cervical branches. These branches arborize and get distributed over the face and the upper neck to supply the muscle of facial expression. Facial nerve branching is very variegated and even the extracranial main bifurcation into temporofacial and cervicofacial branches may not be respected. Davis[11] reviewed 350 cervicofacial halves and categorized facial nerve patterns within parotid gland into six subtypes. Later, the surgical anatomy of the marginal mandibular nerve was studied by Dingman and Grabb[12] and of the frontal branch was studied by of the facial nerve was investigated by Pitanguy and Silveira.[13]

Extratemporal Branches

As the nerve exits stylomastoid foramen, it gives following branches before the main trunk enters parotid gland:

- Posterior auricular nerve
- Nerve to stylohyoid muscle
- Nerve to posterior belly of digastric muscle

The main trunk gives classically five terminal branches into the face and neck, in the form of pes anserinus:

1. Temporal
2. Zygomatic
3. Buccal
4. Mandibular
5. Cervical

A main branch for the orbicularis oculi is often present, and its origin comes from the frontal, temporofacial branch, or zygomatic branch. These give innervation to 18-paired muscles of face. Each division has several branches. Even the cervical division, often described as a single branch, gives origin to several smaller branches. In summary, any attempt to classify extratemporal facial nerve branching may fail to represent a particular pattern because of its extreme variability.

ETIOLOGY OF FACIAL PALSY

Facial paralysis may be congenital or developmental, but may also result from blunt and penetrating trauma to the head and neck, as well as surgical injury. There are also other causes including infection and metabolic disorders; however, cases are often idiopathic.

It is relatively common in patients with head and neck cancer, either primary or metastatic. The cause of facial nerve paralysis here includes a primary parotid mass or iatrogenic sacrifice of the facial nerve during removal of a parotid mass, metastatic lesions of the parotid gland of solid tumor or hematologic origin, perineural invasion of the facial nerve, infectious causes such as Ramsay Hunt syndrome in an immunocompromised host, ischemic events, and idiopathic causes such as Bell's palsy.[14-17] Bell's palsy, largely the most common type of facial paralysis, accounts for 1 in 65 people during their lifetime, and may be associated with herpes virus simplex infections, pregnancy, psychological and physical stress, and general anesthesia.

POTENTIAL SITES OF INJURY

Upper Motor Neuron versus Lower Motor Neuron Palsy

Although the injury to the intracranial part of the facial nerve is less common, it can happen in cases of severe head injury. It is important to differentiate upper motor neuron (UMN) from lower motor neuron (LMN) lesions, which can easily be done clinically. Involvement of forehead suggests LMN palsy of ipsilateral side, whereas a spared forehead and affected lower face suggest that the lesion is in contralateral upper motor neuron.

Trauma to the facial nerve is the second most frequent cause of facial paralysis.[18]

The injury is usually due to a temporal bone fracture or penetrating facial wound. Most fractures occur in the labyrinthine segment of the facial nerve and are readily identified by computed tomography (CT) scan.[19]

Iatrogenic injury to various extratemporal facial nerve branches can occur while operating in the parotid and submandibular regions. Apart from nerve disruption, spirited retraction may cause compression and/or stretching of nerve fibers resulting in neuropraxia (loss of nerve function without axonal/nerve severing). Accidental suture ligation of nerve branches, especially those in close proximity of vessels, may also result in nerve injury.

The temporal and zygomatic branches of the facial nerve might get injured commonly during surgery on temporomandibular joint (TMJ) through a preauricular approach, as these nerves lie in a confluence of superficial fascia, temporalis fascia, and periosteum. Facial nerve injury following TMJ surgeries can occur in 1–32% of patients. Maxillofacial surgeries can also result in facial nerve injuries in up to half of patients.[20-23] The marginal mandibular branch is generally related to as single but, again, several other minor branches run parallel to it, completing and partially substituting its function. This nerve runs forward below the angle of the mandible in a subplatysmal plane, then turning up and forward across the body of the mandible to supply the lower lip musculature. Therefore, incisions in the submandibular region are planned at least 1.6 cm below the lower border and angle of the mandible to avoid injury to the marginal mandibular nerve. In a study done by Batra,[24] the marginal mandibular branch of the facial nerve was always superficial to the facial pedicle (100%). Thus, the facial artery can be used as an important landmark in locating the marginal mandibular nerve during surgical procedures.

Seckel[25] described the most likely sites of facial nerve injury and suggests techniques to avoid damage to specific nerve branches. He arbitrarily divided the face into seven facial danger zones based on known anatomic locations of the branches of facial nerve and the site where they are most susceptible to injury while facial dissection **(Table 1 and Fig. 1)**.

CLINICAL FEATURES

There is a broad spectrum of signs and symptoms a patient with facial paralysis may present with. The common presenting complaints are asymmetry of face (ptosis of soft tissues), loss of facial expression, inability to smile, eye symptoms (dryness, excessive tearing, incomplete closure, and corneal ulceration), inability to eat/drink/speak properly, buccinators paralysis (food tends to collect in buccal sulcus of paralyzed side), lagophthalmos and issues related to psychosocial functioning and social interactions.

A proper history is crucial to determine the etiology and prognosis. This includes duration of paralysis, onset, inciting factors if any, previous facial paralysis, a family history of facial paralysis, and systemic medical conditions such as autoimmune disorders prodromal symptoms related to Bell's palsy or Ramsay Hunt syndrome (sore throat, otalgia, or fever)

Table 1: Danger zones of the facial nerve.

Facial danger zones	*Location*	*Nerve*	*Relationship to SMAS*	*Sign of zonal injury*
1	6.5 cm below external auditory canal	Greater auricular	Posterior to	Numbness of inferior two-thirds of ear and adjacent cheek and neck
2	Below a line drawn from 0.5 cm below the tragus to 2 cm above and lateral eyebrow and above zygoma	Temporal branch of facial	Beneath	Paralysis of forehead
3	Mid-mandible 2 cm posterior to oral commissure	Marginal mandibular branch of facial	Beneath	Paralysis of lower lip
4	Triangle formed by connecting dots of malar eminence, posterior border of mandibular angle and oral commissure	Zygomatic and buccal branches of facial	Beneath	Paralysis of upper lip and cheek
5	Superior orbital rim above mid-pupil	Supraorbital and supratrochlear	Anterior to	Numbness of forehead, upper eyelid, nasal dorsum and scalp
6	1 cm below inferior orbital rim below mid-pupil	Infraorbital	Anterior to	Numbness of side of upper nose, cheek, upper lip and lower eyelid
7	Mid-mandible below second premolar	Mental	Anterior to	Numbness of half lower lip and chin

(SMAS: superficial musculoaponeurotic system)

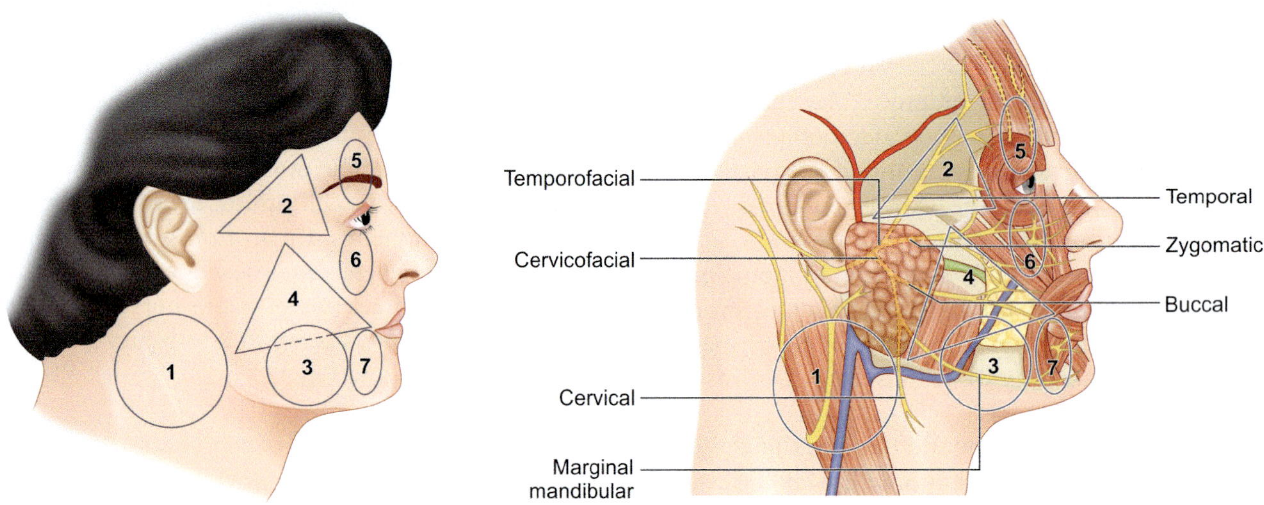

Fig. 1: External topographic outline of 7 facial danger zones and underlying nerves running through each facial danger zone after skin and superficial musculoaponeurotic system (SMAS) layers have been removed.

or otologic symptoms (drainage, hearing loss, vertigo, otalgia, and aural fullness).

In the patients with long-standing facial paralysis, aesthetic concerns go along with the main functional one: The lack of corneal lubrication. In patients with a slow progressive (several months) onset of facial palsy symptoms, the suspicion of underlying tumors (malignant or benign in the facial nerve canal) is mandatory and additional radiologic investigations [such as magnetic resonance imaging (MRI), high-resolution CT] are required.

The sequelae of chronic facial nerve paralysis are highly variable. Some of the resultant features are nasal airway obstruction, oral incompetence, aberrant facial nerve regeneration resulting in involuntary or uncoordinated facial movements (synkinesis), visual disturbances (ocular irritation, lagophthalmos, dry eye syndrome, epiphora, corneal ulceration, and blindness), facial asymmetry due to flaccid atrophic muscles, loss of tone or volumetric loss, loss of dynamic furrows, brow ptosis and asymmetry, effacement or deepening of nasolabial folds, drooping or elevation of oral commissure, and dimpling of the chin.

The features suggested of a neoplastic entity are slowly progressive paralysis, additional cranial neuropathies, suspicious skin lesion or malignancy, parotid mass, facial twitching, absence of facial nerve recovery ≥4 months, concurrent sensorineural hearing loss, aural fullness or tinnitus, concurrent vestibular symptoms, or ipsilateral recurrence of facial paralysis.

The examination is divided into general head and neck examination, facial nerve functional assessment, and other cranial nerve examination. While examining the head and neck region as whole, one should focus on the ear, mastoid, parotid gland, and facial skin. Examine for any scar suggestive of previous surgery or trauma; any evidence of an erythematous or vesicular rash is suggestive of Ramsay Hunt syndrome. Other middle ear pathologies such as acute or chronic otitis media, middle ear effusion, hemotympanum, tympanic membrane perforation, neoplasm, and cholesteatoma should also be ruled out. In cases of acute trauma, ecchymosis over the mastoid process (Battle sign) is suggestive of a basilar skull fracture. The parotid should be palpated for any mass. Also the neck should be examined for any metastatic nodes.

The functional assessment of facial nerve should be done in a systematic manner starting from the brow, the ocular region, the mid-face and nasolabial folds, the oral commissure region, and the lower lip. Ask the patient to perform various facial movements including forehead elevation, eye closure, nasal wrinkling, whistling, pursing of lips, soft smile, full smile, and showing of all dentition. Various points to be noted are:

- *Forehead:*
    - Presence or absence of furrows
    - Position of brow at rest and with movement
- *Eye:*
    - Visual acuity in each eye
    - The height of the palpebral aperture should be measured and compared with the nonparalyzed side
    - The degree of lagophthalmos and the presence of Bell phenomenon

- The lower eyelid position and tone in the lower eyelid (snap test)
- The position of the inferior canalicular punctum
- Any corneal irritation or ulceration

- *Nose:*
  - Medially collapsed ala
- *Extraoral examination:*
  - Philtral deviation
  - Absence or reduced depth of the nasolabial fold
  - Amount of commissure depression and deviation
  - Degree of upper lip drooping and the presence of vermilion inversion
  - Amount of bilateral commissure movement with animation
  - Note how much of the upper incisors show when the patient is smiling.
- *Intraoral examination:*
  - Dental hygiene and evidence of cheek biting.
  - Speech assessment (bilabials—b, p, m)

Position of the eyebrows should be assessed for symmetry as well as location in relation to the supraorbital rim. Bell phenomenon is the upward rotation of the eye on attempted eye closure. It is an important reflex to protect the cornea, and the patient with poor Bell phenomenon are prone to develop corneal ulceration and subsequently blindness if proper measures to protect the cornea are not taken. Normal palpebral fissure and ocular width are around 12 mm and 29 mm, respectively. Patients with total facial paralysis have poor eye closure leading to lagophthalmos. On the other hand, patients with synkinesis and muscular hypertonia at rest often have narrowing of their palpebral fissure leading to asymmetric eyes.[26]

To evaluate the lower lid retraction, *margin* reflex distance-2 is measured. It is the distance between the light reflex and central portion of the lower lid when a patient's eye is in the neutral position. Lower lid position should always be compared to the healthy side. To assess the lower lid laxity, the lower eyelid tone and support should be verified by the snap and lid retraction test **(Fig. 2)**. If the lid does not snap back into its anatomical position within 1 second, the puncta displaces >3 mm or the lid distracts >7 mm, and lid laxity is diagnosed.

Dynamics of Smile

Smiling is primarily performed by the levators of the upper lip. There are two stages in which smile takes place:

- *Stage 1:* Contraction of levators and nasolabial fold muscles elevating upper lip to nasolabial fold against cheek resistance.
- *Stage 2:* Levator superior, zygomaticus major, and caninus muscles raise lip and nasolabial fold upward.

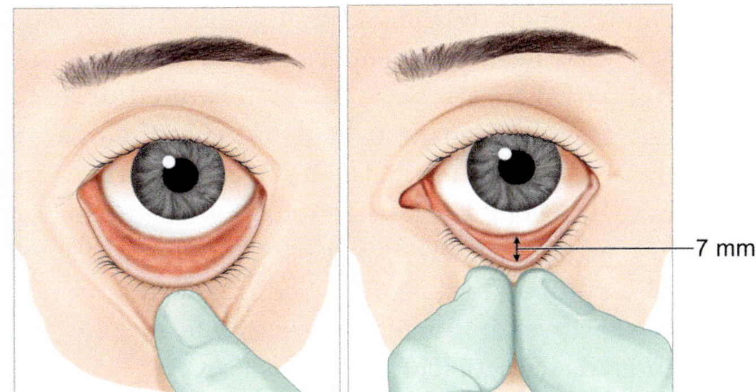

Fig. 2: Snap and lid retraction test.

There are three basic smile patterns noted:

1. *Zygomaticus major smile:* It is the most common type of smile (67%) dominated by zygomaticus major and buccinator muscle. In this type of smile, the angles of mouth elevate first.
2. *Canine smile:* It is the second most common type of smile (31%), mainly controlled by levator labii superioris contracting prior to zygomaticus major and buccinators. There is a dominant upward elevation of lip followed by elevation of corners of the mouth.
3. *Full-denture smile:* This type of smile is the least common (2%). It displays the mandibular and maxillary teeth due to contraction of elevator and depressors of the lips and angles of the mouth.

Knowing the characteristics of the smile allows the surgeon to better understand what procedures are necessary to create a natural appearing smile; however, seldom is it possible to replace one's original smile. Zygomatic smile is the standard goal of surgery.

It is essential to examine clinically and by electromyography other cranial nerves as well. Examine the nerve supplies to the temporalis and masseter muscles (trigeminal nerve), spinal accessory and hypoglossal nerves to determine their utility as donor nerves. Additionally, palpate the superficial temporal and facial vessels or use a hand-held Doppler to assess their suitability as recipient vessels if free-tissue transfer is planned.

TOPOGNOSTIC TESTS

Topognostic tests are done to localize the site of facial nerve lesions. But they often remain unreliable due to the variable anatomy of the facial nerve and its branches, the fact that lesions often fail to localize to one site of the nerve, and the variable recovery rates of differing neural segments.[27] These tests do not have much role in clinical practice and are used only to supplement other diagnostic tests. The tests used are:

1. *Schirmer's test:* This test evaluates the function of the greater superficial petrosal nerve, which supplies

secretory fibers to the lacrimal gland. To perform this test, a sterile filter paper strips is placed in the conjunctival fornix and the tear production after 5 minutes is measured. The obtained value is compared to the normal side. A 25% decrease in tearing or <25 mm of lacrimation on the pathological side is an abnormal test suggesting a lesion proximal to the geniculate ganglion. Schirmer's test is not very sensitive and its results are significant only for high-grade reduction of tear production.

2. *Stapedial reflex:* The stapedial reflex tests the integrity of the stapedial nerve, a branch arising from the mastoid segment of facial nerve innervating the stapedial muscle. This bilateral reflex is elicited by either ipsilateral or contralateral acoustic stimulation. A 50% decrease in the amplitude of the reflex is considered abnormal, signifying a lesion proximal to the stapedial nerve.
3. *Taste tasting:* To test the chorda tympani branch of facial nerve which carries taste fibers to the anterior two thirds of the tongue and secretory fibers of the submandibular and sublingual glands. Taste testing involves application of stimuli to different sites of the tongue and qualitatively compares responses.
4. *Salivary flow test:* This test measures the salivary secretion rates of the submandibular and sublingual glands. The Wharton ducts are cannulated and collected saliva is compared to the normal side. Reduced flow suggests a lesion proximal to chorda tympani branching. Salivary flow testing can be both uncomfortable for the patient and time consuming.

EVALUATION

Radiographic tests such as CT and MRI are indicated to detect the exact site of lesion when a tumor is suspected. It is required to study a specific segment of the nerve, or preoperatively to determine whether the lesion is distal or proximal to the geniculate ganglion. High-resolution, thin-section CT scans may reveal intracranial, intratemporal, or extratemporal tumors, in addition to the fine bony detail of the facial nerve canal within the temporal bone.[28]

Magnetic resonance imaging has been used with gadolinium contrast to differentiate between pathologic and nonpathologic conditions of the facial nerve.[29] Millen[30]and Murphy[31] studied the effectiveness of gadolinium-enhanced MRI of the facial nerve in a number of acute and chronic processes such as facial nerve neuromas, traumatic facial paralysis, and facial paralysis due to inflammation (Bell's palsy and Lyme disease). Gadolinium-enhanced MRI is of no benefit in evaluating the facial nerve after temporal bone fractures because of enhancement of virtually the entire temporal bone.

Electrophysiological testing of the facial nerve may provide additional information. Electroneurography can provide objective quantitative measurement of nerve function, comparative summation potentials, reflect the number of functioning nerve fibers and hence the likely degree of recovery. Electromyography is complementary and can determine if the nerve in question is in continuity, identify fibrillation potentials (evidence of Wallerian degeneration at 2–3 weeks) and polyphasic innervation (may precede clinical signs of recovery by 6–12 months). It can also be used to identify potential donor nerves such as masseteric, deep temporal, hypoglossal, and contralateral facial nerve branches.

Facial Nerve Paralysis Grading Systems

- *House-Brackmann grading system:*[32] This is a standard method to measure and grade the function of facial nerve, given by House and Brackmann in 1983, and endorsed by the Facial Nerve Disorders Committee of the American Academy of Otolaryngology in 1984. It is also used to monitor the status of facial nerve over time to assess the course of recovery and the efficacy of treatment. Although concise and useful for rapid assessment, it is subjective. Another drawback is that it inadequately considers the secondary defects of hemifacial spasm, contractures, synkinesis, crocodile (gustatory) tears, decreased lacrimation, and dysgeusia. It remains the most widely accepted facial nerve grading system.
- *eFACE:*[33] It is becoming the standard tool among reconstructive surgeons because it applies well to parameters that the surgeons want to correct and is applicable also to postoperative results. It is applicable only to unilateral paralysis. This system is proposed by Bell's Society and is based on 16 items divided in three domains:
  1. *Static (5 items):* Brow height at rest, palpebral fissure width at rest, nasolabial fold orientation at rest, and oral commissure position at rest
  2. *Dynamic (7 items):* Brow elevation, palpebral closure (gentle and full eye closure), oral commissure movement, nasolabial fold depth and orientation, and lower lip movement
  3. *Synkinesis (4 items):* Ocular, midfacial, mentalis dimpling, and platysmal synkinesis

For each item of the three domains, a score of 0 indicates the worst condition in terms of extreme malposition, absence of movement, and severe synkinesis. A score of 100, on the other hand, indicates the normal condition in terms of normal balance, normal movement, and absence of synkinesis. The scales run to the score of 200 for variables in which the abnormal state can manifest itself in two directions. The final subscores for each specific area of facial function, static, dynamic and synkinesis, are calculated and assessed the effects of interventions reliably. It is possible to complete an eFACE evaluation based on patient photographs and videos.

PRINCIPLES OF RECONSTRUCTION

Preoperative evaluation and planning is the key to achieve a good result while treating facial paralysis. Selection of the appropriate method depends on the location of the injury, the cause and duration of the paralysis, coexistent functional and cosmetic defects, patient comorbidities, and prognosis of the disease. Additionally, the patient's concerns and expectations must be sought.

The aims of treatment are to protect the eye, to provide symmetry at rest, and then to provide movement. The main areas of concern are the eyelids and zygomaticobuccal region. The goals of treatment for the eyelids are to lubricate the cornea by blinking and to maintain vision, while attempting to improve cosmesis. The goals for the zygomaticobuccal region are to provide symmetry at rest as well as gaining the ability to smile, provide oral continence, and improve speech. The ultimate goal should be restoration of both voluntary and spontaneous mimetic facial expression.

Various factors influencing the surgical strategies and prognosis are the patient's age, denervation time, the cause of lesion, the availability of proximal facial nerve, whether paralysis is complete or partial, the availability of motor donor nerves and likely patient compliance toward postoperative rehabilitation.

Nonsurgical Management

It is mainly focused on protection of cornea and preservation of vision. These are the temporary measures used while waiting for the spontaneous recovery in cases of Bell's palsy, or while the surgery is being planned. Bell's palsy is considered as idiopathic and is usually a diagnosis of exclusion, though several studies have demonstrated an association with herpes simplex virus (HSV). In these cases the treatment regimen includes steroids, antivirals, and eye protection. The following methods protect cornea from exposure keratitis and ulceration, and maintain eye lubrication:

- Lid taping (particularly while sleeping)
- Soft contact lenses
- Moisture chambers (taped to the skin around the orbit)
- Modification of spectacles to provide a lateral shield
- Forced blinking exercises in a patient with weak eye closure
- Eye patches
- Temporary tarsorrhaphy

These methods are also used as an adjunct to the surgical treatment. Eye lubricants used contain either hydroxypropyl methylcellulose or polyvinyl alcohol along with other agents including preservatives. These should be instilled frequently in the affected eye. Thicker ointments contain soft paraffin, mineral water, or lanolin alcohol that are retained longer and can be used at night to protect and seal the eyelids during sleep. The patient who presents with reduced tearing may in fact have a dry eye and may benefit from the use of artificial tears. Corneal ulceration should be managed with prompt referral for ophthalmologic assessment.

Surgical Management

Selecting an appropriate procedure most of the time is difficult and confusing because of lack of consensus in scientific literature. It is important to get a complete and detailed history and examination, in order to find out most troubling areas of face. The procedure should be selected as per the patients' needs and the facial areas should be prioritized accordingly. Selection of the procedure depends on the location of the injury, the etiology and duration of the paralysis, coexistent functional deficiencies and aesthetic defects, associated comorbidities, disease prognosis, and patient needs. It is also influenced by the condition of facial muscles and availability of the donor nerves. The operative procedures can be static or dynamic. The most commonly implemented procedures are: (1) direct nerve repair, (2) cranial nerve substitution techniques, (3) regional reanimation, (4) static suspension, and (5) free-muscle transfer. In most of the cases, both static and dynamic procedures should be employed to obtain static symmetry and dynamic restoration.

Adynamic Reconstruction

Adynamic or static procedure does not produce animation of the facial muscles. It provides corneal protection, improves the nasal airway, prevents drooling and, first of all, it improves facial asymmetry at rest. That is important because the face is at rest most of the time, and stigmata of the paralysis are well hidden by a symmetric static symmetry. Moreover, if the starting position of face components is symmetric, the excursion during movements arrives to a better position in comparison to the same movement when the starting point is lower. An example might be a ptotic angle of the mouth: Smiling will be asymmetric even in case of a good excursion, because the beginning of it, and consequently its end point, is asymmetric. So, a good static symmetry at rest also influences dynamic symmetry.

Static procedures should always be added to dynamic ones to enhance results, primarily and secondarily. Static procedures alone might be considered in cases of minimal residual palsy following incomplete recovery. Static procedures to correct functional disabilities include temporary or permanent tarsorrhaphy, insertion of lid weights, palpebral springs or lid magnets, Müllerectomy, brow lift or suspension, forehead skin excision, unilateral facelift-type procedures, and several fascia lata suspension slings. The procedures are discussed below according to the region.

- *Brow:* Eyebrow ptosis on the paralyzed side produces upper lid ptosis with partial vertical reduction of the visual field. As the paralyzed frontalis muscle cannot work, eyebrow vertical asymmetry results from the difference in position between the elevated healthy side and the ptotic position on the paralyzed side. The brow height discrepancy may be up to 12 mm. This can be easily corrected by brow lift, in which an ellipse of skin, subcutaneous tissue, and a strip of frontalis muscle are excised. During the procedure, care must be taken to preserve supraorbital nerves as they run just beneath the frontalis muscle. Brow lift can be done through three approaches: (1) Direct excision of the tissue above the brow (direct brow lift), (2) open brow lift performed through a coronal incision, and (3) endoscopic brow lift. The healthy side will immediately be lower than the paralyzed side after surgical correction; this slight overcorrection is necessary as a little postoperative ptosis is to be expected.
- *Upper eyelid:* Facial nerve palsy disrupts blinking, making the cornea prone to drying and ulceration. This can be dealt with one of the following procedures:
- *Lid weight implant:* Lid loading with gold implant is the most common procedure because of its ease. Generally, a small prosthesis made of 24-carat gold of weight, ranging from 0.8 to 1.8 g, is used. As 24-carat gold is inserted, allergic reactions are rare. The configuration of patient's eyelid is important in determining whether the bulge of the gold weight will be visible when the eye is open. If the amount of exposed eyelid skin above the lashes is >5 mm with the eyes open, the gold weight is likely to be noticeable. If the distance is <5 mm, the gold weight will roll back and hide in the supratarsal crease. The common method to determine the appropriate weight is by taping the trial prostheses to the upper eyelid over the tarsal plate with the patient in sitting position and looking forward. The lightest weight that will bring the upper eyelid within 2–4 mm of the lower lid and cover the cornea should be used. However, the more recent concept is that the target of surgery should not be eyelid closure but blinking enhancement. Blinking is produced spontaneously 10–20 times per minute[34] by relaxing levator muscle (innervated by 3rd cranial nerve) and activating the orbicularis oculi (7th cranial nerve). The latter is inactive in case of facial palsy, so reanimation should improve the relaxation time. It is important to utilize a light weight (lower than the one needed to close completely the eyelids) because the levator muscle would always be contracted in order to maintain vision: Consequently it will not be able to relax during blinking. So, a weight of 0.6–0.8 g is more appropriate. The gold weight should be fixed to the upper part of tarsal plate through the small holes in the gold weight, taking care not to injure the Müller's muscle. Weights may be dislocated along time, extrude through the skin, and have bad aesthetic appearance. 20% of patients also develop vertical astigmatism. Platinum weights partially avoid those odds because of a lower profile.
- *Palpebral spring:* It is an alternative method to correct lagophthalmos. Originally described by Morel-Fatio, it has the advantage that it is not dependent on gravity. However, there are certain problems that have made it less popular. These are malpositioning of the spring, spring breakage or weakening, pseudoptosis due to excessive spring force, and skin erosion.
- *Lateral tarsorrhaphy:* Moderate lagophthalmos may be addressed by lateral tarsorrhaphy. This procedure narrows the palpebral fissure by approximating parts of the eyelids. Medial tarsorrhaphy is at high risk of injury of the lacrimal punctum and gives an odd appearance to the eye: it should seldom be considered. There are many different variants of lateral tarsorrhaphy, the McLaughlin procedure[35] is the most popular and gives reasonably good results. This procedure consists of resection of a segment of lateral skin, cilia, and orbicularis from the lower lid and a matching segment of conjunctiva and tarsus from the upper lid. It is a lash preserving procedure, where flaps are elevated from the lateral thirds of the eyelids. The flaps are posteriorly based on the lower lid and anteriorly based on the upper eyelid and are sutured together.
- *Lipofilling:* Fat harvesting can be done from the abdominal or gluteal region or in case of simultaneous harvesting of fascia lata, from lateral thigh, usually

after infiltration of a saline-based solution of lidocaine and adrenaline into the donor site. According to standard Coleman procedure,[36] harvested fat is then placed into a centrifuge for 2 minutes at 2,000 rpm in order to separate fat from oil, infiltrative solution, cellular residues, and local anesthetic. The procedure is then completed by injecting the fat in the upper eyelid via a blunt cannula in to a small cutaneous incision of 2 mm in the lateral part of the upper eyelid. About 2 mL of fat (1.6 g), is injected. At the end of the procedure, the injected amount should be insufficient to close the eyelids, but should help relaxation of the levator of the lid during blinking.[37] If they still have discomfort, a second lipofilling is indicated.

- *Lower eyelid:* Normally, the lower eyelid is held firmly against the globe and the eyelid margin rests at the level of the limbus of the eye. Due to paralysis of the orbicularis, the resting tone of the muscle is lost, the lower eyelid stretches and sags, resulting in scleral show, lagophthalmos. Eventually the lid and inferior canalicular punctum roll away from the globe, resulting in an ectropion. This also disrupts the even distribution of tear film. This situation requires support of the entire length of the eyelid. Static sling is the best method to achieve this. A sling is sutured to the lateral orbital margin in the region above the zygomaticofrontal suture and tunneled subcutaneously along the lid anterior to the tarsal plate, 1.5–2 mm inferior to the gray line of the eyelid and then passed around the anterior limb of the medial canthal ligament and sutured to itself. Usually 1.5 mm-wide strip of tendon graft (palmaris or plantaris) or tensor fascia lata is used. Gore-Tex/polytetrafluoroethylene slings have also been described but are associated with higher complication rates. Subcutaneous tunneling of the tendon graft is facilitated by the use of a curved Keith needle. Lateral fixation of the tendon graft may need to be through a drill hole whereby the tendon is woven back to itself and sutured, 2–3 mm posterior to the lateral orbital margin, because fixation to the frontal periosteum may lift the lateral eyelid away from the globe. Minimal lower lid laxity and minimal scleral show may be treated with lateral canthoplasty. Various techniques of canthoplasty have been described by Jelks[38] such as the tarsal strip, dermal pennant, and inferior retinacular lateral canthoplasty. It is important to reapproximate the canthal ligament to the position of Whitnall tubercle, i.e., above the horizontal midpupillary line and 2–3 mm posterior to the lateral orbital margin.

- *Static slings:* These can also be used to recreate the nasolabial fold, elevate the corner of the mouth, and elevate the cheek and nasal ala laterally to open the external nasal valve.

Dynamic Reconstruction

Dynamic procedures provide reanimation in form of synchronous facial movement and improved facial symmetry in repose. The aim of dynamic reanimation is to restore symmetry during voluntary and spontaneous expressions, better enhanced by associated static procedures, and to provide competent ocular and oral sphincter. Some of the goals of dynamic reconstruction are to restore symmetry and coordinated dynamic animation, normal appearance at rest, symmetry during voluntary and involuntary expression, competent ocular and oral sphincters, preservation of existing facial functions, and minimal loss of function in other donor motor nerves.

The reconstructive modalities of facial nerve can be classified broadly into two: nerve-based and muscle-based. The presence of mimetic musculature, depending on the duration of the paralysis, is the principle determinant when deciding the method of reconstruction to be used. Other factors are: Availability of distal and proximal nerve stumps, viability of the motor end plate of the recipient muscle, and availability of the donor nerve. The prerequisite for neurotizing mimetic muscles is viability of the motor end plate of the muscles. If the duration of paralysis is <12 months, it is assumed that the motor end plate on the facial muscle is still viable.

In case of a second paralysis or more, timing may be reduced because the previous impairment of facial musculature may lead to its quicker degeneration. In case of recent paralysis, where electromyography shows fibrillations of the musculature, new neural input from a motor source must be provided. However, it should be kept in mind that the regeneration of the nerve itself will require 3–9 months following repair. When the patient presents later, i.e., >24 months, then muscle transfer is the preferable option left, as by that time mimetic muscles have high chances to be irreversibly atrophied. Combining also static procedures as fascia lata graft and others together to facial reanimation techniques allows more complete results.[38]

The various surgical options for dynamic reconstruction of the face are:

- *Direct nerve repair:* Facial nerve has great capacity to regenerate. If the nerve endings are approximated and matched without any tension, the axons sprout readily. Primary neurorrhapy, the immediate reconstruction of sharp transected facial nerve, is the most effective method of reconstruction and gives the best result. Repair may be planned during surgery for tumor excision; soon after it, in trauma setting, or much later. It is a commonly held belief that the earliest possible repair, optimally within 30 days after the onset of the paralysis, will result in the best functional outcome because of higher axonal regrowth potential closer in time to the lesion.[39] Primary repair is possible in cases of recent facial nerve injury and when both the distal and proximal nerve stumps are available without significant nerve gap. The inner axons regenerate at the rate of 1–1.5 mm/day.

- *Nerve grafting*: At the time of primary repair when the nerve gap is wide and a direct neurorrhaphy cannot be achieved, a sensory nerve interposition graft is used. The most common donor grafts are taken from the sural, great auricular, thoracodorsal, and medial antebrachial cutaneous nerves. Alternative sensory nerves that can also be used as grafts are supraclavicular, lateral cutaneous nerve of thigh, saphenous nerves, and others **(Table 2)**.
  - *Greater auricular nerve:* It is ideal for repair if the gap is <6 cm. The advantages of taking it as a donor nerve graft are that it is available in the same operative field, sensory loss of donor area is well tolerated, the nerve is of adequate diameter and caliber to provide a suitable graft, and it gives off two or three branches suitable for neurorrhaphies. Its use is contraindicated when there is a neurotrophic malignancy nearby. The greater auricular nerve bisects the line drawn from angle of mandible and mastoid tip. It passes from behind the posterior border of sternocleidomastoid and runs behind the external jugular vein. It is easily found underneath the platysma, 5–6 cm beneath the earlobe, where it crosses the anterior margin of the sternocleidomastoid muscle. Additional length can be obtained by dissecting the nerve behind the posterior border of sternocleidomastoid up to the subcutaneous area over the parotid region. While dissection, care should be taken to not injure the XIth cranial nerve, which might otherwise cause shoulder drop.
  - *Sural nerve:* It is harvested from the leg via multiple step-ladder incisions, from behind the lateral malleolus up to the popliteal fossa. It provides much more length than greater auricular nerve, leaving minimal donor-site morbidity (inconspicuous scar in leg and sensory loss of the posterior and lateral border of foot). The diameter of the sural nerve matches well with that of trunk of the facial nerve. Sural nerve leaves the tibial nerve in the popliteal fossa and descends between two heads of gastrocnemius muscle. It then pierces the deep fascia in the posterior middle of the upper third of leg. At this point, the sural communicating branch of common peroneal nerve joins it.
  - *Thoracodorsal nerve:* For total facial nerve reconstruction from the main trunk to peripheral branches, the thoracodorsal nerve is among the most appropriate.[40,41] There are up to six reliable branches, and it has adequate length to perform grafting of the entire facial nerve branching, even when the distal stumps lie at the anterior border of the parotid gland. Morbidity after nerve sacrifice is generally low, with the function of latissimus dorsi muscle being supplemented by one of the rhomboid muscles.

  Coaptation should be accurate, tension free, and should be done with minimal epineural sutures. Perineural stitches have no place because of the absence of significant inner fascicles. There should be no tension at the site of repair. If there is tension due to wide gap then nerve grafts should be used to bridge the gap. The interposition nerve graft should form a "C" or "S" to avoid any tension. Nerve ends should be debrided minimally to expose the epineurium. Repair should be performed with minimal epineural stitches using a 10-0 or 11-0 gauge suture.
- *Direct neurotization of the muscle:* Direct neurotization of the muscle is done when the distal nerve stump is not available and proximal stump is available. Using a cable graft, the muscle is directly neurotized by burying the cut end of the nerve into the substance of the muscle. It is not performed commonly.
- *New motor source neurorrhapies:* When the ipsilateral proximal facial nerve stump is not available, connecting another cranial nerve such as the hypoglossal or the masseter to the distal stump of a transected facial

Table 2: Choice of donor nerves for nerve grafts.

Donor sensory nerves	*Length*	*Area of numbness*
Greater auricular nerve	7–10 cm	Ear lobe
Supraclavicular nerve	10–15 cm	Lower neck
Thoracodorsal nerve	12–16 cm	Lateral thoracic wall
Lateral cutaneous nerve of thigh	15–20 cm	Lateral thigh
Saphenous nerve	25–40 cm	Medial leg
Sural nerve	Up to 40 cm	Lateral foot

nerve is an option. The various nerves that can be used for nerve transfer are usually ipsilateral motor donor nerves such as hypoglossal, masseteric, deep temporal, accessory, and phrenic nerves and the root of C7. The advantage of nerve transfer is that the regeneration has to take place only over single neurorrhaphy, preventing the loss of axons. As a clinical rule, as the nerve cross coaptation site, around half of the nerve fiber density is lost. Therefore, when a nerve graft is used, only 25% of the axons will successfully regenerate. Moreover, the reduced distance to be covered by regenerating axons coming from the same pathological side, compared to the long distance, required regenerating from the contralateral facial side in cross-face nerve grafting, leads to a lot more powerful new innervation. At the same time, it must be underlined how less close to "natural" is a neural stimulus given from a nerve other than the facial one: Chewing to activate facial movements in case of the masseteric, lifting the shoulder in case of the spinal, etc. Summarizing, neural input other than the facial nerve give a powerful but somehow unnatural stimulus; the contralateral facial nerve stimulus via cross-face nerve grafting gives the correct natural stimulus, but with a reduced power to produce movements.

Babysitter and Double/Triple Innervation Concepts

It was proposed by Terzis[42] to avoid atrophy of the affected side facial muscles while the facial nerve is in process of regeneration. As the regeneration occurs at rate of 1 mm/day, there are chances that the motor end plate of the affected facial muscles might atrophy by the time the axons reach it. Terzis suggested that an ipsilateral motor nerve (a section of the hypoglossal) could be transposed as a temporary innervator or "babysitter." This preserves the muscle tone and gives a better restoration of smile following cross-face nerve graft (CFNG). While performing CFNG, at the first surgery, two nerve grafts are connected to the upper and lower trunks of the unaffected contralateral facial nerve. The grafts are tunneled across the face through the upper lip and banked on the paralyzed side pretemporal region. The stumps of the grafts are marked with a 3-0 blue prolene suture, so that they can be easily identified later. At that same time, a short nerve cable graft is used to coapt the nerve to masseter or the hypoglossal nerve to the distal stump of the affected facial nerve. The paralyzed muscle regains its tone in 2–3 months, producing mass movement. About 6–9 months after the initial procedure, at the second surgery, the two CFNGs are identified and coapted to the facial nerve branches distal to the prior masseter-facial nerve repair. Spontaneous facial movements can be observed within 3–6 months of the second stage surgery.

- *Cross-face nerve grafting:* When a proximal stump of the facial nerve trunk of branches is not available, using the opposite side facial nerve to reinnervate the affected facial muscles leads to the best neural stimulus. The advantage of using a CFNG is that the resultant facial movements will be symmetric, mimetic, and spontaneous. However, a CFNG alone is usually not powerful enough to produce an adequate smile. CFNG may be done as a single or two-stage procedure, the first one avoiding a second surgery, but with less of a guarantee of neural axons regrowth into the paralyzed facial nerve branches. In fact, by the time newborn axons arrive at the distal neurorrhaphy, it may be cicatrized and less receptive to neural intake. In case of two-step surgery, the second neurorrhaphy is accomplished only when Tinel's sign is positive (touching the skin overlying the distal end of the nerve graft evokes sensation at proximal neurorrhaphy on the healthy side), generally after 6–10 months. So, no scar may hidden axonal in growth when the distal neurorrhaphy is accomplished. On the other hand, two surgeries are required:
  1. *Single-stage CFNG:* Both the nerve ends are coapted in a single stage.
  2. *Two-stage CFNG:* In the first stage, the buccal branches of contralateral facial nerve are connected with nerve grafts to reach the affected side of face. The donor branches are chosen right in front of the parotid anterior margin, with a good caliber in order to guarantee a minimal count of 800 axons. If more than one cross-face is accomplished, at least one facial nerve branch must be left intact between the donor one in order to avoid a partial paralysis on the healthy side of the face. The nerve grafts are tunneled across the face through the subcutaneous tissue of the upper lip or the front, in reverse, in order not to lose axons through the collateral branches of nerve graft during the nerve regeneration. In the second stage, when a positive Tinel's sign is registered at the buried end of the nerve graft that indicates that axonal regeneration has completed: The terminal neuroma of the buried nerve graft stump is excised and it is coapted to the homologous distal nerve stump on the affected side. A clinical example of the triple innervation technique is shown in **Figures 3 to 8**.

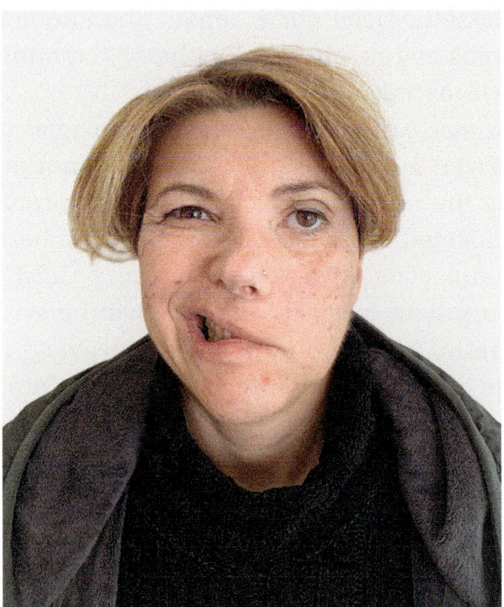

Fig. 3: Patient with a history of left facial palsy for 10 months attempting to smile, with evident deformity.

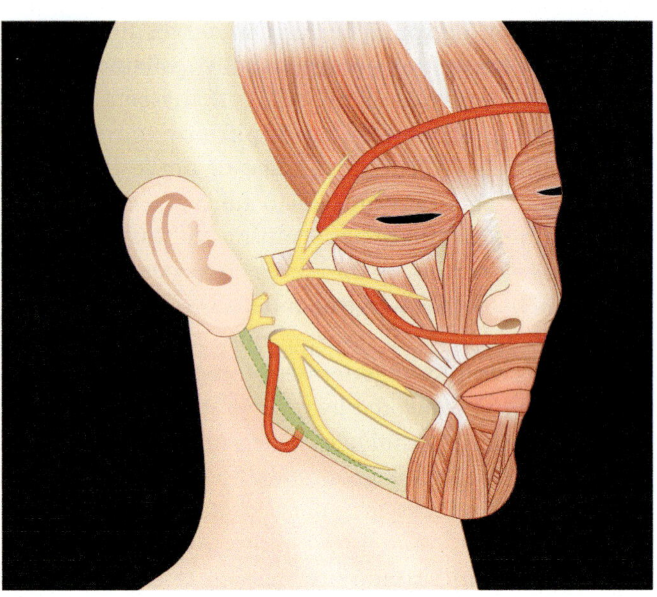

Fig. 5: Schema of the surgery using triple innervation technique.

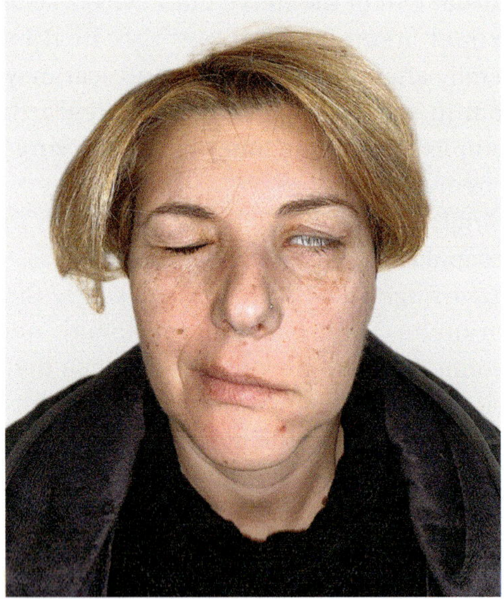

Fig. 4: Incomplete voluntary eyelid closure preoperatively.

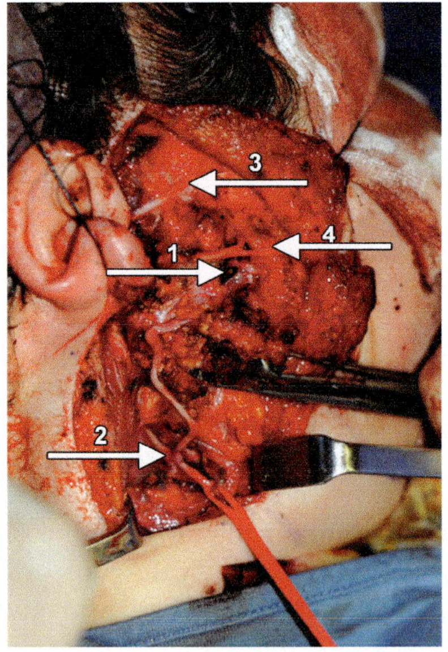

Fig. 6: Intraoperative view of the triple innervation technique: masseteric to upper facial nerve division end-to-end neurorrhaphy (1), 30% hypoglossal to lower facial nerve division end-to-side neurorrhaphy by interpositional nerve graft (2), cross-face nerve grafting to carry contralateral facial nerve stimulus (3 and 4).

- *Free-muscle transfer:* Dynamic reanimation of smile, after mimetic muscles are irreversibly atrophied is performed by free-muscle transfer. Preoperatively smile analysis is essential when smile reanimation is planned. The position of the nasolabial fold on the healthy side must be determined and drawn preoperatively: A symmetrical mark must be reproduced on the paralyzed side where inner stitches will be placed to anchor the free-muscle flap caudally. That will allow production of a symmetrical smile during free-flap activation. An underling fascia lata graft must be placed from the new nasolabial sulcus to the infraorbital rim to guaranteed symmetry at rest. The free-muscle flap is placed from the nasolabial sulcus to the zygomatic prominence to mime zygomaticus major muscle function. Neurorrhaphy between the donor nerve/nerves as the masseteric and the proper free-muscle flap one are accomplished, followed by vascular anastomosis to the facial or temporalis vessels. The same concept of multiple innervation proposed for reversible paralysis

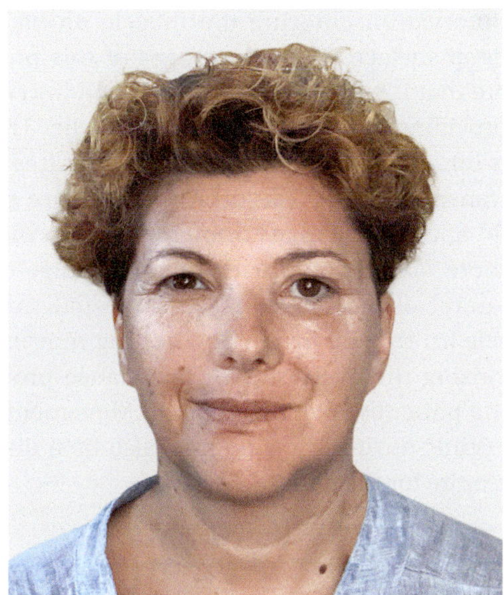

Fig. 7: Good facial symmetry while smiling at 12 months postoperatively.

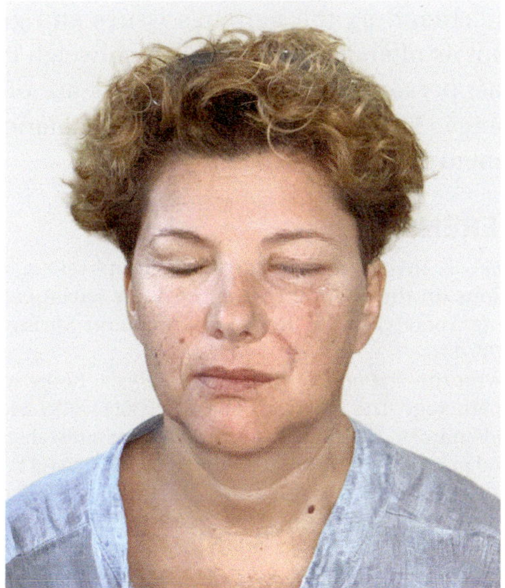

Fig. 8: Complete voluntary eyelid closure at 12 months postoperatively.

reanimation, was applied by Biglioli in long-standing cases to enable gracilis with double innervation to create a powerful and emotional smile.[43] The motor nerve is selected from ipsilateral/contralateral facial, hypoglossal, masseteric, or spinal accessory nerves. The muscles commonly used as gracilis, latissimus dorsi, or rectus abdominis.

Free-muscle transfer can be in a single or double stage. Double stage is accomplished by a first CFNG surgery, followed by a second free-flap transfer surgery. The advantage is a more guaranteed natural smile function because of utilizing the contralateral facial nerve as the main neural source (or adjunctive nerve source—in case of double innervation free-flap).

In case of one-stage surgery, the most utilized nerve source is the masseteric (or the contralateral facial nerve also in case of a double innervation free-flap); spontaneous smiling is seldom possible, more likely in case of double innervation, though with less percentages of success compared to a two-stage procedure. The strongest point in favor of a single-stage procedure is avoiding two surgeries. Latissimus dorsi and rectus abdominis provides a longer nerve segment, therefore nerve graft is not required and may be done. However, even gracilis has been used without a nerve graft,[44] with some concern about its contralateral adequate innervation and proper free-flap setting due to a reduced nerve length. When the contralateral nerve is unavailable, as in Moebius syndrome, other cranial nerves can be used to reinnervate the transplanted muscle. Most commonly used is the nerve to masseter muscle. This has been shown to provide symmetric smile with good muscle excursion.

When a two-staged muscle transfer is planned then the first stage is same as of cross face nerve grafting. Intraoperative facial mapping is done. The various branches are stimulated to find out specific the branches responsible for smile. Sometimes it is difficult to find a smile branch that does not have any orbicularis oculi function. There are usually between two and four nerve branches that activate the zygomaticus and levator labii superioris, out of which one or two branches can be used for nerve graft coaptation. The sural nerve graft is harvested and its proximal end is coapted to the selected facial nerve branches. The distal end of the nerve graft is banked in the upper buccal sulcus or in front of the tragus. During the second operation, the free-flap is transferred and a neurorrhaphy between the previously grafted sural nerve and the nerve of the muscle flap is accomplished in the upper vestibule or in the cheek, according to where the cross-face graft was settled.

The movement in the transplanted muscle is expected 3–8 months after surgery, depending on the length of the free-flap nerve and personal axonal regrowth speed. Coaptation to CFNG provides mimetic, symmetric, and spontaneous smile. However, when nerve to masseter is used, the patient needs to re-train initially. Patient has to take conscious efforts to clench the teeth in order to smile initially. After other 2–3 months, smiling is automatic and the patient does not require clenching of teeth. Emotional smiling or laughing is different; that is seldom achieved with the masseteric nerve as neural source, while it is constant with a CNFG as the sole nerve or coupled to the masseteric in case of double innervated free flap.[45]

- *Muscle transposition:* These are classified as:
  - *Regional muscle transfer for smile:* In patients who are not suitable for free-muscle transfer, regional muscle transfer can be a good option. But, this would not provide spontaneous movements. Temporalis and masseter muscle has been used for smile re-animation. Antidromic temporalis transfer,[46] first described by Gilles, involved detaching the origin of the muscle from the temporal fossa and flipping it over the zygomatic arch and suturing to the oral commissure. The main disadvantage of this procedure was that it caused significant hollowing of the temporal fossa and a bulge over the zygomatic arch. To avoid these problems, various modifications of temporalis transfer were described. Baker and Conley[47] left the anterior portion of the temporalis behind to reduce the temporal hollowing. McLaughlin[48] described orthodromic temporalis transfer where the temporalis muscle is detached from its insertion at coronoid process and anchored to the oral commissure using fascial grafts. Later, Labbè and Huault modified this procedure without the use of fascial grafts.[49] Masseter muscle transfer provides good static control of the commissure but the excursion is not sufficient to produce a full smile. Rubin[50] has advocated transplanting the temporalis and masseter muscles together. The temporalis provides upper lip movements and nasolabial fold, and the masseter provides support to the commissure and lower lip.
  - *Regional muscle transfer for eyelid closure:* Temporalis muscle transposition may also be utilized for eyelid closure. An inferiorly based 1.5 cm-wide flap of temporalis muscle is raised along with the overlying temporalis fascia. The overlying fascia is then lifted off the muscle from caudal to cranial direction and divided into two strips. The superior edge of the muscle is reinforced to the fascia using prolene. The muscle with the two fascial strips is then transposed anteriorly, passing subcutaneously to the lateral canthus. The fascial strips are tunneled along the upper and lower lid margins and sutured to the medial canthal ligament.[51] The flap is based on the blood supply and motor nerve innervation entering the muscle on its inferior deep surface. The advantages of this procedure are that it addresses both upper and lower eyelids providing a static sling for lower eyelid. The result is immediate unlike nerve transfer or free-muscle transplantation. The disadvantages are that, the lid aperture changes from an oval to a slit shape; there may be an obvious muscle bulge over the lateral orbital margin. Also, the patient has to relearn that he has to do chewing movement for closing the eyelids. This may cause problem to the patient while having food. Movements of the eyelids during chewing may also be a disturbing feature for the patient.

CONCLUSION

Facial nerve disorders in the context of head and neck cancer are complex and multifactorial. Appropriate management of facial nerve dysfunction is crucial to avoid a devastating impact on a patient's quality of life. Understanding the patient's issues and goals are important as often functional issues outweigh cosmetic concerns; personalized treatment plans are of utmost importance. Multidisciplinary care and planning are important to optimize outcomes.

REFERENCES

1. Esslen E. Investigations, Part II: Electrophysiologic Investigations on the Natural History of Acute Facial Palsies. The Acute Facial Palsies. Berlin, Heidelberg: Springer; 1977. pp. 39-116.
2. Cawthorne T. Peripheral facial paralysis. Some aspects of its pathology. The Laryngoscope. 1946;56(11):653-64.
3. Lindeman H. The fallopian canal: an anatomical study of its distal part. Acta Otolaryngol Suppl. 1960;158:204-11.
4. Saito H, Takeda T, Kishimoto S. Facial nerve to facial canal cross-sectional area ratio in children. The Laryngoscope. 1992;102(10):1172-6.
5. Fisch U. Total facial nerve decompression and electroneuronography. Neurological Surgery of the Ear; 1977. pp. 21-33.
6. Fowler ÉP. The pathologic findings in a case of facial paralysis. Actaoto-laryngologica. 1963;56(2-6):113-25.
7. Sunderland S, Cossar DF. The structure of the facial nerve. The Anatomical Record. 1953;116(2):147-65.
8. Harris WD. Topography of the facial nerve. Archives of Otolaryngology. 1968;88(3):264-7.
9. Thomander L, Aldskogius H, Grant G. Motor fibre organization in the intratemporal portion of cat and rat facial nerve studied with the horseradish peroxidase technique. Actaoto-laryngologica. 1982;93(1-6):397-405.
10. Gacek RR, Radpour S. Fiber orientation of the facial nerve: An experimental study in the cat. The Laryngoscope. 1982; 92(5):547-56.
11. Davis RA, Anson BJ, Budinger JM, Kurth L. Surgical Anatomy of the Facial Nerve and Parotid Gland Based upon a Study of 350 Cervico-facial Halves. Plast Reconstr Surg. 1958;21(1):84.

12. Dingman RO, Grabb WC. Surgical anatomy of the mandibular ramus of the facial nerve based on the dissection of 100 facial halves. Plast Reconstr Surg. 1962;29(3):266-72.
13. Pitanguy I, Ramos AS. The frontal branch of the facial nerve: the importance of its variations in face lifting. Plast Reconstr Surg. 1966;38(4):352-6.
14. Gordin E, Lee TS, Ducic Y, Arnaoutakis D. Facial nerve trauma: evaluation and considerations in management. Craniomaxillofac Trauma Reconstr. 2015;8(01):001-13.
15. Roob G, Fazekas F, Hartung HP. Peripheral facial palsy: etiology, diagnosis and treatment. European Neurology. 1999;41(1):3-9.
16. Mansour AM, Bailey BJ. Ocular findings in Ramsay Hunt syndrome. J Neuroophthalmol. 1997;17(3):199-201.
17. Catalano PJ, Bergstein MJ, Sen C, Post K. Management of the eye after iatrogenic facial paralysis. Neurosurg. 1994;35(2):259-63.
18. Glasscock III ME, Wiet RJ, Jackson CG, Dickins JR. Rehabilitation of the face following traumatic injury to the facial nerve. The Laryngoscope. 1979;89(9):1389-404.
19. Fisch U. Facial paralysis in fractures of the petrous bone. The Laryngoscope. 1974;84(12):2141-54.
20. Prabhu RK, Sinha R, Chowdhury SK, Chattopadhyay PK. Evaluation of facial nerve function following surgical approaches for maxillofacial trauma. Ann Maxillofac Surg. 2012;2(1):36.
21. doEgitoVasconcelos BC, Bessa-Nogueira RV, da Silva LC. Prospective study of facial nerve function after surgical procedures for the treatment of temporomandibular pathology. J Oral Maxillofac Surg. 2007;65(5):972-8.
22. O'Brien CJ. Facial nerve localization in parotid surgery. ANZ J Surg. 2002;72(5):370.
23. Toure S, Vacher C, Bertrand JC. Anatomy of the marginal mandibular branch of the facial nerve. Rev Stomatol Chir Maxillofac. 2004;105(3):149-52.
24. Batra AP, Mahajan A, Gupta K. Marginal mandibular branch of the facial nerve: An anatomical study. Indian J Plast Surg. 2010;43(01):060-4.
25. Seckel BR. Facial danger zones: Avoiding nerve injury in facial plastic surgery. Can J Plast Surg. 1994;2(2):59-66.
26. Azizzadeh B, Murphy MR, Johnson CM, Massry GG, Fitzgerald R. Master Techniques in Facial Rejuvenation E-Book. Elsevier Health Sciences; 2018.
27. May M, Schaitkin BM. The facial nerve: May's second edition. Verlag: George Thieme; 2000.
28. Anderson R, Olson J, Merkle M, Dowart R, Schaefer S. CT air-contrast scanning of the internal auditory canal. Ann Otol Rhinol Laryngol. 1982;91(5):501-5.
29. Harnsberger HR, Davis RK, Parkin JL, Osborn AG, Smoker W. The tailored CT evaluation of persistent facial nerve paralysis. The Laryngoscope. 1986;96(4):347-52.
30. Millen SJ, Daniels D, Meyer G. Gadolinium-enhanced magnetic resonance imaging in facial nerve lesions. Otolaryngol Head Neck Surg. 1990;102(1):26-33.
31. Murphy TP. MRI of the facial nerve during paralysis. Otolaryngol Head Neck Surg. 1991;104(1):47-51.
32. House WE. Facial nerve grading system. Otolaryngol Head Neck Surg. 1985;93:184-93.
33. Banks CA, Bhama PK, Park J, Hadlock CR, Hadlock TA. Clinician-graded electronic facial paralysis assessment: the eFACE. Plast Reconstr Surg. 2015;136(2):223e-30e.
34. Sforza C, Rango M, Galante D, Bresolin N, Ferrario VF. Spontaneous blinking in healthy persons: an optoelectronic study of eyelid motion. Ophthalmic Physiol Opt. 2008;28(4):345-53.
35. McLaughlin CR. Epiphora in facial paralysis. Br J Plast Surg. 1950;3(2):87-95.
36. Coleman SR. Long-term survival of fat transplants: Controlled demonstrations. Aesthetic Past Surg. 1995;19(5):421-5.
37. Biglioli F, Rabbiosi D, Bolognesi F, Cucurullo M, Dessy M, Ciardiello C, et al. Lipofilling of the upper eyelid to treat paralytic lagophthalmos. Br J Oral Maxillofac Surg. 2020;58(5):558-63.
38. Jelks GW, Glat PM, Jelks EB, Wood M, Gadangi P, Longaker MT. Evolution of the lateral canthoplasty: techniques and indications. Plast Reconstr Surg. 1997;100(6):1396-405; discussion 1406-8.
39. Terris DJ, Fee WE. Current issues in nerve repair. Arch Otolaryngol Head Neck Surg. 1993;119(7):725-31.
40. Biglioli F, Tarabbia F, Allevi F, Colombo V, Giovanditto F, Latiff M, et al. Immediate facial reanimation in oncological parotid surgery with neurorrhaphy of the masseteric-thoracodorsal-facial nerve branch. Br J Oral Maxillofac Surg. 2016;54(5):520-5.
41. Biglioli F, Colombo V, Pedrazzoli M, Frigerio A, Tarabbia F, Autelitano L, et al. Thoracodorsal nerve graft for reconstruction of facial nerve branching. J Craniomaxillofac Surg. 2014;42(1):e8-14.
42. Terzis JK: Pectoralis minor: a unique muscle for correction of facial palsy. Plast Reconstr Surg. 1989;83(5):767-76.
43. Biglioli F, Colombo V, Tarabbia F, Pedrazzoli M, Battista V, Giovanditto F, et al. Double innervation in free-flap surgery for long-standing facial paralysis. J Plast Reconstr Aesthet Surg. 2012;65(10):1343-9.
44. Zuker RM, Goldberg CS, Manktelow RT. Facial animation in children with Möbius syndrome after segmental gracilis muscle transplant. Plast Reconstr Surg. 2000;106(1):1-8; discussion 9.
45. Biglioli F, Colombo V, Tarabbia F, Autelitano L, Rabbiosi D, Colletti G, et al. Recovery of emotional smiling function in free-flap facial reanimation. J Oral Maxillofac Surg. 2012;70(10):2413-8.
46. Gillies H. Experiences with fascia lata grafts in the operative treatment of facial paralysis. Proceedings of the Royal Society of Medicine, London, England, August 1934. London, England: John Bale Sons and Danielsson Ltd.; 1935.
47. Baker DC, Conley J. Regional muscle transposition for rehabilitation of the paralyzed face. Clin Plast Surg. 1979;6(3):317-31.
48. McLaughlin CR. Surgical support in permanent facial paralysis. Plast Reconstr Surg. 1953;11(4):302-14.
49. Labbe D, Huault M. Lengthening temporalis myoplasty and lip reanimation. Plast Reconstr Surg. 2000;105(4):1289-97.
50. Rubin L. Re-animation of total unilateral facial paralysis by the contiguous facial muscle technique. In: Rubin L (Ed). The Paralyzed Face. St Louis: Mosby-Year Book; 1991. p. 156.
51. Frey M, Giovanoli P, Tzou CH, et al. Dynamic reconstruction of eye closure by muscle transposition or functional muscle transplantation in facial palsy. Plast Reconstr Surg. 2004;114(4):865-75.

Post-treatment Care and Rehabilitation

CHAPTER 42

Swallowing Rehabilitation in Head and Neck Cancer

Smita Mathias, Sivakumar Vidhyadharan, Narayana Subramaniam

INTRODUCTION

Dysphagia or difficulty to eat is a symptom indicating a delay in the safe passage of food consistently from the mouth to the stomach. It is one among the crucial symptoms of patients suffering from head and neck cancers.[1] About 60–75% of patients may have varying degrees of dysphagia either as a consequence of their head and neck cancer or as the result of the treatment they had undergone.[2] Struggling to swallow, lengthy meal times, and a restricted range of foods which can be swallowed cause interruption of relationships, depression, and loneliness leading to a reduced quality of life.[3] Prompt return to eating and drinking and development toward a normal swallowing function after surgery or chemoradiation treatments may be attained with swallowing rehabilitation therapy.[2,4,5] Usually, skilled professionals such as speech and language pathologists specializing in dysphagia management implement swallowing exercise interventions for patients with head and neck cancers.[2]

NORMAL SWALLOWING FUNCTION

Swallowing is a complicated activity which needs the accurate coordination of over 25 pairs of muscles within the structure such as oral cavity, pharynx, larynx, and esophagus. The neural swallowing control of system has both voluntary and involuntary mechanisms, and is facilitated by connections between cortical centers in both cerebral hemispheres—the brainstem "swallowing center," the cranial nerves (V, VII, IX sensory, IX motor, X and XII), and pharyngeal receptors such as touch, pressure, and chemical stimulus. Generally, the normal swallow is divided into four phases, namely oral preparation phase, oral phase, pharyngeal phase, and esophageal phase.[1,6,7]

Swallowing process involves the mindful effort to swallow food and an instinctive or involuntary effort of preparation of food bolus. The bolus preparation is represented to as the preparatory phase, the passage of the bolus from the oral cavity and pharynx to the esophagus denoted as the transport phase and bolus traversing through the esophagus into the stomach, as the esophageal transport phase. The timing and pattern of the swallowing mechanism are regulated by a central pattern generator situated within the medulla. The food is chewed and prepared for swallowing during the oral preparatory phase. In the oral preparatory phase, the tongue performs a significant role in mixing the food and pushing the bolus to the occlusal surface of the teeth to help with mastication. Sensory innervation within the oral mucosa and the facial muscles tone assist in manipulation of the food bolus and maintaining it in the oral cavity. A glossopalatal seal is created by approximation of the soft palate to the tongue, thereby preventing premature posterior spillage in to the oropharynx, during the process of mastication involving the muscles of the mandible. The oral phase of swallowing commences when the bolus is mixed with saliva in the center of the oral tongue and the tongue forms a trough with the lateral edges curved upward. Within about a second, the tongue then contracts in an anterior to posterior direction moving the bolus posteriorly into the pharynx. The Vth, VIIth, and XIIth cranial nerves play important roles in the oral phase.[7-12] The larynx and pharynx are at rest during the oral preparatory phase of swallowing. The airway is open and nasal breathing is continuous.[8] Pharyngeal phase is reflexive or involuntary, with sensations passing via the IXth and Xth cranial nerves which usually lasts for a second. The pharyngeal phase encompasses the closure of the soft palate to the nasopharynx, the elevation and closure of the larynx, the contraction of the pharyngeal constrictors, and the relaxation of the cricopharyngeus muscle. A three-layered barrier is formed by the closure or constriction of true cords; the false cords, the epiglottis, and the aryepiglottic folds to prevent aspiration into the airway. The suprahyoid muscles contracts to elevate the larynx.[11] The pharyngeal stage normally occurs during a short period of apnea occurring during the expiratory phase of respiration. This apnea continues post swallow, thus accomplishing some amount of natural airway protection.[10] As the larynx elevates superiorly and anteriorly, it causes relaxation of the cricopharyngeus muscle. Hence, because of inhibition of the cricopharyngeus's normal resting tone, a negative pressure is generated in the cervical esophagus which assists in the passage of the bolus further down toward the stomach.[13,14] The laryngeal inlet is closed and protected by the following actions: The action of the aryepiglottic muscles causing deflection of the epiglottis, the true and false vocal fold closure, pressure exerted by the base of the tongue, and by the bolus itself. This phase usually lasts for a second; however, depending on size of the bolus, it can alter.[15] During the esophageal phase, a single primary peristaltic wave travels downward at 3-4 cm/sec. Numerous secondary peristaltic waves happens in an hour enabling residue clearance and reduce gastric reflux.[10]

SWALLOWING FUNCTION FOLLOWING SURGERY FOR CANCER OF THE HEAD AND NECK

Dysphagia is often encountered after head and neck tumors are surgically excised. The oral preparatory, oral propulsive, and pharyngeal stages of the swallow are usually affected.[16-18] The severity of dysphagia depends on the site of the tumor and the extent of surgical resection. The excision of structures important for protection of airway, bolus formation, and transfer vastly impact the postsurgical dysphagia.[16-20]

Oral and Oropharyngeal Surgery

Dysphagia that ensues after oral cancer resections alters with site of resection and nature of reconstruction.[1] When a part of the oral tongue is resected, patients demonstrate severe dysphagia that is depicted by lengthened oral preparatory time, reduced oral transit time, large amounts of oral residue, and increase residue in pharynx.[21-23] As the bolus viscosity rises, the oral stage dysphagia tends to get worse among the patients.[22-24]

With regards to floor of mouth cancers, unless the resection extends down to the suprahyoid muscles, there is generally limited dysphagia. There may be reduced hyolaryngeal elevation resulting in reduced relaxation of the cricopharyngeus giving rise to residue within the pyriform sinuses. Secondary aspiration can occur due to spill over of the residue into the larynx. With resection of the floor of mouth muscles, patients may experience problems with hyolaryngeal elevation, resulting in residue in the pyriform sinuses that may be aspirated after the swallow.[20,22,25,26]

Patients with tumors in the base of tongue had more poor swallowing functions as compared to patients with tumors in the anterior floor of mouth as reported by Logemann and Bytell. Studies also report that as the amount of the resected tongue and tongue base increases, the efficiency of swallowing decreases.[21] Furia CL et al. conducted a videofluoroscopic analysis of 15 patients, who had undergone either total, subtotal (preserving 10% of tongue base), or partial glossectomies and revealed stasis of residue in all regions of the oropharynx predominantly after subtotal and total glossectomies.[23] The oral transit times were greater for food of all consistencies and the laryngeal elevation and reduction in opening of the upper esophageal sphincter. Patients who underwent partial glossectomy required multiple number of swallows to move the residue in valleculae and had increased oral transit times. There was a high risk of aspiration among patients with advanced stage tongue cancer who had undergone total glossectomy. Hence, as a prophylactic measure, total laryngectomy should be considered simultaneously along with total glossectomy.[1,24] There is an inability to trigger a pharyngeal swallow and difficulty to clear the bolus from the pharynx, leading to severe aspiration postsurgery, if the resection of tongue base is >25%.[24,27]

Defects created after resection of tumors involving the middle segment of mandible when not reconstructed lead to poor cosmetic and functional outcomes. However in defects of purely lateral mandible, the interruption of function is not as severe.[28] Christopoulos et al. conducted a study comparing 10 patients who had undergone reconstruction of various defects of the mandible with 10 patients in whom mandibular reconstruction was not performed. They observed a significant benefit in function among patient who had their mandibles reconstructed.[29] While performing oromandibular reconstruction following composite extirpation of oral neoplasms, to help preserve physiological function, a three-dimensional anatomical correlation should be achieved.[30] Studies have shown that resection of mandibular segment resection without reconstruction had a strong adverse influence on efficiency of the oropharyngeal deglutition, residue, and mastication within the oral cavity.[30-33]

A sizable oronasal or oromaxillary fistula and also deficiency of teeth-bearing segment after surgical resection of palatal and maxillary sinus tumors disrupt functioning of oral and pharyngeal phases of swallowing.[34] Anattachable prosthesis or a skin lined flap to provide a seal along with oronasal separation is recommended to enhance deglutition. The prosthesis, however, needs to be cleaned frequently.[35]

It is advantageous to have a prosthodontist working with the speech pathologist for the design of the prosthetic device.[36] In addition to functional rehabilitation, another matter of concern is the malnutrition that is associated with the treatment of the cancer. Factors influencing the development of malnutrition and its severity are the pretreatment nutritional status of the patient, the site of the primary tumor and the type of treatment delivered.[37] In a study of 117 patients who underwent transoral laser microsurgery for stage III/IV glottic or supraglottic carcinoma of the larynx, swallowing was assessed by the functional outcome of swallowing scale (FOSS). Out of the 68 patients alive on latest follow-up, 7% were feeding tube-dependent. About 44% of the patients could be assessed by the FOSS system and it was seen that the overall median post-treatment FOSS stage was stage 1, which is normal function with episodic or daily symptoms of dysphagia. The authors used a definition of FOSS stage 2 or better as the functional endpoint and found that 22/28 patients for whom follow-up data were available met the criteria.[38]

Partial Laryngectomy

Partial laryngectomy procedures were introduced to decrease the functional impact of total laryngectomy on swallowing and speech. A study comparing the dysphagia outcome in 25 total laryngectomy and 11 frontolateral laryngectomy patients found a statistically significant difference between the two, with 36% patients having difficulties of whom 12 had undergone total laryngectomy and 1 frontolateral laryngectomy ($p < 0.027$).[39] The patients were interviewed by a speech language pathologist using a semistructured questionnaire. In a study of functional outcome of 29 male patients undergoing cricohyoidopexy, frontolateral laryngectomy, or laryngofissure cordectomy, it was found that time to return to oral feeding was significantly longer in patients undergoing cricohyoidopexy (Day 20) and frontolateral laryngectomy (Day 6) in comparison to cordectomy (Day 0).[40] There was no statistically significant difference in the swallowing outcomes when these procedures were combined with arytenoidectomy. In a study comparing 17 patients treated by cricohyoidoepiglottopexy (CHEP) with 21 patients of near total laryngectomy with epiglottic reconstruction (NTLER), nasogastric (NG) tubes were removed at a mean of 23.0 (SD 13.6) days in the CHEP group and 17.0 (SD 11.4) days in the NTLER group. The difference was not significant and the swallow function was good on long-term follow-up in both groups. All the patients selected for the study had T1b glottic cancer.[41]

Supraglottic Laryngectomy

Either one or both superior laryngeal nerves, epiglottis, aryepiglottic folds, false vocal cords and sometimes, the superior aspect of the thyroid cartilage are resected in supraglottic laryngectomy, sparing the true vocal folds and arytenoids.[42-44] Hence after the procedure, there is a risk of aspiration because few of the structures involved in airway protection are resected.[42,45-48] This leads to partial closure of the airway secondary to residue within the oropharynx or hypopharynx spilling over into the inlet of the airway. Also, if a portion of base of tongue down to the hyoid bone or the arytenoids is included in the resection, insufficient propulsive force of tongue and laryngeal elevation will also pose a risk of aspiration.

Hence, the proper functioning of the arytenoids (cricoarytenoid unit) and the base of tongue are vital in compensating for the anatomic structures excised during supraglottic laryngectomy.[15] Rademaker et al. observed that patients who had been operated for extended supraglottic laryngectomy had a considerably prolonged rehabilitation to achieve acceptable swallowing function.[48] In extended supraglottic laryngectomy, where the base of tongue is resected, the time taken for the patient to reach a preoperative diet with normal swallow function is longer than in small resections. They also have a high risk of aspiration pneumonia (up to 74% of patients).[49] Among the patients who have undergone supraglottic laryngectomy and those who are able accomplish reasonable contact between the tongue base and the arytenoids have a reduced risk of aspiration.[47]

Supracricoid Laryngectomy

Supracricoid laryngectomy involves excision of the thyroid cartilage, the true vocal cords and false cords of either side, and the paraglottic space; sometimes a cricoarytenoid unit and epiglottis are also resected. Lewin JS et al. reported that all patients who had undergone supracricoid laryngectomy in their study originally had aspiration along with diminished base of tongue movements and laryngeal elevation. The median time to removal of nasogastric tube after surgery was 9.4 weeks. Although, 81% of patients resumed a normal diet, some had complications of pneumonia and subcutaneous emphysema.[50] Some patients who did not have swallowing difficulties after surgery, presented with dysphagia many years later.[52] Normally, patients undergoing a hemilaryngectomy or vertical partial laryngectomy have less episodes of aspiration and quicker return to normal oral diet as compared to those who have undergone a supraglottic laryngectomy.[48] Vertical partial laryngectomy encompasses the resection of vocal process and the thyroid cartilage on the side of tumor, along with the false vocal fold, ventricle, and true vocal cord without the arytenoids on the involved side.[43,44,52] Since the hyoid bone, epiglottis and arytenoids are preserved on the tumor side, if the resulting defect is reconstructed with adequate bulk to help form a pseudocord and to permit the opposite vocal cord to make contact, it assists with airway closure and protects from aspiration.[43,53]

Transoral Robotic Surgery

A majority of patients who underwent transoral robotic surgery (TORS), have dysphagia for a minimum of 4 weeks of the initial postoperative period; however, almost everyone may be commenced on an oral diet.[54] A small number of patient might require temporary placement of the nasogastric tube. In the published literature, the dysphagia-related readmission rate after undergoing TORS about 4.7–7.8%.[55-57] Hutcheson et al. compared the dysphagia profiles between primary transoral robotic surgery patients and those who received primary radiotherapy and reported some difference in the short term but none by 3-6 months of recovery; a majority of patients regained a functional swallow after primary TORS. During the acute postoperative period, moderate-severe pharyngeal dysphagia that did not recover to baseline by 3–6 months was noted in about 22.7%. They concluded that subacute swallowing outcomes were the same, irrespective of initial treatment approach among low- to intermediate-risk oropharyngeal squamous cell carcinoma patients.[58]

Total Laryngectomy and Laryngopharyngectomy

In cases of advanced cancer of the larynx, total laryngectomy may be performed as a primary treatment modality. Generally, aspiration is not a risk for those who have received a total laryngectomy, except for seepage of liquids either through or around the voice prosthesis is situated within a tracheoesophageal fistula.[46] Dysphagia may still occur following laryngectomy in 10–60%, due to pseudoepiglottis, loss of coordination of pharyngeal muscles, benign stricture, recurrence of cancer, or a second primary cancer.[59,60] Also, the reconstructed pharyngoesophageal segment has considerably lower resting pressures and peak pressures as shown by manometric studies. There is also incoordination between pharyngeal constrictor muscle contraction and pharyngoesophageal segment relaxation with decreased pharyngeal clearing force and loss of negative pressure preceding the bolus, necessitating multiple swallows for the passage of single bolus in a laryngectomy patient.[61-65] In an evaluation of lifestyle changes post-total laryngectomy, Ackerstaff concluded that 25% of patients had a modification in method of eating, food consistency, and diet.[66] If the base of tongue is also included in the laryngectomy, then bolus clearance via oral cavity through the pharynx to esophagus is also disrupted.[67-69] To attain bolus transport, sufficient tongue-base propulsive motion is crucial, generating pressures higher than normal during the swallow.[63] When laryngectomy is performed as a salvage procedure, the occurrence of pharyngocutaneous fistula is higher than primary laryngectomy.[70-72] Myocutaneous flaps, visceral transpositions, and free flaps have been used after total laryngopharyngectomy. Tumors situated within the proximal part of hypopharynx are reconstructed using free jejunal flaps and when the extent of resection is past the thoracic inlet, a gastric transposition is utilized. Triboulet et al. conducted a study on patients who had total laryngopharyngectomy along with either gastric anastomosis or jejunal flaps reconstruction. They reported that the dysphagia-free survival was greater for gastric anastomosis (89%) than for jejunalflaps (76%), with gastric transposition having decreased rates of fistula and stricture formation.[73]

Voice Rehabilitation

The main goal of voice therapy after total laryngectomy is to substitute another vibratory source for voice production. The alternative vibratory sources comprise either mechanical vibration using artificial larynx or vibration of the pharyngoesophageal segment (PES) in esophageal or tracheoesophageal speech.[74]

- *Electrolaryngeal speech:* This technique utilizes an artificial larynx or electrolarynx. The apparatus is placed intraorally or placed on the neck and cheek. Identification of appropriate placement where the quality of observed sound is good is a significant step in the use of electrolarynx. The sound occurs on articulation after turning the device on.[74]

- *Esophageal speech:* This technique involves injecting air into the esophagus and then vibrating the pharyngoesophageal segment (PES) while expelling the air out. Postoperative speech therapy after surgery focuses on learning the techniques of injecting air into esophagus, articulatory effort, and improving the quality and length of speech.[74]
- *Tracheoesophageal speech:* This type of a laryngeal speech utilizes a tracheoesophageal voice prosthesis for voice restoration. During laryngectomy, a puncture is made between the wall of trachea and esophagus and the one-way valve, tracheoesophageal prosthesis, is inserted into this puncture. The air enters the esophagus from trachea via the prosthesis on closure of the stoma, vibrating the PES. The ensuing quality of voice depends on the tonicity of PES. The voice quality sounds strained, if the PES is hypertonic.[74]

Dysphagia Following Thyroidectomy

Total or partial thyroidectomy is a challenging procedure due to complicated thyroid gland anatomy; the restricted space within the neck and the risk of damaging the recurrent laryngeal nerves. Dysphonia and dysphagia are the most commonly reported symptoms following thyroidectomy.[74] Patient may suffer from roughness of voice, vocal strain, and trouble producing a higher pitch or volume. The symptoms of dysphagia are coughing, choking or aspiration pneumonia in severe cases. After thyroidectomy, patients may complain of pain as when the larynx elevates during swallowing, the upper trachea crosses the thyroid bed, causing pain which lasts for 2–5 days.[75] Thereis usually no functional change in swallowing. However, there is a loss of supraglottic sensation leading to aspiration if the internal branch of the superior laryngeal nerve is injured. If the external branch of superior laryngeal nerve (SLN) is damaged, there will be a reduced upper range and volume. The symptoms of SLN damage go unnoticed unless the patient is a professional voice user.[76] Vocal fold palsy is caused by injury to the distal recurrent laryngeal nerve (RLN) causing incomplete glottal closure. Symptoms of hoarseness, reduced vocal range, vocal fatigue, and choking while drinking liquids are reported by patients with vocal cord palsy. Additionally, cricopharyngeal relaxation is also affected in RLN injury.[74,75]

Speech Therapy after Thyroidectomy

The primary objective of speech therapy is to improve glottic closure and restore vocal function for improved regular function and quality of life for the patient.[74,75] There are three major techniques in voice therapy.

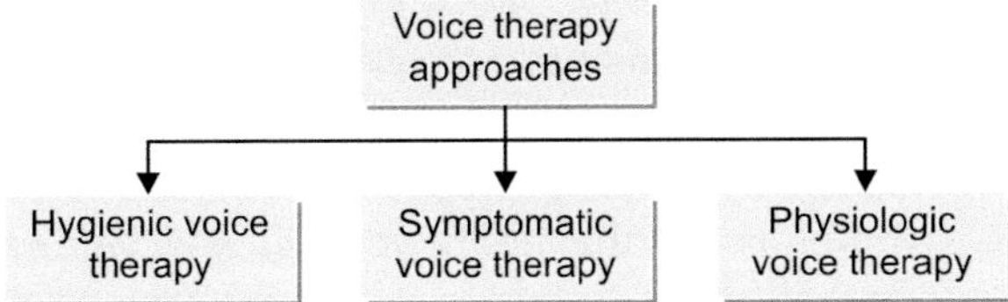

- *Hygienic voice therapy:* The clinician helps the patient to identify the habit of vocal abuse such as shouting, screaming, and throat clearing and aids to modify or terminate these habits.
- *Symptomatic voice therapy:* Focus is on changing the divergent vocal symptoms like pitch which is too high or low, voice that is too soft or loud, and breathy phonation. Some of the symptomatic voice therapy techniques are chant talk, head positioning, and the pushing approach.
- *Physiologic voice therapy:* It is the most holistic of the three approaches, involving the alteration of the laryngeal, respiratory, and resonatory systems with direct physical exercise in an effort to improve voice quality. It is considered the most holistic of three approaches.[4] Examples of physiologic voice therapy include "Vocal Function Exercise" and "Resonant Voice Therapy."[77,78]

Surgery of the Skull Base

The swallowing function in patients with advanced tumors of the skull base adapts well and patients do not complain about significant dysphagia. This is because the cranial nerve palsies occurring in these advanced tumors are generally slow in onset. However, acute dysphagia may occur during the post-treatment period due to injury to the adjoining cranial nerves. Numerous approaches for accessing the skull base affects the swallowing function such as, an anterior cranial approach with maxillectomies may cause nasal regurgitation of food and injury to the V, VII, IX, X, and XII cranial nerves by lateral skull-base approach via the zygoma.[79]

SWALLOWING FUNCTION FOLLOWING RADIOTHERAPY

Among head and neck cancer patients, dysphagia persists as a considerable adverse effect of postoperative radiation or definitive radiation with or without chemotherapy.[80] Although substantial doses are delivered to critical anatomic swallowing structures such as the tongue, pharynx and larynx, the acute and chronic side effects occur indirectly, affecting the patient's quality of life.

Adverse effects which occur in the acute phase of radiation treatment are pain, mucositis, and skin desquamation. The late side effects of radiation are trismus, strictures, osteonecrosis, decaying of teeth, hypothyroidism, hearing loss, fibrosis, and pharyngeal and esophageal stenosis.[81] The occurrence of adverse effects depends on the field, dosage, and timing of radiation received. The deficiency in improving swallow function seen after the initial surgery can be attributed to the extent of tissue damage. Researchers have identified that oropharyngeal muscle function is more often reduced in those receiving radiotherapy than in those receiving surgery.[23,24,82,83]

The oral and the pharyngeal phase of deglutition is affected in irradiated patients, thereby causing prolonged oral and pharyngeal transit times, greater pharyngeal residue, lower oropharyngeal swallow efficiency, and rapid duration of cricopharyngeal relaxation.[8,84] There is also a decrease in propulsive force of the base of tongue due to radiation-induced fibrosis and atrophy, further reducing the period of base of tongue to posterior pharyngeal wall contact.[85,86]

Patients with cancer of the laryngeal and hypopharynx also experience the side effects of definitive or post-operative radiotherapy. Especially amongst patients who underwent adjuvant radiation treatment after supraglottic laryngectomy, there are an elevated number of patients with tracheostomy dependence, late return to normal or independent swallowing and high prevalence of aspiration pneumonia compared to those only receiving surgery.[44] The rates of silent aspiration after head and neck treatment is reported to be 22–42%.[86-89]

Patients who received chemoradiotherapy tend to exhibit similar swallowing disorders,[88] irrespective of the primary tumor site, with at least half of the patients report swallowing dysfunction which manifests clinically as prolonged duration for closure of the laryngeal vestibule, decreased epiglottic inversion, disruption of pharyngeal constrictor muscle contraction, and decreased laryngeal elevation.[90-92] As a result of gradually progressing radiation-induced fibrosis many years after chemoradiotherapy for oropharynx and nasopharyngeal tumors, increased residue in the vallecula and pyriform sinuses are observed due to limited mobility of the oral tongue, tongue base, larynx, and pharynx.[93-99]

Interruption of salivary gland function during radiation treatment leads to xerostomia or reduced flow of saliva, which is also a cause for dysphagia. Doses of radiation in the range of 55–64 Gy cause permanent damage to the parotid gland.[100,101] Patients report complaints of food sticking in the throat, a dry mouth requiring regular consumption of water while eating, and dysgeusia.[102] Mucositis associated with painful ulcers is an acute side effect of radiation treatment affecting the tissue lining in the aerodigective tract within the head and neck radiation field. It normally subsides 2–6 weeks after the treatment.[103,104]

The occurrence of pharyngeal and esophageal strictures after chemoradiotherapy treatment profoundly with incidence rates of between 8 and 24% after chemoradiation.[86,104-107] It has been reported that strictures are formed when doses of radiation to hypopharynx or esophagus are beyond 60–70 Gy.[108]

The European Society for Clinical Nutrition and Metabolism (ESPEN) guidelines on enteral nutrition for nonsurgical oncology state that enteral feeding administered via a tube should be commenced in patients with obstructive head and neck cancer lesions causing dysphagia. There was no evidence identified to substantiate the utility of PEG over NG tubes for enteral nutrition as reported by Corry et al. in a randomized study of chemoradiotherapy for head and neck cancer patients.[109] Stricture formation may also be related to whether the patient was continually taking food orally during and after the course of radiation as this resulted in reduced possibility of significant hypopharyngeal atrophy and muscular fibrosis with the target region as compared to the patients who were on tube feeds.[110,111] Hence if possible, patients must be firmly encouraged to have an oral diet, even if they have a gastrostomy tube or nasogastric tube in place, thereby limiting stricture formation and disuse atrophy. Administration of chemotherapeutic medications influence the ability to swallow normally and alter nutrition status among head and neck cancer patients causing several side-effects such as nausea, vomiting, generalized weakness, fatigue, and neutropenia. Mucositis is reported in about 40% of patients undergoing chemotherapy.[112] Cytotoxic drugs such as methotrexate and 5-fluorouracil most are frequently linked with dysphagia due to oral, pharyngeal, and esophageal symptoms.[113,114] Neutropenia combined with silent aspiration due to chemotherapy may result in aspiration pneumonia, sepsis, and respiratory failure.[69,71]

DIAGNOSIS AND REHABILITATION

A detailed pretreatment assessment, in the form of dysphagia history, clinical and instrumental evaluation of swallowing, is integral for diagnosing the nature of the dysphagia and planning adequate rehabilitation. The rehabilitation is usually conducted by the speech and language pathologist with vital inputs and assistance from the members of the head and neck treatment team. In some complex patients and during difficult assessment, the help of the head and neck surgeon is attained.

The swallowing assessment is done to ascertain the patient's abilities and deficiencies and level to which these deficiencies could be altered.

Clinical assessment or clinical bedside assessment involves a detailed history of the patient's dysphagia and a comprehensive assessment of oral, pharyngeal, and laryngeal anatomy, along with evaluating the sensory and motor functions. If considered suitable, a trial feeding is also done. Crucial information can be history-taking which would encompass questions based on onset, duration, frequency, and patient's narrative of the dysphagia. The water-swallow test (3-oz, 50-mL or 30-mL) is commonly done at the bedside. With the high incidence of silent aspiration among head and neck patients, utilizing an imaging procedure to rule out and assess dysphagia is crucial. The commonly utilized procedures are the modified barium swallow (MBS) and the flexible endoscopic examination of swallow (FEES). These two instrumental evaluations deliver objective evidence about swallowing function and its safety.[115-117] Modified barium swallow objectively assesses the swallowing process, and findings can be graded using several criteria. FEES is another appropriate method to assess dysphagia by using transnasal endoscopy.[1,15]

Measured boluses of radiopaque-contrast material of consistencies ranging from solids to liquids are given during MBS, and the deglutition is observed in the lateral plane with videofluoroscopy. The abnormalities during a swallow are observed and documented. FEES visualizes the pharynx and larynx from above by placing an endoscope transnasally such that the distal end of the tube is suspended over the end of the soft palate, giving a luminal view of the pharynx (which is different from the lateral videofluoroscopic view and allows inspection of closure of true cords). Nonetheless, the information regarding the oral stage of swallow is not visualized in FEES which may be the problematic for patient undergone surgery for oral cavity tumors. MBS is considered as the gold standard technique for observing the swallow, assessing dysphagia, and deriving a treatment plan for patients who have impaired swallow function.[118-120] Cine-MRI directly picturizes the dynamics of swallowing, and abnormal findings, hence it is another tool to assess swallowing function in patients with oral/oropharyngeal cancer.[15,121]

REHABILITATION OF SWALLOWING FUNCTION

Generally, rehabilitation is divided in to three main components—preventative, compensatory, and therapeutic exercises or maneuvers.[122] There is a mounting evidence regarding the importance of commencement of prophylactic swallowing exercises before starting radiotherapy; this is the preventive component of rehabilitation.[123,124] A set of exercises is taught to the patient after the initial clinical and instrumental evaluation. In the setting of surgery as well, some of these exercises are to enhance the strength within the base of tongue after the surgical site has adequately healed or to improve hyolaryngeal elevation and strengthen neck muscles prior to definitive radiation treatment.[125] It is important to note that patients who are more motivated and compliant with their exercises achieved better swallow outcomes after the treatment.[126]

Several studies reported the advantage of continued use of swallowing musculature during chemoradiotherapy ("use it or lose it"). In these studies, patients avoided periods of oral fasting and adhered to targeted swallowing exercise. In the first randomized controlled trial on head and neck cancer patients undergoing chemoradiotherapy with rehabilitation, Van der Molen et al. concluded that preventive exercises were effective in decreasing extent of symptoms at 1 and 2 years post-treatment. They also stressed the importance of pre-treatment swallowing exercises to minimize radiotherapy or atrophy-associated damage to the muscles. Carnaby-Mann et al. showed that prophylactic exercises may result in preservation of oral and oropharyngeal musculature, improving swallowing strength, and reducing the incidence of aspiration pneumonia related to dysphagia. Hence, the role of rehabilitation must be stressed during pretreatment counseling.[127-129]

The key methods for swallowing rehabilitation are postural techniques, sensory techniques, motor exercise, swallowing maneuvers, and changes in diet.[122,130] Alterations made to body position to augment the swallow function and reduce aspiration are referred to as postural techniques of rehabilitation. Logemann described in detail the rationale for the use of various postural techniques based on the disorder observed.[131] Various methods such as stimulation though pressure, changes in temperature, or modifications in taste are referred to as sensory response techniques; different bolus consistencies, bolus placement, or size are the most frequently followed methods. The aim of motor exercises is to improve strength, endurance, and movement of muscles involved in swallowing whenever muscle weakness or reduced range of motion is present.[132,133]

Swallow maneuvers namely, supraglottic swallow, the supersupraglottic swallow, effortful, and the Mendelsohn maneuver are performed to engage specific aspects of swallowing function under voluntary control.[134] With either endoscopic or fluoroscopic assistance, techniques that are most effective for expanding swallow efficacy are taught to an individual with dysphagia. Patients have better results when visual feedback from either MBS, FEES, or manometry is incorporated during therapy.[135,136]

There is insufficient and debatable evidence on the role of neuromuscular electrical stimulation (NES), an addition to swallowing rehabilitation among head and neck cancer patients.[137] Evaluation of dysphagia identifies conditions that have been shown to benefit from surgery for safety, to enhance quality of life, or both. Surgery in indicated patients treated for head and neck cancer is safe and effective in addressing many causes of dysphagia.[138] Oncophagosurgery encompasses the varied surgical procedures performed for improvement or restoration of swallowing function among head and neck cancer patients.

MEASURES OF SWALLOWING

Some of the functional measures of swallowing are comprised of the penetration-aspiration scale (PAS), Performance status scale–head and neck (PSS-HN), National Institutes of Health-Swallowing Safety Scale (NIH-SSS) and MBS impairment profile (MBSImp).[121]

Penetration-Aspiration Scale

It is a validated 8-point ordinal scale which grades safety of a swallow by the extent of entry of bolus within the airway and the patient's response, where "0" signifies no airway entry and "8" signifies silent aspiration.[139]

National Institutes of Health-Swallowing Safety Scale

The NIH-SSS measures safety of a swallow based on seven observations from the Modified Barium Swallow study (laryngeal penetration, aspiration, aspiration response, maximal esophageal entry, residue, and multiple swallows) demonstrating high reliability among patients with in dysphagia.[140]

Performance Status Scale–Head and Neck

Performance status Scale for head and neck cancer patients consists of three subscales namely, eating in public, understandability of speech, and normalcy of diet.[141]

Eating Assessment Tool 10

The Eating Assessment Tool 10 (EAT-10), is a self-administered, symptom-specific, 10-item validated questionnaire for measuring dysphagia severity. The EAT-10 has displayed excellent internal consistency, test-retest reproducibility, and criterion-based validity. An EAT-10 score of 3 or higher is abnormal. The questionnaire may be used to record the initial dysphagia severity and check the treatment response in persons with dysphagia.[142,143]

Modified Barium Swallow Impairment Profile

Modified barium swallow impairment profile (MBSImp) is a validated, standardized measure which rates physiologic constituents of the oropharyngeal swallow. By reviewing an entire MBS video recording, MBSImp ratings for pharyngeal phase components were calculated which includes: soft palate elevation, laryngeal elevation, anterior hyoid excursion, epiglottic movement, laryngeal vestibule closure, pharyngeal stripping wave, pharyngeal contraction, pharyngoesophageal segment opening, tongue base retraction, and pharyngeal residue. Every factor is graded utilizing a 3 to 5-point ordinal scale where "0" indicates, no impairment. Overall pharyngeal impairment MBSImp score is calculated as the sum of the 10 component measures, providing a continuous score (range, 0-28) for which higher ratings show larger physiologic impairment.[144,145]

Quality of Life Questionnaires

Some of the validated patient-reported quality of life (QoL) questionnaires such as EORTC HN 35, FACT-HN, MD Anderson Dysphagia Inventory (MDADI) are used to evaluate functional outcomes in patients with head and neck cancer.[121] The MDADI is validated particularly for Head and Neck cancer patients and is very useful for assessing the impact of dysphagia on QOL among such patients after treatment.[146,147] Similar subjective questionnaires pertaining to certain aspects of swallowing and their influence on QoL include the Sydney Swallow Questionnaire (SSQ), the Swallowing Quality of Life (SWAL-QoL) questionnaire, and the Patient Concerns Inventory (PCI). Although the SSQ was conceived for assessment of problems in neuromyogenic dysphagia patients, it is very useful for evaluation of swallowing in oral/oropharyngeal cancer patients undergone primary surgery.[144] SWAL-QoL is authenticated to detect patients with swallowing problems after treatment for oral, oropharyngeal, and laryngeal cancers.[148] For routine screening of self-reported swallowing dysfunction, the Patient Concerns Inventory is important due to addressed patient's concerns during outpatient clinic visits.[149] The Dysphagia Outcome and Severity Scale is a simple, easy-to-use, clinician-rated performance scale, established to rate severity of functional dysphagia based on objective assessment, and to make recommendations for diet level, independence level and nutrition.[150]

Dynamic Imaging Grade of Swallowing Toxicity (DIGEST) is a validated method to grade the severity of pharyngeal-phase dysphagia from videofluoroscopy based on the safety (using a penetration-aspiration scale) and efficiency (using estimation of the percentage of pharyngeal residue) of bolus clearance. DIGEST grades align to the National Cancer Institute's *Common* Terminology Criteria for Adverse Events framework (Grade 1, mild; Grade 2, moderate; Grade 3, severe; and Grade 4, life-threatening). DIGEST was derived by independent re- view of MBS DICOM files by a trained, blinded speech pathologist who met reliability standards. DIGEST was dichotomized with grade 2 or higher as moderate-severe dysphagia based on published data, suggesting that this is a meaningful split associated with quality of life, diet, and swallow muscle radiotherapy dose.[20] DIGEST Grade 2 or higher dysphagia indicates at least intermittent high-grade penetration or aspiration (penetration-aspiration scale score ≥5) and/or post-swallow residue of a 50% or greater bolus.[147-151]

National Dysphagia Diet

The National Dysphagia Diet (NND) was published by the American Dietetic Association, which aimed to establish standard terminology and practice application of dietary texture alterations in dysphagia management. To increase the nutritional intake of dysphagic patients, the food plan was divided into different levels of solid food and liquid consistency.

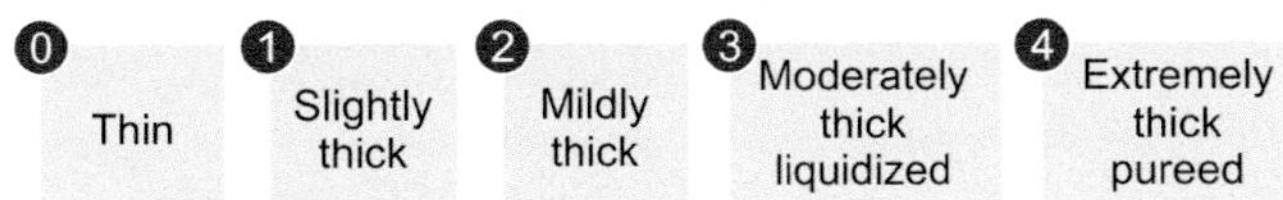

Levels of solids:

- *NDD level 1: Dysphagia pureed*—Foods are thick and smooth and have a moist pudding-like consistency without pulp or small food particle. It needs a minimum amount of manipulation in the mouth and is easy to swallow.
- *NDD level 2: Dysphagia mechanically altered*—Foods are soft, moist, and simple to chew. Moistened ground meats (pieces should not exceed ¼-inch cube), vegetables cooked to a soft mashable texture, soft-cooked or canned fruits, and bananas are included.
- *NDD level 3: Dysphagia advanced*—Foods are very soft. They are in bite-size pieces, and nearly regular in texture. Hard and sticky foods are excluded.

Levels of liquids: Viscosity borders and ranges for thickened liquids.

The NDD has suggested the following viscosity borders and ranges (All measurements were performed at 25°C with a shear rate of 50s^{-1}).

- *Thin liquid:* 1-50 cp*
- *Nectar-like liquids:* 51-350 cp
- *Honey-like liquid:* 351-1750 cp
- *Spoon-thick liquid:* >1750 cp
  (cp*= centipoise, measurement of liquid thickness)

International Dysphagia Diet Standardization Initiative

The International Dysphagia Diet Standardization Initiative (IDDSI) created with the objective of instituting new global standardized definition to describe the texture-modification foods and thickened liquids used for individual with dysphagia of all ages, in all care settings. The IDDSI framework provides detailed description for the five levels of drinks.

Rehabilitative Exercises and Maneuvers

The rehabilitative therapy includes different type of strategies such as shown **Box 1** and **Tables 1 to 3.**

Box 1: Phases of normal swallowing.[6]

Oral preparatory phase:
- Teeth, lips, cheeks, tongue, mandible, and palate grind and manipulate food
- Food mixed with saliva
- Formation of a food bolus consistency appropriate for safe swallow

Oral phase (Duration approximately 1 second):
- Lips and cheeks contract
- Tongue presses the food bolus against the hard palate and soft palate elevates
- Food bolus is moved backward by the tongue
- A central groove is formed in the tongue for passage of bolus
- Bolus is moved to the tonsillar pillars, thus initiating the oral phase of swallowing
- The soft palate moves superior and posterior to close-off nasopharynx

Pharyngeal phase (Duration approximately 1 second):
- Piston-like action of tongue to propel food posteriorly
- Closure of the larynx to the level of the true and false vocal cords
- Retroversion of the epiglottis over the laryngeal vestibule
- Closure of the laryngeal vestibule
- Elevation of the larynx under the tongue base
- Contraction of the pharyngeal constrictors
- Relaxation of the cricopharyngeal muscles
- Opening of the cricopharyngeal sphincter by upward and forward movement of the larynx

Esophageal phase (Duration approximately 3–4 seconds):
Peristaltic contractions of musculature results in movement of the bolus into the stomach

Table 1: Optimal postural techniques and food consistencies for various oropharyngeal swallow disorders.

Disorder	*Optimal postural technique and its effect(s)*	*Optimal food consistency*
Oral stage		
Reduction in cheek tension	Tilt head to stronger side—food flows down stronger side	Thin liquid to puréed
Reduction in tongue elevation	Tilt head back—food flows backward faster	Thin-to-thick liquid
	Tilt head to stronger side—food remains on stronger side	
Reduced anterior to posterior tongue movement	Tilt head back-food flows backward faster	Thin-to-thick liquid
Triggering of pharyngeal swallow		
Delayed or absent triggering of pharyngeal swallow	Chin down—food flows away from airway entrance	Thick liquids, puréed, solid food
Pharyngeal stage		
Reduced base of tongue retraction	Chin down—tongue base pushed posteriorly	Liquids to thin puréed
Unilateral pharyngeal dysfunction	Rotate head to damaged side— food flows down stronger side	Liquids to thin puréed
	Tilt head to stronger side—food remains on stronger side	
Bilateral pharyngeal weakness	Lie down—food does not enter airway; residue remains on pharyngeal wall	Liquids to thin puréed
Reduced laryngeal elevation	Chin down—food flows away from airway entrance	Thick liquid to solid food
Reduced laryngeal closure at entrance	Chin down—food flows away from airway entrance	Thick liquid to solid food
Reduced laryngeal closure at vocal folds	Rotate head—vocal fold adduction improves; food does not flow through vocal folds	Thick liquid to solid food
Cricopharyngeal dysfunction	Rotate head—food flows down opposite side and cricopharyngeal opening widens	Thin liquid

Table 2: Swallowing disorders and their associated interventions.[15]

Swallow-related disorder	*Possible interventions*
Reduced mouth opening	Jaw ROM exercises
Reduced tongue control/ shaping	• Chin-down posture • Supersupraglottic swallow • Tongue ROM exercises • Bolus manipulation exercises • Tongue-strengthening exercises
Reduced vertical tongue movement	• Tongue ROM exercises • Maxillary reshaping prosthesis
Reduced anterior-to-posterior tongue movement	• Head-back posture • Multiple swallows • Alternate liquids and solids • Tongue ROM exercises • Bolus manipulation exercises • Maxillary reshaping prosthesis
Reduced tongue strength	• Effortful swallow • Tongue-strengthening exercises
Delayed pharyngeal swallow	• Chin-down posture • Supersupraglottic swallow • Thermal/tactile stimulation
Reduced tongue-base retraction	• Chin-down posture • Effortful swallow • Supersupraglottic swallow • Tongue-hold maneuver • Mendelsohn maneuver • Tongue ROM exercises • Gargle/yawn for tongue-base retraction

Contd...

Contd...

Swallow-related disorder	*Possible interventions*
Reduced laryngeal vestibule closure	• Chin-down posture • Supersupraglottic swallow • Effortful swallow • Mendelsohn maneuver • Gargle/yawn for tongue-base retraction
Reduced laryngeal elevation	• Mendelsohn maneuver • Chin-down posture • Supersupraglottic swallow • Effortful swallow • Laryngeal ROM exercises • Shaker exercise
Reduced glottic closure	• Head rotation to weaker side • Supersupraglottic swallow • Thickened liquids • Vocal-fold adduction exercises
Reduced pharyngeal constriction/clearance	• Head rotation to weaker side • Effortful swallow • Mendelsohn maneuver • Multiple swallows • Alternate liquids and solids • Gargle/yawn for tongue-base retraction • Tongue-hold maneuver
Reduced/impaired cricopharyngeal opening	• Head rotation to weaker side • Mendelsohn maneuver • Shaker exercise • Effortful swallow

(ROM: range of motion)

Table 3: Examples for exercises and maneuvers for dysphagia.[6]

Mendelsohn maneuver	• Voluntary prolongation of laryngeal excursion and cricopharyngeal opening during swallowing • Participants initiate the swallow and 'hold' the larynx in the elevated position for 5 seconds using the muscles of the neck
Shaker exercises	• Targets upper esophageal sphincter dysphagia • Patients lie flat on their back and lift the head 4 inches and look at their toes without lifting the shoulders • Extended or repetitive format
Effortful swallow	• Targets reduced pharyngeal peristalsis with residue after swallow • Participant swallows hard, squeezing the tongue and walls of the throat together
Supraglottic swallow	Targets decreased airway protection, aspiration by increasing airway protection with closure of true vocal folds dispels residue above the glottis after the swallow
Compensatory positions	• *Chin tuck/chin to chest:* Help with reduced bolus control, premature spillage into larynx decreased tongue base movement • *Head rotation to affected side:* Compensatory measure for unilateral pharyngeal paresis or unilateral vocal fold dysfunction or cricopharyngeal dysmotility
Oral stage exercises	Includes lip closure lingual and jaw ROM
Base of tongue exercises	Includes tongue retraction, yawn/gargle, Masako

(ROM: range of motion)

REFERENCES

1. Manikantan K, Khode S, Sayed SI, Roe J, Nutting CM, Rhys-Evans P, et al. Dysphagia in head and neck cancer. Cancer Treat Rev. 2009;35(8):724-32.
2. Govender R, Smith CH, Taylor SA, Barratt H, Gardner B. Swallowing interventions for the treatment of dysphagia after head and neck cancer: a systematic review of behavioural strategies used to promote patient adherence to swallowing exercises. BMC Cancer. 2017;17(1):43.
3. Rosenthal DI, Lewin JS, Eisbruch A. Prevention and treatment of dysphagia and aspiration after chemoradiation for head and neck cancer. J Clin Oncol. 2006;24(17):2636-43.
4. Kendall K. Anatomy and physiology of deglutition. In: Kendall LA (Ed). Dysphagia Assessment and Treatment Planning. San Diego, CA: Plural Publishing; 2008.pp. 27-34
5. Murray T, Carrau RL. Anatomy and function of the swallowing mechanism. In: Clinical Management of Swallowing Disorders. San Diego, CA. Plural Publishing; 2006. pp. 15-33.
6. Murphy BA, Gilbert J. Dysphagia in head and neck cancer patients treated with radiation: assessment, sequelae, and rehabilitation. Semin Radiat Oncol. 2009;19(1):35-42.
7. Plant RL. Anatomy and physiology of swallowing in adults and geriatrics. Otolaryngol Clin North Am. 1998;31(3):477-88.
8. Jean A. Brain stem control of swallowing: neuronal networks and cellular mechanisms. Physiol Rev. 2001;81(2):929-69.
9. Matsuo K, Palmer JB. Anatomy and physiology of feeding and swallowing: normal and abnormal. Phys Med Rehabil Clin N Am. 2008;19(4):691-707.
10. Martin-Harris B, Brodsky M, et al. Breathing and swallowing dynamics across the adult lifespan. Arch Otolaryngol Head Neck Surg. 2005;131(9):762-70.
11. Kronenberger MB, Meyers AD. Dysphagia following head and neck cancer surgery. Dysphagia. 1994;9(4):236-44.
12. Preiksaitis HG, Mayrand S, et al. Coordination of respiration and swallowing: effect of bolus volume in normal adults. Am J Physiol. 1992;263(3 pt 2):R624-30.
13. Aviv J. The normal swallow. In: Murry CA (Ed). Comprehensive Management of Swallowing Disorders. San Diego, CA: Plural Publishing; 2006. pp. 23-29.
14. Aligiakrishna K Bhaji A, Kurian M. Evaluation and management of oropharyngeal dysphagia in different types of dementia: a systematic review. Archives of Gerontology and Geriatrics. 2013;56(1):1-9.
15. Pauloski BR. Rehabilitation of dysphagia following head and neck cancer. Phys Med Rehabil Clin N Am. 2008;19(4): 889-928.
16. McConnel FM, Logemann JA, Rademaker AW, Pauloski BR, Baker SR, J Lewin, et al. Surgical variables affecting postoperative swallowing efficiency in oral cancer patients: a pilot study. Laryngoscope. 1994;104(1 Pt 1): 87-90.
17. Konsulov SS. Surgical treatment of anterolateral tongue carcinoma. Folia Med (Plovdiv). 2005;47(3-4):20-3.
18. Leder SB, Joe JK, Ross DA, Coelho DH, Mendes J. Presence of a tracheostomy tube and aspiration status in early, postsurgical head and neck cancer patients. Head Neck. 2005;27(9):757-61.
19. Pauloski BR, Rademaker AW, Logemann JA, McConnel FMS, Heiser AM, Cardinale S, et al. Surgical variables affecting swallowing in treated oral/oropharyngeal cancer patients. Head Neck. 2004;26:625-36.
20. Jacobson MC, Franssen E, Fliss DM, Birt BD, Gilbert RW. Free forearm flap in oral reconstruction. Arch Otolaryngol Head Neck Surg. 1995;121(9):959-64.
21. Logemann JA, Bytell DE. Swallowing disorders in three types of head and neck surgical patients. Cancer. 1979;81:469-78.
22. Pauloski BR, Logemann JA, Rademaker AW, McConnel FM, Heiser MA, S Cardinale, et al. Speech and swallowing function after anterior tongue and floor of mouth resection with distal flap reconstruction. J Speech Hear Res. 1993; 36(2):267-76.
23. Furia CL, Carrara-de Angelis E, Martins NM, AP Barros, Carneiro B, Kowalski LP. Videofluoroscopic evaluation after glossectomy. Arch Otolaryngol Head Neck Surg. 2000; 126(3):378-83.
24. Zuydam AC, Rogers SN, Brown JS, Vaughan ED, Magennis P. Swallowing rehabilitation after oropharyngeal resection for squamous cell carcinoma. Br J Oral Maxillofac Surg. 2000; 38(5):513-8.
25. McConnel FM, Logemann JA, Rademaker AW, Pauloski BR, Baker SR, Lewin J, Shedd D, et al. Surgical variables affecting postoperative swallowing efficiency in oral cancer patients: a pilot study. Laryngoscope. 1994;104(1 Pt 1):87-90.
26. Hirano M, Kuroiwa Y, Tanaka S, et al. Dysphagia following various degrees of surgical resection for oral cancer. Ann Otol Rhinol Laryngol. 1992;101(2 Pt 1):138-41.
27. Fujimoto Y, Hasegawa Y, Nakayama B, et al. Usefulness and limitation of cricopharyngeal myotomy and laryngeal suspension after wide resection of the tongue or oropharynx. Nippon Jibiinkoka Gakkai Kaiho. 1998;101:307-11.

28. Marchetta FC. Function and appearance following surgery for intraoral cancer. Clin Plast Surg. 1976;3(3):471-9.
29. Christopoulos E, Carrau R, Segas J, Jonhson JT, Meyers EN, Wagner RL, et al. Transmandibular approaches to the oral cavity and oropharynx: a functional assessment. Arch Otolaryngol Head Neck Surg. 1992;118(11): 1164-7.
30. Haribhakti VV, Kavarana NM, Tibrewala AN. Oral cavity reconstruction: an objective assessment of function. Head Neck. 1993;15:119-24.
31. Schliephake H, Ruffert K, Schneller T. Prospective study of the quality of life of cancer patients after intraoral tumor surgery. J Oral Maxillofac Surg. 1996;54:664-9.
32. Curtis DA, Plesh O, Miller AJ, Curtis TA, Sharma A, Schweitzer R, et al. A comparison of masticatory function in patients with or without reconstruction of the mandible. Head Neck. 1998;19:287-96.
33. Urken ML, Buchbinder D, Weinberg H, Vickery C, Sheiner A, Parker R, et al. Functional evaluation following microvascular oromandibular reconstruction of the oral cancer patient: a comparative study of reconstructed and nonreconstructed patients. Laryngoscope. 1991;101(9):935-50.
34. Wells MD, Luce EA. Reconstruction of midfacial defects after surgical resection of malignancies. Clin Plast Surg. 1995;22(1): 79-89.
35. Brown KE. Peripheral consideration in improving obturator retention. J Prosthet Dent. 1968;20(2):176-81.
36. Gaziano JE. Evaluation and management of oropharyngeal dysphagia in head and neck cancer. Cancer Control. 2002; 9(5):400-9.
37. Nixon DW, Heymsfield SB, Cohen AE, Kutner MH, Ansley J, Lawson DH, et al. Protein-calorie undernutrition in hospitalized cancer patients. Am J Med. 1980;68(5):683-90.
38. Hinni ML, Salassa JR, Grant DG, Pearson BW, Hayden RE, Martin A, et al. Transoral laser microsurgery for advanced laryngeal cancer. Arch Otolaryngol Head Neck Surg. 2007; 133(12):1198-204.
39. Pillon J, Gonçalves MI, De Biase NG. Changes in eating habits following total and frontolateral laryngectomy. Sao Paulo Med J. 2004;122(5):195-9.
40. Kandogan T, Sanal A. Quality of life, functional outcome, and voice handicap index in partial laryngectomy patients for early glottis cancer. BMC Ear Nose Throat Disord. 2005;5(1):3.
41. Oysu C, Aslan I. Cricohyoidoepiglottopexy vs near-total laryngectomy with epiglottic reconstruction in the treatment of early glottic carcinoma. Arch Otolaryngol Head Neck Surg. 2006;132(10):1065-8.
42. Rinaldo A, Ferlito A. Open supraglottic laryngectomy. Acta Otolaryngol. 2004;124(7):768-71.
43. Yeager LB, Grillone GA. Organ preservation surgery for intermediate size (T2 and T3) laryngeal cancer. Otolaryngol Clin North Am. 2005;38:11-20.
44. Wein RO, Weber RS. The current role of vertical partial laryngectomy and open supraglottic laryngectomy. Curr Probl Cancer. 2005;29(4):201-14.
45. Litton W, Leonard J. Aspiration after partial laryngectomy: cineradiographic studies. Laryngoscope. 1969;79(5):888-908.
46. Kreuzer SH, Schima W, Schober E, Pokieser P, Kofler G, Lechner G, et al. Complications after laryngeal surgery: videofluoroscopic evaluation of 120 patients. Clin Radiol. 2000;55(10):775-81.
47. Logemann JA, Gibbons PJ, Rademaker AW, Pauloski BR, Kahrilas PJ, Bacon M, et al. Mechanisms of recovery of swallow after supraglottic laryngectomy. J Speech Hear Res. 1994;37(5):965-74.
48. Rademaker AW, Logemann JA, Pauloski BR, Bowman JB, Lazarus CL, Sisson GA, et al. Recovery of postoperative swallowing in patients undergoing partial laryngectomy. Head Neck. 1993;15(4):325-34.
49. Prades JM, Simon PG, Timoshenko AP, Dumollard J-M, Schmitt T, Martian C, et al. Extended and standard supraglottic laryngectomies: a review of 110 patients. Eur Arch Otorhinolaryngol. 2005;262(12):947-52.
50. Lewin JS, Hutcheson KA, Barringer DA, May AH, Roberts DB, Holsinger FC, et al. Functional analysis of swallowing outcomes after supracricoid partial laryngectomy. Head Neck. 2008;30(5):559-66.
51. Lazarus CL. Effects of radiation therapy and voluntary maneuvers on swallow functioning in head and neck cancer patients. Clin Commun Disord. 1993;3(4):11-20.
52. Ogura JH, Biller H, Calcaterra T, Davis WH. Surgical treatment of carcinoma of the larynx, pharynx, base of tongue and cervical esophagus. Int Surg. 1969;52(1):29-40.
53. Sessions D, Zill R, Schwartz J. Deglutition after conservation surgery for cancer of the larynx and hypopharynx. Otolaryngol Head Neck Surg. 1979;87(6):77996.
54. Albergotti WG, Jordan J, Anthony K, Abberbock S, Wasserman-Wincko Tamara, Kim S, et al. A prospective evaluation of short-term dysphagia after transoral robotic surgery for squamous cell carcinoma of the oropharynx. Cancer. 2017;123(16):3132-40.
55. Iseli TA, Kulbersh BD, Iseli CE, Carroll WR, Rosenthal EL, Magnuson JS. Functional outcomes after transoral robotic surgery for head and neck cancer. Otolaryngol Head Neck Surg. 2009;141(2):166-71.
56. Aubry K, Vergez S, de Mones E, Moriniere S, Choussy O, Malard O, et al. Morbidity and mortality revue of the French group of transoral robotic surgery: a multicentric study. J Robot Surg. 2016;10(1):63-7.
57. Cognetti DM, Luginbuhl AJ, Nguyen AL, Curry JM. Early adoption of transoral robotic surgical program: preliminary outcomes. Otolaryngol Head Neck Surg. 2012;147(3):482-8.
58. Hutcheson KA, Warneke CL, Yao CMKL, et al. Dysphagia after primary transoral robotic surgery with neck dissection vs nonsurgical therapy in patients with low- to intermediate-risk oropharyngeal cancer. JAMA Otolaryngol Head Neck Surg. 2019;145(11):1053-63.
59. Crary MA, Glowasky AL. Using botulinum toxin A to improve speech and swallowing function following total laryngectomy. Arch Otolaryngol Head Neck Surg. 1996;122(7):760-3.
60. Balfe DM, Koehler RE, Setzen M, Weyman PJ, Baron RL, Ogura JH. Barium examination of the esophagus after total laryngectomy. Radiology. 1982;143(2):501-8.
61. McConnel FM, Mendelsohn MS, Logemann JA. Examination of swallowing after total laryngectomy using manofluorography. Head Neck Surg. 1986;9:3-12.
62. Duranceau A, Jamieson G, Hurwitz AL, Jones RS, Postlethwait RW, et al. Alteration in esophageal motility after laryngectomy. Am J Surg. 1976;131:305.
63. Hanks JB, Fisher SR, Meyers WC Christian KC, Postlethwait RW, Jones RS, et al. Effect of total laryngectomy on esophageal motility. Ann Otol Rhinol Laryngol. 1981; 90(4 Pt 1):331-4.
64. McConnel FM, Cerenko D, Mendelsohn MS. Dysphagia after total laryngectomy. Otolaryngol Clin North Am. 1988;21: 721-6.
65. deCasso C, Slevin NJ, Homer JJ. The impact of radiotherapy on swallowing and speech in patients who undergo total laryngectomy. Otolaryngol Head Neck Surg. 2008;139:792-7.

66. Ackerstaff AH, Hilgers FJM, Aaronson NK, Balm AJM. Communication, functional disorders and lifestyle changes after total laryngectomy. Clin Otolaryngol. 1994;19:295-300.
67. Pauloski BR, Blom ED, Logemann JA, Hamaker RC. Functional outcome after surgery for prevention of pharyngospasms in tracheoesophageal speakers. Part II: swallow characteristics. Laryngoscope. 1995;105:1104-10.
68. Lewin JA, Barringer DA, May AH, Gillenwater AM, Arnold KA, Roberts DB, et al. Functional outcomes after circumferential pharyngoesophageal reconstruction. Laryngoscope. 2005; 115(7):1266-71.
69. Lazarus CL, Logemann JA, Shi G. Does total laryngectomy improve swallowing after primary treatment of radiotherapy and chemotherapy? A case study. Arch Otolaryngol Head Neck Surg. 2002;128:54-7.
70. Genden EM, Ferlito A, Silver CE, Jacobson AS, Werner JA, Suarez C, et al. Evolution of the management of laryngeal cancer. Oral Oncol. 2007;43(5):431-9.
71. Grau C, Johansen LV, Hansen HS, Andersen E, Godballe C, Andersen LJ, et al. Salvage laryngectomy and pharyngocutaneous fistulae after primary radiotherapy for head and neck cancer: a national survey from DAHANCA. Head Neck. 2003; 25:711-6
72. Ganly I, Patel S, Matsuo J, Singh B, Kraus D, Boyle J, et al. Postoperative complications of salvage total laryngectomy. Cancer. 2005;103:2073-81.
73. Triboulet JP, Mariette C, Chevalier D, Amrouni H. Surgical management of carcinoma of the hypopharynx and cervical esophagus: analysis of 209 cases. Arch Surg. 2001;136:1164-70.
74. Starmer HM, Tippet DC, Webster KT. Effects of laryngeal cancer on voice and swallowing. Otolaryngol Clin N Am. 2008;41(2008):793-818.
75. Yu W, Wu C. Speech therapy after thyroidectomy. Gland Surg. 2017;6(5):501-9
76. Zealear DL, Billante CR. Neurophysiology of vocal fold paralysis. Otolaryngol Clin North Am. 2004;37:1-23.
77. Beatriz Delgado-Vargas B, Azucena Lloris Romero-Salazar AL, Cobeta I. Vocal changes following thyroid surgery: prospective study of objective and subjective parameters. Journal of Voice. 2019;33(1):27-32.
78. Stemple JC. A holistic approach to voice therapy. Semin Speech Lang. 2005;26(2):131-7.
79. Levine TM. Swallowing disorders following skull base surgery. Otolaryngol Clin North Am. 1988;21:751-9.
80. Nguyen NP, Moltz CC, Frank C, Karlsson U, Nguyen PD, Vos P, et al. Dysphagia severity following chemoradiation and postoperative radiation for head and neck cancer. Eur J Radiol. 2006;59(3):453-9.
81. Rubira CMF, Devides NJ, Úbeda LT, Bortolucci Jr AG, Lauris JR, Rubira-Bullen, Damante IRF JH. Evaluation of some oral postradiotherapy sequelae in patients treated for head and neck tumours. Braz Oral Res. 2007;21:272-7.
82. Nicoletti G, Soutar DS, Jackson MS, Wrench AA, Robertson R. Chewing and swallowing after surgical treatment for oral cancer: functional evaluation in 196 selected cases. Plast Reconstr Surg. 2004;114:329-38.
83. Rogers SN, Lowe D, Patel M, Vaughan ED. Clinical function after primary surgery for oral and oro-pharyngeal cancer: an 11-item examination. Br J Oral Maxillofac Surg. 2002;40:1-10.
84. Pauloski BR, Logemann JA. Impact of tongue base and posterior pharyngeal wall biomechanics on pharyngeal clearance in irradiated postsurgical oral and oropharyngeal cancer patients. Head Neck. 2000;22:120-31.
85. Pauloski BR, Rademaker AW, Logemann JA, Colangelo LA. Speech and swallowing in irradiated and nonirradiated postsurgical oral cancer patients. Otolaryngol Head Neck Surg. 1998;118:616-24.
86. Goguen LA, Posner M, Norris CM, Tishler RB, Wirth LJ, Annino DJ, et al. Dysphagia after sequential chemoradiation-therapy for advanced head and neck cancer. Otolaryngol Head Neck Surg. 2006;134:916-22.
87. Carrara-de Angelis E, Feher O, Barros APB, Nishimoto IN, Kowalski LP. Voice and swallowing in patients enrolled in a larynx preservation trial. Arch Otolaryngol Head Neck Surg. 2003;129:733.
88. Wu C, Hsiao TY, Ko JY, Hsu MM. Dysphagia after radiotherapy: endoscopic examination of swallowing in patients with nasopharyngeal carcinoma. Ann Otol Rhinol Laryngol. 2000;109: 320-5.
89. Chang YC, Chen SY, Lui LT, Wang TG, Wang TC, Hsiao TY, et al. Dysphagia in patients with nasopharyngeal cancer after radiation therapy: a videofluoroscopic swallowing study. Dysphagia. 2003;18:135-43.
90. Eisbruch A, Lyden T, Bradford CR, Dawson LA, Haxer MJ, Miller AE, et al. Objective assessment of swallowing dysfunction and aspiration after radiation concurrent with chemotherapy for head and neck cancer. Int J Radiat Oncol Biol Phys. 2002;53:23-8.
91. Lazarus CL, Logemann JA, Pauloski BR, Colangelo LA, Kahrilas PJ, Mittal BB, et al. Swallowing disorders in head and neck cancer patients with radiotherapy and adjuvant chemotherapy. Laryngoscope. 1996;106:1157-66.
92. Graner DE, Foote RL, Kasperbauer JL, Stoeckel RE, Okuno SH, Olsen KD, et al. Swallow function in patients before and after intra-arterial chemoradiation. Laryngoscope. 2003;113:573-9.
93. Eisele DW, Koch DG, Tarazi AE, Jones B. Aspiration from delayed radiation fibrosis of the neck. Dysphagia. 1991;6: 120-2.
94. Smith RV, Kotz T, Beitler JJ, Wadler S. Long-term swallowing problems after organ preservation therapy with concomitant radiation therapy and intravenous hydroxyurea. Arch Otolaryngol Head Neck Surg. 2000;126:384-9.
95. Kotz T, Abraham S, Beitler JJ, Wadler S. Pharyngeal transport dysfunction consequent to an organ-sparing protocol. Arch Otolaryngol Head Neck Surg. 1999;125:410-3.
96. Kotz T, Costello R, Li Y, Posner MR. Swallowing dysfunction after chemoradiation for advanced squamous cell carcinoma of the head and neck. Head Neck. 2004;26:365-72.
97. Kaneko M, Shirato H, Nishioka T, Okhmori K, Takinami S, Arimoto T, et al. Scintigraphic evaluation of long-term salivary function after bilateral whole parotid gland irradiation in radiotherapy for head and neck tumour. Oral Oncol. 1998; 34(2):140-6.
98. Franzen L, Funegard U, Ericson T, Henriksson R. Parotid gland function during and following radiotherapy of malignancies in the head and neck: a consecutive study of salivary flow and patient discomfort. Eur J Cancer. 1992;28(2-3):457-62.
99. Logemann JA, Smith CH, Pauloski BR, Rademaker AW, Lazarus CL, Colangelo LA, et al. Effects of xerostomia on perception and performance of swallow function. Head Neck. 2001;23(4):317-21.
100. Lalla RV, Peterson DE. Treatment of mucositis, including new medications. Cancer J. 2006;12(5):348-54.
101. Stokman MA, Spijkervet FK, Boezen HM Schouten JP, Roodenburg JLN, de VriesEGE. Preventive intervention possibilities in radiotherapy- and chemotherapy-induced

oral mucositis: results of meta-analyses. J Dent Res. 2006; 85(8):690-700.
102. Nguyen NP, Vos P, Smith HJ, Nguyen PD, Alfieri A, Karlsson U, et al. Concurrent chemoradiation for locally advanced Oropharyngeal cancer. Am J Otolaryngol. 2007;28:3-8
103. Nguyen NP, Moltz CC, Frank C, Vos P, Smith HJ, Karlsson U, et al. Evolution of chronic dysphagia following treatment for head and neck cancer. Oral Oncol. 2006;42:374-80.
104. Bleier BS, Levine MS, Mick R, Rubesin SE, Sack SZ, McKinney K, et al. Dysphagia after chemoradiation: analysis by modified barium swallow. Ann Otol Rhinol Laryngol. 2007;116:837-41.
105. Laurell G, Kraepelien T, Mavroidis P, Lind BK, Fernberg JO, Beckman M, et al. Stricture of the proximal esophagus in head and neck carcinoma patients after radiotherapy. Cancer. 2003;97:1693-700.
106. Corry J, Poon W, McPhee N, Milner AD, Cruickshank D, Porceddu SV, et al. Randomized study of percutanous endoscopic gastrostomy versus nasogastric tube for enteral feeding in head and neck cancer patients treated with (Chemo)radiation. J Med Imaging Radiat Oncol. 2008;52: 503-10.
107. Lee WT, Akst LM, Adelstein DJ, Saxton JP, Wood BG, Strome M, et al. Risk factors for hypopharyngeal/upper esophageal stricture formation after concurrent chemoradiation. Head Neck. 2006;28:808-12.
108. Franzmann EJ, Lundy DS, Abitbol AA, Goodwin WJ. Complete hypopharyngeal obstruction by mucosal adhesions: a complication of intensive chemoradiation for advanced head and neck cancer. Head Neck. 2006;28:663-70.
109. Agarwala SS, Sbeitan I. Iatrogenic swallowing disorders: chemotherapy. In: Carrau RL, Murry T (Eds). Comprehensive management of swallowing disorders. San Diego, CA: Singular Publishing Group; 1999. pp. 125-9.
110. Steel GG. Terminology in the description of drug-radiation interactions. Int J Radiat Oncol Biol Phys. 1979;5:1145-50.
111. Murry T, Madasu R, Martin A, Robbins KT. Acute and chronic changes in swallowing and quality of life following intra-arterial chemoradiation for organ preservation in patients with advanced head and neck cancer. Head Neck. 1998;20: 31-7.
112. Martini DV, Har-El G, Lucente FE, Slavit DH. Swallowing and pharyngeal function in postoperative pharyngeal cancer patients. Ear Nose Throat J. 1997;76:450-6.
113. Tei K, Maekawa K, Kitada H, Ohiro Y, Yamazaki Y, Totsuka Y. Recovery from post-surgical swallowing dysfunction in patients with oral cancer. J Maxillofac Surg. 2007;65:1077-83.
114. Baek S, Lawson W, Biller H. An analysis of 133 pectoralis major myocutaneous flaps. Plast Reconstr Surg. 1982;69: 460-7.
115. Logemann JA. Evaluation and treatment of swallowing disorders, 2nd edn. Austin (TX): Prod Ed; 1998.
116. Mathers-Schmidt BA, Kurlinski M. Dysphagia evaluation practices: in consistencies in clinical assessment and instrumental examination decision-making. Dysphagia. 2003;18:114-25.
117. Doggett DL, Turkelson CM, Coates V. Recent developments in diagnosis and intervention for aspiration and dysphagia in stroke and other neuromuscular disorders. Curr Atheroscler Rep. 2002;4:304-11.
118. Martin-Harris B, Logemann JA, McMahon S, Schleicher M, Sandidge J. Clinical utility of the modified barium swallow. Dysphagia. 2000;15:136-41.
119. Kraaijenga SA, van der Molen L, van den Brekel MW, Hilgers FJ. Current assessment and treatment strategies of dysphagia in head and neck cancer patients: a systematic review of the 2012/13 literature. Curr Opin Support Palliat Care. 2014;8(2):152-63.
120. Mittal BB, Pauloski BR, Haraf DJ, Pelzer HJ, Argiris A, Vokes EE, et al. Swallowing dysfunction-preventative and rehabilitation strategies in patients with head-and-neck cancers treated with surgery, radiotherapy, and chemotherapy: a critical review. Int J Radiat Oncol Biol Phys. 2003; 57:1219-30.
121. Kulbersh BD, Rosenthal EL, McGrew BM, Duncan RD, McColloch NL, Carroll WR, et al. Pretreatment, preoperative swallowing exercises may improve dysphagia quality of life. Laryngoscope. 2006;116:883-7.
122. Carroll WR, Locher JL, Canon CL, Bohannon IA, McColloch AL, et al. Pretreatment swallowing exercises improve swallow function after chemoradiation. Laryngoscope. 2008;118:39-44.
123. Lazarus C. Tongue strength and exercise in healthy individuals and in head and neck cancer patients. Semin Speech Lang. 2006;27:260-7
124. Krisciunas GP, Castellano K, McCulloch TM, Lazarus CL, Pauloski BR, Meyer TK, et al. Impact of compliance on dysphagia rehabilitation in head and neck cancer patients: results from a multi-center clinical trial. Dysphagia. 2017; 32(2):327-36.
125. Kraaijenga SA, van der Molen L, van den Brekel MW, Hilgers FJ. Current assessment and treatment strategies of dysphagia in head and neck cancer patients: a systematic review of the 2012/13 literature. Curr Opin Support Palliat Care. 2014;8(2):152-63.
126. van der Molen L, van Rossum MA, Rasch CR, Smeele LE, Hilgers FJ. Two-year results of a prospective preventive swallowing rehabilitation trial in patients treated with chemoradiation for advanced head and neck cancer. Eur Arch Otorhinolaryngol. 2014;271(5):1257-70.
127. Carnaby-Mann G, Crary MA, Schmalfuss I, Amdur R. Pharyngocise': randomized controlled trial of preventive exercises to maintain muscle structure and swallowing function during head-and-neck chemoradiotherapy. Int J Radiat Oncol Biol Phys. 2012; 83:2109.
128. Martin-Harris B, Brodsky MB, Michel Y, Ford CL, Walters B, Heffner J. Breathing and swallowing dynamics across the adult lifespan. Arch Otolaryngol Head Neck Surg. 2005; 131(9):762-70.
129. Logemann J. Evaluation of swallowing disorders. In: Evaluation and Treatment of Swallowing Disorders. Austin, TX: Pro-ed; 1998. p 181.
130. Leonard R, McKenzie S, Goodrich S. The treatment plan. In: Kendall LA (Ed). Dysphagia Assessment and Treatment Planning. San Diego, CA: Plural Publishing; 2008. pp. 304-8.
131. Murry T. Therapeutic intervention for swallowing disorders. In: Murry CA (Ed). Comprehensive Management of Swallowing Disorders. San Diego, CA: Plural Publishing; 2006. pp. 244-5.
132. Murry T. Nonsurgical treatment of swallowing disorders. Clinical Management of Swallowing Disorders. San Diego, CA: Plural Publishing; 2006. p. 152.
133. Leonard R, McKenzie S, Goodrich S. The treatment plan. In: Leonard R, Kendall LA (Eds): Dysphagia Assessment and Treatment Planning. San Diego, CA: Plural Publishing; 2008. pp. 301-2.

134. Langmore SE, McCulloch TM, Krisciunas GP, Lazarus CL, Van Daele DJ, Pauloski BR, et al. Efficacy of electrical stimulation and exercise for dysphagia in patients with head and neck cancer: a randomized clinical trial. Head Neck. 2016;38(Suppl 1):E1221-31.
135. Carnaby-Mann GD, Crary MA. Examining the evidence on neuromuscular electrical stimulation for swallowing: a meta-analysis. Arch Otolaryngol Head Neck Surg. 2007; 133:564-71.
136. Shama L, Connor NP, Ciucci MR, McCulloch TM. Surgical treatment of dysphagia. Phys Med Rehabil Clin N Am. 2008;19(4):817-35.
137. Dwivedi RC, St Rose S, Chisholm EJ, Georgalas C, Bisase B, Amen F, et al. Evaluation of swallowing by Sydney swallow questionnaire (SSQ) in oral and oropharyngeal cancer patients treated with primary surgery. Dysphagia. 2012;27:491-7.
138. Batth SS, Caudell JJ, Chen AM. Practical considerations in reducing swallowing dysfunction following concurrent chemoradiotherapy with intensity-modulated radiotherapy for head and neck cancer. Head Neck; 2014. pp. 291-8.
139. List MA, Ritter-Sterr C, Lansky SB. A performance status scale for head and neck cancer patients. Cancer. 1990;66:564-9.
140. Belafsky PC, Mouadeb DA, Rees CJ, Pryor JC, Postma GN, Allen J, et al. Validity and reliability of the Eating Assessment Tool (EAT-10). Ann Otol Rhinol Laryngol. 2008;117(12): 919-24.
141. Wang K, Amdur RJ, Mendenhall WM, Green R, Aumer S, Hackman TG, et al. Impact of post-chemoradiotherapy superselective/selective neck dissection on patient reported quality of life. Oral Oncol. 2016;58:21-6.
142. Martin-Harris B, Brodsky MB, Michel Y, Castell DO, Schleicher M, Sandidge J, et al. MBS measurement tool for swallow impairment-MBSImp: establishing a standard. Dysphagia. 2008;23:392-405.
143. Hutcheson KA, Lewin JS, Barringer DA, Lisec A, Gunn B, Moore MWS, et al. Late dysphagia after radiotherapy-based treatment of head and neck cancer. Cancer. 2012;118(23): 5793-9.
144. Chen AY, Frankowski R, Bishop-Leone J, Hebert T, Leyk S, Lewin J, et al. The development and validation of a dysphagia-specific quality-of-life questionnaire for patients with head and neck cancer: the MD Anderson dysphagia inventory. Arch Otolaryngol Head Neck Surg. 2001;127(7):870-6.
145. Hutcheson KA, Barrow MP, Barringer DA, Knott JK, Lin HY, Weber RS, et al. Dynamic Imaging Grade of Swallowing Toxicity (DIGEST): scale development and validation. Cancer. 2017;123(1):62-70.
146. McHorney CA, Robbins J, Lomax K, Rosenbek JC, Chignell K, Kramer AE, et al. The SWAL-QOL and SWAL-CARE outcomes tool for oropharyngeal dysphagia in adults: III. Documentation of reliability and validity. Dysphagia. 2002;17:97-114.
147. Ghazali N, Kanatas A, Scott B, Lowe D, Zuydam A, Rogers SN, et al. Use of the Patient Concerns Inventory to identify speech and swallowing concerns following treatment for oral and oropharyngeal cancer. J Laryngol Otol. 2012;126:800-8.
148. O'Neil KH, Purdy M, Falk J, Gallo L. The Dysphagia Outcome and Severity Scale. Dysphagia. 1999;14:139-45.
149. Goepfert RP, Lewin JS, Barrow MP, Warneke CL, Fuller CD, Lai SY, et al. Grading dysphagia as a toxicity of head and neck cancer: differences in severity classification based on MBS DIGEST and clinical CTCAE grades. Dysphagia. 2018;33(2):185-91.
150. Morrison. Manual Of Clinical Nutrition Management. Inc (A Sector of compass group inc); 2013. pp. 6-8.
151. Logemann JA. Approaches to management of disordered swallowing. Bailliere's Clinical Gastroenterology. 1991;5(2): 269-80.

CHAPTER 43

Rehabilitation of Trismus, Lymphedema, Shoulder Dysfunction and Vocal Cord Palsy

Samskruthi P Murthy, Trupti Kolur, Sivakumar Vidhyadharan, Narayana Subramaniam

INTRODUCTION

With improved treatment and life expectancy, management of treatment-related complications in patients of head and neck cancer (HNC) is an important consideration. Very often these conditions are neglected resulting in poor quality of life (QoL). Although these often cannot be completely eliminated, early and aggressive management of these conditions can limit their severity and the resultant disability that survivors have to deal with. In this chapter we cover the management of secondary lymphedema, trismus, shoulder dysfunction, and laryngeal nerve dysfunction.

SECONDARY LYMPHEDEMA

The head and neck region has a rich plexus of the lymphatic system. Surgery and radiotherapy (RT) form the cornerstone for treating HNC. Commonly both treatment modalities disrupt lymphatic drainage of the head and neck region to cause lymphedema.[1-3] Lymphedema is an abnormal accumulation of protein-rich lymphatic fluid in the interstitial space.[4] Lymphedema is a common complication following HNC treatment and is most often neglected and overlooked. It significantly causes functional impairment, which in turn, results in a lower QoL.[5,6] Primary lymphedema is an inherent congenital malformation or a dysfunctional lymphatic system, while lymphedema that develops as a result of damage to existing normal lymphatic structures is termed as secondary lymphedema.[7] The head and neck cancer-related lymphedema (HNL) can be further divided into external and internal lymphedema. External lymphedema is characterized by involvement of external structures of face and neck while internal lymphedema involves internal structures of the upper aerodigestive tract.[8] Nevertheless, most of HNL secondary to cancer treatment have a combination of both. The following section describes in brief about secondary lymphedema of the head and neck region as a consequence of HNC treatment.

Lymphatic System

The lymphatic system, like the blood circulation system, exists that drains lymphatic fluid from peripheral tissue into a central circulating system. Most superficial lymphatic capillary vessels are nestled between arterial capillaries and venules that are permeable to lymphatic fluid.[9] The superficial system is devoid of valves and hence forms the basis of manual lymphatic drainage therapy, where lymph from one area can be milked to an area of normal lymphatic flow. The vessels progressively become larger (precollecting, collecting, trunks, and ducts) and contain valves to prevent backflow. Lymphatic system lacks a central pump like a heart for blood circulation; hence larger lymphatic vessels propel lymphatic to larger vessels and deeper system. These segmented contracting regions are called lymphagions.[4] Muscle contraction and compression of soft tissue facilitate lymph flow. About 75% of the body's lymphatic drain into left venous angle (junction of subclavian and jugular vein).[9] The other 25% of the body lymph drain into right venous angle (right upper limb, right upper chest, right neck, and head). The primary function of lymphatic capillaries is to maintain fluid balance in the interstitial space, and they carry the capacity to pump fluid ten times the normal if the need arises. Capillary pressure, negative interstitial pressure, interstitial fluid colloid osmotic pressure and plasma colloid osmotic pressure play an essential role in absorbing fluid from interstitial space.[9] Lymphatic system additionally regulates lipid absorption, removes cellular debris, and performs immune cell trafficking.

Causes and Pathophysiology

All treatment modalities used in the management of HNC can cause lymphedema. The head and neck contains approximately 300 lymph nodes to effectively drain lymphatics of the region effectively.[10] HNL has been reported in 75% of cases treated with surgery or radiotherapy.[5,11] Neck dissection, depending on extent of nodal clearance, can remove up to 30–40 lymph nodes during neck dissection. The postsurgery fibrosis can hinder the lymphatic pump mechanism by impending muscle movement. Surgery causes direct anatomic disruption of lymphatic and venous drainage system and lead to HNL.[5,11] The surgical incisions cause watershed areas for lymphatic drainage. The scar tissue acts as a barrier for drainage and can cause HNL above the level of the scar but not below.[12] Surgery by virtue of the removal of the lymphatic system and poor drainage mechanism can alone cause lymphedema. The boundaries of flap inset can hamper lymphatic drainage.

Radiotherapy also includes lymphatic drainage area at risk into the treatment field—the postradiation fibrosis of lymphatic channels and reduced muscle movement due to fibrosis causes lymphedema.[11] RT causes tissue fibrosis that impairs lymphatic drainage by reducing tissue elasticity and constricting vascular flow. It takes 8–12 weeks postradiotherapy treatment for HNL to develop; this could be related to the time RT-induced fibrosis sets in.[11] The mild edema that occurs acutely during the radiation course is most often inflammatory and subsides in a few weeks; however, in due course of time, the reparative process is pathological, resulting in new collagen synthesis by myofibroblasts, which exceeds degradation resulting in overproduction of extracellular matrix and permanent fibrosis and/or lymphedema. Combined lymphatic and venous disruptions can cause mixed edema, which is more resistant to treatment.[4]

Taxane-based chemotherapy is associated with lymphedema of breast cancer while there is no reported evidence of this in HNL.[13] However, taxane-based chemotherapy is uncommonly used in the curative treatment of HNC.

Clinical Presentation

The disease manifestation is a dynamic process, which in early phases presents with heaviness and tightness with no visible edema. Later stages presents with edema, which pits on pressure and in final phases results in severe fibrosis and functional impairment.[4] External HNL is commonly detected as diffused swelling which may be generalized or limited to an area in head and neck based on the extent of cancer-related treatment. On palpation, the swelling may be boggy, soft, or firm, based on duration of HNL.[4] The diagnosis of HNL must be a diagnosis of exclusion. Various disorders can cause edema that mimic HNL-like inflammation, venous thrombosis, hypothyroidism, and localized infection.[4] Tumor relapse can be associated with significant edema and must always be ruled out before making a diagnosis of lymphedema. Internal HNL present with varied symptoms such as dysphagia, breathing difficulty, and voice changes.

Impact on Quality of Life

An HNL impacts QoL at various domains. HNL may result in severe functional dysfunction in communication, alimentation, and respiration.[6] Respiratory impairment can be a consequence of internal laryngeal lymphedema and external HNL can lead to stomal narrowing impeding stomal hygiene, voice prosthesis management, and respiration in postlaryngectomy patients.[14,15] The facial disfigurement due to significant HNL can result in psychological distress. Management of HNL in early phases is essential to improve patients QoL. Deng et al. evaluated QoL in 103 HNC patients in 3 months post-treatment period, reporting that the severity of internal and external lymphedema correlated with physical and psychological domain. The overall severity of HNL was associated with symptom burden, functional status, and QoL.[6]

Assessment

Most evaluation methods are well defined concerning lymphedema of extremities. Assessment modalities of head and neck region are sparse. The measurement modalities can be broadly classified into patient-reported outcomes, clinician reported outcomes, and technical capacity/measurement techniques.

Patient-reported Outcome Measures

Measuring patient-reported outcomes in all cases of suspected HNL is essential to capture the full spectrum of symptoms and functional impacts of lymphedema. Various symptom-specific measurement tools such as MD Anderson symptom inventory-head and neck module, Vanderbilt Head and Neck Symptom Survey, Head and Neck Distress Scale, Head and Neck Symptom Checklist and the National Comprehensive Cancer Network—Functional Assessment exists in the literature but fail to incorporate symptoms domain that is related to HNL. Symptoms such as neck tightness, restricted range of movements of neck are specific to HNL, which are often missed out in the most QoL questionnaires.[16] The Lymphedema Symptom Intensity & Distress Survey-Head & Neck (LSIDS-H&N) is the only existing patient-reported outcome available.[17] It consists of a 65-item symptom tool. The study has validated the tool, which is feasible, readable, and convenient to use. The tool efficiently captures critical and unique symptoms of HNL; however, further testing in a larger sample size is needed.

Clinician-reported Outcome Measures

- *External lymphedema:* Stages of lymphedema (Földi's Scale) are one of the most commonly used grading systems to evaluate lymphedema at any site in the body.[11] Common Terminology Criteria for Adverse Events (CTCAE) and the American Cancer Society (ACS) Scale are specific to head and neck subsites.[18] While their comparison in assessing HNL has shown that they capture features that are specific to HNL, they do not assess edema and fibrosis that commonly coexist and have been not validated. The MD Anderson Cancer Center (MDACC) Head and Neck Lymphedema (MDACC-HNL) Rating Scale has been developed to overcome the limitations of measurement tools mentioned above.[19] However, the MDACC-HNL rating scale also lacks validity and reliability. Edema and fibrosis are intricately linked and commonly coexist. Intense fibrosis can result in lymphedema and long-standing untreated lymphedema progress to fibrosclerotic changes. Hence, a recent publication in 2015 has reported clinician-reported outcome measure that captures both edema and fibrosis.[20] The preliminary report of the measurement tool has been represented in **Table 1**.[20] The tool involves assessment of involved site followed by evaluation of type and grade of changes. However, further validation of this grading system is required for its routine clinical use.
- *Internal lymphedema:* The Radiation Therapy Oncology Group (RTOG), the European Organization for Research and Treatment of Cancer (EORTC) system, and the Late Effects Normal Tissues–Subjective Objective Management Analytic (LENT–SOMA) system have been described to grade laryngeal edema secondary to radiation toxicity.[21-23] However, they fail to evaluate other areas that are also affected by internal lymphedema. The Patterson scale **(Table 2)** uses endoscopic evaluation to grade internal edema and covers eleven structures and two spaces **(Fig. 1)**.[24] This is more comprehensive as multiple sites are evaluated and graded. The inter-rater rating reliability was better between normal versus severe edema than between mild and moderate grades. The reliability was higher in aryepiglottic folds, arytenoids, epiglottis, false cords, and inter arytenoid region,[24] while other subsites had a lower agreement

Table 1: External lymphedema grading system.[22]

Subsite	*Type*	*Grade*
• Left periorbital region • Right periorbital region • Left cheek • Right cheek • Submental region	*Type A:* No visible tissue swelling; palpable thickening; and/or tightness of dermis	–
	Type B: Visible soft tissue swelling; involved tissues are soft to touch; tissue swelling is reducible and fluctuates in severity	*Grade:* • *Mild:* Visible soft tissue swelling on close inspection • *Moderate:* Easily visible swelling that significantly alters • Normal tissue contours • *Severe:* Extreme or massive tissue swelling
	Type C: Visible soft tissue swelling; involved tissues are firm to touch; tissue swelling is non-reducible and persistent	*Grade:* • Mild • Moderate • Severe
	Type D: Firm skin with increased density and decreased compliance in the absence of swelling	*Grade:* • Mild • Moderate • Severe
Smith et al. (MDACC-HNL rating scale) and Földi's scale[10,19]		
0: No visible edema but patient reports heaviness 1a: Soft visible edema; no pitting, reversible 1b: Soft pitting edema; reversible 2: Firm pitting edema; not reversible; no tissue changes 3: Irreversible; tissue changes		

Table 2: Patterson scale for measuring internal lymphedema.[24]

Components	Structures	Spaces
	• Posterior pharyngeal wall • Epiglottis • Pharyngoepiglottic folds • Aryepiglottic folds • Interarytenoid space • Cricopharyngeal prominence • Arytenoids • False vocal folds • True vocal folds • Anterior commissure	• Valleculae • Pyriform sinus
Grade	• Normal • Mild • Moderate • Severe	• Normal • Mildly reduced • Moderately reduced • Severely reduced

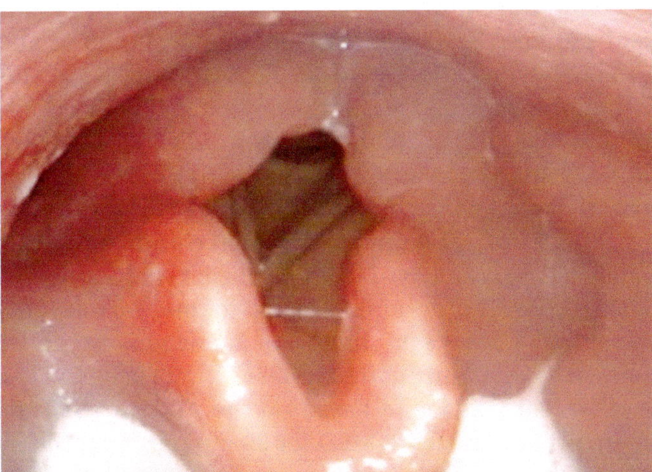

Fig. 1: Endoscopic image showing internal laryngeal edema.

between the observers. The inter-rater reliability needs to be higher for routine clinical use, and additional oral cavity structures will make the assessment more comprehensive.

Technical Capacity/Measurement Techniques

Tape measurement: Tape measurement has been a standard in assessing lymphedema of extremities. While their use in assessing HNL is limited due to variable measuring references. The MDACC-HNL rating scale utilizes various landmarks in the face and neck.[19] The ALOHA trial utilized MDACC-HNL rating scale measures and reported good inter-rater reliability.[25] The trial also described various circumferential measurements, which also showed excellent inter-rater reliability. **Table 3** represents various tape measurement protocols.

Digital photography: Digital photography is effective in documenting external lymphedema over time. The external lymphedema is most often asymmetrical and develops insidiously and may not be perceived by the patient or patient family. Hence, documenting digital photography serves as an excellent reference to compare. The photos must be taken in the same position each time for accurate comparisons. Photography allows for multiple inter- and intra-rater measurements. However, it lacks to add on textural data and quality of skin and soft tissues.

Imaging techniques: Imaging techniques are rarely used to make a diagnosis of HNL, while imaging modalities aid in evaluating response to treatment and supplement data gathered by history and clinical examination.

Table 3: Various tape measurement protocols for head and neck lymphedema.

MDACC-HNL rating scale[19]	*ALOHA trial protocol*[25]

• Facial circumference
  – *Diagonal:* Chin to crown of head
• *Submental:* <1 cm in front of ear, vertical tape alignment
• Point to point
  – Mandibular angle to mandibular angle
  – Tragus to tragus
  – Facial composite
    - Tragus to mental protuberance
    - Tragus to mouth angle
    - Mandibular angle to nasal wing
    - Mandibular angle to internal eye corner
    - Mandibular angle to external eye corner
    - Mental protuberance to internal eye corner
    - Mandibular angle to mental protuberance
Neck circumferences
• *Superior neck:* Immediately beneath mandible
• *Medial neck:* Midway between point 1 and 3
• *Inferior neck:* Lowest circumferential level
	• *Lower neck circumference:* Lowest possible neck circumference taken superior to the angle of the neck and shoulder
	• *Upper neck circumference:* Highest neck circumference measured inferior to the mandible
	• *Length from ear to ear:* Inferior junction of ear lobe and face on the left to inferior junction of ear lobe and face on right intersecting a point 8 cm inferior to the lower lip edge
	• *Length from lip to lower neck circumference:* Inferior lower lip edge to lower neck circumference in midline

Modalities to evaluate functional lymphatic structures: Lymphangiography, lymphoscintigraphy, and NIR (near-infrared) fluorescence imaging aid in mapping functionality of lymphatic structures. Their use is well defined in extremities while their application in HNL is limited. Lymphangiography and lymphoscintigraphy are both invasive methods, and their routine use in HNL has little value. NIR fluorescence, even though noninvasive their role in HNL is not established.

Modalities to evaluate tissue changes: The role of computed tomography (CT) and magnetic resonance imaging (MRI) has been well defined in evaluating lymphedema of extremities. They aid in evaluating fluid accumulation, tissue changes, and fibrotic changes. They also help in evaluating internal edema in HNL. A report has shown that CT scan is reliable in evaluating lymphedema changes in critical structures such as epiglottis and prevertebral tissue.[26] However, methodological protocol in assessing and grading HNL using CT/MRI needs validation.

High-resolution ultrasound: It is an effective method in assessing skin and soft-tissue changes in breast cancer patients. Ultrasound is useful in identifying normal versus abnormal tissue changes and scar thickness. Strain elastography allows for estimation and imaging tissue elasticity distribution within tissue. Elastography uses conventional real-time ultrasonography with elastography software.[27] The fibrotic soft-tissue changes that occur in HNL do affect tissue elasticity, and assessing the same can be invaluable. Strain elastography can objectively measure tissue changes; however, its routine use needs further validation.

Moisture Meter D (MMD): Moisture Meter D (MMD; Delfin Technologies Ltd, Kuopio, Finland) objectively measures tissue dielectric constant (TDC). An ultrahigh-frequency (300 MHz) probe is placed on the skin, which measures TDC, which represents the amount of free and bound water contained within the volume of tissue being measured. The electromagnetic energy emitted is partially absorbed by the water, and the rest is reflected coaxially.[7] Pure water has a TDC reading of 78.5. The TDC reading ranges from 1 to 80 based on the amount of water content with higher reading representing higher water content. MMD shows excellent correlation with HNL, with good intra-rater and inter-rater reliability.

Management

Manual Lymphatic Drainage

Emil Vodder first described manual lymphatic drainage (MLD) in 1930s.[28] MLD consists of circular gentle massage strokes that are applied to the skin to direct lymph to the area of lymphatic drainage area. At present MLD is used along with complete decongestive therapy.

Complete Decongestive Therapy

Complete decongestive therapy (CDT) is the current standard of care in the management of lymphedema. Földi is credited for combining MLD, compression bandages, skincare and physical exercises that comprise components of CDT. CDT consists of two phases; the initial phase consists of intensive phase that will be at the outpatient department for 3–5 days a week for 2–4 weeks, followed by a continuation phase that slow transit from outpatient setting to at-home therapy. Patient and patient caregiver responsibility and strict adherence to the treatment regime at home are essential for best response. The primary aim in CDT is to allow decongestion of the edematous area, prevent refilling, and promote drainage. MLD allows decongestion and promotes lymphatic flow, while physical exercise that aids lymph drainage and compression therapy that prevents refilling of edema in the affected area. The efficacy of CDT in HNL was evaluated by Smith et al., who reported a response of 60% in patients with soft pitting lymphedema. Treatment adherence independently predicted response to CDT. A recent pilot study evaluated HNL therapy program in ten patients.[29] The study included 4 weeks of intensive management phase followed by continuation phase for 22 weeks. The assessment was made based on the ALOHA trial; the therapist administered MLD for 30 minutes followed by application of kinesio tape to promote pattern of drainage development for self-lymphatic drainage. Patient was provided with adequate education about HNL and a self-administered therapy program. Neck exercises included flexion, extension, rotation and lateral flexion. Compression bandage (lipomed face compression with foam inserts) was used for 4 hours during the day and gradually increased to overnight use as tolerated. The study showed significant reduction in HNL with the therapy program.[29] However, the study included only 10 patients and further validation of the program is necessary.

Pharmacotherapy

Use of pharmacotherapy in the management of HNL is limited. The efficacy of sodium selenite in management of HNL at 350 $\mu g/m^2$ body surface area of sodium selenite orally daily for 4–6 weeks was administered. 75% showed an improvement in lymphedema and also better QoL.[29,30] Anti-inflammatory drugs (corticosteroids, D-Penicillamine, and colchicine), vascular-targeted therapies [pentoxifylline, hyperbaric oxygen therapy, and angiotensin-converting enzyme (ACE) inhibitors], and antioxidants (liposomal superoxide dismutase, and vitamin E) have been tested in clinical studies in the management of radiation-induced fibrosis, their role in managing HNL has not been evaluated.[31]

Low-level Light Therapy

Low-level light therapy (LLLT) utilizes low power laser or light-emitting diode (LED) to promote tissue repair, reduce inflammation, and edema. The device emits light in the red/infrared light spectrum (600–1,000 nm) with irradiance in the range of 5 μW–5 W/cm^2. Treatment is recommended weekly or more frequent setting based on severity with treatment time per point of 30–60 seconds. HNL approximately requires ten or more sessions to achieve adequate response. Lee et al. have reported efficacy of LLLT in management of HNL however, further validation is necessary.[32]

Surgical Management

Surgical management is advocated when nonsurgical methods fail. Lymphaticovenous anastomosis can be created with functional dilated lymphatic vessel and venous circulation. The lymphatic vessel is identified using fluorescent lymphangiography with indocyanine green dye for near-infrared fluorescence labeling. The anastomosis is challenging, as the vessel wall thickness is approximately 0.3–0.5 mm. About 8–12 months may be required to observe visible changes after surgery.[33,34] The therapeutic response is not rapid and prolonged period of follow-up is required various studies have shown good response with lymphaticovenous anastomosis. A lymphatic bridge can be used as a last option in severe unresponsive cases. An area that drains into the normal lymphatic system is harvested and transferred on to upper part of lymphedema area, and then CDT/MLD is initiated to drain lymph from the collection area to normal area of drainage.[35]

TRISMUS

Introduction

Trismus refers to inability to open mouth. The term trismus is derived from the Greek word "trismos," which means grinding, grating, or squeaking.[36,37] Various definitions exist to describe trismus; the most accepted definition is a tonic contraction of the muscles of mastication, and as mandibular hypomobility, which results in a limited ability to open the mouth.[38,39] Trismus is caused by varied reasons, which include pathology that affects the mandible and muscles of mastication. The following section briefly describes the management of trismus secondary to treatment of HNC.

Prevalence

The reported rates of prevalence of trismus are a wide range from 0 to 100% depending on the site of the tumor and its extension.[40-42] The definitions of trismus and assessment methods are varied across existing literature, and this makes interpretation of prevalence of trismus difficult. A mouth opening of <35 mm is generally considered as trismus in HNC patients.[43] The prevalence of trismus ranges from 0 to 69% in patients with oral and oropharyngeal cancer,[44,45] 5–32% in maxillary sinus cancer,[43,45] 0–36% in nasopharyngeal cancer patients,[42,46] 44% of hypopharyngeal cancer patients, and 31% of laryngeal cancer patients[47] and <9% in pediatric patients with rhabdomyosarcoma.[42,43] Trismus is reported in 3–26% and 2–61% in patients with large unresectable HNC and recurrent tumors, respectively.[48,49]

Pathophysiology

Intra-articular and extra-articular causes can result in trismus. Most cancer-related trismus, are extra-articular affecting muscles of mastication. The normal mandibular movement is guided by muscles of mastication; mandibular elevation by lateral pterygoid muscles, mandible elevation by temporalis, masseter, and medial pterygoid muscles, mandibular protrusion by lateral pterygoid, masseter, temporalis muscles, mandibular retraction by posterior fibers temporalis and deep fibers masseter muscles and lateral mandibular movement by contralateral lateral pterygoid and bilateral temporalis muscles. Pretreatment trismus is most often due to direct involvement of masseter and pterygoid muscles by tumor and neural invasion. In later stages, the extension of disease above the mandibular notch in oral cancers can lead to involvement of the temporomandibular joint (TMJ). Advanced parotid tumors can present with trismus (72%) due to involvement of TMJ and muscles of mastication.[50] Advanced oropharyngeal and nasopharyngeal cancers involve parapharyngeal space and infratemporal fossa and consequently muscles of mastication resulting in trismus. Coexisting oral submucosal fibrosis can result in trismus in the pretreatment period. Pain and reflex muscle spasm can result in significant trismus, especially in tumors involving retromolar trigone area.[51]

Post-treatment-related trismus is a consequence of progressive fibrosis in muscles of mastication.

Various mechanisms play a role in the causation of trismus such as cellular damage, regional loss of vascularization, and abnormal fibroblast proliferation.[5,50] Mandibular hypomobility is a consequence of surgery or radiation effects can result in degeneration of muscles and TMJ. A TMJ that is immobile even for as short as 3 days can set in degenerative changes, which is evident by thickening of synovial fluid and thinning joint cartilage. The fibrosis and contracture in the post-treatment setting is progressive and is based on the dose of radiation and/or extent of surgery. Surgeries for oral/oropharyngeal cancers commonly involve muscles of mastication and as a consequence, result in postoperative trismus. Appropriated reconstruction of the mucosal defect with patent upper and lower gingivolabial sulcus, lax retromolar trigone area is essential to prevent postoperative trismus. Adjuvant radiation can further compound risk and recovery of trismus.

Radiation-induced trismus is caused by various factors.[52,53] In an acute setting, severe mucositis can lead to trismus due to pain and reflex muscle spasm that may progress to mucosal/submucosal fibrosis in few cases leading to trismus. Muscles of mastication are most often included in tumor irradiation field, which cause progressive fibrosis of muscles leading to restricted mouth opening. The grade of trismus is directly related to the dose received by muscles of mastication, type of radiation technique, duration from radiation and site of tumor.[50,53] Mouth opening after radiation reduces on an average by 18–32% when compared to pretreatment mouth opening.[54] Mouth opening reduces at an average 2.4% per month during the first 9 months.[55] The reduction is at the rate of 0.2% and 0.1% per month during the second year and >2 years, respectively.[15] Two-thirds of total mouth opening reduction occurs during the first 9 months of treatment. Studies have shown a significant correlation between absorbed dose to muscles of mastication and prevalence of trismus. The risk of developing trismus increases by 24% for every 10 Gy additional radiation delivered to the medial pterygoid muscles.[56] Better conformal radiation techniques such as intensity-modulated radiotherapy (IMRT) can help in reducing radiation dose to masticatory muscles. A systematic review has reported a prevalence of trismus in 25.4% and 5% in conventional radiation techniques and IMRT, respectively.[43] However, the prevalence of trismus following primary surgery is underreported in the literature. Alcohol consumption acts as a muscle relaxant and counteracts collagen deposition. Hence, patients with alcohol consumption have reported a lower prevalence of trismus before treatment.[45,57]

Impact

Trismus results in restriction to maintain good oral hygiene, difficulty to examine, and monitor for recurrence and also chewing, deglutition, and speech. Patients using palatal obturator will find it hard to insert a prosthesis. Formation of the bolus is essential for effective swallowing; most patients with trismus are unable to form a bolus and swallow food that is poorly ground and results in subsequent aspiration and significant oral residue.[44] Trismus significantly impacts the QoL of the patient. Tools to measure patient-reported outcomes are limited. Gothenburg Trismus Questionnaire (GTQ) is an instrument with 21 items covering three domains.[58] The tool assesses jaw-related problems, eating limitations, muscular tension, pain and effects of restricted mouth opening. Trismus affects various aspects of patient life due to poor alimentation, loss of weight, depression, and also speech impairment.[44] Although studies evaluating the isolated impact of trismus in HNC patients are limited, most available evidence has shown a significant impact on QoL, including psychosocial domain.[40,44,59,60]

Assessment

Eyeballing mouth opening and number of fingers inserted between teeth lack precision and unreliable. Objective measurement of mouth opening must be done with tape or sliding callipers with 1 mm graduations for accuracy. The maximum interincisor distance (MID) between maxillary and mandibular incisors must be measured, if possible twice and the higher reading is taken into consideration.[58] The MID of ≤3.5 mm has been proposed as the objective cut-off to diagnose trismus based on patient's experiences of limitation of mouth opening and mandibular function impairment questionnaire. The subjective, objective, management, analysis (SOMA) classification for late cancer therapy toxicities has classified trismus into MID from 20 to 30 mm, 10 to 20 mm, 5 to 10 mm, and <5 mm is classified as grade 1,2,3 and 4, respectively.[61,62] Longitudinal measurement of trismus from before treatment, after each treatment and during follow-up visits aids in identifying patients at risk and management planning. A patient who presents with new-onset or rapid progression of trismus after treatment, a recurrence must be considered. Imaging evaluation to rule out local recurrence may aid in further management of trismus. Patients who are treated for recurrence are at a higher risk of developing trismus than a patient being treated for first cancer.

Treatment

Trismus is a progressive phenomenon, and hence early initiation of treatment and prevention strategy can help in halting the progress and prevent potential consequences of trismus. The roadblocks in the management of trismus are poor adherence to conservative therapy and associated pain, which limits patient's ability to undergo physical therapy.

Conservative Medical Management

Botulinum toxin injection into masticatory muscles has been reported in the management of radiation-induced trismus; however, it is an effective analgesic modality. Studies have shown that botulinum toxin injection has not shown improvement in trismus, and hence it must not be chosen as a primary treatment modality.[63,64] Other modalities such as microcurrent electrotherapy, hyperbaric oxygen therapy, and pentoxifylline have been tried but with no improvement.[65,66]

Physical Therapy

Physical/exercise therapy, with or without the aid of jaw opening devices, forms the mainstay in managing trismus. Active and passive jaw exercises are recommended based on the grade and acceptance of patient. Active jaw exercises include opening and closing mouth repeatedly, opening the mouth slightly and then followed by a sideward movement of the mandible, stretching the chin downward and forward and back to original position.[67] Passive jaw opening exercises included the opening of mouth by patient's own hands placed between maxillary and mandibular alveolus guarded by a gauze piece. Increasing range of movement and adding resistance during movement can increase mobility, flexibility, and elasticity of muscles and TMJ. Jaw exercises must be initiated as early as possible during or after the treatment and must be continued during the follow-up period for maximum benefit.[42] The exercises must be repeated as many times as possible.

Jaw Opening Devices

Stacked wooden tongue depressors, corkscrew devices, the TheraBite Jaw Motion Rehabilitation System, and the Dynasplint Trismus System (DTS) are commonly used devices.[41] These devices are used in conjunction with physical exercises. The response to treatment with jaw opening devices is similar to physical therapy. However, the extent of mouth opening is greater with jaw opening devices. Therabite exercises on an average increase mouth opening by 5.4 mm while DTS has shown an improvement of up to 6.2–13.6 mm.[68] A recent systematic review included studies that evaluated the effect of physical therapy in radiation-induced trismus. The review reported a significant increase in MID in after exercise therapy with jaw opening devices.

Surgical Management

When there is pretreatment trismus and patient undergoes surgery as the primary modality of treatment, then factors responsible for trismus must be addressed during surgery. Coronoidectomy, adequate mucosal defect reconstruction, released of fibrotic bands secondary oral submucosal fibrosis with flap insertion into areas of severe fibrosis are recommended. In maxillary sinus cancer, reconstruction with flap must be planned when post-treatment trismus is suspected as use of obturator in this subgroup of patients is challenging. Surgical management is restricted to cases that fail conservative treatment in post-treatment trismus. Coronoidectomy is the most effective surgical treatment with increases in MID of up to 20–30 mm. Post-treatment fibrosis is not limited to temporalis muscle, and hence some patients may require additional reconstruction to correct compounding factor. Postcoronoidectomy and physical therapy must be initiated as early as possible to achieve MID. Forced mouth opening under general anesthesia is not advocated as the effect is short-lived and can lead further fibrosis or lead to alveolar fracture further complicating the situation.

Prevention

Adequate reconstruction during surgery and precise dose planning during radiation therapy is paramount in preventing trismus. Identifying patients at risk and initiation of physical therapy before fibrotic sequence sets in is essential. Patients must be encouraged for oral alimentation as much as possible during radiation therapy and at the earliest after surgery to prevent hypomobilization of mandible. Chewing gum will theoretically encourage all range of jaw movements. However, a randomized controlled study has shown no differential effect between physical therapy and chewing gum.[69]

SHOULDER DYSFUNCTION

Background

Neck dissection (ND) is a surgical procedure that is routinely implemented in the management of HNC. The type of ND performed has been associated with the prevalence of subsequent shoulder pain and dysfunction, most notably due to involvement of the accessory nerve.

Presently, although nerve-preserving NDs are more frequently performed than nerve-sacrificing procedures; there is often occurrence of shoulder and upper limb functional deficits, along with shoulder pain. Evidence indicates ND is linked with shoulder pain, reduced health-related QoL specifically related to ND, and impaired shoulder function.[70]

Shoulder function is associated with various activities of daily living such as dressing, writing, driving, lifting objects and reaching for things; therefore, making it an important aspect of health-related QoL. Several domains of QoL may be affected due to the influence of impaired shoulder function on work, and social and leisure activities. Adjustments of the radical neck dissection were created to limit the extent and frequency of shoulder dysfunction. Spinal accessory nerve sparing neck dissections are associated with better preservation of shoulder function as compared to nerve-sacrificing neck dissections. However, considerable shoulder dysfunction continues to arise even when the spinal accessory nerve is spared during the neck dissection procedure. The concept of the selective neck dissection was introduced in which only the levels at risk for occult lymph node metastases are dissected, so as to diminish shoulder morbidity. Shoulder morbidity increased when attempts are made to clear nodes from the posterior triangle (level V). This is probably caused by damage of the cervical nerve rootlets and other motor supply in the posterior triangle of the neck, the unavoidable effect of devascularization of the spinal accessory nerve and scarring. Undeniably various studies have showed that patients had a better shoulder function after selective neck dissection than modified radical neck dissection.[71] In a study by Cappiello et al., comparison of the results of clinical and electrophysiological investigations of shoulder function in patients affected by HNC, treated with concomitant surgery on the primary and the neck with different selective neck dissections was done. They found abnormalities of shoulder abduction in about 50% with a neck dissection including level V, as compared to only 5% when level V was not dissected. To a much lesser extent, the anteflexion and external rotation were affected. They also reported that in 30% of patients, drooping of the shoulder occurred after dissection of levels II-V, 15% had shoulder protraction, and there was scapular flaring in 5%. If only levels II-IV were dissected, only shoulder droop was found in only 5% of the patients. They confirmed that clearance of the posterior triangle of the neck increases shoulder morbidity.[72] Accessory nerve injury is unique to head and neck surgery and deliberate sacrifice of the nerve is specific to patients requiring neck dissection for HNC.[73]

Accessory nerve damage in patients occurring after radical neck dissections described as "shoulder syndrome," initially in 1952 by Ewing and Martin.[74] They defined the classic clinical picture of shoulder syndrome, which included chronic and nonspecific shoulder pain, drooping of the involved shoulder, with acromion prominence and a marked rhomboid muscle profile, limited lateral abduction of the shoulder, impaired forward shoulder flexion, aberrant scapular rotation, a constant dull ache with a sensation of stiffness or soreness in the involved side, and abnormal electromyographic recordings.[75]

These symptoms and signs can also be observed after selective neck dissection with lesser severity and chronicity. The occurrence of shoulder syndrome is thought to be secondary to neural stretch injury, decompression injury or devascularization of the spinal accessory nerve during extensive dissection (possibly due to segmental demyelinization and consequent neuropraxia), seen more with dissection of level 5, leading to temporary or permanent accessory nerve weakness. Rehabilitation for this dysfunction comes in the form of stretching exercises, occupational therapy, or physical therapy (PT).[74]

Injury to the cervical plexus also adds to the pathogenesis of the shoulder syndrome, due to lesions of the cervical motor branches for the trapezius muscle (C2–C4) and for the levator scapulae (C3–C5), and lesions of the sensitive supraclavicular nerves (C3–C4). From a literature review, a variable degree of shoulder dysfunction is reported to occur even in 30–40% of patients who underwent modified neck dissection (MND) with anatomic sparing of the XI nerve or functional neck dissection (FND), suggesting that other factors other than the sole accessory nerve injury are involved in the etiology of the shoulder syndrome and in its variable clinical presentation.[75]

In 1983 Leipzig et al. presented data from a prospective study of 109 patients who had undergone different types of neck dissections in which they objectively measured shoulder function before and after surgery. They reported that shoulder syndrome occurred in 30% of patients who have undergone FND, in 50% of MND, and 60% of RND.[76]

Anatomic preservation of the spinal accessory nerve does not necessarily adds to normal functioning of the nerve, for the reason that intraoperative situation (extent of nerve dissection, stretching or compression by retractor, burning from electrocautery, accidental ligature done for hemostat purposes) and/or postoperative situations (hemorrhages, hematomas, malpositioned suctioning, drainage, infection, and scarring), respectively, could lead to neuropraxia or axonal injury (axonotmesis). In effect, abnormal electromyograms were often reported after nerve-sparing procedures which tend to improve or normalize with time. Regeneration of spinal nerve fibers that were traumatized, but not cut may explain the improvement in shoulder pain and function that Leipzig et al. reported in their prospective study of shoulder disability in MND between 6 months and 1 year after surgery. Alternatively, the finding of a normal or close-to-normal shoulder function, as shown by electromyography in 25% of patients who had undergone RND can be attributed to a trapezius subfascial innervation pattern of the cervical plexus, which has a deep course in the neck and is able to maintain an adequate motor supply; hence muscle dysfunction is less pronounced.[76]

Adjuvant treatment may be correlated with upper limb function. Undergoing surgery and postoperative radiation treatment was associated with an increased level of upper limb dysfunction compared with surgery alone as soft-tissue fibrosis is a known side effect of radiation treatment. The subsequent contraction of skin, underlying fascia, and the surgical scar in the anterolateral neck may alter the resting position or impair movement of the shoulder girdle, potentially limiting upper limb function. Other possible explanations include radiation-induced damage to neural structures, such as the accessory nerve.[70]

The trapezius is responsible for shoulder joint stability by confirming proper scapular alignment and movement. Inadequate trapezius muscle function leads to scapular dyskinesis. This in turn, limits the ability of the humerus to elevate with respect to the trunk because the scapula is unable to fully upwardly rotate, retract, and elevate. Moreover, trapezius muscle weakness causes the scapula to be protracted, downwardly rotated, and depressed at rest making the affected shoulder appear longer and lower than the affected side. These biomechanical factors may result in soft-tissue injury and pain. Left untreated, this may progress to further activity limitation, participation restriction, and disability.[77] The transient disability of trapezius, resulting from spinal nerve damage, and the weakness of the other muscles of the scapulohumeral girdle innervated by the cervical plexus (rhomboids, levator scapulae, anterior and middle scalene, and sternocleidomastoid), whose branches can be resected during neck dissection, impairs the biomechanical balance between the glenohumeral and scapulothoracic joints (that is crucial for the elevation of the arm) causing pain and functional impairment of superior parts. Paresthetic pain involving the neck (resulting from sensitive cervical branches being sectioned) and the cervical stiffness (caused by the forced immobility of the head in the immediate postoperative period) aggravate these symptoms leading to a secondary glenohumeral stiffness better known as glenohumeral adhesions. This pathologic condition is the result of loss of extensibility of capsular structures (periarticular connective tissue) subsequent to the forced immobilization and the initial arm pain, which favors fibrosis to occur. Postoperative physical therapy is reported to be of benefit by many authors; even though in these studies the patients were not enrolled in any standardized rehabilitative program and the influence of therapy on pain and scapulohumeral girdle dysfunction was not clearly assessed.[75] The spinal accessory nerve is usually referred to as solely a motor nerve providing innervation to the sternocleidomastoid muscle and upper trapezius muscles. After loss of nerve function, both muscles are paralyzed. The loss of upper trapezius muscle activity is more important than with sternocleidomastoid denervation, causing the complex clinical picture of shoulder syndrome. About 60–80% of patients receiving treatment with RND have severe upper extremity impairment with functional motor deficits, stiffness of the neck, or shoulder pain that may radiate to the face, or a combination of these.[3]

Assessment

- *Electrodiagnostic tests:* These are the most sensitive for detection of nerve conduction impairment, which is usually obvious in any type of neck dissection, and in monitoring recovery of function during follow-up.[3] In a prospective study with 109 patients, Leipzig et al. found that patients who had the spinal accessory nerve, jugular vein, and sternocleidomastoid muscle spared had a clinical dysfunction rate of 30% compared with 50% when only the SAN (i.e., MRND) was spared and 60% with radical neck dissection.[76,77] A study by Sobol et al. found that at 16 weeks post-surgery, moderate-to-severe EMG abnormalities were seen in 65% of patients who underwent MRND compared with 22% after supraomohyoid neck dissection.[78] Witt's study demonstrated less electrophysiologic threshold shift and shoulder syndrome with SND compared with MRND. No patient with SND had an electrophysiologic threshold shift, and only 1 of 11 (9%) patients had shoulder syndrome. Higher rates in MRND were discovered. Electrophysiologic integrity of the SAN does not completely correlate with clinical outcome measures for shoulder syndrome. It is significant that 89% patients without an electrophysiologic threshold increase did not develop shoulder syndrome.[79] Shone and Yardley showed that despite SAN sparing surgical techniques available at the time, 80% of patients with HNC and had radical neck dissection within the previous 6 months reported difficulty with everyday tasks, and 46% failed to return to previous employment because of neck dissection-related shoulder dysfunction.[80] Similarly, 77% of patients undergoing selective neck dissection reported mild to severe shoulder dysfunction.[81]

- *Clinical scoring systems:* Goldstein et al. in a systematic review of shoulder disability questionnaires used after neck dissection for HNC highlighted seven outcome measures previously used in the HNC patient population, including the NDII, SPADI, SDQ, Constant's Shoulder Score, the Modified American Shoulder and Elbow Surgeons standardized assessment form (ASES), DASH, and the simple shoulder test (SST).[80,82]
    - The Constant-Murley Shoulder Outcome Score is a validated clinical assessment of shoulder function that has established usefulness and accuracy across many diseases affecting the shoulder. This validated, widely used clinical test has been shown to be an accurate and sensitive measure of shoulder function, detecting subtle changes in shoulder function. The assessment takes approximately 10 minutes to perform. It is a weighted test that combines patient symptom scores and objective measures of active shoulder function. The symptoms score assesses pain, sleep, recreation, and vocational activities. The objective score measures active shoulder range of motion, combined internal rotation, combined external rotation, and shoulder strength in the plane of the scapula. Scores range from 0 to 100, with higher scores indicating better shoulder function.[83,84]
    - The modified Constant-Murley Shoulder Outcome Score is a validated clinical assessment of shoulder function shown to be accurate and sensitive. Scores range from 0 to 100, with higher scores indicating better shoulder function. The scoring system includes both a subjective (35% of total score) and an objective (65% of total score) component. It is calculated from a patient questionnaire.[80]
    - Disabilities of the Arm, Shoulder and Hand (DASH) questionnaire was identified as a potential patient-reported outcome measure to study for use in patients who have undergone neck dissection. It is one of the most extensively developed and evaluated upper extremity disability questionnaires, which has the ability to discriminate between patients with and without neural injury, as well as between those with and without recovery after nerve injury. It has undergone extensive cross-cultural adaptation.[73]
    - The Disabilities of the Arm, Shoulder and Hand (DASH) and Shoulder Pain and Disability Index (SPADI) questionnaires, have been heavily used in the clinic and in research and are robust measures of upper extremity and shoulder dysfunction. Although the Quick Disabilities of the Arm, Shoulder, and Hand (QuickDASH) is easy to administer, the inferior sensitivity and specificity compared to the DASH makes the DASH more attractive. QuickDASH is an 11-item tool addresses symptoms (e.g., pain), functional performance (e.g., carrying bags), and impact on life domains (e.g., work, recreation, social) due to upper limb musculoskeletal conditions.[85] QuickDASH has been deemed applicable for this patient population, and it has favorable evidence supporting its internal consistency and test-retest reliability in breast cancer survivors and construct validity in orthopedic populations.[86] Scores range from 0 (no functional impairment) to 100 (total functional impairment).
    - Neck Disability Index (NDI) is a 10-item questionnaire measures the impact of neck pain on functional tasks such as reading, driving, and sleeping, generating a percentage score from 0% (no functional impairment) to 100% (total functional impairment). The NDI has evidence supporting its test-retest reliability, internal consistency, construct validity, and concurrent validity (e.g., with the McGill Pain Questionnaire) based on populations with whiplash-associated and idiopathic neck pain. The NDI has been used extensively as a self-reported measure of neck disability in studies investigating musculoskeletal disorders of the neck, including among cancer survivors. This is an important finding as patients with cancer with neuropathic pain are likely to benefit from a different approach to rehabilitation than patients without neuropathic pain.[87,88]
    - Neck Dissection Impairment Index (NDII) is heavily weighted toward shoulder-specific questions recommended for use by physical therapists.

Treatment

The rationale of rehabilitative protocol is to prevent or attenuate the capsular and ligaments stiffness of the scapulohumeral girdle, facilitating the early recovery of the passive mobility and to relieve the pain resulting from cervical branches damage and the forced immobility of the neck. Once the passive range of motion is completely achieved, the active motility will spontaneously recover, depending, of course, on the entity of the spinal nerve damage. The goal of rehabilitation was to first recover passive range of motion, considering the scapulohumeral girdles in our patients, such as simple stiff painful shoulder, in accordance with the protocols of Codman and Neer, emphasizing the importance of achieving the "zero position."[88] The zero position consists of the humerus being elevated to 165° in the plane of the scapula; this position allows alignment on the same axis of the humerus, the scapular spine, and the muscles that move the humerus. The forward elevation on the scapular plane is the most frequent act during common daily activities, and the acquisition of such a position is extremely important in rehabilitation because it is the expression of the lack of retraction involving the inner and middle glenohumeral ligaments, i.e., absence of capsulitis.

The rehabilitative protocol includes the following exercises:

- Passive forward elevation of the arm in the plane of the scapula in supine and half-sitting positions
- Passive forward elevation with the hands locked in supine and half-sitting positions and subsequent stretching movements
- External rotation with the elbow at the side and flexed at 90°
- Internal rotation with the hand placed behind the back

The rehabilitative treatment aims to reduce pain and to early recovery of passive motion has been shown to have a real contributory role in decreasing shoulder complaints and ameliorating the patients' QoL. Such a physical therapy protocol should have a place in the postoperative treatment of all patients with HNC undergoing neck dissection when an RND is planned.[75] McNeely et al. recently reported that the progressive resistance exercise program significantly reduced shoulder pain and disability and improved upper extremity muscular strength and endurance in patients who survived HNC who had shoulder dysfunction because of spinal accessory nerve damage. The current evidence suggests that all patients should undertake active shoulder rehabilitation postoperatively. Taking these measures will save both the patient and doctor possible morbidity.[89]

LARYNGEAL NERVE PALSY FOLLOWING THYROIDECTOMY

Introduction

The incidence of temporary and permanent recurrent laryngeal nerve (RLN) palsy following thyroid surgery is 3–8% and 0.3–3%, respectively.[90] Superior laryngeal nerve (SLN) injury has been reported to be as high as 58%.[91] A detailed discussion on laryngeal innervation with respect to thyroidectomy has been covered in the thyroid malignancies.

Clinical Features

Superior laryngeal nerve injury is subtler and is problematic in professional voice users. It results in reduced fundamental frequency, lowering and devoicing of speech. RLN palsy when unilateral can be asymptomatic; however, patients can have breathy dysphonia, dysphagia, or aspiration of liquids. When RLN injury is bilateral, it results in aphonia, aspiration, and a loss of cough reflex. In some patients, bilateral RLN palsy can result in life-threatening stridor necessitating intervention. The British Thyroid Association recommends that voice dysfunction should be evaluated if dysfunction persists beyond 2 weeks after surgery.[92] It has been noted that most cases of temporary dysfunction resolve within 6 months and in the absence of severe symptoms, patients may be observed.

On flexible laryngoscopic examination, there may be reduced or absent movement of the vocal cords. Unilateral RLN palsy results in a fixed cord with a mobile contralateral cord that do not approximate, while bilateral palsy results in both cords remaining fixed in the median position. Previous theories such as Semon's law and Wagner and Grossman theory have been replaced by the belief that the final position of the cord is not static and depends on the degree of muscle atrophy and fibrosis in the cords, the degree of reinnervation and synkinesis of muscles. Other visual abnormalities include mucosal thickening, edema, or subluxation of the arytenoid cartilage, some of which can also result from anesthetic complications.

Treatment

- *Unilateral RLN palsy:* The goal is to improve voice quality and prevent aspiration. In most cases, patients are observed for the first 6–12 months after injury.

Speech and swallowing therapy can help gradually relieve these symptoms. Laryngeal electromyography can help prognosticate patients and monitor recovery. For temporary RLN palsy after initial observation, vocal fold injection can be performed with Teflon, bovine collagen, human collagen, micronized alloderm, fat, or hyaluronic acid. Most of these undergo resorption over 6 months to 2 years in case nerve function recovers. Injection results in medialization of the paralyzed cord that allows better contact with the normal contralateral vocal cord, improving voice quality and preventing aspiration by reducing the glottic chink. In permanent RLN palsy (>12 months) are treated with vocal cord injection with a durable material, injection laryngoplasty or medialization thyroplasty. Injection laryngoplasty involves transcutaneous injection of any of the abovementioned materials lateral to the vocal cord process through the transthyroid membrane, transthyroid cartilage or transcricothyroid membrane; this results in rotation of the arytenoid medially and medialization of the true vocal cord, with a second injection if indicated anteriorly at the midcord level. The amount of injection is determined by endoscopic appearance and if performed under local anesthesia the patient's voice quality is used as a guide. Medialization thyroplasty involves removing a window in the thyroid cartilage with placement of a silastic implant, hydroxyapatite implant or Gore-tex strips, which permanently displace the cord medially. Arytenoid adduction is rarely performed in current practice.

- *Bilateral RLN palsy:* Here the goal is to improve patient's respiration. In an acute setting if the patient has stridor, a tracheostomy may need to be performed. However, it is associated with a lower QoL and should be avoided if other techniques can be performed effectively in an acute setting. Cordotomy, usually with laser, can improve the glottic chink and allow adequate respiration. Another approach is the arytenoid abduction, where there is a laterofixation suture placed over the arytenoid cartilage to simulate posterior cricoarytenoid contraction and keep the glottic airway open.[93] Additional treatment options include botox injection (which temporarily blocks aberrant reinnervation of adductor muscles), laryngeal pacing and functional electrical stimulation and laryngeal innervations.[94] Laryngeal innervation is performed to prevent denervation of the true vocal cord, to prevent loss of bulk and tone. It is performed when chance of spontaneous recovery is low. The reinnervation is performed with nerve-to-nerve anastomosis or a neuromuscular pedicle. The neuromuscular pedicle allows transfer of omohyoid muscle motor units innervated with ansa cervicalis to the lateral crico-arytenoid muscle. Alternatively, the ansa cervicalis or the phrenic nerve is anastomosed to the RLN stump. All of these procedures have shown good outcomes in experienced hands.

CONCLUSION

Although potentially devastating, early and aggressive management of treatment-related complications could result in reasonable outcomes and acceptable quality of life. Sustained multidisciplinary care is imperative in managing these patients.

REFERENCES

1. Rockson SG, Rivera KK. Estimating the population burden of lymphedema. Annals of the New York Academy of Sciences. 2008;1131(1):147-54.
2. Murphy BA, Gilbert J. Dysphagia in head and neck cancer patients treated with radiation: assessment, sequelae, and rehabilitation. In: Seminars in radiation oncolo UK: WB Saunders; 2009. pp. 35-42.
3. Deng J, Murphy BA. Lymphedema self-care in patients with head and neck cancer: a qualitative study. Supportive Care in Cancer. 2016;24(12):4961-70.
4. Smith BG. Lymphedema in head and neck cancer. In: Clinical Care and Rehabilitation in Head and Neck Cancer. Cham: Springer; 2019. pp. 377-96..
5. Deng J, Ridner SH, Dietrich MS, Wells N, Wallston KA, Sinard RJ, et al. Prevalence of secondary lymphedema in patients with head and neck cancer. Journal of Pain and Symptom Management. 2012;43(2):244-52.
6. Deng J, Murphy BA, Dietrich MS, Wells N, Wallston KA, Sinard RJ, et al. Impact of secondary lymphedema after head and neck cancer treatment on symptoms, functional status, and quality of life. Head & Neck. 2013;35(7):1026-35.
7. Anand A, Balasubramanian D, Subramanian N, Murthy S, Limbachiya S, Iyer S, et al. Secondary lymphedema after head and neck cancer therapy: a review. Lymphology. 2018; 51(3):109-18.
8. Deng J, Ridner SH, Aulino JM, Murphy BA. Assessment and measurement of head and neck lymphedema: state-of-the-science and future directions. Oral oncology. 2015;51(5):431-7.
9. Feely MA, Olsen KD, Gamble GL, Davis MD, Pittelkow MR. Cutaneous lymphatics and chronic lymphedema of the head and neck. Clinical Anatomy. 2012;25(1):72-85.
10. Földi M, Földi E, Strößenreuther R, Kubik S. Földi's Textbook of Lymphology: For Physicians and Lymphedema Therapists. Germany: Elsevier Health Sciences; 2012.
11. Deng J, Ridner SH, Dietrich MS, Wells N, Wallston KA, Sinard RJ, et al. Factors associated with external and internal lymphedema in patients with head-and-neck cancer. International Journal of Radiation Oncology* Biology* Physics. 2012;84(3):e319-28.
12. Szolnoky G, Mohos G, Dobozy A, Kemény L. Manual lymph drainage reduces trapdoor effect in subcutaneous island

pedicle flaps. International Journal of dermatology. 2006;45(12):1468-70.

13. Cariati M, Bains SK, Grootendorst MR, Suyoi A, Peters AM, Mortimer P, et al. Adjuvant taxanes and the development of breast cancer-related arm lymphoedema. British Journal of Surgery. 2015;102(9):1071-8.
14. Piso DU, Eckardt A, Liebermann A, Gutenbrunner C, Schäfer P, Gehrke A. Early rehabilitation of head-neck edema after curative surgery for orofacial tumors. American Journal of Physical Medicine & Rehabilitation. 2001;80(4):261-9.
15. Poulsen MG, Riddle B, Keller J, Porceddu SV, Tripcony L. Predictors of acute grade 4 swallowing toxicity in patients with stages III and IV squamous carcinoma of the head and neck treated with radiotherapy alone. Radiotherapy and Oncology. 2008;87(2):253-9.
16. Deng J, Ridner SH, Dietrich MS, Wells N, Murphy BA. Assessment of external lymphedema in patients with head and neck cancer: a comparison of four scales. In: Oncology nursing forum. Oncol Nurs Forum. 2013;40(5):501-6.
17. Deng J, Ridner SH, Murphy BA, Dietrich MS. Preliminary development of a lymphedema symptom assessment scale for patients with head and neck cancer. Supportive Care in Cancer. 2012;20(8):1911-8.
18. American Cancer Society. Lymphedema: Understanding and managing lymphedema after cancer treatment. American Cancer Society; 2014.
19. Smith BG, Lewin JS. The role of lymphedema management in head and neck cancer. Current opinion in otolaryngology & head and neck surgery. 2010;18(3):153.
20. Deng J, Ridner SH, Wells N, Dietrich MS, Murphy BA. Development and preliminary testing of head and neck cancer related external lymphedema and fibrosis assessment criteria. European Journal of Oncology Nursing. 2015;19(1):75-80.
21. Trotti A, Colevas AD, Setser A, Rusch V, Jaques D, Budach V, et al. CTCAE v3. 0: development of a comprehensive grading system for the adverse effects of cancer treatment. In: Seminars in radiation oncology. UK: WB Saunders; 2003. pp. 2003
22. Denis F, Garaud P, Bardet E, Alfonsi M, Sire C, Germain T, et al. Late toxicity results of the GORTEC 94-01 randomized trial comparing radiotherapy with concomitant radiochemotherapy for advanced-stage oropharynx carcinoma: comparison of LENT/SOMA, RTOG/EORTC, and NCI-CTC scoring systems. International Journal of Radiation Oncology* Biology* Physics. 2003;55(1):93-8.
23. Budach V, Zurlo A, Horiot JC. EORTC Radiotherapy Group: achievements and future projects. European Journal of Cancer. 2002;38:134-7.
24. Patterson JM, Hildreth A, Wilson JA. Measuring edema in irradiated head and neck cancer patients. Annals of Otology, Rhinology & Laryngology. 2007;116(8):559-64.
25. Purcell A, Nixon J, Fleming J, McCann A, Porceddu S. Measuring head and neck lymphedema: The "ALOHA" trial. Head & Neck. 2016;38(1):79-84.
26. Chen MH, Chang PM, Chen PM, Tzeng CH, Chu PY, Chang SY, et al. Prolonged facial edema is an indicator of poor prognosis in patients with head and neck squamous cell carcinoma. Supportive Care in Cancer. 2010;18(10):1313-9.
27. Gheorghe L, Iacob S, Gheorghe C. Real-time sonoelastography-a new application in the field of liver disease. J Gastrointestin Liver Dis. 2008;17(4):469-74.
28. Kasseroller RG. The Vodder school: the Vodder method. Cancer: Interdisciplinary International Journal of the American Cancer Society. 1998;83(S12B):2840-2.
29. Pigott A, Nixon J, Fleming J, Porceddu S. Head and neck lymphedema management: Evaluation of a therapy program. Head & Neck. 2018;40(6):1131-7.
30. Bruns F, Büntzel J, Mücke R, Schönekaes K, Kisters K, Micke O. Selenium in the treatment of head and neck lymphedema. Medical Principles and Practice. 2004;13(4):185-90.
31. Micke O, Bruns F, Mücke R, Schäfer U, Glatzel M, DeVries AF, et al. Selenium in the treatment of radiation-associated secondary lymphedema. International Journal of Radiation Oncology* Biology* Physics. 2003;56(1):40-9.
32. Lee N, Wigg J, Carroll JD. The use of low level light therapy in the treatment of head and neck oedema. J Lymphoedema. 2013;8(1):35-42.
33. Mihara M, Uchida G, Hara H, Hayashi Y, Moriguchi H, Narushima M, et al. Lymphaticovenous anastomosis for facial lymphoedema after multiple courses of therapy for head-and-neck cancer. Journal of Plastic, Reconstructive & Aesthetic Surgery. 2011;64(9):1221-5.
34. Ayestaray B, Bekara F, Andreoletti JB. π-Shaped lymphaticovenular anastomosis for head and neck lymphoedema: A preliminary study. Journal of Plastic, Reconstructive & Aesthetic Surgery. 2013;66(2):201-6.
35. Withey S, Pracy P, Wood S, Rhys-Evans P. The use of a lymphatic bridge in the management of head and neck lymphoedema. British Journal of Plastic Surgery. 2001;54(8):716-9.
36. Jablonski S. Illustrated dictionary of dentistry. Philadelphia: WB Saunders; 1982.
37. Landau SI. International dictionary of medicine and biology (In three volumes). US: John Wiley & Sons; 1986.
38. Bensadoun RJ, Riesenbeck D, Lockhart PB, Elting LS, Spijkervet FK, Brennan MT. A systematic review of trismus induced by cancer therapies in head and neck cancer patients. Supportive Care in Cancer. 2010;18(8):1033-8.
39. Melchers LJ, Van Weert E, Beurskens CH, Reintsema H, Slagter AP, Roodenburg JL, et al. Exercise adherence in patients with trismus due to head and neck oncology: a qualitative study into the use of the Therabite®. International Journal of Oral and Maxillofacial Surgery. 2009;38(9):947-54.
40. Kent ML, Brennan MT, Noll JL, Fox PC, Burri SH, Hunter JC, et al. Radiation-induced trismus in head and neck cancer patients. Supportive Care in Cancer. 2008;16(3):305-9.
41. Estilo CL, Huryn JM, Kraus DH, Sklar CA, Wexler LH, Wolden SL, et al. Effects of therapy on dentofacial development in long-term survivors of head and neck rhabdomyosarcoma: the memorial sloan-kettering cancer center experience. Journal of Pediatric Hematology/Oncology. 2003;25(3):215-22.
42. Rapidis AD, Dijkstra PU, Roodenburg JL, Rodrigo JP, Rinaldo A, Strojan P, et al. Trismus in patients with head and neck cancer: etiopathogenesis, diagnosis and management. Clinical Otolaryngology. 2015;40(6):516-26.
43. Dijkstra PU, Huisman PM, Roodenburg JL. Criteria for trismus in head and neck oncology. International Journal of Oral and Maxillofacial Surgery. 2006;35(4):337-42.
44. Thomas F, Ozanne F, Mamelle G, Wibault P, Eschwege F. Radiotherapy alone for oropharyngeal carcinomas: the role of fraction size (2 Gy vs 2.5 Gy) on local control and early and late complications. International Journal of Radiation Oncology• Biology• Physics. 1988;15(5):1097-102.
45. Qin D, Hu Y, Yan J, Xu G, Cai W, Wu X, Cao D, Gu X. Analysis of 1379 patients with nasopharyngeal carcinoma treated by radiation. Cancer. 1988;61(6):1117-24.

46. Weber C, Dommerich S, Pau HW, Kramp B. Limited mouth opening after primary therapy of head and neck cancer. Oral and Maxillofacial Surgery. 2010;14(3):169-73.
47. MacKenzie R, Balogh J, Choo R, Franssen E. Accelerated radiotherapy with delayed concomitant boost in locally advanced squamous cell carcinoma of the head and neck. International Journal of Radiation Oncology* Biology* Physics. 1999;45(3):589-95.
48. McNeese MD, Fletcher GH. Retreatment of recurrent nasopharyngeal carcinoma. Radiology. 1981;138(1):191-3.
49. Katsantonis GP, Friedman WH, Rosenblum BN. The surgical management of advanced malignancies of the parotid gland. Otolaryngology—Head and Neck Surgery. 1989;101(6):633-40.
50. Toljanic JA, Heshmati RH, Bedard JF. Dental follow-up compliance in a population of irradiated head and neck cancer patients. Oral Surgery, Oral Medicine, Oral Pathology, Oral Radiology, and Endodontology. 2002;93(1):35-8.
51. Goldstein M, Maxymiw WG, Cummings BJ, Wood RE. The effects of antitumor irradiation on mandibular opening and mobility: a prospective study of 58 patients. Oral Surgery, Oral Medicine, Oral Pathology, Oral Radiology, and Endodontology. 1999;88(3):365-73.
52. Wang CJ, Huang EY, Hsu HC, Chen HC, Fang FM, Hsiung CY. The degree and time-course assessment of radiation-induced trismus occurring after radiotherapy for nasopharyngeal cancer. The Laryngoscope. 2005;115(8):1458-60.
53. Teguh DN, Levendag PC, Voet P, van der Est H, Noever I, de Kruijf W, et al. Trismus in patients with oropharyngeal cancer: relationship with dose in structures of mastication apparatus. Head & Neck: Journal for the Sciences and Specialties of the Head and Neck. 2008;30(5):622-30.
54. Lee R, Slevin N, Musgrove B, Swindell R, Molassiotis A. Prediction of post-treatment trismus in head and neck cancer patients. British Journal of Oral and Maxillofacial Surgery. 2012;50(4):328-32.
55. Johnson J, Carlsson S, Johansson M, Pauli N, Rydén A, Fagerberg-Mohlin B, Finizia C. Development and validation of the Gothenburg Trismus Questionnaire (GTQ). Oral Oncology. 2012;48(8):730-6.
56. Johnson J, Johansson M, Rydén A, Houltz E, Finizia C. Impact of trismus on health-related quality of life and mental health. Head & Neck. 2015;37(11):1672-9.
57. Pauli N, Johnson J, Finizia C, Andrell P. The incidence of trismus and long-term impact on health-related quality of life in patients with head and neck cancer. Acta Oncologica. 2013;52(6):1137-45.
58. Shulman DH, Shipman B, Willis FB. Treating trismus with dynamic splinting: a cohort, case series. Advances in Therapy. 2008;25(1):9-16.
59. Soma LE. LENT SOMA tables. Radiother Oncol. 1995;35:17-60.
60. Stubblefield MD, Levine A, Custodio CM, Fitzpatrick T. The role of botulinum toxin type A in the radiation fibrosis syndrome: a preliminary report. Archives of Physical Medicine and Rehabilitation. 2008;89(3):417-21.
61. Dana MH, Cohen M, Morbize J, Marandas P, Janot F, Bourhis J. Botulinum toxin for radiation-induced facial pain and trismus. Otolaryngology—Head and Neck Surgery. 2008;138(4):459-63.
62. King GE, Scheetz J, Jacob RF, Martin JW. Electrotherapy and hyperbaric oxygen: promising treatments for post-radiation complications. Journal of Prosthetic Dentistry. 1989; 62(3):331-4.
63. Chua DT, Lo C, Yuen J, Foo YC. A pilot study of pentoxifylline in the treatment of radiation-induced trismus. American Journal of Clinical Oncology. 2001;24(4):366-9.
64. Tang Y, Shen Q, Wang Y, Lu K, Peng Y. A randomized prospective study of rehabilitation therapy in the treatment of radiation-induced dysphagia and trismus. Strahlentherapie und Onkologie. 2011;187(1):39-44.
65. Kamstra JI, Roodenburg JL, Beurskens CH, Reintsema H, Dijkstra PU. TheraBite exercises to treat trismus secondary to head and neck cancer. Supportive Care in Cancer. 2013; 21(4):951-7.
66. Barañano CF, Rosenthal EL, Morgan BA, McColloch NL, Magnuson JS. Dynasplint for the management of trismus after treatment of upper aerodigestive tract cancer: a retrospective study. Ear, Nose, & Throat Journal. 2011;90(12):584-90.
67. Scherpenhuizen A, van Waes AM, Janssen LM, Van Cann EM, Stegeman I. The effect of exercise therapy in head and neck cancer patients in the treatment of radiotherapy-induced trismus: a systematic review. Oral Oncology. 2015;51(8):745-50.
68. Bhrany AD, Izzard M, Wood AJ, Futran ND. Coronoidectomy for the treatment of trismus in head and neck cancer patients. The Laryngoscope. 2007;117(11):1952-6.
69. Høgdal N, Juhl C, Aadahl M, Gluud C. Early preventive exercises versus usual care does not seem to reduce trismus in patients treated with radiotherapy for cancer in the oral cavity or oropharynx: a randomised clinical trial. Acta Oncologica. 2015;54(1):80-7.
70. Gane EM, O'Leary SP, Hatton AL, Panizza BJ, McPhail SM. Neck and Upper Limb Dysfunction in Patients following Neck Dissection: Looking beyond the Shoulder. Otolaryngol Head Neck Surg. 2017;157(4):631-40.
71. van Wouwe M, de Bree R, Kuik DJ, de Goede CJT, Verdonck-de Leeuw IM, Doornaert P, et al. Shoulder morbidity after non-surgical treatment of the neck. Radiother Oncol. 2009; 90(2):196-201.
72. Cappiello J, Piazza C, Giudice M, De Maria G, Nicolai P. Shoulder disability after different selective neck dissections (levels II-IV versus levels II-V): a comparative study. Laryngoscope. 2005;115(2):259-63.
73. Goldstein DP, Ringash J, Irish JC, Gilbert R, Gullane P, Brown D, et al. Assessment of the Disabilities of the Arm, Shoulder, and Hand (DASH) questionnaire for use in patients after neck dissection for head and neck cancer. Head Neck. 2015;37(2):234-42.
74. Watkins JP, Williams GB, Mascioli AA, Wan JY, Samant S. Shoulder function in patients undergoing selective neck dissection with or without radiation and chemotherapy. Head Neck. 2011;33(5):615-9.
75. Salerno G, Cavaliere M, Foglia A, Pellicoro DP, Mottola G, Nardone M, et al. The 11th nerve syndrome in functional neck dissection. Laryngoscope. 2002;112(7 Pt 1):1299-307.
76. Leipzig B, Suen J, English J, Barnes J, Hooper M. Functional evaluation of the spinal accessory nerve after neck dissection. Am J Surg. 1983;146:526-30.
77. Eden M, Flores A, Galantino M, Spinelli B. Recommendations for Patient-reported Outcome Measures for Head and Neck Cancer-related Shoulder Dysfunction: A Systematic Review. Rehabilitation Oncology. 2014;32(3):6-19.
78. Sobol S. Objective comparison of physical dysfunction after dissection. Am J Surg. 1985;150:503.
79. Witt RL, Rejto L. Spinal accessory nerve monitoring in selective and modified neck dissection. Laryngoscope. 2007;117(5):776-80.
80. Shone GR, Yardley MP. An audit into the incidence of handicap after unilateral radical neck dissection. J Laryngol Otol. 1991;105(9):760-2.

81. Carr SD, Bowyer D, Cox G. Upper limb dysfunction following selective neck dissection: a retrospective questionnaire study. Head Neck. 2009;31(6):789-92.
82. Goldstein DP, Ringash J, Bissada E, Spinelli B. Evaluation of shoulder disability questionnaires used for the assessment of shoulder disability after neck dissection for head and neck cancer. Head Neck. 2014;36(10):1453-8.
83. Constant CR, Murley AHG. A clinical method of functional assessment of the shoulder. Clin Orthop. 1987;214:160-4.
84. Chepeha DB, Taylor RJ, Chepeha JC, Teknos TN, Bradford CR, Sharma PK, et al. Functional assessment using Constant's Shoulder Scale after modified radical and selective neck dissection. Head Neck. 2002;24(5):432-6.
85. Beaton D, Wright J, Katz J. Upper Extremity Collaborative Group. Development of the QuickDASH: Comparison of three item-reduction approaches. J Bone Joint Surg Am. 2005; 87:1038-46.
86. Vernon H, Mior S. The Neck Disability Index: a study of reliability and validity. J Manipulative Physiol Ther. 1991; 14:409-15.
87. Pietrobon R, Coeytaux R, Carey T, Richardson W, DeVellis R. Standards scales for measurement of functional outcome for cervical pain or dysfunction. Spine. 2002;27:515-22.
88. Neer CS. Shoulder rehabilitation. Shoulder Reconstruction, 1st edition. Philadelphia: W.B. Saunders; 1990. pp. 487-533.
89. McNeely ML, Parliament MB, Seikaly H, Jha N, Magee DJ, Haykowsky MJ, et al. Effect of exercise on upper extremity pain and dysfunction in head and neck cancer survivors: a randomized controlled trial. Cancer. 2008;113:21422.
90. Steurer M, Passler C, Denk DM, Schneider B, Niederle B, Bigenzahn W. Advantages of recurrent laryngeal nerve identification in thyroidectomy and parathyroidectomy and the importance of preoperative and postoperative laryngoscopic examination in more than 1000 nerves at risk. Laryngoscope. 2002;112:24-33.
91. Barczyński M, Randolph GW, Cernea CR, Dralle H, Dionigi G, Alesina PF, et al. External branch of the superior laryngeal nerve monitoring during thyroid and parathyroid surgery: International Neural Monitoring Study Group standards guideline statement. The Laryngoscope. 2013;123:S1-4.
92. Perros P, Boelaert K, Colley S, Evans C, Evans RM, Gerrard BAG, et al. Guidelines for the management of thyroid cancer. Clinical Endocrinology. 2014;81:1-22.
93. Echternach M, Maurer C, Mencke T, Schilling M, Verse T, Richter B. Laryngeal complications after thyroidectomy: is it always the surgeon? Archives of Surgery. 2009;144(2): 149-53.
94. Li Y, Garrett G, Zealear D. Current treatment options for bilateral vocal fold paralysis: a state-of-the-art review. Clinical and experimental otorhinolaryngology. 2017;10(3):203.

CHAPTER 44

Principles of Dental Oncology and Maxillofacial Prosthodontics

Trupti Kolur, PC Jacob

PRETREATMENT DENTAL EVALUATION AND IMPLICATIONS[1-3]

The purpose of the dental examination prior to cancer treatment is to identify any dental conditions that need to be addressed in order to reduce morbidity and increase a patient's quality of life during active cancer treatment and throughout survivorship. It is also an important opportunity to educate the patient about the changes that may occur in the oral cavity due to treatment such as changes in salivary flow, trismus, and increased risk for dental caries. Also it is important to inform the patient about the risk of osteoradionecrosis (ORN) due to radiation or medication and increased risk for infection.

The time frame from when the dental provider first examines the patient until the cancer therapy is to begin is critical. A patient that presents with multiple dental needs will require an extensive treatment plan and may not have the ability to restore the dental condition given the time requirements. If this is the case, the decision may have to be made to sacrifice part or all of the patient's dentition in order to clear the patient for cancer therapy from a dental standpoint. Good communication with the head and neck surgeon, radiation oncologist, and medical oncologist is crucial to determine this time frame.

The dental examination should consist of all aspects of a standard comprehensive examination. At the initial examination, all head and neck soft and hard tissues should be evaluated and any deviations from normal documented. Appropriate radiography must be obtained to completely evaluate the patient's dental condition. **Figures 1 to 3** show characteristic findings on routine radiography. In charting of the patients, existing dental restorations and previously extracted or missing teeth, a complete periodontal evaluation including periodontal probing and a complete disease control treatment plan are provided to the patient. Impressions should be taken and models of the maxillary and mandibular arch

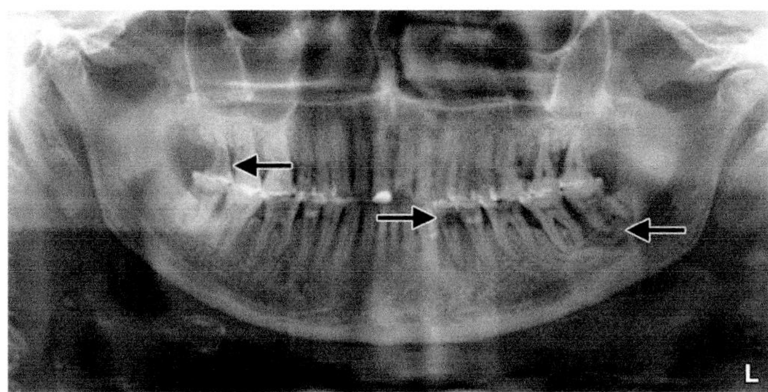

Fig. 1: Carcinoma of oropharynx planned for radical chemoradiotherapy. Patient has periapical abscess on the left lower third molar region; deep caries in relation to left lower first premolar and right upper third molar.

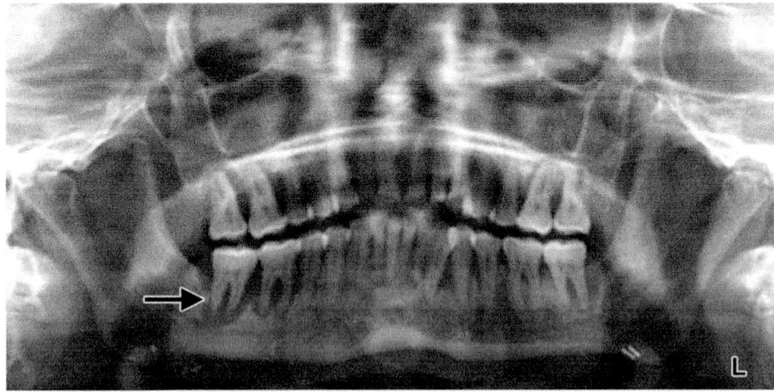

Fig. 2: Tooth with bone loss, mobility and furcation involvement.

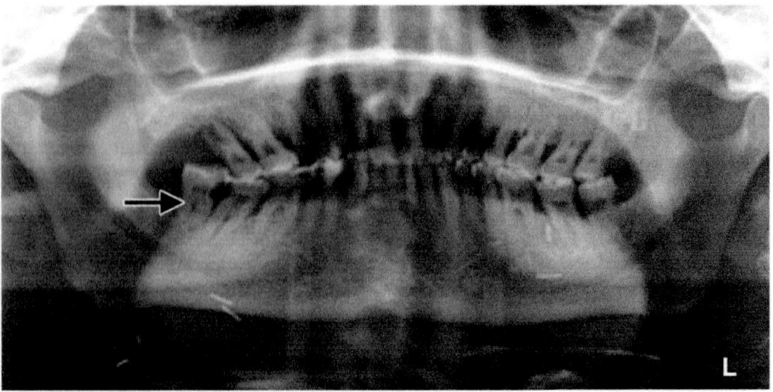

Fig. 3: Patient with carcinoma of left lateral border tongue having multiple caries on the right side lower molars.

should be created as they may be needed to create intraoperative devices and can be a very important resource in reconstruction postoperatively. The dental provider may also want to include intra and extra oral photographs to further document the patient's pretreatment status. An orthopantomograph may serve as an initial screening radiograph.

Dental factors that must be taken into consideration are periodontal disease, dental caries, root canal therapy, impacted teeth, teeth with large restorations, fractures and severe occlusal wear, pain, periapical radiolucency, unopposed teeth, and supraerupted teeth. Teeth that will be in or very near the proposed radiation field should be considered for extraction prior to radiation therapy if the teeth exhibit greater than 50% bone loss, mobility, 5 mm or greater pockets, furcation involvement, history of bleeding, and/or inflamed gingival tissue around the tooth.

Teeth in or around the proposed field of radiation should be considered for preradiation therapy extraction, if they have deep caries approaching the pulp and deep caries extending the deep subgingival or subosseous. Any tooth with dental caries that would make for a difficult or questionable restoration should be extracted. Deep caries in teeth that are in the field of radiation, patients that have multiple carious lesions throughout the mouth, carries high risk need to be considered for extraction prior to radiotherapy. Root canal therapy should be considered for teeth in the proposed field of radiation if the tooth in need of root canal therapy has an adequate periodontal support, a high degree of restorability, and an adequate time frame exists between the root canal therapy and commencement of radiation therapy to allow for evaluation of success of root canal therapy. Teeth having existing root canal therapy in the proposed field of radiation should be considered for preradiation therapy extraction if they have been obturated with silver points, radiographic evidence of internal or external resorption, or periodontal disease.

Teeth in the field of radiation should be extracted if any evidence of endodontic failure exists such as pain, swelling, or apical radiolucency or apical periodontitis. Teeth with large restorations, fractures, and severe occlusal wear that are in the proposed field of radiation should be closely inspected by the dentist, and if the dentist does not have a high degree of confidence that these teeth can be maintained or further definitively restored, then consideration should be given for extraction prior to radiation therapy. The teeth that are unopposed and/or supraerupted should not be impinging on the buccal mucosa or any flap. Unopposed teeth and supraerupted teeth causing traumatic ulcers should be extracted before starting of radiation.

RADIATION CARIES[4,5]

Patients of head and neck cancer who received radiotherapy are at significant risk of developing radiation caries, a progressive carious process involving all the teeth. It can present as early as a month after completion of treatment. One of the earliest signs is demineralization and resultant susceptibility to acid attack. Disruption of salivary production also aids in this process. Alteration in salivary composition, microflora, and composition also contribute to radiation caries. A severe case is seen in **Figures 4A and B**. Some of the measures to prevent and manage radiation caries are:

- Use of artificial saliva substitutes help with lubrication, restoration of salivary pH balance, and inhibiting bacterial growth.

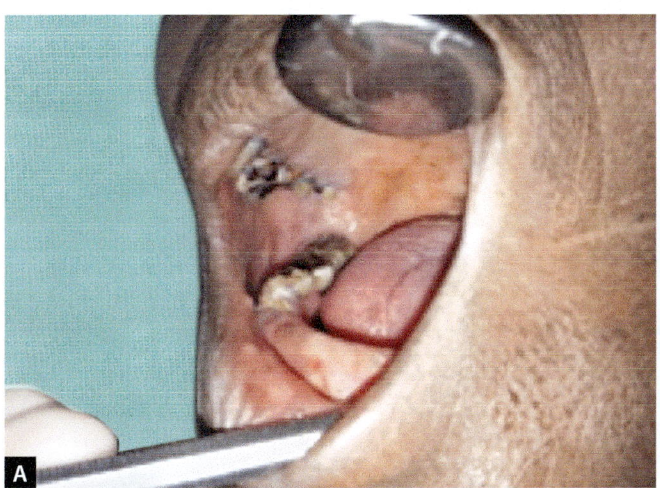

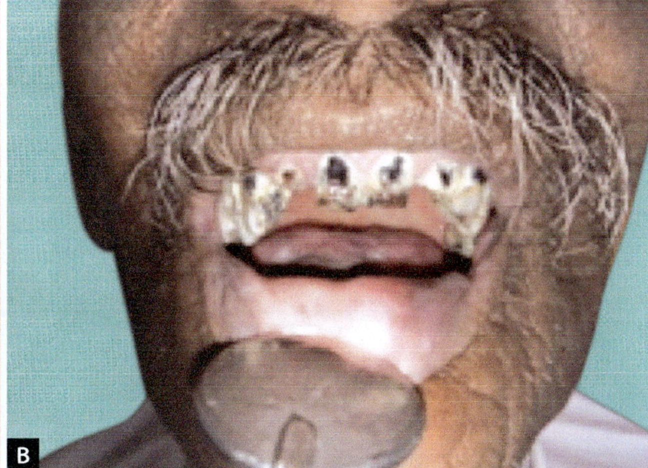

Figs. 4A and B: Patient with generalized radiation caries.

- Systemic sialogogues such as pilocarpine can help stimulate saliva production in early stages where there is hyposalivation. However, these will not be useful if radiation fibrosis occurs in the glands.
- Fluoride applications (commonly 1.1% sodium fluoride gel) for 3–5 minutes using trays can reduce subsequent risk. A fluoride varnish can also be applied before radiotherapy and then once in 3 months.
- Good oral hygiene during radiotherapy with soft brushing, warm saline, and peroxide rinses.
- Early treatment of oral candidiasis with nystatin mouth paint.
- If extractions need to be performed after radiotherapy, prophylaxis with pentoxifylline 400 mg twice a day and tocopherol 400 mg once a day for a month may prevent ORN.

OSTEORADIONECROSIS

This is one of the dreaded complications of head and neck radiotherapy which results in the devascularization of irradiated bone. ORN is defined as presence of exposed bone within an irradiated field that fails to heal within a 3-month period. Early presentation (<2 years) is believed to be a direct result of radiation-induced damage while delayed presentation is believed to occur as a result of secondary trauma or bone damage superimposed on this radiation-induced damage. Although ORN is also possible in the maxilla, it is more common in the mandible due to its supply from the inferior alveolar artery, an end artery, and the minimal contribution from the periosteal attachments. Additionally, the maxilla and mandible are the only bones exposed to the atmosphere through the gingival attachment to the teeth. All patients who receive radiotherapy do not develop ORN; there are patient-related factors (age, atherosclerosis, oral hygiene, and smoking), radiation-related factors (dose of radiotherapy >50 Gy, fractionation, and technique of radiotherapy), and inciting factors (dental extraction or surgery after radiotherapy) that result in this complex interplay.[6,7] There are several theories propounded to explain the pathogenesis of ORN, with Marx's[8] being the most popular **(Flowchart 1)**. In this theory, tissue damage from radiotherapy results in hypocellularity, while endarteritis and vascular disruption result in hypovascularity and ischemic damage result in hypoxia **(Flowchart 2)**. Another theory was proposed by Delanian,[9] which described radiation-induced fibrosis. Clinical features include dry mouth with mucosal

Flowchart 1: Marx's hypoxic hypocellular theory of osteoradionecrosis.

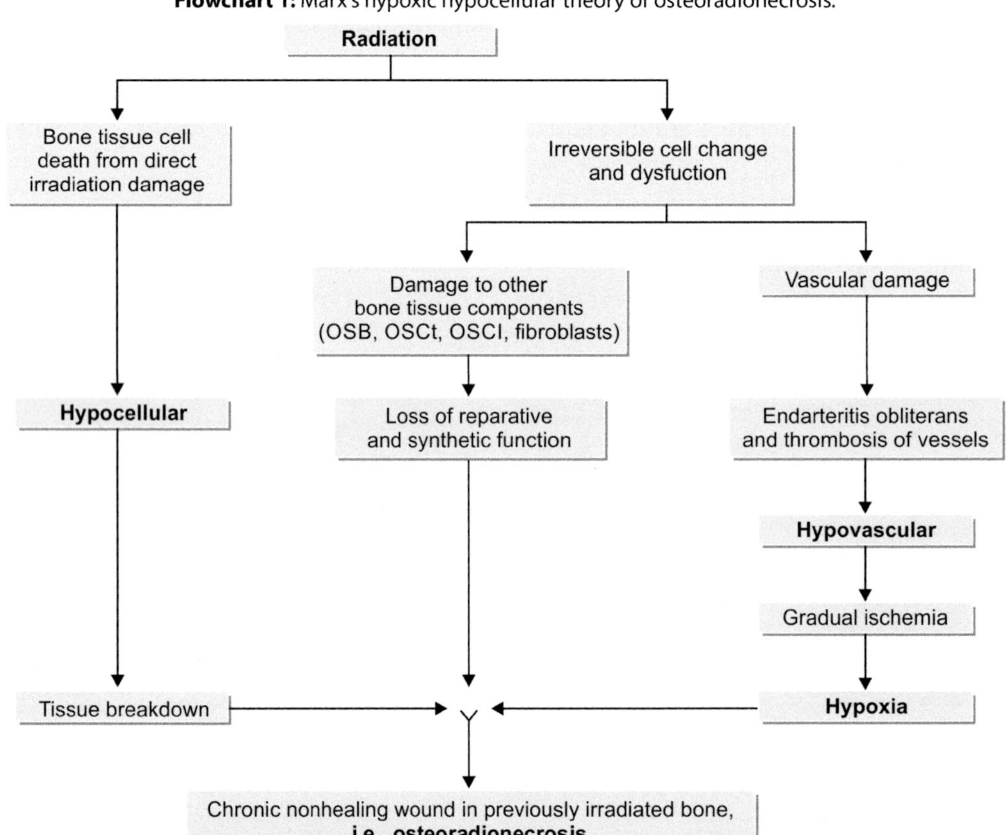

(OSB: osteoblast; OSCt: osteocytes; OSCl: osteoclasts; OSB: osteoblasts)

Flowchart 2: Delanian's radiation-induced fibrosis theory of osteoradionecrosis.

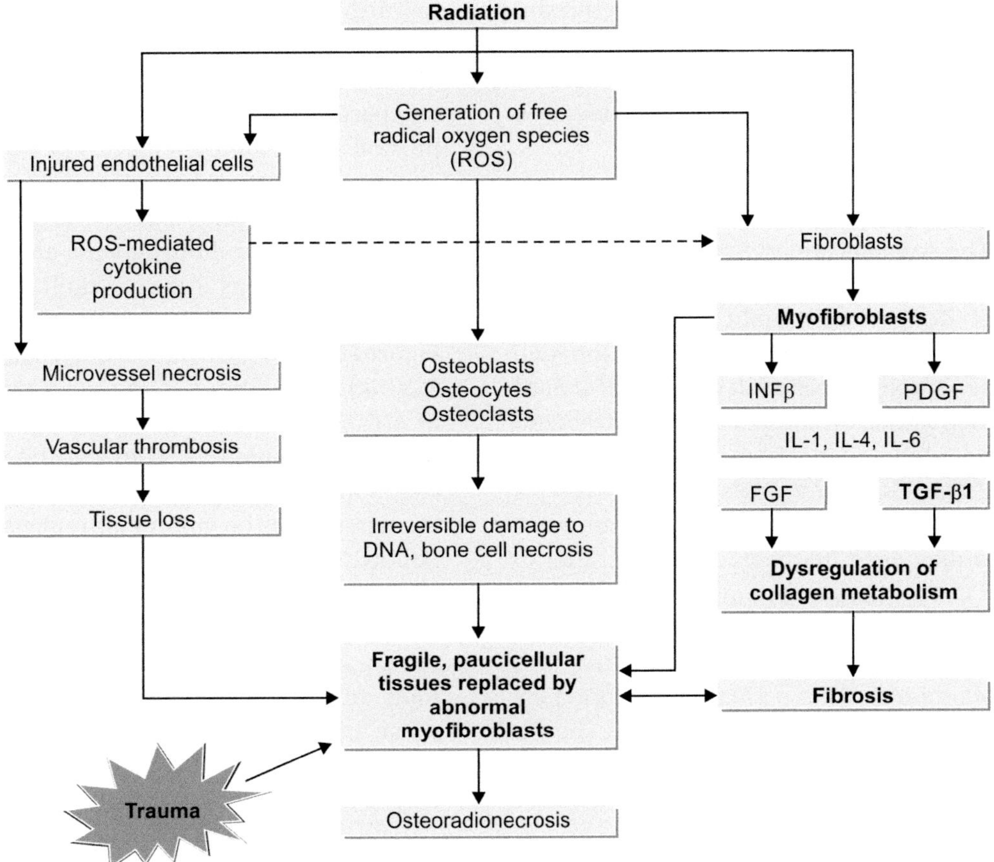

ulceration yielding exposed bone. As the disease progresses, it results in external soft-tissue involvement with formation of orocutaneous fistulae or pathological fracture. Computed tomography (CT) shows focal lytic lesions, loss of trabeculae, and cortical disruptions. Bone scan is highly sensitive and can show nonviability of bone. Medical management is supportive with management of pain and prevention/treatment of infection. Pentoxifylline and tocopherol are the only agents, when administered together have shown therapeutic benefit.[10] Hyperbaric oxygen therapy (HBOT) has shown to have some benefit in early stages, however its role is controversial; recent literature has shown no benefit with this modality of treatment.[11] For advanced stages, where there is fracture, extensive bone, and soft-tissue involvement, surgery is the treatment of choice; dead bone needs to be removed in entirety and replaced with vascularized tissue. It is crucial before surgery for ORN to rule out recurrence, which can be challenging.

REHABILITATION

Resection of the facial bones leads to significant patient morbidity. Loss of support to the teeth, tongue, and lip causes dysfunctional mastication, swallowing, speech, airway protection, and oral competence. Patients also suffer disfigurement following resection. The degrees of dysfunction and disfigurement depend on the extent of tissue loss. Rehabilitation of the oral cancer patient is a coordinated, multidisciplinary effort that requires keen attention to medical, surgical, and humanistic aspects of patient well-being. Although the roles of surgery, radiation, and chemotherapy in extirpation are well-defined for the treatment of oral cancer, understanding of treatment-related sequelae, and how to manage them, continues to emerge.

- *Mandible:* The mandible provides crucial architecture for dentition, mastication, articulation, deglutition, respiration, and facial contour. Satisfactory functional outcomes can be achieved after mandibular resection with appropriate management of the surgical defect. Studies have demonstrated relatively high rates of speech intelligibility, deglutition, and dental rehabilitation after mandibular resection with free-flap reconstruction. When a segmental mandibulectomy has been done, the disruption of bony continuity by segmental mandibulectomy typically necessitates a combination of plating, osseous and/or soft free tissue transfer. Options for osseous-free tissue transfer include the fibula, ilium, and scapula. Dental restoration with conventional dentures or osseointegrated dental implants is often necessary to restore dentition and occlusion following mandibulectomy.

- *Palate and maxilla:* The subsite of the oral cavity that requires attention to functional outcome is the palate or maxilla. The palate is imperative for the oral, oral preparatory, and pharyngeal phases of swallowing, and palatal defects can yield velopharyngeal insufficiency, nasal regurgitation, and dysphagia. Palatal cancers may involve the soft palate and/or hard palate, and depending on the extent of involvement, reconstruction may be performed with a palatal obturator or free flap. Small maxillectomy defects permit the use of obturators, which provide for quick recovery but may need frequent adjustment due to postsurgical tissue changes. Preoperative evaluation with a prosthodontist allows for preparation of the obturator in advance, which can be fitted with prosthetic dentition to aid in occlusion. Appropriately fitted obturators can substantially improve speech intelligibility. Moderate defects can be reconstructed with either obturator or free flap with similar functional outcomes. However, extensive palatal resection may be more appropriately managed with free-tissue reconstruction, as this has been associated with superior functional preservation compared with use of an obturator. This obturator prosthesis is used to fill defects of the soft palate and restore function of the palatopharyngeal sphincter. A pharyngeal obturator allows for effective oronasal separation. Edentulous patients are likely to require dental implants as it is very unlikely that there will be satisfactory retention of conventional prostheses. **Figures 5 and 6** show successful palatal obturation.
- *Zygomatic implants:*[12] These have changed the face of prosthodontic rehabilitation following head and neck cancer ablation. They can be combined with free-flap reconstruction depending on the size of the defect and the volume of replacement required. Following maxillectomy, obturator placement can often be challenging, due to difficulties with retention, fit, and comfort. Zygomatic implants provide a robust alternative. The development of specialized tools and techniques has allowed early loading of these implants in a cancer setting for effective rehabilitation. The Brånemark zygomatic implant was introduced for rehabilitation of the resorbed or

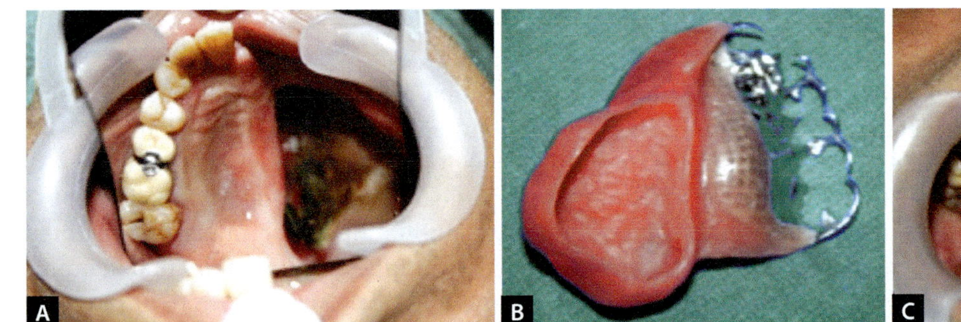

Figs. 5A to C: (A) Maxillectomy defect; (B) Obturator; (C) Obturated defect.

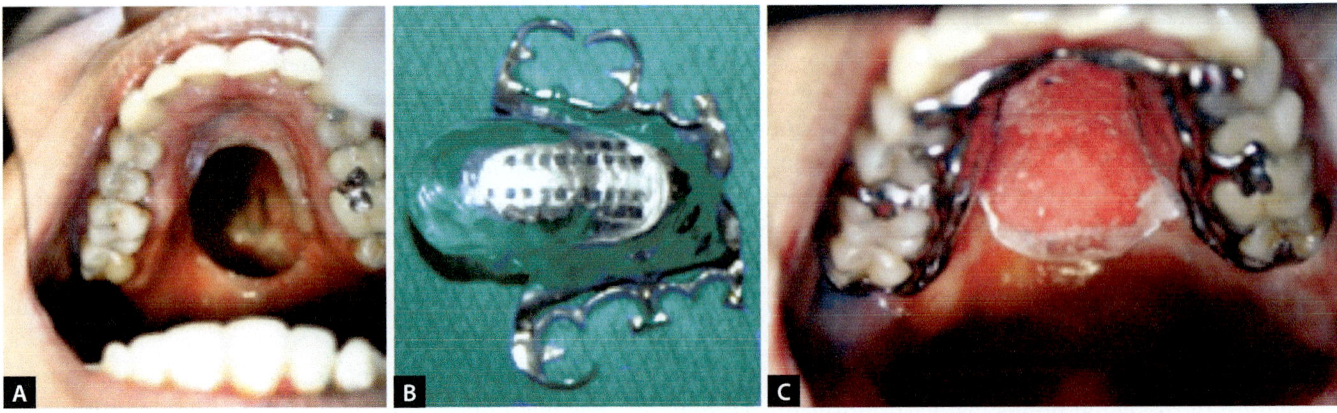

Figs. 6A to C: (A) Hard and soft palate defect; (B) Pharyngeal obturator; (C) Obturated defect.

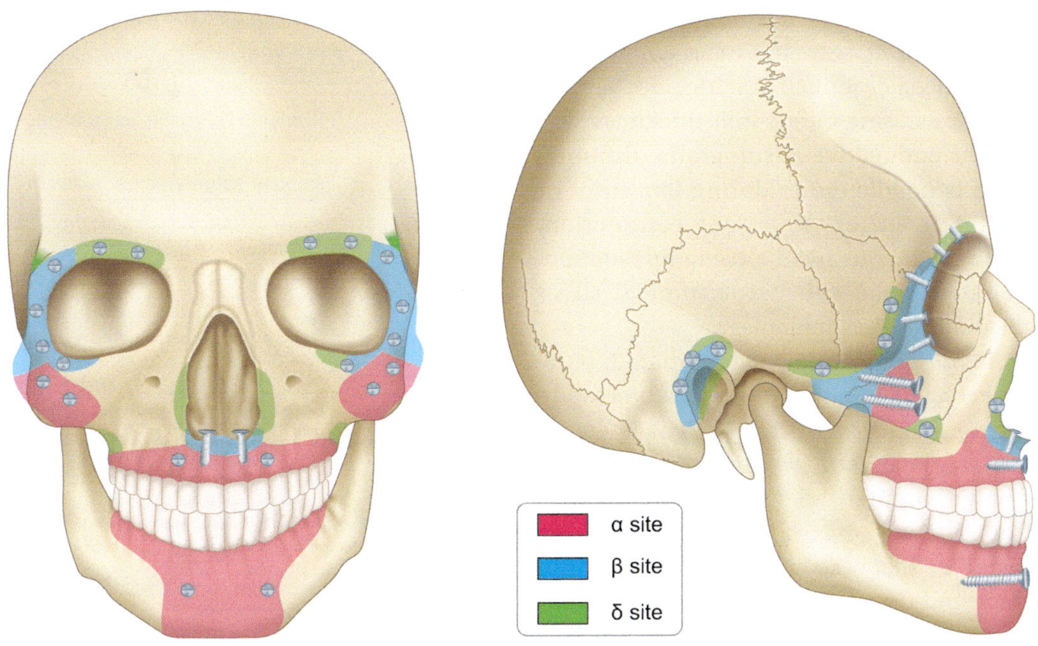

Fig. 7: Craniofacial implant classification.

ablated maxilla where the zygomatic bone could be used to anchor the long implant to allow anchoring prosthesis or obturators. They are also an effective alternative to free-flap surgery in the elderly that can be associated with prolonged anesthesia exposure and its accompanying health risks.

- *Osseointegrated implants:*[13-15] These are endosteal implants that contain pores into which migration of osteoblasts and supportive connective tissue can occur. This biological process of integration ensures greater mechanical stability to withstand the biomechanical forces on them. These implants are most common intraoral, allowing for replacement of dentition, but can also be extraoral to replace the nose, eyes, or ears. They also improve functioning and cosmesis, resulting in improved patient's quality of life **(Fig. 7)**. **Figure 8** shows a fibula free flap with primary osseointegrated implants.
- *Vestibuloplasty:* In patients who undergo large ablative surgeries of the maxilla or mandible, the free-fibula flap is the reconstructive option of choice. Implant-supported dental rehabilitation improves oral health-related quality of life in these patients. Although the volume and density of bone in the free-fibula flap are ideal for implant rehabilitation, the quality of the peri-implant soft tissues is often not optimal. Previous studies have shown that the quality and quantity of the fibula flap used for reconstruction of the mandible is favorable for the placement of osseointegrated dental implants. However, the quality of the overlying soft tissues that form the denture-bearing area of prospective dental rehabilitation is often not optimal. In patients reconstructed with free-fibula flap, in view of oral rehabilitation of these patients, fibula skin flap is a poor substitute for the attached oral mucosa as they are excessively bulky, mobile, and of poor texture (often with the presence of hair appendages). Moreover, in between the fibula bone and the outer surface of the skin flap, there are layers of fat and muscle, which forms a compressible bed (much like a multilayered mattress) when used as a support for prosthetic rehabilitation. Hence, it is extremely important that the soft tissue overlying

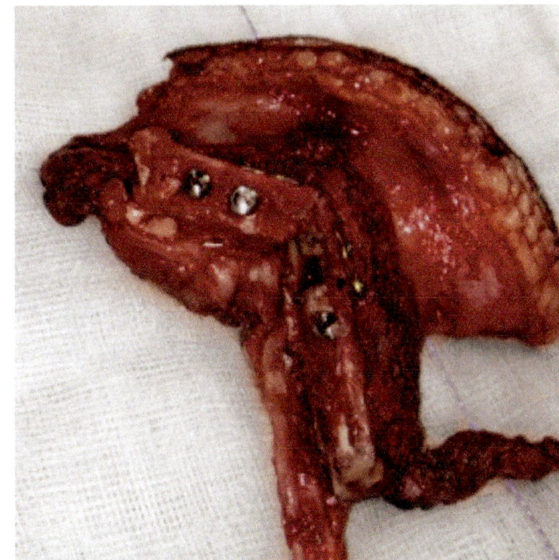

Fig. 8: Fibula free flap with primary dental implant placement.

the reconstructed mandible is modified prior to implant rehabilitation. To solve this issue, a number of techniques have been described that include: Various grafting procedures using either split-thickness skin grafts or palatal connective tissue grafts, thinning of the cutaneous paddle either during flap inset or during implant insertion/abutment connection, thinning of the cutaneous paddle using liposuction, laser resurfacing of the soft tissue, topical silver nitrate application, and vestibuloplasty.

- *Timing of implant placement:* Once irradiated, bone is at risk of necrosis and implant loss if subjected to implant surgery. Hence when the patient is considering implant placement, whether it should be performed before or after radiotherapy is a relevant consideration. The advantages of placement during ablative surgery are that osseointegration occurs prior to radiotherapy and the implant-related complications are significantly lower than those after radiotherapy **(Flowchart 3)**. Patients can benefit from early rehabilitation and avoids an additional intervention. However, the disadvantages are the risk of improper positioning of implants (often even with planning, if the extent of resection changes this can alter the surgical planning irrevocably), risks of delay in wound healing and radiotherapy, and possibility of early recurrence precluding implant use. In patients who receive secondary implant placement, planning is crucial **(Flowchart 4)**. Adequate bony- and soft-tissue volume is required for dental rehabilitation. Risk of wound complications is high and implant loss has been shown to be as high as 35%. Prophylactic hyperbaric oxygen therapy may be of some value.

Flowchart 3: Algorithm for dental implant placement.

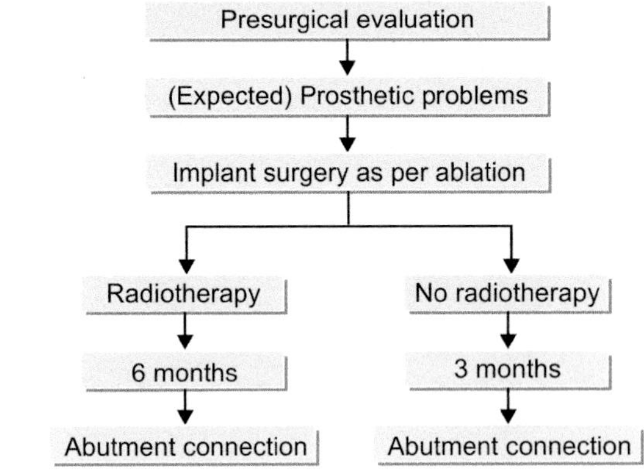

Flowchart 4: Algorithm for dental implant placement after radiotherapy.

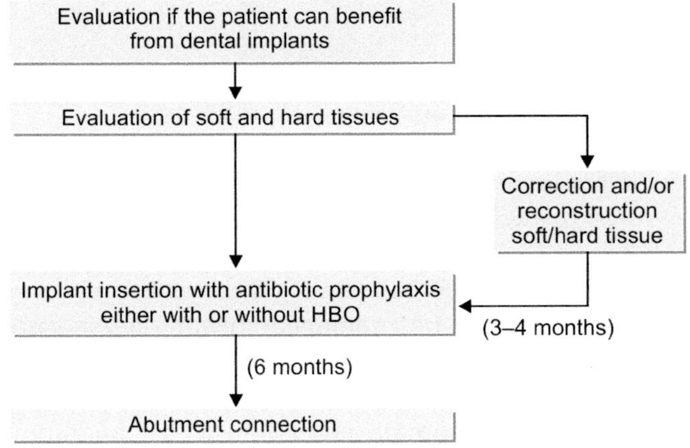

COMPUTER-AIDED SURGERY[16,17]

Although a relatively recent addition to head and neck reconstruction, computer-aided surgery (CAS) has revolutionized the field due to its ability to overcome trial and error issues and drastically reduce operative time. Perfected for fields such as orthognathic surgery, the major challenge in oncology remains planning tumor margins; these often change intraoperatively, impacting the quality of the entire digital plan. It has four components:

1. *Planning:* This involves acquisition of thin slice (<1 mm) high-resolution CT of the head and neck and donor site. These are then converted into 3D images to allow planning for resection margins, osteotomies, and placement of bony segments.
2. *Modeling:* This involves stereolithographic models that are produced using 3D printing. These models are used for planning of the surgery in various ways; the reconstructed model can be used to prebend the reconstruction plate to save intraoperative time, or cutting guides can be printed out for assistance in ablative and reconstructive surgeries.
3. *Surgery:* This is performed using the cutting guides or prebent plates for improved efficiency and accuracy.
4. *Evaluation:* This involves repeating imaging and comparing the results to the preoperative virtual plan.

The advantages of CAS are that it allows for mock surgery and planning, improves accuracy, and reduces ischemia and the operating time. The limitations are the potential cost and expertise required to perform the process, issues related to tumor margins, and disruption of the plan and time taken for planning which can delay the surgery.

REFERENCES

1. Toth BB, Frame RT. Dental oncology: the management of disease and treatment-related oral/dental complications

associated with chemotherapy. Current Problems in Cancer. 1983;7(10):7-35.
2. Maureen S. The expanding role of dental oncology in head and neck surgery. Surgical Oncology Clinics of North America. 2004;13(1):37-46.
3. Garg A, Guez G. Head and neck cancer, dental implants, and dental oncology. Dental Implantology Update. 2011;22(1): 1-8.
4. Barclay SC, Turani D. Current practice in dental oncology in the UK. Dental Update. 2010;37(8):555-61.
5. Meraw SJ, Reeve CM. Dental considerations and treatment of the oncology patient receiving radiation therapy. J Am Dent Assoc. 1998;129(2):201-5.
6. Raggio BS, Winters R. Modern management of osteoradionecrosis. Current Opinion in Otolaryngology & Head and Neck Surgery. 2018;26(4):254-9.
7. Strojan P, Hutcheson KA , Eisbruch A, Beitler JJ, Johannes AL, Lee AWM, et al. Treatment of late sequelae after radiotherapy for head and neck cancer. Cancer Treat Rev. 2017;59: 79-92.
8. Marx RE. Osteoradionecrosis: a new concept of its pathophysiology. J Oral Maxillofac Surg. 1983;41(5):283-8.
9. Delanian S, Lefaix JL. The radiation-induced fibroatrophic process: therapeutic perspective via the antioxidant pathway. Radiother Oncol. 2004;73(2):119-31
10. Rivero JA, Shamji O, Kolokythas A. Osteoradionecrosis: a review of pathophysiology, prevention and pharmacologic management using pentoxifylline, a-tocopherol, and clodronate. Oral Surg Oral Med Oral Pathol Oral Radiol. 2017;124(5):464-71.
11. Bennett MH, Feldmeier J, Hampson NB, Smee R, Milross C. Hyperbaric oxygen therapy for late radiation tissue injury. Cochrane Database Syst Rev. 2016;4:CD005005.
12. Kim DD, Ghali GE. Dental implants in oral cancer reconstruction. Oral and Maxillofacial Surgery Clinics. 2011;23(2):337-45.
13. Ch'Ng S, Skoracki RJ, Selber JC, Yu P, Martin JW, Hofstede TM, et al. Osseointegrated implant-based dental rehabilitation in head and neck reconstruction patients. Head & Neck. 2016;38(S1):E321-7.
14. Schoen PJ, Raghoebar GM, Bouma J, Reintsema H, Burlage FR, Roodenburg JL, et al. Prosthodontic rehabilitation of oral function in head-neck cancer patients with dental implants placed simultaneously during ablative tumour surgery: an assessment of treatment outcomes and quality of life. Int J Oral Maxillofac Surg. 2008;37(1):8-16.
15. Pace-Balzan A, Rogers SN. Dental rehabilitation after surgery for oral cancer. Curr Opin Otolaryngol Head Neck Surg. 2012; 20(2):109-13.
16. Deek NF, Wei FC. Computer-assisted surgery for segmental mandibular reconstruction with the osteoseptocutaneous fibula flap: Can we instigate ideological and technological reforms? Plast Reconstr Surg. 2016;137(3):963-70.
17. Han HH, Kim HY, Lee JY. The pros and cons of computer-aided surgery for segmental mandibular reconstruction after oncological surgery. Arch Craniofac Surg. 2017;18(3):149.

CHAPTER 45

Management of Pain and Palliative Care in Head and Neck Cancer

Shabala Paul, Narayana Subramaniam

INTRODUCTION

Pain is defined as an unpleasant sensory and emotional experience associated with actual or potential tissue damage, or described in terms of such damage.[1] Based on the duration of pain, it can be characterized as acute pain and chronic pain.

- *Acute pain* is a symptom, which serves as a biological alarm that contributes to etiologic diagnosis and resolves on treatment.[2] Patients with head and neck cancer may suffer from acute cancer-related, or acute anticancer treatment-related pain. Acute cancer-related pain may occur as a result of inflammatory and tumorigenic pain mechanisms such as local tumor pressure, or infiltration of tissues or bone, which may cause subsequent obstruction or compression of visceral structures or nerves and also paraneoplastic effects at distant sites.[3] It can also be seen immediately postsurgery and even as a side effect of chemotherapy and radiation therapy.
- *Chronic pain*, on the other hand, is a multidimensional syndrome. The term "chronic pain" applies in case of several of the following criteria: persistence or recurrence, lasting longer than usual for the presumed initial cause, especially when evolving for >3 months; insufficient response to treatment; significant progressive deterioration due to pain in functional and relational capacity in daily activity, at home or at work.[4]

ETIOLOGY OF PAIN

- *Nociceptive pain:* Pain due to excessive nociception can arise from overstimulation of the head and neck nociceptive system, due to tumor expansion and inflammation and to the specific type of treatment (surgery, radiation therapy, and chemotherapy). Compression, ischemia, infection, and destruction of tissue structures can release algogenic substances. Chemotherapy and radiation therapy cause severe pain (mucositis, postradiation necrosis, etc.). Nociceptive pain responds to analgesia, which reduces or interrupts the transmission of nociceptive messages at peripheral (NSAIDs and corticosteroids) and/or central level (paracetamol and opioids).[5]
- *Neuropathic pain:* Neuropathic pain is secondary to a peripheral or central nervous system lesion, altering the nociceptive transmission and/or control processes. In head and neck cancer, it is mainly peripheral. It can also be caused by distal demyelinization in certain curative treatments (platinum- or taxane-based chemotherapy). Pain may be localized or projected exhibiting as hemicrania continua, reflex otalgia, neck pain, etc. It may be exacerbated by neurovascular or cerebral mechanisms. This convergence also explains the reflex muscular responses (contracture, trismus, etc.) and the involvement of the vigilance and emotional systems (tension headache, anxiety, depressive syndrome, etc.). Ortho- and parasympathetic innervation, depending on the cranial nerves, explains vasomotor headache.[6,7] Some common symptoms of neuropathic pain experienced by the patients include spontaneous continuous burning (81%), shooting pain (69%), and allodynia (88%), which describes abnormal pain elicited by light touch.[8]
- *Psychological component:* Correlated with such psychological vulnerability, the patient may catastrophize, showing a pattern of pessimistic thought, expectation, and representation that mediates the attention paid to the pain. The representations common to head and neck cancers (disfiguration, asphyxia, and hemorrhage) are associated with a fear of suffering and the expectation of fatal outcome.[9,10]

ASSESSMENT OF PAIN

The European Society for Medical Oncology (ESMO) has published clinical practice guidelines for the management of cancer pain[11] that entails the following:

- *Assess and reassess the pain:*
  - Causes, onset, type, site, absence/presence of radiating pain, duration, intensity, relief and temporal patterns of the pain, number of BTcPs (breakthroughs of cancer pain), pain syndrome, inferred pathophysiology, and pain at rest and/or moving
  - Presence of trigger factors and signs and symptoms associated with the pain
  - Presence of relieving factors
  - Use of analgesics and their efficacy and tolerability
  - *Description of the pain quality:*
    - *Aching, throbbing, pressure:* Often associated with somatic pain in skin, muscle, and bone
    - *Aching, cramping, gnawing, sharp:* Often associated with visceral pain in organs or viscera
    - *Shooting, sharp, stabbing, tingling, ringing:* Often associated with neuropathic pain caused by nerve damage
- *Assess and reassess the patient:*
  - Clinical situation by means of a complete/specific physical examination and the specific radiological and/or biochemical investigations
  - Interference of pain with the patient's daily activities, work, social life, sleep patterns, appetite, sexual functioning, mood, well-being, and coping
  - Impact of the pain, the disease, and the therapy on the physical, psychological, and social conditions
  - Presence of a caregiver, psychological status, degree of awareness of the disease, anxiety and depression and suicidal ideation, his/her social environment, quality of life (QoL), spiritual concerns/needs, problems in communication, and personality disorders
  - Presence and intensity of signs, physical and/or emotional symptoms associated with cancer pain syndromes
  - Presence of comorbidities (i.e., diabetic, renal and/or hepatic failure)
  - Functional status
  - Presence of opiophobia or misconception related to pain treatment
  - Alcohol and/or substance abuse
- *Assess and reassess your ability to inform and communicate with the patient and his family:*
  - Spend time with the patient and the family to understand their needs.

MANAGEMENT OF ACUTE PAIN

- *Postoperative pain:* Treatment of acute postsurgical pain is initiated in the preoperative period and continued into the postoperative period. Head and neck cancer surgery can cause intense postoperative pain, peaking in the first hours after surgery then gradually decreasing over the following 48–72 hours.[12] Preemptive analgesia can be administered. Immediate postoperative pain following resection surgery to the mid-third of the face or oral cavity is often due to deafferentation of a branch of the trigeminal nerve (V2 or V3), in which case there is hypoesthesia leading to discomfort exacerbated by large edema. Neck and shoulder pain is frequent after neck dissection, directly impairing QoL. The causes remain poorly elucidated, but partly implicate neural lesions (spinal nerve and cervical plexus roots) inducing involvement of the trapezius and other scapulohumeral belt muscles, which tend to cause shoulder stiffness that may evolve toward retractile capsulitis.[13] Management of acute pain follows the same protocols used all over the world. The World Health Organization (WHO) pain ladder forms the basis of pharmacological management of pain[14] **(Fig. 1)**. The principles on which this is based are shown in **Table 1**. The 4th step is a modification applied to the original aimed at using alternate modalities of pain relief.
  - *Step 1:* Step 1 drugs on the WHO ladder consist of paracetamol (acetaminophen) and nonsteroidal anti-inflammatory drugs (NSAIDs) only. Paracetamol is used widely for mild-to-moderate pain with a well-established safety profile. Its mechanism of action is surprisingly not well defined for such a prevalent drug, but it is thought that paracetamol acts as a centrally acting cyclooxygenase (COX) enzyme inhibitor, with suggested modulations of the serotoninergic system and interference with peripheral delivery

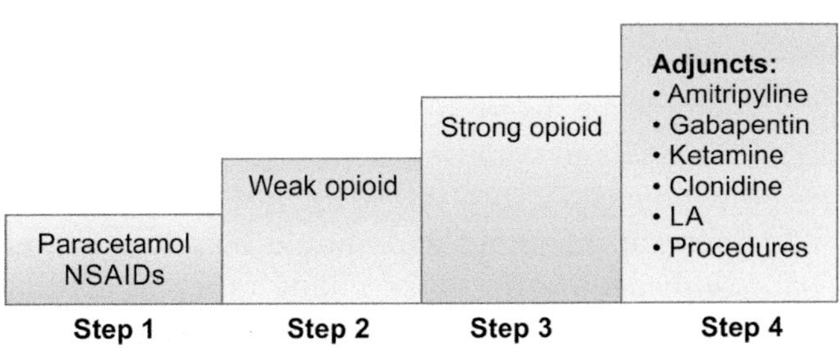

Fig. 1: WHO pain ladder. (LA: local anesthetic; NSAIDs: nonsteroidal anti-inflammatory drugs)

Table 1: Principles of pain relief.

WHO recommendations	*Comments*
By mouth	Use the oral route unless contraindicated. In head and neck cancer, drugs can still be taken enterally by nasogastric or gastrostomy tubes or rectal administration. If not possible, subcutaneous, intravenous, or transdermal routes may be used
By the clock	Regular administration to be given before the previous dose wears off. Breakthrough analgesia is not a substitute but is given in addition to regular
By the ladder	Follow the WHO 3rd step ladder
For the individual	There are no standard doses—the correct dose is one that relieves pain. Titrate dose and add adjuvant therapy as necessary
Attention to detail	Timings, side effects, response, follow-up, weaning, etc. Regular reviews

(WHO: World Health Organization)

of β-endorphins.[15] Paracetamol acts synergistically with NSAIDs and an intravenous preparation can be used in patients who cannot take the drug orally. NSAIDs act on COX enzyme. They can be either nonselective COX inhibitors such as aspirin, ibuprofen, diclofenac, ketorolac, or selective COX II inhibitors such as celecoxib and parecoxib. COX produces prostaglandins, which is one contributor to the peripheral inflammatory response, as well as playing a part in thrombosis, body salt and water homeostasis, blood pressure, and gastric protection.[16] COX II inhibitors have been shown to have lesser incidence of gastrointestinal disturbances than the nonselective NSAIDs.

- *Step 2:* Weak opioids +/– nonopioids are administered in this step. Commonly used drugs are tramadol, codeine, and hydrocodeine. Tramadol is a synthetic opioid, chemically unrelated to morphine with monoaminergic properties. It produces a different analgesic effect compared with simple opioids and has less risk of respiratory depression and addiction potential. However, one should be aware of the increased incidence of nausea and vomiting, dizziness, and orthostatic hypotension with this drug. It also reduces the seizure threshold and should be administered with caution in those taking other drugs that reduce the seizure threshold [e.g., tricyclic antidepressants (TCAs)]. Tramadol is contraindicated in epileptics and in individuals taking serotonergic medication due to serotonin toxicity. Codeine is a prodrug that is metabolized to morphine.
- *Step 3:* These drugs are used for moderate-to-severe pain. This group includes strong opioids such as morphine, oxycodone, and fentanyl. Strong opioids are available in various pharmacological forms—intravenous, oral, elixirs, lozenges and lollipops, transdermal, etc. They also carry known side effects such as constipation, nausea and vomiting, and sedation in diverse degrees. Hence, these drugs should be given their due consideration when being administered.
- *Step 4:* This step involves the usage of adjunct drugs and therapies, which are commonly used for chronic and neuropathic pain. The drugs may include antidepressants (amitriptyline and nortriptyline), anticonvulsants (gabapentin and pregabalin), N-methyl-D-aspartate (NMDA) receptor antagonists (ketamine), steroids, capsaicin, and so on. Local anesthetics are also included as part of interventions for pain relief. The *trigeminal* (CN V) and *facial* (CN VII) are by far the most frequently affected nerves, alone or in combination, explained by their wide anatomic distribution and rich anastomotic connections.

  The commonly used nerve blocks and ancillary interventions are as follows:
  - Sphenopalatine ganglion block
  - Trigeminal ganglion block
  - Glossopharyngeal nerve block
  - Stellate ganglion block
  - Intrathecal drug delivery
  - Occipital nerve block
  - Botulinum toxin injection[17]

  Pain intervention specialists also resort to the use of ultrasound and fluoroscopy guidance to improve the safety and efficacy of these procedures.

- *Postradiotherapy pain:* The most frequent cause of pain is chemo/radiation-related oral mucositis, which involves 80% of the patients and worsens their QoL inhibiting speaking, eating, drinking, or swallowing and sometimes reducing the treatment compliance, the maximum dose intensity, and thus the potential efficacy of treatment. It is also associated with dermatitis and with late pain arising from radiation-induced fibrosis. Pain is involved in a vicious cycle, consisting of dysphagia, malnourishment, reduced treatment compliance, that may hesitate in a lower dose intensity of systemic therapy or in radiation treatment breaks, so ultimately with a possible interference on chance of tumor control.[18] Pain correlates with radiation treatment fields, dose and its fractioning; concomitant chemotherapy or cetuximab results in increased frequency, severity, and duration of mucositis pain. To limit early and late toxicity, radiotherapy should at least be conformal and, if indicated, intensity-modulated, to deliver a homogeneous dose to target volumes and spare healthy tissue as far as possible.[19] When making the treatment plans, the ability of a patient to tolerate increased oral pain and higher doses of opioids should be considered. Once started, the clinician should regularly assess Numerical Rating Scale, Verbal Rating Scale, or Visual Analog Scale to elucidate background, breakthrough, and swallowing-associated pain. Swallowing efforts should be continued during and after radiation treatment as there is increasing evidence that it prevents disuse atrophy and fibrosis and optimizes long-term swallowing function.

The following measures have been used to counter pain related to radiation-related mucositis:

- Basic oral care
- To prevent and treat radiation-induced mucositis, it is recommended to:
    - Assess and eradicate dental infection sites ahead of radiotherapy and transmit irradiated volumes to the dentist.
    - Use a soft toothbrush, replacing it regularly.
    - Apply fluoride to the dental splints.
    - Perform regular mouth rinse with nonalcoholic saline solution.
    - Ensure early diagnosis and treatment of any bacterial, fungal, or viral superinfection.[19]
- *Topical:* Local anesthetics mouthwashes and morphine-based mouthwashes
- *Systemic:* Transdermal fentanyl and intranasal transmucosal fentanyl for odynophagia
- NSAIDs and antispasmodics for musculoskeletal pain

An effective pain regimen should include a fixed and rescue medication (short-release opioids) with an appropriate dose and schedule for each. Often, neuropathic pain requires the addition of adjunct drugs as it responds poorly to narcotics alone.[18] Opiates and gabapentin are believed to interact favorably through a simultaneous decrease in hyperexcitation and increased inhibition of nociception[20] in a synergistic effect[21] that even enhances analgesic effect of morphine and better relieve neuropathic pain in cancer patients than opioid escalating doses with a beneficial effect on daily activity, mood, sleep, and QoL.[22,23]

- *Postchemotherapy pain:* Chemotherapy-induced pain relates to the onset of neuropathy or mucositis. The neuropathy may be irreversible and is secondary to platinum-based (cisplatin); vinca alkaloids (vinorelbine) or taxane-based (docetaxel, paclitaxel) chemotherapeutic agents. Cisplatin can cause late-onset neuropathy, i.e., cumulative and acts mainly on large sensory fibers, primarily due to the effect of platinum. With *paclitaxel*, a reversible distal, predominantly sensory, sensory motor polyneuropathy is seen.[19] Therapy is purely preventive; dose accumulation has to be monitored and the culprit drug withdrawn subsequently. The treatment is symptomatic with neuropathic drugs given at progressively increasing doses. Gabapentin and pregabalin, carbamazepine (anticonvulsants), and amitriptyline (TCA) are the commonly used drugs for neuropathic pain. Where an inflammatory cause of pain is suspected, steroids are also added to the regimen. Ketamine is also an option when pain can be managed in a specialist setting.[24]

PALLIATIVE CARE

Palliative care is interdisciplinary care that provides support for the physical, emotional, and psychological suffering of patients with any advanced illness, regardless of age, diagnosis, or life expectancy. The primary aim is to prevent and relieve suffering and to improve QoL in those dealing with severe, complex illness. It differs from traditional hospice or end-of-life care in that patients who receive palliative care can also continue to receive curative or life-prolonging treatments. This distinction is particularly important in the case of patients with head and neck cancers because these patients often have a relapsing course that is marked by periods of freedom from disease and symptoms, interspersed with bouts of serious illness, debility, and numerous physical and psychological symptoms including pain, dysphagia, weight loss, disfigurement, depression, and xerostomia.[25]

Treatment options for patients with head and neck cancer are diverse and this has increased the duration of disease-free intervals. As a result, patients live longer with the consequences of the disease and its treatment and primary care physicians have to be aware about common side effects and how to treat them.[25]

It is the role of the multidisciplinary team (MDT) to discuss treatment options in all patients. An MDT may include physicians, nurses, and social workers. The purpose of this care is to optimize outcomes. For example, dentists can create prostheses for the teeth and jaw if they are resected. Speech and language pathologists provide voice rehabilitation, including acoustic assistive devices, and teach patients modified swallowing techniques. They can help families in meal preparation and helping them understand the effects of disease and treatment. Physical therapists and occupational therapists help patients adapt to reconstructive procedures involving the use of flaps. Clinical social workers can help coordinate care across settings; nutritionists help assist patients obtain adequate nutrition and hydration. When there is a low chance of cure, the palliative pathway is chosen. This may include surgical and nonsurgical interventions with the aim being slowing disease progression, controlling symptoms, and essentially extending life with a focus on symptom control.[24] The patient and family should have a detailed understanding of the prognosis and likely sequence of events, and if possible a rough timeline. They have to be given the sense of hope and this can be maintained within the context of the patient's own life—be it physical, psychological, or social.[25]

Although physical symptoms must be considered in the care of patients with head and neck malignancies, the constellation of these symptoms and their impact on patient's body image and overall QoL are equally important to consider. It would be in the interest of the patient to seek out medical centers that practice procedures that would maintain cosmetics and function. A patient's best achievable QoL is dependent on factors such as current pathology, stage at diagnosis, and surgical or medical interventions used. In spite of this eventual return to satisfaction with their QoL, the period from diagnosis to full recovery may be marked by symptoms of frustration, hopelessness, and depression. There are instances where specific antidepressant medications may show benefit. Eating is a major social, cultural, and religious ritual in society, and these patients are unable to eat in public. Facial disfigurement—even if only temporary—can turn patients into social recluses. Negative feelings in patients with head and neck cancer can also extend to the impact the illness has on the QoL of their loved ones. Addressing some of these complex issues can often have a positive impact on these patients and improve their QoL.[25]

As with all cancer patients, predicting when an individual is nearing the end of life can be difficult. Signs may include being bed bound, semicomatose, unable to take oral medications, or tolerate artificial feeds.[26] Artificial feeds may be beneficial during the early days of the disease; toward the end of life, it may make patients more uncomfortable and lead to edema, pulmonary congestion, and so on.[27-29] Often a carotid blowout may lead to rapid, massive blood loss from the neck. Ideally those with an impending blowout can be identified and managed in an inpatient setting. If the caregiver can understand this complication and wishes to keep the patient at home, as a practical tip, dark towels (red, green, and black) should be kept near the patient's bedside to absorb the significant amount of blood that may be lost.[25]

Oral morphine has historically been the drug of first choice for the management of moderate-to-severe cancer pain due to its background and for being the most widely used and field-tested clinically. It is also available in various other forms such as tablets, elixirs, and intravenous solutions.

REFERENCES

1. Merskey H. Classification of chronic pain: description of chronic pain syndromes and definitions of pain terms. Pain. 1986;3:216-21.
2. Guy-Coichard C, Rostaing-Rigattieri S, Doubrère JF, Boureau F. Conduite à tenir vis-à-vis d'une douleur chronique. EMC-Anesthésie-Réanimation. 2005;2(1):1-22.
3. Portenoy RK, Lesage P. Management of cancer pain. The Lancet. 1999;353(9165):1695-700.
4. Haute Autorité de Santé. Douleur chronique: reconnaître le syndrome douloureux chronique, l'évaluer et orienter le patient. Douleur analg. 2009;22:51-68.
5. Navez ML, Prades JM. Prise en charge des cancers ORL. La lettre d'ORL et de chirurgie cervico-faciale. 2011;326.
6. Chopra K, Tiwari V. Alcoholic neuropathy: Possible mechanisms and future treatment possibilities. Br J Clin Pharmacol. 2012;73(3):348-62.
7. Perkins FM, Kehlet H. Chronic pain as an outcome of surgery. A review of predictive factors. Anesthesiology. 2000;93(4):1123-33.
8. Lossignol D, Razavi D, Delvaux N. Douleur et analgésie. Précis de psycho-oncologie de l'adulte; 2008. pp. 351-67.
9. Sist T, Miner M, Lema M. Characteristics of postradical neck pain syndrome: a report of 25 cases. J Pain Symptom Manage. 1999;18(2):95-102.
10. Merskey H. PART III pain terms, a current list with definitions and notes on usage. Classification of chronic pain-Descriptions of chronic pain syndromes and definitions of pain terms; 1994. pp. 207-14.
11. Fallon M, Giusti R, Aielli F, Hoskin P, Rolke R, Sharma M, et al. Management of cancer pain in adult patients: ESMO Clinical Practice Guidelines. Annals of Oncology. 2018;29(Suppl 4):iv166-91.
12. Mom T, Bazin JE, Dubray C, Eschalier A, Derbal C, Avan P, et al. Assessment of postoperative pain after laryngeal surgery for cancer. Arch Otolaryngol Head Neck Surg. 1998;124(7):794-8.
13. Espitalier F, Testelin S, Blanchard D, Binczak M, Bollet M, Calmels P, et al. Management of somatic pain induced by treatment of head and neck cancer: postoperative pain. Guidelines of the French Oto-rhino-laryngology-head and neck surgery society (SFORL). Eur Ann Otorhinolaryngol Head Neck Dis. 2014;131(4):249-52.
14. Agulnik M (Ed). Head and Neck Cancer. BoD-Books on Demand; 2012.
15. Remy C, Marret E, Bonnet F. State of the art of paracetamol in acute pain therapy. Curr Opin Anesthesiol. 2006;19(5): 562-5.

16. Grosser T, Fries S, FitzGerald GA. Biological basis for the cardiovascular consequences of COX-2 inhibition: Therapeutic challenges and opportunities. J Clin Invest. 2006;116(1):4-15.
17. Piagkou M, Demesticha T, Troupis T, Vlasis K, Skandalakis P, Makri A, et al. The pterygopalatine ganglion and its role in various pain syndromes: from anatomy to clinical practice. Pain Practice. 2012;12(5):399-412.
18. Mirabile A, Airoldi M, Ripamonti C, Bolner A, Murphy B, Russi E, et al. Pain management in head and neck cancer patients undergoing chemo-radiotherapy: Clinical practical recommendations. Crit Rev Oncol Hematol. 2016;99: 100-6.
19. Blanchard D, Bollet M, Dreyer C, Binczak M, Calmels P, Couturaud C, et al. Management of somatic pain induced by head and neck cancer treatment: pain following radiation therapy and chemotherapy. Guidelines of the French Otorhinolaryngology Head and Neck Surgery Society (SFORL). Eur Ann Otorhinolaryngol Head Neck Dis. 2014;131(4): 253-6.
20. Keskinbora K, Pekel AF, Aydinli I. Gabapentin and an opioid combination versus opioid alone for the management of neuropathic cancer pain: a randomized open trial. J Pain Symptom Manage. 2007;34(2):183-9.
21. De la O-Arciniega M, Díaz-Reval MI, Cortés-Arroyo AR, Domínguez-Ramírez AM, López-Muñoz FJ. Anti-nociceptive synergism of morphine and gabapentin in neuropathic pain induced by chronic constriction injury. Pharmacol Biochem Behav. 2009;92(3):457-64.
22. Gilron I, Bailey JM, Tu D, Holden RR, Weaver DF, Houlden RL. Morphine, gabapentin, or their combination for neuropathic pain. NEJM. 2005;352(13):1324-34.
23. Backonja M, Beydoun A, Edwards KR, Schwartz SL, Fonseca V, Hes M, et al. Gabapentin for the symptomatic treatment of painful neuropathy in patients with diabetes mellitus: a randomized controlled trial. JAMA. 1998;280(21):1831-6.
24. Cocks H, Ah-See K, Capel M, Taylor P. Palliative and supportive care in head and neck cancer: United Kingdom National Multidisciplinary Guidelines. J Laryngol Otol. 2016;130(S2):S198-207.
25. Goldstein NE, Genden E, Morrison RS. Palliative care for patients with head and neck cancer:"I would like a quick return to a normal lifestyle". JAMA. 2008;299(15):1818-25.
26. Ellershaw J, Neuberger RJ, Ward C. Care of the dying patient: the last hours or days of life. Commentary: a "good death" is possible in the NHS. BMJ. 2003;326(7379):30-4.
27. Emanuel LL, von Gunten CF, Ferris FE. Module 11: withholding/withdrawing Treatment. The EPEC curriculum: Education for physicians on end-of-life care. Chicago, IL: The EPEC Project™; 2005.
28. Meier D, Monias A. Palliative medicine and care of the elderly. In: Doyle D, Hanks G, Cherny N, Calman K (Eds). Oxford textbook of palliative medicine, 3rd edition. Oxford: Oxford University Press; 2004.
29. Ganzini L, Goy ER, Miller LL, Harvath TA, Jackson A, Delorit MA. Nurses' experiences with hospice patients who refuse food and fluids to hasten death. NEJM. 2003; 349(4):359-65.

Survivorship and Quality of Life in Head and Neck Cancer

Samskruthi P Murthy, Sivakumar Vidhyadharan, Narayana Subramaniam

SURVIVORSHIP

Introduction

With the advent of advances in various treatment modalities of cancer, the number of cancer survivors has increased dramatically from 3 million in 1971 to 15.5 million in 2016.[1-3] With the change in etiologic pattern of cancer causation in subsites such as oropharynx, the projected incidence rate of the oropharynx in 2030 is as high as 70% of all head and neck cancers (HNCs).[4] The overall survival of human papillomavirus (HPV)-associated oropharyngeal tumors across all stages is approximately 90% and commonly presents at an early age.[5] HPV-related HNC will bring in a wave of survivors who are in their active workforce and play a vital economic role in their families. The needs of cancer patient were often neglected until Mullan's letter "Seasons of survival,"[6] in which he urged that survivorship should be studied as a phenomenon rather than just as a byproduct of cancer treatment and that the challenge in overcoming cancer is not only in finding therapies that will prevent or arrest the disease, but also to map the middle ground of survivorship and minimize its medical and social hazards. Newer perspectives in survivorship have seen a series of initiatives and research to improve and care for special needs during and after cancer treatment. The seminal publication "Lost in transition" has brought the concept of survivorship into the forefront of the cancer treatment spectrum.[7]

Definition

The definition of a cancer survivor is varied. The most accepted definition is "an individual is considered a cancer survivor from the time of diagnosis, through the balance of his/her life. Family members, friends, and caregivers are also affected by the survivorship experience and are therefore included in this definition."[8] Caregivers, relatives, and friends of cancer patient play an essential role in the journey of the cancer treatment; however, the term survivor in this chapter is restricted to the index person diagnosed with cancer.

The terms acute survival, extended survival, and permanent survival were first coined in Mullan's article.[6] Acute survival is the period from diagnosis to end of cancer treatment; this period is marked by fear and anxiety of cancer diagnosis, diagnostic and therapeutic procedural consequences, and psychological burden to deal with their mortality. Extended survival starts from the end of cancer treatment. The endpoint of extended survival is varied based on the cancer; commonly 5 years of disease-free interval is considered the endpoint.[9] The concerns during the extended survival in HNC patients primarily consist of surveillance for recurrence and second primary tumors and functional sequelae of therapy. Permanent survival is considered from point of cure (5 years of disease-free interval) to the end of life. This period of survivorship involves fear of second primary cancer, coping up with new social and familial roles, and also extended treatment sequelae.

Survivorship Care

Various components of survivorship care have been described and are represented in **Table 1**.

Broadly the survivor care plan must consist of following aspects, and the survivor must be supported during the phases of cancer survival:

- *The effects of cancer and its treatment:* HNCs have the potential to affect various vital functions such as speech, chewing, and swallowing. Both surgical and radiotherapy treatment modalities can affect swallowing and breathing functions. Postoperative defects and their sequelae are described in their respective chapters. Reconstruction in the present era

Table 1: Summary of essential components of survivorship care.

Institute of Medicine and The National Research Council (2005)[7]	• Prevention of second primary and recurrent cancer • Surveillance of cancer spread • Assessment of late psychosocial and physical effects • Intervention for cancer treatment-related effects • Coordination of care between primary care providers and cancer specialists
LIVESTRONG Foundation (2011)[10]	• Survivorship plan, psychosocial care plan, treatment summary • Screening and surveillance of second primary and recurrent cancers • Coordination of care between primary care providers and cancer specialists • Health promotion education • Symptom management and palliative care

is most often done during the initial surgery. While rehabilitation is continued for prolonged periods. Reconstruction is aimed at replacing the defect while rehabilitation is primarily focused on strengthening the normal remnant structures and utilizing these to gain normal functioning. Postradiation effects such as xerostomia, altered taste sensation, silent aspiration, post-RT dysphagia, osteonecrosis, and dental hygiene must be cared for during the period of survivorship. Almost 50% of survivors suffered from cancer treatment-related sequelae.[11]

- *Physical effects:* These constitute effects that are related to cancer therapy but are not direct consequences of treatment. These include loss of stamina, loss of weight, and fatigue. Almost 38% of cancer survivors have physical effects that are most often unrecognized by the treating physician.[12]
- *Second primary cancers:* The risk of developing a second primary cancer is based on various factors such as genetic susceptibility, shared causative factors, and mutagenic effects of cancer treatment. About 8.1% of cancer survivors develop second primary cancer in a mean time of 7.1 years, and 55% of them die as a result of second primary cancer.[13] In HNC, the rate of second primary per year is 3.7–6%, and the risk is persistently high even after 10 years with a cumulative risk of 36% at 20 years.[14] Most of the second primary tumors are found in the upper aerodigestive tract (40–59%), lungs (31–37.5%), and esophagus (9–44%).[14] The prognosis of second primary tumor is poor, and hence various strategies such as chemoprevention and routine screening methods have been proposed but with variable results. Lifestyle modifications play an essential role in preventing recurrence and second primary cancer. Tobacco and alcohol cessation forms an essential component of survivorship care.
- *Psychosocial effects:* A good number of cancer survivors have a positive attitude with a heightened sense of gratitude, strengthened relationships, and increased appreciation for life. However, most patients do suffer psychological distress, especially during the early phases of cancer. The distress arises from fear of death, fear of recurrence, financial burden, lack of caregivers, and various social and practical reasons that are particular to the respective culture of the geographical area the patient lives. 19% of cancer survivors fit the diagnostic criteria of post-traumatic stress disorder.[15,16] Psychosocial support during and after cancer therapy is essential in maintaining compliance of the patient with cancer treatment completion and regular surveillance visits.
- *Fear of recurrence:* About 70% of cancer survivors have reported fear of recurrence, which can cause significant psychological distress and also result in more intense surveillance than routinely recommended.[17,18] Cancer survivors with increased fear of recurrence are shown to have a lower quality of life (QoL) and are more often depressed.
- *Employment issues:* Return to work after cancer treatment is based on socioeconomic factors, cultural influences, and cognitive status of the survivor, morbidity resultant from the cancer treatment, and also the psychological status of the patient. In India, where most of the HNC patients are from low-middle income background have shown a 65.6% of return to work rate at 6 months and 81.2% at a median of 19 months.[19] The study showed an increased trend of return to work in patients with fewer male children and the oldest child <20 years, suggesting a financial crisis and need for earlier return to work. However, more research is needed to understand the factors that influence return to work.
- *Financial burden:* The LIVESTRONG survey in 2012 has shown that 33% of working-age survivors were in debt and 3% file for bankruptcy.[20] A medical expenditure panel survey of 16,771 cancer patients has shown that HNC patients had a higher median annual expenditure and also a higher out of the pocket expenses than cancers of other subsites.[21] Financial burden plays a vital role in the psychological status of the patient, maintaining a good QoL and also adherence to treatment and surveillance.

Survivorship Care Guidelines

Various associations have recommended survivorship guideline that have been summarized in **Table 2**.

Table 2: Recommended survivorship guideline by various associations.

Recommendations	*American Cancer Society guidelines*[22]	*Cancer Care Australia guidelines*[23]	*UK guidelines*[24]
Surveillance	No specified minimum *Year 1:* 1–3 monthly *Year 2:* 2–6 monthly *Year 3–5:* 4–8 monthly Annually after that	Minimum 5-year follow-up *Year 1–2:* 3 monthly *Year 3:* 4 monthly *Year 4–5:* 6 monthly	Minimum 5 years, >5 years for high-risk group *Year 1–2:* 4–8 weekly *Year 3–5:* 3–6 monthly
Long-term physical and treatment-related side effects	PCP screen for described side effects listed in the guideline and refer to HNC multidisciplinary team when necessary	PCP or HNC multidisciplinary team screen for side effects using NCCN checklist	HNC multidisciplinary team should assess treatment-related side effects regularly at each follow-up
Long-term psychosocial effects	PCP screen for described psychosocial effects listed in the guideline and refer to HNC multidisciplinary team when indicated	PCP or HNC multidisciplinary team screen for psychosocial effects using NCCN checklist	HNC multidisciplinary team should assess psychosocial effects regularly at each follow-up, guided by a map of medicine
Health promotion	Includes healthy nutrition and weight gain strategy. Oral care, physical activity, and tobacco cessation	Cessation of tobacco and alcohol consumption, healthy body weight, healthy diet, healthy lifestyle	Healthy nutrition, oral care, physical activity, and tobacco cessation
Care coordination	No recommendation	Care plan and treatment summary is provided to patient caregiver and PCP	Clinical nurse liaise between caregivers and HNC multidisciplinary

(HNC: head and neck cancer; NCCN: National Comprehensive Cancer Network; PCP: primary care physician)

Conclusion

The needs of the patient and their caregiver are varied, and a personalized approach is encouraged. The needs and expectations of cancer survivor depend on treatment factors, site of primary cancer, and sociocultural factors, which all must be factored in survivorship care.

QUALITY OF LIFE

Introduction

The outcomes of cancer have always been measured by survival outcomes and tumor response. The concept of QoL originates from a study conducted by Karnofsky in 1948, who recognized the value of nonsurvival outcomes in cancer.[25] His concept of patient well-being has evolved into the modern concept of QoL, as we know today. HNCs are associated with a wide array of treatment-related effects involving vital functions. Like other cancers, socioeconomic factors, psychological status, financial assistance, and caregiver's assistance all influence QoL of the patient.

Definition

The World Health Organization (WHO) definition is most widely accepted and defines QoL as the perception of their position in life in the context of the culture and value systems in which they live and about their goals, expectations, standards, and concerns. It is a broad-ranging concept affected in a complex way by the person's physical health, psychological state, level of independence, and social relationship to salient features of their environment.[26] QoL is a concept where response is personalized to the patient and cannot be deemed similar for all patients. QoL is the perceived discrepancy between the realities of what a person has and the concept of what that person wants, needs, or expects.[27] The three aspects that critically define QoL are based on subjectivity, multidimensionality, and sociocultural context. Every person reacts differently to the same illness, and hence the reported experience of every patient will be subjective. QoL frequently encompasses various domains (multidimensional) such as physical health, psychological, level of independence/functionality, and social, environmental, and spiritual belief.

Overall Quality of Life versus Health-related Quality of Life

Overall QoL is influenced by factors such as finance and housing issues that cannot be related to health care systems and does not represent the influence of the health care system on the patient.[28] Hence, health-related QoL, which is a more limited concept, is more easily applied.

Relation between Symptom, Function Impairment, and Quality of Life

Perfect health is defined by WHO as a state of complete physical, mental, and social well-being and not merely absence of disease.[29] A symptom is perceived as alteration in function or sensation; functional impairment may be apparent or subclinical.[30] Based on the type of QoL administered and symptoms or functional impairment patient is experiencing, various relationships have been described. Firstly, there may be no correlation between symptoms, QoL, or functional loss. Secondly, with increasing intensity of symptoms or functional loss, there may or may not be decreasing QoL. Thirdly, low-intensity symptoms or functional loss can notably affect QoL. In some scenarios, the patient adapts to symptoms or functional loss and hence will report an improved QoL even in the persistence of symptoms or functional loss.

Where does Quality of Life Fit in Cancer Treatment?

Quality of life is used to capture the patient's perspective of the cancer experience. The outcome of cancer has always been measured with survival outcomes. When two treatment options are available for a given patient with equal survival outcome and rate of recurrence, then the treatment with reported higher QoL is chosen. At no point in cancer treatment should QoL be used solely in curative treatment decision-making. In a palliative setting, the treatment option that provides the best QoL and tumor response is chosen.

Basic Methodology of Quality of Life Estimation

Quality of life is based on the science of psychometrics, which includes the science of indirect measurement through questionnaires and other related instruments.[28] QoL is based on the following parameters:

- *Item generation:* This involves the incorporation of information of importance to patients and health professional extracted from literature review, health expertise, and input from the target population.
- *Item reduction:* This refers to a questionnaire of adequate length that is sufficiently sensitive to change.
- *Questionnaire design:* This must factor in readability and clarity.

Indices and Profiles of Quality of Life

- *Reliability:* This refers to the ability to reproduce the scores repeatedly. This is often tested with test-retest reliability.
- *Validity:* This refers to the ability of QoL to reflect the actual area of interest. The questionnaire must ideally not be influenced by the passing mood of the patient but represent the status of the patient during a defined period.
- *Responsiveness:* Responsiveness is a measure of the sensitivity of the QoL to changes over time. It is directly related to the specificity of items and length of the instrument employed.
- *Minimal clinically important difference (MID):* MID is defined as the smallest change in value on a measurement instrument that is of importance to the patient. A 5–10% change in instrument range generally represents MID.[31,32]

Types of Quality of Life

The major categories of QoL are as follows:

- *General health QoL:* Examples are EuroQoL five dimensions questionnaire (EQ-5D)[33], Medical Outcomes Study (MOS), Short Form (SF-36), and Sickness Impact Profile (SIP).[34,35]
- *Disease-specific QoL:* Examples are The Cancer Rehabilitation Evaluation System (CARES),[36] European Organization for Research Treatment of Cancer (EORTC) Quality of life (QLQ-C30),[37] and Functional Assessment of Cancer Therapy General (FACT-G) Version 4.[38]
- *Site-specific QoL for HNC patients:* University of Washington QOL Questionnaire (UWQOL),[39] EORTC-Head and Neck Quality of Life Questionnaire,[40] FACT-Head and Neck; Performance Status Scale for Head and Neck Cancer Patients,[41] MD Anderson Symptom Inventory-Head and Neck (MDASI-HN),[42] and Vanderbilt Head and Neck Symptom Survey (VHNSS) version 2.0[43]
- *Domain-specific QoL:*
  - *Pain:* Brief Pain Inventory (BPI)[44]
  - *Xerostomia:* Six-item linear analogue scale (LAS)[45] and Eight Item University of Michigan XQ[46]
  - *Speech:* Swedish self-evaluation of communication experiences after Laryngeal Cancer (S-SECEL)[47] and Voice Handicap Index (VHI)[48]
  - *Swallowing:* MD Anderson Dysphagia Inventory (MDADI),[49] the wallowing quality of life (SWAL-QOL),[50] and the swallowing quality of care (SWAL-CARE)[51]
- *Treatment-specific QoL:* UWQOL for surgical patients,[52] Head and Neck Radiotherapy Questionnaire (HNRQ),[53] Quality of Life Radiation Therapy Instrument Head and Neck Module (QOL-RTI/H&N),[54] and Liverpool Oral Rehabilitation Questionnaire[55]

Interpretation of Quality of Life Results

Quality of life conceptualizes the experience of the patient, which is based on the psychological state of the patient. Hence, an individual's change in QoL over time is advocated to prevent measurement noise secondary to the psychological state of the patient influencing QOL value during a single cross-sectional value.[28] Most often, the baseline measurement of QoL is taken at the cancer diagnosis, which does not represent a person's QoL when healthy.

Response Shift (Change in Internal Standards)

A response shift represents a modification of value and standards by the patient that leads to a reconceptualization of QoL.[28] For example, patient-reported QoL is rated better than relative-derived QoL values. Response shift is an adoptive process but results in QoL value measurement error. Quantification of response shift is difficult and cumbersome to perform. Use of QoL in a randomized control trial (RCT) model can balance response shift between the arms.

Survivor Effect

When QoL is used in longitudinal studies, there could be an overestimation of long-term QoL values.[28] Survivors of cancer treatment are more likely to comply with QoL measurement, which results in better QoL scores.

Factors Affecting Quality of Life

- *Symptoms that affect QoL:*
  - *Disfigurement:* Cancers of the head and neck region are associated with disfigurement of face and neck region that is difficult to hide, with an additive effect of functional impairment, most HNC are associated with poorer QoL.[56,57] A contradiction to this finding concerns total laryngectomy, where patients have not shown poorer QoL even with loss of speech and permanent stoma.[58]
  - *Dysphagia:* Dysphagia affects 50% of the patients, among whom 15% have severe dysphagia after 6–12 months of treatment for HNC.[59] Dysphagia affects global QoL.
  - *Lymphedema:* Lymphedema is one of the most neglected complications of HNC treatment. External lymphedema can cause disfigurement and internal lymphedema can cause functional defects that affect overall well-being of the patient.
  - *Systemic symptoms:* Systemic symptoms such as fatigue, generalized pain, anxiety, depression, neuropsychiatric symptoms, and neurocognitive dysfunction commonly occur in clusters in cancer patients undergoing treatment. About 50% of patients (post 12 months of treatment) report at least one of the systemic symptoms.[60,61] These are associated with decreased QoL.
- *Functional performance and QoL:* Contrary to the belief, functional deficits in speech, swallowing, and chewing do not impair QoL in the long term, as most patients adapt to their functional deficits and report pretreatment QoL scores. Few patients continue to experience lower QoL scores, which is most often due to emotional distress than solely functional deficit. The Veterans' Affairs larynx trial has shown that improved QoL was associated with freedom from pain, emotional well-being, and lower levels of depression than voice preservation.[62,63]
- *Tumor factors:*
  - *Disease site:* Oral cavity cancers are associated with lower QoL scores than other subsites.[64]
  - *Stage of disease:* Higher stage disease is associated with lower QoL scores which could be attributed to multimodality treatment and higher treatment-related functional deficits.
- *Treatment-related factors:*
  - *Surgery:* Highest QoL values are seen in early disease patients, treated with surgery alone.[65] Larger resections are associated with bigger defects and hence higher functional deficits, which eventually reduce QoL.
  - *Radiotherapy:* Radiation-induced changes such as hyposalivation, taste changes, lymphedema and fibrosis, and their consequences such as poor oral health, trismus, and functional defects due to internal lymphedema are all known to cause reduction in QoL values. Intensity Modulated Radiation Therapy is the current standard of radiation therapy in HNC due to accurate conformity.[66,67] Carcinoma larynx is associated with higher QoL values than other head and neck subsites managed with radiotherapy.[68] Adjuvant radiotherapy has an additive effect that complexes with surgery-associated complications worsen QoL.
  - *Chemotherapy:* Chemotherapy is often used with combination with radiation therapy in HNC. Evidence had shown no improved QoL when treatment comparison was between surgery with adjuvant radiotherapy and chemoradiotherapy.[69]
  - *Immunotherapy:* Checkmate 141 trial, which evaluated the role of nivolumab in cisplatin-resistant recurrent/metastatic HNC, has shown better QoL in the nivolumab arm.[70]

Trajectory of Quality of Life

Quality of life from the time of diagnosis decreases over time gradually, such that QoL values improve toward baseline at approximately 6–12 months following treatment. The general trends noted in QoL are:

- A gradual decrease in global QoL over 6 months after treatment with gradual improvement till 1 year post-treatment
- The emotional domain shows maximum improvement during the first year of cancer treatment
- The physical domain shows maximum deterioration in value over the first year
- Most domains recover to near baseline at 12 months of treatment.[71]

Most studies include follow-up data up to 2 years after treatment. Evidence on the long-term trajectory of QoL is limited. One of the prospective studies has shown an 11% drop and 15% drop in QoL values over long-term compared to baseline and 1 or 2 years' post-treatment respectively.[72] Significant worsening was noticed in emotional and social domains of QoL, swallowing, speech, taste, smell, dry mouth, sticky saliva, and coughing.[73] When compared among survivors and nonsurvivors, survivors experienced better QoL than nonsurvivors during first 2 years post-treatment.

Quality of Life and Survival

Global QoL, functional domains, and symptoms score are known predictors of survival in oncology.[74-76] Poor pretreatment QoL scores are associated with lower survival. Physical domain of QoL has shown to predict survival. The possible explanations for these are follows:

- Poor QoL is a surrogate for advanced disease.
- Patients with low QoL scores are less likely to tolerate and complete cancer treatment.
- Symptoms associated with tumor relapse are associated with lower QoL during the post-treatment period.

Conclusion

With improved survival among HNC patients, QoL plays a pivotal role in the life of cancer patients. Various QoL assessment tools are available, and selection of appropriate QoL tool must be guided by the appropriate research or clinical question. Routine implementation of QoL evaluation and assessment in the clinical setting has been limited, despite increasing evidence of its importance.

REFERENCES

1. Centers for Disease Control and Prevention (CDC). Cancer survivors—United States, 2007. MMWR. Morbidity and mortality weekly report. 2011;60(9):269.
2. Miller KD, Siegel RL, Lin CC, Mariotto AB, Kramer JL, Rowland JH, et al. Cancer treatment and survivorship statistics, 2016. CA Cancer J Clin. 2016;66(4):271-89.
3. Bluethmann SM, Mariotto AB, Rowland JH. Anticipating the "silver tsunami": prevalence trajectories and comorbidity burden among older cancer survivors in the United States. Cancer Epidemiol Biomarkers Prev. 2016;25(7):1029-36.
4. Gillison ML, Chaturvedi AK, Anderson WF, Fakhry C. Epidemiology of human papillomavirus-positive head and neck squamous cell carcinoma. J Clin Oncol. 2015;33(29): 3235-42.
5. Masterson L, Moualed D, Liu ZW, Howard JE, Dwivedi RC, Tysome JR, et al. De-escalation treatment protocols for human papillomavirus-associated oropharyngeal squamous cell carcinoma: a systematic review and meta-analysis of current clinical trials. Eur J Cancer. 2014;50(15):2636-48.
6. Mullan F. Seasons of survival: reflections of a physician with cancer. N Engl J Med. 1985;313(4):270-3.
7. Institute of Medicine. From cancer patient to cancer survivor: Lost in transition. Committee on Cancer Survivorship: Improving Care and Quality of Life; 2006.
8. Twombly R. What's in a name: who is a cancer survivor? J Natl Cancer Inst. 2004;96(19):1414-5.
9. Miller MC, Shuman AG, American Head and Neck Society's Committee on Survivorship. Survivorship in head and neck cancer: a primer. JAMA Otolaryngol Head Neck Surg. 2016;142(10):1002-8.
10. Rechis R, Beckjord E, Arvey SR, Reynolds K, McGoldrick D. The essential elements of survivorship care: a LIVESTRONG brief. Austin, TX: Lance Armstrong Foundation; 2011.
11. Valdivieso M, Kujawa AM, Jones T, Baker LH. Cancer survivors in the United States: a review of the literature and a call to action. Int J Med Sci. 2012;9(2):163-73.
12. Burg MA, Adorno G, Lopez ED, Loerzel V, Stein K, Wallace C, et al. Current unmet needs of cancer survivors: Analysis of open-ended responses to the American Cancer Society Study of Cancer Survivors II. Cancer. 2015;121(4):623-30.
13. Donin N, Filson C, Drakaki A, Tan HJ, Castillo A, Kwan L, et al. Risk of second primary malignancies among cancer survivors in the United States, 1992 through 2008. Cancer. 2016;122(19):3075-86.
14. Priante AV, Castilho EC, Kowalski LP. Second primary tumors in patients with head and neck cancer. Curr Oncol Rep. 2011;13(2):132-7.
15. Bellizzi KM, Miller MF, Arora NK, Rowland JH. Positive and negative life changes experienced by survivors of non-Hodgkin's lymphoma. Ann Behav Med. 2007;34(2):188-99.
16. Hodgkinson K, Butow P, Fuchs A, Hunt GE, Stenlake A, Hobbs KM, et al. Long-term survival from gynecologic cancer: psychosocial outcomes, supportive care needs and positive outcomes. Gynecol Oncol. 2007;104(2):381-9.
17. Boyes AW, Girgis A, D'Este C, Zucca AC. Prevalence and correlates of cancer survivors' supportive care needs 6 months after diagnosis: a population-based cross-sectional study. BMC Cancer. 2012;12(1):150.
18. Koch L, Jansen L, Brenner H, Arndt V. Fear of recurrence and disease progression in long-term (≥5 years) cancer survivors—a systematic review of quantitative studies. Psychooncology. 2013;22(1):1-11.

19. Agarwal J, Krishnatry R, Chaturvedi P, Ghosh-Laskar S, Gupta T, Budrukkar A, et al. Survey of return to work of head and neck cancer survivors: A report from a tertiary cancer center in India. Head Neck. 2017;39(5):893-9.
20. Banegas MP, Guy Jr GP, de Moor JS, Ekwueme DU, Virgo KS, Kent EE, et al. For working-age cancer survivors, medical debt and bankruptcy create financial hardships. Health Aff (Millwood). 2016;35(1):54-61.
21. Massa ST, Osazuwa-Peters N, Boakye EA, Walker RJ, Ward GM. Comparison of the financial burden of survivors of head and neck cancer with other cancer survivors. JAMA Otolaryngol Head Neck Surg. 2019;145(3):239-49.
22. Cohen EE, LaMonte SJ, Erb NL, Beckman KL, Sadeghi N, Hutcheson KA, et al. American Cancer Society head and neck cancer survivorship care guideline. CA Cancer J Clin. 2016;66(3):203-39.
23. National Cancer Expert Reference Group (NCERG). Optimal care pathway for people with head and neck cancers. Cancer Council Australia; 2016. p. 60.
24. Paleri V, Roland N. Introduction to the United Kingdom national multidisciplinary guidelines for head and neck cancer. J Laryngol Otol. 2016;130(S2):S3-4.
25. Karnofsky DA, Abelmann WH, Craver LF, Burchenal JH. The use of the nitrogen mustards in the palliative treatment of carcinoma. With particular reference to bronchogenic carcinoma. Cancer. 1948;1(4):634-56.
26. World Health Organization. WHOQOL: Measuring Quality of Life. Programme on mental health. Division of Mental Health and Prevention of Substance Use. Geneva, WHO (WHO/MSA/MNH/PSF/97.4); 1997. pp. 1-5.
27. Morton RP, Izzard ME. Quality-of-life outcomes in head and neck cancer patients. World J Surg. 2003;27(7):884-9.
28. Ringash J. Survivorship and quality of life in head and neck cancer. J Clin Oncol. 2015;33(29):3322-7.
29. Leppo NE. The first ten years of the World Health Organization. Minn Med. 1958;41(8):577-83.
30. Gilbert J, Murphy BA, Jackson L, Ganz PA, Brizel DM, Fried MP. Health-related quality of life in head and neck cancer. BMC Cancer. 2019;19:425.
31. Ringash J, O'Sullivan B, Bezjak A, Redelmeier DA. Interpreting clinically significant changes in patient-reported outcomes. Cancer. 2007;110(1):196-202.
32. Norman GR, Sloan JA, Wyrwich KW. Interpretation of changes in health-related quality of life: the remarkable universality of half a standard deviation. Med Care. 2003; 41(3):582-92.
33. www.euroqol.org/eq-5d-products.html (Accessed on March 2, 2020).
34. Ware Jr JE, Gandek B. Overview of the SF-36 health survey and the international quality of life assessment (IQOLA) project. J Clin Epidemiol. 1998;51(11):903-12.
35. Gilson BS, Gilson JS, Bergner M, Bobbit RA, Kressel S, Pollard WE, et al. The sickness impact profile. Development of an outcome measure of health care. Am J Public Health. 1975;65(12):1304-10.
36. Ganz PA, Schag CA, Lee JJ, Sim MS. The CARES: a generic measure of health-related quality of life for patients with cancer. Qual Life Res. 1992;1(1):19-29.
37. Bjordal K, De Graeff A, Fayers PM, Hammerlid E, van Pottelsberghe C, Curran D, et al. A 12 country field study of the EORTC QLQ-C30 (version 3.0) and the head and neck cancer specific module (EORTC QLQ-H&N35) in head and neck patients. Eur J Cancer. 2000;36(14):1796-807.
38. Weitzner MA, Meyers CA, Gelke CK, Byrne KS, Levin VA, Cella DF. The functional assessment of cancer therapy (FACT) scale. Development of a brain subscale and revalidation of the general version (FACT-G) in patients with primary brain tumors. Cancer. 1995;75(5):1151-61.
39. Rogers SN, Gwanne S, Lowe D, Humphris G, Yueh B, Weymuller Jr EA. The addition of mood and anxiety domains to the University of Washington quality of life scale. Head Neck. 2002;24(6):521-9.
40. Bjordal K, Ahlner-Elmqvist M, Tollesson E, Jensen AB, Razavi D, Maher EJ, et al. Development of a European Organization for Research and Treatment of Cancer (EORTC) questionnaire module to be used in quality of life assessments in head and neck cancer patients. Acta Oncologica. 1994;33(8):879-85.
41. List MA, D'Antonio LL, Cella DF, Siston A, Mumby P, Haraf D, et al. The performance status scale for head and neck cancer patients and the functional assessment of cancer therapy-head and neck scale: a study of utility and validity. Cancer. 1996;77(11):2294-301.
42. Rosenthal DI, Mendoza TR, Chambers MS, Asper JA, Gning I, Kies MS, et al. Measuring head and neck cancer symptom burden: the development and validation of the MD Anderson symptom inventory, head and neck module. Head Neck. 2007;29(10):923-31.
43. Cooperstein E, Gilbert J, Epstein JB, Dietrich MS, Bond SM, Ridner SH, et al. Vanderbilt Head and Neck Symptom Survey version 2.0: report of the development and initial testing of a subscale for assessment of oral health. Head Neck. 2012;34(6):797-804.
44. Mathias SD, Crosby RD, Qian Y, Jiang Q, Dansey R, Chung K. Estimating minimally important differences for the worst pain rating of the Brief Pain Inventory-Short Form. J Support Oncol. 2011;9(2):72-8.
45. Johnson JT, Ferretti GA, Nethery WJ, Valdez IH, Fox PC, Ng D, et al. Oral pilocarpine for post-irradiation xerostomia in patients with head and neck cancer. N Eng J Med. 1993; 329(6):390-5.
46. Eisbruch A, Kim HM, Terrell JE, Marsh LH, Dawson LA, Ship JA. Xerostomia and its predictors following parotid-sparing irradiation of head-and-neck cancer. Int J Radiat Oncol Biol Phys. 2001;50(3):695-704.
47. Blood GW. Development and assessment of a scale addressing communication needs of patients with laryngectomies. Am J Speech Lang Pathol. 1993;2(3):82-90.
48. Jacobson BH, Johnson A, Grywalski C, Silbergleit A, Jacobson G, Benninger MS, et al. The voice handicap index (VHI) development and validation. Am J Speech Lang Pathol. 1997;6(3):66-70.
49. Chen AY, Frankowski R, Bishop-Leone J, Hebert T, Leyk S, Lewin J, et al. The development and validation of a dysphagia-specific quality-of-life questionnaire for patients with head and neck cancer: the MD Anderson dysphagia inventory. Arch Otolaryngol Head Neck Surg. 2001;127(7):870-6.
50. McHorney CA, Bricker DE, Kramer AE, Rosenbek JC, Robbins J, Chignell KA, et al. The SWAL-QOL outcomes tool for oropharyngeal dysphagia in adults: I. Conceptual foundation and item development. Dysphagia. 2000;15(3): 115-21.
51. McHorney CA, Robbins J, Lomax K, Rosenbek JC, Chignell K, Kramer AE, et al. The SWAL-QOL and SWAL-CARE outcomes tool for oropharyngeal dysphagia in adults: III. Documentation of reliability and validity. Dysphagia. 2002;17(2):97-114.

52. Kazi R, Johnson C, Prasad V, De Cordova J, Venkitaraman R, Nutting CM, et al. Quality of life outcome measures following partial glossectomy: Assessment using the UW-QOL scale. J Cancer Res Ther. 2008;4(3):116-20.
53. Browman GP, Levine MN, Hodson DI, Sathya J, Russell R, Skingley P, et al. The Head and Neck Radiotherapy Questionnaire: a morbidity/quality-of-life instrument for clinical trials of radiation therapy in locally advanced head and neck cancer. J Clin Oncol. 1993;11(5):863-72.
54. Trotti A, Johnson DJ, Gwede C, Casey L, Sauder B, Cantor A, et al. Development of a head and neck companion module for the quality of life-radiation therapy instrument (QOL-RTI). Int J Radiat Oncol Biol Phys. 1998;42(2):257-61.
55. Pace-Balzan A, Cawood JI, Howell R, Lowe D, Rogers SN. The liverpool oral rehabilitation questionnaire: a pilot study. J Oral Rehabil. 2004;31(6):609-17.
56. Fingeret MC, Vidrine DJ, Reece GP, Gillenwater AM, Gritz ER. Multidimensional analysis of body image concerns among newly diagnosed patients with oral cavity cancer. Head Neck. 2010;32(3):301-9.
57. Maurer J, Hipp M, Schäfer C, Kölbl O. Dysphagia. Strahlentherapie und Onkologie. 2011;187(11):744-9.
58. Ramírez MJ, Ferriol EE, Doménech FG, Llatas MC, Suarez-Varela MM, Martínez RL. Psychosocial adjustment in patients surgically treated for laryngeal cancer. Otolaryngol Head Neck Surg. 2003;129(1):92-7.
59. Platteaux N, Dirix P, Dejaeger E, Nuyts S. Dysphagia in head and neck cancer patients treated with chemoradiotherapy. Dysphagia. 2010;25(2):139-52.
60. Low CA, Kalinski P, Bovbjerg DH. Neurocognitive impairment as one facet of cancer-related sickness behavior symptoms. J Natl Cancer Inst. 2015;107(8):djv176.
61. Wulff-Burchfield EM, Dietrich MS, Murphy BA. Late systemic symptom (SS) frequency in head and neck cancer (HNC) survivors as measured by the Vanderbilt Head and Neck Symptom Survey-General Symptoms Subscale (GSS). 2016;34(15):6094.
62. Department of Veterans Affairs Laryngeal Cancer Study Group. Induction chemotherapy plus radiation compared with surgery plus radiation in patients with advanced laryngeal cancer. N Eng J Med. 1991;324(24):1685-90.
63. Terrell JE, Fisher SG, Wolf GT. Long-term quality of life after treatment of laryngeal cancer. Arch Otolaryngol Head Neck Surg. 1998;124(9):964-71.
64. Leung SW, Lee TF, Chien CY, Chao PJ, Tsai WL, Fang FM. Health-related quality of life in 640 head and neck cancer survivors after radiotherapy using EORTC QLQ-C30 and QLQ-H&N35 questionnaires. BMC Cancer. 2011;11(1): 128.
65. Broglie MA, Soltermann A, Haile SR, Röösli C, Huber GF, Schmid S, et al. Quality of life of oropharyngeal cancer patients with respect to treatment strategy and p16-positivity. Laryngoscope. 2013;123(1):164-70.
66. Rathod S, Gupta T, Ghosh-Laskar S, Murthy V, Budrukkar A, Agarwal J. Quality-of-life (QOL) outcomes in patients with head and neck squamous cell carcinoma (HNSCC) treated with intensity-modulated radiation therapy (IMRT) compared to three-dimensional conformal radiotherapy (3D-CRT): evidence from a prospective randomized study. Oral Oncol. 2013;49(6):634-42.
67. Marucci L, Marzi S, Sperduti I, Giovinazzo G, Pinnarò P, Benassi M, et al. Influence of intensity-modulated radiation therapy technique on xerostomia and related quality of life in patients treated with intensity-modulated radiation therapy for nasopharyngeal cancer. Head Neck. 2012;34(3): 328-35.
68. Guibert M, Lepage B, Woisard V, Rives M, Serrano E, Vergez S. Quality of life in patients treated for advanced hypopharyngeal or laryngeal cancer. Eur Ann Otorhinolaryngol Head Neck Diseases. 2011;128(5):218-23.
69. Bottomley A, Tridello G, Coens C, Rolland F, Tesselaar ME, Leemans CR, et al. An international phase 3 trial in head and neck cancer: quality of life and symptom results: EORTC 24954 on behalf of the EORTC Head and Neck and the EORTC Radiation Oncology Group. Cancer. 2014;120(3):390-8.
70. Harrington KJ, Ferris RL, Blumenschein Jr G, Colevas AD, Fayette J, Licitra L, et al. Nivolumab versus standard, single-agent therapy of investigator's choice in recurrent or metastatic squamous cell carcinoma of the head and neck (CheckMate 141): health-related quality-of-life results from a randomised, phase 3 trial. Lancet Oncol. 2017;18(8):1104-15.
71. So WK, Chan RJ, Chan DN, Hughes BG, Chair SY, Choi KC, et al. Quality-of-life among head and neck cancer survivors at one year after treatment–a systematic review. Eur J Cancer. 2012;48(15):2391-408.
72. Mehanna HM, Morton RP. Deterioration in quality-of-life of late (10-year) survivors of head and neck cancer. Clin Otolaryngol. 2006;31(3):204-11.
73. Oskam IM, Verdonck-de Leeuw IM, Aaronson NK, Witte BI, de Bree R, Doornaert P, et al. Prospective evaluation of health-related quality of life in long-term oral and oropharyngeal cancer survivors and the perceived need for supportive care. Oral oncology. 2013;49(5):443-8.
74. Østhus AA, Aarstad AK, Olofsson J, Aarstad HJ. Prediction of survival by pretreatment health-related quality-of-life scores in a prospective cohort of patients with head and neck squamous cell carcinoma. JAMA Otolaryngol Head Neck Surg. 2013;139(1):14-20.
75. Karvonen-Gutierrez CA, Ronis DL, Fowler KE, Terrell JE, Gruber SB, Duffy SA. Quality of life scores predict survival among patients with head and neck cancer. J Clin Oncol. 2008;26(16):2754-60.
76. Aarstad HJ, Osthus AA, Olofsson J, Aarstad AK. Level of distress predicts subsequent survival in successfully treated head and neck cancer patients: a prospective cohort study. Acta Otolaryngol. 2014;134(2):211-9.

Index

Page numbers followed by *f* refer to figure, *fc* refer to flowchart, and *t* refer to table.

C

D

I

J

K

L

M

N

Q

R

S

T

U

V

W

X

Z